CURRENT PEDIATRIC THERAPY 12

SYDNEY S. GELLIS, M.D.

Professor and Emeritus Chairman, Department of Pediatrics,
Tufts University School of Medicine;
Pediatrician-in-Chief Emeritus, Boston Floating Hospital
for Infants and Children,
New England Medical Center, Inc., Boston

BENJAMIN M. KAGAN, M.D.

Director and Chairman, Department of Pediatrics,
Cedars-Sinai Medical Center, Los Angeles;
Professor and Vice Chairman,
Department of Pediatrics,
University of California at Los Angeles

W. B. SAUNDERS COMPANY

Philadelphia   London   Toronto   Mexico City   Rio de Janeiro   Sydney   Tokyo   Hong Kong

W. B. Saunders Company: West Washington Square
                           Philadelphia, PA 19105

The Library of Congress Cataloged the
First Issue of This Serial As Follows:

RJ52   Current pediatric therapy.   1964–
C8   Philadelphia, Saunders.

    v. 28 cm. biennial.

    Editors: 1964–   S. S. Gellis and B. M. Kagan.

    I. Pediatrics—Collected works.   2. Therapeutics—
    Collected works.   I. Gellis, Sydney S., ed.
    II. Kagan, Benjamin M., ed.

    RJ52.C8   618.9/2006   64–10484 rev

    Library of Congress   [r66i3]

Editor: Carroll Cann
Editorial Coordinator: Carolyn Naylor
Developmental Editor: Ken McNally
Designer: Karen O'Keefe
Production Manager: Pete Faber
Manuscript Editor: Susan Thomas
Indexer: Mark Coyle

Current Pediatric Therapy 12   ISBN   0-7216-1574-0

Last digit is the print number: 9   8   7   6   5   4   3   2   1

Contributors

James M. Adams, M.D.
Associate Professor of Clinical Pediatrics, Department of Pediatrics, Baylor College of Medicine; Director, Neonatal Intensive Care Unit, Texas Children's Hospital, Houston, Texas
Tetanus Neonatorum

Robert Adler, M.D.
Associate Professor, Department of Pediatrics, University of Southern California School of Medicine; Medical Education Director, Children's Hospital of Los Angeles, Los Angeles, California
The Child and the Death of a Loved One

Laurie S. Ahlgren, M.D.
Assistant Professor of Surgery, Tufts University School of Medicine; Lecturer in Surgery, Boston University School of Medicine; Attending Pediatric Surgeon, Boston Floating Hospital, New England Medical Center; Chief of Pediatric Surgery, Boston City Hospital, Boston, Massachusetts
Burns

A. Loren Amacher, M.D., F.R.C.S.(C)
Professor of Neurosurgery, University of Connecticut School of Medicine, Farmington; Neurosurgeon, Hartford Hospital, Hartford, and John Dempsey University Hospital, Farmington, Connecticut
Brain Tumors

Frederic P. Anderson, M.D., M.P.H.
Associate Clinical Professor of Pediatrics, Yale University School of Medicine; Attending Physician, Yale-New Haven Hospital and Hospital of St. Raphael, New Haven, Connecticut
Lyme Disease

John A. Anderson, M.D.
Clinical Associate Professor, University of Michigan Medical School, Ann Arbor; Chairman, Department of Pediatrics, and Head, Division of Allergy and Clinical Immunology, Henry Ford Hospital, Detroit, Michigan
Physical Allergy

Warren A. Andiman, M.D.
Associate Professor of Pediatrics and Epidemiology and Public Health, Yale University School of Medicine; Attending Pediatrician, Yale-New Haven Hospital, New Haven, Connecticut
Infectious Mononucleosis

Bascom F. Anthony, M.D.
Professor of Pediatrics, UCLA School of Medicine, Los Angeles; Chief, Pediatric Infectious Diseases, Harbor-UCLA Medical Center, Torrance, California
Group B Streptococcal Infections

Robert M. Arensman, M.D.
Assistant Clinical Professor of Surgery, Louisiana State University Medical School; Chief, Division of Pediatric Surgery, Ochsner Clinic, New Orleans, Louisiana
Chylothorax; Pneumothorax and Pneumomediastinum

Kenneth A. Arndt, M.D.
Associate Professor of Dermatology, Harvard Medical School; Dermatologist-in-Chief, Beth Israel Hospital, Boston, Massachusetts
Topical Therapy: A Dermatologic Formulary for Pediatric Practice

Stephen S. Arnon, M.D.
Senior Investigator, Infant Botulism Research Project, California Department of Health Services, Berkeley, California
Infant Botulism

Stephen C. Aronoff, M.D.
Assistant Professor in Pediatrics, Case Western Reserve University School of Medicine; Assistant Pediatrician, Division of Pediatric Infectious

Diseases, Rainbow Babies and Children's Hospital, Cleveland, Ohio
The Management of Septic Shock

Edward Austin, M.D.
Attending in Surgery, Cedars-Sinai Medical Center, Los Angeles, California
Hernias and Hydroceles

Felicia B. Axelrod, M.D.
Associate Professor of Pediatrics, New York University School of Medicine; Associate Attending in Pediatrics, New York University Medical Center, New York, New York
Familial Dysautonomia

Parvin H. Azimi, M.D.
Clinical Associate Professor of Pediatrics, University of California, San Francisco, California; Director, Infectious Diseases, Children's Hospital, and Chief, Microbiology Laboratories, Children's Hospital, Oakland, California
Malaria

Robert L. Baehner, M.D.
Professor and Chairman of Pediatrics, University of Southern California School of Medicine; Chairman of Pediatrics and Academic Affairs, Children's Hospital of Los Angeles, Los Angeles, California
Aplastic Anemia

Irving W. Bailit, M.D.
Clinical Instructor in Pediatrics, Harvard University Medical School; Senior Associate in Medicine and Associate in Allergy, Children's Hospital Medical Center, Boston, Massachusetts
Anaphylaxis

Robert S. Baker, M.D., F.R.C.P.(C), F.R.C.S.(C)
Assistant Professor of Ophthalmology, Neurology, Neuro-Surgery, and Pediatrics, University of Kentucky College of Medicine; Attending Ophthalmologist and Director of Pediatric and Neuro-Ophthalmology, Albert B. Chandler Medical Center; Attending Ophthalmologist, Good Samaritan Hospital, Lexington, Kentucky
Benign Intracranial Hypertension

Gabor Barabas, M.D.
Chief, Division of Pediatric Neurology, and Associate Professor, Pediatrics and Neurology, University of Medicine and Dentistry of New Jersey-Rutgers Medical School, New Brunswick; Consulting Pediatric Neurologist, Middlesex General University Hospital, New Brunswick, Monmouth Medical Center, Long Branch, Riverview Medical Center, Red Bank, and St. Peter's Medical Center, New Brunswick, New Jersey
Childhood Sleep Disturbances and Disorders of Arousal

Giulio J. Barbero, M.D.
Professor and Chairman, Department of Child Health, University of Missouri School of Medicine, Columbia, Missouri
Pyloric Stenosis; Pylorospasm

Lewis A. Barness, M.D.
Professor and Chairman, Department of Pediatrics; University of South Florida College of Medicine; Attending Pediatrician, University of South Florida Affiliated Hospitals, Tampa, Florida
Fluid and Electrolyte Therapy

Louis Bartoshesky, M.D., M.P.H.
Assistant Professor of Pediatrics, Tufts University Medical School; Assistant Pediatrician, Boston Floating Hospital, Boston, Massachusetts
Neurocutaneous Syndromes

Dorsey M. Bass, M.D.
Clinical and Research Fellow in Pediatric Gastroenterology and Nutrition, Harvard Combined Program at Massachusetts General Hospital and Children's Hospital Medical Center, Boston, Massachusets
Acute and Chronic Nonspecific Diarrhea Syndromes

James W. Bass, M.D., M.P.H.
Professor of Pediatrics, Uniformed Services University of the Health Sciences, Bethesda, Maryland; Clinical Professor of Pediatrics, University of Hawaii School of Medicine, and Chairman, Department of Pediatrics, Tripler Army Medical Center, Honolulu, Hawaii
Toxoplasmosis

David Bateman, M.D.
Assistant Clinical Professor of Pediatrics, Columbia University College of Physicians and Surgeons; Director of Newborn Services, Harlem Hospital, New York, New York
Management of the Newborn Infant at Delivery

Mark L. Batshaw, M.D.
Associate Professor of Pediatrics, Johns Hopkins University School of Medicine; Developmental Pediatrician, John F. Kennedy Institute, Johns Hopkins Medical Institutions, Baltimore, Maryland
Mental Retardation

Charles R. Bauer, M.D.
Associate Professor of Pediatrics, University of Miami School of Medicine; Associate Director, Division of Neonatology, Jackson Memorial/University of Miami Medical Center; Director, High-Risk Follow-up Research Program, Mailman Center for Child Development, Miami, Florida
Necrotizing Enterocolitis

Arthur L. Beaudet, M.D.
Professor of Pediatrics and Cell Biology, Baylor College of Medicine; Investigator, Howard Hughes Medical Institute; Chief, Genetics Service, Texas Children's Hospital, Houston, Texas
Lysosomal Storage Diseases

Marc O. Beem, M.D.
Professor of Pediatrics, University of Chicago Pritzker School of Medicine; Attending Physician and Chief, Section of Infectious Diseases, Wyler Children's Hospital, Chicago, Illinois
Chlamydia

Douglas W. Bell, M.D.
Clinical Instructor, Harvard Medical School; Staff Otolaryngologist, Beth Israel Hospital, and Children's Hospital, Boston, Massachusetts
Branchial Arch Cysts and Sinuses; Salivary Gland Tumors; Thyroglossal Duct Cysts

Bruce O. Berg, M.D.
Professor of Neurology and Pediatrics, and Director, Child Neurology, University of California Medical Center, San Francisco, California
Congenital Muscular Defects

Ira Bergman, M.D.
Associate Professor of Pediatrics and Neurology, University of Pittsburgh Medical School; Attending Pediatrician, Children's Hospital of Pittsburgh and Magee Women's Hospital, Pittsburgh, Pennsylvania
Guillain-Barré Syndrome

Kerry S. Bergman, M.D.
Assistant Instructor of Surgery, Tufts University School of Medicine; Attending Physician, New England Medical Center, Boston, Massachusetts
Head Injury

Stanley Berlow, M.D.
Associate Professor of Pediatrics, University of Wisconsin Medical School; Director, Metabolic Program, Waisman Center on Mental Retardation and Human Development, University of Wisconsin; Consultant, Pediatrics, University of Wisconsin Hospital, Madison General Hospital, and St. Mary's Hospital, Madison, Wisconsin
Hyperphenylalaninemias

Eugene K. Betts, M.D.
Assistant Professor of Anesthesia, University of Pennsylvania School of Medicine; Senior Anesthesiologist and Director, Anesthesia Operating Room Service, Children's Hospital of Philadelphia; Staff Anesthesiologist, Hospital of the University of Pennsylvania, Philadelphia, Pennsylvania
Malignant Hyperthermia

Leonard Bielory, M.D.
Director, Allergy and Immunology Division, Department of Medicine, University of Medicine and Dentistry of New Jersey-Rutgers Medical School, Newark, New Jersey; National Institutes of Health, National Heart, Lung and Blood Institute, Bethesda, Maryland
Serum Sickness

C. Warren Bierman, M.D.
Clinical Professor of Pediatrics, University of Washington School of Medicine; Chief, Division of Allergy, Children's Orthopedic Hospital and Medical Center, Seattle, Washington
Allergic Gastrointestinal Disorders

Jeffrey A. Biller, M.D.
Assistant Professor in Pediatrics, Tufts University School of Medicine; Assistant Professor in Pediatrics, Division of Pediatric Gastroenterology, New England Medical Center, Boston, Massachusetts
Recurrent Abdominal Pain; Ulcerative Colitis and Crohn's Disease

Harry C. Bishop, M.D.
Professor of Pediatric Surgery, University of Pennsylvania School of Medicine; Senior Surgeon, Children's Hospital of Philadelphia; Consulting Pediatric Surgeon, Hospital of the University of Pennsylvania, Pennsylvania Hospital, and Lankenau Hospital, Philadelphia, Pennsylvania
Intussusception

Virginia D. Black, M.D.
Assistant Professor of Pediatrics, Wayne State University School of Medicine; Associate Neonatologist, Hutzel Hospital and Children's Hospital of Michigan, Detroit, Michigan
Hyperviscosity Syndromes

Cynthia Black-Payne, M.D.
Fellow in Pediatric Infectious Diseases, Louisiana State University Medical Center, Shreveport, Louisiana
Histoplasmosis

Joseph A. Bocchini, Jr., M.D.
Associate Professor of Pediatrics, Louisiana State University School of Medicine; Chief, Section of Infectious Diseases, Louisiana State University Medical Center, Shreveport, Louisiana
Histoplasmosis

Marjorie A. Boeck, Ph.D., M.D.
Assistant Professor of Pediatrics, Albert Einstein College of Medicine; Assistant Attending Pediatrician, Montefiore Medical Center, and Adjunct Attending Pediatrician, North Central Bronx Hospital, Bronx, New York
Obesity

E. Thomas Boles, Jr., M.D.
Professor and Director, Division of Pediatric Surgery, Department of Surgery, Ohio State University College of Medicine; Chief, Department of Pediatric Surgery, Children's Hospital; Attending Staff, Children's Hospital and University Hospital, Columbus, Ohio
Foreign Bodies in the Gastrointestinal Tract; Malformations of the Intestine

Earl J. Brewer, Jr., M.D.
Head, Rheumatology Section, and Clinical Professor, Department of Pediatrics, Baylor College of Medicine; Director, Pediatric Rheumatology Center, Texas Children's Hospital, and Division of Maternal and Child Health, HHS Texas Bureau of Crippled Children's Services, Houston, Texas
Collagen Vascular Disease

Itzhak Brook, M.D.
Professor of Pediatrics and Surgery, Uniformed Services University for the Health Sciences; Attending Physician and Consultant in Infectious Diseases, National Naval Medical Center, Bethesda, Maryland, and Walter Reed Army Medical Center, Washington, D.C.
Aspiration Pneumonia; Listeria monocytogenes Infection; Infections Due to Anaerobic Cocci and Gram-negative Bacilli

H. Leon Brooks, M.D.
Assistant Clinical Professor in Orthopedic Surgery, University of Southern California School of Medicine; Active Attending, Cedars-Sinai Medical Center, Children's Hospital of Los Angeles, Los Angeles County–USC Medical Center, and Midway Hospital of Los Angeles, California
Orthopedic Disorders of the Extremities

David R. Brown, M.D.
Associate Professor of Pediatrics, University of Pittsburgh School of Medicine; Attending, Magee-Women's Hospital and Children's Hospital of Pittsburgh, Pittsburgh, Pennsylvania
Meconium Aspiration Syndrome

Gerald L. Brown, M.D.
Staff Investigator, Biological Psychiatry Branch, National Institute of Mental Health, Bethesda, Maryland
Attention Deficit Disorder

John F. Brown, Jr., M.D.
Emeritus Assistant Professor of Medicine, University of Southern California School of Medicine; Attending Staff, Pulmonary Disease Service, Los Angeles County–University of Southern California Medical Center; Consultant, Barlow Hospital, Los Angeles, California
Mucormycosis

Kelly D. Brownell, Ph.D.
Associate Professor, Department of Psychiatry, University of Pennsylvania School of Medicine, Philadelphia, Pennsylvania
Obesity

Richard C. Bryarly, Jr., M.D.
Assistant Professor, Louisiana State University School of Medicine, Shreveport, Louisiana
Nasal Injuries

Kevin A. Burbige, M.D.
Assistant Professor of Urology, Columbia University College of Physicians and Surgeons; Associate Director, Pediatric Neurology, Babies Hospital, New York, New York
Vesicoureteral Reflux

Stephen Burstein, M.D., Ph.D.
Assistant Professor of Pediatrics, University of Chicago Pritzker School of Medicine; Attending Pediatrician, Wyler Children's Hospital, Chicago, Illinois
Short Stature

Victor E. Calcaterra, M.D.
Assistant Professor of Otolaryngology, Tufts University School of Medicine; Senior Surgeon, Department of Otolaryngology, New England Medical Center, Boston, Massachusetts
Foreign Bodies in the Ear; Injuries of the Middle Ear

Gail H. Cassell, M.S., Ph.D.
Professor of Microbiology, University of Alabama School of Medicine, Birmingham, Alabama
Mycoplasma Infections

Elias G. Chalhub, M.D.
Associate Professor of Pediatrics and Neurology, University of South Alabama Medical Center, Mobile, Alabama
Subdural Hematoma and Epidural Hematoma

Nancy J. Charest, M.D.
Fellow, Pediatric Endocrinology, University of North Carolina at Chapel Hill and North Carolina Memorial Hospital, Chapel Hill, North Carolina
Tall Stature

Robert R. Chilcote, M.D.
Associate Professor of Pediatrics, University of Southern California School of Medicine; Attending Pediatrician, Los Angeles County–USC Medical Center, Los Angeles, California
Hemolytic Diseases of the Neonate

J. Julian Chisolm, Jr., M.D.
Associate Professor of Pediatrics, Johns Hopkins Medical School; Director, Lead Program, Kennedy Institute, Johns Hopkins Hospital; Senior Staff Pediatrician, Francis Scott Key Medical Center, Baltimore, Maryland
Increased Lead Absorption and Acute Lead Poisoning

Thomas G. Cleary, M.D.
Associate Professor, University of Texas Medical School at Houston; Attending, M. D. Anderson Hospital and Hermann Hospital, Houston, Texas
Endocarditis

William W. Cleveland, M.D.
Professor and Chairman, Department of Pediatrics, University of Miami School of Medicine; Attending Pediatrician, Jackson Memorial Hospital, Miami, Florida
Gynecomastia

Wallace A. Clyde, Jr., M.D.
Professor of Pediatrics and Microbiology, University of North Carolina at Chapel Hill; Attending Physician, North Carolina Memorial Hospital, Chapel Hill, North Carolina
Viral Pneumonia

Bernard A. Cohen, M.D.
Assistant Professor of Pediatrics and Dermatology, University of Pittsburgh; Director of Pediatric Dermatology, Children's Hospital of Pittsburgh, Pittsburgh, Pennsylvania
Arthropod Bites and Stings

Kenneth L. Cox, M.D.
Associate Professor of Pediatrics, University of California, Davis, School of Medicine; Chief, Pediatric Gastroenterology and Nutrition, and Associate Director of Cystic Fibrosis Center, University of California, Davis, Medical Center; Attending, University of California, Davis, Medical Center, Davis, California, University of Nevada Medical Center, Reno, Nevada
Pancreatic Diseases

Henry G. Cramblett, M.D.
Warner M. and Lora Kays Pomerene Chair in Medicine, Professor of Pediatrics, and Professor of Medical Microbiology and Immunology, The Ohio State University; Attending Staff, Children's Hospital and University Hospitals, Columbus, Ohio
Systemic Mycoses

Helen Cvejic, M.D.
Assistant Professor, McGill University Faculty of Medicine; Staff Psychiatrist, Montreal Children's Hospital, Montreal, Quebec
Psychiatric Disorders

J. Michael Dean, M.D.
Assistant Professor, Departments of Anesthesiology and Critical Care Medicine and Pediatrics, Johns Hopkins University Medical School; Attending Physician, Pediatric Intensive Care Unit, Johns Hopkins Hospital, Baltimore, Maryland
Near-Drowning

Joan DiPalma, M.D.
University of Missouri Department of Child Health Fellow in Pediatric Gastroenterology; Fellow in Pediatric Gastroenterology, Department of Child Health, University of Missouri–Columbia School of Medicine, Columbia, Missouri
Pyloric Stenosis; Pylorospasm

W. Edwin Dodson, M.D.
Associate Professor of Pediatrics and Neurology, Washington University School of Medicine; Attending, St. Louis Children's Hospital and Barnes Hospital, St. Louis, Missouri
Cerebral Edema; Seizure Disorders

Suzanne Dongier, M.D.
Associate Professor, Department of Psychiatry, McGill University Faculty of Medicine; Director,

Consultation Services, Psychiatry Department, Montreal Children's Hospital, Montreal, Quebec
Psychiatric Disorders

Henry L. Dorkin, M.D.
Assistant Professor of Pediatrics, Tufts University School of Medicine; Chief of Service, Pediatric Pulmonary Division and Cystic Fibrosis Center, New England Medical Center, Boston, Massachusetts
Lobar Emphysema; Neonatal Pneumothorax and Pneumomediastinum

John N. Duckett, M.D.
Professor of Urology, University of Pennsylvania School of Medicine; Director, Pediatric Urology, Children's Hospital of Philadelphia, Philadelphia, Pennsylvania
Tumors of the Bladder and Prostate

John M. Dwyer, M.D., Ph.D.
Professor of Medicine, University of New South Wales; Professor of Medicine and Clinical Director, Prince of Wales and Prince Henry Hospitals, Sydney, Australia.
Primary Immunodeficiency Disease

Heinz F. Eichenwald, M.D.
William Buchanan Professor, Department of Pediatrics, The University of Texas Health Science Center at Dallas; Attending Physician, Children's Medical Center of Dallas and Parkland Memorial Hospital, Dallas, Texas
Plague

Arnold Einhorn, M.D.
Professor and Associate Chairman, Department of Child Health and Development, George Washington University; Chairman, Department of Pediatric Medicine, and Director, Residency Training Program, Children's Hospital National Medical Center, Washington, D.C.
Iron Poisoning

Robert W. Emmens, M.D.
Attending Pediatric Surgeon, Strong Memorial Hospital, Rochester General Hospital, Genesee Hospital, St. Marys Hospital, Rochester, New York
Intrathoracic Cysts

Hugh E. Evans, M.D.
Professor and Chairman, Department of Pediatrics, University of Medicine and Dentistry of New Jersey, Newark, New Jersey
Congenital Syphilis

Jon Matthew Farber, M.D.
Assistant Professor of Pediatrics, The Johns Hopkins University School of Medicine, The Kennedy Institute for Handicapped Children, and The Johns Hopkins Hospital Medical Institutions, Baltimore, Maryland
Autism

Ralph D. Feigin, M.D.
J. S. Abercrombie Professor of Pediatrics and Chairman, Department of Pediatrics, Baylor College of Medicine; Physician-in-Chief, Texas Children's Hospital; Physician-in-Chief, Pediatric Service, Harris County Hospital District; and Chief, Pediatric Service, Methodist Hospital, Houston, Texas
Bacterial Meningitis and Septicemia Beyond the Neonatal Period; Leptospirosis

Sandor Feldman, M.D.
Associate Member, Division of Infectious Diseases, St. Jude Children's Research Hospital, and Associate Professor, Department of Pediatrics, University of Tennessee for the Health Sciences; Attending, St. Jude Children's Research Hospital and LeBonheur Children's Medical Center, Memphis, Tennessee
Salmonellosis; Typhoid Fever

James Feusner, M.D.
Assistant Clinical Professor of Pediatrics, University of California School of Medicine, San Farncisco; Associate Hematologist, Children's Hospital and Medical Center of Northern California, Oakland, California
Neuroblastoma

Robert M. Filler, M.D.
Professor of Surgery, University of Toronto Faculty of Medicine; Surgeon-in-Chief, The Hospital for Sick Children; Consultant (Pediatric Surgery), The Princess Margaret Hospital; Consultant (Pediatrics), Women's College Hospital, Toronto, Ontario
Pulmonary Sequestration; Middle Lobe Syndrome; Neonatal Intestinal Obstruction; Tumors of the Chest

Jo David Fine, M.D.
Associate Professor of Dermatology and Director of Dermatologic Research, University of Alabama at Birmingham School of Medicine; Chief, Dermatology Service, Birmingham Veterans Administration Medical Center; Staff Dermatologist, University of Alabama Hospitals, Children's Hospital, and Cooper Green Hospital, Birmingham, Alabama
Skin

Alfred J. Fish, M.D.
Professor, Department of Pediatric Nephrology, University of Minnesota Medical School; Attending, University of Minnesota Hospitals, Minneapolis, Minnesota
Glomerulonephritis

Susan S. Fish, Pharm. D.
Associate Professor of Clinical Toxicology, Massachusetts College of Pharmacy and Allied Health Sciences; Assistant Director, Massachusetts Poison Control System; Research Assistant, The Children's Hospital, Boston, Massachusetts
Acetaminophen Poisoning

David R. Fleisher, M.D.
Clinical Professor of Pediatrics, UCLA School of Medicine; Attending Pediatrician, Cedars-Sinai Medical Center; Visiting Pediatrician, UCLA Center for the Health Sciences, Los Angeles, California
Nausea and Vomiting

Alberto Fois, M.D.
Professor of Pediatrics, Siena University; Director of the Institute of Clinical Pediatrics, University of Siena, Siena, Italy.
Infantile Spasms

Thomas P. Foley, Jr., M.D.
Professor of Pediatrics, University of Pittsburgh School of Medicine; Director, Clinical Research Center, Children's Hospital of Pittsburgh, Pittsburgh, Pennsylvania
Thyroid Disease

Sandra L. Forem, M.D.
Assistant Professor of Clinical Pediatric Neurology, New York University School of Medicine; Assistant Attending Pediatric Neurologist, New York University-Bellevue Medical Center; New York, New York
Chronic Relapsing Polyneuropathy

Marc A. Forman, M.D.
Professor of Psychiatry and Clinical Professor of Pediatrics, Tulane University School of Medicine; Director of Child Psychiatry, Tulane Medical Center, New Orleans, Louisiana
Psychosomatic Illness

Laurie S. Fouser, M.D.
Medical Fellow, Department of Pediatric Nephrology, University of Minnesota School of Medicine and University of Minnesota Hospitals, Minneapolis, Minnesota
Glomerulonephritis

Lawrence A. Fox, D.D.S., M.P.H., M.Ed.
Associate Professor, Department of Community Dentistry and Applied Behavioral Sciences, Case Western Reserve University, Cleveland; Staff, Lake County Memorial Hospital, Willoughby, Ohio
Congenital Epulis of the Neonate

Bishara J. Freij, M.D.
Research Fellow, Pediatric Infectious Disease, Southwestern Medical School, The University of Texas Health Science Center at Dallas, Dallas, Texas
Neonatal Septicemia, Meningitis, and Pneumonia

Louis Friedlander, M.D.
Clinical Professor of Pediatrics, University of Southern California School of Medicine, and Los Angeles County–University of Southern California Medical Center, Los Angeles, California
Uterus, Tubes, and Ovaries; Vulva and Vagina

Bruce Furie, M.D.
Professor, Department of Medicine, Tufts University School of Medicine; Chief, Coagulation Unit, New England Medical Center, Boston, Massachusetts
Pediatric Hemostasis

Stephen L. Gans, M.D.
Clinical Professor of Surgery (Pediatric), UCLA School of Medicine; Attending in Surgery, Cedars-Sinai Medical Center, Los Angeles, California
Hernias and Hydroceles

Lawrence M. Gartner, M.D.
Professor and Chairman, Department of Pediatrics, University of Chicago Pritzker School of Medicine; Director, Wyler Children's Hospital, Chicago, Illinois
Hemolytic Diseases of the Neonate

Robert H. Gelber, M.D.
Associate Clinical Professor, Departments of Epidemiology and International Health and Dermatology, University of California, San Francisco; Associate Clinical Professor, Department of Dermatology, Stanford University, San Francisco; Medical Director, Hansen's Disease Program, Seton Medical Center, Daly City, California
Leprosy

Stephen E. Gellis, M.D.
Assistant Professor of Dermatology and Pediatrics, Tufts Medical School; Dermatologist,

New England Medical Center, Boston, Massachusetts
Miscellaneous Dermatoses

Michael A. Gerber, M.D.
Assistant Professor of Pediatrics, University of Connecticut School of Medicine, Farmington; Attending Staff, John Dempsey Hospital; Consulting Staff, Hartford Hospital, Hartford, and Newington Children's Hospital, Newington, Connecticut
Streptococcal Infections

Anne A. Gershon, M.D.
Professor of Pediatrics, New York University School of Medicine; Attending Physician, Bellevue Hospital Center, New York, New York
Varicella and Herpes Zoster

Welton M. Gersony, M.D.
Professor of Pediatrics, Columbia University College of Physicians and Surgeons; Director, Division of Pediatric Cardiology, Columbia-Presbyterian Medical Center and Babies Hospital, New York, New York
Cardiac Arrhythmias

Hubert L. Gerstman, D.Ed.
Associate Professor of Otolaryngology and Associate Professor of Rehabilitation Medicine, Tufts University School of Medicine; Chief, Speech, Hearing and Language Center, New England Medical Center Hospitals, Boston, Massachusetts
Hearing Loss

Frances M. Gill, M.D.
Associate Professor of Pediatrics, University of Pennsylvania School of Medicine; Senior Physician, Children's Hospital of Philadelphia, Philadelphia, Pennsylvania
Hemolytic Anemia

Herbert E. Gilmore, M.D.
Assistant Professor of Pediatrics (Neurology), Tufts University School of Medicine; Pediatric Neurologist, New England Medical Center, Boston Floating Hospital, Boston, Massachusetts
Congenital Hypotonia

Janet R. Gilsdorf, M.D.
Assistant Professor of Pediatrics, University of Michigan Medical School; Hospital Staff, C.S. Mott Children's Hospital, University of Michigan Medical Center, Ann Arbor, Michigan
Haemophilus influenzae Infections

Wallace A. Gleason, Jr., M.D.
Associate Professor of Pediatrics and Director, The Children's Fund, Inc., Gastrointestinal Unit, The University of Texas Medical School at Houston; Medical Director, The Children's Center, University Children's Hospital at Hermann, Houston, Texas
Chronic Diarrhea and Malabsorption Syndrome

Arnold P. Gold, M.D.
Professor of Clinical Neurology and Professor of Clinical Pediatrics, Columbia University College of Physicians and Surgeons; Attending Neurologist and Pediatrician, Columbia-Presbyterian Medical Center, New York, New York
Chronic Relapsing Polyneuropathy

Richard B. Goldbloom, M.D., F.R.C.P.(C)
Professor and Head, Department of Pediatrics, Dalhousie University Faculty of Medicine; Physician-in-Chief and Director of Research, The Izaak Walton Killam Hospital for Children, Halifax, Nova Scotia.
Nasopharyngitis; Pica; The Tonsil and Adenoid Problem

David Goldring, M.D.
Professor of Pediatrics, Emeritus, Washington University Medical School; Director of Pediatric Cardiology, Emeritus, St. Louis Children's Hospital, St. Louis, Missouri
Systemic Hypertension

Gary M. Gorlick, G.M.G., M.D., M.P.H.
Assistant Clinical Professor of Pediatrics, University of California at Los Angeles School of Medicine; Attending Pediatrician, Pediatric Dermatology Clinic, Cedars-Sinai Medical Center, Los Angeles, California
Eruptions in the Diaper Region

Samuel P. Gotoff, M.D.
Professor of Pediatrics, Pritzker School of Medicine, University of Chicago; Chairman, Department of Pediatrics, Michael Reese Hospital and Medical Center, Chicago, Illinois
Immunization Practice

Jeffrey B. Gould, M.D., M.P.H.
Deputy Director of Maternal and Child Health, School of Public Health, University of California at Berkeley; Neonatologist, Children's Hospital of San Francisco; Pediatric Consultant, Health Department, Contra Costa County, California
Preparation of the Neonate for Transfer

David F. Graft, M.D.
Clinical Instructor of Pediatrics, University of Pittsburgh School of Medicine; Director, Allergy Clinic, St. Francis General Hospital; Attending Staff, Children's Hospital of Pittsburgh, Mercy Hospital, and St. Clair Hospital, Pittsburgh, Pennsylvania
Insect Stings

Nahman H. Greenberg, M.D.
Professor of Psychiatry, University of Illinois School of Medicine; Attending Psychiatrist, University of Illinois Hospital, Illinois Masonic Medical Center, Chicago, Illinois
Child Abuse

Sylvia P. Griffiths, M.D.
Professor of Clinical Pediatrics, Columbia University College of Physicians and Surgeons; Attending Pediatrician, Columbia-Presbyterian Medical Center, New York, New York
Acute Rheumatic Fever

Robert C. Griggs, M.D.
Professor of Neurology, Medicine, Pediatrics, and Pathology, University of Rochester School of Medicine and Dentistry; Director, Neuromuscular Disease Clinic, Strong Memorial Hospital, Rochester, New York
Periodic Paralysis

James Santiago Grisolía, M.D.
Adjunct Assistant Professor, Department of Neurosciences, University of California, San Diego, School of Medicine; Staff, Mercy Hospital and Medical Center, Sharp Memorial Hospital, and Bay Hospital, San Diego, California
Cysticercosis

Moses Grossman, M.D.
Professor of Pediatrics, University of California, San Francisco, School of Medicine; Chief of Pediatrics, San Francisco General Hospital, San Francisco, California
Brucellosis; Rat Bite Fever

Warren E. Grupe, M.D.
Associate Professor of Pediatrics, Harvard Medical School; Chief, Division of Nephrology, The Children's Hospital, Boston, Massachusetts
The Nephrotic Syndrome

Joyce D. Gryboski, M.D.
Professor of Pediatrics, Yale University School of Medicine, New Haven, Connecticut
Disorders of the Esophagus; Gastroesophageal Reflex and Hiatus Hernia

Warren G. Guntheroth, M.D.
Professor of Pediatrics, Head, Division of Pediatric Cardiology, University of Washington School of Medicine; Attending Physician, University of Washington Hospital, Children's Orthopedic Hospital; Consultant, Harborview Medical Center, Pacific Medical Center, Seattle, Washington
Peripheral Vascular Disorders; Sudden Infant Death Syndrome (SIDS) and Near-Miss SIDS

Sue Y. E. Hahm, M.D.
Assistant Professor, Division of Genetics, Department of Pediatrics, Albert Einstein College of Medicine, Bronx, New York
Genetic Diseases

Kevin E. Halbert, M.D.
Fellow in Neonatology, University of Cincinnati College of Medicine, University of Cincinnati Medical Center and Children's Hospital Medical Center, Cincinnati, Ohio
Parathyroid Disease

J. Alex Haller, Jr., M.D.
Robert Garrett Professor of Pediatric Surgery, The Johns Hopkins University School of Medicine; Children's Surgeon-in-Charge, The Johns Hopkins Hospital, Baltimore, Maryland
Peritonitis

Jerome S. Haller, M.D.
Associate Professor of Pediatrics (Neurology), Tufts University School of Medicine; Pediatric Neurologist, Boston Floating Hospital, New England Medical Center, Boston, Massachusetts
Injuries to the Brachial Plexus, Facial Nerve, and Sciatic Nerve

K. Michael Hambidge, F.R.C.P.(Ed.)
Professor of Pediatrics, University of Colorado School of Medicine; Attending Physician, University of Colorado Health Sciences Center, Denver, Colorado
Breast-Feeding

Steven D. Handler, M.D.
Assistant Professor, Department of Otorhinolaryngology and Human Communication, University of Pennsylvania School of Medicine; Associate Director, Division of Otolaryngology and Human Communication, Children's Hospital of Philadelphia, Philadelphia, Pennsylvania
Labyrinthitis; Tumors and Polyps of the Nose

Ronald C. Hansen, M.D.
Associate Professor of Internal Medicine (Dermatology) and Pediatrics, University of Arizona

College of Medicine, Tucson; Staff Dermatologist, University Medical Center, Tucson; Consultant, Dermatology, Tucson Medical Center, Tucson, Phoenix Children's Hospital, St. Joseph's Medical Center, Maricopa Medical Center, Phoenix, Arizona
Discoid Lupus Erythematosus

James Barry Hanshaw, M.D.
Professor of Pediatrics, Interim Vice Chancellor, Academic Dean, University of Massachusetts Medical School; Active Staff, University of Massachusetts Hospital; Consultant, Worcester Memorial Hospital, Worcester City Hospital, St. Vincent Hospital, Worcester, Massachusetts
Cytomegalovirus Infections

Herbert S. Harned, Jr., M.D.
Professor of Pediatrics, University of North Carolina School of Medicine; Attending Physician, North Carolina Memorial Hospital, Chapel Hill, North Carolina
Hypotension

Burton H. Harris, M.D.
Professor of Surgery, Tufts University School of Medicine; Chief, Division of Pediatric Trauma and Director of The Kiwanis Pediatric Trauma Institute, New England Medical Center, Boston, Massachusetts
Head Injury

H. Robert Harrison, D. Phil., M.D., M.P.H.
Clinical Associate Professor, Department of Pediatrics, Emory University School of Medicine; Attending Physician, Grady Memorial Hospital, Emory University Hospital, and Henrietta Egleston Children's Hospital, Atlanta, Georgia
Coccidioidomycosis

Lily Hechtman, M.D.
Associate Professor of Psychiatry, McGill University Faculty of Medicine; Clinical Director, Department of Psychiatry, The Montreal Children's Hospital, Montreal, Quebec
Psychiatric Disorders

Douglas C. Heiner, M.D., Ph.D.
Professor of Pediatrics, UCLA School of Medicine; Chief, Immunology and Allergy, Harbor-UCLA Medical Center, Los Angeles, California
Primary Pulmonary Hemosiderosis

Terry W. Hensle, M.D.
Associate Professor of Urology, Columbia University College of Physicians and Surgeons; Director, Pediatric Urology, Babies Hospital and

Columbia Presbyterian Medical Center, New York, New York
Vesicoureteral Reflux

Layne Hersh, M.D.
Clinical Instructor, University of California, San Francisco; Attending Staff, Children's Hospital and French Hospital, San Francisco, California
Warts and Molluscum Contagiosum

Fred S. Herzon, M.D.
Professor of Surgery, University of New Mexico Medical School; Chief, Division of Otolaryngology, University of New Mexico Hospital, Albuquerque, New Mexico
Retropharyngeal and Peritonsillar Abscess

Frank Hinman, Jr., M.D.
Clinical Professor of Urology, University of California, San Francisco; Chief of Urology, Children's Hospital, San Francisco, California
Patent Urachus and Urachal Cysts

Horace L. Hodes, M.D.
Distinguished Service Professor and Herbert Lehman Professor and Chairman, Department of Pediatrics, Emeritus, Mount Sinai School of Medicine; Attending Pediatrician, Mount Sinai Medical Center, New York, New York
Diphtheria

Joan E. Hodgman, M.D.
Women's Hospital, Los Angeles, California
Bronchopulmonary Dysplasia; Neonatal Atelectasis; Skin Diseases of the Neonate

Lewis B. Holmes, M.D.
Associate Professor of Pediatrics, Harvard Medical School; Chief, Embryology-Teratology Unit, and Associate Pediatrician, Massachusetts General Hospital, Boston, Massachusetts
Lymphedema

Paul J. Honig, M.D.
Associate Professor of Pediatrics and Dermatology, University of Pennsylvania School of Medicine; Senior Physician and Director, Pediatric Dermatology, Children's Hospital of Philadelphia, Philadelphia, Pennsylvania
Headache; Rickettsial Diseases

Debra A. Horney, M.D.
Clinical Assistant Professor, Department of Dermatology, University of California, Davis, Medical Center, Davis, California
Papulosquamous Disorders

Walter T. Hughes, M.D.
Professor of Pediatrics, University of Tennessee Center for Health Sciences; Director, Division of Infectious Diseases, St. Jude Children's Research Hospital, Memphis, Tennessee
Pneumocystis carinii Pneumonitis; Tularemia

Sidney Hurwitz, M.D.
Clinical Professor of Pediatrics and Dermatology, Yale University School of Medicine; Attending Physician in Pediatrics and Dermatology, Yale–New Haven Medical Center and Hospital of St. Raphael, New Haven, Connecticut
Disorders of Pigmentation; The Genodermatoses; Scabies and Pediculosis

Carol B. Hyman, M.D.
Attending in Pediatric, Hematology/Oncology, Cedars-Sinai Medical Center and Children's Hospital of Los Angeles, Los Angeles, California
Thalassemia

Laura S. Inselman, M.D.
Assistant Professor of Pediatrics, Cornell University Medical College; Chief, Pediatric Pulmonary Division, North Shore University Hospital, Manhasset, New York
Tuberculosis

Silvia Iosub, M.D.
Associate Professor of Pediatrics, New York Medical College, Valhalla, New York; Attending Physician, Metropolitan Hospital Center, New York, New York, and Lincoln Medical and Mental Health Center, Bronx, New York
Gianotti Disease

Mira Irons, M.D.
Fellow in Genetics, Harvard Medical School and Children's Hospital and Massachusetts General Hospital, Boston, Massachusetts
Galactosemias

Shunzaburo Iwatsuki, M.D.
Professor of Surgery, University of Pittsburgh School of Medicine; Presbyterian-University Hospital and Children's Hospital of Pittsburgh, Pittsburgh, Pennsylvania
Disorders of the Hepatobiliary Tree; Tumors of the Liver

Jan T. Jackson, M.D., F.R.C.S., F.A.C.S.
Professor of Plastic Surgery, Mayo Medical School; Chief of Plastic Surgery, Mayo Clinic, Rochester, Minnesota
Craniofacial Malformations

Alvin H. Jacobs, M.D.
Professor of Dermatology and Pediatrics, Emeritus, Stanford University, School of Medicine, Stanford, California
Atopic Dermatitis

George A. Jacoby, M.D.
Associate Professor of Medicine, Harvard Medical School; Associate Physician, Massachusetts General Hospital, Boston, Massachusetts
Babesiosis

L. Stanley James, M.D.
Professor of Pediatrics and of Obstetrics and Gynecology, Columbia University College of Physicians and Surgeons; Attending Pediatrician, Presbyterian Hospital in the City of New York at Columbia-Presbyterian Medical Center, New York, New York
Management of the Newborn Infant at Delivery

Catherine V. Jewett, M.D.
Instructor, Department of Pediatrics, University of Alabama at Birmingham, Birmingham, Alabama
Mycoplasma Infections

Stuart D. Josell, D.M.D., M. Dent. Sci.
Associate Professor, Department of Pediatric Dentistry, School of Dentistry, University of Maryland at Baltimore; Staff, University of Maryland Hospital and James Lawrence Kernan Hospital, Baltimore, Maryland
Dental Caries

Michael A. Kaliner, M.D.
Head, Allergic Diseases Section, National Institutes of Health, Bethesda, Maryland
Allergic Rhinitis

Samuel Kaplan, M.D.
Professor of Pediatrics and Professor of Medicine, University of Cincinnati College of Medicine; Director, Division of Cardiology, Children's Hospital Medical Center, Cincinnati, Ohio
Congestive Cardiac Failure

Sheldon L. Kaplan, M.D.
Associate Professor, Baylor College of Medicine; Chief, Infectious Disease Service, Texas Children's Hospital; Associate Attending Medical Staff, Harris County Hospital District, Houston, Texas
Aseptic Meningitis

Maria Kapuscinska, M.D.
Assistant Professor in Psychiatry, McGill University Faculty of Medicine; Staff Psychiatrist, The Montreal Children's Hospital, Montreal, Quebec
Psychiatric Disorders

Lawrence I. Karlin, M.D.
Assistant Professor of Orthopaedic Surgery, Tufts University School of Medicine; Orthopaedic Surgeon, Tufts–New England Medical Center, Boston, Massachusetts
Disorders of the Spine and Shoulder Girdle

Evan J. Kass, M.D., F.A.A.P., F.A.C.S.
Associate Professor of Urology and Child Health and Development, George Washington University School of Medicine; Associate Director, Department of Pediatric Urology, Children's Hospital National Medical Center, Washington, D.C.
Hydronephrosis and Disorders of the Ureter

Arnold E. Katz, M.D., M.S.
Associate Professor of Otolaryngology, Tufts University School of Medicine; Senior Surgeon, New England Medical Center; Senior Attending Staff, Boston Veterans Administration Medical Center, Boston, Massachusetts
Hearing Loss

Rae-Ellen W. Kavey, M.D.
Associate Professor of Pediatrics, Division of Pediatric Cardiology, SUNY-Upstate Medical Center; Pediatric Staff, University Hospital, SUNY-Upstate Medical Center, and Crouse-Irving Memorial Hospital, Syracuse, New York
Mitral Valve Prolapse

Panayotis P. Kelalis, M.D.
Professor of Urology and Chairman, Department of Urology, Mayo Medical School; Consultant, Department of Urology, Mayo Clinic and Mayo Foundation, Rochester, Minnesota
Exstrophy of the Bladder

Edwin L. Kendig, Jr., M.D., D.Sc. (Hon.)
Professor of Pediatrics, Medical College of Virginia, Health Sciences Division of Virginia Commonwealth University; Director, Child Chest Clinic, Medical College of Virginia Hospitals; Director, Department of Pediatrics, St. Mary's Hospital, Richmond, Virginia
Atelectasis; Sarcoidosis

Joseph L. Kennedy, Jr., M.D.
Associate Professor of Pediatrics, Tufts University School of Medicine; Director of Nurseries, St. Margaret's Hospital for Women; Attending

Neonatologist, Floating Hospital for Infants and Children and New England Medical Center, Boston, Massachusetts
Birth Injuries; Disturbances of Intrauterine Growth

Fiona Key, M.B., Ch.B., F.R.C.P.(C.)
Assistant Professor of Psychiatry and Paediatrics, McGill University Faculty of Medicine; Director, Adolescent Treatment Program, Department of Psychiatry, Montreal Children's Hospital, Montreal, Quebec
Psychiatric Disorders

Kwang Sik Kim, M.D.
Assistant Professor of Pediatrics, UCLA School of Medicine, Los Angeles; Attending Pediatrician, Harbor-UCLA Medical Center, Torrance, California
Group B Streptococcal Infections

Melanie S. Kim, M.D.
Instructor in Pediatrics, Harvard Medical School; Assistant in Medicine (Nephrology), The Children's Hospital, Boston, Massachusetts
The Nephrotic Syndrome

George T. Klauber, M.D., F.A.A.P., F.R.C.S.(C.)
Professor of Urology and Pediatrics, Tufts University School of Medicine; Chief of Pediatric Urology, Boston Floating Hospital for Infants and Children and New England Medical Center, Boston, Massachusetts
Circumcision and Disorders of the Penis and Testis; Malignant Tumors of the Kidney

Jerome O. Klein, M.D.
Professor of Pediatrics, Boston University School of Medicine; Director, Division of Pediatric Infectious Diseases, Boston City Hospital, Boston, Massachusetts
Otitis Media

William J. Klish, M.D.
Associate Professor of Pediatrics, Baylor College of Medicine; Chief, Nutrition and Gastroenterology Service, Texas Children's Hospital, Houston, Texas
Total Parenteral Nutrition in Infants

Susan E. Koch, M.D.
Chief Resident, Dermatology, University of California, San Francisco; Staff, University of California, San Francisco, Hospitals, Moffet Hospital, Veterans Administration Hospital, and San Francisco General Hospital, San Francisco, California
Photodermatoses

Steve Kohl, M.D.
Professor of Pediatrics, Program of Infectious Diseases, University of Texas Medical School; Attending Pediatrician, Hermann Hospital; Pediatric Infectious Disease Consultant, M.D. Anderson Hospital and Tumor Institute, Houston, Texas
Endocarditis

Anne Kolbe, M.B., B.S.
Assistant Professor of Pediatric Surgery, Johns Hopkins School of Medicine; Attending Pediatric Surgeon, Johns Hopkins Hospital, Baltimore, Maryland
Peritonitis

Peter K. Kottmeier, M.D.
Professor and Chief, Pediatric Surgery, State University of New York, Downstate Medical Center; Attending Physician, Kings County Hospital Center, Brooklyn, New York
Gastritis; Peptic Ulcers

Stephen A. Kramer, M.D.
Assistant Professor of Urology, Mayo Medical School; Consultant, Department of Urology, Mayo Clinic and Mayo Foundation, Rochester, Minnesota
Exstrophy of the Bladder

John W. Kulig, M.D.
Assistant Professor of Pediatrics, Tufts University School of Medicine; Director, Adolescent Medicine, New England Medical Center, Boston, Massachusetts
Adolescent Sexuality, Contraception, Pregnancy, and Abortion; Sex Education

Peter O. Kwiterovich, Jr., M.D.
Professor of Pediatrics, Professor of Medicine, and Chief, Lipid Research-Atherosclerosis Unit, Johns Hopkins University School of Medicine; Active Staff, Pediatrics, and Director, Lipid Clinic, Johns Hopkins Hospital, Baltimore, Maryland
Hyperlipoproteinemia

Philip Lanzkowsky, M.D., F.R.C.P., D.C.H.
Professor of Pediatrics, School of Medicine, Health Sciences Center, State University of New York at Stony Brook; Chief-of-Staff and Chairman of Pediatrics and Chief, Division of Pediatric Hematology and Oncology, Schneider Children's Hospital of Long Island Jewish Medical Center, New Hyde Park, New York
Megaloblastic Anemia

Emanuel Lebenthal, M.D.
Professor of Pediatrics, School of Medicine, State University of New York at Buffalo; Chief, Division of Gastroenterology and Nutrition, Children's Hospital of Buffalo; Director, International Institute for Infant Nutrition and Gastrointestinal Disease, Buffalo, New York
Malnutrition

Thomas J. A. Lehman, M.D.
Assistant Professor of Pediatrics, University of Southern California School of Medicine, and Division of Rheumatology, Children's Hospital of Los Angeles, Los Angeles, California
Familial Mediterranean Fever

Lucille A. Lester, M.D.
Assistant Professor, Department of Pediatrics, Pritzker School of Medicine; Co-Director, Cystic Fibrosis Center, The University of Chicago Medical Center, Chicago, Illinois
Cystic Fibrosis

Jeremiah Levine, M.D.
Assistant Professor of Pediatrics, School of Medicine, State University of New York at Stony Brook; Attending Physician, Division of Gastroenterology, Schneider Children's Hospital of Long Island Jewish Medical Center, New Hyde Park, New York
Intractable Diarrhea of Infancy

Lenore S. Levine, M.D.
Professor of Pediatrics, Columbia University College of Physicians and Surgeons; Deputy Director, Pediatrics, and Chief, Pediatric Endocrinology Section, St. Luke's–Roosevelt Hospital Center, New York, New York
Disorders of the Adrenal Gland

Melvin D. Levine, M.D.
Professor of Pediatrics, and Director, Division for Disorders of Development and Learning, University of North Carolina School of Medicine, Chapel Hill, North Carolina
Disorders of Learning and Attention

Harvey L. Levy, M.D.
Associate Professor of Neurology, Harvard Medical School; Associate Pediatrician, Massachusetts General Hospital; Senior Associate in Medicine, Children's Hospital, Boston, Massachusetts
Galactosemias

Michael B. Lewis, M.D.
Associate Professor of Surgery, Tufts Medical School; Chief, Division of Plastic Surgery, New England Medical Center, Boston, Massachusetts
Lymphangioma

Robert W. Lingua, M.D.
Assistant Professor of Ophthalmology, University of Miami School of Medicine; Staff, Bascom Palmer Eye Institute, Miami, Florida
The Eye

Frederick H. Lovejoy, Jr., M.D.
Associate Professor of Pediatrics, Harvard Medical School; Associate Physician-in-Chief, The Children's Hospital; Director, Massachusetts Poison Control Center, Boston, Massachusetts
Acetaminophen Poisoning

Anne W. Lucky, M.D.
Associate Professor of Dermatology and Pediatrics and Director, Division of Pediatric Dermatology, University of Cincinnati College of Medicine; Director, Division of Pediatric Dermatology, Children's Hospital Medical Center, Cincinnati, Ohio
Disorders of the Hair and Scalp

John N. Lukens, M.D.
Professor of Pediatrics, Vanderbilt University School of Medicine; Director, Division of Pediatric Hematology-Oncology, Vanderbilt University Children's Hospital, Nashville, Tennessee
Anemia of Iron Deficiency, Blood Loss, Renal Disease, and Chronic Infection

Wallace W. McCrory, M.D.
Professor of Pediatrics, Cornell University Medical School; Director of Pediatric Nephrology, New York Hospital-Cornell Medical Center, New York, New York
Renal Hypoplasia and Dysplasia

Daune L. MacGregor, M.D.
Associate Professor of Paediatrics (Neurology), University of Toronto Faculty of Medicine; Staff Physician, Hospital for Sick Children, Toronto, Ontario
Degenerative Diseases of the Central Nervous System; Spinal Diseases

James G. McNamara, M.D.
Clinical Immunology Fellow, Yale University School of Medicine; Associate, Howard Hughes Medical Institute, New Haven, Connecticut
Primary Immunodeficiency Disease

Ian T. Magrath, M.B, B.S., M.R.C.P., M.R.C.Path.
Visiting Professor, University of Madras, India; Senior Investigator and Attending Physician, National Cancer Institute, Bethesda, Maryland
Burkitt's Lymphoma

Catherine S. Manno, M.D.
Clinical Assistant Professor of Pediatrics, University of Pennsylvania School of Medicine; Clinical Affiliate, Children's Hospital of Philadelphia, Philadelphia, Pennsylvania
Hemolytic Anemia

Herbert C. Mansmann, Jr., M.D.
Professor of Pediatrics and Associate Professor of Medicine, Jefferson Medical College of Thomas Jefferson University; Director, Division of Allergy and Clinical Immunology, Thomas Jefferson University Hospital, Philadelphia, Pennsylvania
The Croup Syndrome

Andrew M. Margileth, M.D.
Professor and Vice Chairman, Department of Pediatrics, F. Edward Hébert School of Medicine, Uniformed Services University of the Health Sciences; Consultant and Pediatrician, Naval Hospital, Bethesda, and Walter Reed Army Medical Center, Washington, D.C.
Cat Scratch Disease

Melvin I. Marks, M.D.
Professor of Pediatrics and Adjunct Professor of Microbiology/Immunology, University of Oklahoma Health Sciences Center; Director, Pediatric Infectious Disease Service, Oklahoma Children's Memorial Hospital, Oklahoma City, Oklahoma
Pertussis

Marian E. Melish, M.D.
Associate Professor of Pediatrics, Tropical Medicine, and Medical Microbiology, John A. Burns School of Medicine, University of Hawaii; Infectious Disease Consultant, Kapiolani Children's Medical Center, Honolulu, Hawaii
Kawasaki Syndrome

Gregory Milmoe, M.D.
Assistant Professory of Surgery (Otolaryngology), George Washington University Medical School; Associate in Otorhinolaryngology, Children's Hospital National Medical Center, Washington, D.C.
Malformations of the Nose

Sylvester L. Mobley, M.D.
Assistant Professor of Pediatrics, Jefferson Medical College of Thomas Jefferson University; Medical Director, Pediatric Intensive Care Unit, Thomas Jefferson University Hospital, Philadelphia, Pennsylvania
The Croup Syndrome

Daniel L. Mollitt, M.D.
Associate Professor of Surgery and Pediatrics, University of Florida College of Medicine; Attending Surgeon, University Hospital of Jacksonville, Jacksonville, Florida
Peritonitis

Ralph E. Moloshok, M.D.
Emeritus Clinical Professor of Pediatrics, Mount Sinai School of Medicine; Emeritus Attending, Pediatrics, Mount Sinai Hospital, New York, New York
Familial Dysautonomia

Beverly C. Morgan, M.D.
Professor and Chair, Department of Pediatrics, University of California, Irvine, California College of Medicine; Chief of Pediatrics, University of California, Irvine, Medical Center; Attending Physician, Children's Hospital of Orange County, Miller Children's Hospital, and Memorial Medical Center, Orange, California
Cardiomyopathies and Pericardial Disease

Joan E. Morgenthau, M.D.
Adjunct Professor, Psychology, Smith College; Professorial Lecturer in Pediatrics and Community Medicine, Mt. Sinai School of Medicine; Attending Pediatrician, The Mount Sinai Hospital, New York, New York
Adolescent Syphilis

Edward A. Mortimer, Jr., M.D.
Elisabeth Severance Prentiss Professor of Epidemiology and Biostatistics, Vice Chairman, Department of Epidemiology and Biostatistics, and Professor of Pediatrics, Case Western Reserve University School of Medicine; Associate Pediatrician, University Hospitals of Cleveland and Cleveland Metropolitan General Hospital, Cleveland, Ohio
Measles

Michael J. Muszynski, M.D.
Fellow in Pediatric Infectious Diseases, Children's Memorial Hospital, University of Oklahoma Health Sciences Center, Oklahoma City, Oklahoma
Infections Due to Escherichia coli, Proteus, Klebsiella-Enterobacter-Serratia, Pseudomonas, and Other Gram-Negative Bacilli

Gary J. Myers, M.D.
Professor, Department of Pediatrics, University of Alabama School of Medicine, The University of Alabama at Birmingham; Director, Chauncey Sparks Center for Developmental and Learning Disorders; Pediatric Neurologist, The Children's Hospital; Neonatologist, University Hospital, Birmingham, Alabama
Myelodysplasia

Alexander S. Nadas, M.D.
Professor of Pediatrics, Emeritus, Harvard Medical School; Chief, Emeritus, Department of Cardiology, and Senior Associate in Cardiology, The Children's Hospital, Boston, Massachusetts
Congenital Heart Disease

Joseph P. Neglia, M.D.
Medical Fellow, Pediatric Hematology-Oncology, University of Minnesota School of Medicine and University of Minnesota Hospitals and Clinics, Minneapolis, Minnesota
Bacterial Meningitis and Septicemia Beyond the Neonatal Period

Marianne R. Neifert, M.D.
Assistant Professor of Pediatrics, University of Colorado School of Medicine; Attending Physician, University Hospital, University of Colorado Health Sciences Center, Denver, Colorado
Breast-Feeding

Lawrence S. Neinstein, M.D.
Associate Professor of Clinical Pediatrics and Medicine, University of Southern California School of Medicine; Coordinator, Teenage Health Center, Childrens Hospital of Los Angeles, Los Angeles, California
Homosexual Behavior

David B. Nelson, M.D., M.Sc.
Associate Professor of Clinical Pediatrics, Medical College of Wisconsin; Director, Graduate Medical Education, Milwaukee Children's Hospital, Milwaukee, Wisconsin
Bronchitis and Bronchiolitis

John D. Nelson, M.D.
Professor of Pediatrics, University of Texas Health Science Center at Dallas; Active Attending Physician, Children's Medical Center, and Parkland Memorial Hospital, Dallas; Consulting Staff, John Peter Smith Hospital, Forth Worth, Texas
Neonatal Septicemia, Meningitis, and Pneumonia; Osteomyelitis and Suppurative Arthritis

Naomi D. Neufield, M.D.
Assistant Professor in Residence, Department of Pediatrics, University of California at Los Angeles School of Medicine; Head, Section of Endocrinology, Department of Pediatrics, Cedars-Sinai Medical Center; Attending Physician,

Pediatrics, UCLA Center for the Health Sciences, Los Angeles, California
Infants Born to Diabetic Mothers

Maria I. New, M.D.
Professor and Chairman, Department of Pediatrics, Cornell University Medical College; Pediatrician-in-Chief, The New York Hospital, New York, New York
Disorders of the Adrenal Gland

Victor D. Newcomer, M.D.
Clinical Professor of Medicine/Dermatology, University of California, Los Angeles, School of Medicine; Attending Physician, UCLA Hospital, Los Angeles, California
Urticaria

Harold M. Nitowsky, M.D.
Professor, Division of Genetics, Department of Pediatrics, Albert Einstein College of Medicine, Bronx, New York
Genetic Diseases

Michael J. Noetzel, M.D.
Assistant Professor, Edward Mallinckrodt Department of Pediatrics and Department of Neurology and Neurological Surgery, Washington University School of Medicine; Director, Birth Defects Center, St. Louis Children's Hospital; Assistant Pediatrician and Neurologist, Barnes and Allied Hospitals; Consultant in Child Neurology, Irene Walter Johnson Institute of Rehabilitation, St. Louis, Missouri
Intracranial Hemorrhage; Hydrocephalus

James J. Nora, M.D., M.P.H.
Professor of Pediatrics, Genetics, and Preventive Medicine, University of Colorado School of Medicine; Director of Preventive Cardiology, University Hospital; Director of Genetics, Rose Medical Center, Denver, Colorado
The Child at Risk of Coronary Disease as an Adult

Antonia Coello Novello, M.D., M.P.H.
Clinical Associate Professor of Pediatrics, Georgetown University School of Medicine; Attending Physician, Georgetown University Hospital, Washington, D.C.; Executive Secretary, General Medicine B Study Section, Division of Research Grants, National Institutes of Health, Bethesda, Maryland
Hemodialysis; Hemolytic Uremic Syndrome; Renal Transplantation

Robert Nudelman, M.D.
Assistant Clinical Professor of Pediatrics, University of California, Los Angeles, School of

Medicine; Associate, Cedar-Sinai Medical Center, Los Angeles, California
Pulmonary Embolism

Edward J. O'Connell, M.D.
Professor of Pediatrics, Mayo Medical School; Consultant, Department of Pediatrics, Mayo Clinic and Mayo Foundation, Rochester, Minnesota
Recurrent Acute Parotitis

William Oh, M.D.
Professor of Medical Science in Pediatrics and Obstetrics, Brown University Program in Medicine; Pediatrician-in-Chief, Women and Infants Hospital, Providence, Rhode Island
Respiratory Distress Syndrome

Edgar Y. Oppenheimer, M.D.
Associate Clinical Professor of Pediatrics and Neurology, Boston University School of Medicine, Boston; Pediatric Neurology Department, North Shore Children's Hospital, Salem, Massachusetts
Maternal Alcohol Ingestion Effects on the Developing Child

Gary D. Overturf, M.D.
Professor of Pediatrics, University of Southern California School of Medicine; Head Physician, Communicable Disease Service, Los Angeles County–University of Southen California Medical Center, Los Angeles, California
Legionella Infections

Seymour Packman, M.D.
Associate Professor of Pediatrics, Department of Pediatrics, Division of Genetics, University of California, San Francisco, School of Medicine; Attending Physician, University of California, San Francisco, Hospitals and Clinics, San Francisco, California
Amino Acid Disorders

Dachling Pang, M.D., F.R.C.S. (C)
Associate Professor of Neurosurgery, University of Pittsburgh School of Medicine; Staff Neurosurgeon, Children's Hospital, Pittsburgh, Pennsylvania
Rhinitis and Sinusitis

John S. Parks, M.D., Ph.D.
Professor of Pediatrics and Associate Professor of Biochemistry, Emory University School of Medicine; Director of Pediatric Endocrinology, Henrietta Egleston Hospital and Henry F. Grady Hospital, Atlanta, Georgia
Endocrine Disorders of the Testis

Nicholas A. Patrone, M.D.
Assistant Professor of Medicine and Pediatrics, East Carolina School of Medicine; Clinical Assistant Professor of Pediatrics, Duke University School of Medicine; Attending Physician, Pitt County Memorial Hospital, Greenville, and Duke University Medical Center, Durham, North Carolina
Eosinophilic Fasciitis

Robert Penny, M.D.
Professor of Pediatrics, University of Southern California School of Medicine; Endocrine Consultant, Newborn Screening, Los Angeles County–University of Southern California Medical Center, Los Angeles, California
Undescended Testes

Carol F. Phillips, M.D.
Professor and Chairman, Department of Pediatrics, University of Vermont College of Medicine; Associate Dean of Academic Affairs, University of Vermont; Attending Pediatrician and Chief of Pediatric Service, Medical Center Hospital of Vermont, Burlington, Vermont
Psittacosis

Larry K. Pickering, M.D.
Professor of Pediatrics, Program in Infectious Diseases and Clinical Microbiology, University of Texas Medical School of Houston; Director, Pediatric Infectious Diseases, University of Texas Medical School at Houston, Houston, Texas
Chronic Diarrhea and Malabsorption Syndromes; Shigellosis

Rosita S. Pildes, M.D.
Professor of Pediatrics, University of Illinois College of Medicine; Chairman, Division of Neonatology, Cook County Children's Hospital, Chicago, Illinois
Infants of Drug-Dependent Mothers

Stephanie H. Pincus, M.D.
Associate Professor of Dermatology and Medicine, Tufts University School of Medicine; Associate Dermatologist-in-Chief and Vice Chairman, New England Medical Center Hospital, Boston, Massachusetts
Contact Dermatitis

Donald Pinkel, M.D.
Professor of Pediatrics, Temple University School of Medicine; Chief of Hematology/Oncology, St. Christopher's Hospital for Children, Philadelphia, Pennsylvania
Acute Leukemia

R. Marshall Pitts, M.D., F.A.A.P., F.A.C.S.
Clinical Assistant Professor of Surgery, Medical College of Alabama; Attending Pediatric Surgeon, The Children's Hospital of Alabama, The University of Alabama Hospital, St. Vincent's Hospital, Brookwood Hospital, and Carraway Methodist Hospital, Birmingham, Alabama
Ambiguous Genitalia

Philip A. Pizzo, M.D.
Chief of Pediatrics and Head, Infectious Disease Section, National Cancer Institute, The National Institutes of Health; Attending Physician, The Clinical Center, National Institutes of Health, Bethesda, Maryland
Leukopenia, Neutropenia, and Agranulocytosis

Jeffrey J. Pomerance, M.D., M.P.H.
Associate Professor of Pediatrics, University of California, Los Angeles, School of Medicine; Director of Neonatology, Cedars-Sinai Medical Center, Los Angeles, California
Disorders of the Umbilicus

Stephen R. Preblud, M.D.
Medical Epidemiologist, Division of Immunization, Centers for Disease Control; Assistant Clinical Professor, Department of Pediatrics, Emory University School of Medicine; Attending Physician, Henrietta Egleston Hospital for Children and Grady Memorial Hospital, Atlanta, Georgia
Mumps

Roy Proujansky, M.D.
Clinical and Research Fellow, Department of Pediatric Gastroenterology and Nutrition, Massachusetts General Hospital and Children's Hospital, Boston, Massachusetts
Irritable Bowel Syndrome

Dane G. Prugh, M.D.
Emeritus Professor of Psychiatry and Pediatrics, University of Colorado School of Medicine, Denver, Colorado
The Children of Divorcing Parents

Paul G. Quie, M.D.
Professor of Pediatrics and Microbiology and American Legion Research Professor, University of Minnesota Medical School; Attending Physician and Chief, Pediatric Infectious Diseases, University of Minnesota Hospital, Minneapolis, Minnesota
Staphylococcal Infections

Edward F. Rabe, M.D.
Professor of Pediatrics and Neurology, Tufts University School of Medicine; Head, Section of Pediatric Neurology, New England Medical Center Hospitals, Boston, Massachusetts
Cerebrovascular Disease in Infancy and Childhood; Febrile Convulsions

Daniel D. Rabuzzi, M.D.
Clinical Professor of Otolaryngology and Communication Sciences, State University of New York, Upstate Medical Center; Attending Physician, St. Joseph's Hospital and Crouse-Irving Memorial Hospital, Syracuse, New York
Disorders of the Larynx

Max L. Ramenofsky, M.D.
Meisler-Ripps Professor of Pediatric Surgery, University of South Alabama; Chief of Pediatric Surgery, University of South Alabama Medical Center, Mobile, Alabama
Congenital Diaphragmatic Hernia; Lymph Node Infections; Lymphangitis

James E. Rasmussen. M.D.
Professor of Dermatology and Pediatrics, University of Michigan Medical School; Attending Physician, University of Michigan Hospitals, Ann Arbor, Michigan
Erythema Multiforme

Owen M. Rennert, M.D.
Professor and Chairman, Department of Pediatrics, Chief, Division of Genetics, Endocrinology and Metabolism, University of Oklahoma College of Medicine; Chief of Staff, Oklahoma Children's Memorial Hospital, Oklahoma City, Oklahoma
Hepatolenticular Degeneration

Thomas S. Renshaw, M.D.
Associate Professor of Orthopedic Surgery, University of Connecticut School of Medicine, Farmington; Director of Orthopaedic Surgery, Newington Children's Hospital, Newington, Connecticut
Torticollis

Sylvia Onesti Richardson, M.A., M.D.
Clinical Professor of Pediatrics and Professor of Communicology and Special Education, University of South Florida, Tampa, Florida
Voice, Speech, and Language Disorders

Robert A. Richman, M.D.
Associate Professor of Pediatrics, State University of New York Upstate Medical Center; Attending Pediatrician, State University Hospital and Crouse-Irving Memorial Hospital, Syracuse, New York
Diabetes Insipidus

Harris D. Riley, Jr., M.D.
Distinguished Professor of Pediatrics, University of Oklahoma College of Medicine; Attending Physician, Children's Memorial Hospital, University of Oklahoma Health Sciences Center, Oklahoma City, Oklahoma
*Infections Due to **Escherichia coli, Proteus, Klebsiella-Enterobacter-Serratia, Pseudomonas,** and Other Gram-Negative Bacilli*

Marie F. Robert, M.D.
Assistant Professor of Pediatrics and Epidemiology and Public Health, Yale University School of Medicine; Attending Pediatrician, Yale-New Haven Hospital, New Haven, Connecticut
Infectious Mononucleosis

Francis Robicsek, M.D.
Chairman, Department of Thoracic and Cardiovascular Surgery, Charlotte Memorial Hospital and Medical Center, Charlotte; Clinical Professor of Surgery, University of North Carolina School of Medicine, Chapel Hill, North Carolina
Congenital Deformities of the Anterior Chest Wall

Alan M. Robson, M.D., F.R.C.P.
Professor of Pediatrics, Washington University School of Medicine; Director, Division of Nephrology, St. Louis Children's Hospital, St. Louis, Missouri
Systemic Hypertension

Gerald Rosen, M.D.
Associate Clinical Professor, University of California, Los Angeles, School of Medicine; Attending Physician, Departments of Pediatrics and Medicine, UCLA Center for Health Sciences and Cedars-Sinai Medical Center, Los Angeles, California
The Treatment of Malignant Bone Tumors

Philip Rosenthal, M.D.
Assistant Professor of Pediatrics, University of Southern California School of Medicine; Attending Physician, Division of Gastroenterology and Nutrition, Children's Hospital of Los Angeles, California
Disorders of Porphyrin, Purine, and Pyrimidine Metabolism

N. Paul Rosman, M.D.
Professor of Pediatrics and Neurology, Boston University School of Medicine; Director of Pe-

diatric Neurology, Boston University School of Medicine and Boston City Hospital, Boston, Massachusetts
Maternal Alcohol Ingestion Effects on the Developing Child

Richard M. Rothberg, M.D.
Professor of Pediatrics and Pathology, University of Chicago Pritzker School of Medicine; Head, Section of Allergy, Immunology, and Pulmonology, Wyler Children's Hospital and University of Chicago Hospitals, Chicago, Illinois
Cystic Fibrosis

Alexandra Roussos, M.D.
Assistant Professor, Department of Psychiatry, McGill University Faculty of Medicine; Director, Day Treatment Centre, Department of Psychiatry, The Montreal Children's Hospital, Montreal, Quebec
Psychiatric Disorders

Barry H. Rumack, M.D.
Professor of Pediatrics, University of Colorado School of Medicine; Director, Rocky Mountain Poison and Drug Center, Denver General Hospital; Attending Physician, Denver General Hospital and University of Colorado Health Sciences Center, Denver, Colorado
Acute Poisoning; Botulinal Food Poisoning

Ruth C. Russell, B.Sc., M.D.C.M., F.R.C.P.(C)
Assistant Professor of Psychiatry and Pediatrics, McGill University Faculty of Medicine; Child Psychiatrist, Consultation Service, Montreal Children's Hospital, Montreal, Quebec
Psychiatric Disorders

Nell J. Ryan, M.D.
Associate Professor Pediatrics, Louisiana State University School of Medicine at Shreveport; Attending Physician, Louisiana State Medical Center, Shreveport, Louisiana
Meningococcal Disease

Hernan Sabio, M.D., M.S.
Associate Professor of Pediatrics and Pathology, University of Virginia School of Medicine; Attending Pediatrician and Pediatric Hematologist/Oncologist, University Hospital, Charlottesville, Virginia
Pediatric Cardiac Tumors

David A. Sack, M.D.
Associate Professor of Medicine, Division of Geographic Medicine, Johns Hopkins University School of Medicine, Baltimore, Maryland; Associate Director, International Centre for

Diarrhoeal Disease Research, Bangladesh Dhaka, Bangladesh; Infectious Disease Consultant, Francis Scott Key Medical Center, Baltimore, Maryland
Cholera

Joseph W. St. Geme, Jr., M.D.
Professor of Pediatrics and Dean, University of Colorado School of Medicine; Attending Physician, University Hospital, University of Colorado Health Sciences Center, Denver, Colorado
Herpes Simplex Virus Infections

Mounir Samy, M.D.
Assistant Professor of Psychiatry, McGill University Faculty of Medicine; Staff Psychiatrist, Montreal Children's Hospital, Montreal, Quebec
Psychiatric Disorders

Julio V. Santiago, M.D.
Professor of Pediatrics, Washington University School of Medicine; Co-Director, Division of Endocrinology and Metabolism, St. Louis Children's Hospital, St. Louis, Missouri
Systemic Hypertension

Robert A. Saul, M.D.
Associate Director, Greenwood Genetic Center, Greenwood, South Carolina
Idiopathic Cortical Hyperostosis

Lawrence Schachner, M.D.
Associate Professor of Dermatology, Associate Professor of Pediatrics, and Director, Pediatric Dermatology, University of Miami School of Medicine; Attending Physician, University of Miami School of Medicine/Jackson Memorial Hospital, Miami, Florida
Drug Reactions and the Skin; Erythema Nodosum; Fungal Infections

Gilbert M. Schiff, M.D.
President, James N. Gamble Institute of Medical Research; Professor of Medicine, University of Cincinnati College of Medicine; Attending Physician, The Christ Hospital and University Hospital; Consulting Staff, Childrens' Hospital Medical Center and Jewish Hospital of Cincinnati, Cincinnati, Ohio
Enteroviruses

Virginia E. Schuett, M.S.
Assistant Clinical Professor, University of Wisconsin; Nutritionist, Metabolic Clinic, Waisman Center on Mental Retardation and Human Development, University of Wisconsin, Madison, Wisconsin
Hyperphenylalaninemias

Richard H. Schwartz, M.D.

Associate Clinical Professor of Child Health and Development, George Washington University School of Medicine; Associate Clinical Professor of Pediatrics, Georgetown University School of Medicine; Attending Physician, Fairfax Hospital, Falls Church, Virginia, and Children's Hospital National Medical Center, Washington, D.C.
Management of a Drug-using Adolescent

Susan M. Scott, M.D.

Assistant Professor of Pediatrics, University of New Mexico School of Medicine; Attending Physician, University of New Mexico Medical Center, Albuquerque, New Mexico
Rickets; Tetany

John H. Seashore, M.D.

Professor of Surgery and Pediatrics, Yale University School of Medicine; Attending Physician, Yale-New Haven Hospital, New Haven, Connecticut
Disorders of the Anus and Rectum

Aileen B. Sedman, M.D.

Assistant Professor, Pediatric Nephrology, University of Michigan Medical School; Attending Physician, University Hospitals at the University of Michigan Medical School, Ann Arbor, Michigan
Chronic Renal Failure

Donald H. Shaffner, M.D.

Chief Resident, Department of Pediatrics, Rainbow Babies and Childrens Hospital, Cleveland, Ohio
The Management of Septic Shock

Alan R. Shalita, M.D.

Professor and Chairman, Department of Dermatology, State University of New York Downstate Medical Center; Chief of Dermatology, State University Hospital, Kings County Hospital Center, and Brookdale Hospital Medical Center; Consultant in Dermatology, Brooklyn Veterans Administration Medical Center and Long Island College Hospital, Brooklyn, New York
Disorders of Sebaceous Glands and Sweat Glands

Bruce K. Shapiro, M.D.

Associate Professor of Pediatrics, Johns Hopkins University School of Medicine; Director, Child Development Clinic, The Kennedy Institute for Handicapped Children, Baltimore, Maryland
Mental Retardation

Sheila Sherlock, D.B.E., M.D.

Professor of Medicine, School of Medicine, University of London; Consultant Physician, Royal Free Hospital, London, England
Chronic Active Hepatitis; Portal Hypertension

Bennett A. Shaywitz, M.D.

Associate Professor of Pediatrics and Neurology, and Director, Child Neurology Section, Yale University School of Medicine; Attending Physician, Yale-New Haven Hospital, New Haven, Connecticut
Hypoxic Encephalopathy

Ira A. Shulman, M.D.

Assistant Professor of Pathology, University of Southern California School of Medicine; Blood Bank Director, Los Angeles County-University of Southern California Medical Center, and Kenneth Norris, Jr. Cancer Hospital and Research Institute, Los Angeles, California
Adverse Reactions to Blood Transfusions

Robert J. Shulman, M.D.

Assistant Professor of Pediatrics, Baylor College of Medicine; Director, Nutritional Support Team, Texas Children's Hospital; Attending Physician, Nutrition and Gastroenterology Service, Texas Children's Hospital and the Harris County Hospital District, Houston, Texas
Total Parenteral Nutrition in Infants

William K. Sieber, M.D.

Clinical Professor of Surgery, University of Pittsburgh School of Medicine; Attending Staff, Children's Hospital of Pittsburgh; Consulting Staff, Mercy Hospital of Pittsburgh and Western Pennsylvania Hospital, Pittsburgh, Pennsylvania
Hirschsprung's Disease

Irwin M. Siegel, M.D.

Associate Professor, Department of Orthopaedic Surgery and Neurological Sciences, Rush-Presbyterian-St. Luke's Medical Center; Attending Physician and Chairman, Louis A. Weiss Memorial Hospital; Assistant Attending Physician, Rush-Presbyterian-St. Luke's Medical Center, Chicago, Illinois
Muscular Dystrophy and Related Myopathies

Richard H. Sills, M.D.

Associate Professor of Pediatrics, State University of New York at Buffalo; Pediatric Hematologist-Oncologist, Children's Hospital of Buffalo, Buffalo, New York
Disseminated Intravascular Coagulation and Purpura Fulminans

Frank A. Simon, M.D.
Associate Professor of Pediatrics, the University of Texas Medical School at Houston; Active Staff, Hermann Hospital and Methodist Hospital; Courtesy Staff, Memorial Hospital, Houston, Texas
Salicylate Poisoning

William D. Singer, M.D.
Associate Professor of Pediatrics (Neurology), Tufts University School of Medicine; Pediatric Neurologist, New England Medical Center; Director, Boston Muscular Dystrophy Association Clinic, Lakeview Hospital, Lakeville, Massachusetts
Spasmus Nutans

Lucius F. Sinks, M.D.
Chief, Cancer Centers Branch, National Cancer Institute, National Institutes of Health, Bethesda, Maryland
Malignant Lymphoma

Jay E. Slater, M.D.
Medical Staff Fellow, National Institutes of Allergy and Infectious Diseases, National Institutes of Health, Bethesda, Maryland
Allergic Rhinitis

R. Michael Sly, M.D.
Director of Allergy and Immunology, Children's Hospital National Medical Center; Professor of Child Health and Development, The George Washington University School of Medicine and Health Sciences, Washington, D.C.
Asthma

Fred G. Smith, Jr., M.D.
Professor and Head, Department of Pediatrics, University of Iowa College of Medicine, Iowa City, Iowa
Perinephric and Intranephric Abscess; Urinary Tract Infections

Howard G. Smith, M.D.
Instructor in Otolaryngology, Harvard Medical School; Senior Associate in Otolaryngology, Boston Children's Hospital; Assistant Surgeon in Otolaryngology, Massachusetts Eye and Ear Infirmary, Boston, Massachusetts
Epistaxis; Foreign Bodies of the Nose and Pharynx

Margaret H. D. Smith, M.D.
Professor of Pediatrics, Tulane University School of Medicine; Senior Visiting Physician, Charity Hospital of Louisiana at New Orleans, New Orleans, Louisiana
Pneumonia

O. Carter Snead, III, M.D.
Professor of Pediatric Neurology, University of Alabama at Birmingham School of Medicine; Attending Physician, University Hospital and The Children's Hospital, Birmingham, Alabama
Myasthenia Gravis

Arthur J. Sober, M.D.
Associate Professor of Dermatology, Harvard Medical School; Associate Dermatologist, Massachusetts General Hospital, Boston, Massachusetts
Nevi and Nevoid Tumors

Robert T. Soper, M.D.
Professor of Surgery, University of Iowa College of Medicine; Director of Pediatric Surgery, University of Iowa Hospitals and Clinics, Iowa City, Iowa
Preoperative and Postoperative Care of Patients Undergoing Gastrointestinal Surgery

Mark A. Sperling, M.D.
Professor of Pediatrics and Associate Professor of Medicine, University of Cincinnati College of Medicine; Director, Department of Endocrinology, Childrens Hospital Medical Center, Cincinnati, Ohio
Hypoglycemia

Adrian Spitzer, M.D.
Professor of Pediatrics and Director, Division of Nephrology, Albert Einstein College of Medicine; Attending Pediatrician, Hospital of the Albert Einstein College of Medicine, Montefiore Hospital and Medical Center, and Bronx Municipal Hospital Center, Bronx, New York
Renal Venous Thrombosis

Mary K. Spraker, M.D.
Assistant Professor of Dermatology and Pediatrics, Emory University School of Medicine; Chief of Dermatology, Henrietta Egleston Hospital for Children; Medical Staff, Emory University and Grady Memorial Hospitals, Atlanta, Georgia
Chronic Nonhereditary Vesiculobullous Disorders of Childhood; Other Skin Tumors

Gopal Srinivasan, M.D.
Associate Professor of Pediatrics, University of Health Sciences/Chicago Medical School; Attending Physician, Cook County Children's Hospital, Chicago, Illinois
Infants of Drug-Dependent Mothers

Lynn T. Staheli, M.D.
Professor, Department of Orthopedics, University of Washington School of Medicine; Director, Department of Orthopedics, Children's Orthopedic Hospital and Medical Center, Seattle, Washington
The Hip

F. Bruder Stapleton, M.D.
Professor of Pediatrics and Head, Section of Pediatric Nephrology, University of Tennessee Center for Health Sciences; Le Bonheur Children's Medical Center, Memphis, Tennessee
Idiopathic Hypercalcemia; Urolithiasis

Kenneth A. Starling, M.D.
Professor and Chairman, Department of Pediatrics, West Virginia University Medical Center, Charleston Division; Attending Physician, Charleston Area Medical Center-Memorial Division, Charleston, West Virginia
The Histiocytosis Syndromes

Thomas E. Starzl, M.D., Ph.D.
Professor of Surgery, University of Pittsburgh School of Medicine; Attending Surgeon, Presbyterian-University Hospital and Children's Hospital of Pittsburgh, Pittsburgh, Pennsylvania
Disorders of the Hepatobiliary Tree; Tumors of the Liver

Robert C. Stern, M.D.
Professor of Pediatrics, Case Western Reserve University School of Medicine; Associate Pediatrician, Rainbow Babies and Children's Hospital, Cleveland, Ohio
Pleural Effusion

Leon Sternfeld, M.D.
United Cerebral Palsy Associations, Inc., New York, New York
Cerebral Palsy

Eugene Strandness, Jr., M.D.
Professor of Surgery and Head, Section of Vascular Surgery, University of Washington School of Medicine; Attending Physician, University Hospital and Veterans Administration Medical Center, Seattle, Washington
Peripheral Vascular Disorders

Richard H. Strauss, M.D.
Instructor, Department of Pediatrics, Albany Medical College; Assistant Attending Pediatrician, Albany Medical Center Hospital; Clinical Assistant, Department of Pediatrics, St. Peter's Hospital, Albany, New York
Brain Abscess; Head Injury; Spinal Epidural Abscess

Fred J. Stucker, Jr., M.D.
Professor and Chairman Department of Otolaryngology/Head and Neck Surgery, Louisiana State University School of Medicine in Shreveport; Consultant, Veterans Administration Hospital, Shreveport, Louisiana
Nasal Injuries

David A. Stumpf, M.D., Ph.D.
Professor of Pediatrics and Neurology, Northwestern University Medical School; Director, Division of Pediatric Neurology, Children's Memorial Hospital, Chicago, Illinois
Acute Ataxia

Se Mo Suh, M.D., Ph.D.
Professor of Pediatrics, University of Hawaii School of Medicine; Director, Endocrine Clinic, Kapiolani Women's and Children's Medical Center; Director, Bone and Mineral Research Laboratory, Shriner's Hospital for Crippled Children, Honolulu, Hawaii
Magnesium Deficiency

Jean W. Temeck, M.D.
Assistant Professor of Pediatrics, Cornell University Medical College; Assistant Attending Pediatrician, The New York Hospital, New York, New York
Disorders of the Adrenal Gland

M. Michael Thaler, M.D.
Professor of Pediatrics and Director, Pediatric Gastroenterology and Nutrition, University of California, San Francisco School of Medicine; Attending Physician, University of California, San Francisco, Medical Center, San Francisco, California
Cirrhosis; Disorders of Porphyrin, Purine, and Pyrimidine Metabolism; Nonhemolytic Unconjugated Hyperbilirubinemia; Reye's Syndrome

Jane Todaro, M.D.
Clinical Professor of Gastroenterology, Department of Pediatrics and Adolescent Gastroenterology, Children's Hospital and Medical Center, Seattle, Washington
Allergic Gastrointestinal Disorders

Myron J. Tong, Ph.D., M.D.
Professor of Medicine, University of Southern California School of Medicine, Los Angeles, California; Chief, Liver Center, and Director, Internal Medicine Residency Program, Huntington Memorial Hospital, Pasadena, California
Viral Hepatitis

Daniel E. Torphy, M.D.
Associate Professor of Pediatrics, Medical College of Wisconsin; Medical Director, Ambulatory Services, Milwaukee Children's Hospital, Milwaukee, Wisconsin
Campylobacter *Infections*

Reginald C. Tsang, M.B.B.S.
Professor of Pediatrics and of Obstetrics and Gynecology, University of Cincinnati College of Medicine; Attending Physician, University of Cincinnati Medical Center and Children's Hospital Medical Center, Cincinnati, Ohio
Parathyroid Disease

J. A. Peter Turner, M.D.
Professor Emeritus of Pediatrics, University of Toronto Faculty of Medicine; Senior Consultant, Division of Chest Diseases, Hospital for Sick Children, Toronto, Ontario
Bronchiectasis

John N. Udall, Jr., M.D., Ph.D.
Assistant Professor, Harvard Medical School; Associate in Medicine, Children's Hospital, Boston, Massachusetts
Vitamin Deficiencies and Excesses

Louis E. Underwood, M.D.
Professor of Pediatrics, University of North Carolina at Chapel Hill School of Medicine, Chapel Hill, North Carolina
Hypopituitarism

Timos Valaes, M.D.
Professor of Pediatrics, Tufts University School of Medicine; Director of Neonatology, New England Medical Center Hospitals, Boston, Massachusetts
Neonatal Ascites

Judson J. Van Wyk, M.D.
Kenan Professor of Pediatrics, University of North Carolina at Chapel Hill School of Medicine; Senior Staff Attending, University of North Carolina Memorial Hospital, Chapel Hill, North Carolina
Tall Stature

Elliott Vichinsky, M.D.
Assistant Clinical Professor of Pediatrics, University of California, San Francisco, School of Medicine; Division Chief, Hematology/Oncology, Children's Hospital Medical Center of Northern California, Oakland, California
Sickle Cell Disease

Theodore P. Votteler, M.D., F.A.A.P., F.A.C.S.
Clinical Associate Professor of Surgery, University of Texas Health Science Center, Southwestern Medical School; Director of Surgical Services, Children's Medical Center, Dallas, Texas
Nontuberculous (Atypical) Mycobacterial Infections

Ken B. Waites, M.D.
Research Associate, Department of Microbiology, University of Alabama School of Medicine, Birmingham, Alabama
Mycoplasma Infections

Ellen R. Wald, M.D.
Associate Professor, Department of Pediatrics, University of Pittsburgh School of Medicine; Associate Medical Director, Ambulatory Care Division; Member, Division of Infectious Diseases, Children's Hospital of Pittsburgh, Pittsburgh, Pennsylvania
Rhinitis and Sinusitis

W. Allan Walker, M.D.
Professor of Pediatrics, Harvard Medical School; Chief, Combined Program in Pediatric Gastroenterology and Nutrition, Children's Hospital, Boston, Massachusetts
Acute and Chronic Nonspecific Diarrhea Syndromes

Philip A. Walravens, M.D.
Assistant Clinical Professor, University of Colorado Health Science Center, Denver, Colorado
Zinc Deficiency

H. James Wedner, M.D.
Associate Professor of Medicine, Washington University School of Medicine; Associate Physician, Barnes Hospital, St. Louis, Missouri
Adverse Reactions to Drugs

Paul F. Wehrle, M.D.
Los Angeles, California
Rabies

Marvin L. Weil, M.D.
Professor of Pediatrics and Neurology, University of California, Los Angeles, School of Medicine; Chief, Division of Pediatric Neurology, Harbor-UCLA Medical Center, Los Angeles, California
Encephalitis Infections—Postinfectious and Postvaccinal; Myositis Ossificans

Gabrielle Weiss, M.D.
Professor of Psychiatry, McGill University Faculty of Medicine; Director, Department of Psychiatry, The Montreal Children's Hospital, Montreal, Quebec
Psychiatric Disorders

Marc Weissbluth, M.D.
Assistant Professor, Department of Pediatrics, Northwestern University School of Medicine; Active Attending Pediatrician, The Children's Memorial Hospital, Chicago, Illinois
Colic

Willis A. Wingert, M.D.
Professor of Pediatrics, Community Medicine, Public Health, and Emergency Medicine, University of Southern California School of Medicine; Director, Pediatric Ambulatory Services, Los Angeles County University of Southern California Medical Center, Los Angeles, California
Animal and Human Bites and Bite-Related Infections

Jerry A. Winkelstein, M.D.
Professor of Pediatrics and Associate Professor of Molecular Biology and Genetics, Johns Hopkins University School of Medicine; Director of the Division of Immunology, The Department of Pediatrics, The Johns Hopkins Hospital, Baltimore, Maryland
Postsplenectomy Syndrome

Joseph I. Wolfsdorf, M.D.
Instructor in Pediatrics, Harvard Medical School; Associate in Endocrinology, The Children's Hospital, Boston; Associate Physician, New England Deaconess Hospital; Senior Physician, Youth Unit, Joslin Diabetes Center, Boston, Massachusetts
Diabetes Mellitus

Robert E. Wood, Ph.D., M.D.
Associate Professor of Pediatrics, University of North Carolina School of Medicine; Chief, Pediatric Pulmonary Medicine, and Medical Director, Pediatric Intensive Care, University of North Carolina at Chapel Hill, North Carolina
Emphysema; Pulmonary Edema

Gordon Worley, M.D.
Assistant Professor, Department of Pediatrics, Duke University School of Medicine; Chief of Pediatrics, Lenox Baker Children's Rehabilitation Hospital; Attending Physician, Duke University Medical Center, Durham, North Carolina
Toxocara canis *Infections (Including Visceral Larva Migrans)*

Gary P. Wormser, M.D.
Professor of Medicine, New York Medical College; Chief of Infectious Diseases, Westchester County Medical Center, Valhalla, New York
Yersinia enterocolitica *Infections*

Jen Wung, M.D.
Associate Clinical Professor of Anesthesiology, Columbia University College of Physicians and Surgeons; Associate Attending Anesthesiologist, Presbyterian Hospital in the City of New York at Columbia-Presbyterian Medical Center, New York, New York
Management of the Newborn Infant at Delivery

Erik L. Yeo, M.D., F.R.C.P.(C.)
Instructor, Tufts University School of Medicine; Fellow, New England Medical Center, Boston, Massachusetts
Pediatric Hemostasis

Carolyn Young, M.N.S., R.D.
Research Nutritionist, International Institute for Infant Nutrition and Gastrointestinal Disease, Children's Hospital of Buffalo, Buffalo, New York
Malnutrition

John M. Zahradnik, M.D.
Assistant Professor of Microbiology/Immunology and Pediatrics, Influenza Research Center, Baylor College of Medicine; Attending Pediatrician, Harris County Hospital District; Courtesy Staff, Infectious Disease Service, Texas Children's Hospital; Consulting Pediatrician, The Methodist Hospital, Houston, Texas
Influenza

Harvey A. Zarem, M.D.
Professor of Surgery (Plastic and Reconstructive Surgery) University of California, Los Angeles, School of Medicine; Chief, Division of Plastic and Reconstructive Surgery, UCLA Medical Center, Los Angeles, California
Diseases and Injuries of the Oral Region

Ekhard E. Ziegler, M.D.
Professor of Pediatrics, University of Iowa College of Medicine; Staff Physician, University of Iowa Hospitals and Clinics, Iowa City, Iowa
Feeding the Low Birth Weight Infant

William H. Zinkham, M.D.
Distinguished Service Professor of Pediatrics and Professor of Oncology, The Johns Hopkins University School of Medicine; Director of Pediatric Hematology, The Johns Hopkins Hospital, Baltimore, Maryland
Indications for Splenectomy

Philip R. Ziring, M.D.
Associate Clinical Professor of Pediatrics, Columbia University College of Physicians and Surgeons; Chairman, Department of Pediatrics, Morristown Memorial Hospital; Associate Attending, Babies Hospital and Columbia Presbyterian Medical Center, New York, New York
Rubella and Congenital Rubella

Preface

The interest shown in earlier publications of this book has been a gratifying indication of the objective need for a reliable text on the treatment of disorders of infancy and childhood.

In this twelfth edition we have made an intensive effort to incorporate all significant advances of the past two years in the management of ill children. To this end we have invited material from contributors who were not in the last edition and have asked all others to bring their material completely up to the minute. This rotation of authors does not in any way reflect dissatisfaction with original contributors, but rather a desire to present variations in points of view. We hope that each volume in the series will have a fresh approach to important therapeutic measures in pediatrics as well as a personality of its own. For this reason, we urge those who own copies of previous editions to retain them for comparison and for reference to previous modes of therapy that were in use at earlier dates.

The art of medicine changes rapidly, and in no area is there more frequent change than in therapy. New antimicrobial agents, new vaccines, new drugs confront the physician almost daily, and it is difficult to reliably determine the effectiveness and safety of these preparations. He must, and should, rely on the experience of qualified clinical investigators to evaluate the usefulness of new agents in a controlled setting.

Actually the vast bulk of childhood illnesses require little in the way of medication, and most of us are guilty of overtreatment. The fewer drugs we utilize, the less harm we are likely to do. There are, however, numerous conditions that require careful administration of specific drug therapy and/or certain newly discovered and relatively unusual methods of surgical intervention; these conditions may be infrequently encountered in an individual's practice, and the physician then requires a careful and detailed guide to their management.

The reader will find footnotes that indicate that the dose of a drug as listed in the text has not been established for infants and children or that the use of a drug recommended by the author is not listed by the manufacturer or that the dose of a drug recommended by the author for a particular purpose exceeds that recommended by the manufacturer or other similar comments. These footnotes present important information for your consideration and your judgment.

Once again we tender deep appreciation to the contributors. Their effective cooperation has been absolutely edifying.

And, finally, a word of appreciation to our wives for continued tolerance.

It is our earnest hope that Current Pediatric Therapy has proved helpful and will continue to prove beneficial not only to the physician but, most important of all, to the patient.

SYDNEY S. GELLIS, M.D.
BENJAMIN M. KAGAN, M.D.

Contents

5   CARDIOVASCULAR SYSTEM

6   DIGESTIVE TRACT

7   BLOD

8   SPLEEN AND LYMPHATIC SYSTEM

9   ENDOCRINE SYSTEM

10   METABOLIC DISORDERS

11   CONNECTIVE TISSUE

12   GENITOURINARY TRACT

16 THE EYE

17 THE EAR

18 INFECTIOUS DISEASES

1

Nutrition

Malnutrition

EMANUEL LEBENTHAL, M.D.,
and CAROLYN YOUNG, M.N.S., R.D.

Malnutrition has long been recognized as a primary health concern in developing countries. When accompanied by diarrhea and intercurrent infection, it is a primary killer of young children in many areas of the world. Only in recent years, however, has the prevalence of malnutrition among persons living in well-developed countries been appreciated. Infants suffering from intra-uterine growth retardation, alone or in combination with postnatal malnutrition, may have suboptimal brain development and may also be more susceptible to infectious diseases and intestinal malabsorption. Malnutrition during childhood in developed countries is often secondary to a chronic underlying disease (e.g., cystic fibrosis, congenital heart disease, renal disease, inflammatory bowel disease, cancer), and the long-term prognosis in these children may often be dependent on an improvement in their nutritional status. In order to prevent or treat malnutrition in any area of the world, it is important to accurately assess nutritional status and to ascertain the most appropriate method for refeeding. In addition, consideration must be given to the influence of malnutrition on liver and intestinal function and the resulting effects on drug metabolism.

An accurate assessment of nutritional status requires evaluation of anthropometric, biochemical, clinical, and dietary criteria. Accurate determination of height and weight is the first step toward determining the nutritional status of a child. Gomez, in 1956, was the first to develop criteria for assessing the degree of malnutrition based on the percentage of expected weight for age. Malnutrition is classified as mild (1st degree), moderate (2nd degree), or severe (3rd degree) based on the percentage of expected weight for age (89–75%, 74–60%, < 60%, respectively). While the Gomez classification is still in use in some areas, it has the primary disadvantage of assuming that appropriate weight for age is independent of height. In addition, children suffering from kwashiorkor (protein-deficiency with adequate caloric intake) may be of appropriate weight for age due to significant edema. A more appropriate method of classification of protein-energy malnutrition (PEM) includes consideration of height for age (stunting) as well as weight for age (wasting). The National Center for Health Statistics (NCHS) has developed standards for growth that are used commonly in the United States. Although some countries have developed standards for growth with data obtained from within their own population, it has been suggested that the differences in attained height and weight observed between populations are due primarily to socioeconomic rather than genetic factors. Thus, use of the NCHS standards or a similar standard appears appropriate for all areas of the world. The 50th percentile is used as the standard for children in developed countries, but in areas of the world where malnutrition is endemic, a lower percentile may be required as the standard for growth, in order to distinguish those children most critically in need of nutritional rehabilitation.

An additional means of distinguishing kwashiorkor from marasmus has also been developed and may be useful in areas of endemic malnutrition. A scoring system designates points for the presence of edema (3 points), dermatosis (2 points), edema and dermatosis (6 points), hair changes (1 point), hepatomegaly (1 point), and the degree of serum albumin deficiency (< 1 gm/100ml = 7, > 4.0 gm/100ml = 0). A score of 0–3 indicates marasmus, 4–8 marasmic-kwashiorkor, and 9–15 kwashiorkor.

Other anthropometric measurements can be of

value in assessing the severity of malnutrition and evaluating recovery during refeeding. The most useful and accessible site for measurement is the mid-arm; tricep skinfold measurements, performed with a Lange or Hapenden caliper, can give a reasonable estimate of body fat (in the absence of edema), and arm muscle circumference has been shown to correlate with lean body mass. Arm muscle circumference can be estimated by the following formula: arm circumference (cm) − (triceps skinfold (mm) = 0.314). Arm circumference and tricep skinfold should both be measured at the point midway between the acromial process and the olecranon process at the back of the arm. These measurements have the primary advantage of being easy to obtain with little equipment. Standards are available for children and adults. Significant amounts of intraobserver and interobserver error may exist with such measurements, however, and it also must be assumed that the upper arm is circular with equal compressibility of fat and that bone density decreases at the same rate as muscle during malnutrition.

Biochemical assessment of protein-energy malnutrition has, in the past, been limited largely to serum total protein and albumin measurements as an indication of visceral protein status. Recent evidence suggests that measurement of plasma proteins with a shorter half-life would be more useful, however, since they more rapidly reflect changes associated with nutrient deprivation and refeeding. Commonly measured proteins include transferrin (normal level = 180–260 mg/dl; < 100 mg/dl indicates severe depletion), retinol-binding protein (RBP) (normal level = 37 meq/ml; ≤ 3 meq/dl indicates severe depletion) and thyroxine-binding-prealbumin (PA) (normal level = 20–50 mg/dl; < 10 mg/dl indicates severe depletion). The PA-RBP complex has been shown to have the highest sensitivity to visceral protein status, and can be assessed by most clinical laboratories.

The creatinine-height index, which involves measurement of 24-hour urinary creatinine excretion, may also be a useful means for assessing lean body mass in cases in which an accurate collection of urine can be made. Creatinine excretion is a function of muscle mass, and standards have been developed to correlate 24-hour urine creatinine excretion with height. A creatinine excretion that is below that expected for height indicates a reduced lean body mass. A high intake of creatine-containing foods (e.g., meats) may influence creatinine excretion, though this does not appear to significantly affect results in most cases. Other more highly technical means for assessment of body composition, such as whole body potassium 40 counting, underwater weighing, and computed tomography of the thigh with assessment of the area of fat and muscle are potentially useful tools

Table 1. VITAMIN DEFICIENCY

Vitamin	Clinical Signs of Deficiency
Vitamin A	Night blindness; rough, dry skin; xerophthalmia
Vitamin D	Rickets; soft bones; bowed legs; poor teeth
Vitamin K	Prolonged clotting time
Vitamin C	Scurvy; sore mouth; bleeding gums; weak-walled capillaries; impaired wound healing
Thiamin (B_1)	Beriberi; anorexia; congestive heart failure; neuropathy
Riboflavin (B_2)	Cheilosis; glossitis; diarrhea
Niacin	Pellagra; dermatitis; dementia; diarrhea
Folate	Megaloblastic anemia; glossitis; diarrhea
Vitamin B_{12}	Macrocytic anemia; pernicious anemia

but at present are available only in a research setting.

Clinical assessment of nutritional status must be undertaken by a professional well versed in the signs and symptoms of various nutrient deficiencies. The clinical differentiation of kwashiorkor from marasmus is an important distinction, for example, since the appropriate dietary therapy may differ. Various vitamin deficiencies may also most easily be recognized by their clinical signs, and physicians and nutritionists both in developing countries and in well-developed areas of the world should be familiar with these signs. A list of common vitamin deficiencies and their clinical signs is provided in Table 1.

Dietary assessment is another important aspect of a complete nutritional assessment. Weighing of foods prior to consumption and nutrient analysis of samples of these foods provide the most accurate determination of intake, but this method is impractical for other than research purposes. Alternatively, a careful dietary history, or preferably, a 3- or 7-day food record can provide a good estimate of the total intake of calories, protein and specific vitamins and minerals. Care must be taken to obtain a complete record of all foods and beverages consumed, along with an accurate estimate of quantities and method of preparation. In the case of malabsorptive disorders particularly, an accurate assessment of intake can be valuable in determining appropriate requirements during refeeding. If malabsorption is suspected, further studies should be performed when possible. These should include (1) a 72-hour measurement of fecal fat excretion, by the following equation:

$$\text{Coefficient of absorption} = \frac{\text{dietary fat} - \text{fecal fat}}{\text{dietary fat}} \times 100$$

Normal values = premature 60–75%; newborn

80–85%; 10 mo to 3 yr 85–95%; >3 yr 95%; (2) a D-xylose test (provide 0.5 gm/kg body weight of D-xylose in a 10% solution; measure xylose in serum fasting and at 60 minutes. A rise of 25 mg/dl is normal. A rise of < 20 mg/dl may indicate mucosal injury); (3) a serum carotene level (provide foods high in carotene—carrots, squash, sweet potatoes, pumpkin; serum carotene ≤ 50 mg/dl = steatorrhea, 50–100 mg/dl = slight steatorrhea; 71–100 mg/dl = normal); and (4) an intestinal biopsy for measurement of disaccharidases and mucosal integrity.

Enteral Refeeding. When an accurate assessment of the severity of malnutrition has been made, it is important to determine the appropriate method for refeeding as well as the appropriate foodstuffs to be used. While there may be practical constraints limiting options, in general the philosophy should be to use a functioning intestinal tract. Thus, for patients with malnutrition not associated with severe gastrointestinal disease, oral feeding or nasogastric tube feeding should be attempted initially. Other methods of enteral feeding, such as nasoduodenal tube feeding or use of a jejunal catheter, may be useful in some patients, especially those who are vomiting.

It should be noted that in developing countries, malnourished children often suffer from frequent episodes of acute diarrhea, and the first mode of therapy for these children is often oral rehydration solutions. While such solutions are of great value in restoring fluid and electrolyte balalnce, they are of very little caloric value. The standard composition of oral rehydration solutions as recommended by the World Health Organization is: NaCl 3.5 gm/l, NaHCO₃ 2.5 gm/l, KCl 1.5 gm/l; and glucose 20 gm/l. This solution provides 90 millimoles per liter of sodium, 80 millimoles of chloride, 30 millimoles of bicarbonate, 20 millimoles of potassium, and 111 millimoles of glucose. It provides only 68 kilocalories per liter. Thus, more substantial feeds must be initiated rapidly to prevent further exacerbation of the malnutrition in such children. The composition of foods most appropriate for refeeding will depend on the tolerance of the individual patient. Breastfeeding mothers should be allowed to continue nursing their infants when oral rehydration therapy is being provided.

Malnutrition often predisposes infants and young children to frequent episodes of diarrhea and intercurrent infection. These episodes can cause significant intestinal mucosal injury, with subsequent malabsorption due to impaired hydrolysis and transport of nutrients in the brush border membrane of the mature epithelial cell. Lactase is often the first and most severely affected enzyme, and thus transient lactose malabsorption is often observed in malnourished children pre-senting with episodes of diarrhea or infection. Children with malnutrition secondary to gastrointestinal disorders will often tolerate lactose-containing products poorly. Thus, while lactose-containing formulas are advantageous for refeeding owing to their ready availability, relative low cost, and the evidence that the presence of lactose significantly improves calcium absorption, their use in severely malnourished children must be approached with caution so as not to aggravate the diarrhea and consequently worsen the nutritional status of the child.

In theory, the ideal composition of the diet for a child recovering from malnutrition would be to provide nutrients in their most readily absorbable form. Thus, the use of formulas containing medium-chain triglycerides (MCT oil), which are partially absorbed directly via the portal circulation, as well as glucose or glucose polymers and protein hydrolysates or amino acid mixtures (with emphasis on essential amino acids) would be the preference for refeeding. However, such formulas are not readily available in developing countries, and while their use is relatively common in developed countries, their high cost makes further research into the advantages of such formulas and possible less expensive alternatives to their use an important priority. Rice water, coconut oil, and boiled chicken provide an example of a simple feeding that may be well tolerated by malnourished children.

In severely malnourished children, feeds should be initiated to provide approximately 50 kcal/kg body weight and 0.5 gm protein/kg per day, with feeds advanced daily, if well tolerated, to 150–200 kcal/kg/day with 3–6 gm protein/kg/day. An adequate ratio of protein to nonprotein calories is required to allow optimal utilization of protein. A ratio of approximately 24 nonprotein calories to 1 gram of protein is necessary to prevent use of protein as a caloric source at the expense of body protein accretion.

Worsening of diarrhea, malabsorptive stools, and poor weight gain should each be considered cause for reevaluation of the type of formula being provided. If such symptoms appear, a more elemental diet may be required. Patients should remain under clinic care until the appropriate weight for height is attained. Care must be taken to provide adequate intake of vitamins and minerals during refeeding, including trace elements, since inadequate micronutrient intake may slow recovery from malnutrition. Intramuscular or intravenous administration of vitamin and mineral supplements should be provided if oral intake is inadequate. If antibiotics are being used, iron should be included (100–200 mg of elemental iron per day).

Parenteral Refeeding. When enteral feeding is

not possible because of a poorly functioning gut (e.g., intestinal obstruction, excessive vomiting, or diarrhea) or an extensive mucosal injury, parenteral feeds should be initiated. Peripheral parenteral nutrition may be of value if some oral intake can be achieved, but the low concentration of dextrose (10%) and amino acids that can be safely infused through a peripheral vein severely limits the number of calories that can be provided. For long-term therapy, parenteral nutrition through a central line, providing dextrose, amino acids, lipids, vitamins, minerals, and electrolytes may be the optimal choice for feeding.

Dextrose infusions should be initiated at a rate of 7–8 gm/kg/min and advanced to 12–14 gm/kg/min. Urine should be checked at every void for glucose. Amino acids can be added when the patient is tolerating 10 gm/kg/day of 10% dextrose. The protein intake should not exceed 3.5 gm/kg/day.

Home parenteral nutrition has allowed nutritional rehabilitation and maintenance of nutritional status in children with chronic disease without significant disruption of their lives. Total parenteral nutrition is not without deleterious effects in some children or when used for a prolonged time, and thus other methods of feeding should always be considered prior to its initiation, and periodically during the course of treatment. However, parenteral nutrition has been shown to be an invaluable technique for allowing rapid rehabilitation of severely malnourished children in whom enteral feedings are insufficient or impossible.

Frequent follow-up at an outpatient clinic for all patients with a history of malnutrition is a vital component of their care, since socioeconomic or environmental factors, as well as possible underlying disease, may predispose these children to recurrent episodes of malnutrition.

Drug Metabolism in Malnutrition. The gastrointestinal and liver dysfunction that often accompanies malnutrition may have marked effects on drug pharmacokinetics. A decrease in plasma protein carriers such as albumin may decrease drug binding, while reduced liver, kidney, and small intestinal function may slow drug excretion. Drug oxidation rates are variably affected by starvation and protein deficiency. For example, antipyrine and theophylline clearance is decreased, and the half-life is increased. Chloramphenicol glucoronidation and clearance is decreased, while the half-lives of isoniazid and salicylate are increased. These variable effects of malnutrition on drug metabolism must be considered in the clinical treatment of patients who suffer from malnutrition superimposed on another disease state.

The prevalence of malnutrition in both developing and well-developed countries requires that aggressive therapy to prevent or treat malnutrition be undertaken. Further research is required to develop methods to better assess nutritional status and to recognize early malnutrition as well as to determine the most appropriate means of treatment and the proper supply of nutrients needed for optimal recovery.

Obesity

KELLY D. BROWNELL, Ph.D.

Overweight children tend to become overweight adults, so physicians and parents who hope the child will "grow out of it" await an unlikely event. The probability increases the longer a child is overweight. The chances that an overweight child will remain overweight as an adult are 14% in infancy, 41% at age 7, and 70% at age 12.

These facts argue for aggressive management and for intervention even when children are mildly overweight. However, pediatricians and parents must deal with children in a calm and rational manner. Children who internalize excessive concern about dieting and body shape can develop serious eating disorders (bulimia and anorexia nervosa) in adolescence.

One must resist the cultural bias against obese persons. This bias has been documented in the public, in physicians, and in obese persons themselves. The obese person is held responsible for a condition that is actually a complex interaction of physical, emotional, and social factors. The parents of overweight children are often blamed because they are overweight themselves. Some physicians sense defeat and give up before trying. Fortunately, new methods and materials are available, and the gloomy picture is changing.

There are four essential elements to the management of childhood obesity: diet, exercise, behavior modification, and involvement of the parents. These are discussed in detail in a 100-page clinical manual prepared by the author for use by health professionals and parents. Copies may be obtained by writing to the author.

Diet is the first concern because of the nutritional needs of growing children. The degree of calorie restriction depends on the degree of obesity, but it must never exceed the level needed for adequate nutrition. For children who are less than 30% overweight, reducing calories until weight stabilizes permits height to "catch up" to weight. For each 20% the child is overweight, approximately 1½ years of weight maintenance are needed to attain ideal weight.

For children in excess of 30% overweight,

greater calorie restriction is indicated. Calories should be reduced to the lowest level without compromising a balanced diet. This can sometimes be accomplished by reducing high-fat foods and eliminating "junk foods." It is useful for a dietitian to work with parents to insure adequate nutrition. Since calories are reduced, foods must be chosen carefully to keep calories low and nutrient density high. A multivitamin with minerals can prevent some deficiencies, but dietary counseling is still necessary.

Very-low-calorie diets of less than 600 to 800 calories per day have been used extensively with adults, and in a limited number of cases, with severely overweight adolescents. More research is needed to determine the safety of such diets with children. These diets must be administered in speciality clinics where precise monitoring can be done.

Exercise is one key to the long-term maintenance of weight loss. Compliance is the major challenge. Overweight children are often embarrassed by their performance in sports and games and avoid exercise. Overweight parents may feel the same. Compliance is best if children are prescribed "lifestyle" activities such as riding a bicycle, walking to a friend's house, and spending more time in active play. We also prescribe a walking program in which time and distance are increased gradually.

Behavior modification and parent involvement are also important. Children need to learn new lifestyle habits regarding eating, exercise, and attitudes. Dietary instruction alone usually fails in the absence of a structured program of habit change. Parents can be given instructional material to implement such a program from the manual mentioned above. They can assist their children by making prudent food purchases, exercising with their children, modeling healthy habits, and providing support and encouragement during the long and difficult process of weight change.

Referral can be the best course for difficult cases. This is true when serious family problems exist or when weight of the child or one parent is a central issue in family conflict. A counselor skilled in family therapy can be useful. Commercial and self-help groups such as Weight Watchers and Overeaters Anonymous are sometimes useful for older children, either as the sole form of treatment or as an adjunct to monitoring by the physician. Speciality clinics for overweight children are an excellent choice, but few exist.

The pediatrician's office is an ideal place to treat childhood obesity. In addition to managing existing cases, the pediatrician can identify children in the early stages of obesity. Preventive efforts are crucial for the control of this serious and prevalent problem.

Vitamin Deficiencies and Excesses

JOHN. N. UDALL, Jr., M.D., Ph.D.

Health professionals who deal with children should be aware of the recommended daily allowances for vitamins (Table 1). A knowledge of the signs/symptoms of vitamin deficiencies and excesses is also important so treatment may be instituted before severe and permanent functional impairment of vital organs occurs.

FAT–SOLUBLE VITAMINS

The fat-soluble vitamins A, D, E, and K are insoluble in water and therefore must circulate in association with lipid-solubilizing carrier systems. Diseases of the pancreas (cystic fibrosis), liver (biliary atresia), or intestine (celiac disease) that impair fat digestion and/or fat absorption may result in a deficiency of one or more of these vitamins.

Vitamin A (Retinol). This vitamin is important for growth, healthy skin, and vision. Deficiency of vitamin A results in growth failure, apathy, mental retardation, skin and corneal changes, and occasionally intracranial hypertension. Xerophthalmia, the term in general use to cover all the ocular manifestations of vitamin A deficiency, is the most common cause of blindness in young children throughout the world.

The treatment of xerophthalmia may be divided into emergency treatment and maintenance therapy. Emergency treatment consists of the oral administration of 100,000 IU of vitamin A (retinyl palmitate in oil) given immediately and repeated on the second day. The response may take several days to appear, but this regimen is adequate to obtain maximal effect. If there is vomiting or severe diarrhea, the dose should be administered intramuscularly, but the preparation must be water dispersible because oily preparations are not absorbed from the injection site. A final dose of 200,000 IU should be given before discharge to boost liver storage. Maintenance therapy consists of administration of the recommended dietary allowance of the vitamin.

Vitamin A intoxication, with resultant intracranial hypertension (vomiting, headache, stupor), skeletal changes, and skin rash, has been reported in infants, from an excessive number of vitamin A tablets or from dietary excesses. Regular daily ingestion of retinol supplements exceeding 3000 retinol equivalents (RE)(10,000 IU) by infants and children is recommended only under the direction of a physician. Toxicity in adults is seen with daily intakes of more than 15,000 RE for long periods. The goal of treatment of vitamin A toxicity is

Table 1. 1980 RECOMMENDED DAILY DIETARY ALLOWANCES*

Age (years)	Weight (kg)	Fat-Soluble Vitamins			Water-Soluble-Vitamins				
		A† (μg RE)	D‡ (μg)	E§ (mg α-TE)	B1 (mg)	B2 (mg)	B3 (mg NE)	B6 (mg)	C (mg)
Infants									
0.0–0.5	6	420	10	3	0.3	0.4	6	0.3	35
0.5–1.0	9	400	10	4	0.5	0.6	8	0.6	35
Children									
1–3	13	400	10	5	0.7	0.8	9	0.9	45
4–6	20	500	10	6	0.9	1.0	11	1.3	45
7–10	28	700	10	7	1.2	1.4	16	1.6	45
Males									
11–14	45	1000	10	8	1.4	1.6	18	1.8	50
15–18	66	1000	10	10	1.4	1.7	18	2.0	60
Females									
11–14	46	800	10	8	1.1	1.3	15	1.8	50
15–18	55	800	10	8	1.1	1.3	14	2.0	60

* Adapted from the National Academy of Sciences–National Research Council. The allowances are intended to provide for individual variations among most normal persons as they live in the United States under usual environmental stresses. Diets should be based on a variety of common foods in order to provide other nutrients for which human requirements are well defined.

† One retinol equivalent (RE) is equal to 1 μg of retinal; 6 μg of beta carotene, or 12 μg of other provitamin A carotenoids. In terms of IU, 1 retinal equivalent is equal to 3.33 IU of retinol or 10 IU of beta carotene.

‡ As cholecalciferol; 10 μg cholecalciferol = 400 IU of vitamin D.

§ See the National Academy of Sciences—National Research Council 1980 Recommended Daily Dietary Allowances for calculation of vitamin E activity of the diet as α-tocopherol equivalents.

obviously to eliminate the dietary source of the excessive vitamin A. Symptoms rapidly subside on withdrawal of the vitamin, and complete recovery always results.

A comment should be made in regard to vitamin A analogs such as isotretinoin and 13-cis-retinoic acid. The use of these analogs for the treatment of acne has been accepted enthusiastically by teenagers because of their effectiveness. However, there is concern regarding the use of large doses of these analogs in teenagers who could become pregnant. Recently it has been recognized that there is a relationship between maternal consumption of large doses of vitamin A and multiple congenital abnormalities in offspring.

Vitamin D. Rickets results in children when vitamin D deficiency occurs before the epiphyses of bones have closed. Rickets has been found in premature infants consuming formulas containing 400 IU vitamin D/liter, probably because of low intake of nutrients in general. Black infants who are infrequently exposed to the sun and who are breast-fed by mothers with impaired vitamin D intake may be at risk for the development of rickets, especially during the winter months. Some patients with nephrotic syndrome may also develop vitamin D deficiency. Vitamin D–dependent rickets may be due to a recessively inherited deficiency of the renal 1α-hydroxylase enzyme or a receptor defect. In mild cases of vitamin D deficiency, 1600 IU/day of vitamin D is the recommended therapy; in advanced cases 5000 IU/day should be administered. Treatment of vitamin D–dependent rick-

ets consists of pharmacologic amounts of vitamin D or physiologic amounts of $1,25\text{-}(OH)_2\text{-}D_3$.

Excessive doses of vitamin D result in the mobilization of calcium and phosphorus from bony tissues, and their redeposition in soft tissues. This occurs principally in the walls of blood vessels but also in kidney tubules, bronchi, and the heart. Vitamin D intoxication may be fatal. Preliminary symptoms of toxicity include anorexia, thirst, urinary urgency, vomiting, and diarrhea. When hypervitaminosis is present, the first step in management is to stop administration of all forms of vitamin D immediately and restrict dietary calcium intake. It is also important to maintain good hydration and urine output and correct any deficiency in serum sodium or potassium. Furosemide may be required (0.5–1.0 mg/kg initially, given orally or parenterally). This may be repeated at 6 to 12 hours if necessary. Prednisone (2 mg/kg/24 hr) may also be used in refractory cases.

Vitamin E (Tocopherol). Vitamin E deficiency has been implicated in hemolytic anemia of preterm infants and glutathionine synthetase deficiency. A dietary intake of 3–5 mg α-TE (tocopherol equivalents) should avoid deficiency states during infancy. Data concerning toxicity are confusing. However, recently the use of a commercially available parenteral vitamin E preparation was associated with several infant deaths. The reason for the toxicity of this preparation has not yet been determined.

Vitamin K. Newborn infants represent a special case when considering vitamin K nutrition because the placenta is a relatively poor organ for the transmission of lipids, and the gut flora important for vitamin K production is meager during the first few days of life. Therefore, vitamin K–dependent factors (plasma prothrombin concentration) may be only 30% of normal on the second and third days of life. Premature infants are even more susceptible than full-term infants to vitamin K deficiency. If prothrombin values fall below 10%, hemorrhagic disease of the newborn may occur. It is for this reason that 0.5 to 1.0 mg of phylloquinone is administered intramuscularly on the first day of life. This is an effective way of preventing hemorrhagic disease. It should also be noted that broad-spectrum antibiotics that dramatically suppress or alter intestinal flora may put an infant or child at an increased risk for vitamin K deficiency.

WATER–SOLUBLE VITAMINS

The water-soluble vitamins include thiamine (B_1), riboflavin (B_2), niacin (B_3), pyridoxine (B_6), folic acid, cyanocobalamin (B_{12}), and several others. These vitamins act primarily as cofactors in biochemical reactions. The entire group is widely distributed in plants and animals. Because they are found so extensively in nature, a vitamin deficiency of any one of them is unusual. When deficiencies occur in industrial nations, they are commonly associated with chronic illness, food faddism, or the chronic use of alcohol or drugs that interfere with the normal absorption or metabolism of a specific vitamin. In contrast, deficiencies of water-soluble vitamins in underdeveloped countries usually coexist with protein-calorie malnutrition.

Thiamine (B_1). Patients with simple thiamine deficiency can be treated orally with 5 mg of thiamine daily. Severely ill children should receive 10 mg IV twice a day. In the management of fulminant heart disease, 100 mg thiamine hydrochloride plus vigorous treatment of congestive heart failure is necessary. No toxic effects of thiamine administered by mouth have been reported. However, there have been reports of hypersensitivity to thiamine given parenterally.

Riboflavin (B_2). Riboflavin-deficient infants respond to 0.5 mg twice daily. Children who are deficient should be treated with 1.0 mg given orally three times a day for several weeks. Since dietary protein influences riboflavin status, it is important that protein and calories in the diet be adequate. Riboflavin toxicity has not been demonstrated in man or animals.

Niacin (B_3). Pellagra, the disease of niacin deficiency, is characterized by the classic "three D's": dermatitis, diarrhea, and dementia. Early symptoms include glossitis, stomatitis, insomnia, anorexia, weakness, irritability, abdominal pain, for-

getfulness, morbid fear, and vertigo. Treatment of the deficiency is usually more effective with oral rather than parenteral niacin, since blood levels remain elevated longer following oral treatment. The usual daily dose is about 10 times the RDA, or 100 mg in an adult. Additionally, a high-calorie, high-protein diet supplemented by the administration of the entire B vitamin group should be instituted. Ingestion of large amounts of nicotinic acid but not nicotinamide may produce vascular dilation. This is associated with "flushing'" and headaches. The effect comes on within 7–10 minutes of nicotinic acid administration and lasts about 30 minutes.

Pyridoxine (B_6). Inborn errors in pyridoxine metabolism require a dose of pyridoxine several times the usual requirement, in some instances as much as 200–600 mg of pyridoxine/day to effect a clinical response. Pyridoxine-dependent convulsion in the neonate usually responds to 5–10 mg of pyridoxine intravenously. These infants can then be maintained on 10–25 mg daily. Toxicity from excessive amounts has not been reported until recently. This has been noted in adults who have been shown to develop severe sensory nervous-system dysfunction after chronic daily megadoses of pyridoxine.

Cyanocobalamin (B_{12}). Vitamin B_{12} deficiency (megaloblastic anemia) is rare in infants because amounts acquired from the mother during fetal life are usually sufficient to carry the infant through the first year of life, especially since those amounts are generally supplemented by additional supplies from mother's (or other) milk. The RDA for children 1–3 years old is 2.0 μg/day, for 4- to 6-year olds it is 2.5 μg/day, for 7- to 10-year olds it is 3.0 μg/day, and for adolescents and nonpregnant adults it is 3.0 μg/day.

Deficiency occurs in pernicious anemia. Although congenital and juvenile pernicious anemias are rare, both require treatment for life. The use of vitamin B_{12} in megatherapy for various conditions is not valid. The only legitimate need for megatherapy with vitamin B_{12} is for the rare patient with a congenital defect in vitamin B_{12} metabolism, such as vitamin B_{12}-responsive methylmalonic acidemia.

Folacin. Folacin is the generic term for compounds having nutritional properties and a chemical structure similar to folic acid. Folic acid deficiency is the most common cause of megaloblastic anemia in infants and children. An appropriate maintenance dose to prevent folate deficiency in a premature infant is 0.05 to 0.1 mg per day. The RDA for infants up to 6 months of age is 30 μg/day; for infants 6 to 12 months it is 45 μg/day; for 1- to 3-year olds it is 100 μg/day; for 4- to 6-year olds it is 200 μg/day; for 7- to 10-year olds it is 300 μg/day; and for older children and adults it is 400 μg/day. Since less than 5 μg of folacin/kg body weight produces hematologic response in children with vitamin B_{12} deficiency. However, 1–5 mg orally given daily is recommended for children with folacin deficiency.

Vitamin C. Deficiency of vitamin C causes scurvy, which is characterized by weakness, petechial hemorrhages in the skin, ecchymosis, gingival and subperiosteal hemorrhage, and defects in bone development in children. It is prevented by 10 mg ascorbic acid per day. In order to attain better tissue saturation, however, the RDA is 45 mg per day in children and 60 mg per day in adults. The usual treatment of infantile scurvy is 25 mg four times a day for 4–5 days and then 25 mg twice a day until healing occurs.

Excessive quantities of ascorbic acid, 2.0–5.0 gm/day*, have been suggested for prophylaxis or treatment of upper respiratory tract infections. There is no substantial evidence that these large amounts consistently affect the incidence and severity of this illness. These amounts will acidify the urine and may lead to nephrolithiasis.

Total Parenteral Nutrition in Infants

ROBERT J. SHULMAN, M.D.,
and WILLIAM J. KLISH, M.D.

INDICATIONS

Parenteral nutrition has become a mainstay in the treatment of infants who are unable to sustain or to replenish their nutritional status enterally. Parenteral nutrition also may be administered as a supplement to infants who are able to take only a portion of their nutritional needs enterally. Patients who have diarrhea or anorexia or have had gastrointestinal surgery can receive a portion of their nutritional requirements by the administration of peripheral vein parenteral nutrition.

All nutritional requirements may be provided by total parenteral nutrition (TPN) via a peripheral vein (peripheral vein TPN) or through a silicone catheter placed into the superior vena cava (central vein TPN). Because of the uncertainties and the discomfort in the maintenance of long-term peripheral venous access, peripheral vein TPN may not be the optimal choice for infants who are severely malnourished or who need more than 2 weeks of parenteral support, e.g., infants with gastroschisis or short bowel syndrome.

TECHNIQUES

Peripheral vein TPN can be administered through either a steel needle or a short silicone catheter. The skin should be prepared with alcohol

and an iodophor solution. After placement, an iodophor ointment should be applied. The incidence of infection and thrombophlebitis increases with the duration of placement. Thus, the needle or catheter should be changed to a different vein every 48 hours. A change in the placement site before the IV becomes infiltrated also allows the vessel to be reused at a later time. Although any vein can be used, the TPN solution is hypertonic and may cause irritation to the vein. Thus, careful observation of the site is necessary so that the needle or the catheter may be removed at the first sign of extravasation.

The administration of central vein TPN usually involves one of two techniques. The first is a surgical approach in which a Silastic catheter is placed via a cutdown into the external jugular vein and then threaded so that the tip lies in the superior vena cava. The other end of the catheter is then tunneled under the skin so that it exits on the chest or behind the ear. The second is a technique (percutaneous method), most commonly used in preterm infants, in which a brachial vein is cannulated with a 19-gauge needle through which a silicone catheter is threaded. The catheter is advanced to the superior vena cava, and the needle is withdrawn. The area is cleaned with iodophor solution and the catheter and needle are taped to the skin. The percutaneous technique is attractive because it is relatively simple. Additionally, it permits the use, if necessary, of the external jugular vein at a later time. At present, the length of time the percutaneous catheter can remain in place without increased risk of infection is unclear. When either method is used, the catheters should be placed only by a person experienced in the techniques. Care of the catheters should also be undertaken by experienced personnel. The percutaneous method requires no dressing changes. Dressings on the surgically placed catheters should be changed every 2 to 3 days. Using sterile technique, the area around the catheter should be cleaned with acetone and alcohol and then with iodophor solution. Iodophor ointment should be applied, and a new dressing placed.

The catheters should be used only for the administration of TPN solutions. The use of the catheters for blood drawing and administration of other medications is likely to increase the risk of infection.

COMPONENTS

Energy. The recommended parenteral energy intake sufficient to provide for growth in a full-term infant is 90 to 110 kcal/kg/day. These needs will be increased in infants who are malnourished or stressed. As a general guideline, energy intake should be calculated on the basis of ideal weight. Thus, a 2-month-old infant who weighs 3 kg should

---

* Two to 5 gm exceeds the manufacturer's recommended dose.

Table 1. RECOMMENDED DAILY PARENTERAL INTAKE OF NUTRIENTS (per kg)

Nutrient	Infant*	Preterm Infant
Fluid (ml)	100	120
Energy (kcal)	90–110	75–85
Amino acids (gm)	2.5	2.5
Glucose (gm)†	25	19
Fat (gm)‡	0.5	0.5
Na (meq as NaCl)	3	4
K (meq)	2	3
PO_4(mM as K_2PO_4)§	2	2
Ca (meq)	2	2
Mg (meq)	1	1
Zn (μg)	100	300
Cu (μg)	20	20
Mn (μg)	8	8
Cr (μg)	0.15	0.15
Vitamins‖		

* Birth through 1 year of age.
† Intake will be less if fat is used as an energy source.
‡ Amount to supply essential fatty acids (see text).
§ 1.0 mM K_2PO_4 provides 1.5 meq K.
‖ >3.0 kg: 5 ml/day MVI-Pediatric; <3.0 kg: 2 ml/day.

Table 2. STANDARD TPN SOLUTIONS*

| Nutrient | Type of Administration | |
	Peripheral†	Central‡
Glucose (gm/dl)	12%	20%
Amino acids (gm/dl)	2.2%	3%
NaCl (meq)	26	38
KCl (meq)	2	6
K_2PO_4 (mM)	15	15
Ca gluconate (meq)	25	25
$MgSO_4$ (meq)	6	8
Trace minerals§‖		
Vitamins‖		
Kcal/ml	0.5	0.8

* Concentrations are per liter except where noted.
† Assumes fat is used as an energy source.
‡ Central strength solution for prematures is the same as peripheral strength solution except for increased concentration (20%) of glucose.
§ Supplied as PTE-4, Multitrace Pediatric, or similar product.
‖ The amount added per liter should supply the levels of intake shown in Table 1.

be given 550 kcal/day (ideal weight of 5 kg × 110 kcal/kg/day).

The requirements for premature infants is 75 to 85 kcal/kg/day. The energy requirements for growth will increase over the first 2 to 3 weeks of life to those of the term infant.

Fluid. Fluid intake should be dictated by the normal fluid requirements for the age of the infant; i.e., approximately 100 ml/kg/day for full-term infants and 120 ml/kg/day for premature infants. In infants with fluid restriction (e.g., infants with renal, heart, or lung disease), the concentration of central vein TPN solutions can be increased so that adequate nutritional intake is provided in a smaller volume of solution.

Protein. Protein is not administered as such but in the form of synthetic amino acids. Recommended parenteral intake is 2.5 to 2.7 gm/kg/day. Infants with malnutrition or protein loss may require up to 3.5 gm/kg/day. The amino acids have an energy density of 4 kcal/gm.

Carbohydrate. Glucose (dextrose) is used as the carbohydrate and prime energy source. The carbohydrate intake will depend upon the amount of fat infused but generally will range from 15 to 25 gm/kg/day (Table 1). In pharmaceutical solutions, the hydrated dextrose used is equivalent to 3.4 kcal/gm rather than the usual 4 kcal/gm normally associated with carbohydrates.

Fat. Intravenous fat solutions consist of triglycerides, egg phosphatides to stabilize the emulsion, and glycerol to make the fat emulsion isotonic with blood. The fat particles and natural chylomicrons are metabolized similarly.

Fat emulsions can be used not only as a source of the essential fatty acids, e.g., linoleic and linolenic, but also as an energy source. Commercial fat emulsions supply either 1.1 (10%) or 2 kcal/ml (20%).

Electrolytes, minerals, and vitamins should be administered according to the recommendations in Table 1. Oral administration is the safest route for patients who require iron supplementation. If this is not possible, the iron may be administered intramuscularly as iron dextran. The use of iron as an additive in TPN solutions, particularly for infants, remains controversial.

ADMINISTRATION

Peripheral Vein TPN. Because of the high osmolarity of TPN solutions, the maximum concentrations of amino acids and glucose that should be used in peripheral vein TPN are 2.2% and 12%, respectively. As shown in Table 2, these concentrations provide 0.5 kcal/ml. Thus, in order to provide 110 kcal/kg/day, 220 ml/kg/day of solution would have to be administrered, obviously an excessive amount of fluid. By necessity, therefore, fat emulsion must be used, in addition to the glucose/amino acid solution, to provide adequate energy intake without an excessive fluid load. An additonal benefit of the fat emulsion is that it is isotonic with blood and, when infused simultaneously with the glucose/amino acid mix, decreases the tonicity of the TPN.

Lipids should be started at a rate of 1.0 gm/kg/day (10 ml/kg/day of 10% or 5 ml/kg/day of 20%) and increased by 1.0 gm/kg/day up to a maximum of 4.0 gm/kg/day. Young infants and particularly premature infants may not tolerate more than 3.0 gm/kg/day. Serum triglycerides should be measured 4 hours after the infusion of fat has begun and with any increase in rate in order to prevent the development of hyperlipidemia. The infusion rate should be decreased if the triglyceride level is over 100 mg/dl (or 150 mg/dl if the ACA enzymatic method is used).

Shown below is a sample calculation for a 5-kg infant who is to receive 90 kcal/kg/day:

1. 5 kg × 90 kcal/kg/day = 450 kcal/day.
2. 5 kg × 3 gm/kg/day of lipid = 15 gm/day = 75 ml/day of 20% emulsion = 150 kcal/day.
3. 450 kcal/day − 150 kcal/day (from lipid) = 350 kcal/day.
4. 300 kcal/day ÷ 0.5 kcal/ml (see above) = 600 ml/day of peripheral vein TPN solution.
5. Lipid infusion rate, 3 ml/hr; TPN solution infusion rate, 25 ml/hr.

The 600 ml will supply 2.6 gm/kg/day of amino acids (600 ml × 2.2 gm/100 ml TPN = 13.2 gm; 13.2 gm ÷ 5 kg = 2.6 gm/kg). As outlined earlier, the lipid should be started at a dose of 1 gm/kg/day so that adequate energy intake (see example above) is achieved in 3 days.

Central Vein TPN. Central vein TPN solution is diluted quickly because it is infused into a vessel with a high blood flow. Therefore, high concentrations of glucose and amino acids may be used. On the first day of central vein administration, the concentrations of glucose and amino acids should be the same as those used in the peripheral vein solutions. On the following day, the concentrations can be increased to those shown in Table 2. The calculations for administration are the same as those outlined for peripheral vein TPN except that the energy density of the solution is 0.8 kcal/ml.

The concentrations of glucose and amino acids can be increased further in patients for whom fluid has been restricted, but the maximum is limited to approximatley 40% and 4%, respectively. In patients who are stressed (i.e., sepsis or trauma), the introduction of the TPN solution should be more gradual; administration should be started 24 to 48 hours after the insult, and full intake should be attained 3 to 5 days after initiation.

To supply adequate essential fatty acids, 0.5 gm/kg/day (5 ml of 10% or 2.5 ml/gm/day of 20%) of fat should be administered. If fat is used as an energy source, the guidelines given under peripheral vein administration should be followed.

In both peripheral and central vein TPN, the lipids and glucose/amino acid solutions can be infused together using a "Y" or "T" connector. Lipids cannot be infused through the 0.22-micron filter used for the administration of the glucose/amino acid solutions. The use of the filter is recommended to decrease the risk of air embolism, the incidence of thrombophlebitis, and the possibility of infection.

MONITORING

It should be borne in mind that the guidelines given in Tables 1 and 2 will meet the needs of most, but not all, infants. Appropriate changes in the TPN solution can be made only if the patient is observed carefully. The frequency of laboratory tests should depend on the severity of illness and the needs of the individual infant.

Initially, electrolytes should be checked twice weekly; calcium, phosphorus, BUN, albumin, ALT (SGPT), and total and direct bilirubin should be checked weekly. The appearance of significant hyperglycemia can be detected through frequent checks for glucose in the urine. If the patient is stable and requires more than 2 weeks of TPN therapy, the frequence of monitoring can be decreased to once every 2 weeks.

If the patient has a nasogastric tube, an ostomy, or another source of loss, the volume and content of the loss should be measured and replaced. If the loss is fairly constant, the replacement needs can be included in the TPN calculations.

COMPLICATIONS

The majority of complications associated with the administration of TPN are preventable with careful observation of the patient and, in the case of central vein TPN, management of the catheter. In this regard, the involvement of a nutrition support team in the care of TPN patients has been shown to reduce the complicaton rate and cost of care significantly. Because a comprehensive description of the potential complications is beyond the scope of this article, the most common problems will be discussed here.

Infection. In peripheral vein TPN, thrombophlebitis is most often a result of the high osmolarity of the solution rather than the result of infection. Local infections, however, may occur around the administration site.

Infection is more often a problem during the administration of central vein TPN. The more frequently the catheter is accessed, the more likely the development of infection. Common pathogens include *Staphylococcus aureus* and *S. epidermidis*. An infection may be limited to the entry site of the catheter or may be systemic. Antibiotics can be used systemically to treat local infections.

Traditionally, the treatment of bacteremia has been removal of the catheter and administration of antibiotics. Recently, it has been suggested that if the patient appears well clinically, systemic antibiotic treatment can be given through the catheter, with the caution that any change in the patient for the worse or a lack of improvement (e.g., continued fever) within 24 to 48 hours dictates removal of the catheter. If the patient looks ill, the catheter should be removed. Exchange of catheters over a guidewire, along with antibiotic therapy, has also been used for the treatment of catheter infection. Because there is little experience with the use of these methods for the treatment of catheter infections in infants, more studies are required to determine the safety and efficacy of the methods.

Mechanical. Plugging of the central venous catheter is the most common mechanical problem. The likelihood of occurrence is increased by withdrawal of blood or administration of blood products through the catheter. An attempt should be made to aspirate the clot and to flush the catheter gently with 2.5 ml of heparin (100 U/ml). If the effort is unsuccessful, urokinase (5000 U/ml) is available commercially for the specific purpose of clearing clotted catheters. An amount of urokinase equal to the volume of the catheter (0.5–1.0 ml) should be injected. The size of the clot usually will limit the amount that can be injected. After 5 minutes, an attempt should be made to aspirate blood from the catheter using a 5-ml syringe. If unsuccessful, repeat aspirations should be made at 5- to 10-minute intervals. After this time, the catheter hub should be plugged, and 60 minutes should elapse before further attempts are made. A repeat dose of urokinase may be necessary. It may take a few hours before the clot is finally removed.

The central venous catheter may become dislodged if it is not securely affixed to the skin. Any evidence of fluid leaking from the skin entry site or evidence of the development of tissue edema strongly suggests that the catheter is no longer in place. These signs necessitate prompt removal of the catheter. A chest radiograph may confirm the dislocation.

Metabolic. The infusion of large quantities of nutrients in severely malnourished patients during the first few days of TPN adminstration can lead to critical metabolic derangements and result in death. Hypophosphatemia and hypokalemia can be particular problems during this period.

Close observation will decrease the likelihood of the development of metabolic abnormalities that may result from any nutrient that is infused in the TPN solution and may occur at any time during the TPN therapy. Such problems as hypophosphatemia, hyperglycemia, hypoglycemia, and trace mineral deficiencies almost always are preventable if watched for. Prerenal azotemia and acidosis may occur if the amino acid intake is too great.

Essential fatty acid deficiency will occur if in-

adequate amounts of lipid are administered. Failure to check triglyceride levels, however, can cause hyperlipidemia, with resultant diminution in oxygenation or blood coagulation.

SPECIAL CIRCUMSTANCES

There have been few studies in infants to examine the safety and efficacy of the special amino acid solutions available for use in patients with renal or liver disease or in patients who are severely stressed. An amino acid mix that is low in aromatic amino acids and enriched in branched chain amino acids may help to lower an abnormally elevated serum ammonia in patients with liver disease. Whether the use of this type of solution in infants is of benefit, compared with a standard amino acid solution, is unknown. Similarly, solutions that consist solely of essential amino acids may offer no advantage to patients with renal disease. Indeed, essential amino acid solutions that do not include arginine probably should not be used in infants. Standard amino acid solutions at a slightly lower intake level may be just as efficacious.

HOME TPN

Patients who require TPN for extended periods of time can be managed successfully at home. In the 2 to 3 weeks before discharge from the hospital, however, the family must be trained in the care of the catheter and in the techniques of administration. A number of companies will deliver supplies to the patient's home and will provide nursing support, including blood drawing for laboratory studies, if the hospital does not offer this service.

An attempt can be made to decrease the time the infant receives the infusion of the TPN solution in order to increase the mobility of the patient. This may be accomplished by "cycling" the TPN. Instead of a 24-hour infusion, the TPN solution may be administered over 18 hours (or 12 hours in older infants). One hour before termination of the infusion, the rate of delivery is decreased by one-half; 30 minutes later, again by one-half; 15 minutes later, by one-half; and 15 minutes later the infusion is stopped. This gradual reduction of the infusion obviates the development of hypoglycemia. The catheter is filled with heparin (100 U/ml) and capped. To restart the infusion, the procedure is reversed. Urine glucose and blood glucose (by Dextrostix) levels must be obtained when cycling first is attempted, to insure patient tolerance. A small portable pump (Cormed), which allows greater mobility for the family, also can be used to infuse the TPN solution.

2

Mental and Emotional Disturbances

Mental Retardation

BRUCE K. SHAPIRO, M.D.
and MARK L. BATSHAW, M.D.,

Mental retardation is defined as significant sub-average general intellectual functioning associated with impairment of adaptive behavior and manifested during the developmental period (AAMD, 1973). Treatment is palliative, as the underlying defect cannot be corrected. However, there are many ways pediatricians can help the mentally retarded child reach his potential, aid the family in coping and, in some cases, prevent the occurrence of mental retardation in future children. The first step is correct and early diagnosis to provide genetic counseling. Next, the pediatrician needs to advise the parents about appropriate expectations. Then, therapy must be directed at the child's educational needs, behavioral problems, and other associated deficits. Finally, there needs to be a periodic review of progress.

Early Diagnosis. Early diagnosis allows for the easing of parental anxiety, realistic goal setting, and greater acceptance of the child. Severely retarded children demonstrate major developmental delays at an early age, making the diagnosis straightforward. However, many mildly retarded children will not have significant developmental delays during the first year of life. Certain groups of children are at increased risk: premature infants, children who are small for gestational age, and infants who have suffered perinatal insults. However, most retarded children do not fall into an identifiable "at risk" group. Thus, taking a complete developmental history is important for all children with developmental delays.

The parents will usually bring the retarded child to a pediatrician because the child is failing to fulfill developmental expectations. In early infancy, these include questions about hearing or vision and problems in feeding or swallowing. After six months of age, motor delay is the most common complaint. Language and behavior problems become prominent between two and four years, and school failure becomes evident in nursery school or in the early primary grades. Once identified, the child should be referred to an interdisciplinary evaluation center—e.g., school, university affiliated facility (UAF), or state diagnostic and evaluation center. Evaluation should include an examination by a developmental pediatrician and formal psychological testing. In addition to medical consultations, evaluations may be required from experts in behavioral psychology, special education, social work, speech, language and audiology, nursing, and physical and occupational therapies.

Etiology. Most cases of mental retardation remain idiopathic, especially in the mildly retarded group, which composes over 85% of the total mental retardation population. However, among retarded individuals with IQ <50, determination of etiology is often possible. A diagnosis allows the parents to known why their child is retarded. It helps to reduce the guilt of "what could I have done differently to prevent this child's handicap" and allows association with other parents who have children with a similar diagnosis. It also permits prediction of future outcome based on reported experience with other children having similar diagnoses. Finally, it is important for genetic counseling. Among idiopathic cases of severe-profound mental retardation, the empiric recurrence risk is 3–5%. However, in chromosomal or single gene defects, recurrence risks can be as high as 25–

50%. Because of the diversity of conditions leading to mental retardation, there is no screening evaluation possible. A complete history and physical may give leads which should then be fully investigated, but fishing expeditions should be avoided. For example, skull x-rays, metabolic screens, and CT scans have not proved useful as diagnostic screening techniques in children with mental retardation. Various techniques of prenatal diagnosis are available for families with children having mental retardation of genetic origin.

Genetic Counseling. There are even a few examples of fetal therapy that may prevent mental retardation. For prenatal diagnosis to be successful, three conditions must be met. First, a correct diagnosis must be established. Second, the mother must be known to be at an increased risk for having a handicapped child; e.g., the increased risk of Down syndrome in a mother over 35 years old, the recurrence risk in a mother who has borne a Down child or a child with fragile-X syndrome, or a mother who is a translocation carrier. Third, the disorder must be identifiable by amniocentesis or other prenatal diagnostic techniques. For example, classic phenylketonuria cannot be diagnosed prenatally because phenylalanine hydroxylase, the deficient enzyme, is not expressed in amniocytes.

The most common form of prenatal diagnosis involves amniocentesis. The amniotic fluid can be used for alpha-fetoprotein determination of neural tube defects. The amniocytes are cultured for karyotyping, to determine the sex of the fetus or to detect chromosomal anomalies. Enzyme assays for inborn errors of metabolism can also be performed on the amniocytes. A second technique of prenatal diagnosis involves fetoscopy, which allows direct visualization of body parts so that syndromes associated with absent or deformed limbs can be identified. Fetal skin and liver biopsy have also been performed during fetoscopy. Fetal ultrasound, a method of indirect visualization, is now being used for definition of neural tube defects, microcephaly, and congenital heart defects.

The primary purpose of prenatal diagnosis has been to identify an affected fetus and offer therapeutic abortion. However, it may also influence the timing and mode of delivery or the perinatal care of the infant. For instance, a child with a complete urea cycle enzyme deficiency, organic acidemia, or maple syrup urine disease will become comatose during the first week of life. If diagnosed prenatally or at birth, the child can be started on appropriate therapy, and coma can be avoided. We are even approaching a time when fetal therapy may be possible. The classic example is the use of intrauterine transfusion for erythroblastosis fetalis. However, recently ventricular shunts have been placed in hydrocephalic fetuses, thyroxine has been injected into a hypothyroid fetus, and vitamin B_{12} has been given to a fetus with methylmalonic acidemia.

Associated Dysfunctions. Mental retardation is often accompanied by associated deficits that further limit the child's adaptive abilities. In their most obvious forms, associated dysfunctions can be considered additional diagnoses—cerebral palsy, visual deficits, seizure disorders, speech disorders, autism, and other disorders of language, behavior, and perception. *Formes frustes* of these disorders have also been recognized—clumsiness, attentional peculiarities, articulation disorders, hyperactivity, and school underachievement. The severity and frequency of the associated dysfunctions tend to be proportional to the degree of mental retardation but may be more incapacitating than the mental retardation itself. Failure to appreciate the effects of associated deficits usually results in unsuccessful habilitation and may heighten behavioral problems.

Educational Placement. If a mentally retarded child is placed in an inappropriate educational setting, his progress will be slowed, and behavioral problems are likely to increase. In 1975, Public Law 94-142, the Education for all Handicapped Children's Act, came into force to ensure education for the retarded. The provisions of this law include identification, location, and evaluation of all handicapped children; provision of a full appropriate public education for all handicapped children; and preparation and implementation of an individualized educational plan (IEP).

The goals for education should be based on the child's developmental level and the future goals for independence. If the child is mildly retarded (IQ 55–69), his prognosis for independence is good. Most of these individuals marry and hold jobs, although they are generally the last hired and first fired. Social-adaptive skills are also impaired, and this results in greater risks of deviant behavior and the need for assistance from social agencies. In school, these children need to gain basic academic and vocational skills and training in social interactions. Some may attain functional literacy (defined as a fourth grade education). The moderately retarded child (IQ 40–54) can look toward independence in self-care skills and partial social independence in a sheltered environment. Education needs to stress "survival" vocabulary and arithmetic and self-care skills. These children will not read for information. The severely–profoundly retarded child (I.Q. less than 40) may develop some language and self-help skills; however, he will remain basically dependent throughout life. If the child has associated deficits such as cerebral palsy or seizures, his function will be further impaired.

The appropriate placement for each of these groups of children should primarily be guided by their developmental level rather than by their chronological age. Although mainstreaming into homeroom, art, music, and physical education may be appropriate for the mildly retarded child, it has little benefit for children with more severe handicaps. The pediatrician should examine the individual educational program (IEP) to see if it appears appropriate in relation to the child's developmental level, especially if behavioral problems or poor school performance become evident.

Recreation is important to the mentally retarded child. Athletics should be encouraged. In general, retarded children do better in individual or small group activities than in the more complicated team sports. Activities requiring gross motor skills rather than fine motor coordination are most appropriate. Examples include track and field, swimming, and hiking. Although some physical limitations may be medically necessary, they should be as few as possible.

Behavior Management. Behavioral problems occur with greater frequency in retarded children than in normal children. The causes are complex and may result from the interaction of a variety of factors, including 1) inappropriate expectations of the child's developmental level; 2) organic behaviors: hyperactivity, short attention span, lack of perseverance, self-injurious or self-directed behaviors; and 3) family problems.

These factors are not mutually exclusive and multiple causes are the rule. The majority of behavioral problems can be ameliorated by altering the child's environment, e.g., changing him to a more appropriate classroom setting and helping the parents understand that although he is 15 years old, he may not have the judgment to cross the street unsupervised. However, behaviors arising from organic deficits are less amenable to treatment by simple means. Two additional methodologies are employed to treat behavioral problems: behavior modification and/or psychotropic drugs.

Behavior modification has proved effective in the control of various behavioral problems: hyperactivity, self-stimulatory, self-injurious, aggressive, and noncompliant behaviors. The basic premise in behavior modification is that behavior is controlled by its consequences. Thus, if a behavior is reinforced, it will occur with greater frequency in the future. If it is not reinforced, it will be less likely to recur. This theory leads to three basic methods of controlling behavior: reinforcement, punishment, and extinction.

Reinforcement leads to an increase in the frequency of a desired behavior. In positive reinforcement, food or social reinforcers, such as hugs, food or money, are given contingent on compliant behavior. Punishment differs from reinforcement in that it reduces the frequency of a behavior by use of aversive consequences or by the withdrawal of positive reinforcement. Aversive approaches, ranging from shouting "No" to electric shock, are used to control noncompliant or self-injurious behaviors. The other form of punishment, "timing out," involves placing the child in a situation or room that lacks anything of interest to him. This isolates him for 5–10 minutes from any social activity that would provide positive reinforcement.

Extinction involves the removal of positive reinforcement from a situation that was previously rewarding. In effect, the prior relationship between the behavior and the consequence is disconnected. An example is ignoring self-stimulatory behavior while providing positive reinforcement as soon as the child stops. Usually, the targeted behavior will increase initially and then gradually diminish. Often extinction is paired with a procedure called differential reinforcement of other behaviors (DRO). While the self-stimulatory behavior is being extinguished, an incompatible behavior such as stringing beads, is being reinforced. As a group, these behavioral approaches appear to be as effective as psychotropic drugs, although they obviously take more time and effort and long term outcome studies have not been performed.

Mental retardation does not necessarily mandate the use of *psychotropic agents*. Drugs should not be used as a substitute for programming but rather to facilitate learning and social interactions or to suppress behaviors that are harmful to the patient or others. The drugs most commonly used to control behavior fall into the groups of phenothiazines, butyrophenones, and amphetamines. Phenothiazines include chlorpromazine (Thorazine), thioridazine (Mellaril), and trifluoperazine (Stelazine). These drugs act as dopamine antagonists. They result in sedation and decreased levels of motor activity, anxiety, combativeness, and hyperactivity. They also impair attention span. The usual dose in childhood for chlorpromazine or thioridazine is 25–200 mg/day but this dosage needs to be individually titrated. The peak drug levels following oral intake occur in 2–3 hours. The half-life varies from 2–5 days. Common side effects include hyperphagia and lethargy. Uncommon toxic effects include blood dyscrasias, cholestatic jaundice, dermatitis, and increased seizure frequency. After long term therapy, tardive dyskinesia and akathesia may occur. These symptoms do not always disappear following termination of drug therapy. Haloperidol (Haldol), a butyrophenone, has similar therapeutic effects. However, it produces more frequent extrapyramidal side effects. The usual dosage range is 0.5–7.5 mg/day.

Stimulants such as methylphenidate (Ritalin) or dextroamphetamine (Dexedrine) have been shown to be effective in the short term control of hyperactivity and attentional problems in children with normal intellectual functioning. However, they are much less effective in controlling hyperactivity in mentally retarded children. Because they have fewer or less severe side effects than phenylthiazines, stimulants are still worth trying in the mentally retarded child. Dosage ranges from 0.5–2.0 mg/kg/day for methylphenidate* and 0.25–1.0 mg/kg/day for dextroamphetamine.† Peak levels occur in 2 hours, and the half life is 2–4 hours.

A 1–2 week trial should be sufficient to evaluate the effectiveness of a medication in controlling behavior. Preferably, the study should be done with the teacher remaining unaware of the drug condition and keeping records of attention, behavior, and hyperactivity. Drug holidays should be attempted at least yearly to evaluate the need for continued medication. Psychotropic approaches using antihistamines, megavitamin therapy, and caffeine have been found to be ineffective.

Thus, the benefits of psychotropic drugs in mentally retarded children are modest and the risks, especially of phenothiazines and butyrophenones, are not inconsiderable. The risk-benefit ratio is not clearly positive in many children. Psychotropic drugs should then be used as a last resort, on a short term basis, and only in combination with an appropriate behavior modification and educational program.

Family Counseling. The emotional impact of having a mentally retarded child is enormous. The stages of grief the family passes through are similar to those of parents who have lost a child. The initial response is one of disbelief. The parents will rarely hear what you say after the words mental retardation are mentioned. Thus, the parents may find it difficult to absorb medical information about their child at this time.

After the initial shock and denial, the parents start to feel guilty. The mother especially may feel that she could have done something during her pregnancy to prevent the handicap or could have given better care to the child or sought medical attention sooner. Accompanying these are feelings of anger, "Why us?" The parents may direct their anger at each other, at God, at the pediatrician, or even at their child. The risk of child abuse is increased. The parents also feel isolated. They may feel they are the only ones with this problem. They need reassurance from the pediatrician and may also benefit from a parents' support group.‡

The next step in coping involves bargaining: "If only we try harder, perhaps he will be normal."

The pediatrician needs to help the parents maintain realistic expectations during this time. Some parents may intellectualize, accumulating a great deal of medical information about the child instead of confronting their own feelings. Some parents remain in this stage forever. Others move on eventually to a stage of acceptance.

Having a mentally retarded child also affects the stability of a marriage and the emotional health of the siblings. It is not uncommon for parents to be at different stages of coping. Further, one parent may want to talk about his or her feelings while the other does not; this leads to feelings of frustration and isolation. The siblings may share this anxiety. They are stigmatized as being the brother or sister of the "mental kid" and they may worry that they can "catch" the mental retardation. While feeling relieved that they are not retarded themselves the siblings may also feel guilty about being normal. They may also feel resentful that the parents spend more time with the mentally retarded child than with them. They may even be worried that they will have to care for their handicapped sibling when they grow up. The grandparents need also to be considered as they may assume some of the care of the child and will certainly influence the attitudes of the parents. Thus, counseling of the entire family is needed.

Re-evaluations. Although mental retardation is considered a static encephalopathy, there is a need for periodic review. As the child and family grow, new information must be imparted, goals readjusted, and habilitation programming altered. A review requires information about health status, family functioning, child functioning at home and at school, and the nature of the school programs. Other information, such as formal psychological or educational testing, may be needed. Annual reviews are generally necessary until school age. These reviews should also be undertaken any time the child is not meeting previous expectations.

As the child grows, he moves from one service provision system to another. This also marks the time for a review. Re-evaluation is necessary with the move from preschool to primary grades, from primary to intermediate grades, from intermediate to senior programming, and at the conclusion of school. By this time, the child has been abandoned by other adolescents. The disparity between cognitive abilities and chronologic age prevents the retarded adolescent from fitting in. This isolation promotes social awkwardness and diminishes the adolescent's self-esteem. Many parents feel incompetent to deal with issues of emerging sexuality in their retarded children.

The teaching of sexuality, dealing with menses, masturbation, and inappropriate closeness are some of the more common issues brought up by parents of retarded adolescents. In the severely retarded patients, sexual drive is limited, and few

---

* Manufacturer's warning: Safety and efficacy in children under 6 years of age have not been established.

† Dextroamphetamine is not recommended for children under 13 years of age.

‡ Batshaw M, Perret Y: *Children with Handicaps*, Brookes Publishing Co., 1985.

problems other than masturbation develop. These youngsters should be taught that masturbation is acceptable behavior in the privacy of their room but not in public. In the moderately retarded patient, sexual drive may be normal, although late in developing. As judgment is limited, close parental supervision is essential. Contraception should be afforded to all retarded individuals who are sexually active. Although controversy regarding reversible versus irreversible methods of contraception continues to exist, the present legal climate precludes irreversible contraception in most cases.

Late adolescence coincides with the transition from intermediate to senior programs. School will be ending, and long term planning concerning vocation, living situation, and independence should be in progress. Such planning needs to be based more on achievement than on potential. It is not uncommon to see a leveling off of academic abilities, and this should not be confused with a progressive neurologic disorder. Heterosexual activities, marriage, contraception, and social integration are all common concerns at this age. With the completion of school, there is no clearly identified service system for the retarded person. Plans for living arrangements and vocational pursuits should be in place and able to be activated when school is completed.

In the past, the answer to placement for the retarded patient was institutionalization. Many of those individuals are now being de-institutionalized and placed into group homes or smaller institutions or returned to their families. In general, the only patient who will be institutionalized in the foreseeable future is the multiply handicapped child whose parents cannot cope with the combined medical, behavioral and intellectual problems. Most moderately–severely retarded individuals will remain at home and attend activity centers or sheltered workshops. Alternate living situations, such as group homes, are gaining acceptance but are still few in number.

General Pediatric Care. Besides these special services, the mentally retarded child requires the same basic pediatric supervision as the child with normal intelligence. This includes following immunization schedules, growth parameters, and treating intercurrent infections. However, there may be additional concerns under certain circumstances. Mentally retarded children in classes or institutions where hepatitis B antigen has been identified may require the hepatitis B vaccine. Multiply handicapped children with recurrent respiratory infections may benefit from influenza vaccine. Weight gain may be deficient or excessive and requires nutritional intervention. Also counseling of parents concerning reduced growth potential is necessary. Dental hygiene needs to be addressed, especially for children receiving phenytoin or who are incapable of self-brushing. Preventive dental measures include decreasing the intake of sucrose-containing sweets by substituting noncariogenic snacks such as fruits and potato chips for candy and sugar-laden cereals. Toothbrushing and the use of fluoride should also be emphasized.

Psychiatric Disorders

GABRIELLE WEISS, M.D.

The treatment of psychiatric disorders of childhood and adolescence is somewhat less specific in relationship to the diagnosis than is the treatment of medical conditions. For some psychiatric disorders the treatment is quite specific and will be described under that diagnosis; for others the treatment chosen will depend as much on the nature of the difficulties existing in the family, the age of the child, the willingness of the family to engage in the treatment of choice, and the availability of skilled therapists as it does on the diagnosis itself.

Some of the reasons for this seeming lack of specificity are interesting. A child tends to react to various environmental stresses in ways that are characteristic of him and that may be related to his sex and genetic endowment. For example, one child may react to his parents' separation by becoming sad, withdrawn, or phobic while another child (more commonly a boy) will react to the same stress by becoming oppositional or developing conduct problems. Yet another child may express distress by developing physical symptoms, e.g., enuresis or pains.

Therapeutic Aspects of the Individual Assessment. As part of a comprehensive assessment, the child or adolescent is interviewed alone. Achieving a therapeutic alliance with a young patient, in the context of which confidential or painful issues can be discussed (e.g., suicidal ideation) is in part a learned skill in which motivated pediatricians can excel. In a facilitating environment in which encouragement is given and the appropriate questions are asked, a child or adolescent will begin to express himself freely and describe the nature of the stresses (internal and external) to which he is reacting. He may also, if asked, be quite willing to share his fantasies, dreams, and wishes. The material thus elicited is crucial to understanding the deviant behavior or emotional stress and to making a correct diagnosis.

Young children express themselves best through play. Some pediatricians have been trained to use diagnostic play sessions and will have various toys in their office for this purpose (e.g., puppets, doll families, crayons, paper, wooden animals, and so on). Small children may become quite uncommunicative in pediatricians' offices if asked questions about their difficulties directly. For example, asking a preschooler why he cannot go to sleep or why he goes to his parents' bed in the night is not productive. A preschooler or even a school-aged child will be more communicative either through the use of play or by selected indirect questions, e.g., "Do you ever worry about Mom or Dad?" or "When do you feel most scared?" A child or adolescent will feel relieved and understood when the physician succeeds in getting at the basis of the anxiety.

The aim of any treatment is to attempt, as far as is possible, to return the child to a normal developmental path, from which, as the disorder indicates, he has deviated. This involves understanding the interplay of biological, psychological, and social factors that have resulted in a deviation from this path and in the subsequent manifestation of internal emotional distress and/or deviant behavior. How this is accomplished depends on the treatment modality chosen. The following are examples of treatments used for psychiatric disorders of children and adolescents: family therapy, parent counseling or therapy, marriage counseling, play therapy, brief, time-limited and focused family or individual child therapy, behavior modification, group therapy, medication, hypnosis, and milieu therapies. Not infrequently more than one treatment modality is required. Rarely is the child or adolescent treated without parental involvement.

The treatment preferred for a given disorder depends on various factors. However, some key principles (or guidelines) exist for selecting the most appropriate form of help for a given child in a given family.

Family Therapy. For families who recognize or who will agree that some of the child's difficulties stem from maladaptive family interactions, family therapy is particularly useful. In reality it takes a great deal of motivation on the part of all family members to come together regularly at a specified time. This alone rules out many families from this modality. In carrying out family therapy the family is viewed as a system in which each member influences every other member and change in one member is contingent on and instrumental in producing change in other members. Occasionally a child's symptom can be seen as a metaphor for the expression of key family dynamics. (For example, a child presenting with elective mutism may come from a family that has an unsharable "secret").

Parent Counseling or Therapy. This treatment is indicated when the child's problem is seen to be directly related to difficulties in parenting. The nature of this treatment may be based on learning theory or on dynamic theories or both.

Marital Therapy. This treatment is preferred when the child is caught up in parental conflicts. For parents to consent to marital therapy, they have to agree that their marriage is a major problem for the child and, in addition, wish to change their interaction.

Play Therapy. This form of therapy (which is nearly always combined with some form of help for the parents) makes use of the notion that through play small children communicate important issues that adults or older children would talk about. Play therapy is indicated when the child's difficulties are perceived as internalized and as not being helped sufficiently by family therapy or parent counseling alone.

Brief, Time-Limited and Focused Therapy. This form of therapy may be used with a family or with an individual child. It is goal oriented, with a focal aim being selected and agreed upon by the family (or child) and therapist from the start. In addition, the number of sessions is limited, and this is agreed upon from the onset. While the efficacy of this form of therapy remains to be researched, it seems to offer some help to families who live far away or who are unwilling to engage in longer therapies. Use is made of the family's or child's existing strengths, and it is made clear at the beginning that they will be able to continue working themselves on the focal issues after treatment is concluded. Follow-up visits are required to reinforce gains made and to evaluate durability of the improvement.

Behavior Modification. This treatment is valuable for many types of disorders. It is most commonly used in conduct disorders and for mentally retarded and autistic children in whom other treatments have been relatively ineffective. It is based on learning theory and presumes that under specifically controlled environmental conditions learned maladaptive behaviors can be unlearned. Various methods are employed to accomplish this. The treatment is based on a prior careful behavioral analysis of the child during which the behavior therapist looks for situations in which the behavior typically occurs or fails to occur as well as for current maintaining conditions.

Group Therapy. Whatever their theoretical underpinning, all forms of group therapy make use of the group's therapeutic potential. Group therapies have been used effectively with disturbed adolescents and with parents who may have common problems, for example, single parents, parents of chronically ill or handicapped children, those who have parenting difficulties, and so on. The members of the group are generally supportive of one another and share their different coping styles. Analytic group therapies make use of interpretations of group interactions to produce insight.

Medication and Hypnosis. The use of medications for specific conditions will be described under the condition, as will hypnosis, which is utilized mainly for conversion symptoms.

Milieu Therapy. The child is admitted to a day center or to an inpatient ward. Professionals from various disciplines make up the staff, and the total milieu is expected to have a therapeutic effect. After a careful assessment of the strengths and deficits of the child, a special program is worked out for him, with the aim of improving the various ego deficits, be they difficulties in socialization, poor impulse control, educational lags, and so on. Usually one worker is assigned as the primary caretaker of the child, and it is to this person that the child relates most intimately. This special relationship may be very influential in helping the child to improve. Milieu therapy is used for the more severe disorders and for those children who require temporary or permanent removal from severely deviant parents. Parents as well as their children are involved in the treatment programs.

INFANTS AND TODDLERS

RUTH RUSSELL, M.D.

Early recognition of disturbances in parent-infant relationships is important because it allows for earlier therapeutic intervention. Recent data show that parents have concerns about difficulties with their child at least a year before a diagnosis and treatment plan are made. The parents had difficulty successfully communicating their concern to pediatricians, nurses, or family doctors. When the coping abilities of mother and her supports are stressed, her distress may sometimes be presented directly to the pediatrician or family doctor or indirectly through the symptoms in the infant or toddler. The common complaints by parents are about their child's feeding habits, sleeping habits, or other behaviors that are discrepant from the parents' expectations. Examples include insomnia, hypersomnia, excessive crying or whining, irritability, breathholding, temper tantrums, failure to thrive, pica, and irregularity of eating and sleeping schedules.

Treatment of problems in the infant and toddler stages involves working mainly with the child's environment, which includes the parents, the family, the extended family, and sometimes the community network around these families. For the parents, the groundwork for their capacity to parent was laid in their own childhood. Their marital interaction and their relationships with extended family and friends also affect their parenting abilities. A major aim of therapy with the parents would be to increase their sense of competence and their pleasure in parenting. The adaptations that have to be made by the parent for improved parent-child interactions would also be a focal point of the therapeutic work. Parents may need to understand and change their own temperamental characteristics and expectations in order to deal with the varied temperamental characteristics in their child. Unique to therapeutic work with infants and toddlers and their families is both the vulnerability of a developing child and also the adaptability and plasticity of a child.

Appetite, Sleep, Behavior. Minor Complaints. A parent or parents complaining of minor frustrations and difficulties adapting to the changing needs of their growing infant and toddler may respond to reassurance and guidance. These parents can be encouraged to respond to the cues given by their infant. For example, long tender holding by the mother and perhaps the use of a snugli greatly reduces crying. Feeding problems also frequently respond to educational suggestions or perhaps modeling by a sensitive nurse. This may include methods of holding the baby that allow eye contact between mother and child as well as better relaxation for both. These parents may also need to work with a psychotherapist on conflicts remaining from how they had been parented.

More Severe Complaints. A combined treatment approach may be necessary for more severe feeding, sleeping, or behavioral difficulties. Such complaints might include pica, failure to thrive, rumination or regurgitation, toilet training struggles, uncontrolled aggressive outbursts, and sleep disruptions resulting in excessively fatigued parent(s) and child. An educative and behavioral approach may help parents with age-appropriate expectations of their child, with consistency of their own behaviors, and with practical plans to change maladaptive behaviors in themselves and in their child. Modeling techniques may again be helpful. These approaches may be used in conjunction with some interpretive therapy to better understand factors that are inhibiting the parents' sense of competence.

Multisystem Complaints. Infants and toddlers may be brought to the physician with several symptoms, such as rashes, colds, diarrhea, poor appetite, temper tantrums, and sleeplessness. If parental anxiety and frustration are severe, incapacitating the parental system or perhaps arousing danger of abuse, the child may need to be removed from the dangerous or nonfunctioning environment. Short-term hospitalization, emergency foster care, or brief placement of the child with caring and capable relatives may be options. Immediate attention to careful future planning is necessary. Such intense incapacity to parent may require that the parent(s) have minimal contact with their child. The child of such parents may be put into a selected nursery or day care center where there is a caring, stimulating, and individualized approach to each child. Home visits may also be included in the treatment plan.

Developmental Deviations. Parents of children with developmental deviations face upheavals within themselves in trying to deal with hopes for a healthy child dashed by daily reminders that they have produced a defective child. Helping these parents to feel competent and experience pleasure in parenting may require a few visits, longer counseling, or referral to a child psychiatrist.

Single Parents. A group of parents growing in number who require increased support are single parents. They have markedly increased stress and responsibility. Environmental assistance involves calling upon extended family, foster grandparents, selected nurseries and day care centers, and babysitters. Individual and/or couple (parent-child) therapy includes educational approaches to a child's biological, psychological, and social development and needs as well as more supportive and psychological approaches that address the parent's capacity to parent and to provide for the child. Another helpful resource for these parents are parent support groups or self-help groups.

Neglected or Abused Parents. Infant stimulation programs are a growing resource, particularly for parents who themselves were neglected or abused. This stimulation can be in the physical, cognitive, and emotional spheres. These programs may be offered by various hospital departments, in community organizations, or in drop-in centers for mothers and infants and toddlers. In these group settings, mothers learn from professionals as well as from each other.

THE PRESCHOOL YEARS (3–5)

ALEXANDRA ROUSSOS, M.D.

The classification of behavioral disorders in the preschool years, that is 3–5-year-old children, is very difficult. This is due to the rapid growth and development during these years, which on the one hand results in some uncertainty of the limits of what constitutes normal development and its vicissitudes and on the other hand leads to lack of crystallization of the behavioral patterns into specific disorders. An additional problem pertains to the assessment of whether a behavior that does not fit the chronological expectations for the child is nevertheless appropriate for his global development level. If we exclude pervasive developmental disorders, mental retardation, and language disorders, which are dealt with elsewhere in this chapter, the most common remaining disorders of preschool age can be best classified under DSM III as falling under the following three

categories: (1) oppositional disorder, (2) anxiety disorders of childhood or adolescence, and (3) parent-child problem. This classification system does not include developmental deviations. The diagnosis of these disorders is of primary importance for this age group, especially since they often constitute a significant factor in the genesis of the behavioral problem the parents are seeking medical consultation for.

Oppositional Disorder

The oppositional disorder may begin as early as 3 years of age, but it also occurs in later childhood and adolescence. The essential feature is a pattern of disobedient negativistic and provocative opposition to authority figures. The oppositional behavior is towards family members, particularly the parents, and towards teachers but may well include other children. The most striking feature is the persistence of the oppositional attitude even when it is destructive to the interest and well being of the child. This behavior may, in fact, deprive the individual of productive activity and pleasurable relationships.

A general distinguishing feature of behavior disorders of preschool children is that they are global in nature rather than being focal or specific, and are generally expressed through the body (poor eating, sleeping, restlessness) or through behavioral deviance (oppositional behavior) rather than through any verbal complaints of distress.

Preschool children with oppositional behavior may present with the following symptoms: kicking, biting, hitting, throwing at, temper tantrums, sleep and eating difficulties, toilet training difficulties, self-mutilation, running away, or destructive behavior. Older children and adolescents with these disorders use negativism, stubbornness, dawdling, procrastination, and passive resistance to external authority. In this age group, the oppositional disorder must be differentiated from conduct disorder in which the basic rights of others or major age-appropriate societal norms or rules are violated.

Prerequisite to a comprehensive treatment of behavioral disorders in preschool children is a thorough assessment of the child and his environment. The need for a complete assessment is accentuated by the fact that for many young children this is the first time their problems are given medical attention and that in many cases there is the possibility of prevention of a chronic or permanent disorder. The evaluation of the child includes assessment of his emotional and social development, his temperament, the level of his skills (motor, perceptual, self-help, language) as well as investigation for any organic factors that might contribute to the genesis of the behavioral problem (e.g., neurologic abnormalities, hearing deficits, eyesight problems). It is important to underline the fact that, the assessment of young children relies heavily on direct observation. Owing to the variability of children's behavior, it is necessary that these observations take place over a period of time and, if possible, in the different settings to which the child is exposed.

Once referred for psychiatric evaluation, family assessment, and direct observation of the child in his home environment are essential parts of the process. If the child is attending nursery school or a day care center, contact with the teacher with a visit for direct observation helps to further clarify the nature and the extent of the problems of the child. The treatment of the child depends on the results of the assessment, and it should always include the parents in the dual role of parents and valuable members of the therapeutic team.

Children with emotional problems who live in a supportive environment may best be treated by individual psychotherapy, which is called play therapy for this age group. Behavior modification is the treatment of choice either when the symptoms require primarily management or when early control of the immediate problem is warranted. These two types of treatment often supplement each other.

Children who present with a multitude and variety of severe problems and who come from multiproblem families require more intensive intervention by a multidisciplinary team. These preschoolers are best treated by milieu therapy in a day treatment center or as inpatients. Remediation of the cognitive deficits that may occur together with their behavior or emotional difficulties is required and is a necessary part of their psychiatric treatment.

SCHOOL AGE CHILDREN

GABRIELLE WEISS, M.D.

For over 50 years, before any sophisticated method of classifying childhood disorders existed, a distinction was made between two main types of nonpsychotic disorders commonly seen in childhood: those in which the child feels some kind of internal distress (anxiety, guilt, and so on) and those in which the child, through his nonconforming behavior, upsets and distresses others. We would now subsume the former under "internalized disorders," in which we include the various types of anxiety disorders, depression, and obsessive compulsive disorders, and the latter are termed conduct or oppositional disorders. These two main groups, which together with the somatizing disorders make up the main body of childhood psychiatric problems, have different symptom clusters, probably different genetics, and different sex ratios and may require different therapies and have different outcomes.

Anxiety Disorders

These will be described under the following three headings: overanxious disorders, separation anxiety, and avoidant disorder.

Overanxious Disorders. Overanxious disorders are characterized by excessive worry and fearful behavior not focused on a specific situation or object or on separation from a person. Nor is this disorder reactive to a recent stress in the child's life. As the child gets older, the anxiety may focus on fears of failure in school, in sports, and in social relationships. These children are often perfectionistic and may have concomitant symptoms such as insomnia, motor restlessness, picking at themselves, pulling their hair, and so on. In the families of these children there is often a high level of anxiety and ambition for the children. At least one parent may have the adult form of the disorder.

Treatment requires assessment of the whole family, to determine "who else" is nervous in the family, who is most worried and what about, and so on. After ascertaining the family dynamics, the preferred treatment is family therapy. In severe cases, the child or adolescent may, in addition, require individual therapy, the nature of which may be supportive or interpretative.

Separation Anxiety. The clinical picture is characterized by excessive anxiety, which may reach panic proportions on separation from major attachment figures or from home. The reaction is beyond that normally expected for the child's age. These children often refuse to play alone in a room and follow a parent everywhere around the house. They often have difficulty in going to sleep unless they come into the parents' bed, and may have repeated nightmares with separation as a theme. Not infrequently, headaches, stomach aches, or vomiting is complained of, particularly on school days.

This disorder occurs equally frequently in boys and girls. "School phobia" is a misnomer for this condition. These children are often intelligent and come from excessively close families or from families in which chronic conflict or depression exists.

The treatment of choice is family therapy, at times combined with individual therapy of the child. In cases of school refusal the child should be returned to the school as quickly as possible. Cooperation of school personnel is required to facilitate this. Behavior modification techniques may be employed initially to get the child back into the classroom. I have not found that medication is required, even though tricyclic antidepressants are said to have a role for this disorder.

Avoidant Disorder. This clinical disorder is characterized by persistent and excessive shrinking from contact with strangers of sufficient severity as to interfere with social functioning and peer relationships. These children show a desire for affection and acceptance with family members and selected others with whom they feel secure. Usually these children are unassertive and have poor self-esteem.

This disorder is relatively rare, and treatment is not simple. Some of these children come from families in which more than one member has the disorder, and some families are isolated from the community and from other families. For these families, an "after school or evening program" where they are exposed to a trained professional in the context of interacting with other children is the treatment of choice. It should never be taken for granted that these children will "grow out" of this disorder without treatment. If the disorder is relatively mild, the pediatrician should nevertheless closely follow the child to determine progress.

Phobic Disorders. The clinical picture in phobic disorders is characterized by an irrational avoidance of certain objects or situations. A diagnosis is warranted only if the avoidance behavior is a significant source of distress to the child and interferes with his functioning. If the child is monosymptomatic, behavior modification is likely to be helpful. Family therapy is indicated in children who have several different phobias and change from one to the other (e.g., the dark, monsters, break-ins at night, and so on). This condition may coexist with overanxious disorders.

Obsessive Compulsive Disorder

The child with an obsessive compulsive disorder shows the following initial features: intrusive ideas, images, and impulses; a subjective feeling that these "mental events" are forced; and a feeling at the same time that the compulsion must be resisted.

The most common therapeutic approach has been toward a comprehensive treatment plan that includes both the child and his family. The child is treated with dynamic psychotherapy, and the family is involved in a variety of therapeutic modalities ranging from family therapy and counseling of the parents to individual treatment for the parents. Since most of these children are reserved, controlling, and unwilling to discuss their symptoms, the establishment of the therapeutic alliance represents a challenge for the therapist. To date no psychotropic medication is available for the treatment of this disorder.

Conduct Disorders

The essential feature of this group of disorders is a repetitive and persistent pattern of behaviors that violate the rights of others and break the normal rules of society. At present these disorders are subdivided on the basis of failure to establish a normal degree of affection, empathy, or bonding with others, which may or may not be present. They are also distinguished on whether direct expression of physical aggression is present.

While the disorder is fairly common and follow-up studies indicate that the prognosis is not encouraging, since about half develop antisocial personality disorders in adulthood, the treatment is difficult. Certainly every form of treatment listed has been tried and may work for some individual children. For the most severely conduct-disordered children, milieu treatment or placement into a group foster home is indicated. There is no evidence that medications are helpful except for those children who have a concomitant attention deficit disorder, although lithium, propanolol, carbamazepine, and haloperidol have been used with some success to reduce aggressive outbursts in severely conduct disordered inpatients.

Since about one third of conduct-disordered children have reading lags, this as well as overall school achievement should be carefully assessed. When specific cognitive impairments are found, remediation for these should be initiated. School failure and conduct problems can interact to create vicious circles.

Attention Deficit Disorder

LILY HECHTMAN, M.D.

Attention deficit disorder has previously been known as minimal brain damage, minimal brain dysfunction, minimal cerebral dysfunction, minor cerebral dysfunction, hyperkinetic reaction of childhood, hyperkinetic syndrome, and hyperactive child syndrome. These various terms represent changes over time in what was thought to be the central problem of the condition. The renaming of the condition by the recent Diagnostic Statistical Manual of Mental Disorders (DSM III) reflects the belief that attentional problems are central and virtually always present in children with this diagnosis, whereas hyperactivity may or may not be present. The key features of this condition are developmentally inappropriate inattention, impulsivity, and hyperactivity.

Associated features vary with age and can include poor social skills (e.g., bossiness, bullying), temper tantrums, stubbornness, negativism, increased mood lability, low frustration tolerance, low self-esteem, and lack of response to discipline. Many children with attention deficit disorder also have specific learning disabilities that need to be assessed and treated. Nonlocalized 'soft' neurological signs, motor-perceptual dysfunctions, and EEG abnormalities may also be present. Usually significant neurologically impaired children, e.g., children with cerebral palsy or epilepsy, are excluded from this diagnosis.

Some of the symptoms of attention deficit disorders can be seen in children with other conditions, e.g., mental retardation, schizophrenia, autism, affective disorders with manic features, conduct disorder, age-appropriate overactivity, and in children in inadequate, disorganized, or chaotic environments. Differentiating the retarded or psychotic child may be easy, whereas separating attention deficit disorder from conduct disorder or a disorganized child due to a chaotic environment may be extremely difficult and at times both diagnoses may be warranted. The disorder is relatively common (1–5%), and males are affected more frequently than females.

Children with attention deficit disorder may have multiple problems. Some of these difficulties are primary to the condition while others arise secondarily. Thus to adequately treat these children, comprehensive assessments and treatment plans are required. These have to address the physical, educational, social, and emotional spheres.

Physical Spheres. A careful comprehensive history of pregnancy, delivery, and the child's development from infancy on will help establish the diagnosis and rule out other conditions such as significant retardation, brain damage, and allergies. A complete physical examination, including neurologic examination and electroencephalography, will further rule out significant neurologic lesions (e.g., epilepsy, cerebral palsy). Soft neurologic signs, such as right-left confusion, clumsy gait, and diffuse electroencephalographic abnormalities, are not unusual in children with attention deficit disorder. Stimulant treatment has been known to exacerbate tics (e.g., Gilles de la Tourette's syndrome) and underlying epileptic seizures; thus neurologic assessment is important, alerting the physician to the need to modify (or discontinue) stimulant treatment if these conditions are present. Careful medical assessment is valuable in monitoring the subsequent appetite suppression and growth effect of stimulant treatment.

Educational Sphere: Remedial Education, Optimal School Setting. Comprehensive educational assessment may include determination of I.Q., testing for specific learning disabilities, and pinpointing the level of academic achievement the child has acquired in various basic school subjects. Assessment of the school setting is crucial to determine whether the environment and teacher can provide adequately for the needs of this child or whether a more specialized program is required, whether remedial help is available, whether there is flexibility in the program, and whether the setting is sufficiently structured.

Social Sphere: Behavior Therapy, Social Skills Training, Cognitive Therapy. Behavioral and social skills programs may help the child gain greater social acceptance, thus decreasing his sense of rejection and isolation and increasing his feelings of acceptance and improving his self-esteem. Cognitive therapy has been used with some success in helping the child shape his own problem solving and social behavior via a stepwise process of verbal self-directing and monitoring. The long-term efficacy of this intervention and how it compares with other treatments is yet to be firmly established.

Emotional Sphere: Psychotherapy, Individual and Family Psychotherapy, and Parental Counseling. Assessment of the child's emotional state, and how he views himself, his family, his peers, and his school is necessary as is evaluation of his personality strengths and how they can best be used to cope with his difficulties. Individual psychotherapy for the child may be required. Assessment of interaction of the child's family and helping the parents interact constructively are most important. Parental counseling or parenting training is sometimes very effective. At times, family therapy is indicated.

Pharmacotherapy. Drug treatment of attention deficit disorder is only one component of the comprehensive treatment plan and is therefore rarely sufficient alone but must usually be combined with one or more other interventions, e.g., behavior therapy, parental counseling, educational therapy, social skills training, or individual and/or family psychotherapy, depending on the requirements of the particular child.

STIMULANTS (METHYLPHENIDATE, AMPHETAMINE). Stimulants, such as amphetamine and methylphenidate, are the most effective medications for this condition, and positive drug response ranges from 70 to 80 percent of children with attention deficit disorder. Stimulants help improve attention and decrease hyperactivity and impulsivity and thus can improve behavior. However, they do not improve academic skills, though they may help the child be more receptive to learning. Before beginning a child on medication, a clear view of which symptoms are targets of treatment and how these are best monitored should be specified. In general, the school and particularly the child's main teacher are best suited to assess the stimulant's effect on attention and behavior. Generally a baseline of the target symptoms is established and then stimulant medication is gradually titrated to obtain optimal response at the lowest possible dose with fewest side effects. This monitoring can be done by close contact with parents and/or teachers with or without formal rating scales, e.g., Conners' Teacher or Parent Rating Scale.

Methylphenidate* has somewhat fewer side ef-

---

* Manufacturer's warning: Safety and efficacy of methylphenidate in children under 6 years of age have not been established.

fects than amphetamine and is therefore the drug of choice. Initial dosage begins at 0.3 mg/kg/day and is gradually increased by 0.1 mg/kg every week or two if no positive clinical effect is reported. The usual upper dose is 0.6 mg/kg/day to a maximum of 1 mg/kg/day. The medication is often given in two divided dosages in the morning before breakfast and at noon. This is done to provide optimal attention during the school day as methylphenidate has a 30-minute to 1-hour long lag phase and peaks in about 2.5 hours after administration. It also will decrease appetite suppression for the larger evening meal and hopefully not interfere with sleep. The long-acting form of methylphenidate is coming into increasing use. It is too early to say how much advantage it has over the shorter-acting pill. When possible, the child should have drug holidays on weekends and when school is not in session, e.g., summers. This practice decreases side effects (e.g., any growth suppression) and tolerance. A trial of several weeks off medication during the school year is also recommended to see if the child still requires medication.

Recently there has been a tendency for physicians to use a lower dose of methylphenidate, e.g., 10–20 mg in the morning (or approximately 0.3 mg/kg/day) in an effort to specifically improve attentional difficulties, since a higher dose may positively affect social behaviors but be less than optimal for sustained attention. Stimulant medication for preschoolers seems to be less useful than for older hyperactive children and may have side effects of whining and clinging behaviors. Other types of treatment such as parent counseling or good management in a nursery setting are often used for this age group.

Side Effects. Insomnia, sleep disturbance, and decreased appetite are the most frequent side effects. Weight loss, irritability, and abdominal pains are less frequent, with headaches, nausea, dizziness, dry mouth, and constipation occurring occasionally. Side effects usually disappear as the child becomes tolerant to the medication, or abate if the dosage is decreased.

There has been concern regarding growth and weight suppression. This effect appears minor and is related to higher doses given over a prolonged period of time. Thus, drug holidays (weekend, summer) are always recommended.

The precipitation of Gilles de la Tourette's syndrome has been reported. Some clinicians therefore do not recommend stimulant use for children whose parents or siblings have Gilles de la Tourette's syndrome or a pronounced history of tics.

PEMOLINE.† This drug is structurally different from methylphenidate or amphetamine. It has been found to be as effective in some studies as methylphenidate and amphetamine in doses of 2.25 mg/kg/day, but it is still a less preferred medication, possibly because of the delayed onset and increased side effects. The main advantage of pemoline is its prolonged duration of action, enabling a single morning dose to be used without the need for a noon dose. However, this longer duration of action may result in no effect being evident in the first two to three weeks and a persistent effect several weeks after the drug is discontinued. Reports of hypersensitivity reactions involving the liver and occurring after several months of treatment present a major concern. The need to periodically check liver function further adds to the disadvantage of this drug. Pemoline should not be the first drug of choice for this condition, but it can be tried if other stimulants are ineffective.

TRICYCLIC ANTIDEPRESSANTS. These drugs have shown some effectiveness in treating attention deficit disorder but not to the same degree as stimulants. Dosage ranges from 5-14 mg/kg/day in divided dosages. However, the anticholinergic and cardiotoxic side effects make them less indicated for this condition, and they should never be the medication of first choice.

OTHER DRUGS. A wide variety of pharmocologic agents have been tried in the treatment of attention deficit disorder. These include haldoperidol, phenothiazine, lithium, dianol, levodopa, caffeine, minor tranquiljzers, and anticonvulsants. To date none has been shown to be superior to stimulants and all have significant side effects, which limit their usefulness.

Disorders with Physical Components
MARIA KAPUSCINSKA, M.D.

Enuresis. Enuresis, a common symptom in childhood and adolescence, has been a concern for parents and physicians since antiquity. Enuresis is described as primary if bladder control has never been fully attained. It is defined as secondary if urinary incontinence reappears after at least one year of dryness. Boys are affected two to three times more frequently than girls. The enuresis is often familial and usually disappears in adolescence, and only in about 1% of children does it persist into adulthood. Functional enuresis is considered to be a variation in normal bladder control, rather than a disease, and most enuretic children do not exhibit any emotional problems. A small functional bladder capacity and a maturational delay, as supported by a high rate of spontaneous cure, appear to be the relevant causes. Some children with primary enuresis do show evidence of emotional or behavioral problems. These should be referred for psychiatric consultation.

† Manufacturer's warning: Pemoline is not recommended for use in children under 6 years of age.

Physiological mechanisms are more likely to contribute to primary enuresis; secondary enuresis is most frequently of psychogenic origin as a response to stress. Any organic cause has to be carefully ruled out in either case.

Bladder control is a developmental skill and as such has to be seen by a child as a challenge and his personal responsibility. Although enuresis as such is not inherently harmful, it may contribute to problems for the growing child. Ensuing tensions in the family, scapegoating, lowered self-esteem, and impaired peer relationships may result. In considering treatment, patience and restraint are advocated for a younger child, to allow him to develop control of his own function without coercion and exposure to potentially harmful methods.

After the age of seven, there is an increase in social demands and potential ostracism and exclusion from important activities. At this stage a more active therapeutic approach is warranted. The first step consists of reassurance and information to the child and his parents about the enuresis in order to remove guilt, prevent blame, and provide hope by giving data about the high rate of spontaneous cure. Active participation of the child should be encouraged by suggesting record keeping of his progress. Family support is needed to elicit verbal praise for dry nights and rewards for major breakthroughs in the form of increasing consecutive dry nights. All punishments for wet mornings should be discontinued.

Restriction of fluids, particularly those with diuretic properties, prior to bedtime and encouraging urination may be of some value but seem to have little effect in more problematic cases. Bladder stretching exercises are helpful to increase functional bladder capacity as well as to improve the child's control over the urination reflex. The procedure is based on encouraging the child to hold the urine as long as possible between voidings. Stream interruption exercises and increased intake of fluids in the morning have a similar aim.

The highest success rate is ascribed to enuresis alarms, which are based on the principle that the child will eventually learn to 'beat the buzzer,' which is a device that rings a bell when moistened by urine at night. There is, however, also a high rate of relapse.

Imipramine‡ remains the most popular drug for enuresis because of its anticholinergic effect on the bladder, which inhibits urination. The starting dose of 10 mg at bedtime is increased weekly to a maximal dose of 40–50 mg for younger children (8–12) and to 75 mg for teenagers. The high toxicity of imipramine and the relatively

modest success rate with its use raise serious doubts about the value of using this medication. Some clinicians use imipramine for periods when dryness becomes very important, as when the child goes to camp.

The less toxic antispasmotic agent oxybutynin (Ditropan) has been tried, but additional studies are needed before this can be recommended. Medications suppress symptoms but do not cure.

Psychotherapy is not a treatment of choice for enuresis, but it can be of value for treatment of secondary emotional problems or if these coexist with enuresis.

Encopresis. Encopresis is defined as repeated voluntary or involuntary passage of feces of normal or near normal consistency into places not appropriate for that purpose in the individual's own sociocultural setting, after the age of four years. While it is tacitly assumed by some to be phychogenic in origin because no organic pathology is found, this does not necessarily follow. Primary or continuous encopresis refers to a child who has never achieved bowel control. This type is more frequently seen as a result of neglect, lax training methods, mental subnormalities, and familial causes. Secondary or discontinuous encopresis refers to a child who was previously trained but who has lost the acheived bowel control, often in response to stress. Sometimes a history of a coercive mother and early and punitive pot training is obtained. In the battle over bowel control, the child withholds his feces, which, in turn, may result in phychogenic megacolon with retention of hard fecal masses and an overflow diarrhea. Occasionally, a painful local lesion such as a fissure may start a similar sequence. Characteristically, an encopretic child is often constipated, refuses to use a pot or toilet, or delays such use, producing instead misplaced and mistimed evacuations. The child seems to fail to respond to his rectal cues, and in cases of soiling, is often unaware of the need to defecate when the watery material is seeping around the impacted mass producing little sensation. Although encopresis is viewed as an ominous symptom, by and large encopretic children are developmentally normal and neurologically intact. However, the encopretic child is neither a popular patient nor is he well liked by his peers due to the odor caused by the symptom. He may be severely rejected by his parents as a result of his symptoms. Not infrequently, the parents are convinced that the child is doing this on purpose. While various personality traits have been ascribed in psychiatric literature to both the child and his parents, they lack specificity for the condition.

A holistic approach to treatment of soiling involves psychological and often physiological treatment of the child and treatment of the parents. Issues over control during attempted toilet training

---

‡ Manufacturer's warning: Not for use in children under 6 years of age.

("the potting couple") are addressed, and an attempt is made to reduce various pressures on the child. It is important to help the child change the negative attitude he has towards his symptom. The parental reaction of anger or helplessness to the soiling should be enquired about and appropriate help given to the parents. Normal intestinal functions should be explained to the child in a simple language, stressing the need for the muscle building aspect in control of the bowel; thus the necessity of daily 'exercises' of going to the toilet.

As part of an assessment of the possible physiological factors in the initial stages of the management program, a plain x-ray film of the abdomen is obtained to assess the degree of stool retention caused by chronic constipation, and to determine whether a functional megacolon exists. If the latter is present, a complete evacuation of the bowel is required as a necessary step to initiation of muscle training. The usual procedure consists of a three-day cycle of catharsis in the following order: on the first day, two hyperphosphate (Fleet) enemas are given in succession; on the second day, the child receives a bisacodyl (Dulcolax) suppository after school and early in the evening, and on the third day, he is given two 10-mg bisacodyl tablets. In milder cases and in children under seven, half of the above dose is usually sufficient. Repeated x-ray films of the abdomen are taken to document the change and to determine whether further catharsis is necessary. The maintenance program consists of mild laxatives or stool softeners, which are usually required for a period of about six months. The training component involves habituating the child to feel comfortable on the toilet, at regular times and at least twice a day for about 10 minutes. Praise and positive reinforcement from the parents are important factors in establishing regular bowel habits.

Since cleansing enemas are frightening for the child, the parents should be urged strongly to avoid any anal manipulations for possible relapses after the initial catharsis. If parents are unable to give up coercive bowel training methods, or if the child does not respond to bowel retraining as outlined, a psychiatric consultation should be requested. This is also true for those children who have concurrent psychological problems as well as symptoms of soiling.

Play therapy with the child is based on establishing a positive relationship in order to allow expression of unconscious negative attitudes. An important task is to help the child achieve a moderate disgust reaction to his feces as contrasted to a too weak reaction or alternatively to a reaction of extreme disgust. Work with the parents often involves resolution of issues of control and reduction of anger that the child is soiling willfully to punish them.

Gilles de la Tourette's Syndrome. A revived interest in this obscure and poorly understood condition resulted from the first reports of successful treatment with haloperidol in the early to mid 1960's. Although the pathophysiology and psychopathology are unknown, most authors agree that an interplay of organic, intrapsychic, and environmental factors exist. Recent studies have called attention to the frequency of associated problems such as attention deficit disorder, obsessive compulsive symptoms, and learning disorders. In some cases treatment with stimulants has been said to trigger the manifestation of the disorder. The natural course of the disease of spontaneous remissions and exacerbations may cause confusion regarding the efficacy of prescribed treatment.

Haloperidol (a butyrophenone) is still regarded as the drug of choice. Medications for this condition do not cure but result in fair to good suppression of symptoms. The starting dose of 0.25–0.5 mg is recommended, with weekly increments of 0.5 mg until the maximum benefit is obtained with minimum side effects. Only if parkinsonian side effects appear is it necessary to add anticholinergic medication to the neuroleptic. To avoid the danger of tardive dyskinesia, which is associated with long-term use of neuroleptics, the lowest dose possible is being recommended. The newer drugs, such as the neuroleptic pimozide and the alpha-adrenergic agonist clonidine have been reported effective for cases resistant to haloperidol. Clonazepam as an adjunct to haloperidol or clonidine may also produce some benefit to alleviate more resistant symptoms.

Mild cases, particularly in very young children, are however best managed without chemical interference at all, until the latter is truly appropriate, as when the child stops functioning at school and is very distressed.

The usefulness of behavioral therapy for Gilles de la Tourette's syndrome seems to be quite limited. The only observable benefit has been seen in training patients to substitute a less obvious symptom for one that is socially objectionable.

Other developmental difficulties often affiliated with the syndrome should be treated properly. Problems of family acceptance and the secondary symptoms of poor self-esteem, social isolation, and depression require psychotherapeutic intervention to decrease the amount of psychic tension and environmental stress, both of which are well known to exacerbate the primary condition. Family therapy and individual child therapy are often helpful, for a condition that is so frightening for the child and his parents.

Somatoform Disorders

SUZANNE DONGIER, M.D.

DSM III lists the following elements as the essential criteria: a loss of alteration in physical functioning suggesting a physical disorder, which is not explained after appropriate investigations by a known physical disorder or pathophysiological mechanisms and is not under voluntary control. Another essential criterion is the presence of psychological factors judged to be etiologically involved in the symptom. This is evidenced by one of the following: (1) relationship between the symptom and an environmental stimulus apparently related to a psychological conflict or need, (2) the use of the symptom in search of secondary gains, and (3) a crisis situation with a feeling of lack of hope for its possible resolution. The goals of the management and treatment will be both stopping the symptom and elucidating the psychodynamics at its roots. Reduction of secondary gains, which can achieve rapid symptom remission, is accomplished by behavior modification techniques. The appearance of a substitution symptom after the first one has disappeared is rare, and if it occurs, a more intensive investigation of emotional factors is indicated.

Clarification of many of the underlying psychological factors will help the child to understand how he felt pushed to "choose" bodily symptoms to express distress. Involvement of the family is a must in view of frequent collusion in regard to secondary gains and because of the major role played by the family in the emotional life of the child.

A thorough assessment will permit a decision as to the best mode of intervention. With the family, the choice will be family crisis intervention or family therapy (short-term or long-term). With the child, it is important to restore a sense of hope and control. A concomitant individual approach can foster alliance with the therapist and permit more active involvement of the child in both the family sessions and in individual work. When the symptom itself appears as potentially dangerous (for example, the risk of chronic contractures) it can be useful to use hypnosis in which suggestion is used in a context of a positive therapeutic alliance and a feeling of active self-control.

A conversion symptom can be an isolated and short-term disorder in reaction to an acute stress and will have no serious consequences. It can also develop in a child with a weak ego and a limited ability to change defensive maneuvers or as part of a long-standing disorder of the developing personality, and is sometimes associated with very serious complex and secret family conflicts. As the child is overwhelmed by the intensity of affects, the body is used like a theatre where fantasies, sometimes related to secret events in reality, can be expressed. In such cases, the approach will have to be multifaceted and the goals set at various levels. Sometimes it will be wise to decide on reasonable limited goals. A short-term hospitalization in a well-structured child psychiatry milieu will permit the work to begin.

In all cases the assessment of the response of the child to the crisis and to the treatment will be of major importance in evaluating further long-term plans. The motivation of the child and of the family for long-term therapy, when this is indicated, can decrease drastically after the symptom is removed. Supportive measures can be very useful (support at school, group activities, after-school program) if more extensive psychological work cannot be done because the family does not wish it.

Pain. Pain is by definition a highly subjective state; its perception and psychological integration and interpretation by the patient are of outstanding importance.

Beside the pure "psychogenic pain" there are a number of pathological pain states that complicate medical problems either acutely or subacutely by the intensity or the prolongation of the pain or in a chronic way when associated with anxiety and depressed mood. In this case, the possibility for narcotic dependence increases and will add to the management problem of the case. When no organic cause has been found to explain the pain, it is important for the family and the patient not to receive the message that the pain is not valid and does not exist. The reality of the pain cannot be denied, and the first goal will be to give back a sense of control to the patient by a better definition of his pain and by having something to do to control it or to cope with it.

Relaxation and hypnotic techniques and self-regulation of pain perception have added new dimensions to the antipain arsenal. Pediatric oncology has recently used and developed the techniques of progressive muscle relaxation, breathing, and guided imagery techniques, which tackle at the same time the perception of the pain itself and the anxious and overwhelming reaction to the pain. These approaches have permitted a substantial decrease in the amount of antipain medication and have contributed to the overall improvement of the functioning and well-being of the child. Antidepressant medication (amitriptyline) has been used with success in adult patients and sometimes with children to break chronic pain syndromes (even in the absence of a depressive state).

Abdominal pain, limb pain, and recurrent headaches are especially frequent in the child. The importance of the environment, the search for secondary gains, and stresses at the origin of pains are consistent elements of the diagnosis of psychogenic pain. For example, it has been found that children of adults with abdominal pain are more likely to suffer from abdominal pain themselves. In these states, as in conversion disorders, the first task will be to stop the vicious circle of secondary gains by at the same time giving the child other ways of expressing his needs. It will be important as well to understand the meaning of the symptom through individual and family approaches. These will explore recent life stress, changes in family structure, habitual ways of coping with life stress as modeled by parents and siblings, and the ability of the child and of the family to work on affective aspects of their functioning.

The best approach is an association of such psychodynamic exploration with more technical methods of coping with the pain. It is important, however, to know that these children can be very difficult to treat, partly as a result of the emotional reactions of the family and staff who face a child in pain, with whom they may identify. This is a field in which a multidisciplinary approach is necessary.

Elective Mutism

RUTH RUSSELL, M.D.C.M.

Treatment of elective mutism requires an evaluation of the possible causes, which may relate to current and past family relationships, character traits of the child, and secondary gain from the symptom. These children (more commonly girls) have begun talking normally and have normal speech and comprehension but have elected to stop talking or to talk to only a few selected people and to remain silent in the presence of most others. There appears to be an emotional charge attached to sound production, which may contain elements of passive aggression and of controlling others through the symptom. Sometimes elective mutism is related to family secrets of which the child is aware, and which family members consider shameful, for example, mental illness or antisocial behavior of a parent or sexual problems between the parents. The condition seems to occur more frequently in immigrant families who may be isolated from the larger culture. A few children showing this disorder had articulation problems during their development.

Elective mutism can be quite resistant to therapy, particularly when there is strong secondary gain for the child or his parents; an example of the latter would be an overprotective and isolated mother who feels less anxious when her child plays in the home rather than mixing with rough children on the street. Family therapy is the treatment of choice. When family secrets exist, the family sessions are used to promote open discussion and free the child from maintaining the silence. Where coercive measures have been used in an attempt to force or shame the child into speaking, behavior therapy is very helpful in replacing punishments with positive reinforcement for spontaneous talking, for example, in the classroom situation.

Psychological Reactions to Chronic Illness and Handicap

HELEN CVEJIC, M.D.

The way in which an individual responds and adjusts to permanent physical damage due to disease or injury is the most important aspect of a rehabilitation program. Any attempts to assist the chronically ill or disabled child and his family has to be tempered by the family's and child's emotional reactions to the situation, plus their acceptance and adaptation to the condition.

Outline of an Optional Treatment Plan

1. Parents have to be given a clear and definitive diagnosis, and a follow-up plan should be outlined. The impact of the illness on the child's lifestyle and that of the parents has to be explained. Familiarization of the child with the treating doctor, the institution, the equipment, and the procedures reduces fear.

2. The diagnosis of a severe chronic illness will precipitate a state of crisis in the family. There is a potential for disorganization in both instrumental and emotional functioning. The physician who is already known to the family can help in minimizing the destructive effects and aid in the reintegration and better adaptation of the family. It should be kept in mind that with the extra demands on parents of caring for a sick child, normal siblings may become neglected. In addition, marital disharmony is a common consequence, which a pediatrician can detect if aware of this possibility. Often a pediatrician can help parents not to blame one another or to displace anger onto each other or siblings. Physicians must be careful not to impose their own coping styles onto the patient and his family.

3. Parents need guidance in order to ensure that the chronically ill child can gain an independent life. Increasing responsibility for his self-care improves his self-image and helps him to feel that he is an active participant in the control of the diseased part that is functioning poorly. Medical supervision helps to ensure that the illness is not minimized or maximized. Dependency needs are easily exaggerated by illness.

4. The continued maintenance of school and peer relationships is very important and has to be stressed. This is important in countering the egocentricity (which is a natural consequence) of the chronically ill child.

5. Parent groups are very supportive and educational. They encourage parents to learn about the illness at their own rate and enable them to share coping techniques. Parent groups have also been instrumental in helping to provide better medical services from government organizations. They also help to counteract the social isolation

that these families almost invariably face in taking care of a chronically ill child.

6. The demands of the child and the family on the treating physician may become excessive and he should feel comfortable in requesting a consultation and/or follow-up treatment program from a child psychiatrist, who is trained to deal with the emotional aspects of the illness on the child and his family.

7. A multidisciplinary team approach is important in cases of chronic illness, particularly when complicated by multiproblem families. The various individuals involved, e.g., child, parents, teacher, nurse, doctor, psychiatrist, need to be in constant and open communication.

The pooling of the stresses and sharing of the resources of the individuals involved provide a wealth of information and strength unavailable to the solitary professional.

Adolescent Years

FIONA KEY, MB.Ch.B.

Adjustment Disorders

Severe behavior problems are not an intrinsic part of the adolescent process. The adolescent who presents with significant conflict towards his family, drug abuse, or school failure is recognized to be having difficulty and in need of help. Adjustment disorders are the most common problems of adolescence and also occur frequently in younger children. Their symptomatology varies widely, but implicit in the diagnosis is the recognition that the adolescent is responding in a maladaptive way to a clearly defined recent stressful situation, the intensity of which may vary considerably. The stressors may be within the individual, associated with a normal developmental task, or from the environment. Sometimes the link between the stressful event and the symptom is evident to the adolescent and at other times clarification of this is an important part of treatment. Adjustment disorders usually occur in previously healthy individuals, but they may also present in adolescents with underlying character disorders and have then to be distinguished from the chronic fluctuating symptoms that are part and parcel of the character disorder.

The first step in treatment is to be able to work with the patient. When the adolescent is himself in sufficient distress, he may ask for help. More commonly parents or teachers notice that there is a problem and have to find a way of encouraging the young person to seek help. Assessment generally involves both an individual and family interview and an evaluation from the school. The diagnostic interview in itself may be sufficient treatment in that there is recognition that the

adolescent is under stress and some association is made between the stressful event and the patient's symptoms. The goal of therapy is to enable the adolescent to find a healthier response to stress and to ensure subsequent normal development. In most cases, brief intervention at the individual or family level should suffice, with consultation with the school when necessary. When this is unsuccessful, there is a possibility of either more serious psychopathology in the adolescent, e.g., affective disorder, identity disorder, or character disorder, or disturbance in the family functioning such that the adolescent's symptom maintains some kind of balance within the family system and cannot be easily given up. In these areas the treatment goals need to be redefined and psychiatric intervention is indicated.

Group therapy is a treatment modality particularly suited for adolescents who are highly invested in relationships with their peers. The issues of separation and individuation with which the young person is dealing in his family are brought into the group, where an opportunity is given to work them through in an atmosphere of support. Groups with adolescents can be very intense and require active participation on the part of the leader. Support groups for adolescents with particular problems, e.g., physical illness, alcoholic parents, divorcing parents, or to teach specific social skills may be helpful. For adolescents who develop drug or alcohol abuse, a combined behavioral and group approach is used.

Brief Reactive Psychosis

Like adjustment disorders, acute reactive psychosis also occurs in reaction to a recent known stressful event. It is the most frequent cause of acute psychotic symptoms among adolescents. Prior to the onset of the psychotic episode, there is no evidence of personality change, as would be expected in a schizophrenic disorder, and the symptoms themselves last anywhere from a few hours to a maximum of two weeks. The symptoms consist of acute emotional distress and presence of either delusions, hallucinations, looseness of associations, or disorganized behavior. A brief period of hospitalization is generally indicated, and symptoms may abate without the use of antipsychotic medication. It is important to rule out any organic cause of the psychosis. Differential diagnosis will include affective disorders (manic episode or psychotic depression), schizophreniform disorder, schizophrenia, and transient psychotic episode in borderline character disorder. Family assessment can contribute to the understanding of the role of the symptom in the family system and eliciting stresses within the family. If antipsychotic medication is prescribed, it is usually given for a few weeks only, as a return to normal level of function is expected. Treatment of the individual focuses on understanding his reaction to the stress and enabling him to find other ways of coping. Should the symptoms persist for more than two weeks, the diagnosis should be revised, as a schizophreniform disorder becomes more likely at this point and antipsychotic medication will have to be continued for several months at least. More intensive rehabilitation is also likely to be necessary.

Identity Disorder

Identity formation is one of the central tasks of adolescence, and trials of identification in a variety of areas are common. However, when there is a profound confusion over identity in several areas of the adolescent's life associated with feelings of distress lasting several months and when this also affects his or her functioning in social, academic, or work situations, the diagnosis of identity disorder is given. The level of disturbance of function is variable. Treatment, either in individual or group psychotherapy, aims at resolving the conflicts preventing the adolescent from proceeding with the task of identity formation. The therapist may also function as a role model. Family therapy is indicated when problems in family functioning are contributing to the youngster's difficulties, for example, in a single parent family in which the adolescent becomes the emotional partner of the parent.

Symptoms of identity disorder may also herald the onset of a more serious disorder such as borderline personality disorder, schizophrenia, or affective disorder. They may also present at times of life other than adolescence, e.g., midlife crisis.

Character Disorders

Although character disorders are not generally diagnosed until adulthood, it is often possible to pick up a consistent pattern of behavior in the adolescent and sometimes even the younger child that would predict these conditions. Character disorders are thought to have their origins in disturbances of early infantile relationships that result in difficulties of various severity in resolving all the developmental crisis points of childhood and adolescence. Thus they pervade many areas of functioning and symptoms tend to be chronic, although with acute decompensations at particular times of stress, either external or developmental.

Sometimes the individual may not be aware of problems, and it is those around him who complain of the way they are treated. More commonly, however, there are subjective complaints that may be quite vague, e.g., anxiety or mood disturbance. Character difficulties are likely to stay with the individual for life. Some studies have indicated that long-term intensive psychotherapy may result

in some improvement in symptomatology. A cognitive behavioral approach has also been found useful in helping the individual cope with symptoms that are seen as chronic. Periodic brief hospitalizations may be necessary for the individual with borderline personality disorder who may become suicidal or acutely psychotic. Medications are not generally useful in treating these conditions.

Affective Disorders

It is only within the past twenty years that affective disorders have been diagnosed in children and adolescents and relatively recently that this diagnosis has been made on the basis of much the same symptomatology as is found in adults.

Affective disorders may be classified as major affective disorders, unipolar and bipolar, cyclothymic disorders, and dysthymic disorders. Manic episodes have been described in adolescence but are rare. They may presage the onset of bipolar affective disorder. Major depressive episodes have been described in childhood and adolescence. Dysthymic disorders are quite common. According to DSM III criteria, major depressive episodes present with a persistent and pervasive feeling of sadness or dysphoric mood and four of the following (three of the first four in children under six) lasting at least 2 weeks: (1) poor appetite or significant weight loss (unless dieting) or increased appetite with significant weight gain, or failure to make expected weight gains in young children; (2) insomnia or hypersomnia; (3) psychomotor retardation or agitation; hypoactivity in young children; (4) loss of interest or pleasure in usual activities, signs of apathy in young children; (5) loss of energy, fatigue; (6) feelings of worthlessness, self-reproach, or excessive guilt; (7) slowed thinking or indecisiveness; and (8) suicidal thoughts or attempted suicide or wishes to be dead.

Dysthymic disorder presents with similar symptoms but they are less severe, occurring over the course of a year, either persistently or with periods of normal mood lasting up to a few weeks at a time.

There is an association between symptoms of depression and separation anxiety disorder (most commonly manifest as school phobia) in young children and with symptoms of conduct disorder in adolescent males. Depression may also be part of the anorexia syndrome. Whether these conditions predispose to depression or vice versa is unclear.

Treatment of affective disorders is generally multimodal. For major affective disorders, a brief period of hospitalization may be effective. Individual psychotherapy is generally indicated, with the aims of improving self-esteem and relieving feelings of guilt and helping the individual to cope with the depressive, more rarely manic, episode. When the family dynamics are considered to be playing an important part in either initiating or maintaining the symptoms, for example, when the child or adolescent is being scapegoated, family therapy is indicated. Parental counseling around management issues may be useful in the treatment of the young child with depression. As a significant number of depressed children come from families with at least one parent suffering from depression, treatment of other affected family members is essential. For children with dysthymic disorder, these measures should be sufficient. For those children and adolescents with a diagnosis of major depressive episode, a trial of antidepressants may be indicated.

The tricyclic antidepressants are preferred over the monoamine oxidase inhibitors and although all of these drugs have sympathomimetic side effects, desmethylimipramine (desipramine)§ appears to have the fewest and would be the drug of choice. The drug is usually given in two or three divided doses, and the dosage is increased gradually over a period of 10 to 14 days to a maximum of 4.5 mg/kg/day for a period of at least 6–8 weeks. There is some controversy over the upper level of drug dosage, as some studies show that these levels are necessary to have a therapeutic effect but that there is a risk of cardiovascular toxicity. Patients on tricyclic antidepressants should regularly be monitored for these side effects by measuring heart rate, blood pressure, and EKG. An increase in heart rate above 130/minute, systolic blood pressure $\geq$ 115 mm Hg, diastolic blood pressure $\geq$ 95 mm Hg, PR interval $\geq$ 0.18, or QRS interval $\geq$ 130% of baseline would indicate a need to reduce dosage as would the presence of unacceptable clinical side effects. Once a satisfactory clinical response is obtained, the drug should be continued for several months and then gradually reduced and stopped unless symptoms recur.

In the rare cases when a manic episode is diagnosed in adolescence, lithium may be tried in addition to individual therapy. Lithium has proved to be very effective in the treatment of manic episodes in adults and in the prevention of both manic and depressive episodes in bipolar major affective disorders. Dosage should be such as to maintain a blood level between 0.6 and 0.9 meq/l. Response appears to be best when there is a positive family history of affective disorder and a strong affective component to the presenting symptoms. Renal and thyroid function should be monitored. Once started on lithium, a patient may have to be maintained on it for life; this should be taken into account in view of the well-documented side effects of the drug.

Eating Disorders

MOUNIR SAMY, M.D.

Anorexia Nervosa. Anorexia nervosa is not a homogeneous clinical entity. It is a developmental syndrome of adolescence and early adulthood that appears within a wide variety of emotional symptoms. Primary anorexia nervosa has to be distinguished from similar conditions that are secondary to a psychotic process, a severe depressive state, or a conversion reaction. Further subclassification of anorexia nervosa is of little value to management.

Hospitalization is necessary if the weight loss is considerable (for example, more than 20 percent of the body weight) or if it relieves the family from the great stress that this condition places on them. Disease of the central nervous system must be ruled out in every case by routine skull x-ray and electroencephalogram. The results of laboratory investigations are usually normal or may display a prepubertal hormonal profile. If the weight drops below 30 percent, tube feeding is indicated.

The management of anorexia nervosa is multimodal. The primary concern is the restoration of body weight not only to prevent medical complications but also as a prerequisite to any other type of therapy. This is effectively achieved by behavioral modification based on reinforcement of *gradual* weight gain. Rapid weight gain should be prevented, as it may worsen the patient's fear and depression. Family and individual therapies should deal with the relational and emotional aspects of the illness and leave the behavioral contract management to the ward staff.

In the family dynamic, one is likely to find a fragile equilibrium that does not tolerate any changes (e.g., the patient's need to grow up and be emancipated) and an excessive intrusiveness and/or closeness between the patient and the mother. The individual therapy should stress the patient's capacity to recognize needs and feelings, to acquire a sense of separateness and self-esteem, and to diminish guilt over appropriate psychosexual development and emancipation. The technique of the therapy should be relational and supportive and based on better reality testing rather than dynamic or interpretative.

A number of drug therapies (e.g., neuroleptics, stimulants, and insulin) have been attempted with no convincing results. Antidepressants are indicated whenever there is evidence from the personal or family history to suspect a relationship between anorexia nervosa and an affective disorder (e.g., anorexic episodes alternating with periods of severe depression with or without binge eating).

---

§ Manufacturer's warning: Not recommended for use in children.

The general prognosis of anorexia nervosa is poor, as two thirds of the patients continue to have anorexic symptoms. Five to 10 percent die from starvation or suicide. Good prognostic signs include an early onset, absence of bulimia and vomiting routines, and a less than severe weight loss on first admission. Therefore, vigorous early intervention is essential in the treatment of anorexia nervosa.

Bulimia. The general management of bulimia is similar to that for anorexia nervosa. One should be prepared for a longer hospitalization with behavior modification and if possible milieu and group therapies to foster peer interactions. The patient's motivation tends to diminish with the slow progress and has to be frequently rebuilt. The prognosis indicates that intermittent relapses occur over many years.

Evaluation and Treatment of Suicide Risk
MOUNIR SAMY, M.D.

The number of adolescents who attempt or commit suicide has increased steadily during the past decade. Children between 10 and 14 years of age are now also considered to be at risk of suicide. But suicide may also occur in much younger children. Suicidal behavior is not specific to any physical or mental disorder, any personality type, or any social class. Therefore it should be ruled out whenever any doubt exists. Sometimes a simple direct question to the patient and the family as part of the routine assessment will suffice.

There are two main characteristics of adolescent suicidal syndrome that affect evaluation and treatment. First, most adolescents who attempt suicide do not seek their death in any active or conscious way. (For children and early adolescents the death concept may even be confused or concrete, e.g., "going away" or "just going to sleep"). The use of self-destructiveness is a maladaptive ultimate effort to make changes in a human environment that is perceived as unreceptive. Second, irrespective of the severity of the suicidal attempt, these adolescents are in a great deal of emotional distress, which warrants immediate active intervention. Therefore, a suicidal gesture should never be disposed of as "hysterical" or "manipulative" just because it has not endangered life seriously. Parents may tend to underestimate the seriousness of the act of their adolescent as part of coping with their own distress. A suicidal threat is clinically equivalent to an attempt. The management requires careful evaluation of the adolescent and his family. The evaluation of the circumstantial factors alone is not sufficient to make management decisions. A review of the patient's life and its general quality as well as a survey of his stresses and recent life changes are important aspects of risk evaluation. Existing personality disorders or other psychopathology should be diagnosed. It is also imperative to meet with family members and assess their cooperation and their capacity to provide support.

All suicide threats, gestures, or attempts have to be taken seriously either for their true potential or for the intense emotional distress that is being conveyed. The most efficient approach in a suicide crisis is rapid and multidisciplinary crisis intervention as soon as the patient is medically clear. The adolescent receives the message that caring physicians or other professionals are attending to his emotional pain and that this crisis presents a golden opportunity to make a change in his life; that even though he/she remains ultimately in control of his/her life, the professionals will not remain passive when presented with threats or attempts at suicide. There is a tendency among certain professionals to disregard mild or moderate suicidal behavior for fear of reinforcing it. Such an attitude may have the opposite results, namely repeated attempts and an escalation of their severity.

If the suicide risk is high, the patient should be hospitalized and put under constant observation. The psychiatric illness, if any, has to be treated with the appropriate medication. The areas of stress have to be dealt with (e.g., reassessing the school assignment with his teachers or reconsidering his living arrangements with the social agencies or getting the family involved in therapy). Finally, time-limited individual psychotherapy with the focal aim of restoring a sense of hope and mastery based on an improved ability to share feelings and express needs is very important.

If the suicide risk is low or moderate, the patient may still have to be hospitalized, as this is often the only way family and community involvement can be ensured. Crisis intervention here should aim at a restoration of a family and social support system that has been inadequate or nonexistant. For example, insist on family involvement and participation, require the help of social agencies, attempt his school or work reintegration, stress the need for follow up by psychiatry or social service. These interventions are at times anxiety provoking and resisted by the patient. His or her suicide threats should not be allowed to blackmail the physician and render him inefficient. In a short time the same patient becomes appreciative of the help offered.

Family intervention, whenever possible, is the rule. It aims at diminishing the patient scapegoating, which is often the case, and at helping family members acknowledge and attend to their conflicts. Often these adolescents have received the implicit or explicit message that the family would be much happier without them. The parents should be helped in understanding the meaning of the suicide behavior and its impulsive nature. This makes it easier for them to understand why all pills or other dangerous objects should be locked away and kept out of reach.

The success of crisis intervention rests frequently on the ability of the physician to establish a good therapeutic alliance with the adolescent that is based on a sense of trust and dependability.

The patient should be given the hospital or office phone number and told that he can call anytime to speak to the physician or his replacement. As well, he should be encouraged to use the emergency room whenever the need arises.

Autism

JON MATTHEW FARBER, M.D.

Our understanding of autism has come full circle since Kanner first described the disorder in 1943. Originally felt to be an organic disturbance, by the 1950s it was viewed as an emotionally based disorder. This misperception began to fade by the late 1970s but is still unfortunately widely held despite recent work that has overwhelmingly documented the organic nature of the condition.

The family pediatrician is usually the first professional to deal with the autistic child, either because the parents come to him with their concerns or because he notices the abnormalities himself. The diagnosis is not difficult to entertain if the pediatrician is alert and does not simply dismiss the cognitive delays and bizarre behavior as something that will be outgrown; autism is generally not a subtle condition.

Once autism has been considered, the work-up is best done using a multidisciplinary approach, for purposes of both diagnosis and treatment. This can be done by referring the child to a university affiliated facility (UAF) or mental retardation diagnostic center. The multidisciplinary team should include a developmental pediatrician, psychologist (for cognitive testing), audiologist, and others as needed. It is important that the team evaluating the child have experience with autistic children, as autism can fool even the expert professional.

Treatment of the autistic child, as with children with other cognitive impairments, is primarily through the school system, using an educational and behavioral approach. Federal Law PL 94-142 entitles educationally handicapped children to special education services beginning at age 5, and in most states this has been lowered to age 3 or younger. Most school districts have services and classrooms set aside for autistic children as a specific category of handicap. The multidisciplinary evaluation is used as a springboard for de-

veloping an individual educational program (I.E.P.) for each child. The program will look at the child's functioning in different areas and develop educational goals, with objective criteria for determining when they are reached. The program will generally emphasize socialization, self-care skills, and development of language, with individualization to the child's level of functioning. Behavioral modification techniques will usually be incorporated in the program to help deal with the behavioral problems.

Unfortunately little traditional medical (e.g., pharmacologic) treatment of autism is available at present. For severe behavioral problems, the major tranquilizers such as haloperidol* (0.5–3.0 mg daily) and thioridazine† (up to 3.0 mg/kg daily) are sometimes helpful; the former has been reported to be more effective. Both presumably work because of their sedating properties and not because of any "antipsychotic" effects. The medications do have side effects, including oversedation, parkinsonian features (particularly with haloperidol), polyphagia (thioridazine), and tardive dyskinesia. Because of this, they should be used only after behavioral approaches have been unsuccessful. Recently, much publicity has been given to the antiserotonin medication fenfluramine, and although early reports are promising, the medication is still in an investigational stage.

A major component of treatment is education of the family. Knowledgeable parent groups, such as the National Society for Children and Adults with Autism, are of value. Books written for parents can also be beneficial, but the material available is variable in quality, and the physician should read a work himself prior to recommending it. The pediatrician himself, in his sessions with the child and parents, will be responsible for much of their education and will need to know both the facts and fictions surrounding autism.

There are many myths concerning autism. Despite the wealth of evidence to the contrary, the following are still widely held *misperceptions*: autism is an emotional disorder, caused by cold, uncaring parents; IQ testing is neither feasible nor useful in autism; and autistic children become schizophrenic adults. It is important to realize the existence of these myths and to understand why they are untrue if one is to properly educate and help the child and his family.

As is common with conditions for which there is no cure, other "therapies" have been advocated in the past, and the pediatrician will need to be familiar with them, even though they are ineffec-

---

* Manufacturer's note: Haloperidol is not intended for children under 3 years old.

† Manufacturer's note: Thioridazine is not intended for children under 2 years of age.

tive, because parents will hear about them and have questions. Milieu psychotherapy was formerly held to be the treatment of choice. However, autism is an organic and not an emotional disorder, and gains seen with this form of treatment were due to the educational/behavioral aspects and not the psychodynamic ones, so that the school system can provide the effective components more conveniently. Orthomolecular approaches, dietary restrictions, vestibular stimulation, patterning, and the rest of the gamut of nonstandard therapies have all been touted as *the* treatment for autism and continue to receive much publicity in newspapers, television, and so forth. None is based on good scientific research, and none has withstood the test of time.

Thus, although the treatment of autism is primarily educational/behavioral, the pediatrician nevertheless has a paramount role to play. He will be the professional parents come to, and even though he may not treat the autism directly, he is vital in the care of the child and his family. He must educate the parents about autism, teaching them to separate the myths from the reality. He must teach them the developmental, organic nature of autism, to remove guilt feelings they may have about somehow having caused it. He must assist them in analyzing the myriad new "cures" that are promulgated daily so that they can be seen from a realistic view. He must also function as a focal point to help them coordinate the care of their child between the school and the multidisciplinary team.

In the therapy of autism therefore, the knowledgeable pediatrician does indeed have much to offer. Autism is a life-long condition, and as such, helping the family and child requires the practitioner to use both his cognitive and interpersonal skills to their fullest. The pediatrician who conducts himself as an educator for parents and advocate for the autistic child will thus be practicing the therapeutic art at one of its highest and most satisfying levels.

Pica

RICHARD B. GOLDBLOOM,
M.D., F.R.C.P.(C.)

The term pica is actually the Latin name for the magpie (*Pica pica*), a bird that is notorious for its habit of collecting all variety of foreign materials. As applied to humans, pica refers to the idiosyncratic craving for and compulsive ingestion of foreign material of any kind, most often material of no food value. An array of "phagia terms" has been coined to denote the particular material craved and ingested, e.g., geophagia (eating earth or clay pica), amylophagia (eating starch), pagophagia (eating ice), geomelophagia) (eating raw potatoes), coprophagia (eating feces), and trichophagia (eating hair). Other foreign substances that have been the objects of pica include plaster, paint, crayons, matches, and specific foods.

Treatment must be directed at both the causes and the effects of pica and at commonly associated problems. In children, pica occurs most commonly in association with iron deficiency, and there is considerable (though not conclusive) evidence to suggest that in such children pica may be the result rather than the cause of iron deficiency. Interestingly, the foreign material craved by the individual with pica is rarely a good source of the deficient nutrient, e.g., iron. It has been repeatedly observed that pica ceases rapidly when the iron deficiency is treated, and iron treatment for pica was recommended as early as 1000 A.D. It has been suggested that pica might be due to depletion of cytochromes or other essential iron-containing enzymes in the brain. However, pica occurs most commonly in lower socioeconomic groups and in families under psychosocial stress. Zinc deficiency has also been found in association with pica.

Depending on the substance ingested, problems resulting from pica may include lead poisoning from ingestion of lead-containing plaster or paint; mercury poisoning from paper pica; trichobezoars or phytobezoars with gastrointestinal obstructions due to the foreign material; parasitic infestations, especially ascariasis and toxocariasis from geophagia; and hypokalemia from clay ingestion. The treatment of each of these conditions is described elsewhere in this book.

To evaluate the overall treatment needs of a child with pica, particular attention should be paid to the following: (1) Socioeconomic status and psychosocial problems. (2) Adequacy of physical growth (growth delay may reflect inadequate caloric intake and /or zinc deficiency). (3) Repeated examination of fresh stool specimens for ova and parasites and examination for eosinophilia if geophagia is present. (4) Determination of iron and zinc status, the latter especially if hypogeusia (decreased taste acuity) is present.

Comprehensive treatment can then be tailored to the problem complex of the particular child. If iron deficiency is present, it may be treated by giving oral iron as ferrous sulfate 25 mg/kg/day (providing 5 mg elemental iron/kg/day) for 2 months. If oral iron therapy is not well tolerated, or if there are problems of compliance, intramuscular iron may be considered, as described in the article on iron deficiency. Milk intake should be severely curtailed or even eliminated for a time. Depending on social conditions, which should be evaluated in detail, a brief hospital admission may be necessary to ensure adequate diagnosis and treatment of all problems that may have caused or resulted from pica.

Psychosomatic Illness

MARC A. FORMAN, M.D.

Psychosomatic disorders specifically may be defined as those in which emotional stress and psychological conflict lead to changes in somatic function. A particular type of stress or conflict is not associated with a specific psychosomatic disorder. Rather, any emotional distress may lead to a psychosomatic disorder in a vulnerable child. Innate constitutional factors and the models of illness available in the child's environment appear to determine the site of the affected organ system. Psychosomatic disorders are of two general types: conversion reactions (or conversion hysteria) and psychophysiological disorders.

Conversion reactions are usually sudden and dramatic in onset. Organs of sensation and the voluntary musculature are the most frequent target sites for the "hysterical" expression of psychological conflict. Symptoms of pain, and certain acute disturbances in autonomic nervous system functioning, such as fainting, nausea and vomiting, may be included as well. While conversion reactions can generally be traced to a precipitating environmental stress, it is at times difficult to assess the impact of the stress on a particular child given the individual variation in the toleration of stress. Examples of common conversion reactions are hysterical blindness, diplopia, gait disturbance, aphonia, and anesthesia. Physical examination fails to reveal objective findings consistent with a pathophysiologic explanation for the complaint, e.g., deep tendon reflexes may be elicited in the paralyzed limb. The supposedly typical characteristic of "la belle indifférence" is inconsistent and unreliable; children with conversion reactions may be just as distressed by their symptoms as children with physical illness. Similarly, "secondary gain" may be found in children with either hysterical or physical illness, as the child unconsciously uses his disability to avoid stressful situations. Children with conversion hysteria may have a history of previous episodes or other psychopathological manifestations. Their families tend to be chronically anxious and hypochondriacal.

Psychophysiological disorders are more insidious in onset and chronic in nature and involve disturbances in the functioning of the autonomic nervous system. Chronic anxiety contributes to the genesis, maintenance, and exacerbation of the disorder. As alteration of organ system function continues, structural damage ensues. Common examples are eczema, asthma, and peptic ulcer. Psychophysiological disorders are not caused solely by anxiety, but are multifactorial in origin. In asthma, for example, other etiologic factors such as genetic vulnerability, allergy, and infection are significant. Children with psychophysiological disorders are reported to be obsessive and inhibited, but this finding is questionable as research data have failed to suport evidence for a specific "psychophysiological" personality type.

For the management of children with psychosomatic disorders the following general principles apply: (1) Do not assume that the complaint, e.g., pain, is not "real" only because a physical cause cannot be found. The diagnosis of conversion reaction should rest on some positive psychological findings—stress factors, premorbid history, familial psychopathology, and models of illness—as well as on the absence of positive physical findings. Follow-up studies of patients originally diagnosed as having conversion hysteria have shown that as many as 30% were subsequently found to have organic illness as the primary cause for the presenting symptom. (2) Children with psychosomatic disorders have "real" symptoms. They are not malingering. The disorder is beyond their conscious control. (3) Psychiatric consultation should be obtained early, rather than after all possible, or even unlikely, physical causes have been ruled out. Referring the patient to a child psychiatrist only after a very long and expensive diagnostic workup has been unproductive often generates resentment and resistance in the family, who feel that the pediatrician has "given up." (4) Joint management by the pediatrician and a mental health professional is especially indicated in the treatment of psychophysiological disorders. (5) The parents must be given a clear explanation of the role of the emotions in the genesis of psychosomatic disorders and should be willing at least to consider psychological factors as one of the determinants of the child's illness. (6) Psychotherapy for the child and counseling for the parents are usually indicated, especially when the illness is persistent and the child's behavior at home, school, or with peers is impaired. Some practitioners prefer a family therapy approach involving siblings as well. Modest doses of tranquilizing medication may be useful as an adjunctive therapy. (7) The pediatrician should be alert to the presence of physical or psychosomatic illness in the parents; the child may unconsciously mimic such illness as the model for his own disorder. The success of the child's treatment may then become dependent on the treatment of the parental illness. (8) Secondary gain must be minimized, and the child should be actively encouraged to return to a full range of academic and social activities as soon as possible.

Childhood Sleep Disturbances and Disorders of Arousal

GABOR BARABAS, M.D.

Abnormalities in sleep behavior and sleep pattern represent a relatively frequent chief complaint in a general pediatric practice. Parents most frequently complain that their children are having difficulty in falling asleep or that they are restless during sleep, with frequent or early awakening. Nightmares also are relatively common. Such sleep disturbances are generally transient and are related to stages in development and certain environmental and psychological factors. For instance, it is not unusual for a young child to develop sleep disturbances upon moving to a new home, starting school, or after the loss of a family member or a close pet. On occasion, sleep disturbances may be symptomatic of more serious psychological conflicts or problems within the family unit.

These "behavioral" phenomena are categorized as sleep disturbances or abnormal sleep behavior patterns. Another group of sleep abnormalities are generally considered to be independent of environmental and psychological factors and are categorized as disorders of arousal. These symptoms tend to occur during specific stages in sleep and are more often thought of as being "organic" and associated with intrinsic biochemical disturbances. This distinction between sleep disturbances and disorders of arousal, however, is in many ways fictitious, for fever, fatigue, emotional tension, depression, and sleep deprivation can affect biochemical changes in the brain and, therefore, can influence the intrinsic organic nature of sleep.

Somnambulism. The management of sleepwalking can pose problems to the physician and family. On rare occasions it can present a physical threat to a child, so that all windows and doors have to be secured. A child may climb out of a window or wander into the street and may risk serious physical harm. In such situations, relocating the child's bedroom to the ground floor when possible is advisable. In children with frequent somnambulism, diazepam, 2.5–5.0 mg before sleep, can dramatically suppress symptoms. While this has been my clinical experience, and while other clinicians also attest to the efficacy of benzodiazepines in individual cases, the few systematic studies that exist on this subject fail to demonstrate a consistent beneficial effect. Benzodiazepines suppress Stage 4 sleep, thereby decreasing the time spent in the sleep state during which sleepwalking characteristically occurs.

Pavor Nocturnus. Night terrors, like sleepwalking, may respond dramatically to diazepam by suppression of Stage 4 sleep. Families need to be reassured of the benign nature of this symptom for to be witness to it can be a frightening experience for a parent. They need to be further reassured that night terrors are usually not associated with psychological problems and that except for rare exceptions, children invariably outgrow the tendency. In contradistinction, persistent nightmares in a child warrant further investigation into family dynamics and potential psychopathology.

In general, pharmacotherapy for sleepwalking or night terrors should be reserved only for severe cases in which the potential for bodily harm exists or when emotional pressures are significant enough to warrant such intervention.

Jactatio Capitis Nocturnus and Sleep-Rocking. Like night terrors, nocturnal head-banging and rocking in sleep tend to affect younger children than sleepwalking does. Therapy does not appear to be necessary. Parents need to be reassured regarding the head-banging. It must be kept in mind that some retarded children engage in stereotypic rocking and head-banging. On rare occasions infants and toddlers suffering from headaches may bang their heads. However, this tends not to be limited to sleep alone, and it is obvious that such a diagnosis is an extremely difficult one to entertain and almost impossible to substantiate. Of assistance is the fact that head-banging from pain is associated with overt evidence of pain while nocturnal head-banging is not accompanied by any apparent discomfort.

Enuresis. The management of enuresis is discussed elsewhere in this book. It suffices to mention that in recent years imipramine has gained the most popularity in the pharmacologic approach to therapy. Its actions are related to parasympathetic effects on the bladder with an increase in bladder capacity. Some effects may also be related to an influence on sleep stages.

Sleeptalking. This appears to be the most frequently encountered "disorder of arousal." Because of its benign nature, it does not pose a management problem and is viewed by most families with amusement.

Bruxism. Nocturnal teeth-grinding can be a bothersome symptom. It has occasionally been linked to temporomandibular joint disease and resultant facial pain. This association, however, has hardly been established. In some children, a dental appliance may be necessary to prevent the teeth-grinding.

Nocturnal Seizures. Some children suffering from epileptic seizures also experience nocturnal seizures. When these are witnessed, the nature of the symptoms is generally apparent. Generalized convulsions associated with urinary incontinence may be seen, as well as various rudimentary motor seizures with tonic spasm, myoclonus, or focal symptomatology. Rolandic seizures begin between 6 and 10 years of age. They frequently present as focal twitching of the face, during which consciousness is often retained, which is followed by slurred speech. The electroencephalogram is often diagnostic.

Some children have only nocturnal seizures. When not witnessed, they may masquerade as enuresis. The presence of tongue biting and postictal somnolence with muscle aches upon awakening may suggest this condition. Sleep lowers seizure threshold, accounting for noctural seizures in susceptible individuals. *Sleep myoclonus* is a benign jerking of the trunk and extremities that occurs commonly upon falling asleep and needs to be differentiated from nocturnal myoclonic seizures. Once again, the electroencephalogram is often helpful in making this distinction.

Voice, Speech, and Language Disorders

SYLVIA ONESTI RICHARDSON, M.D.

Therapy for voice, speech, and language disorders should be administered by qualified speech clinicians (also called speech-language pathologists). The physician's primary responsibilities are in the prevention and early diagnosis of speech, language, and voice problems; in parent counseling; and in the appropriate, timely referral of patients to qualified speech therapists and clinics.

VOICE DYSFUNCTIONS

Hypernasality of voice quality usually is associated with the velopharyngeal incompetence of a child with a cleft palate, even a submucous cleft. Such a child should be followed by a speech therapist who can supervise the home program from the age of 3 months to 2 years, regardless of the type of operative or nonoperative treatment. The parents must be taught how to help the child develop non-nasal speech.

If the hypernasality is not due to anatomic defect (functional) and is serious enough to create a problem for the child, a speech clinician can teach the patient to use the soft palate by doing blowing exercises. Parents also can help at home. To learn to direct the breath stream through the mouth and to help strengthen the palatal muscles, the child should spend several periods a day in blowing activities such as blowing soap bubbles, keeping a feather aloft, blowing boats in the bath-tub, and blowing a Ping-Pong ball across a table.

Hyponasality, or "adenoidal speech," in which "n" sounds like "d," "m" sounds like "b," and "ng"

sounds like "g," can be caused by excessively enlarged adenoids or any nasal or nasopharyngeal obstruction. This usually disappears if the adenoidal mass becomes smaller or if adenoidectomy is performed. If excessive nasality occurs postadenoidectomy and persists for more than 8 weeks, speech therapy should be considered to help the child relearn to use the soft palate correctly.

Hoarseness may appear in children 8 to 10 years of age, especially boys, because of development of tiny nodules between the anterior and middle thirds of the vocal cords. These may be due to prepubescent endocrine changes, allergy, or too much yelling in the Little League outfield. Treating any allergy or requiring the child to stop yelling or singing loudly is usually successful, though difficult to enforce in the latter case. If such hoarseness persists and the nodule shows a slow reduction in size, a speech clinician can teach the child to alter voice pitch until healing is effected. This disturbance usually disappears spontaneously when change of voice occurs around the age of 12 or 13 years.

DISORDERS OF ARTICULATION

Dysarthria is due to neuromotor involvement of the muscles used for articulation, phonation, or respiration. Dysarthria in children is usually due to cerebral palsy. In such a case the child will benefit from an interdisciplinary approach, including the pediatrician, child neurologist, physical and occupational therapists, speech/language pathologist, and infant teacher. The child with *articulatory dyspraxia* is able to carry out the movements necessary for articulation spontaneously but has difficulty in directing them for voluntary imitation of movements (motor planning) or for reproduction of the correct articulatory sounds when hearing is normal. *Dyslalia* includes those defects of articulation which appear to be functional in origin rather than attributable to damage to the brain or failure of neurologic maturation for speech. In this article we are concerned with the latter.

Indications for the physician's referral to a speech and hearing clinic for further evaluation and possible therapy are as follows: 1) Articulation is mostly unintelligible after age 3 years. If the causes appear to be chiefly environmental or functional, a good nursery school can be therapeutic if recommended by a speech clinician. 2) There are many substitutions of easy sounds for difficult ones after age 5 years. In such cases, psychologic evaluation may be sought to determine mental age or reasons for retention of infantile speech patterns. Speech therapy is influenced by the cause of the disorder, as is parent counseling. 3) The child is omitting, distorting, or substituting any sound past age 7 years. Speech therapy consists largely of ear training and teaching the child to produce the sounds correctly in isolation and then in combination with other sounds.

Audiologic evaluation is important in *every* case and is particularly indicated when the speech is characterized by omission of sounds or word endings or if there has been a history of chronic otitis media. Assuming that hearing is normal and the problem is one of dyslalia, the majority of articulatory defects in children under 7 years of age can be handled at home by the mother, in nursery school, or in the classroom. However, such management should be recommended and supervised by a qualified speech clinician.

Home management must be handled skillfully without pressure, or not at all. All members of the family are instructed to use clear, precise speech to provide suitable models. At first, two or three 15-minute periods can be set aside daily when one member of the family reads aloud, leafs through picture books naming the pictures, plays games involving imitation of different animal sounds, and engages in similar activities. As the child begins to identify pictures correctly, these may be cut out and placed in a scrapbook for review. As stated above, the parents should confer with a speech therapist for guidance.

Most children with dyslalia show marked improvement in articulation between the first and second grades and some between the second and third grades. Thus the child's maturation *within a good speech environment* is often the best course of therapy for simple articulatory defects.

A note on "tonguetie": Parents and others still seem to think a child is "tonguetied" if there is any kind of speech problem. If a child can articulate t, d, n, or l; can say "no," "ta-ta," and "da-da"; or can lick a lollipop, the speech problem is not due to tonguetie alone, if at all. If there is a true tonguetie and the lingual frenulum is bound down to the lower central incisors, the treatment is surgical—not a scar tissue–producing snip with a pair of scissors.

STUTTERING

The physician's ability to determine the child's position in the continuum from developmental nonfluency to established stuttering is important in planning treatment.

Effective parent counseling by the physician is the first step in treatment of the problem of nonfluency. He can explain to the parents the developmental nature of early nonfluency and provide instructive reading for them.

Treatment of nonfluency in pre-school children is indirect, aimed at the child's environment rather than the child. The parents must help to change the conditions that precipitate or perseverate stuttering episodes, including problems in the home that tend to produce anxiety in the child. The

parents are advised to encourage the child to speak during fluent periods, to allow ample time for him or her to speak, to maintain eye contact when the child speaks, and to be responsive listeners. Comments like "Slow down, Johnny," or "For heaven's sake, stop and think before you try to talk" are to be discouraged—as is any suggestion that the child modify his speaking.

The effectiveness of the treatment is directly proportionate to the consistency the parents are able to maintain. For this reason, counseling with a speech therapist must be regular and must continue until the problem is resolved.

When nonfluency has progressed to the point at which children think of themselves as stutterers and develop struggle reactions to speech, such as circumlocutions to avoid a sound on which they usually block, facial tics, and grimaces or other evidence of avoidance or anxiety reactions, the treatment is direct and may involve combined speech therapy and psychotherapy.

SPEECH AND LANGUAGE DELAY

Treatment of speech and language delay depends upon definitive diagnosis, and this may be considered one of the most difficult diagnostic problems in pediatrics.

Treatment for delayed speech development may vary from counseling parents to sending the child to a good preschool, or to play therapy in a speech clinic. Psychiatric treatment may be indicated before speech therapy is attempted. Direct speech therapy is usually not recommended before a child has reached a general developmental level of about 4 years.

Deafness and mental retardation must be ruled out. Intervention programs for the child with hearing impairment must be instituted as soon as diagnosis is made. Such programs include amplification, total communication, oral speech/language therapy, and infant stimulation. Mentally retarded children usually present a picture of retardation in all areas of development, especially when the IQ level is below 70. Improvement in speech and language may occur with development and maturation, but training in prelinguistic sensory-motor skills is most helpful. The parents of these children often need to understand that speech therapy per se is of no value to the child until he or she has had adequate prelinguistic experience and has developed the necessary motor coordination of the articulatory muscles to produce speech.

The term language disorder is used to include dysphasia, dyslexia, and dysgraphia. Dysphasia is the inability or limited ability of a child to use spoken symbols for communication. To plan treatment for the young dysphasic child, one must determine whether the primary problem is receptive (understanding speech), expressive (self-expression with speech), some combination of these two, or global (lacking "inner language"). The last condition represents a severe disorder in which the child cannot use symbols internally for thinking, and prognosis is poor regardless of therapy.

The dyslexic child has a problem in the reception of written symbols, and the dysgraphic child has a problem with expression of written symbols. Developmental dysphasia, dyslexia, and dysgraphia are closely related conditions and may be found together in the same patient or in members of the same family. Some children learn to speak adequately and are not recognized to be dyslexic until they fail to learn to read in school.

Therapy for any language disorder requires a total program in which the environment can be suitably structured and the therapy can be tailored to suit the child's individual needs. Speech therapy alone, or any other single kind of therapy, is inadequate and unsuitable for such a child. An experienced team of specialists is usually required for reaching a diagnosis and for recommending appropriate language therapy.

Treatment plans for very young children with language disorders usually include sensory-motor activities: training in the motor bases of behavior, such as posture, the development of laterality and directionality, and the development of body image; training in perceptual skills, such as form perception, space discrimination, stereognosis, and recognition of texture, size, and structure; and training in auditory perception (listening), visual perception (looking), and kinesthetic perception (muscular memory of movements, positions, and posture). The child with a language disorder usually requires assistance in learning these skills, which are developmentally antecedent to language production per se.

Speech and hearing clinicians are now involved in the development and application of new assessment and intervention techniques for high risk and developmentally delayed infants. They are valuable members of the interdisciplinary teams involved with parent-infant programming.

For those with severe communicative disorders, a number of augmentative systems are available. Manual communication using signs has been employed with mentally retarded, cerebral palsied, and autistic children. Communication boards may be used to facilitate communication for those with extensive motor problems. When such systems are used, the speech and language clinician's task is essentially the same as when oral language is taught—to train comprehension and production of language using the augmentative system.

The American Speech-Language-Hearing Association (ASHA) can provide information concerning speech correction facilities throughout the United States. Speech, language, and hearing specialists who are certified by ASHA are listed geographically and alphabetically in its annual directory, which is available at The American Speech-Language-Hearing Association, 10801 Rockville Pike, Rockville, Maryland 20852.

Disorders of Learning and Attention

MELVIN D. LEVINE, M.D.

In recent years there has been growing recognition of a series of central nervous system disabilities affecting children and known to constrain academic performance and, in some cases, behavioral adjustment. These so-called "low severity-high prevalence" disorders consist of a varied group of handicaps that can be described and classified according to different conceptual models. Table 1 shows one such model to delineate the most frequently encountered clinical disorders of learning, including those handicapping conditions that limit the concentration or selective attention of school children. The therapeutics of these disorders necessarily depends upon the antecedent description of individual children. The treatment of a particular deficit depends, at least in part, upon the availability and mobilization of compensatory strengths in other aspects of a child's development. By compiling a broad "functional profile," one can design and implement services that include appropriate counseling, educational intervention, and other forms of treatment.

The management of children with learning attention disorders is intrinsically multifaceted and almost always multidisciplinary. It is becoming increasingly common for general pediatricians or specialists in developmental pediatrics to serve as coordinators of intervention. In doing so, the clinician endeavors to integrate seven levels of service, including 1) counseling and "demystification"; 2) educational intervention; 3) home management; 4) medical treatments; 5) special services; 6) advocacy; 7) follow-up (i.e., assessments of progress and the effectiveness of service).

COUNSELING AND DEMYSTIFICATION

It is common for children who are failing in school to harbor fantasies about why they are doing poorly. Most often they overestimate their degree of handicap, frequently believing they are retarded or "dumb." An even broader array of misconceptions is found in parents who may attribute their child's difficulties to laziness, generalized "slowness," or indifference. Even teachers may misunderstand the plight of a child with a learning

Table 1. COMMON DEVELOPMENTAL DYSFUNCTIONS (LOW SEVERITY DISABILITIES) IN SCHOOL CHILDREN

Dysfunction	Common Cognitive Impacts	Common Academic Impacts	Circumvention	Intervention
Selective attention	Weak reflection, poor planning Poor monitoring Inattention to detail Inconsistency Easy cognitive fatigue Erratic memory	Carelessness Impersistence Poor classroom adjustment Trouble following instructions Inconsistency	Demystification Accommodation Small "chunks" Preferential seating Feedback	Stimulant medication Remedial help—small group or 1:1 Behavioral modification
Visual-spatial	Confusion over: figure-ground size, shape, relative position Poor appreciation of detail	Poor letter, word recognition Possible math problems Phonetic spelling	Auditory inputs Multisensory linguistic approach to reading, spelling	Proofreading for deatil Visual-spatial activities Auditory-visual integration
Temporal-sequential	Poor sequential memory Trouble with multistep processes Secondary inattention	Trouble following instructions Trouble with multisyllable words Poor multiplication, spelling Disorganization	One or two step inputs, repetition Teach to strong channel Note-taking	Diaries, calendars, clocks Mastery over larger chunks Practice recall with feedback
Receptive language	Poor or slow language interpretation Secondary inattention Impaired verbal reasoning	Trouble following instructions Reading, writing weaknesses—math word problem problems	Visual inputs Repetition, short sentences Visual approaches to skills	Language therapy: Use of tapes, other language enhancers
Expressive language	Possible "dysphasia" Diminished vocabulary Articulation problems Poor sentence formulation	Trouble participating in class discussions Delayed reading Poor written expression	Verbal volunteering Strong visual inputs Less stress on oral expression	Speech therapy Dictionary work Expressive exercises
Memory	Difficulty registering, storing, or retrieving specific types of data	Variable, depending on impairment Spelling, math problems Trouble retaining new skills	Subvocalization, mnemonics, rules/generalizations Underlining Note-taking	Specific gradual exercises to enhance weak modality using strong area
Gross motor	None	Social withdrawal Fearfulness Low self-esteem	Avoidance of certain sports Privacy	Adaptive physical education
Fine motor	None	Nonspecific	Reduced output demand More time Prioritization Typing	Overlearning motor patterns, pencil control Extensive writing exercises Work on grasp
Social	Poor feedback from and "titration" of relationships	Indirect	Fostering individuality	Social "tutoring" Parent support Small group work
Higher order cognition	Poor comprehension of new concepts Impaired inference, generalization Concreteness	Delayed acquisition of skill and knowledge, generalized	Use of concrete manipulative materials Use of strengths	"Cognitive Therapy" Work with rules, logic, abstract reasoning

disorder. They may construe the phenomenon as poor motivation, primary emotional disturbance, or an aberration of attitude. Therefore, a critical initial therapeutic step is the process of education or demystification.

First, the child's handicaps and strengths must be carefully delineated and demarcated. Simple explanations, using nontechnical language as well as helpful analogies, should be employed. For example, in describing a child with difficulty in processing language, one might explain: "Although you really don't have any trouble thinking about things or remembering, it is very hard for you to figure things out when people explain them to you in long sentences with a lot of words. This is because you have trouble learning well through your ears. You do much better at understanding what you see. It is as if you were a television set whose picture was very clear but whose sound has too much static." In providing such explanations, the clinician should highlight the youngster's strengths while instilling optimism with respect to the managability of problems. It should be made clear to the child and parents that the deficit is not primarily one of motivation, that the child is not "dumb," and that there *are* ways to help. A nonaccusatory approach that is supportive and sufficiently optimistic is likely to be most effective.

Either by letter, through a conference, or by telephone, the clinician needs also to present his view of the child's disabilities and strengths to school personnel. This too can dispel misunderstandings and establish a good alliance between the health care provider, the school, the parents, and the child.

EDUCATIONAL INTERVENTION

It is obvious that much of the rehabilitation of a child with a learning disorder must take place in an educational setting. Schools have a major role to play, although their effort should not be viewed as the exclusive modality of intervention. Within the school, three delivery systems can be identified: *special education, regular education,* and *special services.*

Special Education. Special education input for children with learning problems includes interventions that generally take place outside of a regular classroom and are aimed at remedying or overcoming the deficits impairing progress. The initial step in such intervention is the selection of a service prototype. Five common prototypes are summarized below in order of their magnitude:

A. SPECIAL ASSISTANCE WITHIN THE REGULAR CLASSROOM. In this model a teacher's aide or some other individual observes and periodically offers assistance to the child with a learning problem. The youngster is not removed from the regular classroom, but is helped during the school day at times when difficulty is noted or anticipated.

B. RESOURCE ROOM OR LEARNING CENTER HELP. In this model, the child receives assistance usually in a small group setting (ranging from 1-7 other students in most cases). A specially trained educator works with the students to remedy specific deficits. Often the effort is aimed at helping a child catch up in areas of delayed skill acquisition. Alternatively, the special educator may wish to work specifically to strengthen a child's developmental weaknesses rather than skill delays. For example, there may be an effort to provide the youngster with exercises aimed at enhancing visual-perception, language, attention, or memory. In such cases, the goal is to work on functions thought to be prerequisites of skill acquisition rather than on the skills themselves. It is not uncommon for both strategies to be employed, namely a combined program of skill-building with

intervention to strengthen areas of developmental weakness.

C. TUTORING. Tutorial services often are provided on a one-to-one basis. For economic reasons, schools may find this impractical to implement. When feasible, parents may seek tutoring outside of school. Most often such intervention is aimed at the enhancement of academic skills. Specific help in spelling, mathematics, reading, or writing may be offered. Some tutors may wish to concentrate on helping a youngster with organization or study skills. This might include techniques of underlining, outlining, summarizing, scheduling work, and note taking.

D. FULL-TIME CLASS FOR LEARNING DISORDERS. Some school systems offer special classes for children with learning problems. Often these contain less students or at least a more favorable teacher: student ratio than do regular classrooms. Special curriculum materials may be employed. Work may be presented at a slower rate, with reduced volume expectations (for homework and tests), and with more repetition. While such classrooms usually offer a considerable degree of expertise geared to the needs of the student, recently there has been some concern about their possible stigmatizing impact.

E. PRIVATE SCHOOLS FOR LEARNING DISABILITIES. In North America there has been a proliferation of private schools that specialize in the management of children with learning disorders. Such schools are staffed by people who have the training, experience, and sensitivity to deal with children afflicted with learning disorders. Specialized curriculum materials often are employed. Classes tend to be small. Because of this, tuition fees are beyond the reach of many families. In some instances, however, school systems will pay the tuition for youngsters whom they feel they cannot teach adequately within the community. Special schools for learning disabilities have the advantage of allowing children to associate with other youngsters who have the same problems, thereby feeling less different. On the other hand, attendance at such an institution could make a child feel that he is not a part of the community or neighborhood, he is in educational "exile." Special schools for learning disabilities may be either residential or day programs.

Many factors enter into the choice of a special educational prototype. Among these are the child's own strengths and weaknesses, the extent of academic delay, the availability and quality of the various prototypes within a community, and the desires and values of the parents and child.

In the United States, Public Law 94-142 has mandated that communities must provide adequate education for children with handicapping conditions, including those with learning disorders. An individualized educational plan is developed, and this specifies the prototype along with specific educational goals and the quantity of service to be offered (e.g., the amount of time per week in a resource room). As part of this law, there has been a growing emphasis on what is called the "least restrictive alternative": while it is deemed important for children to have an appropriate education, serious consideration is given to "mainstreaming" or allowing the youngster to be part of a program that is as close as possible to that of normal children in the community. In this context, sending a child off to a special school for learning disabilities might be considered "restrictive," the least desirable alternative, or "a last resort."

Regular Education. Unless a child is in a full-time learning disability program his or her regular educational program (i.e., the school day minus the special educational component) is just as important, and in some cases more, than the special intervention. Daily management in a regular classroom is critical to ongoing skill development as well as self-esteem and motivation.

It is essential that the regular classroom teacher have a good understanding of the child's problems. Insensitivity of the teacher to the child's plight can result in counterproductive experience marked by diminishing incentive, effort, and self-esteem.

Within the regular classroom, the emphasis is on compensation or "bypass strategies." While the special educational program is geared to help youngsters *overcome deficits*, the regular classroom should be a place where children are encouraged to *circumvent their weaknesses*. For example, a teacher may need to accommodate to the fact that a youngster cannot process a long series of verbal instructions. Succinct directions, visual reinforcement of instructions, and some repetition may be needed. A child who has attention deficits and is highly distractible may need to sit close to the teacher. A youngster who has fine motor problems impairing writing may need to be allowed to type to employ a word processor, to write less, to be spared excessive criticism of his poor handwriting, and to not have to recopy papers. A child with memory weaknesses may need help in taking notes, using mnemonics, and drilling with flashcards to help bypass retention weaknesses. Many other examples of such strategies could be cited. Their selection depends largely upon the child's strengths and weaknesses. Wherever possible, a student's assets should be used in trying to work around handicaps.

The choice of curriculum is another important aspect of regular education for a child with learning difficulties. This is exemplified in reading. A child with language processing problems may need a strong visual approach (a so-called "sight word" method) to reading. Many of these youngsters require a multisensory reading curriculum that uses several modalities simultaneously to reinforce word recognition and analysis. An example is the Orton Gillingham Method, which is widely applied. Some approaches to reading stress language. A child who has difficulty with visual perception or visual memory may benefit from a reading curriculum that emphasizes the *phonetic analysis* of words rather than their *visual configuration*.

Many children with learning disorders require more time to finish tests, to complete assignments, and to assimilate and integrate new skills or knowledge. The classroom teacher must recognize this. In order to accommodate to such time-related constraints, some assignments may need to be shorter. It now is possible for youngsters with learning disorders to take college entrance examinations or secondary school admission tests on an untimed basis. Such allowances can make an enormous difference for an affected student.

Many children with learning problems are dreadfully ashamed of their lack of academic success. In particular, they fear exposure in front of their peers. They are obsessed with maintaining a solid reputation, with looking good. It is important that adults not humiliate disabled students in front of their peers. A certain amount of privacy is critical. For example, if a youngster has a writing problem such that his papers are chronically messy and disorganized, it is cruel to allow other students to correct his work. If a child has expressive language problems, one should be careful and sensitive about calling upon him in a classroom. If a child has difficulty with reading, one may wish to minimize the requirement for oral reading.

As children progress through school, course selection becomes important. Here it is helpful to anticipate the natural history of a child's disability. Many youngsters with language disorders tend to do quite poorly when they are expected to learn a foreign language. One might wish to postpone or even obtain an exemption from such courses. In selecting subjects, however, it is important not to create self-fulfilling prophecies. Many children with learning disorders are extraordinarily resilient and seem to "come to life" academically late in junior high or during high school. One should avoid therefore selection of a curriculum that will constrain future opportunities.

For older adolescents career counseling may be important. Opportunities exist for vocational education, and physicians should be aware of such local resources. Also, increasing numbers of universities and colleges are accepting and making provisions for students with learning disorders.

SPECIAL SERVICES

In addition to special educational input and modifications in regular education, some youngsters with learning disorders require more specialized services. A wide range of options is available, although there is considerable variation from school system to school system, and even between schools in the same community. A practicing physician needs to develop a good understanding of available resources. Among the special services are the following: speech and language therapy for children with either receptive or expressive disorders; guidance or school adjustment counseling for those with social, motivational, or behavioral concomitants of their learning problems; occupational therapy for those with significant motor handicaps; adaptive physical education to enhance motor skills; and social service, particularly useful when family problems complicate the clinical picture.

HOME MANAGEMENT

Frequently parents want to know what *they* can do to help. It is a mistake to minimize their role. Parents can be a reliable "labor force" to help a failing youngster. If they sense their role is minimal, feelings of hopelessness or futility may supervene. Parents can be of direct assistance with homework and with the establishment of study skills. While they should not actually perform the child's assignments, they can be invaluable with regard to organizational skills. Many youngsters with learning problems are disorganized. Parents can help a child "get started" with homework; they can find and prepare the appropriate place to study and set up a work schedule; they can coordinate assignments with teachers; they can help the youngster allocate time effectively; and they can be helpful in pursuing certain games and activities that can enhance a child's learning. For example, reading to a child at bedtime and then asking questions about the story might enhance receptive language abilities. Listening to the child read can be helpful for a youngster with delays in reading skills.

Home management is a major issue for parents of children who have behavioral difficulties along with their learning problems. This is seen most commonly in those with attention deficits. In addition to their poor concentration in school, such youngsters may be overactive, provocative in their behaviors, difficult to satisfy, impulsive, and irresponsible with regard to chores at home. Parents may need help in establishing a system of accountability for such a youngster. Distinct priorities need to be established and short-range incremental goals set. Parents need to be helped to be consistent

with such children, to avoid setting unattainable goals, and to try not to be too moralistic about the youngster's difficulties.

A critical component of home management is the planning and organization of a child's recreational and social life. It is not uncommon to encounter children with learning problems who are seriously "success-deprived." Their parents cannot recall any recent incident in which the child was able to display mastery in any area. This may be the closest thing to a developmental emergency, and there is a serious need for "success induction." Utilizing a child's natural strengths and inclinations, parents should be encouraged to program experiences in which the youngster can feel successful. A child who is failing in school but who likes to draw cartoons might benefit from art lessons and having his works displayed prominently both at home and in school. A youngster whose mechanical skills are excellent but who, because of language difficulties, is having inordinate problems in school, might thrive on computers, on fixing engines, or building model airplanes. Chronic success deprivation is one of the major complications of learning disorders. A critical part of intervention rests in its reversal.

Home computers now offer promise in bolstering academic skills. High motivational software is available to assist children in reading, spelling, and mathematics. Some students with weaknesses of language and/or attention may benefit from the strong visual reinforcement of a computer monitor screen.

A number of children with learning problems also have difficulties with socialization. They may experience undue rejection by peers. In other instances, they seem to isolate themselves. Parents can help by encouraging social experiences at home, by coaching in the formation and maintenance for relationships with peers.

MEDICAL TREATMENTS

The standard medical treatment for a learning problem generally entails two modalities: the correction of any complicating, underlying, or secondary medical problems and pharmacotherapy.

It is important for the physician to recognize and treat any medical disorders or symptoms complicating a child's learning problems. In this group one frequently encounters chronic somatic symptoms, such as enuresis, encopresis, recurrent abdominal pain, tics, or sleep difficulties. These require medical attention, treatment, and followup. In some instances, reassurance can be helpful in alleviating the anxiety these symptoms generate. In some cases direct therapy is necessary.

A number of chronic conditions can complicate learning problems. Most common are seizures, allergies, recurrent ear infections, and sinusitis. Any or all of these can compromise a child's ability to concentrate and acquire skills. Further problems ensue from extended periods of school absence and side effects of medication. The latter is particularly common with the use of antihistamines, theophylline-containing compounds, and some seizure medications (such as barbiturates and primidone).

Various pharmacologic agents are used to help children with learning disorders. Most commonly prescribed are the stimulants. These are summarized in Table 2. Their appropriate use is in children with attention deficits. Stimulant medication appears to strengthen selective attention, diminish impulsivity, curb restlessness and over-activity, and result in some improved learning. Enhanced socialization also can be observed. Stimulants are not beneficial in correcting specific learning disabilities, nor are they appropriately thought of as "tranquilizers." Instead, they appear to affect arousal and alertness probably through regulation of neurotransmission in the reticular activating system of the brain stem. In prescribing stimulant drugs, the clinician should use as small a dose as possible. In most cases, it is best to administer the drug only on school days (the exception being the youngster who is so frenetic that serious behavioral problems occur on weekends and vacations). Periodic "drug holidays" should be attempted. These are days or weeks off medication, designed ultimately to wean the youngster from the drug. It is important that the child, the parents, and the teachers all understand the justifications, therapeutic effects, and possible side effects of the medication.

Medication is never the whole answer. Children with attention deficits have been found to benefit most from multimodal treatments, those that combine psychopharmacotherapy and educational modification (and accommodation) with counseling.

Children with signs of depression accompanying their attentional problems may be helped more with antidepressant drugs (in addition to psychotherapy). Those with prominent tics (suggestive of Tourette's syndrome) should not be treated with stimulants, as these may exacerbate symptoms permanently.

In recent years many forms of poorly evaluated medical therapy and medically related interventions have been advanced and supported (generally by the providers). These include physical exercise programs, optometric training, special diets, allergic hyposensitization programs, and drugs to correct vestibular dysfunction. Varying degrees of research have been directed toward proving the efficacy of such interventions. Although further investigation is warranted, at the time of this writing none of the above has been shown in scientifically replicable and rigorous research to be effective.

OUTSIDE REFERRALS

A child with learning disorders may need services within the community but outside of the school. Selection obviously depends upon what is available in a given area. In addition, the quality and accessibility of interventions *in school* will influence the choice of outside services. Although numerous programs exist, the more common ones include psychotherapy (from a child psychiatrist or psychologist), speech and language therapy, private tutoring, specialized medical help (e.g., neurology, otolaryngology, ophthalmology), and recreational programs.

Table 2. STIMULANT MEDICATIONS FOR USE IN CHILDREN WITH ATTENTION DEFICITS

Generic Name	Brand Name	Preparations	Range of Daily Dose (average)	Onset of Action	Duration of Action	Comments
Methylphenidate	Ritalin	Tablets: 5, 10, 20 mg*	5–60 mg (10–30) (0.3–1.0 mg/kg)	30 min	3–5 hr	Not recommended below 6 years
Dextroamphetamine	Dexedrine	Tablets: 5 mg; sustained release capsules: 5, 10, 15 mg	5–40 mg (5–20)	30 min	3–5 hr (longer in sustained release form)	Not recommended below 3 years
Premoline	Cylert	Tablets: 18.75, 37.5, 75 mg	18.75–112.5 mg (56.25–75)	2–4 hr (may not see clinical results until 3–4 weeks of therapy)	"Long-acting"	Not recommended below 6 years

* Methylphenidate also is available in a sustained release tablet (Ritalin SR 20 mg), which is the equivalent of 10 mg b.i.d of the regular form.

ADVOCACY

The clinician has a crucial role to play in advocating for the rights and needs of children with learning disorders. Helping parents obtain appropriate services, informing them of their legal entitlements (such as those guaranteed under Public Law 94-142), and assisting them to insure that interventions of high quality actually occur are all components of the advocacy role of the clinician. In addition, physicians can be critical in helping parents and schools determine the scientific efficacy (or lack thereof) of various attractive interventions that may tempt them. Scientific consumer advocacy can prevent parents and schools from going to great expense to pursue unsound treatments that replace or delay appropriate intervention.

FOLLOW-UP AND MONITORING

A learning disorder must be thought by the clinician as a chronic disease. Long term follow-up and the monitoring of progress is essential. The physician constitutes an objective professional who has continuity with the child and family and who possesses no conflicts of interest or strong disciplinary biases.

In treating a child with a learning disorder, it is important to agree upon a mechanism for periodic review of progress. If possible, educational testing of skills should be done regularly by an objective specialist *outside* of the school. Based on the results of such periodic re-evaluations, the physician can determine the need for alterations in the amount or type of service, and at the same time be constantly fortifying an alliance with the child and family, which can help to minimize the secondary effects of failure on affect, socialization, self-image, and aspiration.

Attention Deficit Disorder

GERALD L. BROWN, M.D.

The areas of concern in attention deficit disorder (ADD) that are most frequently brought to the physician are school-related difficulties (both academic and behavioral) and difficulties with social relationships in general, the latter of which may involve aggressive behavior and mood lability often resulting in poor peer relationships and difficulty with discipline.

Assessment. The academic difficulties should be assessed in part by baseline educational and clinical psychological testing. The former may include a number of tests that will be useful in prescribing specific remedial courses (e.g., techniques to overcome dyslexia), in assigning special tutoring, and in becoming aware of the child's specific academic strengths and weaknesses, which may aid in the general classroom management, particularly in those instances in which a specialized classroom for learning disabled children would be ideal but is simply not available. Structured classrooms are generally better for children with ADD than "open" classrooms. Specialized personnel, such as physicians, psychologists, nurses, educational consultants or tutors, speech therapists, and social workers, and environmental settings that would be maximally effective are also not usually fully available. Clinical psychological testing similarly provides a baseline assessment to contribute to understanding neuropsychologic functioning, maturity of biopsycho-sexual and -social development or lack thereof, and neuropsychiatric diagnoses. All testing not only provides data to contribute to specific initial treatment and management decisions in individuals with ADD, but also provides one means of longitudinal assessment of the efficacy of such decisions.

Further nonmedical assessments may include home visits by nursing and social worker staff. Such assessments may be useful in determining whether to recommend family counseling. In some cases, there may be major financial and economic difficulties, foster homes, single parent homes, and/or major disturbances within a family such as intense marital discord or substance abuse. Such issues may undermine the most thorough assessment and treatment and management plan; interventions by ancillary personnel can be necessary to allow the most basic treatment and management of ADD. This point is not to imply that family disturbance is necessarily a part of the overall picture, but that some level of family disturbance does seem to be more frequent than one would expect to encounter in a general population of similarly aged children.

Medical assessment should include thorough medical, neurologic, and psychiatric examinations. In a few cases, previously unrecognized medical disorders, usually of a metabolic nature, are noted. In many cases, neurologic findings will consist of no more than soft-signs, such as clumsiness and deficiencies in fine motor coordination; on the other hand, more significant problems such as enuresis, encopresis, and EEG abnormalities (approximately 20%, conservatively) may occur, which in some instances may be associated with various, usually mild, seizure disorders. In some specific individuals, the medical and neurologic evaluation may indicate additional treatment specific to the results of those evaluations.

In addition to the assessment of the family or environmental situation, the psychiatric examination is important in assessing the behavioral disturbance, mood lability, and development of psychological internal and interpersonal functioning of the individual child. This assessment should provide critical data for determining what kind of nonpharmacologic psychiatric treatment would be indicated as well as determining the type and use of pharmacologic interventions.

Behavioral and Psychological Therapy. If the behavioral, mood, and reality-perceptive disturbances are not severe, behavior therapy consisting of a relatively controlled condition or environment from within which intervention variables (positive or negative) are imposed with the expectation of altering the behavioral learning of these subjects in a consistent way may be helpful without the use of medication. However, if the central nervous system functions in a disorganized, deficient, or unpredictable fashion, one might obtain less predictable responses from a stimulus-response paradigm than from medication. In any case, children with relatively mild ADD may respond to nonpharmacological modes of treatment alone, i.e., family counseling, behavior therapy, and/or psychotherapy; occasionally, however, a psychologically capable family might have a child with relatively severe ADD but with few of the ancillary difficulties, i.e., inappropriate social behaviors and mood lability, and thus respond primarily to attention-altering medication with relatively little psychosocial intervention. Some studies have also shown that behavior therapy in conjunction with pharmacotherapy was better than either alone in mild to moderate cases, but that in more severe cases, the pharmacotherapy was the more necessary contributor to the successful results.

The nature of the psychotherapy, if recommended, should result from the psychiatric assessment and be modified appropriately as new data are gleaned from the ongoing experience of working with the child and family. Most individual psychotherapy is likely to be of a supportive, external reality-oriented nature, since it appears that many children with ADD do not evince the ego-strength characteristics that are usually thought to be a prerequisite for favorable responses to a more insight-oriented, psychodynamic form of intense psychotherapy. A few individuals, however, have been reported to have gained considerable benefit from such psychotherapy, either concomitant to taking medication or during adolescence following a period of pharmacotherapy.

Pharmacologic Therapy. With regard to pharmacologic treatment, a number of medications (not all of which will be commented upon) have been used since the initial trial of amphetamine in 1937. Well-controlled studies did not appear until the early 1970s. In general, only methylphenidate*, a cyclisized derivative of amphetamine, has consis-

tently provided as predictable and positive responses as d-amphetamine. Both drugs have strong effects on the CNS dopamine (DA) and norepinephrine (NE) systems, among others. Two other types of medications that have shown promise are (1) magnesium pemoline*, though its onset of action is slower, its effect may appear less marked, and less is known of its neurochemical basis for pharmacological effects; and (2) tricyclic antidepressants, though they are usually more therapeutically effective in the short-term than in the long-term, and cardiac side-effects must be monitored. Other drugs that have indirect and direct pharmacologic effects, primarily on the CNS DA systems, i.e., L-dopa and piribedil, have not been clinically useful in controlled studies. Other compounds, such as tryptophan, which primarily affects CNS serotonin (5HT), and monoamine oxidase inhibitors, which have significant effects on DA, NE, and 5HT systems, have not been studied sufficiently yet to warrant a recommendation for their general use. Though a few diet studies (a special kind of "pharmacologic" input) have been positive, diet regimens generally have not been useful in group controlled studies. Dietary alterations may be useful in specific children with perhaps specific but poorly understood metabolic alterations.

d-Amphetamine and methylphenidate are still the pharmacologic treatments of choice, with methylphenidate apparently deserving first trial since its effects on prolactin and growth hormone are less marked than that of d-amphetamine; therefore, the physician may need to be less concerned with the controversial growth retardation effect. However, the clinician should not automatically rule out pharmacologic treatment even when he knows the patient will lose an "inch(?)" in height, since there are many complicated variables that should influence the use of medication in the complex individual situation. Risks and benefits should be discussed with the family.

Another potentially serious side effect is the development of tics and the possibility that a child with a predisposition for Gilles de la Tourette syndrome may have the onset of that disorder associated with the use of stimulants. If there are early signs of this disorder in the child or a family history of the same, considered caution should be exercised in the decision to use stimulants.

Other, usually transient, side-effects include moodiness, irritability, decreased appetite, and nausea, the last of which can usually be controlled by taking the medication along with food. Though side effects may determine a dose level at a particular time during a treatment course, they are not usually a reliable means of assessing therapeutic response.

Observations of drug response should be as-

---

* Manufacturer's note: Not recommended for use in children under 6 years of age.

sessed in view of the observer's expectation of response, be it child, parent, or teacher; the last usually provides the most accurate response data because of the environmental expectations and the time during which the child is being observed. For the child alone, such parameters as activity level, concentration ability, impulsivity proneness, and distractibility are probably among the best indexes of clinical therapeutic response. Within social group, the child's response to authority and peer relationships are appropriate indexes.

Controlled pharmacokinetic studies appear to support the use of both d-amphetamine and methylphenidate at breakfast and at noon. There is the risk of sleeplessness if used late in the day or in the evening. Controlled pharmacokinetic studies also do not appear to support any advantage of sustained-release preparations. Low starting doses are 2.5 mg bid for d-amphetamine and 5.0 mg bid for methylphenidate.* Observable clinical effects may occur within $\frac{1}{2}$ hour to 2 hours and may last from 2 to 6 hours. Though tolerance in terms of the clinically desirable effects is rather uncommon, and most children do not require beyond 30 mg and 60 mg of d-amphetamine and methylphenidate, respectively, there are no generally agreed upon levels beyond which the physician should not go, nor any generally agreed upon age at which the child should no longer be given stimulant medication. Rebound effects have been reported, usually restlessness and irritability. Some children have also been reported not to respond at one point but later to respond to a trial of the same drug. Some of the more severely disturbed children may respond best to combinations of stimulants and phenothiazines, though one then must also be concerned with the possibility of inducing dyskinetic reactions from the phenothiazines. As a cardinal principle of treatment and management, components of treatment, i.e., environmental manipulations, special academic programs, family counseling, individual behavior therapy, individual psychotherapy, pharmacotherapy, to the degree that some or all may have been used, should not necessarily be terminated at the same time.

There do appear to be theoretical and practical advantages for "drug holidays," such as weekends, summers, beginning of school, other periods of unusual environmental adjustments, and, even some periods of "regular" school. A theoretical advantage for drug-free intervals is that any of the drugs that have shown efficacy in ADD have multiple known CNS effects—and no doubt unknown ones as well. Drug effects can be immediate, short-term, long-term, cumulative, different at different doses and time intervals, different under different concomitant conditions, and so on. One should therefore give such agents in the least amounts that are consistent with the desired response and with ongoing consideration for cause and effect. One realizes from double-blind, controlled trials that observers of clinical response—patients, parents, teachers, and investigators—can be wrong in their possible assumptions that observed changes necessarily are related to a concurrent condition, i.e., pharmacologic treatment. In addition, reliability studies indicate that observers are themselves inconsistent and inaccurate. At the very least, weekend holidays provide a nonblind, short-term, repeated "cross-over design" which may, despite its methodologic limitations, provide some useful comparisons in the individual "N of 1" situation. Furthermore, prolonged periods of drug holidays, whether they are "regular" or "nonregular" environmental situations, provide not only a longitudinal assessment of progress as opposed to the more "on-off" situation of the weekend holiday, but they also provide a "check" system of the clinical assumptions that have been made about drug response versus environmental influences.

Among others, a physician has two major responsibilities in clinical pharmacologic treatment. The first is the primary requirement that he "do no harm" and provide care, amelioration, or cure, where possible; however, a second responsibility, which may at times come into short-term conflict with the first, is to assess the currently advanced basis for use of the drug and effects therefrom and whether observed changes in the patient appear to be causally related to the administration of the drug. Clinical treatment is not controlled clinical research, but the former may be advantageously influenced by the scientific principles of the latter. Not only may the patient benefit from such an investigative approach, but creative ideas may also develop.

In recent years, it has become apparent that ADD does not simply go away at puberty but is often followed by continued difficulty in school, continued difficulty with peers and authority figures, and, sometimes, continued aggressive behaviors (usually aggressive behaviors in the latency years are predictive of similar behaviors as an adolescent). Follow-up demographic studies show higher incidences of alcoholism, personality disorders, affective disorders, and psychoses than one might expect to occur in the maturation of a general population. Children treated for ADD with stimulants are not more likely to use them abusively as adolescents or adults. Some investigators have reported that continued prescription of stimulant medication in adolescents and young adulthood is efficacious, though these treatments perhaps have not come to be generally accepted at this point.

---

* Manufacturer's note: Not recommended for children under 6 years of age.

3

Nervous System

Head Injury

RICHARD H. STRAUSS, M.D.

Five million children suffer head injury in the United States each year, 250,000 of whom are hospitalized; 4000 die and 15,000 have prolonged hospitalization and rehabilitation. Approximately 5% of all hospitalized children are admitted because of head injury. Most of those patients are hospitalized for assessment of neurologic status and for monitoring the development of intracranial complications; less commonly they are hospitalized for immediate treatment of their injuries. Despite these figures, over 99% of children with head injury have normal outcomes, and of children in coma secondary to head injury, at least 60% of the survivors return to their pre-injury condition. Most minor head injuries are treated by pediatricians (or parents, babysitters, or school nurses, who may contact a pediatrician) in emergency rooms or in offices.

EXTRACRANIAL INJURY

Scalp lacerations should be inspected for foreign material, cleaned, and repaired with suture material or sterile tapes, making certain the apposed wound is free of hair. If lacerations extend to the skull or beyond, further investigation may be warranted to check the integrity of the dura and the brain. Tetanus immunization status should be reviewed and appropriate treatment provided.

Hematomas of the scalp usually resolve within several weeks after the injury (although some go on to calcify). Aspiration of subgaleal hematomas or cephalohematomas is not recommended, and may in fact be a cause of further hemorrhage or infection. Some scalp hematomas have sharply edged borders similar to the edges of a depressed skull fracture, so much so that a tangential skull x-ray view may be necessary to differentiate the two.

SKULL FRACTURE

Many patients who have suffered minor head injury have skull x-rays taken, despite the fact that the patients appear normal on examination. Those x-rays sometimes demonstrate linear skull fractures. Unless the history of the accident is unusual or unknown, or the child has abnormal findings on physical and neurologic examinations, hospitalization is not required. (Temporal swelling/fracture and swelling/fracture across the sagittal suture, pathways that cross important blood supplies, are indications for hospitalization in the view of some experts though.) Guidelines for parents ("head injury sheets"), to be used while observing their child at home, and availability of the pediatrician to answer parents' questions are a reasonable alternative to hospitalization. Observation over a period of several hours in an office or emergency room with repeated neurologic examinations before discharge home with a "head injury sheet" is another acceptable alternative to hospitalization. Skull x-ray examinations are not usually necessary or diagnostically helpful for patients with minor head injury. Similarly, lumbar puncture is not a useful procedure for diagnosis or treatment of the child with a head injury.

Depressed skull fracture should be considered when a palpable depression or a large swelling is felt on the skull. Tangential skull x-ray is usually adequate for diagnosis unless there are other abnormalities on exam suggesting intracranial injury, which would make emergency computed tomography a more desirable exam. Surgical elevation of a depressed skull fracture depends on the depth of the depression (greater than 5–10 mm), the presence of a dural tear or compound fracture, and the presence of neurologic abnormalities. Whether elevation of a depressed skull fracture stems the occurrence of post–head injury epilepsy is not known.

Diastatic fractures occur along the lambdoid and

sagittal sutures in young children, and in the absence of other neurologic findings rarely lead to problems; therefore, they require no specific treatment other than the guidelines already mentioned.

Basilar skull fracture involves the basal sections of the frontal, ethmoid, sphenoid, parietal, or occipital bones. Basilar fractures are more often diagnosed from physical findings (mastoid or periorbital ecchymosis, CSF otorrhea; CSF rhinorrhea, and hemotympanum) than from radiographic studies. Basilar skull fracture is associated with dural tear and communication with the paranasal sinuses or the middle ear, so that patients are at risk for the development of meningitis. Studies have not shown that antibiotic prophylaxis (against the commonest infecting organism, *Pneumococcus*) decreases the incidence of meningitis following basilar skull fracture. Most often cerebrospinal fluid rhinorrhea and otorrhea cease spontaneously by 1 week after the injury. Should a cerebrospinal fluid leak persist longer than 2 weeks, radionuclide examination of the cerebrospinal fluid can help localize the leak. Patients with hemotympanum should have tympanographic and audiologic followup after discharge from the hospital or office. Hospitalization is not necessary when basilar skull fracture is unaccompanied by more serious injuries (or CSF leak).

Children with linear, diastatic, and basilar skull fracture associated with dural tear are at risk for the development of "growing fractures" several months after the accident, and they should be followed clinically and radiographically.

INTRACRANIAL INJURY

The child who has sustained a mild closed head injury with a period of unconsciousness not longer than 5 minutes can be observed at home if the results of physical and neurologic examinations are normal and reliable observation at home can be guaranteed over the next day (with "head injury sheets" that tell parents how to monitor changes in level of consciousness, motor activity, pupillary activity, behavior, sleep habits, and breathing patterns). In addition, parents should be told to observe carefully for neurologic and behavior changes and fever over the next few weeks. If reliable observation in the home cannot be guaranteed, hospitalization is necessary. In either situation, hourly observation over a period of 6–24 hours should be instituted, and if the child remains stable, observation may become less frequent. Should a change in the level of consciousness occur, neurologic examination must be repeated, and computed tomography to check for the presence of an intracranial hemorrhage or cerebral edema should be considered. The child with minor closed head injury who has abnormal findings on

neurologic examination even in the absence of obvious head injury should not be sent home; close observation and serial examination in the hospital are mandatory. The decision to admit a comatose child is not a difficult choice. It is much more difficult trying to determine the risk that a healthy looking child has of developing an intracranial complication following minor head injury. Any child who has altered consciousness, focal central nervous system abnormalities, signs of worsening illness, or a poor home situation should be hospitalized.

Severe closed head injury has many anatomic forms, several of which are discussed in other sections of this text. It is frequently associated with prolonged (longer than 5–10 minutes) loss of consciousness, altered state of consciousness (disorientation, unarousability, delirium), seizures, focal neurologic signs, abnormal vital signs, persistent headache, and other physical signs of major trauma. In addition to localizing and describing the intracranial injury by CT scanning, and determining whether it is a surgically remediable lesion, intensive care to the injured brain must be provided to optimize blood flow to the brain and to minimize the possibility of herniation and ischemia. At the same time, support of other body systems must be maintained. Endotracheal intubation provides airway protection and a route for pulmonary toilet and mechanical ventilation as well as a means for hyperventilation (P_{CO_2} approximately 25–30 mm Hg) to decrease arterial P_{CO_2}, thereby avoiding cerebral vasodilatation and increased intracranial pressure (ICP) (normal is less than 15 mm Hg, or 200 mm H_2O). Intubation itself is a noxious stimulus, one that should be performed by the most experienced person present in order to avoid acute severe rises in ICP. Intubation should be preceded by hyperventilation with 100% O_2. Arterial P_{O_2} should be maintained at a level > 100 mm Hg.

Fluid and electrolyte therapy must be titrated to the patient's urine production, insensible water loss, weight change, and degree of cerebral edema/increased ICP, but as a rule, two-thirds fluid maintenance is a reasonable starting point. Serum electrolytes and osmolarity should be monitored frequently in order to avoid (or treat) hyponatremia (caused by inappropriate ADH secretion) or severe hyperosmolarity. There is no conclusive evidence that corticosteroids (dexamethasone 0.1–0.2 mg/kg/dose IV every 4 hours) help reduce cerebral edema/increased ICP secondary to severe head injury. Antacids (0.5 ml/kg via nasogastric tube every 2 hours if gastric pH < 5) should be given to patients with severe head injury irrespective of steroid administration.

Increased ICP can be avoided in some patients and treated in other patients by simple maneuvers designed to maintain cerebral perfusion pressure (CPP) over 50 mm Hg. From the equation, CPP = mean arterial pressure − ICP, it is apparent that if ICP rises or mean arterial pressure falls, cerebral perfusion pressure and cerebral blood flow may become inadequate. (At this stage, direct monitoring of ICP is necessary.) Methods to decrease ICP are elevation of the head to 30 degrees; midline positioning of the head so that venous return is not impeded; avoidance of noxious stimuli; a trial of intravenous lidocaine before endotracheal suctioning; chest percussion and endotracheal suctioning that follow hyperventilation; maintenance of normal temperature to avoid shivering; paralysis with pancuronium (0.1 mg/kg intravenously, then 0.01–0.1 mg/kg/dose, intravenously, given every 1–3 hours as needed) to treat shivering; sedation with diazepam (0.1–0.25 mg/kg/dose IV every 1–2 hours) or morphine (0.05–0.1 mg/kg/dose IV every 2–4 hours) or phenobarbital (15 mg/kg, intravenously as a loading dose no faster than 1.5 mg/kg/min, then 5–7 mg/kg/day divided in 2 doses) unless sedation is felt to interfere with accuracy of the neurologic exam.

Acute ICP elevation over 20 mm Hg can be treated with hyperventilation, hypertonic osmotic agents (mannitol 0.25–2.0 gm/kg/dose IV over 20 minutes every 4 hours; gycerol 10% in a maintenance dextrose-electrolyte solution 0.25–0.50 gm/kg/dose IV over 30 minutes every 2 hours, or by continuous infusion: 0.5 gm/kg glycerol over 30 minutes, then 0.5 gm/kg glycerol over 90 minutes, every 2 hours); and drainage of small aliquots (0.5–1.0 ml) of CSF. Osmotic agents may be given along with furosemide or ethacrynic acid (1 mg/kg/dose IV), especially for treatment of increased intracranial pressure the first day after severe head injury. Craniectomy, hypothermia, and high-dose barbiturate therapy may be considered if other treatments fail. If inadequate mean arterial pressure is the cause of low cerebral perfusion pressure, IV fluid administration and pressor agents may be necessary, as well as measurement of central venous pressure.

Phenytoin (15 mg/kg intravenously as a loading dose, no faster than 0.75 mg/kg/min, then 5–7 mg/kg/day orally or IV over 30 minutes, divided in 2 daily doses) is recommended as an anticonvulsant when seizures occur in children with head injury, and in patients with brain injury, because it does not usually have an effect on the level of consciousness. It is unclear how long anticonvulsant therapy should continue, so patients treated with phenytoin should be followed for subsequent seizures even beyond the 6- to 12-month seizure-free period of suggested anticonvulsant treatment. Patients with early seizures, those occurring in the first week after head injury, are less likely to develop subsequent epilepsy than those patients with seizures developing after the first week.

Nutritional status should be discussed early in the patient's hospitalization, and consideration should be given to hyperalimentation or nasogastric feeding when it becomes clear that the patient will not be able to take food by mouth.

Approximately 10% of survivors of prolonged coma following severe head injury have persistent, severe intellectual and motor deficits. Early diagnosis of intracranial injury, cerebral edema, and increased ICP helps lead to definitive care of those problems, thereby improving the outcome of patients with severe closed head injury.

Head Injury

BURTON H. HARRIS, M.D.,
and KERRY S. BERGMAN, M.D.

Head injury is a frequent indication for hospitalization following blunt trauma. Craniocerebral trauma, a common event, may be an isolated injury or may be seen as a component of the blunt trauma syndrome. Each year 170,000 children are hospitalized for such injuries, and although children fare better than adults, head trauma is a leading cause of death and disability.

The majority of pediatric neurologic injuries are the result of blunt trauma. These injuries can involve the scalp, the skull, the neural tissue, and any combination of these structures.

Scalp Injuries

The passage through the birth canal requires deformation of the skull and scalp. Caput succedaneum is a subcutaneous collection of fluid in the areolar tissue of the scalp, presenting as a large, boggy mass. It usually crosses suture lines, is most commonly seen over the parietal skull, and is resorbed in several days. Cephalohematoma, a subperiosteal blood collection, is usually unilateral and limited by cranial sutures. These are usually accompanied by an underlying fracture, most often of the parietal bone. The collections resolve, and they should not be aspirated unless infection is suspected.

Scalp lacerations are common injuries in older children. The rich blood supply of the scalp results in profuse bleeding. When first seen, the scalp should be palpated with a gloved finger to be certain that no fracture is present. Then the laceration should be thoroughly cleansed to remove debris, since retained dirt, devitalized tissue and foreign material are the most common causes of postrepair infection. Hair is conservatively shaved along the wound margins. Débridement and anatomic suture repair should produce an excellent scar. Scalp lacerations are tetanus-prone wounds, and the child's previous immunizations should be checked.

Skull Fractures

Fractures of the cranial vault can be linear, comminuted, depressed, or basilar. In addition, each fracture should be thought of as open or closed, depending upon the integrity of the overlying soft tissue.

Most linear skull fractures involve the frontal or parietal bones. The most dangerous fractures are those that cross the middle meningeal groove, because the blow or the fracture may disrupt the middle meningeal artery and produce an epidural hematoma. Fractures crossing the sagittal suture also may injure major venous sinuses, and fractures extending to the foramen magnum may be accompanied by brainstem or spinal injury. While all patients with skull fractures require observation, a fracture in these sentinel locations can prompt hospitalization.

Linear fractures wider than 3 mm may be associated with disruption of the underlying dura mater. In such circumstances, herniation of dura or brain tissue may occur and only be discovered several months later ("growing fracture"). Children with wide fracture lines require follow-up skull radiographs 2 to 3 months after injury to evaluate healing.

Depressed skull fractures usually result from high-energy impact with relatively small objects. While the fracture is impressive, the problem is the injury to the brain. Débridement and elevation are indicated for open fractures, or when the depression overlies an area of cortex that corresponds to an observed neurologic deficit, or when the depression of the inner table on tangential skull radiographs exceeds 3–5 mm.

The cardinal signs of basilar skull fractures are ecchymosis of the mastoid, periorbital ecchymosis (raccoon eyes), hemotympanum, or cerebrospinal fluid in the ear or the nose (Battle's signs). These findings should be sought in all head injury patients, since patients with basilar skull fractures may be otherwise asymptomatic. Treatment is aimed at decreasing the flow of CSF by lowering intracranial hypertension. Cerebrospinal fluid leak may be viewed as a pressure-venting mechanism. Antibiotics are withheld unless meningitis is documented or suspected. To prevent superinfection with resistant organisms, prophylactic antibiotics should be avoided.

Closed Head Trauma

Cerebral concussion and the postconcussive syndrome are characterized by a brief loss of consciousness after injury. When the child awakens, lethargy, confusion, vomiting, visual disturbances and amnesia are common. Linear skull fractures are frequently associated with concussions.

A child with a mild concussion can usually be observed at home in anticipation of a short, uneventful recovery. Hospital admission is recommended for children with skull fractures crossing a major arterial or venous route and for those who have suffered prolonged loss of consciousness, confusion, changing levels of consciousness, or persistent vomiting. In addition, all children with seizures following head injury, regardless of degree, should be hospitalized for observation.

Hospitalized children require frequent observation, with special attention paid to level of consciousness, pupillary size, equality and reaction to light, and verbal and motor activity. Careful documentation with flow charting is desirable. Persistent symptoms or changes in the neurologic signs are indications for computed tomography (CT) for diagnosis of surgically correctable conditions.

Severe Brain Injury

The management of severe head trauma begins with attention to the basic elements of emergency care—airway, breathing, and circulation. The neck should be immobilized until x-rays of the cervical vertebrae are performed. Nasogastric intubation is important to treat gastric dilatation and prevent vomiting and aspiration. The neurologic examination includes notations of the level of consciousness, cranial nerve function, motor and sensory abilities, and reflexes. Serial examinations, with special reference to the level of consciousness, are useful in managing severe head injury patients. The Glasgow Coma Scale assesses eye opening and verbal and motor response and assigns a numeric scale to various observations. When corrected for age, the Glasgow Coma Scale provides useful prognostic information and quantitation of neurologic status.

Computed tomography has replaced other imaging studies as both the initial and definitive neurodiagnostic test. All patients with severe head injury, fluctuating or deteriorating neurologic status, or focal deficits should have a CT scan. Intracranial blood collections and parenchymal injuries are well visualized.

If no operable lesion is visualized at CT scan, treatment becomes supportive in anticipation of recovery. Invasive monitoring of intracranial pressure provides valuable information, and treatment of intracranial hypertension may be necessary. Attention to urine output and serum osmolality, which may be altered by inappropriate antidiuretic hormone (ADH) secretion, is important.

The use of steroids, local hypothermia, and barbiturate coma is controversial. These methods of treatment remain unproven despite some anecdotal reports. Seizures can be controlled with intravenous diazepam (Valium), 0.2 mg/kg, followed by intravenous phenytoin (Dilantin) given as a loading doze of 15 mg/kg and a maintenance dose of 6 mg/kg/24 hours.

Children with severe closed head injuries can remain comatose for months and still make a complete recovery. Excellent supportive care directed at both the central nervous system injury and other vital functions is rational therapy in any child with potentially survivable injuries.

Cerebral Edema

W. EDWIN DODSON, M.D.

Cerebral edema has been classified into several types depending on the pathogenesis. The types include cytotoxic, vasogenic, hydrocephalic, and mixed. Cytotoxic edema results from widespread injury to neurones and glia. Common etiologies include hypoxia, infarction, and Reye's syndrome. Vasogenic edema is characterized by increased permeability of brain capillaries to water and serum constituents. It is seen in lead poisoning, meningitis, trauma, brain tumors, and brain abscesses. In hydrocephalus the edema has a unique interstitial and periventricular localization, suggesting that this type of edema has a distinctive pathogenesis. In many situations both cytotoxic and vasogenic mechanisms coexist.

The primary therapy of cerebral edema should be directed at reversing the cause. The symptomatic therapies to be described may produce temporary improvement but will ultimately fail if a progressive pathologic process is not reversed. Mass lesions that produce localized edema should be extirpated by the neurosurgeon. If the edema is diffuse, surgical decompression by means of frontal or subtemporal craniotomy is at best controversial, usually ineffective, and rarely used. When diffuse edema is present and there is no mass lesion, conservative therapy is best.

Time is always required to arrange definitive treatment or for the patient to respond. In the interim, intracranial hypertension is dangerous in and of itself. It must be controlled temporarily by symptomatic and supportive measures.

Immediate supportive measures for treating cerebral edema include positioning the patient in the head up–head midline position. Fluid administration should be restricted to 1000 ml/m²/day or less. Hypotension must be avoided or rapidly corrected to ensure cerebral perfusion pressure. Adequate oxygenation and blood glucose content are essential.

The symptomatic therapy of cerebral edema is directed at reducing the intracranial volume. The

Table 1. SYMPTOMATIC THERAPY OF CEREBRAL EDEMA

Head up–head midline position	
Fluid restriction	<1000 ml/m² day
Hyperventilation	$Paco_2$ 25–30 torr*
Mannitol	1–2 gm/kg q 4 hr or as necessary
Glycerol	1–2 gm/kg q 4 hr or as necessary
Furosemide	1 mg/kg
Dexamethasone	initial dose: 0.5 mg/kg to maximum of 10 mg
	maintenance dose: 0.25 mg/kg q 6 hr, with a maximum dose of 6 mg
Pentobarbital†	loading dose: 2–5 mg/kg
	infusion dose: 1 mg/kg/hr

* 1 torr = 1 mm Hg = 13.6 mm water pressure.
† Should be used only in the intensive care unit in association with monitoring of intracranial pressure and cardiac output. Hypotension due to reduced cardiac output is a common side effect.

approaches are aimed at reducing the cerebral blood volume (hyperventilation), reducing brain water content (osmotherapy), decreasing vascular permeability (corticosteroids), or decreasing the volume of cerebrospinal fluid (lumbar puncture, osmotherapy, diuretics, corticosteroids). Lumbar puncture is the most dangerous intervention and carries the risk of provoking or aggravating cerebral herniation. Lumbar puncture should not be used until it is first established that there is no intracranial mass lesion, that the ventricular and subarachnoid pathways are patent, and that the CSF-containing spaces are capacious.

The most rapid change in intracranial volume is produced by hyperventilation. Hypocarbia produces vasoconstriction of the cerebral arterioles and slightly reduces the intracranial blood volume. Because one is operating on the nonlinear portion of the volume versus pressure curve, the decrease in intracranial pressure is usually significant. The patient should be hyperventilated until the $Paco_2$ is approximately 30 torr. Reducing the carbon dioxide level below 25 torr may produce focal cerebral ischemia.

After hyperventilation, the next step is usually to administer osmotic diuretics. Congestive heart failure is a contraindication to osmotherapy, and other diuretics should be given instead. Several osmotic agents have been used. Mannitol is preferred for intravenous use. Glycerol (glycerin) is administered by mouth or gavage. Intravenous urea was used previously, but mannitol is preferred because there is less rebound increase in intracranial pressure than with urea. The administration of osmotic agents promotes the movement of water from the brain to the intravascular space and thence into the urine. Increased serum osmolality also reduces the rate of CSF production. Other diuretics such as furosemide, ethacrynic acid, and acetazolamide can also reduce brain water, but the primary mechanism is probably systemic dehydration. These agents may also reduce CSF production, but this is probably a minor effect.

Although patients with mass lesions usually improve after diuretic administration, the progressive nature of the underlying process should be remembered. When a mass lesion is causing localized edema, the definitive therapy is surgery. Unnecessary delay predisposes to deterioration of the patient preoperatively and substantially worsens the prognosis for recovery.

The problem with both hyperventilation and osmotherapy is that they affect normally functioning brain more than injured or diseased brain. In fact, osmotic agents may leak into damaged brain and worsen localized edema, particularly after repeated doses. Another complication of osmotherapy is the production of systemic hyperosmolality after repeated doses. Thus osmotherapy is of transient benefit, and its use should be limited.

Corticosteroid therapy, usually dexamethasone, is the mainstay in treating vasogenic cerebral edema. Pharmacologic doses are administered. The onset of action is several hours after the dose; maximal effect usually requires a day. The response is best when a mass lesion such as a tumor or abscess is producing local edema and swelling. If dexamethasone is given for longer than 10 days, it should be tapered slowly and not discontinued abruptly. There is little evidence that steroids help edema caused by hypoxia, trauma, or infection.

Intravenous doses of barbiturates have been used to reduce intracranial pressure. The mechanism of action is thought to be the barbiturate-induced reduction of cerebral metabolic rate, which causes secondary decreases in cerebral blood flow and volume.

Pentobarbital has been used most often. Unfortunately, pentobarbital has a narrow therapeutic index in this situation because the doses that decrease intracranial pressure are close to those that depress the myocardium and reduce cardiac output. Lowered cardiac output causing hypotension is a serious, limiting side effect of pentobarbital when very high doses are needed. Pentobarbital should be administered only when the patient is in an intensive care unit where facilities exist to monitor both intracranial pressure and cardiac output via a Swann-Ganz catheter. The goal of therapy is to keep the intracranial pressure below 15 torr and the cerebral perfusion pressure above 50 torr. Serum pentobarbital levels of 2.5 to 4 mg/dl are usually effective. However, the endpoint of therapy is the reduction of intracranial pressure and not the production of a particular pentobarbital concentration.

The pentobarbital concentrations that are required to reduce intracranial pressure cause the EEG pattern to be burst-suppression or flat. In addition, the patient is rendered neurologically inert and the neurologic examination is lost as a means of patient evaluation. Whereas there is general agreement that barbiturate coma can decrease intracranial pressure, data that indicate an improved outcome are lacking.

Hypothermia reduces intracranial pressure, presumably by the same mechanism as barbiturates. However, hypothermia also produces metabolic acidosis and other problems and thus is rarely used.

Severely ill patients with cerebral edema are candidates for monitoring of intracranial pressure. A monitor device is indicated whenever severe intracranial hypertension requires conservative therapy for more than a day or so. Knowing the intracranial pressure can lead to more judicious administration of osmotherapy and barbiturates than when standard repeated doses are given. It also discloses the effects of body positioning and nursing interventions such as endotracheal suctioning on intracranial pressure. Several types of monitors are available. The specific type that is used is the prerogative of the neurosurgeon who installs it. It is important to remember that monitors can fail. When they do, they usually indicate falsely low readings. Thus it is important to know that the monitor is functioning properly and how to test it. The placement of intracranial pressure monitors has low risk relative to the gravity of inadequately treated, severe intracranial hypertension.

Subdural Hematoma and Epidural Hematoma

ELIAS G. CHALHUB, M.D.

Subdural hematoma and epidural hematoma in infants and children are important clinical problems. They are important because of the high frequency and necessity of immediate diagnosis and treatment. The clinical symptoms and treatment differ from the usual approach in the adult patient, Therefore, it is necessary to review certain important clinical distinctions.

Subdural Hematoma. Subdural hematoma occurs because of disruption or tearing of the bridging meningeal veins and is often associated with an underlying contusion of brain. In the full-term neonate, the convexity subdural hematoma is usually unilateral, while in older infants and children the subdural hematomas are almost always bilateral. Primiparity, cephalopelvic disproportion, and difficult forceps delivery are risk factors that predispose full-term neonates to subdural hematoma. The etiology in neonates as well as older children is usually direct closed head trauma. Child abuse, with direct injury and shaking of a child's head, can result in subdural hematoma. Subdural hematomas above the tentorium are associated with skull fracture in about 30% of the cases.

Generally, subdural hematoma produces few specific symptoms and the clinical presentation varies according to the age of the patient. The full-term neonate with small lesions may show only irritability. Other infants may have focal signs such as hemiparesis opposite the side of the subdural hematoma with focal seizures. Seizures may occur in up to 50–70% of infants. Still another group of children may have few signs early in the neonatal period but develop an enlarging head with delayed motor and intellectual milestones. The older infant and child with subdural hematoma present with a bulging fontanelle, retinal and preretinal hemorrhages, seizures, vomiting, and decreased level of consciousness. Chronic subdural hematoma in the older infant presents with pallor, failure to thrive, irritability, macrocephaly, and low-grade fever.

Epidural Hematoma. Epidural hematoma is less frequent than subdural hematoma. It is associated with fracture of the temporal bone, which causes a laceration of the middle meningeal artery in approximately 75% of the cases. Epidural hematoma occurs almost exclusively unilaterally. It is rarely associated with seizures. Epidural hematomas of venous origin, resulting from injury to the venous sinuses and the diploic veins, are characteristic of approximately 25% of children with this lesion. The predisposing factor is almost exclusively related to traumatic head injury. The clinical symptoms vary in children. The classic history of a mild head injury with loss of consciousness, followed by a lucid interval, followed by progressive signs of clinical deterioration is seldom seen in childhood. Children can manifest mild signs of headache, nausea, and vomiting up to days without progression and still have this clinical entity. More frequently, the extracerebral collection of blood will produce massive, increased intracranial pressure, with diffuse or focal signs. If intracranial pressure rises quickly and diffusely, there will be immediate loss of consciousness with Cheyne-Stokes respirations and bradycardia, necessitating the need for immediate therapy. If pressure is localized, there will be focal signs, such as a third nerve paralysis with contralateral hemiparesis and a decreased level of consciousness. Rarely are retinal and preretinal hemorrhages seen in children with epidural hemorrhages.

Diagnosis. The diagnostic studies in children with subdural hematoma and epidural hematoma are dictated by the clinical situation. If the patient is deteriorating rapidly, then minimal studies are performed and the patient is stabilized and made ready for surgery. The single most useful study for both clinical problems is a CT brain scan. This is especially helpful for acute lesions and lesions above the tentorium. If time allows, skull films may then be obtained to document fractures. Cervical spine x-rays should be obtained to exclude trauma to the cervical area. If CT scan is unrevealing and there is still high suspicion for an intracranial hemorrhage, then magnetic resonance imaging may detect lesions in unusual or difficult-to-visualize areas, such as posterior fossa. Angiography can be utilized for further clarification of the lesion but has been used with decreasing frequency.

Treatment. Treatment of acute and chronic subdural hematoma is directed at decreasing intracranial pressure, removing extracerebral hemorrhage, and treating seizures. The treatment of increased intracranial pressure is best accomplished by removing the extracerebral collection of fluid. However, temporizing measures may be necessary. If the patient is deteriorating rapidly, then endotracheal intubation with hyperventilation to decrease the intracranial pressure may be necessary. In addition, the intravenous infusion of mannitol at 1 to 2 gm per kg should be instituted. It must be emphasized that these measures should be performed only when surgery is imminent because of the possibility of rebound increased intracranial pressure. Steroids can be given at the time of diagnosis. Even though therapeutic effect will be delayed, they may be helpful in the postoperative period. Dexamethasone can be given at a dose of 0.1 to 0.2 mg/kg intravenously or intramuscularly.

It should be emphasized that barbiturate coma and hypothermia are not used routinely, and their usefulness is controversial.

The acute subdural hematoma or the symptomatic chronic subdural hematoma is best removed by subdural taps in children under 2 and by drainage through burr holes of the skull in children over 2. Subdural taps should be performed by physicians experienced in this procedure. Fluid should never be aspirated because of the risks of rebleeding and hypovolemic shock. Repeated subdural taps are often necessary until stabilization of rebleeding follows.

Seizures are frequent and can be difficult to manage. Seizures should be treated with appropriate anticonvulsants. Phenobarbital or phenytoin should be given in a dosage of 10–20 mg/kg if the infant is actively seizing. Maintenance dosage is 5 mg/kg/day intravenously or by mouth, depending on the status of the infant.

The treatment of epidural hematoma is an emergency procedure and is directed at removal of the extracerebral collection of fluid. While the patient is prepared for surgery, careful observation is necessary, as deterioration can be rapid. Craniotomy and direct operative removal of the hematoma should proceed. If the patient is deteriorating rapidly then as with the method of increased intracranial pressure of subdural hematoma, endotracheal intubation with hyperventilation can be instituted. In addition, mannitol and steroids may be also given as with the treatment of subdural hematomas.

Prognosis. The mortality rate in children with epidural hematoma is from 20 to 40%. Survivors tend to be free from residual neurologic damage. The mortality rate in children with subdural hematoma is low as compared with epidural hematoma, but morbidity is greater. This is attributed to the underlying brain contusion or injury. The neurologic sequelae related to subdural hematoma include mental retardation, hemiparesis, seizures, and hydrocephalus.

Intracranial Hemorrhage

MICHAEL J. NOETZEL, M.D.

Intracranial hemorrhage encompasses all forms of bleeding within the head, including bleeding into the parenchyma of the brain as well as subarachnoid, subdural, and epidural hemorrhages. The diverse nature of intracranial hemorrhage is reflected in its multiple etiologies and modes of presentation, although certain specific age-dependent factors and clinical syndromes can be identified.

NEONATAL PERIOD

Intracranial hemorrhage represents a significant problem in neonatal medicine owing to its high frequency and resultant serious neurologic sequelae. Periventricular-intraventricular hemorrhage is the most common and serious hemorrhage in the premature infant, occurring in 40–50% of newborns less than 35 weeks' gestation.

Ideally, management of periventricular-intraventricular hemorrhage would consist of preventative measures, either to eliminate premature birth or to prophylactically minimize those factors responsible for the hemorrhage. At present, however, treatment is for the most part supportive. Every effort should be made to maintain normal cerebral perfusion and thus decrease the possibility that the hemorrhage will be extended. A prerequisite of successful management is the normalization of arterial blood pressure through careful fluid balance. Acidosis, hypoxia, and hypercapnea, all of which may cause cerebral hyperperfusion, must be minimized by controlled respiration. For similar reasons, seizures and apnea must also be recognized early and effectively managed. Elevated intracranial pressure, if documented at the time of CSF exam, may be treated by serial lumbar punctures. This latter form of therapy may also be of benefit in slowly evolving posthemorrhagic ventricular dilatation, as are medications that decrease CSF production, such as acetazolamide* (100 mg/kg/day), furosemide (1 mg/kg/day), and glycerol (1–2 gm/kg q6h).

Newborns with rapidly progressive ventriculomegaly usually require an external ventriculostomy. Since the incidence of infectious complications increases significantly after 5 to 7 days, the ventriculostomy must be removed at that time. Such a temporizing measure may allow resolution of other critical problems that render the child a poor risk for surgical placement of an internal shunt. On occasion the ventriculostomy may actually prevent the development of hydrocephalus. More commonly, however, the progressive nature of the condition necessitates utilization of a ventriculoperitoneal shunt.

Other forms of neonatal intracranial hemorrhage, while not as common as periventricular-intraventricular hemorrhage, have similar pathogenic and clinical features. In incipient herniation, rapid surgical evacuation of a subdural or intraparenchymal hemorrhage may prove lifesaving. Cerebral convexity hematomas can often be treated with only subdural taps, in which a blunt 22-gauge 1/2-inch needle is carefully placed through the lateral edge of the anterior fontanel into the subdural collection of blood. Indications for repeated taps include recurrence of neurologic symptoms or disproportionate head growth. Primary subarachnoid hemorrhage usually requires only the supportive measures previously described, unless the rare complication of hydrocephalus supervenes.

INFANTS AND CHILDREN

Trauma is the major cause of intracranial hemorrhage in infants and children. Unfortunately, many of the traumatic injuries are nonaccidental, resulting from child abuse.

Initially management should be directed towards ensuring adequate ventilation and circulation. Once the patient's condition has been stabilized, a computed tomographic (CT) scan should be obtained. In cases of clear-cut trauma with incipient brainstem herniation, subdural taps prior to CT evaluation may be both diagnostic and lifesaving. Conversely, lumbar punctures have little role in the management of traumatic intracranial hemorrhage unless infection is a consideration. In any event they should be avoided, at least until a mass lesion has been excluded by CT examination.

---

* This use of acetazolamide is not listed by the manufacturer; in addition, this dosage is higher than manufacturer recommends for other uses.

Epidural and, less frequently, subdural hematomas may require surgical evacuation of the blood clot, especially when there is progressive deterioration. Intracerebral hemorrhage can usually be managed conservatively with strict limitation of activity and close observation in an intensive care unit. The fluid status should be monitored carefully, as diabetes insipidus or inappropriate antidiuretic hormone secretion can follow from trauma. A clinically significant increase in intracranial pressure requires placement of a monitoring device. The elevated pressure is then managed initially by controlled ventilation to lower Pco_2 to 22–25 mm Hg and by fluid restriction. High doses of barbiturates can also be employed to reduce cerebral edema, as can hypothermia. In patients with diffuse hemorrhage, osmotic agents such as mannitol (1–2 gm/kg of a 20% solution administered intravenously over 15 to 20 minutes) and furosemide (1 mg/kg IV) may also be helpful in decreasing cerebral edema. Such agents are contraindicated in focal hematomas, unless used as a temporizing measure prior to surgery, since they may cause rebleeding.

In all types of intracranial hemorrhage, the immediate goal of therapy is to stabilize the child. Surgical evacuation of accessible aneurysms is at present the most prudent course producing the lowest subsequent morbidity and mortality. In addition, an infectious source of the aneurysm such as subacute bacterial endocarditis should be sought and treated appropriately. In arterial venous malformations, the indications for surgery are less clear, reflecting to a large degree the often inaccessible location of the malformation.

Another common cause of intracranial hemorrhage in children is bleeding into an area of infarction, usually the result of arterial or venous thrombosis. Such a pattern may be seen in children with sickle cell anemia, congenital cyanotic heart disease, and abnormal lipoprotein metabolism. Treatment consists of supportive measures as previously defined. Careful management of fluid status is especially critical in sickle cell disease, congenital cyanotic heart disease, and other high-viscosity states, since excessive restriction of fluids may produce extension of the hemorrhagic infarction while liberalization may potentiate cerebral edema. In hemorrhage secondary to emboli or a hypercoagulable condition, anticoagulation in the form of heparin (100 units/kg IV q4h) may be of value. Maintenance therapy would then consist of dipyridamole (Persantine), aspirin, or warfarin sodium (Coumadin).

Systemic diseases may produce intracranial hemorrhage, usually as a result of a hypocoagulable state. Approximately 25% of children with hemophilia sustain central nervous system hemorrhage, often following incidental head trauma.

Persistent complaints, usually headaches, should be evaluated with a CT scan. Treatment consists of previously described support and the administration of appropriate clotting factors to achieve a level of 50% of normal. Intracranial hemorrhage is also common in leukemia, although the bleeding may reflect either hyperviscosity (acute leukemia with increased numbers of circulating white cells) or hypocoagulability (advanced stage of the disease with resultant thrombocytopenia). In both situations, fresh frozen plama should be administered to increase the level of circulating platelets, in addition to treatment with standard chemotherapeutic measures.

Hydrocephalus

MICHAEL J. NOETZEL, M.D.

Hydrocephalus is characterized by an increased amount of cerebrospinal fluid (CSF) within the ventricular system, often under elevated pressure. The causes of hydrocephalus are varied, but all result in either an impairment of CSF absorption within the subarachnoid space (communicating hydrocephalus) or in an obstruction of CSF flow within the ventricles (noncommunicating hydrocephalus). Regardless of the cause, early diagnosis and appropriate long-term management of hydrocephalus are imperative given the progressive cerebral damage that can result from this condition.

The management of hydrocephalus centers on three major areas: initial relief of the hydrocephalus, treatment of complications arising from shunting of CSF, and management of problems related to the effects of hydrocephalus on normal psychomotor development. A mass lesion such as a tumor or cyst not uncommonly may cause obstruction to the flow of CSF. In these instances, the hydrocephalus may be corrected by surgical removal of the mass.

Shunt Procedures. Most children with hydrocephalus, however, require primary drainage of the CSF from the ventricles to an extracranial compartment, usually the peritoneum or vascular system. The majority of shunt systems today consist of a ventricular catheter, a flush pump, a unidirectional flow valve, and a distal catheter. A reservoir is often added to allow direct access to the ventricular system for instillation of chemotherapy agents or antibiotics and removal of fluid. The valves open at predetermined CSF pressure levels and are selected to fit an individual patient's need. High-pressure valves (60 to 120 mm H_2O) are utilized to prevent complications from rapid decompression of the ventricles, most commonly subdural hematomas. Long-standing hydrocephalus in most children can be treated with medium-pressure valves (40 to 60 mm H$_2$O). Low-pressure valves (0 to 40 mm H$_2$O) are often used in small infants.

A single shunt procedure is rarely curative; revisions are usually required, since fixed catheter lengths can accomodate only limited growth. The ventriculoperitoneal (VP) shunt is the preferred form of initial management, especially in neonates and young infants, since there is a greater allowance for excess tubing, thus minimizing the number of revisions. The ventriculoatrial (VA) shunt is usually reserved for those older children whose somatic growth is nearly complete. The VA shunt is contraindicated in patients with cardiopulmonary disease or elevated CSF protein (over 250 mg/dl) and should be avoided when the CSF has been recently infected.

Elective lengthening of a shunt should be a routine procedure in the management of all children with extracranial shunts. If the initial shunt is placed within the first 3 to 4 months of age, revisions at 18 to 24 months, 4 to 6 years, and at an age when approximately 80% of adult height is reached (usually 10 to 12 years) are recommended. Compared with emergency shunt revisions, elective procedures are performed with fewer complications and, as part of a management program predicated on frequent clinical and radiologic evaluations, have been shown to control hydrocephalus and preserve brain function better.

SHUNT MALFUNCTION. The most commonly observed shunt complication is mechanical obstruction, which occurs in 20–40% of children with shunts. The obstruction may occur at either end of the catheter, but usually is the result of obstruction within the ventricles. Distally the malfunction is often secondary to thrombosis (VA shunts) or linear growth, which displaces the catheter from the peritoneum (VP shunts). Shunt obstruction may present as an emergency; the clinical manifestations are those of acutely raised intracranial pressure, often with a worsening of a previously noted neurologic deficit. In the more indolent cases, alterations in behavior such as lethargy, irritability, a sudden drop in grades, and episodic emesis are common. In some children, progressive cranial enlargement is the only evidence of obstruction. Once the obstruction is confirmed, surgery should follow promptly even if the site of the obstruction is not perfectly clear. Temporizing measures such as frequent reservoir pumping or irrigation are of little benefit and may in fact accelerate decompensation and adversely affect outcome.

SHUNT INFECTIONS. Infectious complications of extracranial shunts occur with a frequency of 5–15%. Septicemia, bacterial endocarditis, wound infection, shunt nephritis, meningitis, and ventriculitis usually result from concurrent infection at the time of shunt placement or introduction of the organism during surgery. Meningitis and ventriculitis are of greatest concern, since central nervous system infection complicating shunted hydrocephalus is a significant predictor of poor intellectual outcome. The period of greatest risk for infection is 1 to 2 months after shunt placement, but an infection can occur at any time. The most common pathogens isolated are *Staphylococcus epidermidis* and *S. aureus* acting alone or in concert with other gram-positive organisms.

Appropriate antibiotics, as determined by organism sensitivity, are mandatory and should be administered systemically or intraventricularly. Many clinicians agree with the dictum that any infection requires expedient removal of the entire shunt device and, if necessary, institution of an external drainage system through which to instill antibiotics or remove fluid and control intracranial pressure. Recent studies, however, have shown that almost 50% of infected VA shunts can be treated successfully with high-dose combined systemic and intraventricular antibiotics without resorting to shunt removal. Such a regimen requires a reservior through which antibiotics can be instilled and, in most instances, the capability of measuring an antibiotic's minimum inhibitory concentration in both the CSF and blood.

Medical Therapy. Attempts at nonsurgical management of hydrocephalus have been disappointing except in newborns with progressive ventricular enlargement secondary to intracranial hemorrhage. As many as 50% of these infants will spontaneously exhibit stabilization or resolution. Therapeutic measures such as serial lumbar punctures or medications that decrease CSF production may improve this figure. In any event, the decision to proceed with a shunt in this clinical setting must be weighed carefully. In older children, acetazolamide and isosorbide have been of some benefit, both in the treatment of very slowly progressive hydrocephalus and as temporizing measures in acute hydrocephalus when prompt surgery is contraindicated.

Other Problems in Management. On the average, the overall IQ in children with hydrocephalus will be slightly lower than normal, in the range of 90 to 95, although a wide spectrum is seen. Deficits are usually more pronounced in nonverbal intellectual skills. The degree of overall impairment appears to relate to the rate at which hydrocephalus develops, the duration of raised intracranial pressure, the frequency of complications (especially shunt infection), and in all probability the etiology of the hydrocephalus. All children with hydrocephalus should therefore have a psychometric evaluation performed at some time prior to the start of their education with the aim of establishing both realistic goals and an appropriate educational program through which the child's potential might be realized.

A child with hydrocephalus is also at greater risk for developing an emotional problem such as an anxiety neurosis or antisocial-conduct disorder. These difficulties are amenable to treatment through early intervention, especially family counseling.

The management of hydrocephalus in children is a demanding task often requiring a multidisciplinary effort. The aim of the management program should be to maximize the potential of each child. In this regard, an awareness of complications common to hydrocephalus and its treatment by extracranial shunts are essential. Prompt initial treatment, routine shunt revisions, prevention and early treatment of shunt infection, and maximization of intellectual development should be cornerstones of a management program which, if properly enacted, will enable a child with hydrocephalus to experience a normal or nearly normal life.

Myelodysplasia

GARY J. MYERS, M.D.

Abnormal development of the neural tube affecting the spinal cord can occur as an isolated event or can be associated with vertebral abnormalities. Its most severe forms compatible with survival are spina bifida (myelomeningocele) and the caudal regression syndrome. In extreme cases of open spine (rachischisis), those affected do not survive.

Approximately 1 infant in every 1000 live births in the United States has open spina bifida. The recurrence risk in subsequent pregnancies is markedly increased (5%) and rises even higher if one parent has spina bifida. Prenatal counseling of parents at risk should always be offered. Evidence is accumulating that pre- and postconceptual consumption of vitamins may reduce the incidence of spina bifida. However, experimentally hypervitaminosis can also cause spina bifida. Presently this is the only truly preventive measure known.

INITIAL MANAGEMENT BY THE PRACTITIONER

Survival of infants born with spina bifida has increased dramatically and now exceeds 90%. In addition, technological advances have improved their functional abilities and long-term outcome. The early care and attitudes of health professionals may have a profound and lasting effect. Early optimism tempered with realism is a wise course. The outcome for a given child is difficult to predict, and a negative or discouraging attitude is not helpful to a family destined to care for a handicapped child for many years.

Most infants with open spina bifida are born in community hospitals. However, the specialized knowledge and consultants needed to properly care for such children are generally located in regional centers. The diagnosis is usually obvious and transfer to a specialized center is indicated. However, urgent transfer is needed only if the back lesion is actively leaking cerebrospinal fluid or an associated life threatening anomaly is present (cardiac or gastrointestinal malformation). Surgical closure of the back lessens the risk of meningitis, but there is no evidence it improves the outcome in other ways. Initially attention should focus on decreasing the infant's risk of infection and helping the family understand, adjust, and knowledgeably participate in the decisions that need to be made. Infants with spina bifida generally appear normal except for the back lesion and perhaps lower extremity deformities. Both parents need an opportunity to see, hold, and become attached to their infant. They should also be counseled about the problems associated with myelomeningocele and given the opportunity to jointly participate in decisions concerning treatment. The Baby Jane Doe case confirmed the family's right to participate in decisions and stimulated many hospitals to establish a bioethical review committee. Any final decision about how aggressive care and treatment should be, especially if limited intervention seems indicated, requires the opinions of specialists with experience in treating this disorder.

The initial medical assessment should focus on the following: (1) the open spina bifida and its associated problems (hydocephalus, spinal lesion, paraplegia, orthopedic deformities, genitourinary abnormalities; (2) acquired problems, whether associated (meningitis) or not (hypoxia, hemorrhage); and (3) other malformations (cardiac, gastrointestinal).

The spinal lesion should be inspected first. If leakage of cerebrospinal fluid (CSF) is present, early surgical closure should be considered to lessen the risk of meningitis. The sac itself should be kept sterile prior to surgery. It can be covered with gauze and kept moist with sterile saline. A ring placed around the defect made of cotton wadding and gauze will allow the infant to be held and even lie on the back without further damage to the sac. Montgomery straps are used to hold the ring in place. If meningeal infection is suspected, CSF should be aspirated and examined. Aspiration is done by starting the needle lateral to the lesion in normal skin and running it parallel to the back through subcutaneous tissue into the sac. Associated vertebral anomalies above or below the defect are common and scoliosis can be present at birth.

The head is next examined for separation of sutures. The occipitofrontal head circumference should be recorded daily. A cranial ultrasound or CT scan will document any ventricular enlargement. Ultrasonography is an excellent method of following ventriculomegaly serially. Placement of a shunt is not an emergency in the newborn, but shunting should be considered when there is clear evidence that the hydrocephalus is progressive. A cranial CT scan may document the presence of an Arnold-Chiari malformation. Clinically the presence of cranial nerve abnormalitites (abnormal eye movements, laryngeal dysfunction, hyperactive gag) will support this diagnosis.

The level and extent of spinal dysfunction deserve careful evaluation. Most lesions involve the midlumbar region, but high lumbar or sacral involvement is also common. There is marked individual variation. Consequently, specific muscle testing is required. Voluntary muscle movement must be distinguished from reflex activity resulting from an isolated functioning spinal cord segment that is not under voluntary control. The level of sensory loss may differ from that of motor loss. Incontinence of urine and stool is nearly universal except in cases of hemimyelocele. However, the type of bladder or rectal involvement varies widely. Imbalances of muscle innervation can lead to dislocation of the hips, club foot, or other orthopedic abnormalities of the spine, hips or lower extremities.

In addition, a careful evaluation for other abnormalitites shold be performed. The presence of dysgenetic features or cardiac malformations might suggest a chromosomal problem. If inoperable or lethal defects are found, supportive care performed locally may be best for all concerned. The information gained by this initial assessment will help the practitioner in early management, facilitate consultation, and determine the need for and timing of referral.

INITIAL MANAGEMENT BY THE SPECIALIST

Transfer to a specialized center should occur in the first few days of life, generally when the family has had an opportunity to understand the situation, at least partially. Referral should be to the spina bifida team, usually the pediatrician, so that the overall picture will not be lost by a narrow focus of attention. Other team members such as the nurse, social worker, physical therapist, neurosurgeon, urologist, and orthopedist are then called upon to evaluate the infant and make recommendations. After the evaluations, a consensus opinion should be reached. A comprehensive plan is then formulated and presented to the family along with the evaluation results.

First priority should be given to helping the family understand the defect and reach a decision about closure of the back lesion. Inclusion of the mother in this process, even if via telephone, is important, since she will likely be the primary caretaker for many years. Until a decision is reached and surgery performed, the sac should be kept sterile and moist. Occasionally multiple major defects or an extensive back lesion will lead the family and spina bifida team to feel that aggressive treatment is not indicated. Such a decision should be made only after the hospital's bioethical review committee evaluates the situation and concurs. This decision can be reversed later if the infant stabilizes or other considerations become more important. Most infants will have the back surgically repaired.

A shunting procedure for hydrocephalus should be performed if serial cranial ultrasounds or a rapidly increasing head circumference documents progressive hydrocephalus. A daily occipitofrontal head circumference should be measured and plotted. Should elevated CSF pressure lead to CSF leakage through the back repair, an early shunt may be necessary. Shunts successfully reduce intracranial pressure but can lead to shunt dependence and serve as loci of infection; and their malfunction can result in acute life-threatening increases of intracranial pressure. Avoidance of a shunt, if feasible, is in the long-term interests of the child.

The genitourinary tract deserves early and regular evaluation. Preservation of renal function is essential to long-term survival. Infections of the bladder or kidneys and retrograde pressure leading to hydronephrosis need early recognition and aggressive treatment. A urine culture, serum BUN and creatinine, and radiologic studies (IVP, VCUG, renal sonogram) should be done.

Early orthopedic care is indicated, since scoliosis and joint deformities, especially in the lower extremities, may be present at birth. In infancy the deformities may not be so fixed. Consequently, serial casting of such defects as club feet may be more effective and reduce the need for later surgery. Similarly, early treatment may help the hip joint to form properly, and the progressive dislocation that sometimes occurs may be avoided. The longer orthopedic treatment is delayed, the less likely it is that surgical treatment of musculoskeletal abnormalities can be avoided.

MANAGEMENT AFTER INFANCY

Responsibility for Care. Ongoing care by an interdisciplinary team with experience treating children with spina bifida and their families provides optimal medical expertise. However, such a team of experts should not displace or intimidate the primary care physician. Specialized expertise should be neither under- nor overvalued. These experts are often located at some distance and oriented to a single organ system, periodically change responsibilities, and are often very busy. They may not understand the child in the context of his family or local environment. It is in the areas of psychosocial care, a comprehensive overview, and time for counseling and discussion that the primary care physician can and should make a major contribution. The fundamentals of primary care for the chronically ill include the following six basic canons:

Care: genuine, personal, and professional
Communicate: establish mutual trust
Customize: each child is unique
Counsel: help the family understand their choices
Coordinate: guide and assist
Continue: provide longitudinal stability

The primary care physician is in an optimal position to provide these essentials while simultaneously utilizing the expertise of the spina bifida team and its specialists for assistance.

The Head. The majority (approximately 66%) of individuals with spina bifida have intelligence within the normal range. This is a valuable asset for a child handicapped in other ways, and one that should be recognized, reinforced, and built upon. Although CNS infections often lower intellectual capability, it appears that shunt revisions and the rate of early head growth do not. The expectations of parents and others need to be tailored to this ability. Some children with a normal intellect, however, do have learning disabilities. Visuomotor perception problems are prominent. Attention to learning ability and appropriate school arrangements can greatly improve the child's chances for both learning and socialization with peers. Public Law 94-142, which mandated that public schools provide education to all handicapped children, facilitated the correct school placement.

Progressive hydrocephalus generally occurs early and in roughly 75% of children with spina bifida requires shunting. Cranial ultrasound through the anterior fontanelle provides a safe, easy, reliable way to serially document changes in ventricular size and the need for a shunt procedure. Ventriculoperitoneal shunts have reduced complications and the need for frequent revisions. However, blocked shunts do occur and if not promptly recognized and corrected, can lead to death. The main signs of shunt blockage are drowsiness, headache, vomiting, irritability, and changes in neurologic condition. Neurosurgical consultation or evaluation should be promptly obtained if any of these signs are present and especially if they are persistent.

Musculoskeletal System. Skilled orthopedic care is a cornerstone for helping the child with spina bifida. It should begin early and be longitudinal, since deformities may be present at birth or result from growth or prolonged muscle imbalance. Involvement of muscles can result in flaccidity or spasticity. There is great diversity in individual patterns of involvement. In addition, the pattern may change over time. Deterioration of neurologic function may indicate tethering, a lipoma, or other complications. Imbalance of muscles about a joint, such as the hip, can result in dislocation. The dislocation may be present at birth or occur gradually as normal hip flexors and adductors (L1-L3) act unopposed by hip extensors and abductors (L5-S1). Unequal forces acting on knees, feet, or spine can also result in progressive deformities.

Sitting, standing, and mobility all require certain joints to be stable and body parts to be properly aligned. For example, plantigrade feet improve standing balance and more evenly distribute the weight over the soles to lessen the risk of pressure sores. Similarly, if hips or knees are not fully extended, the trunk cannot be balanced, while if the hips cannot be flexed, sitting is difficult. Viewing the world from an upright position such as sitting or standing is important in development. In addition, truncal stability is essential for full use of the upper extremities. Recent developments in bracing using lightweight materials have made standing and independent mobility feasible for most of these children. These are important experiences for them, especially during the developmental years, even though many choose a wheelchair as a more practical solution when they reach their teens.

Many orthopedic procedures such as casting and surgery are prolonged and disruptive of school, family, or social life. Coordination of care and selection of priorities is especially important in this area since the problems being addressed are seldom urgent.

Genitourinary System. Social acceptability, the concept of self, and long-term survival are all affected by how well the genitourinary system is managed. An experienced urologist is needed on the spina bifida team, and regular evaluations, including x-rays, throughout life are indicated.

Continence is needed for socialization and acceptability, as well as prevention of skin damage in the perineal area. Abdominal pressure to empty the bladder (Credé's method) has been replaced by clean intermittent catheterization (CIC), a simple reliable method that ensures total emptying of the bladder. If performed regularly, it prevents overflow incontinence and ureteral reflux secondary to retrograde high pressure. CIC can be performed by parents or learned by young children. Ensuring full bladder evacuation decreases the risk of infection. Medications can be used with CIC to improve bladder storage and continence. The use of CIC has nearly eliminated the need for surgical urinary diversion. However, CIC has limitations (it must be performed regularly in a clean manner). Implanted artificial sphincters have been designed and used, but they need careful regulation to avoid serious problems.

Infections are a significant problem in these children and require prompt, vigorous therapy. Because of the spinal cord dysfunction, signs such as local pain may be absent. A urinary tract infection should be considered anytime a child with spina bifida is ill. A urinalysis and urine culture are needed to rule out this possibility.

Sexual function is possible in many individuals with spina bifida. Most females are fertile, able to have normal sexual activity, and capable of bearing children. Sexual function in males depends on their individual pattern of denervation. Some have erections and ejaculations and can have fairly normal sexual activity. Many are sterile as a result of either chronic prostatitis or retrograde ejaculation. Urologic care may improve male sexual functioning.

Bowel Control. Rectal continence is important for social acceptability and the concept of the self. With time and consistent effort it can be achieved in most children with spina bifida. Regular bowel evacuation with no stool leakage between bowel movements is the goal. It requires good dietary and toileting habits. Constipating or laxative foods must be avoided and systematic toileting procedures developed. Medications may be needed. Achievement of bowel control is often a lengthly procedure, but one that is rewarding to all concerned.

Summary. The outlook for children with spina bifida has steadily improved in recent years. Although they have multiple problems, much can be done to help them and their families. Proper treatment requires the expertise of specialists, preferably in coordination with a spina bifida team. The pediatrician or general practitioner, however, can play a significant role.

Brain Tumors

A. LOREN AMACHER, M.D.

New Techniques. Some recent technologic refinements hold great promise for allowing neurosurgeons to safely biopsy deeply placed mass lesions in the brain. Growing concern for the long-term effects of radiotherapy and chemotherapy upon the immature brain has made us more desirous than ever of having tissue diagnosis of cerebral masses before recommending therapies that may be detrimental to the intellectual development of children who survive treatment of brain tumors. Reliable diagnosis of medulloblastoma may be possible from cerebrospinal fluid cellular sediment obtained from the ventricles of a child with a posterior fossa mass. In like manner, chemical-hormonal markers in raised concentration in the CSF from patients with pineal region masses may indicate a tumor of germinal cell origin. As many such tumors are exquisitely sensitive to radiotherapy or chemotherapy, open biopsy may be obviated.

CT-guided stereotactic biopsy of deeply placed or otherwise poorly accessible lesions is proving to be a safe and reliable technique for determining histology. Examples of tumors that are prime candidates for this procedure are pineal region masses, tumors of the thalamus hypothalamus, and tumors abutting the brainstem. CT-guided stereotactic surgery is applicable for drainage of cysts and for the placement of interstitial radiation carriers for brachytherapy.

Vastly improved resolution of ultrasonic images of discrete cerebral structures, including mass lesions, makes it practicable to consider *ultrasound-guided biopsy* for any lesion that has sufficiently contrasting density from surrounding brain to create a visible image on the viewing screen. The probes containing the image-creating crystals are small enough to allow the surgeon to visualize and biopsy a tumor through a small craniotomy. A substantial advantage of the technique is that the surgeon can view a real-time image while advancing an instrument to the lesion within the plane of the ultrasonic slice. Image resolution is good enough now that it is possible to watch the jaws of a microsurgical biopsy forceps opening and closing within the desired target. Pulsations of nearby larger arteries often are discernible.

Magnetic resonance imaging (MRI) of the brain has a decided advantage over CT scanning for lesions within the posterior fossa or spinal canal. Since bone produces only a faint image with MRI, bone artifact is reduced substantially, making visualization of brainstem and spinal cord tumors in particular more dramatic and convincing. Current progress in finding agents that will enhance the signal between tissues of sufficiently different cellular densities holds promise for reliable differentiation between masses of neoplastic and non-neoplastic histopathology.

Stereotactic technique combined with finely collimated and focused beams of ionizing radiation delivered through several small ports is the basis for *stereotactic radiosurgery* of brain tumors and other lesions, notably arteriovenous malformations. The equipment and procedure were developed and refined at the Karolinska Institute in Sweden, and the equipment has only recently become available commercially. The advantage of this technique is that high tissue doses of radiation can be delivered in a very steep isodense spectrum to small volumes of tissue, thereby minimizing serious radiation damage to surrounding normal tissue.

The substantial pool of experience in craniofacial surgery for traumatic and congenital craniofacial disorders has led to innovative approaches to tumors at the base of the brain and in front of the brainstem. For example, temporary removal of the zygomatic arch permits the surgeon to approach the interpeduncular fossa from a more anterior and inferior aspect. Tumors that may be more accessible as a result include craniopharyngioma and chordoma.

Certain tumors of the central nervous system may be more safely approached through smaller exposures or may be more completely resectable when ancillary equipment such as carbon dioxide laser or an ultrasonic aspirator is used. Intrinsic spinal cord tumors, for instance, may be exposed with less damage to normal tissue by carrying out the myelotomy by laser radiation. Tumor removal is enhanced by either laser evaporation or ultrasonic aspiration.

Brain Tumors in the Very Young. The incidence of cerebral neoplasms in infants has been reported variously as a distinct rarity or as approximately the same as at other times during childhood. At least one observer has expressed concern that tumors in babies may occur more frequently in communities in which certain chemicals are manufactured. No data clearly supports this hypothesis yet.

To qualify as a truly congenital lesion, a tumor must be present at birth, or produce symptoms within a few weeks of birth. Many such neoplasms are of primitive ectodermal origin and were usually classified as medulloblastoma in older taxonomic nomenclatures. These small-celled, extremely cellular tumors may arise at any site where primitive undifferentiated cells occur, including on the surface of the cerebellum, in the posterior medullary velum, in the pineal area, and in or around the third ventricle. They are usually aggressive and difficult to control.

Ependymomas appear to occur with uncommon frequency in infants, and they may be spread diffusely throughout the subarachnoid space at diagnosis. Hydrocephalus and cranial nerve palsies are the common presenting signs for ependymomas and primitive ectodermal tumors.

Malignant gliomas of poorly differentiated origin have a propensity for deep midline structures. The clinical description of an irritable infant with loss of subcutaneous fat, motor delay with or without spasticity, voracious appetite, and large head with a bright-eyed appearance frequently suggests a tumor of the hypothalamus, which gives rise to the diencephalic syndrome.

Treatment of malignant CNS tumors in babies is likely to be frustrating and unrewarding. Seldom are the lesions resectable in their entirety, and vigorous radiotherapy and chemotherapy carry substantial risks of damage to normal tissue. Experience suggests that children who survive the tumor and its treatment pay a price in terms of physical and intellectual development. Nevertheless, long-term survivors are recorded, 10 to 30 or more years from treatment, and some have done very well.

Benign tumors of the CNS presenting in infancy include papillomas of the choroid plexus, neuroglial cysts, dermoids, and benign teratomas. Aggressive surgical therapy for such lesions is usually very efficacious, unless the anatomy at the base of the brain is distorted grossly by such lesions as infiltrative teratomas or dermoids. Antecedent hydrocephalus may require a pre-resection shunt procedure, and the hydrocephalus may remain shunt dependent after the tumor is removed.

Intracranial dermoids may be connected to the skin surface by a dermal track, particularly when the tumor is located in the posterior fossa or at the midline base of the frontal fossa. These tracks may allow entry of skin organisms with abscess formation within the tumor and a great risk of contamination of the subarachnoid space. Meningitis arising from this mechanism is likely to be polybacterial and recurrent. The external os of the track is in or close to the midline and is discernible as a small pit that usually has short, thick protruding hairs. A diligent search over the midline skin of the posterior fossa may necessitate shaving the hair. Tracks presenting on the nose may have their external os between the glabella and the junction of the middle and lower thirds. There may be a visible bulge above the external os, often with a history of recurrent inflammation. Intermittent extrusion of a creamy, thick exudate from the os is not uncommon. Such tumors obviously are congenital, although their clinical presentation may be delayed for years.

Tumors Associated with the Neurocutaneous Syndromes. The genetically related neurocutaneous syndromes of neurofibromatosis and tuberous sclerosis are commonly associated with neoplasms of the CNS. In areas where there is a genetic pool with several family pedigrees having manifestations of these disorders such tumors are frequent. Because the spontaneous mutation rate in the gene responsible for neurofibromatosis is high, sporadic cases are almost as common as familial ones. Tumors of Schwann-cell origin involving lower cranial nerves (especially the eighth), optic nerve gliomas, and meningiomas are the hallmarks of CNS neurofibromatosis. The classic tumor seen with tuberous sclerosis is the giant-cell astrocytoma arising from the environs of the foramina of Monro and obstructing it. Hamartomas of deep grey matter and cortex are extremely common in tuberous sclerosis, perhaps acting as seizure foci. In neurofibromatosis, CNS tumors may be multiple and of varying histology. Bilateral acoustic nerve tumors are of particular note, as removal of both will usually result in permanent deafness. Sarcomatous change in the Schwann-cell derivative tumors may arise in as many as 10% of such lesions.

Intracranial neoplasms in the form of hemangioblastomas are a common finding in patients with the Von Hippel-Lindau syndrome. The tumors may be cystic, commonly occur in the cerebellum and upper spinal cord, are slow growing but frequently multiple, and may be curable.

Hydrocephalus occurring in children with neurocutaneous syndromes is not necessarily due to tumor. Aqueduct stenosis occurs with an increased frequency in these conditions. And it is well to recall that extracranial tissue of neurectodermal origin exhibits a greater than usual incidence of neoplasms such as chemodectomas, pheochromocytomas, and secreting neuroblastomas. Initial symptoms in such cases may mimic intracranial pathology.

The tumors associated with the neurocutaneous syndromes are congenital in the sense that they are preprogrammed by genetic anomalies The symptoms and signs that declare their existence do not frequently arise before later childhood or adolescence.

Brain Abscess

RICHARD H. STRAUSS, M.D.

Brain abscess occurs as frequently now as in the preantibiotic era, yet the mortality from this illness has decreased substantially over the same period owing to the development of sophisticated radiographic procedures resulting in earlier diagnosis, antibiotics that attain significant levels in brain tissue, surgical techniques that lessen risk to the patient, and anti-edema regimens that diminish the severity of associated cerebral edema.

Brain abscess, 2 to 3 times commoner in boys than in girls, affects infants as well as older children. Causes of brain abscess are hematogenous seeding in patients with congenital cyanotic heart disease; local venous extension or hematogenous spread from sinus, dental, and middle ear infections; direct inoculation of organisms from penetrating head injury, meningitis, and dermal sinuses; blood-borne infection from other areas of the body. The organisms most frequently isolated from abscess specimens are staphylococci and streptococci; anaerobic bacteria, fungi, *Haemophilus* species, and gram-negative enteric bacteria are less commonly isolated, and in 10–20% of cases, no organism is isolated. Initial broad antibiotic coverage with methicillin or nafcillin (200 mg/kg/day, divided into 4 to 6 intravenous doses) and chloramphenicol (100 mg/kg/day, divided into 4 intravenous doses) is suggested, with later antibiotic therapy based on culture results. Multiple organisms are found in 25% of patients.

Management of brain abscess depends on the stage of abscess formation, the degree of intracranial hypertension, and the presence of single or multiple abscesses. Nonencapsulated cerebritis has at times been treated with systemic antibiotics alone, without surgery, and with CT followup. A well-circumscribed abscess in a safe area of the brain, albeit an uncommon situation, may be accessible to complete surgical excision. Unless the abscess is well encapsulated and situated in a safe, accessible area of the brain, however, aspiration via a burr hole is the preferred procedure. Contents of the abscess should be sent for aerobic and anaerobic culture (and TB and fungal cultures depending on the patient's history and physical exam). Because the life-threatening aspect of brain abscess may be cerebral edema, dexamethasone (0.1–0.2 mg/kg/dose, intravenously, every 4 hours) is suggested. Careful fluid and electrolyte management must be instituted to avoid iatrogenic fluid overload, which contributes to the problem of cerebral edema. For severely elevated intracranial pressure, intravenous mannitol (0.25–2 gm/kg/dose, over 20 minutes), endotracheal intubation, paralysis, hyperventilation, and ICP monitoring may be necessary. Lumbar puncture is contraindicated in the patient with brain abscess because it may precipitate brain herniation. Antibiotic therapy described above should be continued for 3 to 4 weeks after abscess aspiration/excision. The success of treatment is ultimately determined by resolution of the abscess on CT scan, improvement in the neurologic exam, and absence of signs of infection. Brain abscess may lead to cortical scarring, meningoencephalitis, and cortical vein phlebitis, and because of those phenomena and the associated tissue injury from aspiration/excision of the abscess, patients are at risk for development of seizures. Phenytoin (5–7 mg/kg/day, divided into 2 doses, given orally or by slow intravenous infusion) is recommended as prophylactic anticonvulsant therapy. Should seizures develop earlier in the patient's course, anticonvulsant care as described elsewhere in this text must be begun. Late epilepsy occurs in 10% of survivors.

Mortality from brain abscess has fallen over the last half century from 75–80% to 10–20%, and the continued decrease in mortality will depend on earlier recognition of brain abscess as a diagnostic possibility. The triad of focal neurologic signs, impaired consciousness, and evidence of infection should suggest brain abscess as a diagnosis, and workup with CT scanning should follow. Survival rates increase if brain abscess is discovered and treated before development of increased intracranial pressure. The outcome is directly correlated with preoperative level of consciousness: those patients awake or somnolent on presentation have excellent prognoses, whereas those in coma have grave prognoses despite vigorous therapy. Approximately 70% of survivors have normal neurologic and developmental exams on followup. Mental retardation is commoner in surviving patients whose preexistent risk factor is congenital cyanotic heart disease. Evaluation and treatment of preexistent risk factors must be part of the patient's management.

Spinal Epidural Abscess

RICHARD H. STRAUSS, M.D.

Acute spinal epidural abscess is a neurosurgical emergency requiring immediate operative drainage. Although this condition is rare in patients under 12 years of age, its prompt recognition and treatment may prevent permanent neurologic damage or death.

Any painful, febrile spinal syndrome should be considered an acute spinal epidural abscess until proven otherwise, and such conditions should be evaluated immediately. Location of the abscess by CT scan influences the selection of operative procedure: vertebral body osteomyelitis is more commonly associated with anterior spinal epidural abscess, which requires an anterior or lateral approach for costotransversectomy, whereas the more common posterior/posterolateral abscess requires laminectomy via a posterior approach. Once the diagnosis has been made, the patient should undergo immediate decompressive costotransversectomy laminectomy, which drains the abscess, removes necrotic material, and decompresses the spinal cord. Blood for culture should be drawn before surgery, and antistaphylococcal (or other antibacterials, depending upon the history and upon other sites of infection) antibiotics, such as nafcillin 200 mg/kg/day divided and administered intravenously every 4 to 6 hours, should be begun before drainage of the abscess in order to prevent further spread of infection. Lumbar puncture is not part of the diagnostic workup, and its use may cause inoculation of the CSF with subsequent meningitis. The surgical wound is commonly irrigated during surgery with antibiotic solution or povidone-iodine solution, and drains are placed so that antibiotic irrigation may continue postoperatively. Antibiotic therapy is recommended for 3 to 4 weeks or longer, depending on the presence

of vertebral osteomyelitis, the organism isolated, and the patient's hospital course. Orthopedic evaluation is useful for followup care, since postoperative patients are at risk for spinal instability from kyphosis, scoliosis, and spondylolisthesis.

Postoperative recovery depends largely on the duration, if any, of preoperative loss of spinal cord function or paralysis. Preoperative paralysis below the level of the abscess lasting more than 36 hours is associated with poor recovery of function. Preoperative loss of sensation may also be a predictor for poor recovery of function, but in general, when progression of signs and symptoms has stopped short of impaired spinal cord function, postoperative neurologic recovery is excellent. The key to successful outcome of spinal epidural abscess is its early consideration as a diagnostic possibility before signs of spinal cord dysfunction have occurred.

Cerebrovascular Disease in Infancy and Childhood

EDWARD F. RABE, M.D.

Strokes are spontaneous cerebrovascular events due to thrombosis or embolization of vessels, or to intracranial bleeding in the subarachnoid or intracerebral compartments. Management of these ictal events is dependent upon the diagnosis of what has occurred, and of where and how the events are moving in time. The spectrum of signs and symptoms is wide, ranging from recurrent headaches with or without stiff neck and mild focal neurological deficits to sudden ictus with hemiconvulsions, hemiplegia, and coma. These occur if the pathology is in the anterior or middle cranial fossa. If the pathology is in the posterior fossa, then vertebrobasilar symptoms appear, with headache, dizziness, ataxia, diplopia, dysarthria, and unilateral or bilateral motor and/or sensory symptoms.

The major pathology is cerebrovascular occlusion, spontaneous intracranial bleeding, or vascular spasm. *Arterial occlusions* in children occur most often in the carotid vessels as well as the anterior cerebral and middle cerebral arteries. Less frequently they occur in the vertebrobasilar system. They are often idiopathic and occur on the background of a mild antecedent illness. Occasionally, internal carotid occlusions are secondary to trauma of the pharynx or pharyngomaxillary space infections. Vertebrobasilar occlusions can occur after chiropractic or athletic-induced traction and turning of the neck leading to vertebral artery intimal tears with thrombosis and embolism. The treatment and prognosis of supratentorial arterial occlusions are influenced by the presence or absence of multiple telangiectasias in the region of the basal ganglia. If these are present, the term "moyamoya" disease is affixed, implying that the syndrome is progressive and may be immunologically based. Without telangiectasias, with an onset after 2 years, and without seizures as a presenting complaint, the patient is unlikely to develop epilepsy, intellectual deficit, or a restricting motor deficit.

Cortical vein thromboses may occur secondary to congenital heart disease, and *venous sinus thrombosis*, secondary to dehydration or local infections of the scalp, mastoid, or middle ear in older children (sagittal or transverse sinus disease, respectively). Small vessel occlusions occur in sickle cell disease and homocystinuria, while intracranial arterial occlusions are seen in fibromuscular dysplasia in children. Necrotizing arteritis causing beading of small arteries can occur after ingestion of street drugs, such as the amphetamines and pseudoephedrine.

Spontaneous intracerebral hematomas occur secondary to ruptures of arteriovenous malformations (AVM's), intracranial aneurysms (uncommon in children), as late sequelae of cranial trauma, in association with bleeding diathesis in leukemia, thrombotic thrombocytopenic purpura, or hemophilia, and very uncommonly as the presenting symptom of intracerebral tumor. Multiple small intracerebral perivascular hemorrhages occur with hyperosmolar states, and this may also produce venous sinus thromboses.

Diffuse vasoconstriction, which may be reversible, occurs as the result of ingestion of phencyclidine (angel dust), LSD, or mescaline. This may be reversed or prevented by a Ca antagonist, verapamil.

The holistic approach to infants and children with strokes is important so as to alert the physician to the cause of the stroke. For example, coarctation of the aorta or polycystic kidney suggests intracranial aneurysm, whereas inflammation of the ears and/or mastoids suggests lateral sinus thrombosis. A careful neurologic examination will suggest the vascular area involved, and repeated observations will determine the pace of the evolving pathology.

The major ancillary tests, besides the routine tests of blood count, urine, blood electrolytes, and appropriate blood chemistries, are the CT scan, with and without contrast, followed when indicated by an arch arteriogram to demonstrate all four major cerebral vessels. When vertebrobasilar symptoms occur, visualization of the vertebral arteries must be performed.

The child with a stroke should be closely monitored in an ICU until the cause of symptoms is known and the direction and pace of the physiologic changes are understood. Cardiopulmonary and renal status must be known and supported.

If Hgb S disease is present, the patient should be transfused to reduce the percent of Hgb S to less than 20 before arteriography is performed. Hydration at a rate not to exceed 1200 ml/m²/24 hours, with 0.2 to 0.4% saline and 10% glucose and, when renal function is adequate, 20 mEq per liter of potassium should be started. If febrile, appropriate wide spectrum antibiotics should be used until a definite etiologic diagnosis is reached. Cardiac arrhythmias should be appropriately managed.

Seizures should be stopped as quickly as possible. If status epilepticus occurs, sodium phenobarbital in a dose of 12 mg/kg (300 mg/M² in children larger than 25 kg) should be given slowly intravenously over 5 minutes. If the seizures continue longer than 15 minutes, a repeat dose of 6 mg/kg (in children larger than 25 kg, 150mg/M²/dose) should be given slowly. If the seizure is not controlled within 15 to 20 minutes phenytoin in a dose of 14 mg/kg at a rate not to exceed 50 mg/min in a concentration of 10 to 15 mg/ml should be given. Subsequent doses of phenobarbital should be given at 6 to 8 hour intervals to maintain a level between 30 and 55 μg/ml, and if phenytoin is also used, IV doses should be given every 12 hours to maintain a level between 15 and 20 μg/ml.

Diazepam (Valium) may be used intravenously to treat the seizures initially, in place of phenobarbital, in a dose of 0.2 mg/kg, not to exceed 10 mg/dose in patients 50 kg or more. The dose should be given slowly IV, never diluted. The dose may be repeated if seizures are not stopped in 15 to 20 minutes. If, after this, the seizures are not stopped, intravenous phenytoin or phenobarbital as described above may be given. The combination of diazepam and phenobarbital is alleged to produce respiratory depression, although if each is injected slowly, we have not observed this. If diazepam is used initially and controls the seizures, it will still have to be followed by either long-acting anticonvulsant (phenytoin or phenobarbital as described above), since the t½ of IV diazepam is only 15–25 minutes due to the large volume of distribution (V_D) of this drug.

Some children with strokes will have signs of increased ICP due to the mass effect of the blood and/or the brain swelling, which occurs secondary to free blood in the brain. Immediate reduction of pressure can be obtained with IV mannitol, 20%, in a dose of 0.25 to 1.5 gm/kg, given over 20 to 30 minutes. The dose may be repeated in 4 to 6 hours, and the smaller dose is recommended if repeated administration appears necessary. An effect upon the blood-brain barrier (BBB), which helps to minimize brain edema, occurs with steroid administration. This effect takes up to 12 hours to develop. IV dexamethasone (Decadron) in doses of 0.25 mg/kg q 8 h following a loading dose of 0.5 mg/kg may be used concomitantly with mannitol. Decadron may be used for 7 to 10 days without apparent serious side effects, but the dose should be gradually decreased as soon as increased ICP is no longer a clinical problem.

Further management of strokes in children is handled in conjunction with a neurosurgeon, who may work with the neuroradiologist. Large subdural hemorrhages, ruptured intracranial aneurysms, and accessible AVM's with significant symptoms are best handled surgically. Some large AVM's or AVM's in surgically inaccessible areas are now managed by controlled embolization through the internal carotid artery with plastic spherules, reducing the size of the AVM and then reassessing the value and safety of surgical removal. Some cases of thrombosis of the extracranial common, or internal carotid, artery are surgically amenable to treatment.

Children with strokes have recognized sequelae that must be dealt with as soon as the acute event subsides. Motor deficits with developing spasticity must be treated with PT and OT. In infants with onset under 2 years of age, seizure disorders are often chronic and are sometimes difficult to control medically. Behavior problems, especially the hyperactivity syndrome, may be treated successfully with CNS stimulants. Intellectual assessment, as well as achievement test results, should be used to monitor the progress of these children in school, for it is often irregular, and appropriate intervention can be guided by such repeated testing.

Benign Intracranial Hypertension

(Pseudotumor Cerebri)

ROBERT S. BAKER, M.D., F.R.C.P.(C), F.R.C.S.(C)

Pseudotumor cerebri is characterized by signs and symptoms of increased intracranial pressure in a patient who does not have a mass lesion or hydrocephalus. The sensorium is clear, and true localizing neurologic signs are absent. The condition is often idiopathic, but a long list of causative agents must be considered, e.g., tetracycline or nalidixic acid use, steroid withdrawal, anemia, obstruction of venous outflow of the brain, and endocrinopathies. The peak incidence is said to be in the third and fourth decades and the classic patient is female, is obese, and has menstrual irregularity. However, the condition is not rare in childhood and should be considered in any child with unexplained increased intracranial pressure.

The major goals of therapy in this disease are to relieve headache and prevent visual loss or to prevent the progression of visual loss if it is present at the time of diagnosis. In order to achieve these goals, visual function must be closely monitored in the children with this condition. Assessment of central acuity is inadequate in itself as an indicator of the condition of the optic nerves. As with glaucoma, once central acuity is lost, the damage is extensive and may be irreparable. Signs of optic neuropathy must be detected prior to this stage if serious damage is to be prevented. Careful assessment of visual function is more problematic in the child than in the adult and testing strategies must be adjusted for the patient's age. With experience and patience, considerable information can be obtained. Ideally, the examination would include a test of visual acuity, Amsler grid examination, color vision testing, and a visual field assessment. For continued monitoring, the visual field test is the most sensitive indicator of progression or resolution of optic neuropathy. Some form of visual field testing is possible in most children beyond infancy. Standardized visual field testings such as Goldmann perimetry or automated perimetry can be performed in children as young as 5 years old but is most useful in children beyond 8 years of age. In younger children, more information may be obtained by a tangent screen examination, and if this is unsuccessful, confrontation fields can be performed with finger puppets.

The frequency of assessment depends on the state of the visual system at the time of diagnosis. In a child with severe papilledema (with hemorrhages, exudates, and nerve fiber layer infarcts) and visual field abnormalities already present, ophthalmologic assessment should be performed daily as therapy is introduced. In milder cases, weekly assessment may be adequate, with the introduction of gradually larger intervals as resolution is seen. In all cases, follow-up evaluations should be obtained for several years on a 6-month to one-year basis once the condition appears to be stable. If abnormalities are present at the time of discharge and deterioration is a concern, the child can be taught to use an Amsler grid at home for daily assessments. This is not meant to replace complete ophthalmologic evaluations as it tests only the central and paracentral areas of the visual field.

Treatment of Specific Etiologic Agents. In some children with pseudotumor cerebri, resolution of the signs and symptoms occurs with removal of a causative agent, such as tetracycline or nalidixic acid, or the reinstitution of steroids that have been tapered or discontinued in the course of treating nephrotic syndrome or asthma. In other cases anemia, obesity, hyperthyroidism, or hypoparathyroidism may be causing the elevated intracranial pressure and appropriate treatment will result in resolution. The majority of cases require nonspecific means of lowering intracranial pressure if the condition does not resolve on its own rapidly after diagnosis.

Lumbar Puncture. Diagnosis requires the measurement of cerebrospinal fluid (CSF) pressure after appropriate neuroradiologic investigations have been done. The use of repeated lumbar punctures in the long-term management of this condition or in an attempt to monitor the results of therapy is often suggested. The goals of therapy, as already stated, are to prevent visual loss and relieve headache. These are the parameters that should be assessed in the evaluation of success or failure of treatment. In normal individuals, the CSF pressure returns to normal within 1 to 2 hours after a lumbar puncture. Although there are no similar data for patients with abnormal CSF regulatory mechanisms, there is no justification for assuming that a lumbar puncture provides prolonged normalization of CSF pressure. The danger of adopting a CSF pressure approach to therapy is that attention will be diverted from the visual system and the physician will have a false sense of security that the problem is being adequately managed. Even if lumbar punctures are done on an every-other-day basis, the patient is still probably spending most of the 48-hour period with elevated intracranial pressure, thereby exposing the optic nerves to potential damage. Furthermore, repeated lumbar punctures are traumatic for the child and until evidence is presented that they alter the natural history of the disease, they cannot be recommended in the treatment of this condition.

Steroids. The oral administration of dexamethasone sodium (Decadron) in a dosage of 2 mg four times daily has been found most effective in children requiring medical therapy for pseudotumor cerebri. Dexamethasone reduces intracranial pressure by a mechanism not yet determined. It is dramatically effective on the vasogenic edema that attends some kinds of intracranial tumors and also lowers the intracranial pressure in pseudotumor cerebri. This drug is more effective in pseudotumor cerebri of childhood than it is in adults, and it should be started at the time of diagnosis in any child with a mild or moderate abnormality of the visual sensory system or severe papilledema. Stabilization or resolution of the visual abnormalities and a decrease of the severity of the papilledema should be looked for in the first two weeks of therapy. If a response is seen, the dosage should be tapered over a further two weeks. If no effect is seen within two weeks, an alternative form of therapy should be instituted. If there are no abnormalities other than an increased blind spot at the time of diagnosis but papilledema is moderate and does not resolve in two weeks of observation,

then dexamethasone should be started in the above regimen.

Some patients relapse during the withdrawal phase and require long-term steroid therapy. In this situation we continue to withdraw dexamethasone and switch to prednisone in a dosage of 1 mg/kg/day, moving to an alternate-day regimen as signs and symptoms permit. The steroids are then withdrawn gradually as with other diseases requiring chronic steroid therapy.

Acetazolamide. Acetazolamide is a carbonic anhydrase inhibitor that can diminish the production of CSF. The dosage required to decrease CSF secretion (60 mg/kg/day) far exceeds that used for other conditions.* Many patients are unable to tolerate this medication because of gastrointestinal upset, perioral and digital tingling, loss of appetite, acid-base and electrolyte imbalance, and the development of renal calculi. If a beneficial effect is seen, the lowest dose to maintain relief of signs and symptoms should be used.

There is a theoretical advantage to the use of the carbonic anhydrase inhibitor methazolamide, since it more readily penetrates the blood-brain barrier and can be used in smaller amounts. However, drowsiness is a common side effect of this medication.

Other Diuretic and Hyperosmotic Agents. Furosemide is occasionally used as an adjunct to acetazolamide therapy. Although it is a sulfonamide, like acetazolamide, it is not a carbonic anhydrase inhibitor, and its mechanism is presumably dependent on depletion of total body extracellular fluid. There is little scientific evidence as to its efficacy in pseudotumor cerebri. The starting dosage is 2 mg/kg three times daily. Side effects include acid base and electrolyte abnormalities and allergic reaction.

Surgical Therapy. If medical therapy fails to prevent the development or progression of optic neuropathy or incapacitating headaches, surgical therapy should not be delayed. In the past, subtemporal decompression has been performed, but this procedure has an unacceptably high incidence of failure and complications and is no longer recommended. The two procedures that are now employed are lumboperitoneal shunt and optic nerve sheath fenestration. The criteria for choosing one procedure over another are not yet firmly established. Lumboperitoneal shunting has been shown to arrest progression of optic neuropathy and relieve headaches in pseudotumor cerebri; however, the incidence of complications from the procedure is higher than with optic nerve sheath fenestration. If headaches are the only symptom and optic neuropathy has not developed, then lumboperitoneal shunting remains the procedure

---

* This use of acetazolamide is not listed by the manufacturer.

of choice. If headaches are not a problem and progression of optic neuropathy is the principle concern, then optic nerve sheath fenestration should be performed. This procedure has been shown to be effective in relieving the progression of optic neuropathy and will reverse visual field and acuity loss in some patients. It should be emphasized that if surgical therapy is to be successful, it must be instituted before irreversible visual loss has occurred. Progressive loss of visual field or visual acuity despite medical therapy are both indications for surgical intervention.

Neurocutaneous Syndromes

LOUIS BARTOSHESKY, M.D., M.P.H.

Traditionally, a number of diseases with some overlapping features have been grouped as the neurocutaneous syndromes. These conditions are characterized by discreet neoplastic, usually hamartomatous lesions ("phakomas") located in various parts of the body (notably the central nervous system) along with various skin lesions. Five are considered here, but a number of other conditions might be candidates for inclusion (incontinentia pigmenti, multiple mucosal neuromas, linear sebaceous nevus syndrome, basal cell nevus syndrome). Those discussed here include three that are inherited as autosomal dominant traits (neurofibromatosis, tuberous sclerosis, Von Hippel-Lindau disease), one that is an autosomal recessive trait (ataxia telangiectasia), and one that is sporadic (Sturge-Weber syndrome).

TUBEROUS SCLEROSIS

Tuberous sclerosis (Bourneville syndrome) has traditionally been characterized by a triad of seizures, mental retardation, and adenoma sebaceum. More precisely, however, it is a multisystem disease inherited as an autosomal dominant trait. There is variable expression of the trait among affected individuals, and only some have the classic triad.

There are several characteristic dermatologic features. The hypopigmented macule is present at birth. It is often leaf shaped. It is most readily seen with the aid of a Wood's lamp but usually can be detected with the naked eye. Mandatory Wood's lamp examination of all newborns has been proposed as a screening test for tuberous sclerosis. This is inappropriate because of the poor sensitivity and specificity of the examination and the unavailability of appropriate intervention once the diagnosis has been made.

Adenoma sebaceum responds to local dermabrasion, but it recurs. The subungual and periungual fibromas may be surgically removed if they cause discomfort, interfere with function, or become cosmetically important.

Intracranial tumors should be resected if they are symptomatic. If obstructive hydrocephalus occurs because of tubers around the foramen of Munro, shunting is needed.

Seizure medication is selected according to the clinical and EEG findings, though for most physicians phenobarbital is the drug of first choice. Control may be difficult, and multiple drugs may be required. Infantile spasms are treated with corticotropin. Their management is complicated, and a pediatric neurologist should be involved.

Cardiac tumors may be very difficult to treat, and some are not accessible to the surgeon. Asymptomatic cystic renal masses may not need to be treated; but if obstruction, recurrent infection, or persistent gross hematuria is present, resection is required.

Early identification of mental retardation and early intervention are recommended. Special education programs are required in 60–80% of children.

Tuberous sclerosis can be devastating to a family. Family counseling should be offered. Genetic counseling is essential. An apparently unaffected parent of an affected child may, on close examination, prove to have some features of the disorder. In such a family, the risk of recurrence would be 50%. Therefore, before concluding that an affected child represents a spontaneous mutation, the pediatrician should arrange for both parents to have a careful skin examination with a Wood's lamp, head CT scan, and renal ultrasound. A detailed family history is required as well.

ATAXIA TELANGIECTASIA

Ataxia telangiectasia is an autosomal recessive condition.

No treatment is effective nor is any required for the telangiectasia. Various medications (propranolol, major tranquilizers, and others) have been used for the ataxia, though none has been universally successful.

Vigorous supportive treatment is required for recurrent infections, including antibiotics, pulmonary toilet, and monitoring of pulmonary function. Immunotherapy techniques, including bone marrow transplant, administration of transfer factor, IgA administration, and thymic transplant, have been generally ineffective.

Treatment of lymphoreticular malignant disease is difficult, since patients often respond to radiation or chemotherapy with exaggerated mucosal ulceration, severe dermatitis, and gastrointestinal symptoms.

Genetic counseling is recommended. Family support and counseling are usually necessary and should be provided early in anticipation of the complicated course.

NEUROFIBROMATOSIS

This autosomal dominant trait is probably the most common of the neurocutaneous syndromes, with the prevalence rate estimated at 1 in 3000. There is some heterogeneity, and several distinct forms have been described. The cutaneous hallmark in 99% of affected persons, café-au-lait spots, may be present at birth but may not begin to appear until the first year. Although neurofibromas almost always involve the skin, they also may occur in deeper peripheral nerves and nerve roots as well as in or on viscera and blood vessels.

The café-au-lait spots need no treatment. Neurofibromas are surgically resectable, though resection of cutaneous lesions should be restricted to those that are substantially disfiguring or of functional importance. Tumors of the central nervous system are treated the same way such tumors are treated in other individuals, with specific therapy depending upon location, pathology, age of patient, and so on. There continues to be controversy over proper treatment of the optic gliomas. Kyphoscoliosis should be treated vigorously as it frequently progresses rapidly. Congenital pseudarthroses are difficult to manage and should be handled only by orthopedists with expertise in pediatrics.

Of paramount importance is anticipation of complications. Regular hearing tests, careful monitoring of blood pressure, skilled back examination for kyphoscoliosis, regular monitoring of language and cognitive development with early intervention and special education when indicated, regular skilled eye exams, periodic careful abdominal exam, and CT examination of the head may allow early identification of the treatable features of neurofibromatosis.

Genetic counseling appropriate for an autosomal dominant trait is indicated as well. This includes a family survey for identification of other affected individuals and construction of a pedigree. No prenatal diagnosis is available, but new DNA techniques hold out hope for the future availability of reliable prenatal tests.

The psychologic and emotional burdens of this condition are great. Early involvement of appropriate counselors and family support systems is essential. The pediatrician must provide the affected individual and the family with reliable, correct information and coordinate the many specialists whose skills will be required. Ophthalmologists, orthopedists, speech pathologists, audiologists, family counselors, neurologists, neurosurgeons, and dermatologists to whom patients are referred should have pediatric experience and an understanding of the principles of growth and development.

STURGE-WEBER SYNDROME

Sturge-Weber syndrome (encephalotrigeminal angiomatosis) is a sporadic neurocutaneous syndrome. Clinical findings include a port-wine hemangioma (nevus flammeus) in the distribution of the first, second, and sometimes third division of the fifth cranial nerve.

Skin grafts, excision, and tattooing have been of limited use on the facial lesion. Laser treatment is useful in some of the smaller lesions, and a dermatologist skilled in its use should be consulted. Tinted opaque waterproof creams are available in various shades and are effective cosmetically.

Glaucoma should be anticipated, and early referral to a pediatric ophthalmologist is recommended. Seizures begin in the first year and are treated with phenobarbital first but may be difficult to control; multiple drugs are often required. Surgical removal of the intracranial lesion has been suggested, but has been of limited value and is quite difficult. The high prevalence of delay in cognitive development requires early testing and referral to special needs preschools and to special education programs.

The recurrence risk to the family of an affected individual is presumed to be low.

VON HIPPEL-LINDAU DISEASE

This autosomal dominant condition is traditionally listed among the neurocutaneous syndromes. It is characterized by hamartomas of the central nervous system, as are the other neurocutaneous syndromes, but cutaneous manifestations are rare.

Individuals in whom the diagnosis has been made and those at risk on a genetic basis merit careful neurologic and ophthalmologic followup. CT scan and vertebral angiography are needed if cerebellar signs appear or if there is polycythemia. Intravenous urography, renal ultrasound, and/or renal angiographies may be required. Myelography is indicated if spinal cord signs or symptoms are detected.

Treatment includes resection of the cerebellar tumors and shunting if there is hydrocephalus. The retinal angiomas require special consideration. Some do not require treatment; others may be treated with photocoagulation.

Genetic counseling, including careful pedigree analysis, is indicated.

Acute Ataxia

DAVID A. STUMPF, M.D., PH.D

Acute ataxia has many causes and tests the clinician's diagnostic skills. Accurate diagnosis directs the therapy. Preceding events such as infections, trauma, migraine, or seizures are important in the history. Many disorders produce recurrent bouts of ataxia, and this historical feature should be sought in an effort to narrow the diagnostic considerations. A thorough neurologic examination is essential because disease at any level can produce problems in coordination.

INFECTION AND POSTINFECTIOUS ATAXIA

Postinfectious acute cerebellar ataxia is common. Varicella infection is a frequent antecedent, but respiratory and gastrointestinal viruses are often responsible. Usually there is a delay of 5–10 days from the onset of the infection to the onset of ataxia. The ataxia may worsen, generally over a 24-hour period, and then slowly resolve over several days. This is a mild form of demyelinating disease and is generally benign and untreatable. Attention is directed to excluding other more serious or treatable entities, which are usually suspected by the presence of findings in addition to the ataxia.

METABOLIC ENCEPHALOPATHY

In young children, ataxia is often the principle manifestation of metabolic encephalopathy. Although lethargy is generally present, this may be difficult for parents and physicians to distinguish from that typically present in sick children. A high index of suspicion, followed by laboratory assessment, is necessary. Hypoglycemia and electrolyte disturbances are common causes, but hyperammonemia and organic acidemias occasionally produce ataxia. Drug overdose produces ataxia, and virtually all centrally active drugs are capable of causing this side effect. Anticonvulsants, particularly phenytoin, are commonly involved. Other toxins, such as alcohol, organic solvents, and other "recreational" drugs, should be considered. Therapy is directed at removal (Ipecac, nasogastric intubation, magnesium citrate) and elimination of further absorption (charcoal) of the toxin as well as specific antidotes for some poisons.

PAROXYSMAL DISORDERS

Migraine can be complicated by ataxia. Basilar artery migraine and benign paroxysmal vertigo are related and are characterized by acute ataxia, which is sometimes accompanied by brainstem signs. Therapy is identical to that in other patients with migraine. Counseling concerning patient's anxiety and life style issues related to migraine are very helpful. Drug therapy, including ergots and analgesics, can be given at the time of the episodes. Prophylactic therapies are numerous and include imipramine, propranolol, cyproheptadine, phenobarbital, and many other drugs.

Epilepsy produces ataxia in two settings. First, patients may be unaware of a preceding seizure and notice only the postictal ataxia. Second, some with partial complex or absence seizures have ictal ataxia, vertigo, or dizziness as one manifestation of the seizure; other features lead the clinician to the diagnosis. Minor motor or "atypical petit mal" status epilepticus produces ataxia; a change in mental state and multifocal twitching and eye deviations are clues to the diagnosis. An EEG is diagnostic; diazepam (Valium) or acetazolamide (Diamox) can be given intravenously during the EEG to treat this condition. A careful history is essential in establishing the diagnosis; the EEG is an ancillary study. Anticonvulsant therapy will eliminate ataxia on this basis.

WEAKNESS

Children don't give up easily, and younger children with acute weakness often stagger about in an attempt to overcome their problem. This is a notorious diagnostic trap; muscle strength must be specifically assessed, and this is often overlooked. The Guillain-Barré syndrome frequently presents as an acute ataxia in the young child; reflex loss, weakness, and CSF protein are the critical clues. When acute onset of weakness is observed, other causes should be considered, including tick paralysis, myositis, myasthenic syndromes, transverse myelitis, poliomyelitis, and postdiphtheritic neuropathy. Careful observation of these children is important because of the risk of respiratory compromise and aspiration. Intubation and ventilatory support may be necessary.

NEOPLASMS AND INCREASED INTRACRANIAL PRESSURE

Cerebellar tumors produce gait ataxia (vermis) or appendicular ataxia (hemisphere). The acute onset of symptoms is generally due to hydrocephalus, edema, or hemorrhage into the tumor. Signs of increased intracranial pressure are frequently present. Brainstem gliomas produce associated cranial nerve and pyramidal tract disturbance but usually no increased intracranial pressure. Hydrocephalus of various causes stretches the frontopontocerebellar fibers and produces ataxia. Shunting is sometimes necessary before tumor surgery. Dexamethasone will reduce edema before operation. Therapy is determined by the type of tumor. Biopsy and excision are important in extramedullary tumors. Low-grade cerebellar astrocytomas require no further therapy. Radiation therapy is useful in brainstem gliomas, medulloblastoma, and higher grade cerebellar astrocytomas. Chemotherapy is improving the outlook with medulloblastoma, but morbidity is still high.

Neuroblastoma occasionally produces a paraneoplastic syndrome with ataxia due to opsoclonus (darting conjugate but random eye movements) and myoclonus; this generally responds to tumor removal and ACTH therapy (150 U/M²/day).

STROKE

Vertebral and basilar arterial disease are rare in children. Neck injuries or instability and thoracic surgical procedures can traumatize a vertebral artery. Coagulopathies require serious consideration in pediatric posterior circulation stroke. Sickle cell disease and hypercoagulable states are important, treatable causes. Exchange transfusion programs minimize further strokes in sickle cell patients. Vasculitis produces discrete, usually pontine, strokes that cause ataxia. Embolic disease rarely produces only ataxia. Cerebellar and pontine hemorrhages produce ataxia and often a dramatic, rapidly progressive deterioration. Diagnosis is often difficult and requires a high index of suspicion. Cerebellar hematomas can occur after trauma, with hypertension and arteriovenous malformations. A rapidly swelling cerebellar infarct or enlarging hemorrhage may require urgent and life-saving surgical intervention.

EAR DISORDERS

Acute labyrinthitis produces vertigo, nystagmus, and associated ataxia. However, no specific diagnostic studies are available, and this diagnosis is generally one of exclusion. Dramamine may be helpful. When hearing loss accompanies vertigo and ataxia, the red flags should go up; this implies damage to the inner ear or eighth nerve. Neurologic or otologic referral is generally necessary. After head trauma, basilar skull fracture can damage the vestibular system; hemotympanum and a Battle's sign may also be seen. Perilymphatic fistulas (openings in the perilymphatic system) often appear at the round or oval window and are surgically treatable. Endolymphatic hydrops has many causes: fibrosis or hemorrhage after trauma, postinfectious states, congenital anomalies, and idiopathic disorders (Meniere's disease). Symptomatic relief generally follows surgery for hydrops. Vasculitis can involve small labyrinthine vessels and produce acute ataxia and vertigo.

Degenerative Diseases of the Central Nervous System

DAUNE L. MACGREGOR, M.D.

The degenerative diseases of the nervous system are a diverse group of conditions that can be defined as disorders resulting in a progressive disturbance or loss of neurologic function (intellectual or motor in nature). The presumption is that each of these disorders originates in an abnormality of a structural protein or enzyme function and that as the biochemical definition of each entity is realized, the classification and clinical approach will become clearer. At present, the defects causing a significant number of these conditions (which include over 600 different disorders) remain unknown, and a classification that is standard and clinically useful has not been achieved.

The treatment for these conditions embraces two approaches: those therapies directed at the biochemically defined entities and less specific symptomatic treatment for the child with a chronic, progressive mental and/or physical handicap.

Prevention

Prenatal Diagnosis. The availability of antenatal diagnosis of many of the degenerative disorders has been achieved recently, based on the premise that by using cultured amniocytes (obtained by amniocentesis), accurate diagnosis can be provided. The requirements for such accuracy for a given disorder include a reliable diagnostic test that can be applied to fetal cells and the ability to clearly distinguish the heterozygote or carrier states. Prenatal detection allows counseling for at-risk families, with the possibility of prenatal screening and therapeutic abortion.

Population Screening. Mass screening for the known metabolic disorders is not possible at the present time, but carrier detection can be offered to relatives of known patients. There has, however, been a successful screening program for Tay-Sachs disease. The practicality of any screening program for the foreseeable future will depend on the identification of a high-risk population.

Treatment Possibilities

Enzyme Replacement. Infusion of the disease-related enzyme has been suggested as a possible specific therapy, with the most encouraging results having been seen in the noncerebral form of Gaucher's disease. There is unfortunately no convincing evidence that infused enzymes can pass the blood-brain barrier, and replacement trials in disorders associated with central nervous system damage have been unsuccessful. Current research attempts are focusing on the temporary modification of the blood-brain barrier to allow molecules as large as enzymes to enter the brain.

Organ Transplantation. Attempts have been made to provide patients with known neurodegenerative conditions with a continuous source of enzyme using transplant grafts. Little success has been achieved thus far, however. Patients studied with transplant techniques have included those with Fabry's disease (kidney transplant), Gaucher's disease (splenic transplant), and Niemann-Pick disease (hepatic transplantation). Other trials have included the use of leukocyte infusions.

Genetic Engineering. Genetic modification is currently being considered as a therapeutic possibility, although the technical difficulties and hazards associated with this type of approach presently render genetic engineering impractical as well as impossible.

Dietary Therapies

Commercially prepared diets containing restricted amounts of amino acids are useful in the treatment of several of the amino acidopathies (for example, maple syrup urine disease and phenylketonuria). The diets must be begun within the first days of life, and management is complex, requiring frequent measurements of serum amino acids, vigorous treatment of infection, and close monitoring of growth. Complications of dietary treatment include poor physical growth, hypoglycemia, hypoproteinemia, anemia, and retardation of bony maturation. The termination of dietary restriction is uncertain for many of the amino acidopathies. With phenylketonuria, however, it is possible to discontinue treatment at the end of the first decade. Other metabolic conditions appear to respond to restriction of protein intake (for example, urea cycle disorders such as argininosuccinic aciduria).

Additional dietary treatment involves the administration of cofactors. In some conditions massive amounts are required (an example is the use of large doses of pyridoxine in patients with one type of homocystinuria).

Symptomatic Care

The symptomatic care of a child with a progressive degenerative disorder is basically that required by any patient with a severe physically and mentally handicapping condition.

The physician in charge of the child's care must be aware of the family's involvement and concerns. Parental supports must include ease of access to their child's medical team, and they must be made thoroughly knowledgeable about the degenerative and progressive nature of the diagnosed condition. Other supports include parent relief resources and guidance for parents in seeking out various types of financial assistance (for such needs as wheelchairs and other assisting devices). The problem of the child's eventual placement and the ethical issue of vigorous resuscitation and life support must be discussed before a crisis situation arises for the family.

Basic physical care includes the following:

1. The placement of nasogastric feeding tubes or a permanent gastrostomy tube for feeding if discoordinate swallowing results in recurrent aspiration or extreme difficulty in feeding the child.

2. Positioning and skin care (for the prevention of skin breakdown and the formation of decubitus ulcers).

3. Appropriate caloric and fiber intake (for the management of potential constipation).

Treatment and physician supervision of the child's ongoing medical needs will involve the following:

1. Appropriate management of seizures with anticonvulsant drugs.

2. Provision of behavior management assistance with the addition of psychotropic medications as necessary (for example, thioridazine, chlorpromazine).

3. Basic treatment of intercurrent infections (respiratory and genitourinary).

4. Surgical orthopedic intervention (with the objectives being either ease of nursing care, the prevention of painful joint dislocations, or a temporary increase in mobility) of contractures or bony deformities.

5. Arrangements for active physical therapy and educational programs with ongoing revision of treatment goals.

Physical therapy should address both respiratory problems (by positioning, deep breathing, and postural drainage) as well as neuromuscular function.

There are no uniformly useful medications presently for the treatment of spasticity in patients with degenerative disorders, although drugs to be tried include diazepam, baclofen, and dantrolene sodium.

Cerebral Palsy

LEON STERNFELD, M.D.

Cerebral palsy is the diagnostic label given to a group of conditions characterized by delayed neuromotor development resulting in disordered movement and posture due to an insult to the developing brain. The insult is not progressive and may occur at any time during gestation and the perinatal period (congenital form) or the first five years of life (acquired). Currently the most frequent type of new case seen is spastic diplegia, although the incidence of this type seems to have decreased with the increasing availability of neonatal intensive care units. The frequency of occurrence of spastic hemiplegia apparently remains constant. The most dramatically decreased incidence has been seen with the athetoid form, undoubtedly due to prevention (by Rhogam, for example) or prompt treatment (phototherapy) of hyperbilirubinemia and its resultant kernicterus.

The primary care physician has responsibility for the customary child health services and medical care of intercurrent acute conditions. However, in most instances the primary care physician is not in a position to provide the multiplicity of services needed by the child with cerebral palsy. These services may be available in a child development center, which may be located in a hospital center, in a center operated by a voluntary health agency (such as United Cerebral Palsy or Easter Seal Society), in a university-affiliated center, or in schools. The physician should refer suspect cases of delayed development to an interdisciplinary developmental center for further assessment and evaluation, and formulate and implement an individual program plan of management. A close relationship must exist between the primary care physician and the interdisciplinary staff, and both the physician and a parent should be involved in developing the individual program plan.

Management. Children who are developmentally delayed do grow and develop, albeit at a rate that is measurably slower than that of the growth and development of the normal child. Furthermore, as in normal children, development and maturation in children with a developmental disability occur in several inter-related areas: physical, emotional, cognitive, and social. Children with cerebral palsy will become adults with cerebral palsy, and at this time there are no measures that will "cure" the condition. Therefore, the approach to their care is to provide a management or individual program plan. This plan, which is reviewed and modified at regular intervals, encompasses goals and objectives in the several areas of development within a given period (2 to 6 months for the young child and longer intervals for the older child). It is designed to improve and increase the child's function to the utmost allowed by the type, degree, and extent of the disability. The plan is a synthesis of medical, educational, and psychosocial approaches, and experience has shown that this produces a synergetic effect that is practical and efficacious.

This developmental approach involves two (much discussed) concepts, an interdisciplinary team and normalization of the environment. The interdisciplinary team will involve various professionals and will vary from time to time, as the goals and objectives of the individual management plan are changed. At all times a physician should be involved as a member of the team, although in many instances the physician will not serve as the facilitator or coordinator. Members of the team share their specialized professional skills with each other and with the facilitator. Normalization requires making available to persons with a developmental disability conditions of everyday living that are as similar as possible to those of the general population. Any intervention should be the least intrusive and the least disruptive of the child's life and represent the least possible departure from normal patterns of living.

Frequently overlooked are the needs of the family unit. The primary care physician is in a strategic position to support and counsel the family and help them cope with their feelings of confusion, guilt, grief, anger, despair, rejection, depression, and marital blame and discord, which can lead to family break-up. Social workers and psychologists can provide skilled services for family members who require such specialized services. Also, parental groups have proved to be of great value in providing basic support and practical experience in helping family members to recognize and deal adequately and maturely with the problem of having a long-term handicapped child.

Physical, Occupational, and Speech Therapies. For the infant and young child, physical, occupational, and speech therapies appear to be most useful. There are a number of different modes of therapy, of which the one most generally accepted in the United States and Great Britain is that of neurodevelopmental therapy, advocated by the Bobaths. The major contribution of the therapist is to instruct the mother (or other caretaker) in avoiding abnormal primitive reflexes and in helping to establish more mature reflexes in the child. In so doing the mother learns how to position the infant and young child correctly, and this in turn improves the mother's ability to care for her child in such mundane but important areas as feeding, clothing, diapering, and the like. The therapist should supervise and monitor the exercises and activities demonstrated to the mother, so as to assure that they are being done correctly at home and do not demand excessive time and effort. A useful adjunct is the paperback *Handling the Young Cerebral Palsied Child at Home* by Nancie R. Finnie (E. P. Dutton & Company, New York).

Whatever habilitation method the physical therapist uses, emphasis is placed on developing lower extremity skills, correct posture, and locomotion. Improvement of posture and locomotion requires evaluation of primitive reflexes, tone, and contractures, and a plan to use the information in a constructive manner. The physical therapist also assists in the use of orthotics prescribed by orthopedic surgeons and/or physiatrists.

Speech therapy is important in the young child in promoting feeding patterns and somewhat later in helping to develop speech patterns that are as close to normal speaking as possible, within the limits imposed by involvement of the tongue and oropharyngeal musculature.

Occupational therapy with the young child assists in developing mature reflexes, eye-hand coordination, and appropriate gross and fine motor movements. The therapist is involved with improving upper extremity and self-help skills. These include development of head control and trunk stabilization, which in turn helps in using the upper extremities and developing ambulation. Occupational therapists are skilled in devising special dishes and eating utensils and functional seating arrangements that keep the child flexed and serve to decrease extensor thrust.

All these therapies can be continued throughout childhood and adolescence, although the extent of each varies. Physical therapy is most intensive in the child of preschool age; speech therapy, in the child of school age; and occupational therapy, in the adolescent. However, no hard and fast division should be made, as all the therapies are useful throughout childhood, and the relative "mix" should be determined by the needs of the particular child.

Medications. It is estimated that about 30% of children with cerebral palsy have convulsive seizures. Anticonvulsant medications are used routinely for this group of children. Generally, phenobarbital and phenytoin are the most widely used, and appear to be quite effective in most instances. In selected cases other anticonvulsants or combinations may need to be tried and in such instances the expertise of a pediatric neurologic consultant should be obtained. Whenever anticonvulsants are used, regular periodic monitoring of blood levels should be instituted, the aim being to obtain the anticonvulsant effect with the smallest possible dosage.

Other types of medication have been tried and generally have been found to be ineffective over any period of time and frequently are accompanied by undesirable side effects. Muscle relaxants such as dantrolene sodium, baclofen, and methocarbamol (Robaxin) are used for short periods in older children and adolescents, but if continued over a period of time secondary effects result. Diazepam is used frequently (all too frequently), and its use should be restricted to older children and adolescents with severe hypertonicity and a particularly stressful situation, and even then, it should be prescribed for only a short time, such as three to five days.

Not infrequently children with cerebral palsy exhibit drooling of saliva due to oropharyngeal impediments to swallowing. In some children with excessive drooling there may be excoriation of the skin around the mouth and chin, and this may cause quite a bit of distress, both to the child and particularly to other members of the family. In some instances, surgical procedures have been used (e.g., diversion of the ducts of the sublingual, submaxillary, and parotid glands). Medications, specifically anticholinergic agents, have been tried. Benztropine mesylate (Cogentin) is one of these drugs and is being used experimentally. Because of its side effects, it is advisable that the problem of drooling be handled in ways other than by the use of medications.

Dental Services. Dental care is one of the most overlooked areas in the care of children with cerebral palsy. Dental care can, and should, begin as soon as dentition appears. Dental prophylaxis can be instituted as soon as teething occurs, using a moderately soft toothbrush and a fluoride-containing nonabrasive dentifrice. After several teeth are present, the use of dental floss should be introduced and this pattern of brushing and flossing should be continued for life. The young child should be introduced early to visiting the dentist for a routine examination and correction of dental caries and hyperplastic gums, as necessary. There is no need to subject a child with cerebral palsy to extensive dental surgery under anesthesia provided regular dental supervision has been instituted since infancy.

Orthopedic Surgery and Physiatry. Before the advent of gait analysis, orthopedic surgery and the use of orthoses were frequent in children from 3 years of age into adolescence. Since gait analysis has come into use in the larger medical centers, the amount of orthopedic surgery and the use of orthosis have decreased considerably. Prevention of deformities is of prime importance, and short leg braces (of lightweight plastic material) for the child with a progressive ankle deformity in equinus position may certainly be indicated. Evidence of a hip subluxation may lead to correction by adductor surgery. Other types of orthopedic surgery may be indicated in individual instances. The point is that the orthopedic surgeon should be consulted periodically so that his expertise can be incorporated into the goals and objectives of the individual program (management) plan.

Physiatry and rehabilitation medicine have concentrated on the adult, but there is an increasing awareness of their value in pediatrics. However, there are too few pediatric physiatrists available at present. Where there is such a specialist, the expertise and input can be of considerable value in addition to, and not in place of, the input of the orthopedic surgeon.

Neurosurgery. A number of neurosurgical procedures have been tried in some more severely involved persons during the past 30 years. Dentatomy and thalamotomy were done in the 1950's and have been abandoned. In the 1970's chronic cerebellar stimulation enjoyed a brief vogue, but follow-up studies resulted in an almost complete cessation of this procedure. During the past half-dozen years upper cervical spinal stimulation has been performed by a few neurosurgeons. The results are ambiguous, and it is difficult to see this procedure as being applicable on a wide scale. The efforts of some neurosurgeons in attempting to alleviate the disabilities of persons with cerebral palsy must be appreciated and applauded. However, the neurosurgeons involved in these efforts must realize the importance of good experimental design and not raise possibly unrealistic expectations of persons with cerebral palsy and their families.

Technological Equipment and Aids. There is a wide variety of technological equipment available to improve the functioning of children with physical and sensory disabilities. For young children there are specially designed electromechanical "toys" that employ the concept of biofeedback to improve functioning. For example, a child as young as two can be helped to attain head and trunk balance by using a specially designed headpiece that provides auditory and visual feedback when the head is not appropriately balanced. With appropriate switches, toys such as trains and automobiles can be operated when the head and trunk are in mid-plane. Similarly, hand-eye coordination can be attained, in part at least, by using appropriate toys and games.

In the area of nonvocal communication, there has been a virtual explosion in the development of electronic aids. Combining microcomputer technology with voice synthesizers provides equipment that speaks as well as printing to a monitor screen and providing paper print-outs. Not all commercially available nonvocal communication aids are suitable for each child with cerebral palsy. To the extent possible, equipment should be tested for each child. As more and more nonvocal children use communication aids, it is becoming increasingly evident that many of these children were erroneously considered to be mentally retarded.

Entire systems of electronic aids are now available so that persons with even severe physical involvement can live independently in their own (suitably equipped) apartments. Sensors can be activated and deactivated using, for example, a head-stick, the tongue, eyebrow movement (even voluntary eye movement), which will open and close doors (exterior and interior) and cabinets; move sinks and shelves up and down; and turn telephones, radios, televisions, typewriters, microcomputers, and other electric and electronic household equipment on and off. Children who have become familiar with the use of such systems will, as adults, acclimate themselves more readily to their use. Also, similar systems can be developed for working environments in offices, stores, service establishments, factories. This in turn can lead to more extensive gainful employment of physically disabled adolescents and adults.

The National Institute of Handicapped Research (NIHR) in the U.S. Department of Education funds, in part, a national network of bioengineering and rehabilitation research centers where trained staff are able to provide technical assistance and consultation to physicians and to their disabled clients and their families with respect to appropriate aids and equipment to improve functioning for independent living and working. NIHR and the bioengineering centers are an important resource for physicians who work with disabled children, such as those with cerebral palsy.

Sports, Physical Fitness, and Recreation. Until relatively recent years, many children with cerebral palsy tended to be overprotected, particularly when it came to physical exercise and sports. Young children with cerebral palsy should be exposed to all of the physical activities that are available to nondisabled children. Aquatic activities are particularly suitable for disabled children of all ages. Obviously there must be adequate supervision so that no harmful effects result. A number of developmental centers have both outdoor and indoor playgrounds and gyms which provide, under supervision, physical activities of all kinds designed to appeal to all youngsters.

Increasingly, competitive sports for disabled persons have developed so that now under the aegis of the National Association of Sports for Cerebral Palsy adolescents (and adults) with cerebral palsy can be involved in training and competition on a local, state, regional, national, and international level. The U.S. Olympic Commission in Colorado Springs has a committee on Sports and the Disabled Athlete, from whom information can be obtained. The National Association of Sports for Cerebral Palsy, UCPA, Inc., may be contacted at 66 East 34th Street, New York, NY 10016.

Spinal Diseases

DUANE L. MACGREGOR, M.D.

The spinal cord can be affected by a variety of pathologic conditions, however, clinical presentations of such dysfunctions are limited. Myelopathy is one term for spinal cord dysfunction; it can imply any pathologic situation affecting the spinal cord, but should be used to describe cord disease resulting from compressive, toxic, or altered metabolic states. Myelitis is a nonspecific term for inflammation of the spinal cord.

For the purpose of therapeutic discussion, spinal disorders can be approached by addressing the separate issues of myelopathic conditions and congenital structural or degenerative conditions.

MYELOPATHY/MYELITIS

There are several aspects to therapy for patients with spinal cord dysfunction. The management of spinal cord trauma may be emergency oriented or long term. A rapidly evolving spinal syndrome indicative of cord compression (for example, decompensation with a spinal tumor or hemorrhaging secondary to a vascular malformation) must also be considered to represent a neurologic emergency.

Emergency Care with Spinal Cord Trauma. The principle of treatment is "not increasing the injury." If spinal injury is suspected, the patient should not be moved until transfer can be provided by a team experienced in handling such patients, preferably supervised by a physician. The patient should be placed on a firm, flat surface. When lifting the patient, one person should be responsible for stabilization of the head if cervical injury is suspected. Other considerations are the establishment of adequate ventilation and treatment of shock. Early medical management involves the following: (1) Administration of dexamethasone 5–10 mg IV to reduce edema (studies have also shown mannitol to be effective). (2) Bladder care includes gentle manual massage rectally with initial catheterization after 24 hours to avoid distention; following this the use of the nontouch technique of intermittent catheterization is most physiological and thus probably most effective. (3) Assessment and management of respiratory, gastrointestinal, and vasomotor dysfunction.

Surgical management may include the placement of skeletal traction for cervical injuries as well as dislocation reduction, immobilization (casting), and vertebral fusion, as indicated. Presently, studies of spinal fluid manometry and myelography are not considered to provide any information in addition to that obtained by clinical evaluation and carefully limited radiographs.

The role of laminectomy and the indications for the procedure have been recently reviewed. The present consensus is that a conservative approach is preferred and that there are few if any indications for laminectomy.

Continuing Long-Term Care

BLADDER CARE. Complications involving genitourinary dysfunction include infection, formation of urinary calculi and fistulae and hydronephrosis. Careful ongoing assessment of bladder and renal function is essential, as is the early start of bladder training. Surgical treatment can include the use of presacral neurectomy and pudenal neurectomy (preceded by assessment nerve blocks) and transurethral resection. Electronic devices are being studied for the management of the neurogenic bladder.

Prevention of urinary calculi is best accomplished by activity and proper genitourinary care. Surgical removal is sometimes necessary if there is no response to conservative management.

BOWEL CARE. Lubricants and bulk-forming substances are used initially to treat impacted feces; enemas are to be avoided if possible and, if not, with greater bowel responsivity should be replaced by suppositories.

SKIN CARE/DECUBITUS ULCERS. Careful and repeated turning (keeping the child off pressure points) prevents the formation of decubiti, as does rigorous skin cleanliness. If skin breakdown does occur, various management techniques are employed (compressing, infrared and ultraviolet rays) but the primary factor promoting healing is a good general nutritional status. Plastic surgery is necessary for large deficits.

SPASMS AND SPASTICITY. Active management and prevention of the previously noted complications with early physical therapy may reduce spasms. Drug therapy is not generally effective. Surgical treatment may include subarachnoid injection of alcohol or phenol and neurologic procedures (lumbosacral myelotomy).

In general, long-term management of these patients is best carried out by a rehabilitation team. The psychological effect of spinal cord injury on the child and family must be recognized and supportive psychotherapy should be offered when indicated. Sexuality becomes an important issue for the para- or quadriplegic adolescent.

Spinal Tumors or Mass Lesions. Following appropriate clinical assessment and radiographic investigations, surgical exploration is carried out with the possible goals of complete and/or partial excision or biopsy for pathologic diagnosis. Treatment may then be continued with chemotherapeutic agents or radiation therapy.

CONGENITAL STRUCTURAL AND DEGENERATIVE CONDITIONS

Myelodysplastic conditions (e.g., spina bifida) are discussed in other articles. The major group of the degenerative disorders to be discussed here are the progressive spinal muscular atrophies, including Werdnig-Hoffman disease, Kugelberg-Welander syndrome, distal spinal muscular atrophy, and scapuloperoneal syndrome.

Management of children with spinal muscular atrophy varies depending on the type and rate of progression. The primary methods are rehabilitative and orthopedic.

Medical therapy involves the following: (1) General well child care and maintenance of a well-balanced diet. It is essential to prevent excessive weight gain. (2) Treatment of recurrent chest infection and provision of routine chest physical therapy. (3) Monitoring cardiac status (although cardiac involvement in these syndromes is rare). (4) Ongoing assessment of the development of scoliosis. (5) Treatment of complications secondary to immobilization (decubitus ulcers, constipation, genitourinary disorders, pneumonia, and pulmonary embolism). (6) The psychological and social implications must be considered for both patient and family.

Orthopedic treatment and rehabilitation are based on a classification of a child's maximal physical function. Rehabilitative efforts include physiotherapy and postural drainage, provision of appropriate seating devices, and cognitive and fine motor stimulation. Encouragement of mobility is accomplished through regular swimming activity and range of motion exercises. For less physically involved children, orthotic devices (polypropylene rigid ankle-free or knee-ankle-foot orthoses) as well as rollator walkers are used. Orthopedic management is directed at treatment of scoliosis with early spinal bracing and later spinal instrumentation. For the patient with acute spinal muscular atrophy, spinal deformities are best approached by the provision of a total body contact seating device. In the older child subluxation of the hips is a common complication requiring femoral osteotomy.

Seizure Disorders

W. EDWIN DODSON, M.D.

Seizures result from paroxysmal discharges in cortical neurons. Seizures are symptoms of abnormal brain function. With a sufficient insult to the brain, anyone can have a seizure; therefore, when seizures occur, one must first exclude specifically treatable causes before resorting to long-term antiepileptic therapy.

The urgency of starting therapy is dictated by the seizure frequency. If convulsive seizures are continuous, or nearly so, such that the patient does not reawaken between seizures (convulsive status epilepticus), the situation is an emergency and requires aggressive, intensive medical care. If seizures are less frequent and brief, evaluation and therapy can be initiated more gradually. Starting therapy slowly minimizes the chance of acute side effects, which usually occur when anticonvulsant drugs are initiated in full-strength dosage.

THE EMERGENCY MANAGEMENT OF SEVERE SEIZURES

In status epilepticus generalized convulsive seizures are continuous or recurrent without recovery of consciousness for 1 hour or longer. However, because serious metabolic consequences can begin within the first hour, therapy should be aggressive if the convulsion has lasted 10 minutes. A continuous, nonconvulsive seizure is referred to as minor motor or absence status. Nonconvulsive status is treated less urgently than convulsive status, with avoidance of drug doses that are likely to impair respiratory efforts.

Status epilepticus is a medical emergency and requires aggressive and intensive therapy and support. Concurrent with treating the status, one should seek to determine the cause. Among patients with epilepsy, discontinuation of anticonvulsant medications is a common cause of status. However, patients with epilepsy also develop fever, central nervous system (CNS) infections, obstructed airways, and other metabolic problems that can precipitate status epilepticus. Patients without a history of prior epilepsy should be evaluated as rapidly as possible for potentially damaging but treatable causes.

The initial steps in treating status epilepticus are to obtain vital signs; give oxygen; draw blood for the laboratory determination of glucose, BUN, and electrolyte levels; and rapidly estimate the blood glucose level with a Dextrostix. If this is not available, glucose (25% dextrose, 1 to 4 ml/kg) should be given intravenously. This should be followed by the intravenous infusion of fluid containing 10% dextrose. In patients taking antiepileptic drugs baseline drug levels should be determined. Because oxygenation, blood pressure, and acid-base balance may be disturbed, supportive medical care is vitally important while one uses anticonvulsant drug therapy to stop the convulsion.

Whenever medications are needed to stop seizures, depression of respiration is expected. The airway must be maintained and ventilation assisted before the patient becomes hypoxic. In general, patients should be positioned on their sides so that secretions drain from the mouth by gravity. The patient's mouth should not be forced open, as this is likely to break teeth or injure the patient in other ways. When it is necessary to place an endotracheal airway, the patient should first be well ventilated by mask. It is unusual for patients who are actively convulsing to require intubation. If one is unfamiliar with the administration of muscle relaxants and intubation is essential, the anesthesiologist should be called. Most patients who require more than one drug intravenously to stop convulsions need airway protection and assisted ventilation. In this regard, patients who have status epilepticus are similar to patients in coma due to other causes.

The selection of anticonvulsants in treating status epilepticus is to some extent a matter of personal preference. It is most important that the physician have a plan in mind and use familiar drugs in adequate doses, rather than conform to a particular drug regimen. Furthermore, the primary goal of drug administration is to stop the seizures, not to produce a particular drug level. It is often necessary to administer high doses to interrupt status, particularly if status is prolonged and "refractory" (Table 1).

My preferred sequence of drugs is a benzodiazepine, followed by phenytoin, phenobarbital, and paraldehyde. General anesthesia is recommended if all else fails. The choice of an anesthetic

Table 1. DOSES OF MEDICATION USED TO TREAT STATUS EPILEPTICUS IN CHILDREN.

Drug	Route	Dose
Diazepam	IV	0.3 mg/kg (1 mg/yr of age)
Diazepam	PR	0.5 mg/kg
Lorazepam*	IV	1–4 mg (Adult 4–8 mg)
Phenytoin	IV	20 mg/kg
Phenobarbital	IV	20 mg/kg
Paraldehyde	PR	0.3 ml/kg
Pentobarbital	IV	Loading 2.5–4 mg/kg Infusion 0.5 mg/kg/hr

* This use of lorazepam is not listed by the manufacturer.

Table 2. DOSES OF DRUGS USED TO TREAT NEONATAL SEIZURES

Dextrose (25%)	2–4 ml/kg*
Phenobarbital	20 mg/kg IV in two doses
Phenytoin	20 mg/kg IV slowly
Pyridoxine†	100 mg IV
Calcium gluconate (5%)	4 ml/kg IM
Magnesium sulfate (50%)	0.2 ml/kg IM
Diazepam	0.5 mg/kg IV
Paraldehyde	0.15 ml/kg PR

* Loading doses of dextrose must be followed by infusion of dextrose-containing solutions to avoid rebound hypoglycemia.
† Manufacturer's warning: Safety and efficiency in children have not been established.

agent is a matter of preference. I prefer repeated doses of phenobarbital or diazepam. Other barbiturates such as pentobarbital and inhalation anesthetics can be used, but these are anticonvulsant only at anesthetic, depressant doses. Among all of these drugs, phenobarbital has the most favorable ratio of antiepileptic to hypnotic actions and is thus more likely to stop the convulsion before deep anesthesia is produced. Because phenobarbital is eliminated slowly it is very long acting, and patients awaken slowly after phenobarbital is given in very high doses. Because of the complex biopharmaceutical problems of infusing diazepam in intravenous solutions and the uncertainty about the dose that is actually delivered to the patient, repeated, frequent intravenous bolus doses of diazepam are preferred over continuous drip infusions for pediatric patients.

Diazepam is used widely to stop *status epilepticus*. It enters the brain rapidly, but then exits rapidly as it redistributes into other body tissues. When diazepam is successful, it must be followed by a longer-acting anticonvulsant to maintain seizure control. Usually phenytoin is recommended because it has little additional hypnotic effect. If diazepam is not followed by a longer-acting anticonvulsant, the seizures usually recur in 20 minutes. Lorazepam, a benzodiazepine that has been used less extensively than diazepam, is water soluble, remains in the brain longer, and is thus longer acting.

In most patients, status epilepticus stops after the first or second medication. If not, it often means that a severe cerebral insult has occurred and the search for the cause should be intensified.

Nonconvulsive, *absence status* is not an emergency like generalized convulsive status. If desired, a benzodiazepine, such as diazepam, may be given intravenously while one observes the electroencephalogram (EEG) for a response. Alternatively, high doses of medication can be given orally. Ethosuximide, acetazolamide, valproic acid, and diazepam have been used. Intravenous acetazolamide is available for treating absence status. Valproic acid, 20 mg per kg, may be given rectally.

Because absence status is not life threatening, medication should be administered cautiously to minimize the risk of respiratory compromise.

NEONATAL SEIZURES

Because neonatal seizures are frequently severe and continuous, the approach to management is considered here. Most newborns with seizures require intravenous medications and intensive medical care. Because treatable causes are prevalent, the initial management of the convulsing newborn is directed at metabolic and infectious causes.

The initial steps in treatment are first to estimate the blood glucose level with a blood glucose test tape (Dextrostix) and draw blood for the laboratory determination of glucose and electrolyte levels, including calcium and magnesium. If a Dextrostix test result is either low (less than 40 mg/dl) or unavailable, 25% dextrose should be given intravenously in a dose of 2 to 4 ml/kg. The bolus dose should be followed by the infusion of a 10% dextrose solution. Followup measurements of blood glucose are essential to make sure that it is in the range of 100 mg/dl.

Hypocalcemia and hypomagnesemia are treated only after they are documented by the chemistry laboratory. Pyridoxine should be given to newborns with persistent seizures even though pyridoxine dependency is quite rare (Table 2).

Continuous neonatal seizures that are not reversed by glucose should be treated with anticonvulsant drugs, which are usually given intravenously. The drugs used most often include phenobarbital, phenytoin, paraldehyde, and diazepam. Diazepam is short acting because it is redistributed from the brain into other tissues. Thus it must be either followed by a longer-acting anticonvulsant or given repeatedly. Paraldehyde should be given per rectum and has the potential to produce or worsen metabolic acidosis. Therefore, my preference is to use only phenobarbital and phenytoin (Table 2).

Phenobarbital is given in two doses of 10 mg/kg

separated by 15 to 20 minutes (total dose of 20 mg/kg). If the seizures stop after the first 10 mg/kg, the remaining 10 mg/kg should still be given to provide adequate phenobarbital levels to prevent the recurrence of seizures. If these doses of phenbarbital are ineffective, one may administer either phenytoin or additional phenobarbital.

Because phenytoin is slowly and unreliably absorbed from muscle, it must be given intravenously. The dose is 20 mg/kg given slowly, no more than 3 mg/kg/minute, perferably while observing an electrocardiographic monitor. If phenytoin is infused too rapidly, it may cause hypotension, bradycardia, or asystole.

When convulsions are refractory and continue after loading doses of phenobarbital and phenytoin, my preference is to give additional phenobarbital. Alternatively, one may consider diazepam, 0.5 mg/kg intravenously, or paraldehyde, 0.15 ml/kg per rectum. The combination of diazepam and phenobarbital is highly likely to cause apnea. Additional doses of phenobarbital, 5 to 10 mg/kg every 20 minutes, can be given until the seizures cease or hypotension occurs. These doses cause apnea, and mechanical ventilation is required.

Certain causes of neonatal seizures have relatively good prognosis. Neonatal convulsions that are familial usually abate and require therapy for only a year or less. Seizures caused by hypocalcemia or hypomagnesemia have a good prognosis and do not require antiepileptic drug therapy.

After neonatal seizures are controlled acutely, maintenance therapy should be given with either phenobarbital (initially 3 mg/kg/day) or phenytoin (initially 6 mg/kg/day). Because newborns' drug-eliminating capacity increases during the first weeks of life, it is necessary to reevaluate them frequently. The measurement of drug levels is an essential aspect of adjusting the patient's dosage.

Newborns who have seizures due to metabolic causes and who develop normally and have normal EEG's usually do not require prolonged anticonvulsant therapy. Most authorities recommend withdrawing the anticonvulsant by age 6 months or sooner.

CHRONIC ANTIEPILEPTIC THERAPY

Usually seizures do not begin with an episode of status epilepticus, so that patient evaluation and initiation of therapy can be more gradual.

The first priority of patient evaluation is to identify treatable causes of "nonepileptic" seizures and to treat them specifically. When a treatable cause is not found, antiepileptic drugs are used. In order to select the right drug, one first defines or classifies the type of seizure. Finally, one attempts to diagnose the type of epilepsy or epileptic syndrome. If a specific type of epilepsy can be diagnosed, therapy can often be refined. Whenever possible, therapy should be specific. Mistreatment of cardiac, metabolic, or infectious disorders with anticonvulsants keeps the patient at risk for serious consequences. The importance of identifying and treating remediable causes of seizures specifically cannot be overemphasized. Although reversible causes of seizures do not always lead to permanent brain damage or epilepsy, they are more likely to do so when they are intense and prolonged.

Types of Epileptic Seizures

The seizure type provides an initial basis for the selection of antiepileptic drug. Partial seizures result from localized epileptic discharges in brain tissue. The manifestation of the seizure is determined by the location of the epileptic discharge in brain.

Generalized tonic-clonic (grand mal) seizures are the most common type of seizure in children and occur to a variable degree in most of the epileptic syndromes. Despite reports to the contrary, these are rarely a patient's sole seizure type. More often patients are eventually found to have partial seizures that become rapidly generalized. In many cases, the focal origin of the generalized fit is not recognized until after the patient is treated with antiepileptic drugs and the ictal progression is interrupted. Thus the prevalence of generalized tonic-clonic seizures as a manifestation of a primary generalized epilepsy is probably overestimated.

The generalized seizure types, *clonic* and *tonic*, in many patients seem to be fragments of the complete ictal program of a generalized tonic-clonic seizure. Generally the medications that are effective against generalized tonic seizures are recommended.

Partial and generalized tonic-clonic seizures respond to the same antiepileptic drugs and thus seem to have shared epileptic mechanisms. Effective drugs include phenobarbital, phenytoin, carbamazepine, primidone, and methsuximide. When administered over long periods, these drugs have comparable effectiveness. The primary differences between them relate to issues of neurotoxicity and other side effects.

Other types of generalized seizures seem to have different epileptic mechanisms because they respond to different types of antiepileptic drugs. Absence seizures are characterized by the abrupt alteration of awareness with variable amounts of twitching and automatic, purposeless movements. Posture may change, but the patient does not fall down. Absence seizures are accompanied by diffuse spike and wave abnormalities on the EEG. Detailed studies have shown that when generalized 3 Hz spike and wave discharges occur, responsiveness to stimuli is always impaired. Thus this EEG pattern is an indication for antiabsence drug therapy. The frequency and pattern of the EEG abnormalities vary with the type of absence seizure. Atypical absence seizures have more dramatic and complicated movements and EEG patterns.

Atonic (astatic) seizures are characterized by sudden alterations of posture and are typically difficult to prevent. They are most likely to respond to valproic acid or a benzodiazepine such as clonazepam. In some cases, acetazolamide works. Patients who are refractory to these medications sometimes benefit from the ketogenic diet.

Myoclonic seizures are defined as sudden, brief shocklike jerks, which may be localized to individual muscle groups or generalized. They may arise from diseases that affect the brainstem or spinal cord. Thus an ictal EEG may be particularly helpful in identifying epileptic myoclonus, which is likely to be amenable to anticonvulsant therapy.

Epileptic Syndromes

After classifying the patient's seizure type, one should try to determine if the patient has an epileptic syndrome or a distinctive type of epilepsy. Epileptic syndromes (the epilepsies) should be distinguished from seizure types. The patient's specific type or types of seizures is only one of several factors that contribute to the definition of an epileptic syndrome. Patients with epileptic syndromes often have more than one type of seizure.

Epileptic syndromes are characterized by several factors. These include seizure type(s), etiology, natural history, precipitating factors, the EEG, and the pattern of response to different antiepileptic drugs. A given epileptic syndrome such as infantile spasms may be symptomatic (secondary) of a known brain disorder or idiopathic (primary). The important issue is to recognize the difference between seizure types and epilepsies so that the patient receives optimal treatment. In several instances diagnosing an epileptic syndrome allows the clinician to better determine how long therapy should be continued.

Febrile Seizures

Febrile seizures occur in children aged 3 months to 5 years old who have fever and no evidence of another cause. The evaluation of patients with febrile seizures is directed at excluding treatable causes of seizures, especially meningitis, and at identifying those patients who in fact have epilepsy. The latter problem is not so simple because the only sure test may be time. In general, those patients who have partial or prolonged seizures and focal or diffusely paroxysmal EEG abnormalities are considered to have epilepsy. Patients who are neurologically abnormal or who have prolonged, dangerous seizures are also usually treated as if they have epilepsy and not febrile seizures.

It is unknown if prophylactic anticonvulsant administration averts later epilepsy. However, anticonvulsants frequently cause behavioral and other side effects in these patients. The risk of treatment must balanced against the potential benefits. A majority of patients who have brief febrile convulsions do not need treatment.

The rare patients who develop serious complications of prolonged seizures associated with fever are more likely to do so during recurrent or complicated, complex febrile seizures. Because of this, some authorities recommend treating younger patients (those less than 18 months old) and patients who have more than two risk factors, especially a complex seizure with fever.

Drugs that are effective in preventing febrile seizures include continuously administered phenobarbital and valproic acid and intermittently administered diazepam. Because of the possibility of the rare, but potentially fatal, idiosyncratic hepatotoxicity, valproic acid is not recommended for febrile seizures. When phenobarbital is given, the doses must be sufficient to produce blood levels of 15 μg/ml. At this dose, side effects are expected in 40% of patients. Reports from Europe indicate that diazepam solutions given rectally when fever occurs are also effective. Orally administered benzodiazepines have not been tested systematically. Antipyretic therapy is logical and widely recommended but of unproven value. Phenytoin and carbamazepine are not effective in preventing recurrent febrile seizures.

Atonic Seizures and Juvenile Myoclonic Astatic Epilepsy

Juvenile myoclonic astatic epilepsy is characterized by atonic seizures. The combination of atonic, partial, and generalized tonic-clonic seizures, with mental subnormality and the EEG pattern of slow (2.5 Hz) spike and wave has been called the Lennox-Gastaut syndrome.

The Lennox-Gastaut syndrome is typically difficult to treat. Traditionally, antiepileptic drugs have been selected on the basis of the patient's most common seizure type. Often these patients present initially with a partial or generalized tonic-clonic seizure. After they are begun on a drug such as phenobarbital, phenytoin, or carbamazepine, they begin to have drop attacks, suggesting the eventual diagnosis. When this occurs, the addition of valproic acid with eventual *withdrawal* of the initial medication is sometimes followed by control of both seizure types. Benzodiazepines and acetazolamide may also be helpful. In patients who do not respond to these medications, the ketogenic diet should be considered.

ACTH has also been used to treat Lennox-Gastaut syndrome. But the benefits here are not as well documented as with infantile spasms, which are discussed in a separate article. As with infantile spasms, patients seem to do better if ACTH is given soon after the seizures appear. Benzodiazepines, especially clonazepam, are also useful in Lennox-Gastaut syndrome. The old admonition that combinations of clonazepam and valproic acid might precipitate minor motor status has not been confirmed by experience. Prior to valproic acid, the ketogenic diet was an important and primary therapy in this disorder. It now used among patients who do not respond to the more easily administered drugs.

Absence Epilepsies

Absence epilepsies have absence seizures as a major seizure type. The major absence epilepsies are petit mal epilepsy and juvenile myoclonic epilepsy. Both these disorders are uncommon.

Petit mal epilepsy appears to be a benign self-limited disorder. Generalized tonic-clonic seizures are uncommon, and prophylactic therapy is not recommended until a tonic-clonic seizure occurs. Drugs that are effective in petit mal include ethosuximide, valproic acid, trimethadione, the ketogenic diet, a benzodiazepine such as clonazepam, or a carbonic anhydrase inhibitor such as acetazolamide. Because petit mal is benign, ethosuximide is recommended first; valproic acid is recommended when ethosuximide is insufficient or when the patient also has generalized tonic-clonic seizures.

Juvenile myoclonic epilepsy should be suspected when absence seizures begin in late childhood or at puberty.

Valproic acid is the drug of choice for juvenile myoclonic epilepsy. The generalized tonic-clonic seizures seen here may be refractory to anticonvulsants such as phenobarbital or phenytoin but respond to valproic acid; thus, making the diagnosis of this disorder is important.

Benign Rolandic Epilepsy

Benign rolandic epilepsy is characterized by simple partial and sometimes generalized convulsions. The natural history and familial nature of this epileptic syndrome suggest that it is a primary epilepsy. Despite the usually benign natural history, most authorities believe that therapy is advisable.

Rolandic epilepsy is usually responsive to the antiepileptic drugs that are effective in partial and generalized tonic-clonic seizures, such as carbamazepine, phenytoin or phenobarbital. It is important to recognize this diagnosis so that antiepileptic therapy is not unduly prolonged. Patients who are seizure free for one or two years are candidates for discontinuation of drug therapy.

GENERAL PRINCIPLES OF DRUG THERAPY

The goal of epilepsy therapy is to prevent seizures and avoid side effects. Usually this means that antiepileptic drugs will be taken chronically. Because patients differ considerably from one another, it is necessary to individualize their therapies. The factors to be considered when individualizing include seizure type and frequency, patient characteristics, pharmacokinetics, concurrent drug therapy, duration of therapy, and potential drug side effects.

The process of individualizing chronic drug therapy uses several techniques. The most important of these are repeated history taking and patient examination. Laboratory tests, including drug level monitoring, are adjuncts to the overall process. Drug level measurement provide an important, objective basis for adjusting therapy. If the patient's epilepsy is intense, requiring multiple antiepileptic drugs, monitoring drug levels is essential.

After it is determined that the patient has epilepsy, therapy should be initiated with an antiepileptic drug that is appropriate to the patient's type of seizure(s) and epilepsy (Table 3). The initial dose and route of drug administration are dictated by the gravity of the clinical situation. If status epilepticus is present, it is necessary to give high doses of antiepileptic drugs intravenously and to provide intensive support of the patient's vital functions. The goal in treating status is to stop the seizures. The correct doses are those that work; drug levels are of secondary importance. On the other hand, monitoring drug levels is very helpful during long-term therapy.

If seizures are brief and infrequent, therapy can be initiated more gradually in a manner that minimizes the chance of acute side effects and enhances patient acceptance of the drug therapy. Since epilepsy is a chronic disease, patient education and other factors that facilitate compliance are especially important. Patients who have epilepsy often have other problems that require as much attention as their drug treatment.

When therapy is started, it is optimal if the drug dose is low initially and gradually increased to an average value over approximately three weeks. In many cases, a low initial dose does not work. If the initial dose is ineffective, it should be increased until either seizures are controlled or side effects occur. If significant side effects occur, the dose must be reduced.

If an initial drug remains ineffective at the highest tolerated dose, its dosage level should be tapered while therapy is instituted with a different drug. Whenever possible, patients should be treated with a single antiepileptic drug, so-called monotherapy. Monotherapy can be expected to

Table 3. PHARMACOKINETICS OF FREQUENTLY USED ANTICONVULSANT DRUGS

Drug	Dosage Range (mg/kg/day)	Route of Administration	Therapeutic Range (µg/ml)	Half-life Range (hours)
Used Primarily in Partial and Generalized Tonic-Clonic Seizures				
Phenobarbital	1–5	PO, IV, IM	10–20	30–150
Primidone	10–20	PO	8–?	6–8
Carbamazepine	15–25	PO	4–12	10–30
Phenytoin	4–12	PO, IV	10–20	3–60*
Methsuximide	10–20	PO	10–20†	18–30
Used Primarily in Absence Seizures				
Ethosuximide	10–40‡	PO	45–100	24–42
Valproic acid	10–70§	PO, PR	50–100	4–15
Clonazepam	0.03–0.1	PO	0.02–0.07	16–60
Acetazolamide	10–20	PO, IV		
Trimethadione	30–60	PO	700–1200‖	150–300

* Effective half-life increases with level.
† N-desmethyl metabolite.
‡ Manufacturer's note: The optimal dosage for most children in 20 mg/kg/day.
§ The maximum recommended dose for adults is 60 mg/kg/day. The dose of 70 mg/kg/day is higher than manufacturer recommends.
‖ N-desmethyl metabolite, dimethadione.

control between 50 and 80% of patients. Several studies have shown that when multiple antiepileptic drugs are given simultaneously, side effects are common. Thus drug toxicity is a highly important issue among those patients who might benefit from taking more than one drug.

Adjusting the Dose

Adjusting the dose is necessary in more than half of children. Children vary greatly in their capacity to eliminate drugs, more so than adults. In addition, they require larger relative doses than adults to achieve comparable blood levels and effects. Because this variability is so great, a dosage based on weight is unreliable for approximately half of pediatric patients.

Newborns who are sick and require drug therapy have the largest range of drug clearances and half-lives of any age group. During the first month of life, drug-eliminating capacity and dosage requirements sometimes increase as much as fourfold. After the newborn period, intrapatient changes in dosage requirements are usually not a problem unless the patient develops an illness or takes another medication that alters the drug-eliminating process. Changes in body size due to growth have less effect than expected on the relationship between drug dose and concentration because the relative drug clearance also declines with age. Whereas infants sometimes "outgrow" drug doses, this is an infrequent situation in older children. For most antiepileptic drugs "adult" values for relative clearance and half-life are seen after age 10 to 15 years.

Patients having incomplete seizure control or troublesome side effects should have their drug therapy changed. If the problem is continuing seizures and there are side effects, therapy should be switched to another antiepileptic drug. Before the new drug is added, appropriate baseline laboratory tests should be done and the concentration of the current anticonvulsant drug measured.

The guiding principle for the changing from one drug to another is based on maintaining protective drug concentrations. The new medication is brought up to therapeutic levels slowly to avoid acute side effects. Then the first drug is withdrawn. Throughout the process, periodic measurements of all the drugs involved can help the physician maintain antiepileptic protection for the patient and evaluate symptoms, if they occur.

Minor side effects sometimes occur during the transition, if the first drug was near toxic levels at the outset. These side effects are usually temporary and disappear after the first drug is discontinued. In this situation, compliance is enhanced by warning the patient about the temporary side effects.

Side Effects

Drug side effects have been classified on the basis of the time after initiation of therapy until the occurrence of the side effect (acute versus chronic) and on the basis of the relationship of the dose to the probability of the occurrence of the side effect (dose-dependent versus idiosyncratic). If the side effect occurs at any dose, independent of the concentration, it is idiosyncratic. Many idiosyncratic side effects, especially allergic reactions, are believed to result from genetic predispositions. However, certain neurologic idiosyncratic side effects are related to nongenetic brain abnormalities. These abnormalities are usually dif-

Table 4. MAJOR CHRONIC SIDE EFFECTS OF ANTIEPILEPTIC DRUGS

Concentration-Dependent Side Effects

Phenobarbital	Irritability, hyperactivity, sedation
Primidone	See Phenobarbital
Carbamazepine	Sedation, headache, neutropenia
Phenytoin	Ataxia, hirsuitism, gingival hyperplasia
Methsuximide	Sedation
Ethosuximide	Sedation, nausea and vomiting, ataxia, hiccups, eosinophilia
Valproic acid	Nausea and vomiting, mild alopecia
Clonazepam	Sedation, mood disturbances, minor motor status
Trimethadione	Bone marrow depression, nephrotoxicity, highly teratogenic
Acetazolamide	Metabolic acidosis, sedation,

Idiosyncratic Side Effects*

Phenobarbital	Increased atonic seizures
Primidone	See Phenobarbital
Carbamazepine	Ophthalmoplegia, choreoathetosis, dystonia, increased atonic seizures, hepatotoxicity
Phenytoin	Choreoathetosis, bradykinesia, pseudodementia, pseudolymphoma, cerebellar degeneration, increased atonic seizures
Ethosuximide	Hiccoughs, hallucinations, bone marrow depression
Valproic acid	Hepatotoxicity, pancreatitis, encephalopathy–Reye-like syndrome, hyperammonemia, hyperglycinemia, hypofibrinogenemia
Clonazepam	Behavior disorders

* Allergic rashes may be induced by any of the antiepileptic drugs. They are most common with ethosuximide, phenytoin, and carbamazepine.

fuse encephalopathies, which make patients vulnerable to developing neurological side effects at drug levels that would be tolerated by most patients (Table 4).

Acute side effects are likely if patients are started on full doses. If it is necessary to give high doses initially because of a high frequency of seizures, patients and parents should be warned about the side effects and encouraged to continue taking their medication. When the dose is low initially and gradually increased thereafter, acute side effects may often be avoided. The most common acute side effect of the antiepileptics is drowsiness and sedation.

Idiosyncratic neurologic side effects include behavioral reactions, movement disorders, and worsening of akinetic seizures in children with mixed seizure disorders of the Lennox-Gastaut type. Movement disorders are most common among brain-damaged patients. Examples include dystonia and choreoathetosis induced by carbamazepine or phenytoin.

An allergic reaction is an indication for discontinuation of the drug that caused it. Patients with generalized allergic reactions manifest varying organ involvement. Cutaneous, hepatic, or renal involvement may dominate the picture. Except for the case of valproic acid, hepatotoxicity due to antiepileptics usually occurs in the setting of a generalized hypersensitivity response.

Frequently Used Antiepileptic Drugs

Barbiturates. Barbiturate anticonvulsants, such as phenobarbital, mephobarbital, and primidone, are effective in partial and generalized tonic-clonic seizures and febrile seizures. The advangtes of barbiturates include low cost and a high index of safety. The negative features of barbiturates include a high incidence of sedative and behavioral side effects in children. Concentrations of phenobarbital greater than 20 μg/ml produce reduced scores on tests of motor performance. When therapy is begun, they initially produce sedation, which usually abates with time. Behavioral side effects, especially hyperactivity, are more likely to be permanent and necessitate changing to another drug. Because primidone is metabolized to phenobarbital, the two should not be given simultaneously. Mephobarbital is rapidly metabolized to phenobarbital; its action and side effects are due to phenobarbital.

Phenobarbital can be given by several routes. In treating status epilepticus it should be given intravenously. After intramuscular doses, peak concentrations usually occur in 1 to 2 hours. Phenobarbital can be administered repeatedly, to very high doses, in treating refractory status epilepticus, but patients must be adequately ventilated by artificial means.

Phenytoin. Phenytoin is effective for the treatment of partial and generalized tonic-clonic seizures. It is also useful in treating convulsive status epilepticus, for which its lack of sedative action is a major advantage.

Phenytoin has saturable, nonlinear elimination kinetics, and dosage adjustment requires special attention. As the phenytoin concentration increases, the drug-eliminating mechanisms become progressively saturated and the apparent half-life is prolonged. Thus, as the concentration increases, it is necessary to make smaller increments in dose to avoid unexpectedly large increases in concentration that overshoot the therapeutic range.

The advantages of phenytoin include low cost and a low incidence of serious systemic toxicity. Because of the nonlinear relationship between doses and concentrations, precise adjustment of the level is difficult in some patients.

The principal neurologic side effects of phenytoin are related to concentration. Most patients experience nystagmus with phenytoin levels above 20 μg/ml and ataxia and somnolence with levels above 30 μg/ml. At higher concentrations phenytoin causes choreoathetosis and tonic seizures.

Phenytoin is highly prone to drug interactions, the direction and magnitude of which are often unpredictable. Whenever chronically administered medication is added or deleted, the possibility of changing phenytoin levels must be evaluated.

Phenytoin should not be given intramuscularly because absorption is slow and erratic, although eventually complete. In most children, twice daily dosage is adequate if the dose is sufficient; in older patients, a single daily dose is sometimes sufficient. The different generic brands of phenytoin are not bioequivalent. Patients should be instructed to choose one brand and stick with it to avoid fluctuating drug levels.

Carbamazepine. Carbamazepine is effective in treating partial and generalized tonic seizures. It is available only for oral administration. Sedation is rare unless the dose is increased rapidly. Carbamazepine causes less behavioral toxicity than phenobarbital, primidone, phenytoin, and benzodiazepines. It also has antidepressant actions and is favored for patients with affective symptoms. Cosmetic side effects are uncommon. Carbamazepine causes a usually harmless dose-dependent neutropenia in 10 to 20% of patients. Idiosyncratic aplastic anemia is rare. The neutropenia is rarely severe enough to require discontinuation of the drug, but blood counts with differentials should be checked periodically. Neurologic side effects include initial sedation, to which most patients become tolerant, both idiosyncratic and concentration-related vertigo, and diplopia.

Carbamazepine induces its own metabolism, and its pharmacokinetics have been described as time dependent. Carbamazepine concentrations decline during the first 4 to 6 weeks of therapy if a constant dose is administered. This decline is to be expected and should not be misinterpreted as noncompliance. It is usually necessary to increase the dose after 4 to 6 weeks' therapy.

Patients who take carbamazepine alone in monotherapy tolerate higher concentrations than those who take it with other antiepileptics. When taken with other medication, side effects are common with levels above 8 μg/ml. Patients taking it alone rarely have side effects until the concentration is above 12 μg/ml.

Ethosuximide. Ethosuximide prevents absence seizures but not partial complex seizures. Neurologic side effects include hiccups, which are probably related to high concentrations, and hallucinations, which are idiosyncratic. Systemic toxicity is a moderate problem, due to a 10% incidence of rashes. Less often there may be depression of the white blood cell count.

Methsuximide. Methsuximide is chemically related to ethosuximide but has a different spectrum of activity. Methsuximide is effective in partial and generalized tonic-clonic seizures. Its principal side effects are transient sedation when therapy is initiated and inebriation at high concentrations. It is often used in combination with phenytoin or carbamazepine for refractory partial seizures.

Valproic Acid. Valprioc acid is effective in absence, atonic, and myoclonic seizures. It is the drug of choice for juvenile myoclonic epilepsy and is used as an adjunct in refractory partial seizures. It is recommended for primary generalized epilepsy with tonic-clonic seizures, but this seems to be an uncommon diagnosis. Valproic acid is as effective as phenobarbital in febrile seizures but is not recommended for this purpose because of its potential to produce hepatotoxicity, which may be fatal.

Valproic acid has a low incidence of neurotoxicity. Common side effects include transient alopecia, gastrointestinal upset, skin rash, and alterations of appetite. Drug interactions are common. It consistently causes phenobarbital levels to increase and phenytoin levels to decrease. Because valproic acid has a short half-life, it should be given in three or more daily doses, or a slowly absorbed preparation should be prescribed, such as the enteric-coated sodium divalporex.

The most serious though rare side effect of valproic acid is hepatic failure. This idiosyncratic problem usually occurs in the first 6 months of therapy, most often among young patients who are taking other anticonvulsant drugs. Liver function tests should be done before starting valproic acid and periodically during the first months of treatment. Unfortunately, it is not clear which liver function test is best for the early detection of this side effect. Transaminase determinations are most widely used. Valproate-induced hepatotoxicity usually causes hyperbilirubinemia, hypoalbuminemia, and abnormal coagulation test results when it is diagnosed. Because of dose-dependent reduction in fibrinogen has been reported, patients taking valproic acid should have coagulation studies prior to surgery.

Benzodiazepines. Among the benzodiazepines, clonazepam and diazepam are the most widely used; lorazepam and clorazepate may have advantages in certain situations. Diazepam and lorazepam administered intravenously are effective in stopping status epilepticus. Clonazepam is given orally in the chronic therapy of infantile spasms and atonic, astatic seizures. Benzodiazepines are reported to be effective in treating absence seizures in petit mal epilepsy but are unpopular because of the high incidence of side effects. In Europe, diazepam solutions are given per rectum to prevent recurrent febrile seizures, or to interrupt prolonged seizures. Clorazepate has been used in an adjunctive role to treat refractory complex partial seizures. Benzodiazepines are the drugs of choice for treating status epilepticus and seizures caused by poisoning due to local anesthetics, isoniazid, penicillin, and strychnine.

The principal side effects are sedative and behavioral. Irritability, disobedience, and reduced attention span are common complaints. When clonazepam is given over a long period, it is usually necessary to increase the dose slowly, allowing the patient to develop tolerance to the sedative drug actions. Some patients appear to become tolerant to the anticonvulsant actions. At high concentrations clonazepam can cause absence (minor motor) status. When ineffective, benzodiazepines must be withdrawn slowly over weeks or months, because of the high incidence of withdrawal seizures.

Trimethadione. Trimethadione has been rarely used since valproic acid became available. It is effective in absence seizures. It is highly teratogenic and is contraindicated in women of childbearing potential. Blood counts and urinalysis should be checked periodically. Nephrotic syndrome is a potential complication of trimethadione administration.

Acetazolamide. Acetazolamide is effective in absence and myoclonic seizures. Because it is a sulfonamide, it is contraindicated in patients who are allergic to sulfa. Sedation can be a major problem. Some patients appear to develop tolerance to the antiepileptic action, and thus it is used primarily as an adjunctive medication. Chronic therapy with this drug causes renal tubular acidosis and osteopenia, rarely with clinically important rickets.

Drug Level Measurements

Throughout the process of starting, adjusting, and switching drugs, monitoring drug levels is helpful in determining when and how much the doses should be changed. Drug levels are also helpful in evaluating the cause of symptoms that might be medication-induced side effects. When multiple anticonvulsant drugs are taken, drug levels are highly important, determining which drug dose should be altered. Repeated drug measurements also encourage compliance.

Drug levels should be measured whenever the patient develops symptoms that might be side effects or fails to respond as expected. If an initial low average dose is effective, drug levels are not necessary. However, children vary so much in their capacity to eliminate drugs that average doses based on weight produce reasonable levels only in half the patients. In the other half the dosage must be readjusted. When seizures persist or a patient develops symptoms that may be due to side effects, drug levels allow the physician to individualize each patient's dose with greater insight than can be achieved by clinical examination alone.

When should drug levels be determined? The simplest answer is whenever the physician wants to know the drug level. Most often the question to

be answered is, does the patient have a concentration that is sufficient to prevent seizures? In this case, the best time to obtain the drug level is when it is at its lowest point, usually just prior to the morning dose after the patient has taken the drug long enough for the drug concentration to be stable (at steady state). If the question concerns drug-related toxicity, a level drawn when the patient is symptomatic is most relevant.

To use drug levels effectively, they must be interpreted properly. The basis for understanding the actions of a drug in the body over time is the pharmacokinetics of the drug. Among the various pharmacokinetic measurements, the half-life is most valuable. A general knowledge of a drug's half-life provides a rational basis for prescribing how frequently the drug should be given and predicts how much time must elapse before drug concentrations stabilize after chronic administration is started. Drug doses should generally be taken once each half-life. For drugs with short half-lives such as valproic acid, this means that 3 or 4 daily doses would be needed unless a slow-release formulation of the drug is administered. Valproic acid has a half-life of 6 hours when taken with other medication. By taking the enteric-coated divalproex sodium preparation, twice-daily doses are adequate for a majority of patients.

It is best to check the drug level after sufficient time has transpired for drug concentrations to be stable. Five half-lives are required for the drug concentrations to be stable. Five half-lives are also required for the drug concentration to stabilize after a dosage change is made. In many cases, this is accomplished in 1 or 2 weeks. For phenobarbital or drugs that are metabolized to phenobarbital, the process may take 3 to 6 weeks.

Stopping Antiepileptic Drugs

After seizures are controlled for a period of time, the discontinuation of antiepileptic medication should be considered. It is important to remember that all antiepileptic drugs have side effects that are sometimes subtle. Often patients who were thought to be free of toxicity report feeling and thinking better after drugs are stopped.

The consideration of stopping antiepileptic drugs is especially important for well-controlled adolescent girls who are approaching childbearing age. All antiepileptic drugs have teratogenic potential. Trimethadione is the worst, producing malformations in a majority of exposed offspring; it is contraindicated in women of child bearing potential. Once the patient is pregnant, drug therapy usually should be left alone, because prolonged maternal convulsions, although rare, usually have disastrous consequences for the fetus. Therefore, the possibility of discontinuing antiepileptic drugs is best considered prior to the pregnancy. For most of the antiepileptic drugs besides trimethadione, teratogenic potential is low and the odds greatly favor a normally assembled baby, if drug therapy is needed. Neural tube defects have been associated with maternal valproic acid therapy. Alpha fetoprotein determinations should be considered in these situations.

Except in infancy, children with reasonable drug levels usually do not "outgrow" their drug doses. Therefore, it is necessary to reduce the dose if drug withdrawal is elected.

Infants who had neonatal seizures due to metabolic factors, subarachnoid hemorrhage, or unknown causes rarely require prolonged therapy. Usually it can be discontinued by age 3 months. When there are associated neurologic deficits, drugs are usually given until the young child is seizure free for at least one year.

Older patients who are well controlled for 2 to 4 years should be advised of the possibility of discontinuing drug therapy. Previously it was recommended that anticonvulsants be withdrawn after four seizure-free years. Subsequent studies suggest that the patients who can successfully be withdrawn after 4 seizure-free years can probably succeed after two.

It is difficult to predict who will relapse after drugs are withdrawn. Overall, among all types of seizures, the chance of relapse is around 50%. According to most studies, the EEG is of little or no predictive value. However, certain patients, especially those with rolandic epilepsy, petit mal epilepsy, and primary generalized epilepsy with tonic-clonic seizures have better odds. Probably in excess of 75% succeed. When patients have partial seizures, especially associated with neurologic deficits, or severe epilepsy with multiple seizure types, or prolonged epilepsy before control, the chance of success is lower. Approximately 25% or fewer of these types of patients succeed at withdrawal of all antiepileptics after 4 seizure-free years.

Discontinuation of antiepileptic drugs carries some risk. The major concern is that there will be a prolonged convulsive seizure, i.e., status epilepticus. When drugs are withdrawn, the family should be prepared for this possibility. They should have in mind a nearby medical facility with the capability to care for a convulsing child. Most of the problems that arise consequent to severe convulsive relapse result from inappropriately administering medications without adequate supportive care. Thus drugs should not be withdrawn when the family will be traveling in unfamiliar territory. Also, the period of drug withdrawal should not be a long one, making the time of high risk ill defined and unduly prolonged.

Except for the benzodiazepines, there are no reliable data indicating that tapering over six or more months is safer than shorter tapering periods. Although not extensively documented, it has been shown that patients who have taken benzodiazepines in full antiepileptic doses may have rebound or withdrawal seizures. Thus benzodiazepine dosages are tapered the most slowly, over a period of several months, remaining at each stepped-down dosage for at least two weeks. I generally taper phenobarbital and related drugs in three equal steps over two to three months. Phenytoin levels often decline precipitously after the first reduction in dose; thus the largest change in concentration occurs early in the withdrawal process. I usually withdraw phenytoin over four weeks. Other antiepileptic drugs, such as carbamazepine, ethosuximide, valproic acid, and methsuximide, are tapered in three or four decrements every two weeks, with completion of the process in six to eight weeks.

HABILITATION OF THE CHILD WITH EPILEPSY

Patients with epilepsy have more than their share of psychosocial problems, including behavior disorders and learning problems. In addition, the label of epileptic carries a social stigma despite the efforts of lay and professional groups to dispel misconceptions. The habilitation of children who have associated problems is a major feature of treating patients with epilepsy.

Oversheltering the young patient is detrimental to personality development because the child is not given the opportunity to acquire interpersonal and social skills. Children who have epilepsy should be reared as normally as possible. They should participate in age-appropriate group activities of all types. Behavioral restrictions are few. In some cases this means taking a few extra chances. Although children with epilepsy generally are advised to take showers, not tub baths, most authorities feel that children with epilepsy should be allowed to climb and ride bicycles unless seizures are very frequent. Protective clothing such as a hockey helmet is recommended only when astatic, drop seizures are very frequent. Obviously, judgment and common sense are required, but the rule "Better a broken arm than a broken heart" is usually applied.

In adolescence, driving becomes an important issue. Most states have guidelines that allow patients with well-controlled seizures to drive. The standards vary from state to state, but seizure-free periods of 6 to 12 months usually qualify the patient to apply for a driver's license.

Learning disabilities and other intellectual handicaps have a higher than normal prevalence among children with epilepsy. The physician caring for the child should inquire about academic progress and refer the child to the educational psychologist if there are problems. When test results indicate handicaps to learning or performance, the physician should support the child's getting appropriate help.

Plans for careers or vocations should be considered in adolescence. Counselors, vocational specialists, and social workers are particularly helpful. The schools and lay advocacy groups such as the Epilepsy Foundation of American are good resources. It is better to plan in advance for success than to try to get the patient going after a failure thwarts goals and leaves the patient unemployed and frustrated.

Febrile Convulsions

EDWARD F. RABE, M.D.

Febrile convulsions occur in infants or children with fever due to an infection in any organ or tissue except the brain or meninges. They occur commonly between the ages of 6 months and 5 years, with a peak incidence at 23 months. It is estimated that between 3 and 4% of children 5 years of age and under have had febrile seizures. Twenty per cent of the siblings or parents have also had febrile seizures.

One-third of patients who have had febrile convulsions will have at least one recurrence. The recurrence rate is mainly affected by the age at onset; thus, if the first febrile seizure occurs before 13 months of age, there is a 2.3:1 chance of recurrence; if between 14 and 32 months, a 1:2 chance of recurrence; and if after 32 months, a 1:5 chance of recurrence. It is equally important to know that one third of recurrences appear within 6 months of the first seizure, one half within 13 months, and 88% within 30 months.

The complications most commonly noted are epilepsy, mental retardation, and permanent motor and coordination defects. Death from febrile convulsions occurs only when status epilepticus (seizures lasting more than one hour, or repeated seizures without regaining consciousness between them for more than one hour) complicates the convulsions. Incidence of most of these complications is not definitely known, but they occur more frequently in children with a complicated perinatal course, onset of febrile convulsions before 13 months of age, or in those with an abnormal neurological or developmental status before the first febrile convulsion.

Epilepsy occurs in 2 to 3% of children with febrile convulsions. This is four times the incidence in other children who have not had febrile convulsions. But epilepsy does not occur equally in all children who have had febrile convulsions. Rather, it occurs more frequently in those with certain "high risk factors." These are a family history of afebrile seizures, occurrence of more than one febrile convulsion in the first 24 hours of the febrile illness, or the febrile convulsion being complex, i.e., it was focal, it lasted more than 15 minutes, or the patient had abnormal neurologic or developmental status before the seizure. If two of these factors occur there is a 13% incidence of epilepsy in such children before 7 years of age. Other factors that are reported to cause an increased likelihood of significant sequelae are severe febrile convulsion (more than 30 minutes in length) and multiple febrile convulsions.

Infants and children with febrile convulsions of any duration need systematic medical evaluation. This includes a history and a physical and neurological examination. Infants less than 2 years of age, or any child in whom the cause of fever is not apparent, should have a lumbar puncture. There are rare clinical exceptions. Other laboratory tests may be obtained if deemed appropriate, but none of the "routine tests" in these children have provided evidence not suspected clinically.

The usefulness of the EEG in these children is moot. In a single, widely accepted study on this subject, children with febrile convulsions who developed recurrent afebrile seizures (epilepsy) developed epileptiform EEG tracings *after* the clinical epilepsy. More information is needed.

Children who have had febrile convulsions are treated to prevent recurrence, and by so doing prevent prolonged seizures, recurrent multiple seizures, development of mental retardation or learning disorders, epilepsy, and other chronic debilitating neurological sequelae. In truth, the only proved value of appropriate chronic medication is that it prevents the occurrence of febrile convulsions. The previously cited data imply that more is accomplished by preventing these convulsions and their concurrent sequelae, but this is not proved.

Who should receive chronic anticonvulsant medication to prevent recurrence? Simple, brief febrile convulsions in infants and children over 18 months of age seem to be benign. Since febrile convulsions may appear with the onset of a febrile illness, only chronic ongoing medication would be effective. Based upon the foregoing information, infants and children who have had one febrile convulsion, and any of the following, appear to deserve chronic anticonvulsant medication: infants under 15 to 18 months of age; patients who have had a complex seizure; patients who are neurologically or developmentally abnormal; patients who are neurologically normal but have a family history of afebrile seizures; and patients who are normal but have had two febrile convulsions.

Management is concerned with treatment of the acute convulsion followed by treatment of the potential chronic state, i.e., prevention of recurrent febrile seizures in those who are at high risk for complications. Simple febrile convulsions are usually terminated spontaneously within a few to 15 minutes. Although convulsions longer than 15 minutes have been shown in one study to be almost devoid of serious sequelae, many other reports state that prolonged febrile convulsions are the ones most frequently followed by serious sequelae. It is prudent, then, to treat patients whose seizures have lasted more than 15 minutes, both to stop the seizure and then to prevent recurrent convulsions. A patient with a febrile convulsion lasting more than 15 minutes should receive an anticonvulsant to stop the seizure. Several options exist. They are as follows:

1. *Sodium phenobarbital*, 10 mg/kg IV or IM (250 mg/m^2 in patients weighing more than 25 kg). An IV dose will produce a rapidly attained level, while an IM dose will take from 30 to 90 minutes to reach a therapeutic plateau. The latter route will prevent a recurrent convulsion, but will not quickly terminate an ongoing status epilepticus. The IV dose may be repeated at 15 to 20 minute intervals up to three doses, if needed to stop the convulsions.

2. *Diazepam*, 0.2 mg/kg IV (never IM), not to exceed 5 mg in a patient weighing 25 kg or 10 mg in a patient weighing 50 kg or more. The dose should be given slowly, never diluted. The dose may be repeated every 15 minutes, if needed, up to two or as many as four times.

3. *Phenytoin*, intravenously, 14 mg/kg, at a rate not to exceed 50 mg/min. Blood pressure and cardiac rhythm should be monitored during administration. Rarely, IV phenytoin produces hypotension, which is the result of a high level secondary to too rapid administration. Phenytoin should never be given IM, since it is painful and the absorption from this site is inconstant. If the seizure is not stopped by the IV dose within 20 minutes, another anticonvulsant may have to be used.

4. *Lorazepam*,* a recently issued anticonvulsant, is not available for general use. In doses of 0.05 mg/kg, given IV slowly, it promises to be less toxic and have a much longer t$\frac{1}{2}$ than its benzodiazepine predecessor, diazepam.

The need to treat a prolonged seizure in a patient with febrile convulsions indicates that this is a complex seizure and the patient requires chronic medication. Whatever drug is thereafter used, the necessity to reach a therapeutic plateau level quickly must be recognized and an appropriate dose and route should be used to prevent rapid recurrence of febrile seizures.

Chronic anticonvulsant medication, such as phenobarbital, valproic acid, or rectal diazepam, is given to prevent recurrent febrile convulsions. Rectal suppositories of diazepam are not available

in the United States, and since one report of its use abroad noted poor compliance by parents, this is a poor option for treatment. Valproic acid in a minimum of two divided doses daily and in amounts from 30 to 60 mg/kg/day, aiming at a serum level between 50 and 100 μg/ml, has been comparable in effectiveness to phenobarbital. However, with its tendency to produce as many early side effects as phenobarbital, and its proclivity to produce hepatic toxicity, with death, and with no satisfactory indicators to predict these serious side effects, advocacy for this therapy has not grown rapidly. Phenobarbital is the most commonly used anticonvulsant to prevent recurrent febrile seizures. It is given in two or rarely three divided doses and in amounts to produce a serum level between 15 and 21 μg/ml (4 to 6 mg/kg/day). Chronic treatment has produced hyperactivity and poor sleeping in from 10 to 20% of children, with a tendency to note these effects as an exaggeration of pretreatment personality. There is no convincing evidence that phenobarbital produces adverse effects on intellectual development or school performance in children. Studies of adverse effects of phenobarbital upon the behavior and development of experimental animals are not directly applicable to children.

Whatever anticonvulsant is used to prevent recurrent febrile convulsions, it should be given for a least 2½ asymptomatic years. At the end of this interval, medication, especially phenobarbital, should be gradually discontinued over a period of 4–6 weeks.

If, during the period of chronic treatment, the patient does not tolerate phenobarbital, and valproic acid is either not tolerated or deemed unacceptable, are there other drugs to use? Phenytoin may be considered. It has been shown to decrease the severity of febrile convulsions in young children and possibly prevent them in children over 3 years of age. Its use needs further evaluation. Primidone may be considered, since it is metabolized to phenobarbital and one other effective anticonvulsant metabolite. One should measure and obtain appropriate phenobarbital serum levels when using primidone. A better tolerance to primidone than to phenobarbital alone has been suggested by some, but this has not been proved.

Infantile Spasms

ALBERTO FOIS, M.D.

Infantile spasms is a form of epilepsy with maximum incidence in the first year of life. The frequency of the disease is considered to be about 3–4 cases per 1000 live births. This figure has not noticeably changed in the last 15 years.

---

* Lorazepam (Ativan) is available in the U.S. but use as an anticonvulsant is not listed by the manufacturer.

Not all cases present the triad of Salaam spasms, hypsarrhythmia, and psychomotor retardation. However, in order to make this diagnosis, there must be at least two of these symptoms simultaneously.

Cases with well-defined neurologic disease, such as tuberosclerosis, TORCH syndrome, and phenylketonuria, or clear signs of organic CNS involvement, such as microcephaly, cerebral palsy, and malformations, are classified as secondary cases. Primary cases are those in which neurologic development is apparently normal prior to the onset of spasms. The so-called postinfectious cases, in which symptoms begin shortly after an infectious episode, are now generally considered primary cases.

Since prognosis appears to differ substantially between primary and secondary cases, accurate diagnosis is important and should be aimed at the detection of possible etiologies. Thus, before deciding on treatment, exhaustive neuroradiologic examination (especially computed tomography) and virologic, cytogenetic, and biochemical studies are necessary.

Secondary cases are widely considered to have a poor prognosis mainly in regard to psychomotor development, even if spasms or other types of convulsions are controlled. Benzodiazepines, particularly nitrazepam* and clonazepam, have been shown to be useful in the treatment of infantile spasms. Sodium valproate has also been demonstrated to be effective. ACTH was first used with good results in 1958 by Sorel; corticosteroids have also been employed with good results. Hormonal treatment has, however, been the subject of controversy, and as yet there are no definite guidelines for therapy. This controversy is particularly important in regard to the treatment of the primary cases because a number of authors feel that the prognosis for long-term psychomotor development can be substantially improved if treatment with ACTH or corticosteroids is started soon after the onset of symptoms. The literature is in fact rather inconclusive in this regard because treatment protocols and dosages of ACTH and corticosteroids are considerably different. This may also explain the great variability in the incidence of severe side effects during hormonal therapy.

The great variety of etiologies underlying the secondary cases precludes the possibility of evaluating the result of any particular therapy, but all authors agree that evidence of brain pathology is an ominous prognostic sign. Special reference is made to neurocutaneous syndromes, microcephaly, cerebral palsy, psychomotor retardation, duration of spasms, neuroradiologic abnormalities, or seizures beginning before the third month of life. However, one basic difficulty in evaluating different therapeutic approaches is the paucity of large controlled perspective series and also the tendency not to differentiate secondary from primary cases. Moreover, authors preferring the oral or intravenous administration of benzodiazepines and sodium dipropylacetate have not compared these drugs with hormonal treatment, particularly on a long-term basis. The more recent papers on the subject consider ACTH gel superior to either synthetic steroids, benzodiazepines, or valproic acid, particularly for primary cases, because of a subsequent lower incidence of epileptic syndromes and psychomotor retardation. The main inconvenience of ACTH or corticosteroid treatment is the frequent occurrence of side effects, including hypertension, deaths due to uncontrollable sepsis and pneumonia, skin abscesses, and candidal infections. Complex electrolyte imbalances can also be observed and these can be further aggravated by the not infrequent onset of diarrhea. Therapeutic protocols usually consist of high doses of corticotropin (40–180 IU/day), hydrocortisone (15 mg/kg/day) or prednisone (2 mg/kg/day). These drugs have been administered for periods ranging from several weeks to 12 months with different rhythms of administration. High long-term dosages have been questioned in the light of good results obtained with lower doses. Though no controlled therapeutic trials have been reported, current opinion seems to favor ACTH over corticosteroids.

Since 1954 we have used ACTH in the treatment of 211 patients selected from a group of 256 subjects with infantile spasms. The criteria for evaluation and therapy were the same for all patients. The period of followup was between 3 months and 3 years in 120 cases and more than 3 years in 91 cases. In the group with the shorter followup, the primary cases were 41, and in the group with the longer follow up there were 27 primary cases. Extracted porcine corticotropin gel was used up to 1965 and synthetic corticotropin gel after that year. The therapeutic schedule consisted of daily IM administration of 2 IU/kg for 10 days. A result was considered positive if the spasms disappeared and EEG was substantially improved or normalized. In these cases corticotropin treatment was given two or three times a week for another 3 weeks. If, on the contrary, there was no improvement after the initial 10 days, ACTH was given in a full course for another 10 days, sometimes increasing the dosage to 4 IU/kg. If definite improvement was not obtained, the hormonal treatment was terminated. Nine patients died: 2 were primary cases and 7 were secondary cases. Normal psychomotor development was observed in 39 primary cases. There was a substantial improvement in another 8 subjects. In the other 21 cases psychomotor development and frequency

---

* Nitrazepam is an investigational drug and not currently approved for use in the United States.

of spasms were unchanged in 13 and slightly improved in 8. Among 143 secondary cases normal psychomotor development was observed in only 2 patients, one with neonatal hypoglycemia and the other with congenital hypothyroidism. Disappearance of spasms was noted in 61 and normalization of EEG in 15 children. There was a definite improvement in 10 of 19 tuberosclerosis patients.

The side effects from this therapy were insignificant and consisted in slight hypertension, moderate weight increase, and sometimes diarrhea, which subsided with proper treatment.

The long-term results obtained in primary cases seem to justify the use of low doses and relatively short periods of corticotropin treatment in primary cases of infantile spasms. In secondary cases hormonal treatment was only partially beneficial. Anticonvulsive therapy was associated with corticotropin therapy in most of our cases. Benzodiazepines, sodium valproate, and phenobarbital were more commonly employed. These drugs were the fundamental treatment in secondary cases. In 5 of the more recently observed primary cases we have tried not giving any anticonvulsant after the corticotropin therapy. These children at present have normal psychomotor development, no seizures, and normal EEG.

In conclusion, the following guidelines for the treatment of infantile spasms can be suggested.

1. ACTH treatment can improve the prognosis of primary cases of infantile spasms and should be considered the first therapy. The use of low doses for short periods is suggested, as side effects seem to be dose dependent.

2. Close observation of the patients for side effects is essential. Bacterial infections must be excluded before starting hormonal treatment. It is also advisable to check for unapparent or apparent viral infections, especially from cytomegalovirus or herpes. These would be a contraindication to hormonal treatment.

3. Close monitoring of blood electrolytes, blood pressure, and weight is also very important. A low-sodium diet is recommended, with supplementary potassium salts administered when necessary; diuretics may be used if fluid retention is excessive. Other side effects such as osteoporosis, transient glycosuria, thrombocytosis, hyperaminoaciduria, and aminoacidemia are usually not observed with the low-dose therapeutic regimen.

4. No more than two 10-day courses of ACTH should be administered. Longer periods do not seem to improve the prognosis for psychomotor development. Only conventional anticonvulsants should thereafter be used.

5. Complete therapeutic results are more frequently obtained if treatment is started within a month of the onset of symptoms.

6. More extensive trials seem to be justified in order to evaluate the possibility of therapy with corticotropin alone.

7. Secondary cases must be accurately classified. Besides neuroradiology, extensive biochemical, immunological, cytogenetic, and virological investigations must be performed before starting hormonal therapy. Conventional anticonvulsive treatment, preferably with benzodiazepines or valproic acid, must be used first. ACTH or corticosteroids can be employed in short courses with the aim of obtaining better control of seizures.

Spasmus Nutans

WILLIAM D. SINGER, M.D.

This unusual benign condition begins between 3 and 12 months of age and is characterized by head nodding, nystagmus, and head tilt. For reasons unknown, it begins most frequently during winter months. It is a self-limited disorder with spontaneous remission occurring 4 to 36 months after onset. There is no sex preference. The reported incidence is declining, making this a rare disorder.

Head nodding, often the first symptom noted, may be intermittent or constant and may be either from side to side or forward to back. The nodding is not compensatory for nystagmus. It is accentuated when the child is upright and during ocular fixation, decreasing when supine, and disappearing during sleep. Nystagmus, when present, may be unilateral or bilateral but is more marked in one eye. The movements are rapid and of small amplitude, horizontal, vertical, rotatory or pendular in character. Combinations of these movements may be seen. The abnormal eye movements disappear when the eyes are covered and during sleep. Head tilt is the least constant finding, occurring in approximately one third of cases.

The diagnosis of spasmus nutans should be reserved for children who are neurologically normal and have no structural or functional abnormality of the eyes. It may be differentiated from the bilateral searching nystagmus associated with marked visual impairment and congenital nystagmus. The latter two are bilateral and do not disappear with advancing age. Congenital nystagmus may be accompanied by head nodding compensating for the abnormal eye movements. The head tilt must be distinguished from that associated with structural abnormalities of the neck, cerebellar hemisphere tumors, and abnormalities of extraocular muscles with malalignment of the eyes.

Computed tomography of the head should be performed because of the occurrence of symptoms resembling spasmus nutans associated with optic gliomas and frontal lobe tumors.

Headache

PAUL J. HONIG, M.D.

Headache is a common complaint of school-age children and adolescents. The discomfort is due to involvement of the pain-sensitive intracranial and extracranial structures (blood vessels, meninges, nerve roots, facial sinuses, orbits, teeth, muscles) or on occasion is psychogenic in origin. Children in families where complaints of headaches are frequent may begin to verbalize similar symptoms on a purely imitative basis.

Isolated or intermittent headaches rarely cause concern. However, when they are recurrent or chronic the physician is asked to investigate the situation.

The most commonly encountered situation is the child with a simple viral or minor bacterial infection who has a fever and headache. The pain is usually due to dilatation of intracranial vessels caused by the elevated temperature. These children frequently complain of intensification of the head pain with motion.

Other more serious infections of intracranial and extracranial structures are also associated with headache. Many times the site of the pain is a clue to the location of the infection. This is especially true in the case of sinusitis. The location of the headache helps to pinpoint the infected sinus.

A combination of antipyretics and analgesics generally controls headache due to minor infections. Headaches due to dental abscesses, sinusitis, and other causes disappear with appropriately directed therapy. The more difficult situations include the psychosocially produced headache and the migraine. Counseling or referral for family therapy may be helpful for the psychosocially produced headache.

An acute migraine should be initially treated with mild analgesics and bed rest. Sedatives are more useful than analgesics to promote sleep (e.g., chloral hydrate 25–30 mg/kg/dose, maximum 1 gm). Ergot preparations used early in migraine attacks can be very useful (e.g., ergotamine tartrate* 1–2 mg sublingually at the onset of the attack, repeated at 30-minute intervals; up to 3 tablets in 24 hours but not more than 10 tablets (10 mg) in one week). Sensitivity to ergots may vary, making proper dosage difficult. If migraines are frequent and severe, prophylactic treatment is indicated. Propanolol, cyproheptadine, imipramine, phenytoin, methysergide, and phenobarbital may be prescribed. Cyproheptadine is probably the safest to use (8–12 mg daily). Propranolol* 80–320 mg daily has been used successfully. Remember, this preparation is contraindicated in

patients with asthma. Since the natural history of migraine is variable, prophylactic agents should be given for 6 to 12 months and then stopped. Prophylaxis can be restarted if the attacks recur.

Guillain-Barré Syndrome

IRA BERGMAN, M.D.

The Guillain-Barré syndrome is an idiopathic peripheral neuropathy that often follows a respiratory or gastrointestinal infection and presents most characteristically with areflexic, flaccid, relatively symmetric weakness beginning in the legs and ascending to involve arms, trunk, throat, and face. Progression can occur rapidly, in hours or days, or more indolently, over 2 to 4 weeks. Numbness, paresthesias and crampy muscular pain may be prominent symptoms early in the illness, but objective signs of sensory loss are usually minor compared with the dramatic weakness. Dysfunction of autonomic nerves can lead to hypertension, hypotension, orthostatic hypotension, tachycardia and other arrhythmias, urinary retention or incontinence, stool retention or episodes of abnormal sweating, flushing, or peripheral vasoconstriction. The illness resolves spontaneously and 75% of patients recover to functional normalcy within 1 to 12 months. Twenty percent of patients are left with mild to moderate residual weakness in the feet and lower legs. Mortality is 5% and is caused by respiratory failure or complications of mechanical ventilation, cardiovascular collapse, or pulmonary embolism.

Specific therapy to reverse the pathologic changes of inflammation and segmental demyelination in the peripheral nerve is not available at the present time. ACTH, steroids, and plasma exchange have been recommended, but thus far controlled studies have not supported their efficacy.

Therapy is symptomatic, prophylactic, and rehabilitative and directed to the following areas: ventilation and airway; hypertension, hypotension, and cardiac arrhythmias; venous stasis; nutrition, fluids, and electrolytes; pain; skin, cornea, and joints; bowel and bladder; infection; psychological support and communication. Patients with moderate or severe weakness or rapidly progressive weakness are best managed in a pediatric intensive care unit.

Ventilation and Airway. Endotracheal intubation should be performed electively in patients who exhibit either early signs of hypoventilation, accumulation of bronchial secretions or obtunded pharyngeal or laryngeal reflexes. Ventilation is monitored by frequent spirometric studies, including vital capacity (VC) and maximum inspiratory force (MIF). The indications for intubation include

---

* Manufacturer's warning: Safety and efficacy for use in children have not been established.

VC $<$ 12 to 15 cc/kg; MIF less negative than -20 to -40 cc H_2O; weak cough, voice or cry; difficulty swallowing; drooling; and aspiration. Prolonged airway intubation lasting 3 weeks to 7 months is often required; the care and comfort of the patient may be facilitated by early tracheostomy.

Hypotension, Hypertension, and Cardiac Arrhythmias. All patients with Guillain-Barré syndrome require continuous cardiac monitoring and frequent blood pressure determinations during the acute phase of their illness. Mild to moderate hypertension is common but usually transient, lasting 2 to 21 days, and does not require treatment. Malignant hypertension should be treated with a drug of rapid onset and short duration such as sodium nitroprusside. Blood pressure is often labile, and severe hypotension can strike unexpectedly and be difficult or impossible to reverse in the patient on chronic antihypertensive medication. Maneuvers that decrease venous return to the heart such as sudden elevation of the patient, straining to pass bowel movements or urine, and use of high positive end-expiratory pressure should be avoided.

Venous Stasis. Pulmonary embolism can cause sudden death in either the acute or chronic phase of the illness. All patients must be encouraged to exercise their legs and feet to the limits of their ability, receive passive physiotherapy to the legs when voluntary movement is not possible and wear thigh-length elastic stockings. Treatment with low dose subcutaneous heparin should be strongly considered in older children and adolescents who have very poor or absent voluntary movement of their legs.

Nutrition, Fluids and Electrolytes. Patients who require intubation are also likely to experience prolonged pharyngeal weakness. Adequate nutrition should be ensured immediately with nasogastric or gastrostomy feedings. Hyponatremia caused by the syndrome of inappropriate secretion of antidiuretic hormone is a complication which can be detected promptly by daily assessment of body weight, fluid intake, urine output, and serum and urine sodium concentration and can be managed by restriction of free water. The patients should be provided with a low calcium diet because prolonged immobilization can lead to hypercalciuria.

Pain. Crampy muscular pain is treated with mild analgesics such as aspirin or acetaminophen. Painful dysesthesias or lancinating pain may require continuous prophylactic therapy with carbamazepine* (10–20 mg/kg/day) or phenytoin (5 mg/kg/day).

Skin, Cornea, and Joints. Skin breakdown and pressure palsies in the immobile patient can be avoided by use of a water or air mattress, soft pads at pressure points, frequent turning, and positioning in different postures. Facial palsy may prevent lid closure in some patients with GBS. Patching or treatment with artificial tears during the day and ophthalmic ointment at night is required for protection of the cornea. Physical therapy using exercises and splints to maintain full range of motion and functional positions at all joints is an integral part of therapy.

Bowel and Bladder. Urinary retention or incontinence are usually transient problems which require either the Credé maneuver or intermittent or constant bladder catheterization. Constipation is frequent and requires stool softeners, rectal or oral purgatives or enemas. Adynamic ileus and gastric dilatation are rare complications. Abdominal distension is relieved by continuous nasogastric suctioning.

Infection. Urinary retention and bladder catheterization increase susceptibility to urinary tract infections. Prolonged immobilization, impaired coughing, and low tidal volumes increase the risk of developing pneumonia. Appropriate antibiotic treatment should be promptly instituted where bacterial infection is documented. Chest physical therapy with percussion, postural drainage and appropriate suctioning must be aggressively pursued, both as a prophylactic and as a therapeutic effort.

Psychological Support and Communication. Inability to care for one's own basic needs, inability to communicate easily and effectively, and worry about prognosis pose a tremendous psychological strain on the patient with severe weakness. Frequent reassurance regarding the good long-term prognosis, help in doing as much for himself as possible, and development of an effective means of communication with a communication board or other system will help relieve some of the distress. Constant attendance by family, visitors, nurses, therapists, or "foster" grandparents may reduce anxiety and the sense of isolation. Occasionally professional psychological counseling is necessary.

The responsibility of the primary physician is to ensure that the diagnosis is correct, guarantee the safety of the patient's ventilation and airway, and coordinate a therapeutic team consisting of patient, family, physicians, nurses, respiratory therapists, physical and occupational therapists, play therapists and psychologists.

Chronic Relapsing Polyneuropathy

SANDRA L. FOREM, M.D.,
and ARNOLD P. GOLD, M.D.

Chronic relapsing polyneuropathy is a disease of the peripheral nervous system characterized by the subacute onset of weakness or sensory deficit

---

* Manufacturer's warning: Safety and efficacy in children less than 6 years of age have not been established.

in the lower extremities or upper extremities or both. At initial presentation or early in subsequent relapses, it is advisable to admit the child to the hospital for careful observation of respiratory status, including formal pulmonary function tests and serial bedside vital capacity or peak flow measurements at least once every 8 hours. Chest physiotherapy and incentive spirometry or inflatable balloons can be employed during the acute phases. General physical therapy and occupational therapy also should be instituted as soon as possible. If there is evidence of acute deterioration in pulmonary function or a consistent trend toward deterioration, then prophylactic intubation or tracheostomy should be performed and an arterial catheter inserted for frequent assessment of arterial blood gases. Orthostatic blood pressure changes and urinary output must be monitored and evidence of urinary tract infections evaluated during the acute phase of the illness. Post-void bladder residual is measured; and, if there is significant urinary retention, intermittent straight catheterizations of the bladder are begun.

If the patient's initial course evolves over more than three weeks, or if he or she is a known relapser, we treat with prednisone 1–2 mg/kg/day divided into three to four daily doses for 10 to 14 days, after which an attempt is made to rapidly taper the dose over the next 4 to 7 days. In children who relapse once steroids are withdrawn, a regimen of alternate-day oral prednisone at a dose of 1–2 mg/kg/day is given in once-daily dosage every other morning for 1 to 2 months, and then again a gradual taper is attempted. Others recommend the use of prednisone or ACTH intramuscularly.

In children who do not respond to steroids or show evidence of rapid deterioration, a 1- to 2-week trial of plasmapheresis, preferably before mechanical ventilation may have to be used, can be given 3 to 4 times per week using up to 55 ml/kg exchanges with synthetic replacements. If this is successful, continued, less frequent exchanges are advisable (usually one to two times per week) until the child shows evidence of maximal recovery. Special equipment is commercially available to perform plasma exchange in children weighing over 10 kg. If the patient weighs under 10 kg, or is significantly anemic, or if equipment requiring an extra corporeal volume in excess of 150 ml is used, then the bowl on the apparatus must be primed with donor blood. This will add the risks attendant upon any blood transfusion to this otherwise seemingly benign mode of therapy.

In the minority of patients who manifest continued severe deterioration after steroids and plasmapheresis have been employed, or if "steroid dependency" exists, a trial of azathioprine,* 2–4

* This use is not listed in the manufacturer's directive.

mg/kg/day, should be continued for a period of at least 3 months. Variable success has been reported in treating the severely affected patient with chronic relapsing polyneuropathy with other agents, including high-dose IV methylprednisolone in pulse therapy, nitrogen mustard, cyclophosphamide, chlorambucil, and poly ICLC. The use of gammaglobulin injections has also been reported with some seeming success. It is hard to assess the efficacy of any of these agents used alone or in combination in a disease that may be characterized by spontaneous remissions and exacerbations. It is necessary to monitor closely for evidence of drug toxicity if chemotherapy is used.

Appropriate psychological support of the child and his or her family is essential in this disease as in any other chronic condition. Close followup and monitoring of the patient is important between relapses, especially during periods of intercurrent illness, pregnancy, or emotional stress, all of which have been reported to precede relapses.

Familial Dysautonomia

FELICIA B. AXELROD, M.D., and RALPH E. MOLOSHOK, M.D.

Many of the clinical manifestations of familial dysautonomia are caused by a deficit in autonomic homeostatic function and sensory appreciation of peripheral pain and temperature. Both deficiencies can be accounted for by the decreased number of unmyelinated neurons noted in sural nerve biopsies and autopsies. Prominent early manifestations include feeding difficulties, hypotonia, delayed developmental milestones, labile body temperature and blood pressure, absence of overflowing tears and corneal anesthesia, marked diaphoresis with excitement, recurrent aspiration pneumonia, breath-holding episodes, ataxia, spinal curvature, and intractable vomiting.

Treatment is directed to specific symptoms and complications.

FEEDING

Breastfeeding is usually impossible owing to the infant's poor suck, uncoordinated swallow, and misdirection of liquids. Experimentation with different nipples and thickening feedings should be tried before deciding to eliminate oral liquids completely from the infant's diet. For infants completely unable to suck and thus unable to maintain hydration, gavage feedings are used as a temporary measure. If the infant accepts spoon feedings well, the gavage feedings can be discontinued. However, if the problem persists, a gastrostomy is indicated to maintain nutrition and avoid dehydration and prevent aspiration.

FEVERS

Labile body temperatures result in brief episodic fevers in response to dehydration, mucus plugs in the bronchi, excessive external temperature, and even stress. Fever often is accompanied by shaking chills, cold extremities, and lack of sweating. Antipyretics may not suffice. Cool extremities should be massaged while cooling the trunk by sponging or even with a hypothermic mattress.

A muscle relaxant often is helpful in reducing anxiety and muscular spasms during hyperpyrexia. Diazepam* (0.1 mg/kg/dose) or chlorpromazine (0.5 mg/kg/dose) has been found effective.

A persistent fever lasting more than 24 hours requires a search for a source of infection.

VOMITING

Dysautonomic patients have abnormal gastrointestinal motility patterns, making them prone to vomiting. Vomiting occurs intermittently in some patients as part of a systemic reaction to infection or stress. In another group of patients (40 percent), vomiting assumes a cyclical pattern. These vomiting crises often are associated with hypertension, tachycardia, diffuse sweating, personality changes, and, occasionally, hyperpyrexia. The cyclical pattern can be quite marked and is usually characteristic for that patient. The vomiting may occur once a month or even once a week. The crises can last from 3 to 72 hours and can lead to severe dehydration. Aspiration is an ever-present risk.

Management has five goals: (1) maintenance of adequate hydration; (2) relief of gastric distention to prevent gastroesophageal reflux and aspiration; (3) cessation of clinical vomiting with antiemetics; (4) relief of hypertension; and (5) induction of sleep, which seem to be necessary for resolution of the crisis. Despite the loss of copious amounts of gastric fluid, the dehydration is characteristically isotonic. A volume expander, such as Ringer lactate, should be given rapidly upon hospital admission at 10 ml/kg for mild dehydration and 20 ml/kg for severe dehydration. Maintenance and calculated rehydration are given with a solution of one-third normal saline in 5 percent glucose. Dehydration is best estimated on the basis of weight change. A nasogastric tube should be placed and set on low intermittent suction and continued until the vital signs are stable and nausea has abated.

Diazepam is now considered to be an effective antiemetic for the dysautonomic vomiting crisis. The initial dose is 0.1 to 0.2 mg/kg/dose IV. The dose should be effective in normalizing the blood pressure and producing sleep. *If hypertension is still present 15 minutes after the diazepam,* then chlorpro-

* Manufacturer's Precaution: Oral diazepam is not for use in infants under 6 months of age. IV diazepam is not for use in the neonate.

mazine, 0.5 to 1 mg/kg, IM or by rectal suppository should be given. If hypertension is not present but the patient is not sleeping, then chloral hydrate, 30 mg/kg, can be given as a rectal suppository. Subsequent doses of diazepam are repeated at 3-hour intervals until the crisis resolves. Chlorpromazine and chloral hydrate can be repeated at 6-hour intervals. Frequent monitoring of blood pressure is indicated, because the choice of subsequent antiemetics will be influenced by the absence or presence of hypertension. Cimetidine (20 mg/kg/24 hr) IV is a useful adjunct in reducing emesis volume. The crisis usually resolves abruptly and is marked by normalization of personality and return of appetite. At this point the patient may be allowed to resume a normal diet.

PNEUMONIA

Recurrent pneumonias are frequent. Repeated aspiration is probably the major factor in causing pulmonary disease, with most of the damage to the lung occurring during infancy and early childhood. Gastroesophageal reflux also may be a contributing factor. The signs of pneumonia may be subtle. Cough is not consistently present and is rarely productive. The child is more likely to vomit increased pulmonary secretions. Tachypnea is generally not evident and auscultation may be unrevealing because of decreased chest excursion. Radiographic examination is often necessary for diagnosis. Pathogens cultured from tracheal aspirations are often uncommon agents, such as *Escherichia coli*, *S. proteus*, or *Serratia*. Broad-spectrum antibiotics should be used until bacteriologic study permits more specific therapy. In the seriously ill child, blood gases must be monitored to detect CO_2 accumulation, which may be severe enough to cause coma and require assisted ventilation.

Bronchiectasis is a common sequela of repeated pneumonias. Pulmonary hygiene, consisting of postural drainage and intermittent positive pressure breathing, is helpful not only in the acute situation but also as a daily routine for children with chronic lung disease. Suctioning is often required because of ineffective cough. Chest therapy should be administered at home by the parents on a regular basis. Chest surgery is rarely indicated, as the disease usually is diffuse. In patients with gastroesophageal reflux, fundoplications have been performed if medical management has been unsuccessful.

SPINAL CURVATURE

Spinal curvature (kyphosis or scoliosis or both) will develop in 95 percent of dysautonomic patients by adolescence. Spinal curvature may start as early as 3.5 years or as late as 14 years. There may be rapid progression at any time. The completion of puberty generally halts the progression of scoliosis as it does in the idiopathic adolescent form, but puberty is commonly delayed in dysautonomia. Spinal curvature further compromises respiratory function, adding the component of restrictive lung disease to bronchiectatic disease.

Annual radiographic examination of the spine is recommended after the child starts to walk. Splinting with a brace is the only effective conservative treatment. The brace must be carefully fitted and the skin inspected daily at pressure points because of the risk of ulceration as a result of decreased sensitivity to pain. The brace may also impair pulmonary ventilation. Most patients rely primarily on the use of their abdominal muscles for adequate pulmonary excursion. A high anterior projection on a brace, compressing the epigastric area, may restrict breathing and even contribute to esophageal reflux. The orthopedist should be alerted to the possibility of these problems. If the brace is not successful in halting progression, or if the patient has a severe curve, spinal fusion is recommended.

CORNEAL ABRASIONS

Corneal complications have been decreasing with the regular use of artificial tear solutions containing methylcellulose. Artificial tears are instilled three to six times daily, depending on the child's own baseline eye moisture, environmental conditions, and whether or not the child is febrile or dehydrated. Moisture chamber spectacle attachments help to maintain eye moisture and protect the eye from wind and foreign bodies. If an ulcer occurs, the eye should be patched. Tarsorrhaphy of the medial or lateral part of the palpebral fissure has been reserved for unresponsive and chronic situations. Soft contact lenses have been found recently to be very effective in promoting corneal healing.

BREATH-HOLDING (SEIZURES)

The phenomenon of prolonged breath-holding with crying in the early years can result in actual cyanosis, syncope, and seizure activity. This is due to lack of awareness that it is necessary for the next inspiration to be initiated, i.e., the patients are manifesting insensitivity to hypoxia and hypercapnea. This may become a manipulative maneuver with some children. Such an episode is frightening but self-limited and, in our experience, has never been fatal. The cyanosis of breath-holding must be differentiated from that which occurs with mucus plugs. Both types of cyanotic spells can produce seizure-like movements and decerebrate posturing. Electroencephalograms usually are normal or nonspecific, and the frequency of either type of spell is unaffected by anticonvulsant therapy.

Owing to the lack of appropriate response to hypoxia and hypercapnea, diving, underwater swimming, and air travel at high altitudes are potential hazards. If the plane's altitude exceeds 39,000 feet, the cabin pressure will be equivalent to >6000 feet, and supplemental oxygen probably will be necessary.

AZOTEMIA

A large proportion of patients have a moderate degree of azotemia (20 to 30 mg/dl) and variable values for creatinine clearance. Although these patients do not exhibit clinical signs of dehydration, the urea nitrogen often may be reduced by simple hydration. In four patients whose urea nitrogen was consistently greater than 40 mg/dl and unalterable by IV hydration, renal biopsies were performed. These showed significant ischemic-type glomerulosclerosis. The high prevalence of this renal lesion has been confirmed by retrospective analysis of autopsy material. It has been suggested that these slowly progressive lesions are associated with labile blood pressure. Patients are being encouraged to maintain adequate hydration, especially during warm weather. Treatment of postural hypotension is becoming more aggressive (see below).

POSTURAL HYPOTENSION

Episodes of postural hypotension may be associated with actual syncope, complaints of "dizziness," brief loss of vision, or leg cramps. These episodes may also occur with micturition or with sudden change in position, such as after sitting or extended periods in a car or theater.

In addition to increasing dietary salt and fluids, the addition of caffeinated beverages has been very helpful. Elasticized waist-high stockings also are beneficial.

ANESTHESIA

Anesthesia for surgical procedures is associated with an increased risk because of extreme lability of blood pressure and diminished responsiveness to variations in blood gases. Local anesthesia with diazepam as preoperative sedation is preferred whenever possible. Large amounts of epinephrine should not be infiltrated because of the exaggerated response to sympathomimetic drugs. If general anesthesia is indicated, the gas anesthetics are preferred because of the rapid reversibility of their effects. An intravenous drip is maintained to assure adequate hydration and to permit the rapid administration of volume expanders and/or norepinephrine to combat profound hypotension. The amount and duration of norepinephrine administration is determined by the blood pressure response. In lengthy surgical procedures, an arterial line should be inserted for frequent monitoring of blood gases and blood pressure. If the patient is going to have a prolonged postoperative course, as in spinal fusions, elective tracheostomy may be performed 1 week before the major surgery, as it is during this period of inactivity that the patient is most likely to aspirate and develop mucus plugs and pneumonia.

Because dysautonomia is a multisystem disorder, the physician can render the family a great deal of support and comfort by becoming thoroughly familiar with its varied manifestations. Living with the dysautonomic child imposes a great burden upon the parents, who are aware of the serious prognosis and are faced with the care of a chronically handicapped child with the repeated life-threatening crises. A sympathetic, artful physician can provide needed reassurance.

Injuries to the Brachial Plexus, Facial Nerve, and Sciatic Nerve

JEROME S. HALLER, M.D.

FACIAL NERVE PALSY IN THE NEWBORN

Peripheral facial nerve palsy, partial or complete, in the newborn results from compression of the nerve in utero by dint of facial position against pelvic prominences or from misapplied forceps during the delivery process. Facial nerve electrodiagnostic tests are usually normal during the first 3 days even with complete paralysis. There is no therapy for this form of facial palsy. Spontaneous recovery is the usual course beginning within 3 to 6 weeks of delivery. Rarely will there be a permanent paresis.

Neonatal peripheral facial palsy should not be confused with the asymmetric crying-face syndrome or hypoplasia of the triangularis muscle. In this situation, there is no inferolateral movement of the corner of the mouth with crying, but there is normal deepening of the nasolabial fold. This anomaly is important because of its association with cardiac and renal anomalies.

Bell's palsy, or idiopathic facial paralysis, is an inflammatory neuropathy believed by some to be a component of a cranial nerve polyneuropathy most frequently caused by a viral infection. In adults, the most likely agent is herpes zoster. This may well account for the complaints of facial and retroauricular pain reported commonly in adults but infrequently in children. As with the newborn facial palsy, electrodiagnostic testing will initially be normal and of little value in predicting the degree of recovery. Children tend to recover more completely than adults.

Before considering treatment, it is necessary to have established that the paralysis is not associated with an active otitis media and mastoiditis or one

manifestation of a postinfectious polyradiculoneuropathy or brain stem tumor.

Although touted for use in adults, there is no clear indication for steroid therapy in the pediatric-age patient with Bell's palsy.

A very small percentage of patients have a recurrent facial palsy. Repeated bouts may result in permanent residua. It is conceivable that such a patient might be beneficially treated with prednisone, 2 mg/kg/day, for 10 days, beginning as soon as possible following the appearance of palsy.

BRACHIAL PLEXUS PALSY OF THE NEWBORN

Obstetric injury of the newborn infant's brachial plexus by excessive traction on the shoulder or neck may take one of three patterns, an upper plexus paralysis (C5, C6 and to a lesser degree C7, Erb-Duchenne), a lower plexus palsy (C8, T1 with or without Horner's syndrome, Klumpke), or total plexus palsy. If respiratory distress is present, C3 and C4 spinal nerves may also be involved, with a resultant hemidiaphragmatic paralysis.

The posture of the involved arm indicates the initial acute injury, but not necessarily the eventual recovered state. A flaccid limb without response to pin prick or to Moro reflex corresponds to a total paralysis. An arm inwardly rotated, elbow extended, and with fingers flexed and in the pronated position represents an upper plexus palsy. Abduction of the shoulder and flexion of the elbow are lost; therefore, the Moro response will be asymmetric or even absent. The lower plexus of Klumpke's palsy results in loss of function of the triceps, wrist extensors, and some of the finger flexors. Since the proximal musculature is unaffected, shoulder abduction is possible with a Moro response. X-rays of the involved extremity and the clavicle should be done to exclude fracture of the involved bony structures.

Therapy is directed toward preserving joint function and preventing contractures. Range of motion activity can begin 2–3 days after delivery. Splinting is used only to maintain functional hand position.

Recovery can begin within 2–3 weeks of birth. Limited return can be anticipated with a complete paralysis. Useful functional recovery of an upper or lower plexus palsy depends on intact sensation of the involved hand. Recovery may continue for as much as the first 3 years of life. The upper plexus palsy has the greatest likelihood of recovery, with almost full function, the residua being mild weakness of the most proximal musculature of the shoulder.

A brachial plexus palsy in the older child or adolescent resulting from penetrating injuries of the plexus is best managed by neurosurgical and orthopedic specialists.

Brachial plexopathy is an acute onset paralysis and atrophy of several muscles innervated by trunks, divisions, and nerves of the brachial plexus. Immediately preceding paralysis, there is rather significant, but transient shoulder and arm pain, leaving behind an area of hypesthesia or anesthesia over the deltoid, C5 root. The disorder may be unilateral, bilateral, or present sequentially on one side and then the other. Antecedents to this disorder have been viral infections, immunizations (not necessarily in the afflicted extremity) and surgery. Although steroid therapy has been recommended, it may not be effective and prognosis for a complete recovery is uncertain.

INJURY TO THE SCIATIC NERVE

This injury is most commonly iatrogenic, from a misplaced injection into the gluteal muscles. Irreversible injury to the sciatic nerve may be caused by direct injection of material, usually an antibiotic, into the nerve sheath or into the immediately surrounding tissue.

The sciatic nerve has three major branches: the lateralmost, making up the perineal nerve; the middle branch, the tibial nerve; and the most medial branch, which innervates the hamstring muscles. The least injury to a child may be a foot drop and sensory impairment over the dorsum of the foot and lateral aspect of the leg. Dorsiflexion weakness, sensory loss of the sole of the foot, and hamstring weakness indicate deeper penetration of the neurotoxic substance.

The only treatment of such an injury is to prevent its occurrence. If necessary, injections into the gluteal muscle might be directed into an area bounded by the anterior superior iliac spine, the iliac crest, and the greater trochanter, using the palm of one's hand to locate the latter, and placing the widespread second and third fingertips on the other two points. This area is free of major nerves and vasculature, providing a relatively safe segment of musculature for injections.

Hypoxic Encephalopathy

BENNETT A. SHAYWITZ, M.D.

In pediatric practice hypoxic-ischemic encephalopathy is seen at all ages. In the newborn period its pathogenesis is usually intrauterine asphyxia, though this may be complicated by postnatal difficulties including recurrent apnea, congenital heart disease, sepsis, and, in premature infants, hyaline membrane disease. Intrauterine asphyxia is typically diagnosed by low Apgar scores at birth, depressed level of consciousness, seizures beginning 6–12 hours after birth, and, often, frequent apneic spells. Other clinical features are weakness in the hip-shoulder distribution in full-term newborns and lower limb weakness in premature newborns, and disturbances in feeding and persistent hypotonia. Neuronal necrosis is evident in the cerebral and cerebellar cortices, thalamus, brainstem, basal ganglia, and, perhaps, in the parasagittal and periventricular areas.

While postnatal events may exacerbate pre-existing problems, in most cases hypoxic-ischemic encephalopathy is a consequence of intrauterine factors. Thus, effective treatment depends upon the identification of the woman who is at high risk for the development of hypoxic-ischemic encephalopathy and the subsequent careful intrauterine monitoring of the fetus. If signs of intrauterine asphyxia become evident, measures must be taken to deliver the infant by cesarean section as quickly as possible. After birth, the primary focus is prevention of an exacerbation of the hypoxic-ischemic events. Good supportive care must include maintenance of adequate ventilation; this may necessitate intubation and controlled positive pressure ventilatory support. Measures must be taken to treat such common sequelae of hypoxia-ischemia as seizures, myocardial failure, and acute tubular necrosis. Seizures should be treated with phenobarbital given as an intravenous loading dose (10–20 mg/kg) and then at 5 mg/kg/day to maintain phenobarbital blood levels at 20–30 µg/ml. If seizures continue, phenytoin should be added at an intravenous loading dose of 15 mg/kg and a daily maintenance dose of 5–7 mg/kg, designed to maintain blood levels between 10–20 µg/ml. Myocardial failure is treated with agents to improve cardiac contractility and prevent arrhythmias. Acute tubular necrosis is managed by appropriate fluid therapy, and, at times, dialysis. Sepsis, too, may complicate the immediate postnatal course, and appropriate antibiotics are frequently employed. More specific measures in the treatment of the hypoxic-ischemic insult itself, such as the prevention and treatment of associated brain edema, the use of barbiturates, and the role of glucose therapy, remain controversial in the newborn period. Their role in hypoxic-ischemic encephalopathy in older individuals is discussed below. A significant and often the most difficult part of the management of hypoxic-ischemic encephalopathy in the newborn period is determination of severity of the insult. Such an estimate is critical in providing the physician with a rationale for counseling the parents of the affected infant about the prognosis and potential complications. Thus, the mortality rate ranges between 10 and 20% and the incidence of neurological sequelae in survivors is estimated at 25–45%. These include a variety of spastic motor deficits (cerebral palsy), psychomotor retardation, bulbar difficulties, and seizure disorders. The treatment of each of these complications is formidable and includes, in addition to anticonvulsant agents to treat seizures, physical and occupational therapy, speech therapy, and supportive counseling to the parents. Details of each of these are discussed elsewhere in this volume.

In contrast to hypoxic-ischemic encephalopathy in the newborn period, which nearly always results from intrauterine asphyxia, the disorder in older children may occur after a variety of insults. Thus hypoxic-ischemic encephalopathy is seen in disorders resulting in airway obstruction, such as suffocation and drowning; as a consequence of obstruction of blood flow in the cerebral vessels in strangulation, severe brain edema from a closed head injury, or disseminated intravascular coagulation from sepsis or leukemia; and in sudden decreases in cardiac output, as in myocarditis or hemorrhagic shock. Such an insult immediately deprives the brain of substrate and oxygen for the formation of high energy phosphate, which is necessary for maintenance of the integrity of the brain. The clinical consequences are immediate and are characterized by sudden loss of consciousness, pupillary dilatation, and, often, generalized convulsions. Although survival with good neurologic functioning has been reported in rare instances (associated with drowning in ice cold water) of prolonged asphyxia (10–20 minutes), several minutes (2–4) of anoxia will usually result in significant neurologic sequelae, with damage first to mitochondria and neuronal cell body. The neuronal injury is compounded by the development of brain edema and local circulatory disturbances, which further exacerbate the hypoxic-ischemic insult.

As was the case in the infant with a hypoxic-ischemic insult, prevention of further hypoxia by attention to ventilatory support and maintenance of circulatory parameters is critical in these older children. Management of brain edema often plays a critical role in reducing mortality and minimizing neurologic sequelae. Cerebral edema is often difficult to recognize. Papilledema may be observed, but it is far more common after an hypoxic-ischemic insult for brain edema to be suspected and then confirmed after intracranial pressure monitoring. We accomplish this by insertion of a ventricular catheter lead to a transducer. Intracranial pressures are maintained below 20 mm Hg, a pressure chosen to maintain cerebral perfusion pressure (calcuated as the difference between mean arterial blood pressure, usually approximately 100 mm Hg, and intracranial pressure) above 60–70 mm Hg. Measures taken to reduce intracranial pressure include careful monitoring of fluid intake; administration of Decadron at a loading dose of 1 mg/kg and then a daily maintenance dose of 0.25–0.5 mg/kg; and periodic intravenous infusion of mannitol at doses ranging between 0.25–1 gm/kg. Mannitol infusion usually results in reductions in intracranial pressure within 5–10 minutes and a duration of effect between 30 minutes and 4 hours. We have also employed another diuretic, furosemide, at doses of 1 mg/kg every 3–6 hours as an alternative if mannitol does not produce the desired effect.

In addition to the treatment of the complications of hypoxic-ischemic encephalopathy described, investigators have attempted to mitigate the effects of the insult by measures designed to increase the tolerance of the brain to hypoxia. The first such attempt was the use of hypothermia to reduce the energy requirements of the brain. For example, with body temperatures as low as 16 degrees C, cardiac arrest can be tolerated for as long as 30 minutes; this technique has been employed for many years in patients undergoing open heart surgery. However, such extreme hypothermia is accompanied by major systemic complications, and this is not practical, even in intensive care situations. A less severe degree of hypothermia, though effective in experimental paradigms of hypoxia, has proven to be disappointing in the usual clinical situation.

More recent studies have focused on the observation that administration of barbiturates either before or shortly after an insult may offer some degree of protection against the hypoxic-ischemic episode. Their mechanism of action is not altogether clear. Barbiturates may act to reduce cerebral metabolism and reduce elevated intracranial pressure by reducing cerebral blood flow. Recent evidence suggests that a significant portion of the residua of a hypoxic ischemia may be related to the action of free radicals released during the insult which damage the lipids of cell membranes. Barbiturates are believed to inactivate these free radicals and thus limit the extent of the brain injury. More recent studies, using animal models, suggest that barbiturates have little effect on cerebral metabolism or inactivation of free radicals, but rather help by ameliorating the seizures that often complicate the hypoxic-ischemic episode. Until the issue is resolved in well-controlled clinical studies, we advocate the use of barbiturates in cases of hypoxic-ischemic encephalopathy complicated by increased intracranial pressure. We use pentobarbital at a loading dose of 5 mg/kg with increments of 1–2 mg/kg every 2–3 hours to maintain barbiturate blood levels at 30 μg/ml. This agent is more rapidly cleared after discontinuation than phenobarbital, which may be given at a loading dose of 10–15 mg/kg with maintenance blood levels as for pentobarbital.

Prognosticating the effects of hypoxic-ischemic encephalopathy remains a difficult problem and, to date, such laboratory procedures as computed tomography, EEG, and brainstem evoked responses have provided little help. In general, rapid initial improvement remains the most reasonable gauge of further recovery; children who remain unresponsive to painful stimuli for 2 weeks after the insult have a bleak outcome.

Reye's Syndrome

M. MICHAEL THALER, M.D.

Reye's syndrome should be considered in any child with an ordinary febrile illness, such as influenza A or B or varicella, who develops vomiting and behavioral changes. Hyperexcitability frequently alternates with lethargy in the early stages. The diagnosis is strongly suggested when serum transaminase, blood ammonia, and prothrombin values are elevated. In cases requiring invasive intervention, a definitive diagnosis can be established with a percutaneous liver biopsy, which reveals uniformly distributed fatty droplets.

Treatment of Reye's syndrome is directed toward (1) control of intracranial pressure due to brain edema, which interferes with cerebral perfusion and (2) correction of metabolic derangements, mainly acidosis and hypoglycemia. The treatment selected depends on estimation of neurologic status according to severity of the comatose state (stages 1–5). Initial evaluation also includes serum electrolytes, serum osmolality, blood sugar, BUN, serum amylase, and a toxic screen (blood and urine for salicylates, phenothiazines and acetaminophen).

Management of the Precomatose Patient

All patients with presumptive Reye's syndrome regardless of stage on admission are hospitalized in the intensive care unit and placed on NPO. Intravenous infusion of 10–15% dextrose in 0.3–0.5 normal saline is initiated at maintenance rates and then modified according to serum and urinary electrolytes and intravascular volume estimates. Potassium is provided as the phosphate salt at 2–3 mEq/kg every 24 hours. If serum phosphorus is >5.5 mg/dl or calcium is <8.0 mg/dl, KCl is used. In patients with impending shock the intravascular volume is expanded with a rapid infusion (20–30 min) of 5% dextrose/normal saline at 15 ml/kg or 5% albumin at 0.5–1.0 gm/kg.

Vital signs and pupillary reflexes are monitored every hour; serum osmolality prior to institution of osmotherapy is meaned every 6 hours; and intake, output, body weight, serum electrolytes, BUN and glucose are recorded twice daily.

Clotting studies are obtained (prothrombin time, platelet count, factors V and VIII, fibrinogen, fibrin split products) and deficits are corrected with vitamin K and fresh frozen plasma before invasive procedures are started. Support lines and monitoring devices are placed as follows: nasogastric tube, arterial line, airway intubation set to maintain Pao_2 at 100–120 torr and $Paco_2$ at 20–30 torr, urinary catheter, intracranial pressure (ICP) monitor, and central venous pressure line.

The patient is left as undisturbed as possible. If sedation is required, morphine (0.05–0.10 mg/kg) is recommended.

Osmotherapy to prevent accumulation of excessive fluid in the brain is regulated with an intracranial pressure monitor. Intracranial pressure is maintained at 15 torr with manual hyperventilation, followed by mannitol infusion (0.25 gm/kg over 5 minutes). Doses of mannitol are increased using 0.25 gm/kg increments at 15-minute intervals to a maximum of 2 gm/kg if the intracranial pressure fails to return to 15 torr. The serum osmolality should be maintained below 350 millimoles/liter, measured just prior to the next injection.

Management of the Comatose Patient

In addition to osmotherapy, patients in stages 3, 4, and 5 are often treated with barbiturate anesthesia. Pentobarbital is administered by slow intravenous infusion at a dose of 5 mg/kg per hour for 4 hours to a total loading dose of 20 mg/kg, followed by a maintenance dose of 1–2 mg/kg. Blood pentobarbital levels are checked every 4 to 6 hours until the concentration stabilizes at 30 micrograms/ml for at least 12 hours. Thereafter the blood barbiturate level is tested daily.

Withdrawal of pentobarbital therapy is initiated when neurologic status, intracranial pressure, and cerebral perfusion pressure have stabilized at normal levels for 24 hours.

The efficacy and safety of prolonged pentobarbital-induced anesthesia in Reye's syndrome have not been established, but dose requirements of mannitol for control of refractory intracranial pressure are drastically reduced in such deeply sedated patients.

Currently, the reported mortality of Reye's syndrome is 25–30%; an additional 15–20% suffer from neurologic sequelae. Recent reports link ingestion of aspirin with Reye's syndrome. While this association remains to be firmly established, the results of several studies suggest caution in the use of salicylates in children with varicella or influenza.

4

Respiratory Tract

Malformations of the Nose

GREGORY MILMOE, M.D.

Malformations of the nose, exclusive of cleft lip and palate associations, are uncommon. Their presentation at birth may lead to a constellation of symptoms reflecting airway obstruction and feeding difficulty.

The most distinct malformation is bilateral choanal atresia, for which emergency management of the airway is often needed. Initially, this may respond to simple placement of a McGovern nipple or a large gavage tube to break the seal of the palate and allow for oral respiration. If the infant responds to this, then one can wait several weeks before undertaking surgical repair. This permits the child to grow and also to achieve spontaneous oral respiration. Surgery is done either by a transpalatal approach or by a transnasal approach using the laser and/or curettes. Patency of the choanae is maintained with open tubes as stents for several months as one tries to minimize the tissue trauma of these tubes on the anterior nasal chamber. A transpalatal approach would be favored if the base of skull configuration produces a very shallow and slanted nasopharynx. Unilateral choanal atresia may show constant rhinorrhea but less airway difficulty. Surgery can often be deferred several years.

Encephaloceles and gliomas may prolapse into the nasopharynx and the anterior nasal chamber. Their removal is warranted to relieve the airway and minimize the risk of meningeal infection. A combined surgical approach is often useful and intraoperative radionuclide studies may assist in determining whether there is persistent CSF leakage.

Dermoids of the nose may enlarge with time and have the potential for infection. The presence of hair follicles in a midline pit is a strong clue. Excision is recommended after radiographic stud-ies determine the relation of a dermoid to the crista galli and the dura. One can use a midline rhinotomy or an H-incision for approach, with craniotomy reserved for significant transdural extent.

Congenital dislocation of the nasal septum can be viewed as a malformation or an intrauterine injury. In either event, it gives airway symptoms and rhinorrhea as well as having growth consequences. Replacement in the midline is indicated. However, this must clearly be delineated from molding of the alar cartilages and nasal tip in the birth canal or by traumatic delivery. This circumstance of molding will correct itself in time. The distinction is made by looking at the symmetry of the nasal floor on either side.

Hemangiomas of the head and neck are common and may affect the nose either mucosally or cutaneously. Both types tend to regress over 18 to 24 months. If they are expanding enough to compromise local function or if there is bleeding difficulty then a course of systemic steroids is indicated. This should be kept relatively short (weeks) and repeated if necessary. Surgical control of bleeding may become necessary. After involution is complete, the fibrosis may lead to sufficient distortion to warrant surgical reconstruction.

Malformation of the cribriform plate may lead to a cerebrospinal fluid leak. This may come to attention only after recurrent meningitis. Surgical repair is most assuredly done through a craniotomy, although a rhinotomy approach is feasible for small leaks.

Tumors and Polyps of the Nose

STEVEN D. HANDLER, M.D.

Inflammatory Lesions. The presence of nasal polyps requires a complete search for associated symptoms and any predisposing conditions (for example, cystic fibrosis, foreign body, immotile cilia

99

syndrome, chronic infection, and Kartagener's syndrome). The treatment of nasal polyps is primarily medical, with antihistamines, decongestants, corticosteroids, and allergic desensitization. Anatomic deformities such as septal deviation must be corrected and foreign bodies must be removed as part of the treatment plan. Surgical resection of nasal polyps (together with drainage and debridement of affected sinuses) may be required in children who do not respond to this regimen and who are symptomatic with nasal obstruction or rhinorrhea.

Congenital Lesions. Nasal dermoids are epithelial-lined cysts or tracts that present on the dorsum of the nose. Radiographic evaluation must be performed to make sure that there is no intracranial extension. Complete surgical excision of these cysts is required to prevent recurrence.

Benign Neoplasms. Hemangioma is a common benign tumor of the nose. Since these lesions characteristically undergo a period of rapid growth for 12–18 months before they begin to involute, a period of observation is recommended before considering active intervention. Corticosteroid treatment (20–40 mg/day for 4–6 weeks) or surgical excision is necessary for large lesions that present with hemorrhage, thrombocytopenia, high-output cardiac failure, or necrosis of overlying skin. Lesions that have not involuted by the time the child is 4 or 5 years of age may be excised for cosmetic reasons.

Papillomas are verrucous growths that are most often found on the nasal septum. Simple excision or fulguration is the preferred treatment for these virus-induced neoplasms. Fibro-osseous disorders include osteomas, giant cell granulomas, fibrous dysplasia, fibroma, and the brown tumor of hyperparathyroidism. After blood tests to rule out hyperparathyroidism, treatment consists of simple excision or sculpturing for cosmetic purposes and for relief of nasal or sinus obstruction.

Juvenile nasopharyngeal angiofibroma is an uncommon neoplasm that presents with severe epistaxis in prepubescent males. Surgical excision is the treatment of choice after adequate radiographic evaluation and embolization of the tumor. Radiation therapy is reserved for those lesions that have recurred after multiple procedures or that are unresectable.

Malignant Neoplasms. Malignant tumors of the nose and sinuses in children include rhabdomyosarcoma, lymphoma, esthesioneuroblastoma (olfactory neuroblastoma), and rare metastatic lesions from primary tumors below the clavicle. These lesions can present with clinically apparent cervical adenopathy. Treatment usually involves the combination of surgery, chemotherapy, and radiotherapy.

Inverted papillomas are low-grade malignant tumors that are uncommon in children. Treatment requires complete surgical excision. Since these lesions usually present on the lateral wall of the nose, the surgical procedure most often includes resection of the lateral wall of the nose and affected sinuses via a lateral rhinotomy approach.

Nasal Injuries

FRED J. STUCKER, JR., M.D.,
and RICHARD C. BRYARLY, JR., M.D.

Nasal injuries in children are often considered a normal occurrence of growing up. Unfortunately, the management may not be so routine. Many aspects tend to complicate the treatment of this common problem. An accurate diagnosis in the face of significant swelling and hematoma formation, which is a hallmark in the pediatric age group, is frequently impossible. An uncooperative, frightened child and lack of efficacy afforded by x-rays also impede a correct diagnosis.

Although it is true that injuries in children heal rapidly, a premature diagnosis can contribute to more problems than it solves. Unwarranted general anesthesia and surgical trauma may result from an early incorrect diagnosis. Fear of an inability to reduce a fractured nose after a week's delay may prompt one to avoid treatment, which contributes to a gross deformity and/or obstruction, at least until secondary surgery is carried out.

Nasal injuries in children can be arbitrarily divided into three broad categories. They can exist separately or in any combination. The three entities are nasal skeletal fractures, including those of the septum, septal hematomas, and soft tissue injuries.

Skeletal Fractures of the Nose

The diagnosis of a depressed nasal bone is often masked by hematoma formation in a child. The lateral bony nasal walls are not fused in the midline, and blows can depress these structures. Swelling and hematoma formation can obscure the depressed bone and may actually produce an apparent depression on the opposite side. Our approach for the past 10 years has been to delay any surgical intervention until a secure diagnosis is made. This often means repeated daily examinations until the swelling and hematoma have resolved to allow a more accurate assessment. These delays are usually on the order of 4 or 5 days, after which time most fractures are readily reduced by a closed technique under general anesthesia. If proper alignment is not possible, or there is a prolonged delay before repair, a 2-mm chisel pushed through the endonasal mucosa is utilized to realign the disrupted bony parts. There have been no untoward consequences using this very conservative operative technique in children.

Septal Hematoma

Most children require general anesthesia for adequate treatment of a septal hematoma. The consequences of failure to properly evacuate a septal hematoma are manifested by the severe saddle deformity seen in adolescents who have sustained nasal trauma as a child. This problem must be anticipated and looked for in all cases of nasal trauma. Some of the more severe hematomas are obvious by merely examining the nose from the submental view. More subtle septal hematomas can be diagnosed by bivestibular palpation of the septum with cotton-tipped applicators. The recommended treatment includes a generous dependent incision, evacuation of the hematoma, and obliteration of the dead space by a transseptal running whipstitch of a 4-0 chromic suture. Hematomas can occur on both sides but are usually unilateral. Obviously both must be evacuated in the bilateral variety, but the placement of the transseptal whipstitch is identical for both. It was once thought that the hematoma must progress to an abscess for the dissolution of cartilage to occur with the resulting saddle deformity. It is likely, however, that a hematoma, with its interruption of the nutrient supply from the perichondrium, will cause cartilage dissolution and saddle deformity even in the absence of an infection. All these patients should be placed on antibiotic coverage.

Soft Tissue Trauma

These injuries are broadly separated into animal bites, lacerations, and avulsions. Diagnosis in this group of injuries is obvious, but these injuries can be associated with either septal hematoma and nasal fractures or both.

Bites. Most of these injuries are animal bites and, in contrast to the situation in adults, human bites are very rare. The potential of a bite by a rabid animal must be considered, as should tetanus prophylaxis as in any contaminated wound. Bites are the least likely of all wounds to heal per primary intention because of the large inoculum of bacteria placed in the wound. For this reason, irrigation with saline under pressure is advocated as well as the use of fewer, nonreactive sutures in closure. The possibility of revisional surgery should be explained to the parents.

Avulsion. Full-thickness loss of skin can be associated with a concomitant loss of cartilage and endonasal lining. It is generally a good policy to avoid employing flaps for the primary repair of trauma, but at times they are the only possible source of adequate tissue, especially with the loss of inner and outer epithelial covering. There are few indications for use of split-thickness skin ex-

cept for the lining of a flap when providing two-layer coverage. Loss of skin can be managed by the use of a perichondrial-cutaneous graft from the ear. This graft's survival is very predictable, and there is little or no graft contraction.

Laceration. Lacerations can be either quite simple or very complex, especially when combined with other injuries. All lacerations must be explored to their depths to determine the extent of injury, especially to the underlying bones, and the presence of foreign bodies. The closure is dependent upon the location and extent of the laceration. In general, the policy is to employ the minimum number of nonreactive sutures to affect the proper repair. It is essential to accurately realign the parts without excessive tension, dead space, or foreign material, including sutures. All soft tissue wounds are covered with steroid ointment.

Epistaxis

HOWARD G. SMITH, M.D.

Nasal bleeding is a common childhood event. The thin, vascular, anterior septal mucoperichondrium is easily damaged by crusts or trauma. This most common site of spontaneous epistaxis is readily accessible for treatment by parent and practitioner alike. To treat this condition, proceed, or instruct the child's parents calmly to proceed, through an orderly sequence of first aid to control the bleeding.

Bleeding may cease without treatment following the 5–10 minutes necessary for spontaneous blood clotting. Use of aspirin-containing products and hyperactivity of the cardiovascular system may impede clotting. Application of pressure by squeezing the nasal tip for 7–10 minutes will control active bleeding and allow a clot to seal the torn blood vessel. The child should sit up and lean forward to prevent bleeding into the pharynx.

A cotton pledget soaked in vasoconstricting nose drops, such as 1/8 to 1/4% phenylephrine hydrochloride (Neo-Synephrine hydrochloride), may be introduced into the nostril and additional pressure applied. Leave the cotton in place for 1 hour and then remove it gently to avoid clot disruption.

Recurrent or persistent bleeding from a point on the anterior septum requires attention by pediatric or otolaryngologic clinicians. Chemical cauterization is preferable to electrocautery. The latter is difficult to perform in children and can produce unnecessary tissue damage.

To stop recurrent bleeding have the child sit upright on the parent's lap and face forward, with legs between the parent's knees and the parent holding the child's hands. An assistant positions the child's head. Explain each upcoming step to the child before beginning and be certain to mention those that will produce pain. Hysterical children or developmentally disabled adolescents and adults may require sedation and additional restraints.

Use axial illumination from a headlight or head mirror and open the nostril with a small nasal speculum. If these instruments are unavailable and the child is not actively bleeding, an alternative instrument is a halogen-illuminated operating otoscope with a large speculum tip. A suction source and a 5- to 7-French suction tip should be available. A 16- to 18-gauge angiocath-type plastic catheter may be substituted.

Insert cotton pledgets moistened with an anesthetic vasoconstrictor, such as 4% cocaine or 4% lidocaine with added epinephrine, into each nostril and wait 5 minutes. Remove the pledget and firmly press a silver nitrate stick against the broken blood vessel for 30–40 seconds. Warn the child to expect pressure, then a burning sensation within the nose. Use a cotton applicator stick to remove excess silver nitrate.

Remind the child not to touch the cautery site or wipe secretions from the nose into the eyes. Have the child avoid strenuous physical activity for 1 week. The parents should apply moistening agents such as saline nose drops or petrolatum to the site on a daily basis, use vaporizers to humidify the air in the child's room, and avoid the use of salicylates for several weeks.

The inability to locate a bleeding site poses both diagnostic and therapeutic problems. Active bleeding must be effectively controlled, and a determination of the cause of bleeding must be made. Active bleeding is initially controlled and the nose prepared for examination by gently packing the entire nasal cavity with cottonoid strips or gauze packing moistened with the anesthetic vasoconstrictor solution. After the packing is removed, a search is made for a bleeding site. Maneuvers to induce bleeding include lowering the child's head and the Valsalva maneuver.

Superior, anterolateral, and posterior septal bleeding can be controlled by packing the nasal cavity. Placement of time-honored packing materials like petrolatum gauze packs and iodoform gauze with antibiotic ointment is uncomfortable and requires the systemic administration of analgesics to supplement the topically applied medications. Newer materials such as custom or commercially manufactured balloons (Gottschalk Nasostat) and self-expanding tampons (Merocel) are placed and removed with less discomfort and with less damage to the nasal linings. This is particularly important when treating children with thrombocytopenia.

Packing materials should be firmly anchored to the nasal dorsum, preventing backward motion and possible aspiration. Packing is left in place for 3 days, and systemic antibiotics, often an erythromycin-sulfa compound, are routinely prescribed to avoid sinusitis. Hospitalization is not mandatory. A hemogram and studies of coagulation parameters should be obtained.

If no further bleeding occurs once the packing is removed, the child returns in 4–6 weeks for a repeat examination and sinus x-rays. A careful evaluation will determine the presence of a serious disease.

Hemorrhage from the posterior nasal cavity or nasopharynx is fortunately rare. When it does occur, it should be treated by an otolaryngologist in a hospital setting. It is important to identify the cause of the bleeding as well as to control it.

An intravenous drip is begun. A hemogram and coagulation studies are obtained, and the child is typed and crossmatched for at least two pediatric red blood cell units. Red blood cells and colloid should be administered to stabilize the patient's hemodynamic status.

If bleeding is temporarily controlled with a balloon catheter, an angiogram and radiologic imaging of the sinuses may provide useful diagnostic information. If identified, a highly vascular lesion is embolized to control bleeding and to prepare for an open biopsy and definitive treatment.

Management of continued posterior nasal bleeding requires the placement of a posterior pack. This is frightening and painful to a child or young adolescent. Deep sedation and systemic analgesics pose an unacceptable risk of aspiration, and a general anesthetic with endotracheal intubation is preferred.

During the procedure, the nose and nasopharynx should be examined for a source of bleeding. If a hypervascular neoplastic lesion, such as an angiofibroma, is found, plan the biopsy to avoid excessive hemorrhage. If a bleeding point is located, direct electrocautery may provide hemostasis, obviating the need for packing.

When a posterior pack is placed, always with anterior nasal packing, it remains for 5 days. The patient is hospitalized, maintained on systemic antibiotics, and monitored for signs of hypoxemia. If bleeding occurs through a tight pack, surgical ligation of the internal maxillary and anterior ethmoid arteries may be necessary.

Most cases of epistaxis can be prevented. The dry air of heated or cooled homes can desiccate nasal mucus, producing irritating crusts, natural targets for the probing fingers of children. The nose may be injured by blunt trauma or by the introduction of foreign objects into the nasal cavity. Allergens can produce irritation leading to excessive sneezing and nose blowing. Advise parents to maintain adequate humidification in the household and to remind children to keep their fingers away from their noses. Allergies should be treated, or their symptoms should be controlled.

Foreign Bodies in the Nose and Pharynx

HOWARD G. SMITH, M.D.

Management and successful extraction of foreign bodies in the upper aerodigestive tract requires careful preparation and skillful execution. Major emphasis should be placed upon protection and maintenance of the airway.

The nasal cavities with their scrolled turbinates and often boggy linings make ideal hiding places for objects of various sizes and materials. Diagnosis must precede treatment, but unless the parent or caretaker has knowledge of the foreign body's introduction or the clinician has a high index of suspicion, the foreign body may go undetected. *A unilateral chronic purulent rhinitis with or without sinusitis is caused by a nasal foreign body until proved otherwise.* Nasal discharge can also be bilateral if the foreign body and its associated debris are located posteriorly. Nasal foreign bodies may also be accompanied by epistaxis, nasal manipulation, and complaints of nasal and facial pain.

The inquisitive young child learns as much with the lips and mouth as with the fingers and hands. Small toys and pieces of toys or shiny objects such as coins, paper clips, pins, or metal screws readily escape from the lips and front of the mouth into the pharynx. Many sharp objects such as fishbones may be trapped in the tonsils or the base of the tongue. Other objects drop lower and find niches in the folds of the hypopharynx or larynx. Smooth objects are more often swallowed or aspirated.

If the parents know that a foreign body has been introduced, ask them to bring a duplicate of the item to the examination. If a foreign body is unexpectedly sighted during the examination, describe it or directly show it to the parent. Detailed information about or an exact sample of the object is of help in planning the extraction procedure.

Foreign bodies in the anterior nasal cavity, the tonsils, or the base of the tongue can often be removed successfully in the examining room, particularly with cooperative children and adolescents. Objects known to be in the nasopharynx or the hypopharynx can be safely removed *only* in the operating room under general anesthesia with a protected airway. A radiologic examination of the pharynx should precede the direct examination.

The infant or young child should sit on the parent's lap facing the examiner. The child's legs rest between the parent's knees and the parent holds the child's hands. An assistant gently but firmly holds the child's head. Anxious older children and developmentally delayed adolescents and adults are examined in the semi-recumbent position. They may require sedation with chloral hydrate and diazepam as well as additional restraints. General anesthesia may be necessary, even for an object that can be readily visualized.

The patient's nasal linings should be treated with an analgesic vasoconstrictor solution, such as 4% cocaine or 2% lidocaine with added epinephrine, in order to improve examiner visibility and patient comfort. The pharynx should only be lightly anesthetized with topical lidocaine or benzocaine (Cetacaine) in order not to interfere with sensations that will help locate the object.

A high intensity light source such as a headlight or a spotlight directed into the nose or oral cavity by a head mirror is necessary to provide adequate illumination while freeing both of the examiner's hands. A nasal speculum, tongue blades, small laryngeal mirrors, a suction source, several sizes of suction tips and cerumen wire loops, a wire hook, and a variety of forceps with straight, curved, cupped, or circular jaws complete the list of useful instrumentation.

Many nasal foreign bodies are located near the front of the nasal cavity, since forcing an object backward produces discomfort to the child. If a foreign body is small or fragmented, it may move backward easily, and care must be taken to prevent this from occurring during the preliminary portions of the examination.

Once the object is visualized in the anterior nasal cavity, choose an appropriate grasping instrument for use in removal. In one or multiple moves, draw the object toward the front of the nasal cavity while minimizing its fragmentation and any damage to the nasal linings. Suction will remove excess secretions, but it is usually not strong enough to extract a foreign body of any significant mass. If the object falls backward toward the nasopharynx, abandon efforts to remove it and examine the child under general anesthesia, during which the airway is protected by the endotracheal tube.

Remove foreign bodies with instruments that grasp and hold the object. Balloon catheters such as the Fogarty should not be used. Their introduction past the object may accidentally force it farther toward the nasopharynx. During the extraction process, the object can deviate upward or in a lateral direction, becoming lost.

Materials irritating to the nasal tissues, such as vegetable matter, can induce so much inflammation and friable granulation tissue that visualization may be impossible. A second examination after treatment with systemic antibiotics and topical steroids may be necessary to detect a foreign body.

Foreign bodies trapped in the upper pharynx produce localized discomfort, which helps the clinician locate them. Use the tongue blade to hold down the tongue and the suction tip to touch suspicious areas systematically. Play a game of hot or cold, and the child will guide you to the exact location. Fishbones or other objects with neutral coloration will be difficult to see until you are upon them. Once found, grasp the object with a forceps and remove it. The child's discomfort associated with the foreign body should immediately disappear, confirming that your extraction was successful and complete.

If there is a convincing history of foreign body introduction, but none can be visualized, a radiologic examination of the nasal cavity and pharynx, with or without contrast material, may locate the object. If it cannot be demonstrated by direct examination or by x-ray examination, yet the child's symptoms persist, an examination under general anesthesia is mandatory.

Remember that children may have multiple foreign bodies. After successfully removing a foreign body, take the time while still in the examining or operating room to re-examine the nose or throat and to survey the entire head and neck region for evidence of other foreign bodies.

Nasopharyngitis

(The Common Cold)

RICHARD B. GOLDBLOOM, M.D.

The symptom complex of the common cold may be produced by infection with rhinoviruses, respiratory syncytial virus, adenovirus, influenza virus, or parainfluenza virus. The lack of any specific or particularly effective treatment for these infections or their symptoms is emphasized by the variety of remedies promoted for the purpose.

Very preliminary studies have suggested that rhinovirus colds may be preventable by use of nasal spraying of human interferon alpha-2 from *Escherichia coli*, and that antiviral agents effective against rhinovirus may reduce cold symptoms in infected individuals. At present these are no more than attractive experimental possibilities.

Irrespective of its cause, the common cold is normally self-limited. Younger children in large groups, as in day-care centers, are especially susceptible. Prevalence increases with the opening of school and remains high through winter and spring.

These infections may cause fever, especially in younger patients. Other signs and symptoms are sneezing, sore throat, mucoid or mucopurulent nasal discharge with nasal obstruction, cough, conjunctivitis, headache, chills, and malaise. The acute symptoms usually last 3 or 4 days, often followed by several days of nasal catarrh and cough. Sec-

ondary complications, which may be bacterial, can include otitis media, cervical adenitis, sinusitis, and pneumonia.

The course of the viral illness is completely unaltered by antibiotics, and these should be reserved for infants and children with strong evidence of bacterial infection, such as otitis or pneumonia. Fever alone does not constitute such evidence. Antibiotics are of no value as prophylaxis against the bacterial complications of viral respiratory illness, and the practice of prescribing antibiotics over the telephone for infants and children with nonspecific respiratory illness when the child has not been examined must be condemned.

Treatment is directed at the relief of symptoms, of which nasal obstruction is one of the most bothersome, often interfering with an infant's ability to feed or sleep. Some relief can often be provided by using an inexpensive rubber bulb type of infant nasal aspirator. Parents should be instructed in the correct use of the aspirator, which can be effective in clearing the nasal airway. The procedure is best performed 15 minutes or so before feedings.

If nasal obstruction is severe, the nose can be irrigated with 2 or 3 drops of lukewarm normal saline before using the aspirator. Alternatively or additionally, decongestant nose drops may improve patency of the nasal airway temporarily and facilitate feeding. Phenylephrine (Neo-Synephrine), 0.25%, or xylometazoline (Otrivin Pediatric Nasal Solution), 0.05%, 1 drop in each nostril every 8 hours, may be used in infants over 3 or 4 months of age. In younger infants, it is best to avoid these sympathomimetic decongestants, since they may cause irritability and tachycardia, and to use only saline irrigation and the aspirator. For children over 6 years of age, 0.25% phenylephrine drops may be used, and 0.1% xylometazoline drops or spray may be used for children over the age of 12 years. Decongestant nose drops should never be used for more than 4 or 5 days, because progressively increasing rebound swelling of the nasal mucosa develops with continuing use.

Because otitis media is a complication of viral upper respiratory infection, one should remember that in infants the supine position during feedings (and possibly at other times, such as during sleep) allows fluid direct access via the eustachian tube to the middle ear during the act of swallowing. It follows that infants should never be fed in the supine position, and that moderate elevation of the head may be helpful during respiratory infections in preventing or relieving earache, which occurs most commonly at night.

When the onset of infection is associated with fever and anorexia, mild degrees of ketoacidosis are common, especially in young children and when fever is present. This phenomenon is often evidenced by irritability and acetone breath. The association of ketosis with minor infections is often overlooked, which is a pity, because the symptoms often can be prevented or treated by the temporary administration of any form of concentrated carbohydrate (clear candy, honey, lollipops, soft drinks) and by encouraging a good fluid intake. In this situation the same soft drinks and candy that are looked upon with horror by our dental colleagues may constitute simple but valuable therapeutic adjuncts, which can effectively lessen the crankiness that so often accompanies minor infections in young children.

A cool, humidified atmosphere, best achieved with a cold water home nebulizer, may give some relief, especially if the house is abnormally dry.

Bed rest is advisable only if significant fever is present. Concern has been expressed recently over the use of acetylsalicylic acid in the treatment of influenza virus infections and varicella in children, because of an epidemiologic association that has suggested that salicylates may enhance the susceptibility of young children to the development of Reye's syndrome. The causal significance of such an association is still unsettled. Until the matter is clarified, a conservative approach to antipyretic medication seems prudent, especially if the illness has features suggestive of influenza.

Minor temperature elevations do not require medication, and may be treated if necessary with tepid water sponging and encouragement of a good fluid intake. Pending settlement of the salicylate–Reye's syndrome controversy, acetaminophen may be given orally in the following dosage: under 1 year, 60 mg four times daily; 1–3 years, 60–120 mg four times daily; 3–6 years, 120 mg four times daily; 6–12 years, 150–300 mg four times daily. Or dosage may be calculated on the basis of surface area, giving 700 mg/m^2/24 hours, divided into 4–6 doses.

Alternatively, and in the absence of influenza-like features (and of chickenpox), acetylsalicylic acid may be given in a dose of 65 mg/kg/24 hours, divided into 4–6 doses. Antipyretics are rarely required for more than one or two days.

Innumerable cold remedies are available over the counter and are prescribed widely by physicians. These include assorted combinations of vitamin C, sympathomimetics ("oral decongestants"), antihistamines, antitussives, analgesics and/or belladonna alkaloids.

Vitamin C has not been shown to have significant therapeutic or prophylactic value. Orally administered sympathomimetics are of questionable or limited value in diminishing nasal congestion. The dose sufficient to do so may also cause some degree of general vasoconstriction and a rise in blood pressure.

As for antihistamines, the few studies that have been well designed and controlled show no benefit attributable to antihistamine administration for prevention or relief of the common cold. These compounds may have some drying and inspissating effect on secretions; they also commonly have a pronounced sedative effect—a consideration that may have special importance for adolescents of driving age in whom drowsiness may render driving dangerous. Antihistamines may be expected to provide some relief to nasal congestion only if allergic rhinitis is present.

Oral decongestant mixtures, with or without antihistamines, do not reduce the frequency of otitis as a complication of colds, nor do they improve the course or outcome of otitis itself.

Sympathomimetic-antihistamine mixtures are even available in oral drop dosage form. These may carry particular risks for young infants, in whom we have observed hypercapnia attributable to respiratory depression following their use, especially if the infant happened to be mildly dehydrated. Too often these mixtures are prescribed principally as a result of advertising pressure or as the easiest way to deal with parental pressure to "do something." This sort of parental anxiety is normal and should be dealt with more directly through reassurance and explanation of what can be expected in the normal course of the illness. The emotional tolerance of different families for the normal frequency of respiratory illness in their children is variable. Many parents are unaware of the fact that the average North American preschooler or young school-age child has 5 or 6 minor respiratory infections per year.

Removal of the tonsils and adenoids is without effect on the frequency of viral upper respiratory infections, and the empirical administration of gamma globulin under such circumstances is completely without logical foundation or demonstrated value. Kleenex and "tincture of time" remain the bulwarks of treatment of the common cold.

Rhinitis and Sinusitis

DACHLING PANG, M.D., F.R.C.S. (C), F.A.C.S., and ELLEN R. WALD, M.D.

Infections of the upper respiratory tract are the most common reason for seeking medical care. Most of these infections are caused by viruses and require no specific therapy; symptomatic treatment may increase patient comfort. However, other respiratory infections such as otitis media and sinusitis may be primarily bacterial or may be complicated by impaired local drainage resulting in bacterial superinfection.

RHINITIS

Rhinitis, when acute, is almost exclusively caused by respiratory viruses, and as such requires no antimicrobial treatment. However, in the newborn period rhinitis may be due to congenital syphilis.

Persistent rhinitis in infants or young children (less than 3 years old) suggests the possibility of group A beta-hemolytic streptococcal infection, or "streptococcosis." Streptococcal infection in this age group often fails to localize in the throat and instead causes a clinical picture of a protracted cold. Occasionally an older child (over 5 years of age) with streptococcal infection presents with persistent nasal discharge and cough.

If streptococcal infection is documented by culture of the nasopharynx or throat, treatment with penicillin for 10 days is appropriate. Dosages of phenoxymethyl penicillin of 125 mg three or four times daily for those under 60 pounds and 250 mg three or four times daily for those over 60 pounds are recommended. In penicillin-allergic patients erythromycin at 40 mg/kg/day in four divided doses is a suitable substitute.

In both infants and older children the likelihood of paranasal sinusitis should be considered as a cause of persistent nasal discharge (see next section on sinusitis). Purulent rhinorrhea may also be indicative of an intranasal foreign body, especially if fetor oris is prominent or if the discharge is unilateral or bloody or both.

Whether bacteria other than group A streptococci may cause purulent rhinitis has not been adequately evaluated. The use of antimicrobial preparations cannot therefore be recommended in the management of the routine upper respiratory infection. However, there are data suggesting that antibiotic prophylaxis (daily or during the course of a cold) may be effective in preventing symptomatic episodes of acute otitis media in otitis-prone children.

Children with persistent rhinitis may be demonstrating symptoms of allergic inflammation or vasomotor rhinitis. Children with the former problem may have a positive family history of allergies or the physical stigmata of allergic problems. Symptomatic treatment with oral antihistamines or decongestants or combination agents may result in prompt improvement. Cromolyn sodium and aerosal steroid preparations may be helpful in older patients with chronic allergic nasal symptoms. Reduction of environmental allergens should always be undertaken. If simple measures of avoidance and symptomatic therapy fail, desensitization may be necessary.

SINUSITIS

There is a paucity of literature on the efficacy of antimicrobial therapy for sinusitis in children. However, in adults, although there are conflicting reports regarding the benefit of antimicrobials, several points emerge. (1) Appropriate antimicrobials eradicate susceptible microorganisms in sinus secretions; inappropriate agents fail to do so. (2) In order to accomplish sterilization of the sinus secretions, a level of antimicrobial agent exceeding the minimum inhibitory concentration of the infecting microorganism must be present in the sinus secretions. (3) In some instances in which adequate antimicrobial levels within sinus secretions are documented, sterilization of secretions is still not accomplished. This observation points to the importance of local defense mechanisms (such as ciliary activity and phagocytosis), which may be impaired in the altered environment within the purulent sinus secretions (decreased partial pressure of oxygen, increased carbon dioxide pressure, and decreased pH.) Therefore, irrigation and drainage of sinus secretions may be required in some patients. (4) There does appear to be a decrease in the serious suppurative orbital and intracranial complications of paranasal sinus disease consequent to the systemic use of antimicrobials, and currently medical therapy with an appropriate antimicrobial agent is recommended in children with acute sinusitis. The recommended treatment is amoxicillin (40 mg/kg/day in three divided doses) or ampicillin (100 mg/kg/day in four divided doses). Both these drugs are relatively safe, inexpensive, and active against the common bacterial pathogens as well as most anaerobic organisms found in the sinuses.

Alternative antimicrobials, which may be useful if the patient is allergic to penicillin or if there is a high local prevalence of beta-lactamase–producing *Hemophilus influenzae* or *Branhamella catarrhalis*, are trimethoprim/sulfamethoxazole* (8 and 40 mg/kg/day, respectively, in two divided doses) or erythromycin-sulfisoxazole* (50 and 150 mg/kg/day in four divided doses) or cefaclor (40 mg/kg/day in three divided doses). Trimethoprim-sulfamethoxazole is not optimal therapy for *Streptococcus pyogenes* and is therefore not the best choice as an amoxicillin alternative in the 5 to 15 year age group, an age group in which *S. pyogenes* is most likely to be encountered. Cefaclor, while a reasonable substitute for amoxicillin in selected patients, has been noted to be ineffective in vitro against approximately 40% of the beta-lactamase–producing *B. catarrhalis*. A new drug combination consisting of amoxicillin and potassium clavulanate (Augmentin) is also suitable for use in patients who have sustained a clinical failure with amoxicillin or reside in geographic areas where there is a high prevalence of beta-lactamase–producing bacterial species. Potassium clavulanate is an irre-

---

* Manufacturer's warning: Contraindicated in children less than 2 months of age.

versible beta-lactamase inhibitor. If this drug combination is used in treating an infection with a beta-lactamase–producing bacterial species, the beta-lactamase will be bound by the inhibitor and the amoxicillin restored to its original spectrum of activity.

In pediatric patients who require parenteral therapy for acute sinusitis but who do not have intracranial or intraorbital complications, cefuroxime at 150 mg/kg/day in 3 divided doses given intravenously is ideal. This agent is suitable for *S. pneumoniae* and both beta-lactamase positive and negative *B. catarrhalis* and *H. influenzae*. Cefuroxime is also adequate, although perhaps not ideal for *Staphylococcus aureus* and anaerobes of the upper respiratory tract.

The use of antihistamines and decongestants in the treatment of sinusitis is controversial. There has been no evaluation of the efficacy of these preparations in acute or chronic sinusitis. Although the topical decongestants phenylephrine and oxymetazoline produce potentially undesirable local effects such as ciliostasis, they may provide dramatic relief from symptoms. The effectiveness of these agents with respect to shortening the clinical course of illness in acute sinusitis or preventing suppurative complications is unknown.

Sinus puncture with irrigation and drainage (usually best accomplished by a transnasal approach) often results in dramatic relief from pain and provides material for definitive culture and sensitivity (cultures of the nose and throat correlate poorly with sinus aspirate cultures). In experienced hands and with proper sedation, the procedure is safe and can be accomplished with minimal discomfort. Although a sinus aspiration is not necessary for the management of an uncomplicated case of acute sinusitis, indications for sinus aspiration include clinical unresponsiveness to conventional therapy, sinus disease in an immunosuppressed patient, severe symptoms such as headache or facial pain, and life-threatening disease at the time of clinical presentation.

Orbital Complications

Orbital cellulitis is the most frequent serious complication of acute sinusitis. Despite antimicrobial therapy, it is a potentially life-threatening infection.

Children with stage I disease (see Table 1) can be managed as outpatients by the usual regimen for acute sinusitis, provided the parents are cooperative and cognizant of the serious implication if prompt alleviation of symptoms does not occur. If the infection has progressed beyond stage I, hospitalization and intravenous antibiotics are mandatory. The choice of antibiotics is guided by knowledge of the usual bacteriology of acute sinusitis. Blood cultures and sinus aspirate should be obtained aerobically and anaerobically, and appropriate antimicrobials should be added if unsuspected organisms are isolated. Surgical drainage is required if there is a subperiosteal or orbital abscess, but orbital cellulitis may respond to antimicrobials without surgical intervention. The prognosis for stages I and II is usually good if diagnosis and appropriate therapy are carried out promptly, but residual visual loss due to infarction of the optic nerve may complicate frank abscesses. Severe neurologic sequelae or death may follow cavernous sinus thrombophlebitis.

Intracranial Complications

Intracranial extension of infection is the second most common complication of acute sinusitis. Although the incidence of suppurative intracranial disease in patients with sinusitis is unknown, paranasal sinusitis is the source of 35 to 65% of subdural empyemas. Intracranial infection should be suspected if signs of systemic toxicity and headache do not improve after an adequate course of oral antibiotics and decongestant has been given for the original sinusitis.

Treatment of sinusitis-related intracranial suppuration requires antimicrobials, drainage, and excellent supportive care. There is evidence that preoperative meningitic doses of antibiotics may improve the chances for survival. Since the predominant organisms isolated from sinusitis-related subdural empyema include anaerobic and microaerophilic streptococci, non–group A streptococci, *Staphylococcus aureus*, and a mixture of *Proteus* and other gram-negative rods, the initial antibiotic regimen prior to culture and sensitivity results should be a combination of a penicillinase-resistant penicillin and chloramphenicol. The recently available third-generation cephalosporin cefotaxime (Claforan) may be used in place of chloramphenicol to avoid hemopoietic complications in young infants, although experience with this drug is limited.

Hyperosmolar agents should be given if high intracranial pressure threatens brain herniation. Systemic doses of steroid are prescribed with caution because of the theoretical suppressive effect on granulocytic and immune functions. Anticonvulsants should be given prophylactically to protect against a 79% incidence of associated seizures.

Extradural and subdural empyemas should be drained through a generous craniotomy. The entire collection of pus can be evacuated and the infected bed profusely irrigated with bacitracin solution under direct vision, and, with a judiciously fashioned flap, the opposite parafalcine space can be explored. Extradural and subdural drains are left in place for 3 to 5 days for continuous drainage and intermittent antibiotic lavage. An underlying brain abscess is best handled by intracapsular

Table 1. CLINICAL STAGING OF ORBITAL CELLULITIS*

Stage		
I	Inflammatory edema	Inflammatory edema beginning in medial or lateral eyelid; usually nontender with only minimal skin changes. No induration, visual impairment, or limitation of extraocular movements.
II	Orbital cellulitis	Edema of orbital contents with varying degrees of proptosis, chemosis, limitation of extraocular movement and/or visual loss.
III	Subperiosteal abscess	Proptosis down and out with signs of orbital cellulitis (usually severe). Abscess beneath the periosteum of the ethmoid, frontal, or maxillary bone (in that order of frequency).
IV	Orbital abscess	Abscess within the fat or muscle cone in the posterior orbit. Severe chemosis and proptosis; complete ophthalmoplegia and moderate to severe visual loss present (globe displaced forward or down and out).
V	Cavernous sinus thrombophlebitis	Proptosis, globe fixation, severe loss of visual acuity, prostration, signs of meningitis; progresses to proptosis, chemosis, and visual loss in contralateral eye.

* Modified from Chandler, J. R., Langenbrunner, DJ, and Stevens, EF: The pathogenesis of orbital complications in acute sinusitis. Laryngoscope 80:1414–1428, 1970.

evacuation and catheter drainage to avoid unnecessary brain damage associated with radical excision of deep-seated lesions within eloquent areas of the brain. In some cases of subdural empyema, the underlying brain is so swollen that the bone flap must be left out for external decompression. Following radical débridement of all osteomyelitic sequestra, the frontal sinus is opened widely, its content exenterated, and its cavity drained.

Postoperatively, intravenous administration of antibiotics should be maintained for a minimum of 2 to 3 weeks. Intermittent antibiotic irrigation of the infected cavities can be done through the catheters until their removal in 3 to 5 days. The shrinking of the abscess or empyema can be followed accurately by serial CT scans.

Despite modern diagnostic and surgical capabilities, the mortality associated with subdural empyema and brain abscess remains over 20 percent. Causes of death and permanent morbidity are related to delayed diagnosis, recurrent suppuration, missed concomitant lesions, extensive cortical and dural sinus thrombophlebitis, and fulminant bacterial meningitis in infants. Early diagnosis remains the most effective way for improving survival.

Retropharyngeal and Peritonsillar Abscesses

FRED S. HERZON, M.D.

Retropharyngeal abscess is not an uncommon admission diagnosis in major pediatric centers throughout the country. It is, however, an extremely rare discharge diagnosis for the 1980's.

This is not to say that a child entering with a high fever, stiff neck, drooling, and x-ray evidence of widened retropharyngeal space could not have a retropharyngeal abscess. If an abscess is present,

general anesthesia, intraoral incision, and drainage are indicated, with strict attention to protection of the airway. Parenteral antibiotics would be dependent upon culture results, with broad coverage given until bacterial identification is obtained.

Peritonsillar abscess, on the other hand, is the most common intraoral abscess in children today. The abscess occurs in association with tonsillitis and pus formation in the peritonsillar space between the capsule of the tonsil and the superior constrictor muscle. Diagnosis is made by observing unilateral bulging of the tonsil, deviation of the uvula, and trismus. It is confirmed by needle aspiration of the abscess at a point midway between the base of the uvula and the posterior molar. As much pus as possible is removed by aspiration. In over 90% of the cases this will result in resolution of the abscess within 24 to 48 hours, without further drainage. Penicillin, parenterally or orally, is the drug of choice, and hospitalization is unnecessary for resolution of this disease. In 59 peritonsillar abscesses treated in a 10-year period at the author's institution, at no time did culture results influence the outcome of the disease. Therefore, I do not advise sending the pus for culture and sensitivity. The recommendation for tonsillectomy after resolution of the peritonsillar abscess is still subject to some controversy.

The Tonsil and Adenoid Problem

RICHARD B. GOLDBLOOM, M.D., F.R.C.P. (C.)

The decision to perform or not to perform tonsillectomy and/or adenoidectomy (T&A) remains one of the most subjective in the pediatric family practice and otolaryngologic repertoires, and the tenacity with which individual opinions are held often seems inversely proportional to the volume of supporting scientific evidence. Over the past decade the trend has been toward conservatism in recommending either procedure. This is reflected by a steady decrease in the number of T&A's performed annually. Parenthetically, the declining number of these operations has been paralleled by a progressive increase in the rate of myringotomy and tube insertions. Thus, the total number of pediatric otolaryngologic procedures performed annually under general anesthesia has not changed substantially.

A decision to perform these operations on a child should never be taken lightly. A small but significant number of fatalities associated with T&A continue to occur every year. Postoperative hemorrhage is not uncommon, and other serious unanticipated complications, such as malignant hyperthermia can turn an ostensibly simple intervention into a major catastrophe. Therefore, such surgery should never be looked upon as "minor" and should be carried out in hospitals that offer skilled pediatric anesthesia and postoperative care. In most instances, an elective T&A is a decision in favor of a procedure that carries a small but definite mortality in order to benefit a condition that carries none. Probably the only absolute indication for surgery is the occurrence of obstructive sleep apnea associated with CO_2 retention, hypoxia, pulmonary hypertension, and cor pulmonale—an uncommon syndrome. Antecedent peritonsillar abscess (quinsy) has been considered a strong indication for tonsillectomy in the past, but this assumption has not been adequately tested.

Among children with *severe* recurrent throat infections (representing less than 10% of patients referred for tonsillectomy), a recently reported large-scale controlled study suggests that surgery is followed by significantly fewer throat infections during the first 2 postoperative years as compared with unoperated controls, with the difference tending to disappear in the third year. However, in this study many of the subjects who did not undergo operations also had markedly fewer throat infections during follow-up, and most that did occur were minor. Differences in the number of sore throat days or in the number of days of school absence were modest or insignificant between operated and unoperated children. Thus, even for children with severe recurrent throat infections, the evidence of benefit from tonsillectomy is modest and transient and must be weighed against the risks of the procedure. It has been estimated that at most only one or two children with the frequency and severity of throat infection required for inclusion in this study would be seen annually in a pediatric or family practice.

Despite continuing debate, there is no convincing evidence of benefit from adenoidectomy in the treatment or prevention of recurrent otitis media.

On the other hand, there is good evidence to support the efficacy of daily sulfonamide prophylaxis for this purpose. One absolute contraindication to adenoidectomy is the presence of a cleft palate (typically associated with recurrent otitis media), since removal of the adenoid will further exaggerate the defect in palatopharyngeal closure, thereby increasing the nasal escape of air, which creates serious speech problems for these children. The presence of a bifid or notched uvula should also be regarded as a likely contraindication to adenoidectomy, since it is often accompanied by a submucous cleft or related anomalies.

Physicians sometimes feel pressured by the parents' insistence that something be done for their child who has recurrent throat or ear infections, snores at night, or has other symptoms attributed to enlarged or infected tonsils or adenoids. It has now been well-documented that parental perceptions of the frequency of antecedent sore throats in their child are unreliable guides to the subsequent frequency of sore throats under close observation. From the physician's viewpoint, it is always easier and quicker to recommend surgery than to discuss the pros and cons of surgery with patients (or guardians), defer a decision, or attempt less dramatic alternatives. The temptation to take the expeditious route should be resisted.

Parental tolerance for recurrent respiratory infections in their children varies greatly. The parents' diminished tolerance or exasperation may be conditioned by familial factors unrelated to the child or by anecdotal reports of dramatic improvements following surgery. A thorough understanding of the family is essential to making a decision that is in the child's best long-term interest. If the basis for conservatism is fully explained to parents, they will usually accept and respect such caution.

The natural process of involution of tonsillar and adenoidal lymphoid tissue in the prepubertal years is usually associated with decreasing frequency of throat and ear infections. In this age group, a decision to defer surgery is often rewarded by progressive and spontaneous clinical improvement.

Aside from any beneficial impact that tonsillectomy and adenoidectomy might have on the frequency of throat and ear infections, our knowledge about possible deleterious effects of such surgery on the immune system is fragmentary. Prior to the advent of the polio vaccine, it had been well-established the previously tonsillectomized children who contracted poliomyelitis were at increased risk for bulbar involvement. Children who underwent tonsillectomy have been shown to be at increased risk for colonization by *Neisseria meningitidis*, but it is not yet known whether children thus colonized (or their associates) are at increased risk for invasive meningococcal disease. The presence of virus-specific cellular reactivity in tonsillar lymphocytes is associated with significant clinical protection during close household contact with varicella-zoster virus. These observations are mentioned here simply to underline the possibility that the long-term effects of tonsillectomy and adenoidectomy may extend well beyond the pharynx and are still poorly understood. Taken together, the foregoing considerations favor increasing caution and conservatism in recommending tonsillectomy or adenoidectomy in the majority of children.

Disorders of the Larynx

DANIEL D. RABUZZI, M.D.

More than just a phonatory organ, the larynx also functions as an organ of respiration as well as the guardian of the trachea in the prevention of aspiration. Pediatric laryngeal disorders can cause changes in one or more of these functions through their effect on any of the three endolaryngeal anatomic regions—supraglottis, glottis, and subglottis. There are many causes of dysfunction, but the symptom response of the larynx is such that respiratory problems produce inspiratory stridor; phonatory dysfunction is noted by hoarseness; and sphincteric deglutitory abnormalities are observed by aspiration with coughing and/or pneumonitis.

Congenital Disorders. Laryngomalacia is the most common laryngeal disorder seen in the newborn. Collapse of the supraglottic structures, including the epiglottis, into the laryngeal introitus during inspiration is the most common cause for this difficulty. This is believed to be due to the extreme elasticity and flexibility of infant cartilage. Recent observations have also suggested a muscular dysfunction of the hyomandibular suspension system. Affected infants seem to do best in the prone position. Diagnosis may be made definitively by direct laryngoscopy and elevation of the supraglottic structures. Treatment should be observation and parental reassurance, as symptoms usually subside by 18 months of age. Tracheotomy is rarely necessary.

Congenital cysts are supraglottic and produce stridor without hoarseness. They should either be excised or marsupialized via direct endoscopy. Webs usually occur at the glottic level and will produce hoarseness with or without airway obstruction. Surgical incision, preferably with a carbon dioxide laser, should be done for thin webs. Thicker webs will require both incision and tracheotomy with endolaryngeal stenting for 4 weeks.

Congenital stenoses usually occur in the immediate subglottic region. This is the most narrow portion of the upper airway and the only portion of the trachea surrounded by a complete cartilaginous ring. Most patients can be observed without the need for surgical intervention. These children are particularly vulnerable if struck by laryngotracheobronchitis. Conservative dilatations may be of some benefit.

Unilateral and bilateral vocal cord paralysis occurs in the newborn. The former is usually secondary to recurrent laryngeal nerve injury with the vocal cord in the paramedian position. Symptomatology in these cases is usually minimal, i.e., hoarseness when the problem is acute, with gradual resolution. Aspiration and airway obstruction rarely occur. Bilateral vocal cord paralysis, on the other hand, is an extremely dangerous situation. The voice is normal, but the airway is severely compromised owing to narrowing of the glottis. It is often seen in the Arnold-Chiari syndrome. Tracheotomy is routinely necessary.

Posterior laryngotracheal cleft is caused by a defect in the posterior lamina of the cricoid cartilage. Infants with this problem will have repeated bouts of pneumonitis and "failure to thrive." Since a functioning cricopharyngeal sphincter is absent, esophageal reflux occurs with aspiration. Repair is by lateral pharyngotomy, muscle interposition, and direct closure of the cleft.

Acquired Disorders. With the advent of prolonged endotracheal intubation in the neonate and infant in the late 1960's, acquired subglottic stenosis became a significant pediatric problem. Improved techniques of intubation and the use of smaller endotracheal tubes made of less irritating substances have reduced the incidence of this problem, but such stenosis is still seen routinely in major pediatric centers. The subglottic stenosis begins with exuberant granulation tissue and infection, with or without cricoid chondritis. If the narrowing is not intolerable, conservative measures are first used, including high humidity, steroids, and antibiotics.

Endoscopic evaluation determines when the stenosis is not reversible by conservative measures and when tracheotomy is indicated. This procedure should always be done over an endotracheal tube or indwelling bronchoscope. Steroids and antibiotics should be continued for several weeks after tracheotomy. Inflammatory reaction will subside in about 6 to 8 weeks, and the larynx and subglottic region should be reassessed at that time. An adequate lumen will allow decannulation. If scar tissue has progressed to obstruction, definitive surgery is required. Purely intraluminal stenoses may be handled by endoscopic carbon dioxide laser excision of the scar tissue and soft intraluminal stenting for 4 weeks. If there is cartilage necrosis and collapse or the intraluminal scar is either too thick or too long, then open surgery is indicated. The cricoid must be divided, and the subglottic lumen must be expanded either by stenting with cartilage or by bone interpositioning.

Vocal cord nodules are commonly seen in the preadolescent child. They classically occur at the junction of the anterior and middle thirds of the true vocal cords and are the direct result of vocal abuse. They may be reversible with the introduction of good speech therapy, but this is somewhat difficult in the pediatric patient. They almost always resolve at puberty. Vocal cord nodules should not be operated upon in the child.

Infectious Disorders. Laryngotracheobronchitis (croup) and epiglottitis (supraglossitis) are discussed in another section. It should be noted that croup is routinely a medical problem, whereas epiglottitis is a surgical one. The croup patient responds well to racemic epinephrine, a mist tent, and/or steroids. The epiglottitis patient demands either endotracheal intubation in the operative suite or tracheotomy, depending on the facilities available.

Neoplasms. The most common neoplasm in children is the recurrent juvenile laryngeal papilloma. This lesion seems to begin at the glottic level, but it may also involve the supraglottic and subglottic regions. Endotracheal spread is not uncommon, particularly in the untreated patient. A viral etiology seems most likely, and there appears to be a causal relationship between juvenile laryngeal papilloma and condylomata acuminata in the mother. Meticulous excision of all obstructive tumor is done best with the carbon dioxide laser. A multicenter trial using interferon is now under way. Cure seems evasive, however, since recurrence is frequent, even up to 10 years after therapy. Tracheotomy is often necessary, despite the known propensity for papilloma implantation at the operative site.

Subglottic hemangiomata usually become symptomatic during the first year of life. They are associated with cutaneous hemangioma in 50% of the cases. Steroid therapy may cause some remission and obviate the need for tracheotomy. Recently, endoscopic use of the carbon dioxide laser and direct excision have also been shown to be efficacious. Radiotherapy should never be used.

The Croup Syndrome

(Spasmodic Croup, Laryngotracheitis, Epiglottitis, and Laryngotracheobronchitis)

SYLVESTER L. MOBLEY, M.D.,
and HERBERT C. MANSMANN, JR., M.D.

Croup is defined as a group of signs that are present when there is obstruction or inflammation in the area of the larynx and/or trachea. The signs are stridor, cough, and hoarseness.

Airway obstruction in the croup syndrome is a potential emergency. Therefore, immediately upon presentation to the physician a child has to be evaluated for an adequate, stable, and secure airway. This must be the first step in any decision that leads to further diagnosis or therapy. If the airway is not secure, there must be a preset plan of action (movement from a local physician's office to a hospital emergency room) that mobilizes a team whose goals are safe, rapid transport to the hospital and establishment of a secure airway. This team varies depending on the individual hospital but as a minimum should include experienced ENT and anesthesia personnel. Ideally, there should be pediatric support.

Spasmodic Croup. Spasmodic croup is a condition in which subglottic edema develops in a child who undergoes sudden onset of obstruction. The child usually goes to bed well or with some very mild respiratory symptoms and signs (runny nose and mild cough). There is no fever. The child awakens with acute edematous obstruction that is characterized by barking cough, stridor, and hoarseness.

There is no close association between any infectious agents and spasmodic croup. In fact, some investigators state that this condition has an allergic nature.

The majority of children with this condition will be significantly better by the time they are seen by the physician. These children can be sent home, and the parents should be instructed to use cool mist in the child's room. If symptoms return, steam from the hot tap in the bathroom with the door closed should be used. Close, frequent observation to avoid overheating of the child is necessary.

If the child has moderately severe symptoms when examined, hospital admission for observation and therapy is warranted. Cool mist therapy and racemic epinephrine (see Laryngotracheitis) may be used.

Spasmodic croup is rarely progressive; therefore airway control measures are not necessary. This condition tends to recur in some patients and with each succeeding attack the parents become more experienced at coping with the child.

Laryngotracheitis (Acute Infective Laryngitis). Management should start with assessment of the airway. If the airway is adequate, one can proceed with disposition, diagnosis, and treatment. A child with a typical history who is hoarse and has a barking cough and stridor does not need further work-up. However, in cases that are not as straightforward, a lateral neck x-ray and possibly a chest x-ray may help exclude such conditions as retropharyngeal abscess, early epiglottitis, or foreign body. Children who have no significant stridor at rest, no lethargy, and no significant tachycardia can be sent home. The parents should be instructed to use a cool mist humidifier in the child's room and to use the mist from the steam of hot water in a closed bathroom in case the child's condition becomes exacerbated. The parents should be made aware of signs and symptoms of increasing airway obstruction and should be told to return if these symptoms occur.

The child with stridor at rest but with fair air entry, with or without excessive use of strap muscles or striking lethargy, should be admitted for observation and therapy. Intravenous hydration is usually necessary, and cold mist at least does not cause significant problems and may help. Oxygen may be of benefit for moderate to severe obstruction, but often children will not tolerate a mask or nasal prongs.

Racemic epinephrine by nebulizer can lessen or completely abolish moderately severe symptoms. It should be prepared by adding 0.25–0.5 ml of racemic epinephrine to sterile water or saline to make 2–4 ml of solution. While racemic epinephrine provides relief to many children, the duration of relief is variable, with some children obtaining relief for only 15 to 20 minutes. Because of this variable duration, no child should be treated with racemic epinephrine and sent home. There are those who recommend racemic epinephrine to be delivered by intermittent positive pressure breathing (IPPB) with a face mask. Undoubtedly in some institutions there are personnel who can accomplish this, but in most cases the attempt to maintain a snug mask fit to a struggling child with upper respiratory obstruction will only increase the obstruction and add to the hypoxia and work of breathing. Therefore, delivery of racemic epinephrine by IPPB is not recommended.

The use of corticosteroids is more controversial. However, there are a few statements that can be made based on a knowledge of the action of steroids and on a number of studies. First, no one should rely on steroids to have an immediate effect. Second, there seems to be evidence that steroids decrease the severity and duration of illness. Third, an extension of this is that some children who present with or who are progressing toward severe obstruction may be stabilized, and intubation or tracheostomy can be avoided. The recommended dose is 0.3–0.6 mg/kg of dexamethasone q 6 hr for 1 day.

Very few children will not respond to this combination of treatments. However, those who present or progress to severe airway obstruction should be treated by a team that transports the child to the operating room for bronchoscopy and attempted nasotracheal intubation (tracheostomy if this fails). This will provide a stable airway while the obstruction resolves in 24 to 48 hours. An increasing air leak will indicate the reduction of the edema. After 24 to 48 hours of sustained air leak, the child can be extubated. Some who treat this condition recommend bronchoscopy before extubation. There are some children who will have a return of obstructive symptoms with succeeding viral respiratory infections, but usually these are of lesser severity each time. This is usually a reassuring fact to many parents.

Epiglottitis. Epiglottitis is a condition that causes airway obstruction because the large swollen globular epiglottis has replaced a very thin leaflike structure. With every swallowing motion this obstruction is accentuated. By far the most common cause of acute epiglottitis is *Haemophilus influenzae* b.

The natural history in many children with this condition is ominous. Increasing airway obstruction leads to hypoxia, hypercapnia, and acidosis. As muscular tone and level of consciousness decrease, obstruction becomes more or less complete, and a rather sudden death is the end result. Therefore, a presumptive diagnosis of epiglottitis represents the diagnosis of an emergency.

Physicians practicing outside a hospital setting should have a preset plan to move a child with epiglottitis to a facility capable of handling this situation. The facility should have a working plan to mobilize at the very least an experienced team of airway specialists (ENT and anesthesia) and to alert the operating room personnel. In the meantime, an onsite team of those with the most experience in airway management (emergency care physicians, critical care physicians, and ENT and anesthesia residents) must be in attendance. If there has to be a waiting period, it should take place in the operating room or operating room area, in a well-equipped and staffed ICU, or in the emergency room, in that order. When everything is ready, the child should be moved toward the operating room with a preset plan of movement. Emergency procedures should have been discussed. During that movement, the emergency establishment of a secure airway should be left to the person with the greatest experience.

In general, it is a good idea to transport the child in a parent's lap because children tend to be more calm in this position. The parent is often encouraged to accompany and to comfort the child in this position even into the holding area of the operating room. If epiglottitis is strongly suspected, the guiding principle should be that less is better in regard to testing and manipulation. Attempts to visualize the epiglottis outside the operating room can lead to disaster. Some children voluntarily open their mouths wide for inspection, but at no time should a tongue blade be used. A portable lateral neck film can be made if it does not take up too much time. It should be made in the emergency room or in the ICU while the child sits in the parent's lap and experienced airway management personnel are available. The child should not be taken to the radiology department. Venipunctures, blood cultures, and cultures of the epiglottis can be done, and antibiotics can be started in the operating room. All members of the team can always think of one more thing to do for completeness on their part, but the team leader must keep everyone moving toward the operating room.

Once in the operating room, deep halothane anesthesia is induced in the child in a sitting position and orotracheal intubation is accomplished following bronchoscopy; then, a nasotracheal endotracheal tube is placed.

The child should be returned to an intensive care unit that is capable of managing the pediatric patient with an artificial airway. The patient who is stable at this point can be transferred to another facility that has more expertise in dealing with this situation. The child should be kept well sedated in order to tolerate the endotracheal tube and should be restrained in commercially available arm splints, which work very well.

It is our practice to visualize the epiglottis while the child is sedated or briefly paralyzed each morning. The obvious advantage of this is that as soon as the epiglottis is normal, extubation can be accomplished. However, another advantage is that the knowledge of the size of the epiglottis can be very important in planning the course of action if there is an accidental extubation. If the epiglottis has been observed to be much reduced in size, the child can be observed with the expectation that the airway will be adequate. Usually, the epiglottis undergoes a significant decrease in swelling and inflammation after 24 hours, and in most cases by the third day the shape and thickness of the epiglottis are near normal, and extubation can be attempted. Few children need to be reintubated. We start corticosteroids about 24 hours before extubation if the intubation was traumatic or there was a subglottic inflammatory process found at bronchoscopy. The child can usually be transferred from the intensive care unit in about 12–24 hours to complete the course of antibiotic therapy.

The antimicrobial treatment of *Haemophilus influenzae* b epiglottitis should be either a combination of ampicillin/amoxicillin and chloramphenicol or single-drug treatment with one of the third-generation cephalosporins such as ceftizoxime or cefotaxime.

Laryngotracheobronchitis. Laryngotracheobronchitis (pseudomembranous croup or bacterial tracheitis) is also a true airway management emergency. All studies have pointed out that a high percentage (greater than 90%) of children with this condition need to be intubated. Therefore, these children should be managed in a fashion much like that for those with epiglottitis; however, several studies have pointed to the great difficulty in maintaining a patent endotracheal tube secondary to copious thick secretions and pieces of pseudomembrane that detach very easily. Therefore, the possibilities of tube blockage and tube replacement should be kept in mind by all. If secretions become a significant problem, tracheostomy should be performed. A disturbing number of these children have had to be reintubated when extubated on a sound clinical basis (no fever, good clinical status, and no secretions suctioned from the endotracheal tube). Therefore, it would seem prudent to perform bronchoscopy before extubation.

If disease is suspected, antimicrobial therapy for penicillinase-producing staphylococci and *Haemophilus influenzae* b should be instituted.

The duration of intubation and the length of hospitalization are longer than with epiglottitis and laryngotracheitis. However, children who survive without hypoxia have not as of yet been found to have any significant sequelae.

Pneumothorax and Pneumomediastinum

ROBERT M. ARENSMAN, M.D.

Except in a child already compromised by underlying pulmonary disease, simple pneumothorax is unlikely to cause a great problem. The seriousness of pneumothorax occurs when tension develops within the thoracic cavity. The mediastinal structures of a child are relatively mobile compared with those of an adult. Tension pneumothorax leads to mediastinal shift with partial occlusion of the superior and inferior venae cavae. This occlusion decreases venous return to the heart and produces hypotension, poor tissue perfusion, and cardiac arrest if not corrected.

Tension pneumothorax is a surgical emergency and demands immediate decompression of the affected hemithorax. Initially, this can be done most easily and expeditiously with a needle or small plastic catheter inserted between two ribs high and anterior in the chest wall. A whistling escape of air confirms the diagnosis and solves the immediate problem. A clinical diagnosis of tension pneumothorax based on decreased or absent breath sounds, hyperresonance, and tracheal deviation suffices, and time should not be wasted in waiting for a chest x-ray.

More definitive therapy for the pneumothorax is tube thoracoscopy. A large-caliber chest tube is inserted beneath the third or fourth rib in the auscultatory triangle just lateral to the pectoralis major muscle. Insertion of a chest tube generally converts a partial pneumothorax to a complete collapse until the tube is sealed beneath a column of water. Respiration after the tube is inserted will usually reexpand the lung, but suction applied to the thoracoscopy tube assures reexpansion and allows the pleural surfaces to approximate one another until the source of the air leak seals.

It is common practice to clamp chest tubes just prior to removal to test whether the lung will remain expanded. This appears to be a rather dangerous maneuver when the same information can be obtained by placing the chest tube on a simple water seal system. In the event that an air leak persists the lung may collapse, but without clamping a tension situation cannot develop. Care must be taken upon removal of the chest tube to prevent air from again entering the chest cavity.

Pneumomediastinum is a situation closely associated with pneumothorax, but it is considerably less dangerous. When air collects in the loose connective tissue between the parietal pleura and the mediastinal structures, one sees areas of radiolucency outlining the trachea, heart, and great vessels. Generally this represents an air leak in pulmonary parenchyma without overlying pleural rupture. The air dissects along the bronchi to the mediastinum, where it collects.

Only rarely is pneumomediastinum important clinically. It may be of diagnostic importance, especially after trauma when one needs a high index of suspicion for intrathoracic damage such as an esophageal rupture or a bronchial disruption. In addition, one should always consider the possibility of coexisting pneumothorax or pneumopericardium when air is present in the mediastinum.

Pleural Effusion

ROBERT C. STERN, M.D.

Once the presence of a pleural effusion has been established, thoracentesis must be considered. This procedure can be diagnostic or therapeutic. Although diagnostic thoracentesis is usually indicated when a nonrecurrent pleural effusion is present, there are some important exceptions. One of these, classic lobar pneumococcal pneumonia, is a relatively common cause of pleural effusion in childhood. Sequelae are rare if these patients receive appropriate antibiotic treatment and supportive care. It is generally accepted that thoracentesis can often be omitted in patients who are afebrile, with either congestive heart failure and rapid-onset effusion or hypoproteinemia with pleural effusion and ascites. The majority of other first-time pleural effusions should be investigated with thoracentesis. Thoracentesis can be important diagnostically because a variety of laboratory tests can be performed on the pleural fluid itself and because in patients with large effusions roentgenographic evaluation of the lung is easier after fluid is removed. Specific information of great therapeutic and prognostic importance can often be obtained with minimal difficulty and relatively low risk. Therapeutic thoracentesis is indicated if the patient is in respiratory distress because the effusion is compromising expansion of the lung(s), to remove pus from an empyema, or as part of an evaluation prior to chemical pleurodesis treatment of recurrent malignant effusion.

Thoracentesis. Immediately prior to thoracentesis, arterial blood gases (including pH) and serum LDH and total protein measurements should be obtained for comparison with pleural fluid measurements. In patients whose effusion is not loculated, the 8th intercostal space in the posterior axillary line is usually the best site. In older children, there should be dullness to percussion over the area of proposed thoracentesis. If the effusion is loculated or if there is substantial doubt as to whether the space-occupying pleural lesion is really fluid (as opposed to fibrous tissue, for example), ultrasound can be very helpful. Once the site has been selected, a small-gauge (e.g., #26) needle is used to infiltrate local anesthetic into the skin and superficial subcutaneous tissue. A slightly larger and longer needle can then be used to administer deeper anesthesia and to search for the depth of the pleura. The needle is slowly advanced perpendicular to and just above the rib to avoid injury to the intercostal artery, which generally hugs the undersurface. As this needle is advanced, frequent attempts at aspiration are made. If pleural fluid is not obtained, some anesthetic is injected and the needle advanced farther. When pleural fluid is aspirated, the needle is clamped at the skin line and then withdrawn. A larger-bore needle or a plastic intravenous catheter is then inserted into the pleural space. Before use, this needle is clamped so that it can penetrate $\frac{1}{4}$ to $\frac{1}{2}$ centimeter (depending on the size of the patient) deeper than the anesthetic needle. The fluid obtained during the preliminary procedure, albeit mixed with anesthetic, should not be discarded until fluid is obtained with the definitive procedure. Occasionally, additional pleural fluid will not be obtained and the culture of the original fluid may prove important. Obviously, fluid mixed with anesthetic cannot be used for chemistries. In most cases, a substantial amount of pleural fluid is obtained with the larger needle or catheter. This fluid is then used for laboratory analyses. Two of the samples should be heparinized, one for total cell and differential counts and one in a syringe for pH determination. The sample obtained for pH, if kept anaerobic and on ice, is stable for 2 hours.

There are two major risks of thoracentesis. Occasionally, the underlying lung will not reexpand fast enough as the pleural fluid is removed. The mediastinum can then shift toward the side of the procedure and the patient may develop chest pain or become more dyspneic. Similarly, if intrapulmonary pressure falls, fluid may be drawn into the parenchyma, resulting in pulmonary edema. If the patient develops signs of these complications, the physician should temporarily stop removing additional fluid or should terminate the procedure altogether.

The other major risk of thoracentesis is iatrogenic pneumothorax secondary to injury to the lung by the thoracentesis needle. The patient may move unexpectedly or cough sufficiently hard to allow contact between the needle and the lung. A repeat chest film after the procedure is important to assess efficacy and to rule out iatrogenic pneumothorax. In patients with extensive effusion, the postprocedure film may be the best diagnostic radiograph.

Treatment. Analysis of pleural fluid enables correct diagnosis of the underlying illness in approximately 80–85% of patients. A few of the remaining patients can be definitively diagnosed with pleural biopsy. The results of pleural fluid analysis also determine the subsequent treatment of the pleural effusion itself.

Many parapneumonic effusions do not require specific treatment. If the fluid is sterile and its pH is above 7.30, treatment of the underlying pneumonia is sufficient. Antibiotic doses need not be increased. Patients with sterile parapneumonic effusions rarely develop empyema later in the disease course, provided effective therapy has begun. If the parapneumonic effusion has a pH less than 7.20, chest tube drainage (as will be described) is indicated. The pleural disease in these patients should be treated as if it were empyema.

CHEST TUBE DRAINAGE. In older children and teenagers the management of empyema and other exudative effusions is similar to that in adults. In these younger patients, exudative effusions with very low pH (below 7.0) should be treated with tube thoracostomy; when the fluid pH is above 7.0, tube thoracostomy can often be delayed pending subsequent evaluation of the patient's course with appropriate therapy. Pleural fluid glucose can also be used as a guide in determining which patients require tube drainage, but the fluid pH appears to be more sensitive. In most patients, fluid pH will drop below 7.20 before the fluid glucose falls below the 50 mg/dl level some consider critical for this important clinical decision. Early tube placement, in those patients who will ultimately require it, is probably advantageous, in that drainage is smoother when done before extensive loculation has occurred. Direct insertion of anti-

biotics into the pleural space is unnecessary because penetration of systemically administered antibiotics into the pleural fluid is excellent. Similarly, the use of enzymes such as streptokinase does not appear to be helpful, at least in the majority of patients. Chest tube drainage of pleural exudates should continue until the amount of fluid has drastically diminished (exact amounts vary with age/size of patient) and the fluid is sterile and serous. Nondraining tubes should always be removed; if tube drainage is still thought necessary, a replacement can be inserted, using ultrasonography as a guide to location. When patients with empyema remain febrile, despite antibiotic treatment and apparently adequate chest tube drainage, the following possibilities (among others) should be investigated: (1) A loculated infected area is not being adequately drained; (2) the antibiotic coverage is not sufficient—perhaps there is more than one pathogen; and (3) the patient has developed a drug fever.

Younger children require chest tube treatment for a shorter time; once clinical improvement is evident, the tube can usually be removed. Long-term complications are rare.

CHEMICAL PLEURODESIS. Chemical pleurodesis is used primarily for treatment of recurrent malignant effusions. It is indicated only if recurrent effusions cause dyspnea (i.e., are relieved by thoracentesis) and analysis of pleural fluid reveals a pH above 7.30. Tetracycline is most commonly used, although some physicians prefer talc. These tumors are extremely rare in childhood and therefore this procedure will be discussed only briefly. Following insertion of a chest tube and drainage of as much of the effusion as possible, 5–10 ml of 2% lidocaine is inserted into the tube and the patient is turned to lie on the abdomen, back, and right and left sides. Intravenous narcotics may be used in place of or in addition to local anesthesia. The tetracycline (0.5–1 gm in 30–50 ml of normal saline for an adolescent, smaller amounts for younger children) is then injected slowly into the chest tube. When the entire dose has been given, the tube is clamped and the patient is positioned on the right and left sides, abdomen, and back, with the bed in a head-up, head-down, and flat position. Each rotation is maintained for approximately 3–5 minutes. Dyspneic patients may require additional oxygen during this procedure and generally do better if the head-down rotations are done first. This procedure is performed daily for 3 days unless severe chest pain or fever indicates that adequate inflammatory reaction has already been achieved.

DECORTICATION. A restrictive ventilatory defect is inevitable in patients who have had a pleural exudate. Usually this is transient and resolves in several months. However, if it does not resolve and the impairment of pulmonary status is symptomatic, a decortication procedure may be indicated.

Chylothorax

ROBERT M. ARENSMAN, M.D.

Chylothorax occurs when lymphatic fluid flowing through the thoracic duct empties into the free pleural space rather than into the left subclavian vein. The lymphatic fluid is rich in protein, lymphocytes, immunoglobulins, and lipids. As it accumulates, space occupation may lead to compression of the ipsilateral lung, with consequent respiratory distress. With sufficient accumulation the mediastinum and its structures may shift, leading to decreased venous return to the right heart. These problems, either alone or in combination, may lead to respiratory arrest and death.

In neonates, chylothorax may be congenital or acquired. In neonates who are born with respiratory distress, action is usually required prior to the first feeding; consequently, no lipid appears in the chyle to give it the characteristic milky appearance. In older children, chylothorax may also be spontaneous or acquired.

Therapy for both groups rests on complete drainage of the effusion, an attempt to decrease drainage through the thoracic duct, and good nutritional support of the patient, with repletion of protein stores if the patient is in a debilitated state when first seen (Fig. 1). Once a diagnostic thoracentesis has been undertaken, the chest cavity should be drained as completely as possible. A post-thoracentesis x-ray film will demonstrate how successful this procedure has been. With complete removal of the fluid the parietal and visceral pleura can approximate and obliterate the opening in the thoracic duct responsible for the effusion.

Dietary management involves removing all lipid sources other than the medium-chain triglycerides, which can enter the portal circulation directly and do not require the thoracic duct to enter the general circulation. Unfortunately, medium-chain triglycerides are not a complete source of necessary lipids, and their exclusive use will result in fatty acid deficiency after 2 to 3 weeks. At present, commercially available formulas for infants do not exceed 80% medium-chain triglycerides; consequently one of these formulas should be substituted as the baby's nutrition. In the older individual appropriate dietary selections greatly reduce the offending lipids. However, in both groups continued use of the alimentary tract for nutrition will result in some degree of chylous flow.

In the event that low lipid diet with heavy concentrations of medium-chain triglycerides fails

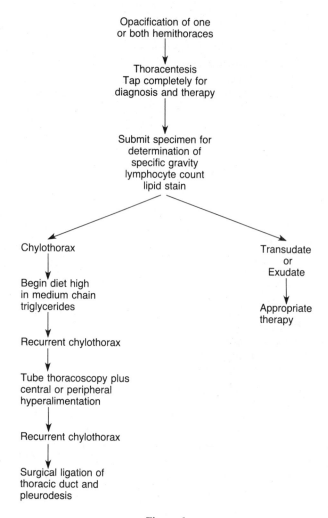

Figure 1.

to control the effusion, peripheral or central hyperalimentation should be considered. Use of 10–13% dextrose solutions, 8.5% protein solutions, and fat emulsions via a peripheral vein can closely approximate required calories, especially in the older and nutritionally stable child. In children with malignant disease and a chronic debilitated state and in neonates it may be necessary to institute central hyperalimentation to achieve carbohydrate levels sufficient for repletion and growth.

Considerable controversy exists over the question of serial thoracentesis versus tube thoracostomy. Certainly this disease process has a mortality in neonates between 15 and 40%. It is reasonable to try to seal the source of the effusion as quickly as possible to reduce this mortality. Coupled with the possibility of pneumothorax and infection attendant on repeated taps, failure to resolve and to control the effusion completely after one or at most two taps should lead to the insertion of a chest tube.

Intrathoracic Cysts

ROBERT W. EMMENS, M.D.

Intrathoracic cysts are an unusual problem, and patients can present with a variety of symptoms. These symptoms may vary from potentially life-threatening respiratory distress to an asymptomatic mass detected on a chest x-ray examination. Intrathoracic cysts may arise from almost any organ within the thoracic cavity. They should all be considered surgical lesions because of their presenting symptoms or potential for producing those symptoms.

Bronchogenic Cysts. Bronchogenic cysts are the most common intrathoracic cysts and occur as the result of abnormal development of the primitive foregut. Most occur in the region of the carina, but it is important to remember that they may occur anywhere within pulmonary tissue. In infants the cyst may cause partial bronchial obstruction with consequent air trapping in peripheral pulmonary tissue. The resultant overinflation may necessitate emergency resection in the infant because of severe respiratory distress due to compression of the surrounding tissue. In the older child the presenting symptoms may include recurrent infections and an intractable pulmonary infiltrate, or the cyst may be picked up on a routine chest x-ray.

Therapy is directed toward surgical removal, and this is usually not a difficult procedure. The mass is found to be a mucus-filled cyst lined by respiratory epithelium that may have bits of cartilage within its wall. Recurrence is almost unheard of, and malignant degeneration has not been seen in the child.

Esophageal Duplications. Esophageal duplications represent the second most common type of malformation arising from the primitive foregut. Since their symptoms are usually caused by dysphagia, diagnosis in the young is rather unusual. As the cyst may infringe on the lumen of the esophagus, mucosal irritation with resultant anemia is a possibility. Esophageal duplications are found most commonly in the lower part of the esophagus in direct continuity with the esophageal wall. Treatment is surgical excision, but since esophageal duplications share a common muscular wall, this may not be possible. Removal of this wall and establishment of a common channel is also an acceptable form of therapy. Histologically, the cysts are generally divided into two types. The rare developmental type of cyst is lined with respiratory epithelium. The more common type is the enteric duplication lined with different types of gastrointestinal mucosa. Removal of the latter is desirable to avoid esophageal ulceration.

Pulmonary Cysts. Pulmonary cysts are generally divided into congenital and acquired types. Differentiating between these two may be very difficult unless an accurate history and good chest x-rays can be obtained.

Simple pulmonary cysts are uncommon lesions, usually located in the upper lobes. They are the result of faulty embryogenesis, with formation of either single or multilocular cystic lesions lined with cuboidal or columnar epithelium. They become symptomatic when overexpansion results in compression of the surrounding pulmonary tissue and in a mediastinal shift away from the side of the lesion. Rupture with resultant pneumothorax is a relatively uncommon complication. Radiologically these cysts appear as a round lucency with a very thin radiopaque border. Therapy is surgical removal of the lesion, which usually requires a lobectomy. In a life-threatening situation, needle decompression of the cyst may be necessary, but this should not be used to avoid surgical removal. Infections within the cyst may make the differentiation from pneumatoceles somewhat difficult. A pneumothorax should be treated in the usual manner.

Lobar Emphysema. Congenital lobar emphysema occurs when air is trapped, usually in a single lobe, apparently because of deficient cartilage in the bronchus leading to that particular lobe. The resultant air trapping with compression of surrounding pulmonary tissue causes respiratory distress, at times life-threatening in the infant. This occurs more commonly in males and is generally seen in the left upper lobe. Patients are almost all less than 4 months of age, and the diagnosis is usually made by chest x-ray. Radiologically it appears as an overinflation of the affected lobe without a radiopaque rim suggestive of a cyst wall. The surrounding lobes are usually atelectatic. Rupture with resultant pneumothorax is very unusual, and therapy is surgical resection of the affected lobe.

Adenomatoid Malformation. Cystic adenomatoid malformation is a congenital lesion usually confined to one lobe, which again frequently results in respiratory distress in the newborn infant. When found in the stillborn, there are other associated abnormalities not found in children born alive with this lesion. If there is a communication with the tracheobronchial tree, the lesion appears radiologically as a multicystic lesion within the thoracic cavity and may be confused with a diaphragmatic hernia. In the older child it may result in recurring infections or in pneumonia that is refractory to therapy. Therapy is surgical excision. The blood supply is in communication with the pulmonary artery and veins, differentiating it grossly from the pulmonary sequestrations. Histologically it is basically a benign hamartomatous lesion that does not recur when totally excised.

Rarely this lesion is associated with anasarca and hypoproteinemia, in which case the prognosis is exceedingly poor.

Acquired Cysts. Acquired cysts are usually related to an infectious process, with the formation of pneumatoceles or lung abscesses. Over the last several years, with the increased use of ventilators in infants with respiratory distress syndrome and the subsequent development of bronchopulmonary dysplasia, formation of cystic disease is being seen with greater frequency.

PNEUMATOCELE. Pneumatoceles are the localized collection of air within the pulmonary parenchyma, usually associated with either staphylococcal or *Haemophilus influenzae* infections. Treatment of these should be concentrated on administration of appropriate antibiotics and insertion of chest tubes when necessary for treatment of pneumothoraces or formation of empyemas. Open thoracotomy is rarely necessary.

LUNG ABSCESS. Lung abscesses occur when infection within the pulmonary parenchyma forms an inflammatory wall around an area of suppuration. If this communicates with the tracheobronchial tree, an air-fluid level will be seen radiologically. Again, treatment is with appropriate antibiotics. Transbronchial aspiration of these lesions may help considerably in obtaining material for culture to guide antibiotic therapy. In addition, this may aid in drainage of the material within the abscess, hastening resolution of the infection. If the abscess does rupture into the pleural space, an empyema will form, and a chest tube should be inserted. Formal surgical resection should not be necessary.

THYMIC CYST. Thymic cysts are located in the superior mediastinum and may present with dyspnea. They can usually be excised without difficulty, with the approach being either from the suprasternal approach or through a median sternotomy.

PERICARDIAL CYSTS. Pericardial cysts are simple cystic structures attached to the pericardium and are usually found on routine chest x-ray. The diagnosis is usually made by echocardiography, and most of these cysts can be removed by elective thoracotomy without difficulty.

CYSTIC TERATOMA AND DERMOID CYST. Cystic teratomas and dermoid cysts of the intrathoracic regions are relatively rare. Teratomas are composed of components from all three embryologic germ layers and frequently have calcification within them. Dermoid cysts, being composed of only two of the germ layers, are not associated with calcifications. They are most frequently located in the midline, more commonly in the upper mediastinal region, and present symptomatically because of compression of the airway or esophagus. Therapy is directed towards total excision,

with the approach best determined by the location of the lesion and its size.

PULMONARY SEQUESTRATION. Pulmonary sequestrations are localized collections of abnormal pulmonary tissue whose blood supply comes from the systemic circulation. In general there is no communication with the tracheobronchial tree, but not uncommonly they will have a connection with the gastrointestinal tract. They are usually found in the left lower lung fields; if they occur within the pulmonary parenchyma, they are termed intralobar sequestrations. These usually require a lobectomy, whereas extralobar sequestrations, ones not within the pulmonary parenchyma, can usually be removed with minimal difficulty and without removing any normal lung tissue.

Tumors of the Chest

ROBERT M. FILLER, M.D.

Neoplasms of the chest that develop in childhood involve the mediastinum and the pulmonary parenchyma.

MEDIASTINAL TUMORS

Neurogenic tumors are the most common mediastinal tumor and present in the posterior mediastinum. Most often they are found incidentally when the infant or child with respiratory symptoms is being evaluated by chest x-ray. Except for massive tumors and those dumbbell-type tumors that involve the spinal canal and cause cord compression, mediastinal neurogenic tumors rarely cause symptoms.

Neuroblastoma. In the younger child, neuroblastoma is the predominant histologic type. The primary treatment is surgical excision. If the tumor is completely excised, no chemotherapy or radiation therapy is given, and cures approaching 100% are reported for children under 18 months of age. For the child with a dumbbell neuroblastoma, treatment varies, depending on the presence of signs and symptoms of spinal cord compression. In those with cord compression, emergency laminectomy is necessary as a first step. At thoracotomy, usually 7 to 10 days later, the intrathoracic portion of the mass is removed. This order of surgery is reversed when the intraspinal component of the tumor is small and there are no signs of cord compression.

Radiation therapy and chemotherapy are employed for those children in whom the entire tumor cannot be excised. Repeated courses of cyclophosphamide and vincristine are used in those with localized residual disease. More complex chemotherapy protocols are being tried in institutional and multicenter group trials for disseminated disease. Radiation doses to areas of residual tumor range from 1000 to 2400 rads, depending on the patient's age.

Ganglioneuroma is the benign variant of neuroblastoma and is usually found in the older child. It may represent maturation of a neuroblastoma. Surgical excision is curative.

Lymphoma. Lymphoma is the commonest tumor in the middle and anterior mediastinum in children. Primary treatment of these tumors is described elsewhere in this book. Surgery is generally not indicated for the treatment of either Hodgkin's or non-Hodgkin's lymphoma, although the surgeon is often called upon to obtain tissue specimens for a histologic diagnosis.

Occasionally a patient with mediastinal lymphoma presents with the "superior mediastinal syndrome" and severe respiratory obstruction. In these high-risk patients intravenous high-dose steroid therapy is instituted at once, and biopsy is delayed. When a therapeutic effect from steroids is obtained (usually in 1 to 2 days), one can proceed with biopsy. In the child with an extremely large mediastinal mass, steroid therapy alone may not relieve the respiratory problems, and emergency radiation therapy may be necessary. Since the rapid resolution of lymphoma may result in hyperuricemia, allopurinol, intravenous hydration, and alkalinization of the urine are advised for these patients.

LUNG TUMORS

Primary Tumors. Primary tumors of the lung are rare in childhood, but *bronchial adenoma* is the most common type. These tumors are recognized as low-grade adenocarcinomas. The carcinoid-type tumor accounts for 80–85% of all adenomas seen in childhood. Children with these tumors present with infection or atelectasis in the lung supplied by the affected bronchus. These lesions can be seen by bronchoscopy and biopsied, but attempts at complete excision via the bronchoscope are not recommended for definitive treatment because most tumors grow through the bronchial wall. Most adenomas require pulmonary resection for cure. Lobectomy is used for lesions localized to a lobar bronchus or peripheral lung. Bilobectomy and pneumonectomy may be necessary when an adenoma in a main bronchus extends into a lobar bronchus or extraluminally to adjacent structures. Sleeve resection of the bronchus without pulmonary resection should be considered for the small adenoma confined to a central bronchial segment, provided infection has not destroyed the distal lung.

Secondary Tumors. Secondary tumors of the lung are relatively common in children, especially those originating from Wilms' tumor and osteogenic sarcoma.

Initial therapy for pulmonary metastases from *Wilms' tumor* includes radiation therapy (1500 rads to both lungs) and chemotherapy (usually actinomycin D and vincristine). More complex chemotherapy is used for those patients whose tumor is of "bad histology." Additional radiation is given to sites of persistent tumor. Resection is undertaken when tumor persists or recurs after medical treatment, provided that complete removal is technically possible.

Recent experience for patients with pulmonary metastases from *osteogenic sarcoma* has shown that by combining an aggressive surgical approach with the standard chemotherapy program approximately 40% of patients can be salvaged. Surgical resection of lung metastases is most effective in those patients with the fewest number of lesions, and in those in whom metastases develop many months after initial diagnosis of osteogenic sarcoma. However, the presence of a large number of metastatic deposits is not a contraindication to surgery per se, since many cures have been reported even after the resection of more than 10 lesions from each lung. The indications and timing for surgery have varied in individual cases and among different institutions. Our feeling is that metastatic lung lesions should be excised prior to the institution of other therapy in the following circumstances: (1) when lesions persist despite adequate staandard chemotherapy; (2) when metastases are isolated (less than 5) and appear late (greater than 6 months from diagnosis); and (3) when the metastatic tumor mass is large and unlikely to respond to chemotherapy. Surgery is delayed in favor of chemotherapy for those who have received inadequate or no prior chemotherapy and for those in whom pulmonary metastases are detected within 3 months of the original diagnosis. In the latter situation, lung metastases are excised as soon as rapidly growing lesions are stablized by chemotherapy. Our experience has shown that there is little hope for the patient who develops multiple metastases soon after diagnosis and in whom chemotherapy fails to halt their growth.

One of the important principles of surgery when dealing with metastatic lung lesions is to preserve as much lung tissue as possible, since most patients usually have more than one metastatic lesion, and others are likely to develop in the future. Wedge resection of the involved lung is usually adequate, but lobectomy and even pneumonectomy are sometimes required. Cure is unlikely unless all gross tumor is excised. When bilateral lesions are present, they can be excised at one operation by exposure through a median sternotomy. Alternatively, bilateral tumor nodules can be resected through two separate lateral thoracotomies spaced 1 week apart. In patients in whom pulmonary metastases recur after successful surgical excision, repeat resection is indicated as long as the volume of residual lung is sufficient to support life.

Pulmonary Sequestration

ROBERT M. FILLER, M.D.

Pulmonary sequestration is an uncommon congenital malformation characterized by the presence of nonfunctioning lung tissue that usually has no communication with the normal bronchial tree. The sequestered lung receives its blood supply from an anomalous systemic artery instead of a branch of the pulmonary artery. Two forms of pulmonary sequestration occur: intralobar sequestration, in which the abnormal pulmonary tissue is incorporated within the normal lung, and extralobar sequestration, in which the abnormal tissue is separate from the normal lung and has its own pleural investment. A fistulous communication from the sequested segment to the esophagus or stomach is occasionally present in both types. The lesions are located on the left side of the chest in approximately two thirds of the cases.

Resection is the treatment of choice. Extralobar sequestration should be totally excised if symptomatic or discovered as an incidental finding. Intralobar sequestration is usually best treated by lobectomy. Segmental resection has been performed, but it is rarely feasible because the associated infection has destroyed the segmental planes. Communications with the gastrointestinal tract are divided when found. Special care should be taken by the surgeon in handling the friable aberrant artery or arteries that supply the sequestration. The results of operation have been excellent.

Middle Lobe Syndrome

ROBERT M. FILLER, M.D.

The diagnosis of middle lobe syndrome is made by the finding of atelectasis of the middle lobe. In children it is usually secondary to lymphoid hyperplasia, which partially obstructs the middle lobe bronchus. Clinically atelectasis is usually asymptomatic, and only rarely is recurrent pneumonia a problem.

Treatment of this syndrome in childhood is based on symptoms rather than x-ray findings, since spontaneous resolution over many weeks or months is the rule. Endoscopy is rarely used except when the presence of a foreign body is suspected. Similarly, bronchography is not useful. Appropriate antibiotic therapy is indicated in the presence of pneumonia. Surgery is almost never indicated, since bronchiectasis or pulmonary abscess almost never occurs, and the atelectasis resolves spontaneously.

Bronchitis and Bronchiolitis

DAVID B. NELSON, M.D., M.SC.

Acute bronchitis, inflammation of the bronchial mucosa, is a mild self-limited disease that has cough as its primary symptom. Viral infections are the primary cause of bronchitis, therefore, specific therapy is limited and treatment is aimed at symptomatic relief. Therapy, when necessary, should be directed at cough control. In most children, fluids alone may be sufficient; however, if the child's cough either keeps him awake at night or results in vomiting, the use of a cough suppressant is indicated. Preparations containing either codeine sulfate or dextromethorphan are the most helpful. Decongestants and antihistamines are of no value.

Bronchiolitis, an inflammation of the bronchioles, results in small airway obstruction. The illness is characterized by tachypnea, wheezing, hyperinflated lungs, and often hypoxia. Like bronchitis, bronchiolitis is usually caused by a viral infection, with the respiratory syncytial virus (RSV) accounting for 50–75% of diagnosed cases. Except for *Mycoplasma* pneumonia, a relatively rare cause of bronchiolitis, there is no specific antimicrobial therapy. If *Mycoplasma* pneumonia is suspected, then erythromycin 30–50 mg/kg/day in four divided doses will help shorten the clinical course. Other antibiotics are useless in the treatment of bronchiolitis and should not be used. The interstitial pneumonia seen in children with bronchiolitis is caused by the infecting virus. Secondary bacterial pneumonia is extremely rare.

Specific viral therapy is unavailable at this time. However, early therapeutic trials with the antiviral agent ribaviran given by aerosol have been encouraging, making this drug a possible candidate for future use in children with RSV infections.

The majority of children with bronchiolitis can be managed as outpatients. Parents should be advised to give their child fluids and be instructed to look for signs of respiratory distress. Decongestants and antihistamines should not be prescribed.

If the child has significant respiratory distress, or is hypoxic, he should be hospitalized. The mainstay of hospital treatment is good supportive care: hydration and oxygen. All hospitalized children should receive sufficient humidified oxygen to maintain their arterial pO_2 at 80–100 mm Hg. This usually requires an FiO_2 of between 30 and 40%. Mist alone is of no value and may actually increase airway resistance.

Intravenous hydration should be given since the

infants have significant respiratory distress and are usually too ill to maintain adequate oral hydration. The child should receive maintenance fluids with correction of any fluid deficit. Overhydration may be harmful and should be avoided.

Although hypercarbia and respiratory failure are rare in bronchiolitis, 1–2% of hospitalized children will require mechanical ventilation. Assisted ventilation should be considered in a child with clinical deterioration as evidenced by increased work of breathing or by increasing pCO_2. Any child requiring mechanical ventilation for bronchiolitis should be cared for in a pediatric intensive care unit experienced in managing severely ill children.

Studies evaluating the efficacy of bronchodilators such as aminophylline for bronchiolitis have been inconclusive. Bronchial smooth muscle is sparse in children younger than one year, the age when children are at greatest risk of having severe bronchiolitis. Because of the relative lack of smooth muscle in young children bronchospasm is not a major component of this disease. Edema, inflammation, mucus, and sloughing of epithelial cells rather than bronchospasm lead to the classic obstructive signs seen in bronchiolitis. With this underlying pathophysiology bronchodilators should theoretically have little effect. However, in selected cases of severe illness aminophylline* may be useful. If used, aminophylline should be administered at a rate of 0.4–0.5 mg/kg/hr following an infusion of 5 mg/kg administered over 30 minutes. Because of aminophylline's relatively low therapeutic index in infants, and its variable and to a degree unpredictable metabolism in young children, it should only be used when blood levels can be monitored closely. The level should be maintained in the 10–20 µg/ml range. Aminophylline should never be used for the outpatient management of bronchiolitis, since the risk of complications far outweigh any possible therapeutic benefit. Steroid therapy has been studied and is of no value in treating bronchiolitis.

Since RSV is contagious, children hospitalized for bronchiolitis should be isolated from other patients. Children hospitalized with certain chronic illnesses, particularly those with lung and cardiac problems, are at particular risk of developing severe disease with this infection.

Aspiration Pneumonia

ITZHAK BROOK, M.D.

Aspiration pneumonia involves an inflammatory reaction in the lung parenchyma following entrance of foreign material. Following aspiration of

chemicals, food, vomitus, or secretions, the initial reaction is chemical, with edema and cellular infiltrations accompanied by acute respiratory distress. In instances in which mucus secretions containing oral flora are also aspirated, these microorganisms may initiate an infectious process that ranges from aspiration pneumonitis to lung abscess.

Milk, Food, and Vomitus. Aspiration of milk, food, and vomitus is common in pediatric patients who tend to aspirate because of debilitation, tracheoesophageal malformations, central nervous system disorders, and altered consciousness. Aspiration of food and vomitus rarely causes asphyxiation and death. More often, there is a short latent period of 1 to 2 hours prior to onset of pneumonia. The pneumonia is characterized by tachypnea, with fever and rarely apnea and hypotensive shock. Prevention of aspiration is of particular importance. Overfeeding should be avoided, and the child should be placed on its abdomen, with the head elevated when the child is supine. Suctioning of the airway, sometimes through intubation and administration of oxygen, should be initiated as soon as possible. Intubation and mechanical ventilation may be required. Bronchodilatory therapy with theophylline and beta agonists may be useful in improving airway patency. The administration of corticosteroids and prophylactic antibiotics is advocated by some; however, their usefulness is not proven. Antimicrobial agents should, however, be used whenever the clinical course, after an episode of aspiration, is protracted or deteriorating.

Saliva and Oropharyngeal Secretions. Since human saliva and oropharyngeal secretions contain many aerobic and anaerobic bacteria, their aspiration may contaminate the lower respiratory tract. Children with periodontal disease are at particularly high risk. The mixed aerobic-anaerobic infection that usually occurs after aspiration of oropharyngeal secretion into a dependent segment of the lung commences as pneumonitis with relatively mild symptoms. If untreated, liquefaction and abscess formation occur within 7 to 14 days. Empyema may also occur in many patients. Excavation may lead to solitary lung abscess or multiple small areas of necrosis of the lung, with or without air-fluid levels (necrotizing pneumonia). Following cavitation, putrid discharge may be noted in about half of patients. The severity of the illness varies considerably. Patients with acute necrotizing pneumonia are often quite ill, and their illness is relatively prolonged. Patients with only parenchymal disease require therapy of 3 to 8 weeks for complete cure. A much longer time—perhaps 4 to 5 months—is required for patients with empyema.

Therapeutic decisions involving the use of an-

---

* Manufacturer's warning: Safety and efficacy for use in children less than 6 months of age have not been established.

tibiotics are best made with the identification of specific organisms causing the infection. The selection of antimicrobial agents for the treatment of pneumonia in children is largely based on age, history, and physical and radiographic findings and by recovering an organism from the blood or directly from the injected lungs of the pleural space. Nasopharyngeal or sputum aspirates cannot provide reliable specimens for the identification of pathogens causing this disease, since the samples so obtained are contaminated by bacteria present in the oropharynx. Attempts should be made to avoid such contamination by sampling the lower respiratory tract by direct lung puncture, transtracheal aspiration (TTA), bronchoscopy, repeated washing of the expectorated sputum, or quantitative culture of the sputum; however, contamination of the specimen by oropharyngeal organisms can occur with all of these techniques except direct lung puncture and TTA.

Because of the small risks (occurring in less than 1% of patients) of bleeding, pneumothorax, and subcutaneous or mediastinal emphysema involved in these procedures, even when done by experienced persons, the decision to perform an invasive diagnostic procedure such as TTA or lung puncture should be weighed against the potential benefit. In most instances selection of antimicrobials can be made without any of these procedures. However, in patients who do not respond to therapy, or who are at risk of harboring unusual or resistant pathogens, obtaining cultures through these procedures should be considered. Transtracheal aspiration is contraindicated in uncooperative patients and in those with bleeding diatheses, severe coughing, and serious dyspnea and hypoxemia requiring positive pressure ventilatory aid.

The organisms recovered from the infected lungs consist of mixed flora of aerobic and anaerobic bacteria. The number of organisms that can be isolated from these infections varies between 3 and 10 (average of 3 anaerobes and 2 aerobes). The predominant anaerobes include anaerobic or microaerophilic streptococci, *Bacteroides melaninogenicus*, *Fusobacterium* and *Clostridium* bacteria, and *Bacteroides fragilis*. The major aerobic pathogens are *Staphylococcus aureus*, *Klebsiella pneumoniae*, and *Pseudomonas aeruginosa*.

Antimicrobial therapy may be guided by Gram's stain of appropriate material but should not be withheld pending culture results in severely ill patients. Parenteral penicillin G is still the drug of choice in the majority of anaerobic pleuropulmonary infections, since most of the anaerobic bacteria isolated, with the exception of the *Bacteroides fragilis* group and some strains of *Bacteroides melaninogenicus*, and *Bacteroides oralis* are generally highly sensitive to penicillin. It should be noted that an increase in the percentage of beta-lactamase–producing *Bacteroides*, other than *B. fragilis*, has occurred. These strains are more often found in patients who have recently been treated with penicillin. Whenever the presence of a penicillin-resistant organism, such as *Bacteroides* or *Staphylococcus aureus*, is suspected, other antibiotics also effective against these organisms should be used.

Clindamycin is an effective alternative to penicillin in the treatment of anaerobic pleuropulmonary infections. In addition to its effectiveness against beta-lactamase–producing *Bacteroides*, it is also effective against various aerobic organisms, including *Staphylococcus aureus*. Carbenicillin and ticarcillin are effective agents against many anaerobic organisms, including *Bacteroides fragilis*, and were successfully used in the treatment of aspiration pneumonia in children. They are also active against many aerobic gram-negative rods and manifest synergy with aminoglycosides against these organisms. This factor should be considered when such organisms, especially *Pseudomonas*, are recovered. The combination of amoxicillin and clavulanic acid (a beta-lactamase inhibitor) is active against most pathogens isolated from this infection, including those that produce beta-lactamase.

Aminoglycosides such as gentamicin should be added to the agents directed against the anaerobes when gram-negative enteric rods are also present. Emergence of resistance to gentamicin has been a concern in recent years, however. Other aminoglycosides, such as amikacin sulfate or tobramycin, are also available for the treatment of such infections.

Hydrocarbons. Aspiration of hydrocarbons, such as kerosene, gasoline, and turpentine in furniture polish, can cause a secondary pneumonitis. Following accidental or intentional ingestion, the child gags, coughs, and sometimes vomits. All these can induce direct aspiration of the ingested hydrocarbon. Pulmonary symptoms in extensive aspiration can be observed within hours; however, in cases of minimal aspiration they may be delayed up to 1 day. These symptoms include tachypnea, dyspnea, cough, and fever. Radiographic changes, which are usually in the lung bases, may also be delayed in appearance up to 48 to 96 hours. No therapy is indicated prior to appearance of symptoms. Induction of vomiting or gastric lavage is contraindicated. If dyspnea or cyanosis develops, supportive therapy is indicated. This includes supplemental oxygen, ventilatory support, physiotherapy, and bronchodilation with intravenous theophylline and inhalation of beta-2 agonist. Antimicrobial therapy is indicated only when secondary bacterial infection develops. This can be suspected when fever reappears and symptoms and signs worsen. Administration of corticosteroids have not been shown to be helpful. Prevention of ingestion by small children should be emphasized to parents.

Bronchiectasis

J. A. PETER TURNER, M.D.

Bronchiectasis occurs when bronchial obstruction persists to the point that distal airways become dilated, secretions are static, and infection supervenes, setting the stage for bronchial wall destruction and a series of events progressing from cylindrical or reversible bronchiectasis to saccular or irreversible bronchiectasis.

Unresolved pneumonia involving one segment of lung is probably the commonest event leading to bronchiectasis. More widespread involvement occurs after infection with pathogenic adenovirus infections. Tuberculous hilar lymphadenopathy with extrusion of caseous material into a contiguous bronchus may eventually produce bronchiectatic change, frequently involving the right middle lobe or either of the upper lobes. Unrecognized foreign body aspiration invariably leads to bronchiectatic change.

Underlying problems commonly associated with bronchiectasis are cystic fibrosis, immune deficiency states, and immotile cilia syndrome. The last category includes cases formerly diagnosed as Kartagener's syndrome.

Although bronchiectasis may be strongly suggested in plain chest radiographs, confirmation depends upon the bronchogram. The extent of involvement determined by this examination is particularly important when surgery is contemplated.

Medical management is indicated for cylindrical bronchiectasis. Chest physiotherapy with the addition of bronchodilator agents such as beta agonists or theophylline is directed against the obstructive component of the condition, so that ectatic change may be reversed. Surgical resection is indicated for segmental saccular bronchiectasis, provided that the remainder of lung is not extensively involved from underlying problems as noted above.

Atelectasis

EDWIN L. KENDIG, JR., M.D.

Atelectasis is a term used to refer to nonaeration of the lung. The condition is more common in young infants because of the smaller bronchial lumen, more easily collapsible bronchi, and less rigid thoracic walls.

The object of therapy in obstructive atelectasis is to locate the cause of obstruction, remove it as promptly as possible, and maintain good pulmonary ventilation. Treatment will depend on the cause of the atelectasis. Postural drainage, physiotherapy, antibiotics, and bronchoscopy may be utilized, and each has its indication. Computed tomography may sometimes aid in establishing diagnosis.

Atelectasis associated with acute infection of the lower respiratory tract is usually short-lived and requires treatment only with appropriate antibiotics. If atelectasis persists, postural drainage and physiotherapy are indicated. If no improvement is noted after 8 to 12 weeks, bronchoscopy should be considered.

In those instances in which atelectasis results from extrabronchial compression, treatment must be directed toward the underlying cause; for example, in pleural effusion, treatment consists of the removal of the fluid.

In nonobstructive atelectasis apparently due to diminished surfactant, aerosol inhalation of synthetic surface-active agent, postural drainage, and physiotherapy are indicated.

Persistent atelectasis is uncommon. When it does occur, surgical removal of the affected portions of the lung should be delayed until there are frequently recurring infections and medical therapy has been ineffective, usually a period of at least 2 years.

Emphysema

ROBERT E. WOOD, Ph.D., M.D.

Emphysema may be defined as (1) alveolar dilation (due to a variety of causes) or (2) the presence of air in the interstitial tissues of an organ. In adults, alveolar dilation due to destruction of elastic fibers in the alveolar septa and small airways by neutrophil elastase is the most common cause of emphysema and is most often associated with chronic inflammation due to cigarette smoking. This form of emphysema is rare in children but may be associated with a genetic deficiency of alpha-1-antitrypsin. Research in progress suggests that replacement therapy with alpha-1-antitrypsin or with synthetic elastase inhibitors may be feasible, but there is at present no specific therapy. Clearly, abstinence from smoking will be helpful, and children identified as having low levels of alpha-1-antitrypsin should be strongly counseled to avoid smoking (as, of course, should all other children). Patients with genetic predisposition to emphysema should receive routine immunizations against influenza and probably against pneumococci. Any pulmonary infection should be promptly and vigorously treated.

"Emphysema" in children is usually a radiographic diagnosis, which refers to a persistent generalized or localized overinflation of the lung. Although these conditions are not truly emphysema, they are discussed in this context for convenience. Radiographic hyperlucency may occur as a result of compensatory overinflation associated with atelectasis or surgical removal of adjacent lung tissue. Hyperlucency may also be associated with hypoplasia of the pulmonary artery. None of these conditions require specific therapy except, of course, for atelectasis.

Air Trapping. Air trapping for mechanical reasons is relatively common in pediatric patients, and the treatment depends on the cause. Generalized air trapping may be associated with diffuse bronchial edema or bronchospasm, as in asthma or bronchiolitis. Air trapping that does not respond to the usual therapy (bronchodilators) within a reasonable period of time should raise questions about the diagnosis and deserves further diagnostic study (sweat testing). Localized air trapping may result from inherent defects in the bronchi (congenital lobar emphysema), intrabronchial lesions (granulation tissue, foreign bodies, mucus plugs, bronchial stenosis, tumors), or extrinsic compression lesions (enlarged great vessels, lymph nodes, tumors). Definitive diagnosis is mandatory in these conditions and should usually include bronchoscopy as well as radiographic studies. The recent development of suitable instruments for flexible fiberoptic bronchoscopy in infants and children has made bronchoscopy a safe and effective diagnostic technique that should be employed with relatively little reservation. The rigid bronchoscope, however, must be used for removal of aspirated foreign bodies.

Lobar Emphysema. Congenital lobar emphysema is a special case, as it may result in a surgical emergency in the newborn, owing to rapid expansion and compression of adjacent lung tissue. Although direct needle aspiration of a distended lobe has been reported, this should be reserved as an emergency measure. Selective intubation of the contralateral mainstem bronchus may bring temporary relief, but if the infant exhibits marked respiratory distress, surgical intervention (lobectomy) is probably necessary. In most cases no therapy will be required.

Interstitial Air Collection. Interstitial collection of air (in the mediastinum or subcutaneous tissues) may occur in a variety of situations in children (e.g., mechanical ventilation, acute asthma, and foreign body aspiration). Careful diagnostic evaluation is required, and the underlying lesion should be treated specifically. Massive subcutaneous emphysema may be treated by aspiration with a large-bore needle and syringe, with manual expression of the air towards the needle. This is rarely necessary, but if the skin is tightly distended,

it can be very helpful in relieving pain and anxiety. Patients with mediastinal emphysema who are receiving mechanical ventilation are at high risk for pneumothorax and must be watched carefully for this complication.

In premature infants receiving ventilator support, interstitial collection of air within the pulmonary lymphatics is not uncommon and may produce mechanical consequences similar to those of a tension pneumothorax. In many patients conservative therapy will be successful, with resolution occurring within several days. Reduction in mean and maximal airway passage may be helpful if consistent with maintenance of adequate gas exchange. If the process is localized, selective intubation of one main bronchus may be helpful. Lobectomy is occasionally performed but should be avoided if possible, as the basic lesion is reversible. The use of 100% oxygen to speed resorption of the interstitial gas is not recommended in premature infants.

Pulmonary Edema

ROBERT E. WOOD, Ph.D., M.D.

Pulmonary edema is the accumulation of abnormal amounts of fluid in the interstices and alveolar spaces of the lungs. In general, two forms of pulmonary edema are recognized: cardiogenic ("hydrostatic") and permeability ("noncardiogenic"). The former results from increased microvascular pressure in the lungs due to poor left ventricular function or obstruction of pulmonary venous return. The latter is associated with a variety of insults to the lung, including aspiration, sepsis, and shock, and is often referred to as the adult respiratory distress syndrome (ARDS). The two mechanisms of pulmonary edema may well coexist in a given patient. In addition, massive fluid overload or severe hypoproteinemia may also contribute to pulmonary edema.

The management of pulmonary edema begins with an assessment of the physiologic status of the patient and the etiology of the edema. Arterial blood gas determinations, chest radiographs, and a careful physical examination are essential. Hemodynamic monitoring with a pulmonary artery catheter (Swan-Ganz) may be helpful in both diagnosis and management of pulmonary edema, although it is not always necessary. Such catheters may be placed through a central venous access in patients of virtually all ages. Placement of an indwelling arterial catheter for continuous measurement of blood pressure and frequent sampling for arterial blood gas determinations will contribute greatly to the effective management of the patient. Further diagnostic measures should be undertaken concurrently with the initiation of therapy to assess and then specifically treat contributing factors such as infection.

The primary goal of therapy is the maintenance of oxygen delivery to the tissues: effective cardiac output and arterial oxygenation. All patients with pulmonary edema will be hypoxic, and should be given oxygen in sufficient concentrations to achieve an arterial oxygen saturation of at least 90% (equivalent under most circumstances to an arterial pO_2 of 60) if possible. Severe anemia should be treated by infusion of packed red cells, in order to increase the oxygen carrying capacity of peripheral blood.

In both cardiogenic and permeability edema, measures to reduce the pressures leading to fluid filtration across the alveolar-capillary barrier are appropriate. Diuretics effectively decrease the driving pressure from the right ventricle by reducing total body water, and they may also increase serum oncotic pressure by the resulting hemoconcentration. Furosemide, 1–2 mg/kg given intravenously, is the most common diuretic used in treatment of acute pulmonary edema. In patients without adequate renal function, hemodialysis or peritoneal dialysis may be required to remove sufficient volumes of water. In some patients, however, hypotension due to low circulating blood volume may itself be a major etiologic factor in the development of increased pulmonary capillary permeability ("shock lung"), and so fluid status must be assessed carefully in all patients. Hypovolemia should be treated by fluid replacement with colloids or blood, as this will result in more effective correction of circulatory status than will crystalloids. However, late in the course of pulmonary edema due to increased permeability, colloid administration may actually worsen the clinical status of the patient by allowing leakage of more protein into the alveolar spaces. Therefore, colloids should not be given except in the patient who is clearly hypovolemic or seriously hypoproteinemic.

Morphine, in a dose of 0.1 mg/kg, may often be beneficial in patients with pulmonary edema. Relief of anxiety may result in more efficient respiratory patterns, and the central vasodilation produced will reduce venous return to the heart.

The presence of fluid in the alveolar spaces and interstitial tissue will result in impairment of alveolar gas exchange, with consequent hypoxemia. Positive pressure ventilation, especially with the addition of positive end-expiratory pressure, will help to maximize ventilation of perfused alveolar-capillary units by increasing functional residual capacity and preventing alveolar collapse. Although intubation and mechanical ventilation will not be necessary in many patients, if there is evidence of alveolar hypoventilation (arterial pCO_2 > 45–50) or severe hypoxemia, the patient should be intubated and ventilated as necessary. Depending on the degree of ventilatory impairment, end-expiratory pressures ranging from 5 to more than 15 cm of water may be required to optimize gas exchange. There is little evidence to support the common notion that increased airway pressure actually results in net movement of fluid back into the vascular space.

In patients with impairment of left ventricular function, the pressure in the pulmonary veins may be increased, thus leading to pulmonary edema. In addition, obstruction of venous return to the heart (e.g., pericardial tamponade, mitral stenosis) may also produce increased pulmonary microvascular pressure and edema, emphasizing the importance of thorough diagnostic studies in addition to initial therapy. Left ventricular function may be improved under most circumstances by inotropic agents such as dopamine or dobutamine (acutely) or by digitalis (in more chronic circumstances). Dopamine* infused in low doses (2–5 µg/kg/min) effectively stimulates renal blood flow and diuresis, while providing a mild inotropic effect on the heart. In higher doses (7–20 µg/kg/min), dopamine has a more pronounced inotropic effect. It also produces increasing degrees of peripheral vasoconstriction and is thus perhaps best used in patients with relative hypotension. Dobutamine infusion (5–20 µg/kg/min) produces an effective inotropic effect without marked increases in peripheral resistance. In pediatric patients, a convenient method for administration of these drugs (dopamine and dobutamine) is to prepare a solution containing 15 mg/kg in 250 ml. The infusion of 1 ml/hr is then equivalent to 1 µg/kg/min. When the myocardium cannot be stimulated more effectively, afterload reduction by vasodilators such as nitroprusside (0.5–8 µg/kg/min) or hydralazine (0.1–0.5 mg/kg every 3–6 hr) may effectively increase cardiac output and relieve pulmonary congestion. Care must be taken to avoid systemic hypotension. When inotropic and vasoactive agents are used in patients with complicated myocardial dysfunction, hemodynamic monitoring (measurement of cardiac output and pulmonary capillary wedge pressure) is very helpful, if not essential.

Pulmonary Embolism

ROBERT NUDELMAN, M.D.

Although pulmonary embolism is rarely diagnosed in childhood, its occurrence may be more frequent. In contrast to adults in whom pulmonary

---

* Safety and efficacy of dopamine in children have not been established.

emboli usually arise postoperatively from the deep venous system of the pelvis or lower extremities, in children embolism is often a complication of a primary disease such as heart disease, neoplasia, or sepsis or from the use of central lines for hyperalimentation or monitoring.

ACUTE THERAPY

Supportive Care. Necessary measures should be taken to support circulation and respiration. Adequate analgesia should be provided, and underlying infections and primary conditions should be appropriately treated. Possible sources of further emboli such as central venous catheters should be removed, if feasible.

Heparin Administration. Since pulmonary embolism is usually a complication of venous thrombosis, unless there is a compelling contraindication, intravenous heparin should be administered as soon as the diagnosis is suspected. A bolus of 50 units/kg is given initially followed by a constant infusion of 20 units/kg/hr in small premature neonates and 25 units/kg/hr in larger premature or term neonates, in infants, and in older children. In adolescents and young adults, an initial bolus of 5000 units is followed by 1000 to 2000 units/hr. Sufficient heparin should be given to maintain the level of anticoagulation test results to $1\frac{1}{2}$ to $2\frac{1}{2}$ times control values. In neonates, the Laidlaw clotting time is preferred, if available, since it can be done by heel stick on small quantities of blood. Otherwise, the activated partial thromboplastin time (APTT) or Lee-White clotting time is used. Initially, one of these tests is measured every 4 hours, and the infusion rate is adjusted by 5 units/kg/hr until the desired clinical and laboratory effects are achieved. Thereafter, once daily monitoring is usually sufficient. Heparin is generally continued a minimum of 7 to 10 days—the time required for the venous thrombus to become firmly adherent to the vascular endothelium. Therefore, recurrent thromboembolism during the first few days of heparin therapy does not constitute a therapeutic failure. In these patients, increasing the dose of heparin to maintain the APTT or clotting time at the upper end of the therapeutic range should be the first maneuver.

Common complications of heparin therapy are bleeding and thrombocytopenia. Bleeding that occurs when clotting studies are excessively prolonged can usually be controlled by discontinuing heparin for a few hours and then resuming it at a lower rate, maintaining the APTT or clotting time at the lower end of the therapeutic range. Platelet counts should be monitored during therapy, and heparin should be discontinued if significant thrombocytopenia occurs.

Thrombolytic Therapy. While thrombolytic therapy leads to a more rapid improvement in pulmonary circulation, there is no documented difference in survival rates compared with heparin, and there is an increased incidence of bleeding complications. Therefore, thrombolytic treatment is recommended presently only for patients with a massive embolus that has caused systemic hypotension in which a small subsequent embolism could be fatal. In this situation, the quicker resolution of the embolism by thrombolytics may be life saving.

Thrombolytic treatment should be given only within 7 days of the onset of the embolism. Prior to the start of therapy, anticoagulants must be withdrawn, baseline anticoagulation tests should be obtained, and the thrombin time (TT) and APTT should be less than twice control values.

Two drugs, urokinase and streptokinase, are available for therapy. Neither is recommended for pediatric use. Urokinase may be preferable in children, since preexisting antibodies to streptokinase may be present, which can cause resistance to its action and a greater incidence of allergic reaction. The loading dose of urokinase is 4400 units/kg over 10 minutes followed by a continuous infusion of 4400 units/kg/hr for 12 hours.

If streptokinase is used in adolescents or young adults, a loading dose of 250,000 units is given over 30 minutes followed by 100,000 units/hr for 24 hours for pulmonary embolism and up to 72 hours for concurrent deep vein thrombosis. (Urokinase is not approved for treatment of deep vein thrombosis.) In younger children, an initial dose of 20 units/ml of blood volume (estimated as 80 ml/kg body weight) is given intravenously over 30 minutes followed by the same dose hourly.

The presence of the lytic state should be confirmed by performing the TT 4 hours after streptokinase therapy is begun. If the result is less than $1\frac{1}{2}$ times the control value, excessive resistance to streptokinase is present and therapy should be changed to urokinase. Laboratory monitoring beyond 4 hours of streptokinase therapy or at any time during urokinase treatment does not seem to be necessary, since results do not reliably predict efficacy or bleeding complications.

During thrombolytic therapy, invasive procedures such as arterial blood gas determinations should be avoided if possible. At the end of treatment, heparin should be resumed once the TT is less than twice control values. This usually takes 2 to 4 hours.

Absolute contraindications to thrombolytic therapy include active internal bleeding and a stroke within the last 2 months. Relative contraindications are recent major operations or trauma, serious gastrointestinal bleeding, obstetrical delivery, and severe arterial hypertension.

Complications of thrombolytic therapy are bleeding and febrile and allergic reactions. Mild bleeding can usually be controlled with compression, while major bleeding usually requires cessation of treatment and, at times, transfusion. Mild allergic reactions can usually be managed with antihistamines and/or corticosteroids. Severe reactions usually require discontinuation of treatment as well. Febrile reactions can be alleviated with acetaminophen.

Surgical Interventions. Surgery can be used either to prevent further emboli to the lungs or to remove emboli already present. These procedures have rarely, if ever, been performed in children.

If the source of embolism can be demonstrated to be from the pelvic or leg veins, the surgical interruption of the inferior vena cava below the renal veins may be indicated. Indications include recurrent emboli despite several days of adequate anticoagulation; a contraindication to or complication of heparin therapy; uncontrolled septic emboli despite 24 to 48 hours of anticoagulants and antibiotics; and paradoxical embolism.

Pulmonary embolectomy should be reserved for the patient who has had a massive embolus with systemic hypotension and in whom either an absolute contraindication to anticoagulation exists or maximal medical therapy has failed to correct inadequate perfusion of the lungs and the left ventricle. Inferior vena cava interruption should be performed at the time of the embolectomy to prevent recurrence if the embolus arose from below the renal veins.

LONG-TERM MANAGEMENT

Oral sodium warfarin is usually begun after the first week of heparin therapy, after which time the thrombus is adherent to the vessel and there is sufficient clinical improvement to allow for ambulation. Heparin is continued while the patient is begun on an average maintenance dose of warfarin of 10 mg for an adolescent or young adult and 2.5 to 5 mg for a child. After 3 to 4 days of combined therapy, the minimum time necessary to deplete vitamin K-dependent clotting factors, and when the PT is $1\frac{1}{2}$ to $2\frac{1}{2}$ times control values, heparin can be discontinued. The PT should be checked every 1 to 2 weeks thereafter. Ideally oral anticoagulation should be maintained for 3 to 6 months after the first episode of thromboembolism and indefinitely in those who had recurrences or are at continued risk.

Finally, despite adequate oral anticoagulation or because of a contraindication to or complication of therapy, a small number of patients may continue to have recurrent thromboemboli. Many will have increased platelet adhesiveness, and the use of antiplatelet agents such as aspirin* (10 mg/kg/

---

* This use of aspirin and dipyridamole is not listed by their manufacturer.

day) or dipyridamole* (3–5 mg/kg/day) may be beneficial.

PREVENTION

There is no data to support the use of low-dose preoperative heparin in children, but it seems reasonable to avoid prolonged immobilization and excessive use of central lines and to exercise the legs following an operation. Warfarin therapy may be helpful in preventing recurrent thromboemboli in patients with antithrombin III deficiency.

Primary Pulmonary Hemosiderosis

DOUGLAS C. HEINER, M.D.

Primary pulmonary hemosiderosis is a severe form of pulmonary disease in which there is diffuse bleeding into the alveoli but no known underlying disease such as heart failure, collagen vascular disease (e.g., pulmonary polyarteritis or disseminated lupus), anomaly of the pulmonary vascular system, elevated pulmonary venous pressure, or a primary bleeding disorder. The diagnosis must be confirmed by the demonstration of iron-laden macrophages in gastric or bronchial washes or in the alveoli at pulmonary biopsy. Unexplained pulmonary hemosiderosis probably has diverse etiologies. In a significant proportion of infants with this diagnosis, there appears to be an abnormal immunologic and clinical response to dietary constituents—most commonly cow's milk proteins. Several subjects have been observed who had both clinical and immunologic evidence of hypersensitivity to soy protein. Peanut and pork have been implicated in a few instances. Rational treatment requires a careful search for etiologic agents that can be eliminated from the diet or from the environment. Contributing factors include (1) upper or lower esophageal dysfunction with aspiration of food or gastric contents and (2) immunologic disturbances, including selective IgA deficiency, IgG subclass deficiencies, and abnormally high levels of antibodies to cow's milk or other specific food proteins. Precipitating antibodies, when present, constitute a strong indication for a trial elimination diet. In infants under 1 year of age, a cow's milk–free diet and/or soy-free diet should be tried whether or not precipitins are present.

Once the diagnosis is established, I recommend a trial on a milk-free diet, since the likelihood of benefit far outweighs the risks of psychologic or nutritional deprivation, problems which can be avoided by skilled physicians. About two thirds of infants with primary pulmonary hemosiderosis respond favorably to the elimination of cow's milk and milk products from the diet. Perhaps one third of patients 4 to 10 years of age also respond to this measure, as do about one tenth of those in later childhood and adolescence. A trial milk-free diet must be maintained for a minimum of 1 month in subjects who are experiencing continuous symptoms, since a favorable response may not be apparent until that time. In addition, strict milk elimination must be continued for a period exceeding the length of any spontaneous remission that has occurred prior to the time of beginning the milk-free diet. Thus, if a patient has had persistent symptoms for many months and there is no response following 1 month of a milk-free diet, it is unlikely that a response will occur, and other measures should be taken. However, if there have been intermittent pulmonary symptoms with remissions, for example, of up to 6 months' duration, the milk-free diet must be continued for at least 7 months in order to provide some assurance that any remission observed is not a spontaneous one, unrelated to the diet. I have seen a number of children who provided no evidence by history or laboratory studies of an etiologic role for milk, yet in 3 of them remissions of greater than 2 years followed the institution of a milk-free diet. On the other hand, I am aware of a greater number of subjects without clues that milk played a contributory role who continued to have persistent or recurrent pulmonary disease in spite of a milk-free diet. Some subjects seem to improve not at all or incompletely on a milk-free diet, yet when milk is reintroduced into the diet it induces an exacerbation. Only by dietary challenge of these patients following a period of milk elimination does it become apparent that milk intake should be prohibited.

The initial period of milk elimination should include all milk-containing products. Beef and gelatin share bovine serum proteins with cow's milk and are to be avoided, as should goat's milk, cheeses of all kinds, chocolate and all products containing milk, casein or whey solids. After prolonged remission has been established, a trial of well-cooked beef and foods containing boiled or canned milk can be made. A food known to aggravate the disease may cause no trouble if eaten in small quantities on infrequent occasions. However, caution must be exercised in ever allowing unrestricted use of a food once shown to cause clinical exacerbations. One must be quite certain that he is not contributing to the insidious development of chronic lung disease. Hence, at least yearly evaluation of pulmonary function by a competent specialist is necessary if milk or another incriminated food is again permitted. Similar comprehensive pulmonary follow-up studies are required in subjects who have had a progression of pulmonary symptoms or infiltrates in the previous

year. If there is an unavoidable exposure to milk or another offending food, symptoms can sometimes be minimized or averted by the administration of antihistaminics or corticosteroids or both for a period of 48 hours.

When a patient is critically ill with respiratory distress or massive bleeding, I recommend treatment with generous doses of corticosteroids. I prefer IV methylprednisolone (Medrol) 1.0 mg/kg every 6 hours, continued until active bleeding has ceased and the patient's condition has stabilized for 48 hours. I follow this by daily, then alternate-day, steroids in the amounts needed to minimize or abolish ongoing symptoms. If fresh bleeding continues after 3 days of adequate corticosteroid therapy, or if the patient's status deteriorates in spite of therapy, either azathioprine,* 3 mg/kg/day po, or cyclophosphomide (Cytoxan),* 2 mg/kg/day IV for 1 week, may be given in addition to continuing the corticosteroids. If either of these drugs is used, WBC and platelet counts should be determined once or twice weekly and the physician must be familiar with the use of the drug, including side effects which might mitigate against its continued use. Oral maintenance therapy with either azathioprine or cyclophosphamide in the above doses may be necessary.

Oxygen is administered when there is hypoxemia. Positive pressure respiration may be helpful during severe exacerbations since it may diminish active bleeding. Whole blood transfusions should be given to replace blood loss and to correct anemia. On two separate occasions following whole blood transfusions, one patient with primary pulmonary hemosiderosis and marked IgA deficiency in both plasma and secretions had dramatic reversal of severe pulmonary bleeding and near fatal respiratory distress. It was tempting to speculate that a deficiency was repaired or a more normal immunologic balance attained following transfusion in this child, yet extensive investigations revealed no deficiency other than a lack of serum and secretory IgA. Plasma or whole blood infusions of 10 ml/kg IV may have particular value in patients with a deficiency of serum IgA (10% of children with primary pulmonary hemosiderosis are IgA deficient). A word of caution should be given against overloading the circulation with large amounts of fluid, particularly saline, since this may aggravate pulmonary congestion. Usually no greater than one quarter normal saline (in 5% dextrose) is used for patients with active pulmonary disease who require IV fluid therapy.

It is always essential that a patent airway be ensured, especially if there is evident airway obstruction due to tracheal blood, secretions or tonsillar or adenoidal hypertrophy, or if cardiomeg-

---

* This use is not listed in the manufacturer's official directive.

aly, pulmonary hypertension or ECG evidence of right ventricular strain is found. An endotracheal tube or a tracheostomy occasionally may be needed.

In patients in whom there is a history of swallowing difficulty or tracheal aspiration in early childhood or in whom there is current clinical evidence of esophageal dysfunction, appropriate studies of lower esophageal sphincter competence and of swallowing function should be made. In infants with postprandial regurgitation or demonstrable esophageal dysfunction, continuous propping in a semi-upright position may help. If simple measures such as propping and frequent small feedings spaced throughout the day are of insufficient value, surgical measures should be considered. Even if the history is negative for esophageal symptoms, it is wise to evaluate esophageal function carefully and institute appropriate treatment in children with primary pulmonary hemosiderosis who fail to respond to dietary measures.

Congenital Diaphragmatic Hernia

MAX L. RAMENOFSKY, M.D.

There are two commonly recognized types of congenital diaphragmatic hernia, the most serious being the hernia through the foramen of Bochdalek, the second being of the foramen of Morgagni.

BOCHDALEK HERNIA

Congenital diaphragmatic hernia through the foramen of Bochdalek continues to be a defect of major importance because of the exceptionally high mortality rate associated with its presence. The foramen of Bochdalek, although a misnomer for the site of the hernia, is taken in context to mean the pleuroperitoneal canal, located anatomically at the posterolateral aspect of the developing diaphragm, and is the last portion of the diaphragm to close, thus separating the pleural from the peritoneal cavity.

Neonates with congenital diaphragmatic hernia are usually full term with anomalies associated only with the hernia. Occasionally an intracardiac defect is present. Anomalies related to the congenital diaphragmatic hernia include bilateral pulmonary hypoplasia (both endodermal and mesenchymal derivates), malrotation of the intestine, and a small peritoneal cavity. Also encountered are pathophysiologic abnormalities such as patent ductus arteriosus and patent foramen ovale. The hernia is located on the left side in 80%, is on the right side in 10–15%, and is bilateral in 5% of cases.

The time at which the hernia causes symptoms is of greatest prognostic value for ultimate outcome. Most patients present at delivery, as soon as the umbilical cord is clamped. Mortality in this group varies from 50–70%. Patients whose symptoms occur after leaving the delivery room but before 24 hours of age have a 40% mortality, and infants presenting after 24 hours of age approach 0% mortality. The mortality appears to be most closely related to the degree of pulmonary hypoplasia. The most severe degrees are manifested by very early presentation and result from inability of the hypoplastic lungs to sustain adequate ventilation.

From the outset, diagnosis and treatment are inseparable. This congenital disease represents the ultimate pediatric surgical emergency! The time from the onset of symptoms to treatment must be minimized to maximize the chances of survival.

Treatment of patients with congenital diaphragmatic hernia can be separated into three phases: preoperative, operative, and postoperative.

Preoperative Treatment. The full-term newborn with respiratory distress in the delivery room when the cord is clamped requires prompt diagnosis and treatment. Typically these newborns have a markedly scaphoid abdomen, barrel-shaped chest, and severe respiratory distress with peripheral to central cyanosis. Once respiratory distress has been noted, oxygen must be started and an orogastric tube (12 F) inserted into the stomach. An immediate upright and lateral chest/abdominal x-ray is obtained. This diagnostic/therapeutic maneuver will show the hernia, frequently with the orogastric tube coursing into the hernia in the chest. The tube will allow evacuation of swallowed air, allowing the intrinsically compromised pulmonary parenchyma more room for expansion and ventilation.

Most of these infants are not born in hospitals where there is pediatric surgical expertise and a neonatal ICU. Consequently, transfer is necessary. Time should not be wasted attempting to resuscitate these infants, as the ultimate resuscitation must occur in the operating room.

Ventilation is difficult. If the infant is able to self-ventilate, oxygen should be continued. However, if the infant remains tachypneic and cyanotic, an endotracheal tube (3.5) should be inserted and assisted ventilation started. Maximal ventilatory pressure should not exceed 25 cm H_2O. It is often necessary to use positive end-expiratory pressure (PEEP) of 4–6 cm H_2O to overcome the high intrapleural and consequently transpulmonary pressures generated by the herniated viscera. All further resuscitative efforts should be performed in the operating room, where conditions can be more rigidly controlled.

An umbilical arterial line is inserted and arterial blood gases obtained. Respiratory acidosis is managed by correcting the ventilatory defect. Metabolic acidosis is often present as well and should be corrected by the use of a buffer, usually sodium bicarbonate. The following formula has proven useful: meq $NaHCO_3$ = BE × weight (kg) × 0.3 BE = a negative base excess. The bicarbonate is diluted and given over a 3–5 minute period. If the PCO_2 is greater than 55 torr, bicarbonate should not be given; rather the ventilatory rate should be increased. There is recent evidence that high-frequency, "jet" ventilation is a better method of ventilating these newborns.

The period of resuscitation should last only as long as the patient shows improvement but not longer than one hour. Should no improvement occur or should the patient start to deteriorate, the operation should be started immediately.

Operative Treatment. Most pediatric surgeons prefer a transverse left upper quadrant abdominal incision for left-sided defects. However, the incision must be made rapidly. If the hernia is on the right side, most prefer a right posterolateral thoracotomy. However, if intestine, in addition to liver, is in the defect on the right side, an abdominal incision is often favored. The herniated viscera are reduced, and a sac, if present, is excised. The lung, as visualized through the hernia defect, appears very small and hypoplastic. The anesthesiologist should *not* try to inflate this lung. A thoracostomy tube is placed into the chest on the side of the defect but *not* attached to waterseal drainage. A second prophylactic chest tube is placed into the opposite pleural cavity at the end of the operation and is attached to waterseal. The hernia defect is closed. The hernia defect itself may be closed primarily, as there is usually a posterior rim of muscle which can be used for closure, but on occasion a silicone coated nylon patch is required.

At the end of the operative procedure, a right radial or right temporal arterial line should be inserted. If an umbilical arterial line was not inserted prior to the start of the procedure, one should be inserted at this point. If technically feasible, a pulmonary arterial catheter should be inserted postoperatively, as this is very helpful in the management of the rapid changes in these patients' pulmonary arterial pressures.

Postoperative Treatment. The postoperative care of the neonate with congenital diaphragmatic hernia requires constant attention to the details of ventilatory therapy, acid-base balance–pulmonary arterial pressure, and mediastinal positioning. In essence, the management involves treatment of a persistent or recurring fetal circulation. Although the details of management will be discussed under the separate topics of ventilatory management, acid-base balance, pulmonary arterial pressure,

and mediastinal stabilization, in practice simultaneous evaluation and treatment is necessary.

VENTILATORY MANAGEMENT. Most neonates will require ventilatory assistance. The most common mistake is the use of an inspiratory pressure that is too high. Because the hemithorax on the side of the hernia is empty due to the hypoplastic lung, the use of high inspiratory pressure causes the contralateral lung to overexpand into the empty hemithorax. The use of a low ventilatory pressure with a rapid ventilatory rate is preferred. Positive end-expiratory pressure is contraindicated.

The initial FiO_2 should be 100%. When the arterial blood gases, both pre- and postductal, are normal, the FiO_2 should be decreased but not at increments greater than 5% per setting change. Too great or too rapid change results in rebound pulmonary hypertension and progressive return of the fetal circulation.

ACID-BASE MANAGEMENT–PULMONARY ARTERIAL PRESSURE. Right-to-left shunting occurs in these patients. Three loci of shunting have been identified, all associated with the development of pulmonary hypertension: the foramen ovale, the ductus arteriosus, and within the lung. Monitoring pulmonary arterial pressure is the ideal way to identify pulmonary hypertension. However, simultaneous pre- and postductal arterial blood gas determinations via the right radial and umbilical arterial catheters can be used to estimate the degree of right-to-left shunting through the ductus arteriosus, which indicates pulmonary hypertension. For example, if a right-to-left shunt through the ductus arteriosus is present, the preductal pH and PaO_2 will be higher than the postductal pH and PaO_2, indicating that the preductal blood has traversed ventilated lung whereas the postductal blood had not. Additionally, a preductal arterial blood gas gives important information regarding the oxygen tension of the blood perfusing the brain.

Simultaneous pre- and postductal blood gases do not give information about shunts through the foramen ovale. A preductal arterial blood gas and the use of a shunt equation or a shunt nomogram provides useful information about the degree of right to left shunting through the foramen ovale. There is normally an 18–20% physiologic right-to-left shunt in the neonate. When a 25% shunt is present the pulmonary arterial hyypertension causing the increased shunt should be treated.

Pulmonary hypertension is treated with dopamine* (10 µg/kg/min) and chlorpromazine (1 mg/kg/8 hours). It is important that the neonate's intravascular volume be in the normal range before

---

*Safety and effectiveness of dopamine in children have not been established.

starting these drugs, as severe systemic hypotension may result if the patient is hypovolemic. Normovolemia can best be estimated by a normal urine output and a normal pulse and blood pressure. Once these drugs have been started they should *not* be stopped abruptly but should be tapered over a period of several days.

Acidosis is one cause of pulmonary hypertension. Thus, if the patient becomes acidotic, it is vitally important to bring the pH back into the appropriate range. If the Pa_{CO_2} is less than 55 torr, sodium bicarbonate can be given by the formula noted previously. However, if the Pa_{CO_2} is greater than 55 torr, another buffer such as THAM or TRIS should be given in addition to vigorous ventilatory resuscitation to bring the Pa_{CO_2} back into line. The use of sodium bicarbonate when the Pa_{CO_2} is elevated results in a further increase of the Pa_{CO_2}. The ideal arterial pH in such a patient is 7.46–7.50. At this pH range the ductus is neither solidly closed or widely patent, owing to the degree of oxygen saturation. This is the ideal situation, since any pulmonary overload can be shunted through the ductus, as the ductus will serve as a "pop-off" valve. For this reason, ligation of the patent ductus in these patients is contraindicated.

MEDIASTINAL STABILIZATION. After repair of the hernia there is a period of relative pulmonary ventilatory stability. This may last up to 18 hours postoperatively and has been referred to as the "honeymoon" period. After that, progressive pulmonary insufficiency may occur. One cause of this deterioration is overexpansion of the contralateral lung. The lung expands because of the void on the side of the repaired hernia resulting from the long-delayed growth and expansion of the lung on that side. Stated another way, the ventilatory pressure needed to expand one lung normally is counterbalanced by the expanding lung on the opposite side. If the opposite side is empty, the lung will overexpand into the empty side, particularly if the mediastinum is mobile, as it is in the neonate. The inspiratory pressure will serve only to overinflate the "good" lung into the empty space. Attaching the thoracostomy tube on the side of the hernia to waterseal serves only to keep the intrapleural pressure on that side negative, thus allowing the overexpansion of the opposite lung. Rather, air should be injected into the empty hemithorax to stabilize the infant's mobile mediastinum in the midline radiographically. Occasionally the mediastinum may appear to be pushed or fixed in the chest opposite to the side of the hernia. In that situation the thoracostomy tube on the side of the hernia should be used to evacuate air from the side of the hernia and to pull the mediastinum toward the midline. This will allow the inspiratory pressure to effectively ventilate the lung instead of causing it to underexpand.

The length of time required for the patient's condition to stabilize and improve is 4–7 days. The end point should be spontaneous ventilation on room air, permanent resolution of the pulmonary hypertension, and stabilization of the mediastinum in the midline, which will occur when the lung on the opposite side of the hernia grows and expands.

MORGAGNI HERNIA

A hernia through the foramen of Morgagni is usually asymptomatic. However, symptoms may result should incarceration of the herniated viscera occur. Operative repair should be carried out when the diagnosis is made.

5

Cardiovascular System

Congestive Cardiac Failure

SAMUEL KAPLAN, M.D.

Goals of treatment remain relief of symptoms by diuresis to alleviate water and salt retention, improvement of myocardial function, a decrease in oxygen requirement while increasing oxygen supply, and correction of metabolic abnormalities. Recognition of the underlying cause is paramount in planning strategies of treatment. In the majority, a surgically treatable structural abnormality is the cause. Medical therapy is instituted prior to surgery to decrease the risk of operation and is continued for a varying period postoperatively. In others, congestive cardiac failure is caused or aggravated by arrhythmias (such as paroxysmal supraventricular tachycardia), anemia, primary or secondary myocardial disease (such as cardiomyopathy or myocarditis), sepsis, or hypertension.

METABOLIC ABNORMALITIES

Hypoglycemia, hypocalcemia, hypomagnesemia, and acidemia are frequent, especially in neonates and young infants. Hypoglycemia of uncertain cause and of temporary duration can present in neonates with signs of congestive cardiac failure. Infants of diabetic mothers, who frequently have cardiomyopathy and in whom the prevalence of congenital heart disease is higher than the general population, may have heart failure, aggravated by hypoglycemia. Infants with congenital cardiac lesions, especially those whose aortic flow is dependent on persistent patency of the ductus arteriosus (such as neonates with symptomatic coarctation of the aorta), frequently develop hypoglycemia when ductal flow is inadequate. In all these instances early recognition and prompt treatment with intravenous doses of glucose are essential. Hypocalcemia of unknown cause must also be recognized

and treated promptly with intravenous calcium. Acidemia may be due to inadequate cardiac output, or inadequate pulmonary or systemic blood flow in neonates with ductal dependent lesions and constriction of the ductus. Acidemia is treated immediately, usually with sodium bicarbonate. When the underlying cardiac anomaly is ductal dependent, infusions of prostaglandin E_1 (0.05–0.1 µg/kg/min) are especially effective to maintain ductal patency prior to and during diagnostic tests and surgical management.

MANIPULATING OXYGEN SUPPLY AND DEMAND

Even in the absence of overt cyanosis, decreased oxygen tension is frequent, especially with intercurrent pulmonary disease. Oxygen supply can be increased by delivering humidified oxygen, most conveniently with nasal prongs. Oxygen demand can be decreased by (1) prompt treatment of infections, with restoration of normal temperatures, (2) prevention of hypothermia, especially in neonates, (3) bed rest in a semireclining position, which is more comfortable, especially in older children, and (4) sedation. Sedation in acutely ill patients reduces oxygen consumption by decreasing apprehension and irritability as well as the work of breathing. This is best accomplished with a small dose of morphine (not to exceed 0.1 mg per kilogram) but chloral hydrate or codeine are alternate choices. In extreme instances tracheal intubation and mechanical ventilation are used.

CALORIC AND FLUID REQUIREMENTS

When congestive cardiac failure is mild or easily controlled with diuretics, fluid restriction is unnecessary. In acutely ill children, however, a delicate balance must be maintained so that adequate calories are supplied to ensure growth while fluid restriction is instituted. These goals are frequently difficult to reach, especially in infants or prema-

132

tures. Initially the desperately ill infant is treated with intravenous fluids (restricted to about 70 ml/kg/day) and oral feedings are discontinued. Aspiration of gastric contents helps to prevent vomiting and aspiration. With clinical improvement, fluids are liberalized and oral feedings started. Frequently adequate calories can be supplied only with continuous nasogastric feedings of high caloric content. In other instances, oral intake is supplemented with nasogastric feeds. Since sodium retention is a major feature of heart failure, the diet must have a low sodium content.

Diuretics. These agents occupy a major role in treatment. They vary in potency and all have side effects that need anticipation, prevention, and immediate treatment. They are used to relieve edema and pulmonary congestion of cardiac failure. Effective therapy results in diuresis, which is monitored by measuring daily fluid intake and output and by noting a daily weight loss until stabilization at a constant level. Furosemide and ethacrynic acid, two extremely potent diuretics, may be given orally or parenterally. Their action is independent of pre-existing serum electrolyte levels. The dosages of the two agents are similar, but there has been greater experience with furosemide in infants and children. In some instances, however, ethacrynic acid will produce a diuresis when prolonged furosemide therapy has lost its efficacy. The reverse is also seen, so that furosemide may be effective when ethacrynic acid is not. In the acute situation furosemide is given intravenously, usually 1 mg/kg. If a diuresis does not occur, a similar dose may be repeated 2–4 hours later. Parenteral therapy may be continued 2–3 times daily with a total maximum dose of 5–8 mg/kg/ day. Oral furosemide is the usual route of treatment and is given one, two, or three times daily. The dosage is individualized from 0.5 to 8 mg/kg/ day. In others alternate-day, or even twice-weekly, diuretic therapy is adequate.

Thiazides are moderately potent, are preferred by some for long-term management of heart failure, and are administered orally one to three times daily. Chlorothiazide is available as a syrup, making it easier to use in infants and small children. The dose of chlorothiazide is 20–40 mg/kg/day and that of hydrochlorothiazide 2–5 mg/kg/day. Spironolactone, the aldosterone inhibitor, is a mild diuretic but is used primarily to decrease urinary potassium wastage (dose 1–2 mg/kg/day in divided doses orally). Usually 2–3 days of therapy are necessary before optimal effects are produced. Metolazone* is a potent diuretic that is reserved for patients who are unresponsive to the conven-

* Manufacturer's warning: Metolazone is not recommended for use in children.

tional therapy. It is used in conjunction with other diuretics (usually furosemide) and is given as a single dose 1 to 3 times weekly. The diuretic response may be massive, so that careful monitoring for electrolyte imbalance is essential. The recommended oral dose is 0.1 mg/kg.

COMPLICATIONS FROM DIURETIC THERAPY. Complications are common, especially electrolyte imbalance, so that repeated monitoring of serum electrolytes is necessary. Increased urinary potassium excretion occurs with the use of furosemide, ethacrynic acid, and thiazides and ultimately leads to depletion of total body potassium. Since hypokalemia is expected, serum potassium is maintained at normal levels by intravenous infusions in the acute situation and for long-term therapy by spironolactone and oral potassium. In the patient receiving digitalis, hypokalemia is a potent cause of digitalis toxicity. *Hypochloremic alkalosis* may also occur with chronic diuretic therapy. Treatment consists of reducing the dose of diuretics or discontinuing them temporarily, treatment of hypokalemia, and addition of spironolactone. More significant electrolyte derangements are treated with chloride replacement, in the form of either potassium chloride or oral ammonium chloride. *Hyponatremia* is usually dilutional and improves with water loss induced by diuretics. In rare instances hyponatremia is due to sodium depletion and is treated with liberalizing sodium intake. Intravenous sodium chloride is seldom needed and is used with great caution, since the diagnosis of sodium depletion is difficult and an increased sodium load can worsen pulmonary edema and generalized congestion. *Prematures* who require prolonged diuretic therapy for treatment of chronic lung disease and heart failure may develop renal calculi (because furosemide is calciuric), soft tissue calcification, ototoxicity, or gall stones.

ENHANCING MYOCARDIAL FUNCTION

Digitalis. Digitalis augments myocardial contractility, and some believe that it is indicated in most forms of heart failure. While these glycosides have been available for two centuries, attainment of optimal effects can be difficult, especially in infants and neonates, side effects are frequent, and reassessment of drug efficacy needs to be individualized in each patient. There is still a lack of unanimity of opinion concerning the use of digitalis in congestive cardiac failure. While clinical benefit occurs in some patients, responders to therapy cannot be predicted before initiation of treatment. Therefore, in the nonacute state, some prefer to rely on diuretic therapy initially and add digitalis if desired symptomatic improvement is not achieved.

Table 1. GUIDE TO ORAL DIGOXIN DOSAGES*

	Total Digitalizing (μg/kg)	Maintenance (μg/kg/day)
Full-term neonates	30–50	5–10
Prematures	30–35	5
Infants <2 years	50–60	10–15
Children >2 years	30–50	10

* See text for important exceptions.

Digoxin. Digoxin is the form used most frequently in pediatric practice. Since digoxin has a relatively short half-life (almost 36 hours), the effect is more easily controllable when the dose is inadequate or toxicity has occurred. The dose of digoxin and the rapidity of administration depend on the severity of cardiac failure, the weight and age of the patient, and the clinical response to digitalizing and maintenance doses. *Any dosage schedule of digoxin is merely a guide* because there are significant individual variations in response to the same dose. Thus, the time of administration and the dose may need to be modified after part or all of the calculated digitalizing dose has been administered. This is especially applicable to prematures and newborns who have an unusual intolerance to digoxin. Some prefer to treat heart failure in very low birth weight infants with diuretics only because of the prevalence of digitalis toxicity in these babies. Digoxin is excreted primarily by the kidney, so that the dosage must be reduced in renal failure to prevent toxicity. There is increased sensitivity to digoxin immediately after surgical procedures and in patients with myocarditis. If quinidine is indicated in a patient taking digoxin, digitalis intoxication occurs with therapeutic doses because quinidine displaces digoxin from its receptors.

Oral digoxin dosages in Table 1 are merely guides to therapy. Parenteral doses are about 75% of the oral dose. Some use the total digitalizing dose in acute situations only and prefer daily maintenance doses without a loading digitalizing dose, especially in prematures or in children with mild symptoms as may occur in cardiomyopathy. The route of administration varies according to the severity of illness. In the very ill child the intravenous route is preferred, whereas oral medication is suitable when symptoms and signs are relatively mild. One third of the total digitalizing dose is given initially followed by another third in 6–8 hours, and the final third 6–8 hours later. Daily maintenance is begun 12 hours later, usually in two equally divided doses. It is imperative that the physician carefully recheck the order sheet to be certain that the dose is correct and that the decimal point is in the correction position. In large older children and adolescents the dose of digoxin

is not weight dependent and adult doses are used. Generally the total digitalizing dose is about 1.5–2.0 mg with a daily maintenance dose of 0.25 mg. Electrocardiographic signs of *digitalis effect* are unusual in infants, but in older children there may be prolongation of the PR interval, shortened QT interval, depressed ST segment, and diphasic or inverted T-waves.

The clinical response is the major determinant of adequate treatment, since the goal of therapy is to reduce heart rate, relieve dyspnea, reduce liver size and venous pressure, and produce a diuresis. *Digitalis toxicity* may occur at any time during treatment and presents most frequently as arrhythmias. These consist of multiple premature ventricular contractions (sometimes bigeminal or trigeminal), premature atrial or junctional beats, intra-atrial block, paroxysmal atrial tachycardia with block, and varying degrees of heart block. Gastrointestinal and neurologic symptoms are less frequent in children than in adults and consist of anorexia, nausea, vomiting, diarrhea, visual symptoms, and dizziness. While gastrointestinal symptoms, especially vomiting, can be a sign of digitalis toxicity, this symptom is also a frequent nonspecific sign of gastric irritation from congestion due to heart failure.

The treatment of digoxin toxicity consists of discontinuing the drug, treatment of hypokalemia, and management of symptomatic arrhythmias. In many instances, signs of toxicity disappear within 24 to 48 hours after discontinuing digoxin, and the drug is cautiously reinstituted at a lower dosage. In children who require long-term management digoxin toxicity may occur when the dose has remained unchanged for many months. Massive digoxin poisoning may occur after accidental ingestion and has been treated successfully with digoxin-specific antibodies. *Digoxin serum levels* are useful as a guide to whether outpatients are compliant with therapy and as a means to determine whether a poor response to treatment for no apparent reason is due to an inadequate dose in patients with renal failure, in those taking quinidine, and in accidental ingestion. The higher dosage of digoxin used in infants results in a high serum level, which is not necessarily accompanied by signs of toxicity. In adults serum digoxin levels exceeding 2 ng/ml are likely to be associated with toxicity. In infants, however, levels as high as 5 ng/ml have been reported without signs of toxicity. Since the therapeutic digoxin concentration in infants has not been clearly defined, toxic serum levels vary but are thought to be in the range of 4–5 ng/ml. In children the level is probably 3 ng/ml.

Other Inotropic Agents. These are reserved for acute, life-threatening situations. A number of drugs are available (Table 2), and personal pref-

Table 2. INOTROPIC AGENTS

Drug	Dose Range	Comments
1. Dopamine*	4–30 μg/kg/min	Moderately potent inotropic effect
2. Dobutamine*	2.5–40 μg/kg/min	Potency similar to that of dopamine
3. Combination:		Administered in ratio of 1:4 as mixture or varied independently as required for blood pressure
Norepinephrine	0.1–2.0 μg/kg/min	dently as required for blood pressure
Phentolamine	0.4–8.0 μg/kg/min	
4. Epinephrine	0.05–1.0 μg/kg/min	Potent inotropic effect, especially in hypotensive states
5. Isoproterenol	0.025–0.5 μg/kg/min	Excessive tachycardia may limit use of higher doses

* Manufacturer's warning: Safety in children has not been established.

erence usually dictates the choice. They are infused intravenously with an infusion pump through a line reserved for the drug because the dose may need frequent adjustment. The goals of treatment are to increase cardiac output, elevate arterial blood pressure to near normal levels, increase urine production, and decrease pulmonary congestion. During infusion, parameters monitored include the electrocardiogram, arterial pressure, urinary output, and central venous and pulmonary arterial wedge pressures. These agents may be supplemented with intermittent intravenous furosemide, small boluses of fluid if venous pressures are low, and sometimes an infusion of a vasodilator such as nitroprusside.

VASODILATORS

Reduction of systemic vascular resistance by vasodilation can increase cardiac output significantly without major effects on heart rate or contractility. In acute heart failure without significant hypotension, infusions of nitroprusside can result in marked clinical improvement since the drug also produces venodilatation with a decrease in pulmonary venous pressure. The usual initial dose is 0.5–2 μg/kg/min; if the response is unsatisfactory, the dose may be slowly increased up to 10 μg/kg/min. Blood cyanide or thiocyanate levels need to be monitored during infusion to detect toxicity.

Vasodilators (in addition to digoxin and diuretics) are also used successfully in the management of refractory chronic congestive heart failure. These include oral prazosin† (10–25 μg/kg/dose, four times daily), which has similar effects as intravenous nitroprusside. A first dose response may occur, presenting primarily as hypotension, so that careful monitoring is necessary at initiation of therapy. Other drugs that have been used include hydralazine, nitrates, and captopril. Tolerance to these drugs may occur after chronic administration.

† Manufacturer's warning: Safety for use in children has not been established.

Congenital Heart Disease

ALEXANDER S. NADAS, M.D.

For the 1980's, the current pediatric therapy of congenital heart disease is cardiac surgery. Not all cardiac surgery is corrective—some operations are still palliative—but there is no *medical* cure for congenital heart disease. Looking into my murky crystal ball, I sometimes see the vague outlines of prevention of congenital malformations of the heart, but this surely will not happen before the millenium.

It may be worth spending a brief paragraph on the significance of the problem. With the virtual disappearance of rheumatic fever from the United States, due to a variety of medical and socioeconomic factors, congenital heart disease is the commonest type of pediatric heart disease in this country today. The ratio of admissions of congenital to acquired heart disease to the Children's Hospital in Boston is close to 100:1 today. This figure is an approximate one and may not be valid for all institutions, but it is the only one available to me. The overall incidence of congenital heart disease in the United States is generally estimated at 8/1000 live births. Other figures for other parts of the Western world are quite similar. Roughly, one-third of these patients become critically ill within the first year of life, another third may get sick later on, while the final third may never experience significant handicaps from their cardiac malformation. It may be said that at present birth rates close to 40,000 babies are born with congenital heart disease in the United States and one-third of these will need urgent attention within days, weeks, or months after birth.

In the following paragraphs the conventional, and largely meaningless, classifications of congenital heart disease will be disregarded. Instead, the malformation will be presented according to age of manifestation and incidence. According to long-established principles of this volume, diagnosis will not be discussed in detail, though where important the tools of diagnosis appropriate for the entity will be identified. Emphasis will be on the course of action to be taken, and the risks and benefits

Table 1. DIAGNOSTIC FREQUENCIES IN INFANTS*

Diagnosis	Infants Number	Infants Percent
Ventricular septal defect*	374	15.7
D-Transposition of great arteries*	236	9.9
Tetralogy of Fallot*	212	8.9
Coarctation of aorta*	179	7.5
Hypoplastic left heart syndrome*	177	7.4
Patent ductus arteriosus*	146	6.1
Endocardial cushion defect*	119	5.0
Heterotaxis (dextro-, meso-, levo-, asplenia)	95	
Pulmonary stenosis*	79	3.3
Pulmonary atresia with intact ventricular septum*	75	3.1
Atrial septal defect secundum	70	2.9
Total anomalous pulmonary venous return*	63	2.6
Tricuspid atresia*	61	2.6
Single ventricle	58	2.4
Aortic stenosis	45	1.9
Double-outlet right ventricle	35	1.5
Truncus arteriosus	33	1.4
L-Transposition of the great arteries	16	0.7
Other heart disease	117	4.9
No significant heart disease	24	1.0
Primary pulmonary disease	106	4.5
TOTAL	2381	100

of surgery in our institution today will be given. We will restrict the discussion to the commonest lesions, both in infancy and in childhood, making up at least 75% of the total.

INFANCY

The following discussion is based on our experience with infants who were so ill that they either died, had to be operated upon, or had to undergo cardiac catheterization within the first year of life in one of the six New England states. Clearly, some babies could be entered by several of these criteria.

Ventricular Septal Defect. This commonest cardiac malformation does not need surgical treatment unless the baby is in congestive heart failure or manifesting respiratory distress or failure to thrive. Without these signs accurate diagnosis and surgery may be safely postponed beyond the first birthday. If a baby in congestive heart failure is suspected to have a ventricular septal defect on the basis of physical examination, the diagnosis should be confirmed by ECG, x-ray, ultrasound, and catheterization. If through vigorous anti-congestive measures, including diuretics (furosemide), digitalis (Digoxin), and oxygen, the respiratory distress can be overcome and the baby starts gaining weight, surgery may be postponed, in the hope that the defect will get smaller or even close

spontaneously. By watching the baby closely, through weekly, later monthly, office visits, the pediatrician is in the best position to monitor the infant's progress. If the clinical course is satisfactory and the baby progresses within an acceptable growth channel, there is no reason why surgery could not be postponed beyond the first year of life, assuming that pulmonary vascular obstructive disease can be excluded with reasonable certainty by electrocardiography and echocardiography. A baby with intractible congestive heart failure needs corrective surgery within the first weeks or months of life. Hospital mortality is about 6%; probability of complete closure among the survivors is 90%.

Transposition of the Great Arteries. The second commonest defect among infants is transposition of the great arteries. It always needs surgical correction or palliation. There are many varieties of transposition, but irrespective of anatomic details, and in contrast to ventricular defect, *all patients have to be operated upon.* The commonest form of the malformation is the patient *without a ventricular septal defect*; these are babies who are quite cyanotic within hours after birth, with unimpressive physical findings, normal chest x-ray, and ECG. The echocardiogram is diagnostic. In most institutions, as soon as the diagnosis is established, the baby is taken to the cardiac catheterization laboratory for physiologic studies, angiography, and balloon septostomy (rupture of the interatrial septum to promote mixing between systemic and pulmonary blood flow). If through the creation of an atrial defect, the baby's resting arterial saturation is no lower than 65% and the pH is satisfactory, a venous switch operation (Mustard or Senning) with an operative risk of about 5% may be postponed until the third month of life, assuming a steady clinical course. If the baby is not thriving, an atrial baffle operation may be performed at any time, with only slightly, if any, higher risks. The long-term outcome of the venous switch operation has not been definitely established; some centers have satisfactory survivors into the second and third decades. Still, enough doubt has been expressed about late development of arrhythmias, and the capacity of the right ventricle to perform systemic work for several decades, that in a few institutions, including our own, an arterial switch operation (transposing the aorta over the left ventricle and the pulmonary artery over the right ventricle) is the procedure of choice for some of these critically ill babies within the first days of life. Initial results are quite encouraging (22/25 operative survivors); no long-term data are available.

Patients with transposition and a ventricular septal defect (with or without pulmonary stenosis) represent complex diagnostic problems with congestive heart failure or cyanosis dominating

Table 2. INCIDENCE OF CONGENITAL HEART DISEASE AMONG CHILDREN SEEN AT CHILDREN'S HOSPITAL IN BOSTON

Diagnosis	Number	Age (years)			
		0–5	*5–10*	*10–15*	*15–20*
Ventricular septal defect*	1950	25%	21%	21%	21%
Pulmonary stenosis*	1066	7	14	16	17
Tetralogy of Fallot*	857	10	9	9	8
Aortic stenosis*	774	3	8	12	17
Patent ductus arteriosus*	678	15	7	3	2
Atrial septal defect secundum*	671	6	13	9	7
Coarctation of the aorta*	464	5	7	7	4
Mitral disease	372	2	4	7	7
Transposition of the great arteries	351	8	3	2	2
Endocardial cushion defect*	315	5	3	3	3
Single ventricle	133	2	2	1	1
Malposition	80	1	1	1	1
Other	943	11	8	9	10
Total cases	8654	3324	1574	1424	1128

the picture. Cardiac catheterization is mandatory for intelligent assessment of the anatomy and physiology. The timing of surgery depends on the baby's clinical course and the status of the pulmonary vascular bed. Surely those without significant pulmonary stenosis need surgery within the first six months of life or much sooner. Operative mortality of unselected cases is between 10 and 15%; results of long-term follow-up are encouraging but incomplete. Patients with transposition of the great arteries, ventricular septal defect, and significant pulmonary stenosis are the most likely to survive, and even thrive, for years without surgery. An arterial shunt operation (Blalock Taussig) may furnish satisfactory palliation for many years. Eventually, they do need corrective surgery (Rastelli). In general, the operative risk and long-term follow-up are similar to those cited for transposition and a ventricular septal defect.

Tetralogy of Fallot. The third commonest lesion manifesting itself in infancy is tetralogy of Fallot. Rarely is cyanosis critical within hours or days of life; in most instances it is noted within weeks and months and may be compatible with reasonable growth and development. The diagnosis may be suspected through physical examination, x-ray and ECG; ultrasound is diagnostic. Corrective surgery is being performed, electively, by one year of age in our institution; other centers prefer to palliate initially with correction at around two years. Operative mortality, through one-stage correction or through a combined two-stage approach, should not be higher than 10%. Long-term results, now encompassing three decades, are excellent, with some concern for late appearance of arrhythmias. Surgery for these patients is also mandatory. Early appearance of hypoxic spells or severe exercise intolerance may force one's hand for early inter-

vention at weeks, months, or even days of life. Pre-operative catheterization is necessary for adequate morphologic and physiologic detail.

Coarctation of the Aorta. In the majority of instances, coarctation of the aorta causes congestive heart failure in infancy. In a minority (20%) it remains dormant through childhood and even adolescence. Although aggressive medical management of congestive failure in infancy may be transiently successful, in our institution we believe today that after initial treatment with diuretics, with or without digitalis, corrective surgery is necessary within days or weeks. Diagnosis is strongly suggested by absent, or delayed, femoral pulses in an infant with congestive failure. Relative hypertension in the right arm with severe cardiac enlargement and right ventricular hypertrophy in the electrocardiogram complete the clinical diagnosis; a two-dimensional echocardiogram clearly localizes the aortic obstruction. Preoperative catheterization for anatomic and physiologic detail is recommended but is not mandatory. Operative mortality is less than 10% and long-term outcome, with the recent modifications of operative technique (Waldhausen), is promising. Reoperation should not be necessary in the majority of those operated upon in infancy today.

Hypoplastic Left Heart Syndrome. This syndrome is a highly lethal combination of valvular atresias and hypoplasias involving the mitral and aortic valve, resulting in more or less underdevelopment of the left ventricle. Babies with this syndrome become critically ill with congestive heart failure, metabolic acidosis, and hypoxia as soon as the ductus arteriosus closes, surely within the first week of life, sometimes even within hours. The outcome is fatal without operative intervention and somewhat better with surgery. The present, largely experimental (Norwood) operative technique involves two stages. The first stage has to be performed within hours or days after birth and carries an approximately 50% mortality. The second stage, with another 50% mortality, has been proposed for the first or second year of life. Experience is quite limited with this approach but given the uniformly fatal outcome of the malformation and a few survivors of the second-stage surgery with good postoperative hemodynamics, it may be worth consideration in a few selected centers with a large patient population. The diagnosis is suspected clinically in a baby with symptoms as described, poor peripheral pulses, and a very large heart with pulmonary vascular engorgement. Characteristically, the electrocardiogram is diagnostic; cardiac catheterization is mandatory for anatomic and physiologic details only for those to undergo surgery.

Patent Ductus Arteriosus. All newborns have an open ductus. In less than 1% of full-term infants the ductus remains open beyond the first week of life. The incidence of a hemodynamically significant patent ductus arteriosus in prematures is 20% overall; the smaller the baby and the more respiratory distress it has, the more likely it is to have an open ductus. On the basis of studies within the past decade, one may state without hesitation that prematures in whom a large ductus arteriosus does not close under usual medical management of congestive failure within approximately 48 hours should be given indomethacin by mouth or, when available, intravenously. If after treatment with indomethacin the ductus remains open, surgery with an operative risk of less than 1% is recommended. The ductus arteriosus in full-term infants usually does not manifest itself within the first month of life. The diagnosis is suspected in a baby with congestive heart failure and bounding pulses, a systolic murmur with or without a diastolic component (rarely is the typical continuous murmur heard), a large heart with pulmonary vascular engorgement, and combined ventricular hypertrophy on the cardiogram. The echocardiogram is diagnostic. Indomethacin is ineffective beyond the first month of life. Surgery with or without preoperative catheterization is safe (hospital mortality less than 1%) and curative.

Atrioventricular Canal. Congestive failure and cyanosis early in infancy are the usual manifestations of atrioventricular canal. The diagnostic feature is the superior axis of the electrocardiogram (between −30 and −90 degrees). There are regurgitant murmurs present and x-ray views show a large heart with pulmonary vascular engorgement. Close to three-quarters of the babies with this defect who come to surgery are infants with Down's syndrome. The question of whether these babies with Down's syndrome ought to be handled as aggressively as babies without chromosomal abnormalities used to be one of the most difficult dilemmas in pediatric cardiology. In the 1980's the law speaks very clearly. Down's babies with congenital heart disease have to be treated without regard for issues of quality of life. Given the propensity of these babies for cardiac failure as well as pulmonary artery hypertension, elective surgery is recommended beyond six months of age and much earlier if congestive heart failure is uncontrollable. Surgical mortality, depending on the age and the complexity of the anatomy, is between 10 and 30%. No good long-term follow-up study of these babies is available.

Valvar Aortic Stenosis. The occurrence of valvar aortic stenosis with critical obstruction in a young infant is a real surgical emergency. Without skillful operative intervention, these babies succumb within weeks or months. The presenting symptoms are congestive heart failure with poor cardiac output, which is not too dissimilar from hypoplastic left heart and even critical coarctation. The principal difference is that in these babies the cardiogram shows severe left ventricular hypertrophy with strain. The echocardiogram is diagnostic. It may be worth noting that the characteristic murmur of aortic stenosis may not be present until the baby's cardiac output has increased through treatment with vigorous anticongestive measures. Surgery through inflow occlusion is life saving though mostly not curative; repeat valvotomy and even aortic valve replacement may not be avoidable within the first one or two decades. Operative risk is less than 10%. Preoperative cardiac catheterization, without attempting to cross the aortic valve, is mandatory.

Valvar Pulmonary Stenosis with Intact Ventricular Septum. Valvar pulmonary stenosis with an intact ventricular septum does not cause symptoms in infancy unless the obstruction is severe enough to result in right ventricular pressure of at least systemic level. In this case, the baby is cyanotic (right-to-left atrial shunt) and has the typical murmur of pulmonary stenosis, and the chest film shows a large globular heart with ischemic lung fields. The ECG indicates severe right ventricular hypertrophy, usually with P pulmonale, and the echocardiogram is diagnostic. Cardiac catheterization is mandatory on clinical suspicion prior to cardiac surgery. Operative risks are below 5% and long-term results are excellent.

Pulmonary Atresia with Intact Ventricular Septum. Pulmonary atresia with intact ventricular septum presents itself with severe, even critical cyanosis as soon as the ductus arteriosus (the only source of pulmonary flow) closes. The clinical picture is quite similar to that of valvar pulmonary stenosis except that the electrocardiogram shows a mean frontal plane axis between +30 and +90 degrees without significant right ventricular hypertrophy. Also, cyanosis is more severe and the murmur is not that of pulmonary stenosis but rather of tricuspid incompetence. Emergency surgery is recommended (a Blalock-Taussig shunt plus opening of the right ventricular outflow tract) as a life-saving measure, but the mortality is high (over 25%) and cure unlikely. At this writing, this is a highly unsatisfactory situation in all but those with only marginally hypoplastic right ventricle.

Total Anomalous Pulmonary Venous Return. This disorder is one of the most difficult diagnostic problems in pediatric cardiology. These babies are very sick very early, within the first few days of life. Their heart size is normal. The lung fields are congestive, but it may be difficult to know whether this in fact is pneumonia or pulmonary venous engorgement. Cyanosis may vary from severe to trivial. Murmurs are unimpressive. The ECG shows severe right ventricular hypertrophy. Sophisticated echocardiogram of the two-dimensional variety frequently pinpoints the diagnosis, but it has to be emphasized, however, that this is the lesion most easily missed, not only by clinical examination and echocardiogram but even at cardiac catheterization unless one's index of suspicion is very high. Surgery is mandatory following diagnosis. In our department, palliative measures like atrial septostomy are not recommended. Corrective surgery is highly effective with a mortality of less than 10% and good long-term outlook.

Tricuspid Atresia. There is no good explanation as to why tricuspid atresia, physiologically not very different from pulmonary atresia with intact ventricular septum, has a so much better prognosis. The clinical picture is similar, except for the usually smaller heart and an ECG with a mean frontal plane axis that is designated as a QRS between -30 and -90 degrees. Surgery, consisting of a Blalock-Taussig shunt within the first weeks or months of life, depending on the severity of the cyanosis and the limitation of exercise tolerance, can be carried out with a risk of less than 5%. The "curative" Fontan operation at a risk of less than 10% can be performed anywhere between 2 and 5 years of age, or even earlier, depending on the effectiveness of the previous Blalock-Taussig shunt. Long-term follow-up extending through 10 to 20 years seems to be satisfactory.

CHILDREN

Ventricular Septal Defect. Patients with a ventricular septal defect seldom present as an emergency with congestive heart failure beyond infancy in the United States today. Mostly they are referred on account of a murmur. How far one should investigate these patients, if they are asymptomatic, is one of the more difficult problems in the field. At the present time, given an asymptomatic child,

I would not proceed beyond obtaining an electrocardiogram and probably (not certainly) a chest x-ray. If the results of both are normal, I would forget about it, though the more timid and trusting of our colleagues may recommend dental prophylaxis. If the ECG or chest x-ray examinations show some abnormality, an echocardiogram is highly recommended. If these studies suggest a ventricular septal defect of significant size, cardiac catheterization should be performed. Surgery for those with pulmonary hypertension (pulmonary arterial mean pressure over 20 mm Hg) and a net left-to-right shunt is mandatory; for those without pulmonary artery hypertension but with a pulmonary to systemic flow ratio arbitrarily beyond 1.6 to 1 surgery may be advisable. In those few patients with pulmonary artery hypertension and no left-to-right shunt, those with the so-called Eisenmenger syndrome, surgery is contraindicated. Operative risks in uncomplicated cases should be 1 to 2%, with elimination of the left-to-right shunt a virtual certainty. The course of pulmonary hypertension, if any, depends on many known and unknown factors.

Secundum Atrial Septal Defect. Patients with this relatively simple anomaly seldom present in infancy. It is the commonest lesion to be discovered in childhood and adolescence or even in adulthood. Sophisticated pediatricians will suspect the diagnosis from the "fixed" splitting of the second sound, in association with the characteristic ejection murmur, modest cardiac enlargement with pulmonary vascular engorgement, and an electrocardiogram showing right intraventricular conduction delay. A two-dimensional echocardiogram will show the size and shape of the opening in the atrial septum, particularly in younger children with thin chest walls. I believe all atrial defects detectable by clinical means should be closed at some time before the end of the second decade. Surgical mortality is less than 1%; long-term results are excellent. Successfully closed atrial defects do not need dental prophylaxis. In our institution, given a clear-cut clinical profile, preoperative cardiac catheterization is omitted.

Endocardial Cushion Defect.

ATRIAL SEPTAL DEFECT PRIMUM. This disorder is a somewhat more complex and potentially more serious defect than the secundum variety, most likely on account of its frequent association with a cleft mitral valve, resulting in mitral incompetence. The diagnosis is based on auscultatory findings, an electrocardiogram with a mean frontal plane axis between -15 and -60 degrees, and cardiac enlargement. There is some urgency about operating on these patients on account of the potential risk of the development of pulmonary hypertension and the effect of mitral regurgitation. Operative mortality is around 1 to 2% and long-term outlook is almost, but not quite, as favorable as that of the secundum variety. Antibiotic prophylaxis is recommended even after apparently successful surgery.

COMPLETE ATRIOVENTRICULAR CANAL. The complete atrioventricular canal variety of the endocardial cushion defect is a more serious problem. These patients have already been discussed in the infant's group, since they frequently present as ventricular defects with a superior frontal plane axis in severe heart failure in a young baby. Surgery is mandatory, with an operative mortality beyond infancy of close to 10%. A "cure" cannot always be expected. Mitral valve replacement may be necessary in the second or third decade and late arrhythmias (atrial fibrillation) are not uncommon.

Patent Ductus Arteriosus. Two or three decades ago this was the commonest congenital cardiac malformation referred to pediatric cardiac centers. These days, many, even most, of the patients are being treated in infancy. Still, an occasional child with a classical ductus murmur does appear in the office of the pediatrician. Surgery is indicated on diagnosis. If the clinical findings, the ECG, and x-ray are classical, no catheterization is necessary. The surgical risk is well below 1%, and one can expect to achieve a perfectly normal circulation for the rest of the child's life.

Tetralogy of Fallot. This is by far the commonest cyanotic defect to present beyond infancy. The typical clinical picture, the murmur, the x-ray, and the electrocardiogram allowed Dr. Helen Taussig to make this diagnosis with great accuracy through many decades without cardiac catheterization. Many thousands of children all over the world benefited from the shunt operation bearing her and Dr. Blalock's name. Today the Blalock-Taussing shunt is rarely indicated for children with tetralogy of Fallot. Since complete correction is the preferred operation, cardiac catheterization is necessary to furnish appropriate anatomic and physiologic details. The operative risk is less than 5% and long-term results are excellent.

Coarctation of the Aorta. Next to atrial defect of the secundum variety, coarctation of the aorta is the commonest congenital cardiac malformation to be discovered in childhood. The reason for this is the reluctance of pediatricians to obtain blood pressure measurements in infants. Also, regretfully, feeling for the femoral pulses, like noting the right radial pulse, is still not an automatic part of pediatric physical examination. Whenever a coarctation of the aorta is discovered, it should be operated upon. The earlier, the better. The long-term results are better the younger the patient is at the time of surgery. At our institution, those with the classical clinical picture do not undergo preoperative catheterization. Operative risks are estimated at 1 to 2% and long-term results are good, though a certain percentage will need re-operation.

Valvar Pulmonary Stenosis. Valvar pulmonary stenosis should be treated surgically if the right ventricular pressure is at least 50% of the systemic arterial pressure. The best clinical tool for estimating the severity of pulmonary valvar obstruction is the electrocardiogram; patients beyond infancy presenting with clear-cut right ventricular hypertrophy in the chest leads almost certainly have a significant increase of right ventricular pressure. Given the characteristic auscultatory and radiologic findings, surgery can be, and has been, performed, without catheterization. The two-dimensional echocardiogram with Doppler flow measurement further improves the accuracy of the clinical assessment. Still, in most cases, traditional cardiac catheterization is performed preoperatively. The recent introduction of the use of balloon angioplasty makes this approach a more logical one. Within the framework of cardiac catheterization, balloon fracture of the pulmonary valve can be accomplished and thoracotomy can be avoided. There is no mortality so far with this noninvasive management of pulmonary stenosis and the surgical mortality is also less than 1%. Long-term results are excellent.

Valvar Aortic Stenosis. Valvar aortic stenosis commonly first presents in childhood. The diagnosis is easily made through the typical murmur of aortic stenosis coupled with left ventricular hypertrophy in the cardiogram. The radiogram contributes relatively little to the clinical picture and is of little use in quantitation in this age group. Echo-Doppler cardiogram is very helpful in determining the gradient across the valve. Still, most centers justifiably perform cardiac catheterization preoperatively. Our policy is to operate on all patients with a resting gradient of over 75 mm Hg with or without left ventricular strain in the cardiogram. Gradients of under 25 mm Hg surely do not need surgery. Those with gradients between 25 and 49 mm also can be managed conservatively under close supervision. Those with gradients between 50 and 75 mm Hg we probably would operate upon because of the virtual certainty that at some point the valve will become more severely obstructed and will eventually calcify. To postpone aortic valve replacement, surely necessary for calcific aortic stenosis, as far as possible, we are inclined to propose a valvotomy even for these patients with moderate aortic valve obstruction. Surgery is safe (between 1 and 2%), but need for re-operation is likely in the third or fourth decade. Very careful, at least yearly, follow-up is mandatory, and careful antibiotic prophylaxis is essential.

The Child at Risk of Coronary Disease as an Adult

JAMES J. NORA, M.D.

Because of lively debate on the issue of pediatric preventive programs for coronary disease, it must be stated that the following recommendations may be opposed by some. In the absence of 70-year longitudinal studies, one can always assert that the evidence for the efficacy of a specific or even a general preventive program is not available. With this disclaimer, I present the approach we follow on our service.

1. For the majority of children and families, specific preventive programs are not required beyond a general commitment to a life-style that embraces exercise, ideal weight, stress control, a reasonably prudent diet (but not necessarily adhering consistently to the prudent diet shown in Table 1), and abrogation of smoking. However, it should be noted that this prudent diet is the diet recommended by the U.S. Senate committee on nutrition for *all* Americans.

2. For high-risk children from high-risk families, the commitment to prevention cannot be casual. Those at high risk should be deliberately sought out at an early age and should have a preventive program designed to attack the specific risk factors. We recommend that at between 1 and 2 years of age (or at later pediatric ages if necessary) the following be done.

   a. Obtain a family history of onset of coronary disease or stroke in first- and second-degree relatives before age 65.
   b. Obtain family history of hypertension in first- and second-degree relatives and begin annual "tracking" of patient's blood pressure.
   c. Obtain serum cholesterol level.
   d. For those with a family history of early-onset coronary heart disease or stroke and a cholesterol level about 190 mg/dl, the cholesterol study should be repeated and the prudent diet initiated if the cholesterol level is found to be above 190 mg/dl on the second determination.
   e. For those without a family history, the cholesterol level may be "tracked" at annual visits for 2 years. If the elevated level persists over 190 mg/dl, the prudent diet should be instituted and consistently adhered to.
   f. Young children *with a positive (or unknown) family history* who do not respond to a prudent diet by lowering cholesterol (being sure that the prudent diet is truly being followed) should receive the following additional evaluation and therapeutic approach.
      (1) A study of total cholesterol, high-density lipoprotein (HDL) cholesterol, triglycerides, and lipoprotein fractions in the child for phenotyping.
      (2) An initial study of cholesterol levels in first-degree family members (parents, siblings) to help distinguish between the dietary-resistant monogenic and the dietary-responsive polygenic forms. This differential diagnosis will be discussed in the next section.
      (3) If the family pattern is compatible with the polygenic forms, diet alone (with the healthful life-style indicated in Item

Table 1. A PRUDENT DIET

1. Avoid overweight, consume only as many calories as you expend: if overweight, decrease calories and increase expenditure.
2. Increase consumption of fruits, vegetables, and whole grains (complex carbohydrates and "naturally occurring" sugars) from the present 28 per cent of calories in the average diet to about half (48 per cent) of your caloric intake.
3. Decrease consumption of refined and other processed sugars and foods high in such sugar by almost half (about 45 per cent) to account for only about 10 per cent of total calories.
4. Decrease consumption of foods high in total fat from 42 per cent of calories to 30 per cent.
5. Specifically reduce saturated fat in the diet (from the present 16 per cent to 10 per cent) and partially replace this with polyunsaturated and monounsaturated fat to account for the remaining 20 per cent of fat intake, by reducing intake of animal fat from meats and high fat dairy products. Eat more fish and poultry, and select lean meats low in fat (e.g., trimmed ground round in place of hamburger). Low fat and non-fat milk may be substituted for whole milk except in those infants whose diet is almost entirely milk.
6. Reduce cholesterol to about 300 mg per day. (The major dietary sources of cholesterol are egg yolks, meats, whole milk, and high fat dairy products.) For children, the major dietary source of cholesterol is whole milk.
7. Decrease your consumption of salt and foods high in salt content.

Table 2. DIET FOR THOSE WITH HIGH CHOLESTEROL LEVELS THAT DO NOT RESPOND ADEQUATELY TO THE PRUDENT DIET

1. Avoid overweight, as in the prudent diet.
2. Increase consumption of complex carbohydrates (fruits, vegetables, grains) to about half (48 per cent) of total caloric intake, as in the prudent diet.
3. Decrease refined sugar and other processed sugar to about 10 per cent of total calories, as in the prudent diet.
4. Decrease total fat intake to 30 per cent of calories, as in the prudent diet.
5. Reduce saturated fat and take twice as much polyunsaturated fat (P/S = 2/1), as in the prudent diet.
6. Reduce cholesterol to 100 mg; this is lower than in the prudent diet.
7. Reduce salt consumption, as in the prudent diet.

Table 3. DIET FOR THOSE WHO HAVE BOTH HIGH CHOLESTEROL AND HIGH TRIGLYCERIDES THAT DO NOT RESPOND ADEQUATELY TO THE PRUDENT DIET

1. Reduce weight to the lower limits of the desirable weight range.
2. Maintain complex carbohydrate consumption (fruits, vegetables, grains) at about half (48 per cent) of total calories, as in the prudent diet.
3. Eliminate as much as possible refined sugars and processed foods high in sugar—certainly hold this to less than 5 per cent of calories. This is lower than in the prudent diet.
4. Decrease total fat intake to 30 per cent of calories, as in the prudent diet.
5. Reduce saturated fat, as done in the other diets, to the point that twice as much polyunsaturated fat is consumed as saturated (P/S = 2/1).
6. Reduce cholesterol to 100 mg per day, much lower than in the prudent diet.
7. Reduce salt intake, as in the prudent diet.

1) is all that is necessary. However, a diet stricter than the prudent diet may be required for some families. These diets are provided in Tables 2 and 3. Diets for elevated triglycerides alone are rarely needed for polygenic forms, and the contribution of high triglycerides to coronary disease is small compared with cholesterol. If a child has elevated triglycerides in spite of being ideal weight, but does not simultaneously have high cholesterol, we do not usually suggest a special diet beyond the prudent diet.

3. Distinguishing monogenic from polygenic forms of hyperlipoproteinemia.
   a. Monogenic forms in heterozygotes generally have the following features.
      (1) Higher levels (e.g., cholesterol in childhood of 260 mg/dl rather than 200 mg/dl).
      (2) Do not respond well to diet alone.
      (3) Show bimodality in cholesterol values in family studies. A "classic" monogenic family of six first-degree relatives (adults and children) would have the following cholesterol values: 300, 290, 310, 180, 195, 175—as though the cho-

lesterol levels were coming from two different populations or families.
   b. A "classic" polygenic family of six first-degree relatives (adults and children) would have the following cholesterol levels: 220, 240, 255, 215, 260, 205—as though the cholesterol levels were all from the same bell-shaped distribution curve.
   c. The monogenic forms should fit comfortably into the lipoprotein phenotype classification of Fredrickson and the W.H.O., with the caution that possible underlying diseases such as hypothyroidism and lupus must be eliminated before concluding that the lipoproteinemia is a primary rather than a secondary disorder. See Table 4 for a classification of phenotypes.
4. Treating monogenic hyperlipoproteinemias in heterozygotes.
   a. This is the most difficult and controversial area.
   b. Even strict dietary measures are usually insufficient.
   c. We do not usually consider medication except for patients with cholesterol levels above 240 mg/dl in children and 270 mg/dl in young adults on a 100-mg cholesterol diet.
   d. If medications are then used, we first consider what medications are showing successful results in the parents and older siblings, because there is doubtless considerable heterogeneity among the monogenic disorders. If a regimen works well for one family member, it is more likely to work in first-degree relatives.
   e. A resin (such as cholestyramine or colestipol) in combination with nicotinic acid, or either agent alone are regimens we use in children (with considerable caution, starting with very low doses, looking for adverse reactions, and being prepared to discontinue if results are unsatisfactory). A dosage schedule will not be offered for these drugs because one has not been established for children. If management with drugs is undertaken as the lesser of two unfavorable alternatives, it may be wise for the primary

Table 4. PHENOTYPING HYPERLIPOPROTEINEMIAS

Phenotype	Cholesterol	Triglycerides	Serum	Electrophoresis	Ultracentrifugation
I	↑	↑	creamy	Chylomicrons	Chylomicrons
II (IIa)	↑		clear	Beta ↑	LDL ↑
III	↑	↑	± cloudy	Broad beta	Intermediates
IV		↑	± cloudy	Pre-beta ↑	VLDL ↑
V	↑	↑	creamy	Chylo, pre-beta ↑	Chylo, VLDL ↑
VI (IIb)	↑	↑	± cloudy	Beta ↑, pre-beta ↑	LDL ↑, VLDL ↑

physician to work with a consultant experienced in this area.

5. Treating monogenic hyperlipoproteinemia IIa in homozyotes. These rare conditions require intensive diagnostic evaluation at the hands of experienced consultants. Portacaval shunt has been the most efficacious approach in our experience.

Cardiac Arrhythmias

WELTON W. GERSONY, M.D.

Childhood cardiac rhythm disturbances are recognized more often now because diagnostic methods have improved. Furthermore, there are more surgical survivors after repair of congenital heart disease, and some of these patients may be prone to rhythm disturbances.

The major risk of a cardiac rhythm disorder is that a severe tachycardia or bradycardia may lead to decreased cardiac output, a more severe arrhythmia, syncope, or sudden death. When there is apparent ectopic cardiac activity, the major issue is whether there may be deterioration into a life-threatening tachyarrhythmia or bradyarrhythmia. Some rhythm abnormalities, however, such as single premature atrial and ventricular beats are common among children without heart disease and in the great majority of instances do not pose a risk. Thus, accurate differential diagnosis of cardiac arrhythmias is critically important prior to most decisions about further studies, pharmacologic treatment, restriction of physical activities, and prognosis.

An increasing number of pharmacologic agents are available for the treatment of significant rhythm disturbances in children (Table 1). Problems with frequency of administration, compliance, side effects, and variable responses remain, and selection of an antiarrhythmic agent still involves a great deal of empiricism. However, for most rhythm disturbances, treatment regimens with single agents that reliably control the abnormal rhythm pattern are available. In recent years, surgical intervention to eliminate bypass tracts associated with preexcitation syndromes or unusually electrically active areas in the heart have become available, but this approach is reserved for situations in which extreme measures are necessary to control a life-threatening rhythm disorder. Finally, implanted pacemakers are presently more reliable and less prone to technical failure than in the past.

BRADYCARDIA

Bradycardia in older children and adolescents is defined as a heart rate of less than 60 beats per minute. Sinus bradycardia may occur because of abnormalities in sinus node automaticity, central nervous system disease, hypoxia, metabolic disease, drug effects, or injury to the sinus node region. However, sinus bradycardia is most often seen as a normal phenomenon, especially in a well conditioned athlete. The cause of bradycardia that is of the most concern is complete heart block. Atrioventricular (AV) conduction is blocked at the level of the AV node or His-Purkinje system. This results in an intrinsic ventricular rhythm that is independent of atrial activity. The atrial rate is always faster than the ventricular rate, and the electrocardiogram shows no consistent relationship between the P wave and the QRS; the P wave is seen to "march through" the QRS. In most instances of complete heart block, the heart rate is between 30 and 40 beats per minute.

Sinus Bradycardia

When sinus bradycardia is secondary to a noncardiac pathologic process, the underlying disorder requires urgent management and no specific therapy is required for the bradycardia. For example, in the presence of a subdural hematoma resulting in central nervous system–mediated sinus bradycardia, successful evacuation of the hematoma will result in the re-establishment of a normal cardiac rate. Similarly, sinus bradycardia as a result of a high degree of physical conditioning is a normal response and requires no attention.

Complete Heart Block

Congenital heart block is a not infrequent abnormality and may be identified in utero. In most instances, no treatment is required during the neonatal period and beyond. Indeed, individuals may live into old age without symptoms or necessity for treatment of any kind. When complete heart block is associated with congenital heart disease, temporary or even permanent cardiac pacing may be required in the newborn period or later in life. However, in most instances, even in the presence of heart disease, a slow, stable cardiac pacemaker arising from the His-Purkinje system, especially with a narrow QRS, tends to be stable for an indefinite period.

Rarely, a patient with congenital heart block will have a syncopal episode. When this occurs, pacemaker therapy should be instituted.

Acquired Complete Heart Block

When complete heart block occurs secondary to surgical repair of a congenital heart defect, permanent pacemaker therapy is virtually always necessary. When heart block is noted immediately after operation, temporary pacing is instituted and is continued for 2–4 weeks. If spontaneous normal AV conduction does not return, permanent pacing is instituted prior to discharge from the hospital.

Table 1.   COMMONLY USED ANTIARRHYTHMIC DRUG SCHEDULES IN PEDIATRIC PATIENTS

Drug	Oral Administration		Intravenous Administration*		Comments and Side Effects	
	Maintenance Dose†	*Maximal Maintenance Dose*	*Loading Dose*	*Maximal Dose*	*Comments*	*Side Effects*
Digoxin	0.01–0.02 mg/kg/day DD‡ q 12 h	0.5 mg	0.025–0.05 mg/kg in 3 DD q 4–8 h	0.5 mg	Oral loading dose 0.04–0.07 mg/kg/day DD q 8 See text for age-related differences	APDs, VPDs, conduction defects, bradycardia, nausea, vomiting, anorexia
Quinidine sulfate	20–60 mg/kg/day DD q 6 h	2.4 gm	—	—		Nausea, vomiting, diarrhea, cinchonism, QRS and QT prolongation, AV block, asystole, syncope, thrombocytopenia, hemolytic anemia, blurred vision, convulsions, allergic reactions, exacerbation of periodic paralysis, enhancement of digoxin effects
Quinidine gluconate	20–60 mg/kg/day DD q 8–12 h	2.0 gm	10–15 mg/kg as 250 µg/kg/min	20 mg/min to 1.0 gm	Oral test dose 2 mg/kg	
Procainamide	50–100 mg/kg/day DD q 4–6 h DD q 6 h†	6.0 gm	10–20 mg/kg as 300 µg/kg/min	20 mg/min to 1.0 gm	Intravenous maintenance 20–40 µg/kg/min	PR, QRS, QT prolongation, anorexia, nausea, vomiting, rash, fever, agranulocytosis, thrombocytopenia, Coombs-positive hemolytic anemia, lupus erythematosus-like syndrome, hypotension, exacerbation of periodic paralysis
Disopyramide	8–12 mg/kg/day DD q 6 h DD q 12 h†	1.2 gm	—	—	—	Anticholinergic effects, urinary retention, blurred vision, dry mouth, QT and QRS prolongation, exacerbation of periodic paralysis, negative inotropic effects
Phenytoin	3–6 mg/kg/day DD q 12 h	600 mg	10–15 mg/kg as 250 µg/kg/min	20 mg/min to 1.0 gm	—	Rash, gingival hyperplasia, CNS manifestations, ataxia, lethargy, vertigo, tremor, macrocytic anemia
Lidocaine	—	—	1 mg/kg repeat q 5 min × 3	50–75 mg	Intravenous maintenance 30–50 µg/kg/min	CNS effects, confusion, convulsions, high degree AV block, asystole, coma, paresthesias, respiratory failure
Verapamil	4–10 mg/kg/day DD q 8 h	480 mg	0.075–0.15 mg/kg q 20 min × 2	5 mg	—	Bradycardia, asystole, high degree AV block, hypotension, congestive heart failure, enhancement of digoxin effects
Propranolol§	1–4 mg/kg/day DD q 6 h	Not established	0.1–0.15 mg/kg	1 mg/min to 10 mg	Long-acting beta-blocking agents (nadolol, atenolol) are preferred for long-term therapy (less frequent administration and CNS side effects)	Bradycardia, loss of concentration or memory, bronchospasm, hypoglycemia, hypotension

From Gersony, W. and Hardof, A. J.: Cardiac arrhythmias. *In* Dickerman, J. D., and Lucey, J. F.: Smith's The Critically Ill Child: Diagnosis and Medical Management. 3rd ed. Philadelphia, W. B. Saunders Co., 1985.

* Intravenous administration of antiarrhythmic drugs should always be given slowly with constant monitoring of blood pressure and electrocardiogram, particularly in patients with compromised cardiac function or compromised renal or hepatic function. Dose must be modified in patients with abnormal renal or hepatic function.

† Sustained-release preparations available for clinical use.

‡ Divided doses.

§ Manufacturer's warning: Safety and efficacy of propranolol for use in children have not been established.

Drug Therapy. Atropine (0.01–0.02 mg/kg/IV; maximim 1.0 mg) is effective in treating supraventricular bradycardias. The same dose is used to enhance AV conduction in transient heart block. However, in unusual circumstances, the acceleration of sinus rate may exceed the improvement of AV conduction caused by the atropine and may result in a rate-related increase in the degree of block with a reduction in the ventricular rate.

Isoproterenol is used for the treatment of supraventricular bradycardia and atrioventricular block. It is the agent of choice for symptomatic complete heart block until a cardiac pacemaker can be introduced. Isoproterenol is titrated to desired effect or until toxic effects are observed. The usual dosage range is 0.05–0.5 µg/kg/min. Beta-adrenergic stimulating agents should be used with caution in patients with hypoxia or acidosis and in those who are taking digitalis preparations.

Cardiac Pacing. Cardiac pacemakers are used for treating patients with bradyarrhythmias, to control the cardiac rate, and recently have also been used to convert cardiac arrhythmias. Many of the modern pacemaker's functions can be controlled by external means after its insertion. In children, the most common indications for cardiac pacing are complete heart block, either postsurgical or congenital, and sick sinus syndrome. The latter is common after open heart surgery for transposition of the great vessels (Mustard procedure). However, most patients do not require a pacemaker.

Pacing is most commonly carried out from the right ventricle; however, recently, atrial pacemakers have been used more frequently, with pacing wires inserted in the right atrium. The pacing wires can be inserted either transvenously or via a thoracotomy on the epicardial surface of the heart. Generally, in infants and young children epicardial wires are employed for long-term pacing. In older children and adults, transvenous pacemaker insertion is the preferred method of electrode implacement.

In addition to having the ability to pace the heart, modern pacemakers have a sensing system that allows them to sense the patient's spontaneous rhythms. The most commonly used ventricular pacemakers are the R-wave–inhibited pacemakers. If the pacemaker senses the spontaneous R-wave of the patient's inherent rhythm, the output of the pacing mechanism is inhibited. The rate at which the pacemaker will discharge and be inhibited is preset. The pacing mode of the noncompetitive stimulation pacemaker will be inhibited at all spontaneous rates that are more rapid than the set pacemaker rate. This inhibition theoretically prevents the occurrence of competitive arrhythmias. Noncompetitive atrial P-wave–inhibited pacemakers are also available.

The newest, most sophisticated type of pacemaker produces atrioventricular sequential pacing at all pacing rates. These pacemakers require two leads, one in the atrium and one in the ventricle. The atrial and ventricular leads are both used for pacing and sensing. In a patient with normal sinus rhythm the pacemaker functions by sensing the atrium and stimulating the ventricle. However, should the patient have severe bradycardia or sinus arrest, these pacemakers function as atrioventricular sequential and synchronous pacemakers at a preset low rate. This pacemaker provides for every contingency of cardiac pacing under all physiologic conditions and is replacing all other types of atrioventricular sequential pacemakers.

Automatic antitachycardia pacemakers are used in extreme circumstances for patients with tachyarrhythmias that are refractory to standard medical or surgical intervention. These pacemakers can be activated by the patient in response to symptomatic tachycardia, or they have automatic devices that sense the tachycardia and deliver a train of impulses or a single defibrillatory shock to terminate the arrhythmia. These devices can be used for intractable atrial arrhythmias, for ventricular arrhythmias, and for the conversion of ventricular fibrillation. Prior to using this type of pacemaker, detailed intracardiac electrophysiologic testing must be carried out to ascertain whether a particular type of pacing will terminate the tachyarrhythmia.

TACHYARRHYTHMIAS

Supraventricular Tachycardias

In most infants and children who have supraventricular tachycardias without associated cardiac diseases, adequate hemodynamic status is maintained for extended periods. Therefore, in a hemodynamically stable patient a gradual approach for termination of the tachycardias can be carried out. The length of time that these arrhythmias will be tolerated is a function of (1) the underlying state of the myocardium, (2) the rate of the tachycardia, and (3) the duration of the abnormal rhythm. It should be emphasized that electrical cardioversion is the treatment of choice in any patient in whom the cardiac output is significantly compromised.

The first measure is that of vagal stimulation. Initiation of a strong vagal discharge by inducing the diving reflex is the most effective maneuver to enhance vagal tone in children. In a neonate or infant, induction of the diving reflex is carried out by suddenly placing an ice-cold wet towel or washcloth on the patient's face and holding it there for several seconds. In older children, facial immersion in ice-cold water is similarly effective. Other vagal maneuvers, such as carotid sinus massage, stimulating the gag reflex, inducing vomiting, or ocular pressure, have not been as effective in infants as in older children and adults. Often a "vagal maneuver of choice" may exist for each patient, even a bizarre method such as a headstand.

Other measures to induce an increase in vagal tone include the intravenous administration of (1) an adrenergic agent such as phenylephrine in order to increase systolic blood pressure and initiate a responding baroreceptor reflex and (2) an acetylcholinesterase inhibitor, such as edrophonium (Tensilon) that enhances vagal tone by inhibiting the breakdown of acetylcholine by the enzyme acetylcholinesterase. Digitalis is the drug of choice for patients in whom antiarrhythmic drug therapy is to be used to convert supraventricular tachycardias. Once again the mechanism of action is that of vagotonic effect. Digoxin is the most versatile agent and can be administered intravenously, intramuscularly, or orally. The mode of administration is dependent upon how rapid an effect is required. It has a relatively rapid onset of action when used intravenously and has a long enough half-life so that it does not have to be given very frequently when administration is long-term. Digoxin is administered intravenously as a total digitalizing dose of 25–50 μg/kg in divided doses, with a maximum total digitalizing dose of 1 mg. The oral dose is 40–70 μg/kg in divided doses with a maximum dose of 1.5 mg. The lower dose is recommended for neonates. Premature infants and patients with renal failure must be evaluated on an individual basis, and even lower doses are required because of decreased rates of excretion.

Digoxin is generally administered in divided doses, with a quarter to a half of the "digitalizing" dose given initially, followed in 2 to 8 hours by subsequent doses. The timing of the doses depends upon how rapidly it is necessary to convert the supraventricular tachycardia to sinus rhythm. The onset of action of intravenous digoxin is approximately 30 minutes, and the peak action occurs within 2 hours. Therefore, if the arrhythmia remains unchanged 2 hours after the initial dose, one can give a second dose of digoxin intravenously at that time.

Once conversion of the tachyarrhythmia occurs, digitalization of the patient can be completed at a more leisurely rate, and even orally rather than intravenously. For an oral dose, a third greater than the intravenous dose should be calculated. Maintenance digoxin dosage is a quarter to a third of the digitalizing dosage and usually is between 10 and 20 μg/kg/day orally, with a maximum maintenance dosage of between 0.25 and 0.5 mg/day. Digoxin has a relatively long half-life of 36 hours, and therefore the maintenance dose is either administered once daily or in divided doses twice daily.

Atrial flutter or fibrillation is also treated with digoxin, which slows the ventricular rate on the basis of the vagotonic effect. Rarely, digoxin will convert atrial flutter to sinus rhythm. However, digoxin often will convert atrial flutter to atrial fibrillation, resulting in a slower ventricular rate.

Digoxin must be used with care in patients with the pre-excitation syndrome in general, and not at all in those who have short antegrade effective refractory periods of the bypass tract. Digoxin may further shorten the antegrade effective refractory period of the bypass tract, resulting in enhanced conduction to the ventricle, particularly in patients with atrial fibrillation. This effect can result in very rapid ventricular rates that can lead to ventricular tachycardia or fibrillation. This mechanism is very uncommon in infants and children. However, it is a significant potential risk in older children and adults. Another concern about the use of digoxin is the potential for post-digitalis cardioversion-induced ventricular arrhythmias. This possibility is only theoretical and in practice is very uncommon in children. It would be of major concern in patients with severe underlying heart disease and would be unlikely to occur in patients with no structural heart disease unless digoxin had been given in near toxic doses.

Verapamil is extremely effective in terminating supraventricular tachycardias, particularly those involving the AV node. Verapamil is a blocker of the slow inward current carried primarily by calcium. Since the action potentials of the AV node are "slow response type" calcium-mediated action potentials, verapamil is very effective in treating rhythm disturbances that originate in this region. Its advantage over digoxin is that it has a very rapid onset of action (3–5 min) and the effects are seen immediately. However, the immediate effects can also dissipate fairly rapidly and subsequent doses may be required. The usual dose of verapamil is 0.075–0.15 mg/kg intravenously, with a maximum dose of 5 mg. It can be repeated between 10 and 30 minutes following the initial dose. Verapamil is also useful in slowing the ventricular response in patients with atrial flutter and fibrillation, particularly as an adjunct to digitalis therapy. However, verapamil has been shown to shorten the effective refractory period of the bypass tract in patients with pre-excitation syndrome, and therefore the same risks are present for these patients that exist with digitalis. Although verapamil has been proved to be more efficacious than digitalis in the immediate pharmacologic conversions of supraventricular tachycardias, it also has a higher incidence of side effects, particularly in infants, including a high degree of AV block, extreme bradycardia, asystole, hypotension, and congestive heart failure. The adverse cardiovascular effects can generally be overcome by treatment with beta-adrenergic agents such as isoproterenol and parenteral administration of calcium. Verapamil is also available as a long-term oral preparation. The starting oral dosage in children is approximately 4 mg/kg/day in 3 divided doses. This dosage can be increased until either therapeutic or early "toxic" effects are seen. The upper limits of the dosage for long-term oral preparation is approximately 10 mg/kg/day in infants and young children but this limit has not been definitely established.

A third antiarrhythmic drug that can be used immediately for the treatment of supraventricular arrhythmias is the beta-adrenergic blocking agent propranolol. As with the other agents, the major effects are on the AV node. The blocking of sympathetic input to the AV node results in an unbalanced parasympathetic (vagal) effect. The intravenous dose of propranolol* is 0.1–0.15 mg/kg. The maximum immediate dose should not exceed 5 mg, and the maximum rate of administration should not be greater than 1 mg/minute. This dose can be repeated in approximately 20–30 minutes if no effect is seen. As with verapamil, side effects can include a high degree of AV block, extreme bradycardia, asystole, hypotension, and congestive heart failure. The adverse cardiovascular effects can be effectively treated with a beta-adrenergic agent such as isoproterenol.

On occasion, supraventricular tachycardia may be detected in utero. If the arrhythmia persists, the fetus may develop congestive heart failure that is manifested by evidence of hydrops fetalis. The administration of an antiarrhythmic drug such as digoxin to the mother at usual therapeutic doses will often convert the arrhythmia to sinus rhythm in utero. Thus, early delivery by cesarean section is avoided.

Electrical cardioversion using defibrillation and DC cardioversion is the emergency treatment of choice for any patient with a supraventricular tachycardia in an unstable hemodynamic state or severe congestive failure. This includes most forms of supraventricular tachycardia, atrial fibrillation, and atrial flutter with rapid ventricular response. Cardioversion is also used for elective conversion of these arrhythmias in stable patients who are refractory to routine long-term antiarrhythmic therapy. Such patients should be "anesthetized" by an agent such as diazepam or thiopental prior to the attempted cardioversion. Electrical cardioversion of an awake, fully alert patient is "unkind." The usual dose for cardioversion is 1–2 watt-seconds/kg.

Electrical conversion of supraventricular arrhythmias can also be carried out by electrical

*Manufacturer's warning: Safety and efficacy of propranolol for use in children have not been established.

pacing. Supraventricular tachycardia can be converted either by inducing properly timed premature atrial beats or by rapid atrial pacing. Atrial flutter or fibrillation is best converted to sinus rhythm by means of electrical cardioversion. Atrial flutter also can be converted using rapid atrial pacing of the atrium at rates significantly faster than the flutter rate (entrainment).

Long-Term Management. Long-term therapy of supraventricular tachycardias can be carried out with a variety of antiarrhythmic drugs either alone or in combination. These include digoxin, beta-blocking agents (propranolol, nadolol, atenolol) verapamil, quinidine, procainamide, and disopyramide.

Long-term treatment of atrial flutter or fibrillation is commonly carried out with either digoxin to control the ventricular rate or a combination of digoxin and quinidine to prevent recurrence of the flutter or fibrillation. When treating atrial flutter, one should "protect the AV node" by digitalizing the patient prior to instituting quinidine therapy. This treatment prevents the occurrence of a more rapid ventricular response, which may follow quinidine administration because of the potential anticholinergic effects of quinidine on the AV node and slowing of the flutter rate. In addition, because of the interaction between digoxin and quinidine, the dose of digoxin must be decreased 25 to 33% when quinidine therapy is prescribed for a "digitalized" patient.

A form of therapy that may be useful in selected refractory cases is surgery. Patients with pre-excitation syndrome who display life-threatening or refractory arrhythmias require careful endocardial and epicardial mapping to determine the location of the bypass tract, which is followed by surgical division. This procedure has been successful in patients with drug-resistant cardiac arrhythmias due to pre-excitation, and recently has also been utilized successfully in patients with refractory atrial tachycardias secondary to ectopic atrial foci. The focus is removed surgically after careful mapping, which locates the area of disease from which the arrhythmia originates.

VENTRICULAR ARRHYTHMIAS

The management of the child with a ventricular arrhythmia is dependent upon the severity of arrhythmia, the associated hemodynamic effect of the arrhythmia, and the presence of associated cardiac and extracardiac disease. Premature ventricular depolarizations in a child with a normal heart, whether they are uniform with fixed coupling, uniform without fixed coupling, multiform, or even couplets, do not require emergency therapy. This applies even if the premature ventricular depolarizations are in a bigeminal pattern unless they are interfering with cardiac hemodynamics or are a precursor to the development of ventricular tachycardia or fibrillation. In patients with abnormal cardiac function or conditions such as the prolonged QT syndrome, suppression of the ventricular ectopy is recommended. Ventricular tachycardia should be treated in most patients regardless of their hemodynamic state. Occasionally, if a child does not have associated heart disease and the tachycardia is "nonsustained" or well tolerated, long-term antiarrhythmic drug therapy may not be required. If the patient with ventricular tachycardia has severely compromised hemodynamics, electrical cardioversion with 1–2 watt-seconds/kg is the treatment of choice. For ventricular fibrillation, it is the only treatment available.

If the patient is stable enough so that emergency electrical cardioversion is not immediately necessary, an intravenous access route should be established and treatment with intravenous lidocaine is instituted. The initial dose should be 1 mg/kg as a rapid bolus. The maximum amount administered in one dose should never exceed 75 mg. Lidocaine is effective in suppressing ventricular arrhythmias in approximately 85% of pediatric patients. When recommended doses are used, lidocaine has no significant electrophysiologic effects on the AV conduction system, and other than suppression of the ventricular arrhythmia, changes in the PR interval, QRS duration, or QT interval are not seen. If the initial dose does not result in conversion of the arrhythmia, a bolus can be repeated every 5 to 10 minutes to a maximum dose of 3 to 5 mg/kg. Generally, if three doses do not convert the arrhythmia, then lidocaine is not going to be useful. Once lidocaine has been demonstrated to be effective, the intravenous bolus should be followed by an intravenous infusion at a rate of 30 to 50 μg/kg/minute. It takes approximately three to five half-lives to reach the steady state of intravenous infusion (lidocaine half-life of approximately 90 minutes). If ventricular ectopy returns after 1 or 2 hours following the start of the intravenous infusion, rather than increasing the infusion rate, one should give another bolus of lidocaine at half the initial dose, or 0.5 mg/kg. Since the infusion may not have reached steady state at this time, the lidocaine level may have fallen below the therapeutic range. In patients with ventricular tachycardia that does not respond to intravenous lidocaine, the drug of choice is intravenous procainamide, given as a loading dose of 300 μg/kg/min and infused at a maximal rate of 20 mg/min to a maximum dose of 20 mg/kg (mixed as 1 gm of procainamide in 100 ml of normal saline). Once procainamide has been demonstrated to be effective, the loading dose should be followed by an intravenous infusion of 20–40 μg/kg/min.

To properly evaluate the efficacy of any of the antiarrhythmic drugs, one should obtain plasma drug levels to ensure that the dose being administered is resulting in therapeutic blood levels for that particular agent. Dosing schedules for children have not been well standardized and in most instances been adapted from adult dosing schedules. Since there are significant differences in both the pharmacokinetics and responsiveness of the developing heart, one has to be very careful in extrapolating adult dosage to the child's dosage.

The choice of antiarrhythmic agent for the long-term suppression of ventricular arrhythmias in children must often be made on an empiric basis. There are no detailed studies of drug efficacy available to help determine the best choice of antiarrhythmic agents and the proper dosages for pediatric patients of different age groups.

Most patients are treated with quinidine or procainamide. Disopyramide has also been an effective agent. The development of sustained-release preparations has been helpful in encouraging compliance in patients taking antiarrhythmic agents. Newer antiarrhythmic drugs such as amiodarone and mexilitene await further evaluation to determine their place as effective and safe alternative therapy in children.

Surgical treatment of ventricular tachycardia in children is rarely required. However, surgical excision of an arrhythmogenic focus located at the right ventricular outflow tract has been carried out successfully. In addition, surgery has been carried out in children with arrhythmogenic right ventricular dysplasia and cardiac tumors.

Mitral Valve Prolapse

RAE-ELLEN W. KAVEY, M.D.

Mitral valve prolapse is a diagnosis that has sprung from obscurity to become the most common cardiac diagnosis of childhood during the last decade. An auscultatory pattern that had been well-described by clinicians was found to be associated with abnormal mitral valve motion imaged with angiography or echocardiography; these findings were unified as the syndrome of mitral valve prolapse. Pathologically, mitral valve prolapse alludes to posterior protrusion of the mitral valve leaflets beyond the boundary of the mitral ring during ventricular systole. There is redundancy of the valve leaflets with lengthening of the chordae, which may be associated with a dilated valve ring; the findings involve one or both leaflets. During peak ventricular contraction, the abnormal leaflets balloon back in the left atrium and may produce late mitral insufficiency. Histologically, myxomatous degeneration of the valve tissue is seen. The etiology of these changes is unknown. The exact incidence in childhood remains undetermined, since the diagnosis is clinically obscure in young children and becomes increasingly manifest with age. Mitral prolapse may be seen in association with various forms of congenital heart disease, most importantly secundum atrial septal defect. It is also considered to be part of the cardiovascular involvement in Marfan's syndrome.

The natural history of isolated mitral valve prolapse in children is usually entirely benign. In a small percentage of patients, there is progressive mitral insufficiency throughout life, but this is not seen during the childhood years. Supraventricular and ventricular arrhythmias occur frequently, and when patients are symptomatic with these, therapy is recommended. In general, beta blockade is the most effective form of treatment for both supraventricular and ventricular arrhythmias. Sudden death has rarely been reported in children with isolated mitral valve prolapse and has been presumed to be due to ventricular arrhythmias. For this reason, treatment of asymptomatic children with documented ventricular tachycardia is often considered appropriate. Bacterial endocarditis has been well described in patients with isolated mitral valve prolapse and the incidence is thought to be about the same as it is in ventricular septal defect. Therefore appropriate antibiotic prophylaxis at predictable times of risk is recommended. Asymptomatic children with mitral valve prolapse do not appear to require regular cardiology followup and should be encouraged to participate in full unrestricted activity. However, infrequent cardiac reevaluation should be performed to document changes in the physical findings and to provide appropriate care should symptoms develop.

Cardiomyopathies and Pericardial Disease

BEVERLY C. MORGAN, M.D.

CARDIOMYOPATHIES

Cardiomyopathies involve the heart muscle itself. They have been classified on etiologic, clinical, functional, and pathologic bases. Important in classification is whether the disease is idiopathic or secondary to one of a number of specific infectious, toxic, or infiltrative agents. A clinically useful classification of idiopathic cardiomyopathy contains three categories: dilated (formerly called congestive), hypertrophic, and restrictive. This classification can be therapeutically useful as well.

Dilated Cardiomyopathy. Dilated cardiomyopathy is associated with dilatation of both ventricles and clinical findings of congestive heart failure. Therapy is supportive. Since all therapeutic agents are potentially hazardous, their use should be selective and cautious. The congestive component may respond to traditional therapy for congestive heart failure: digitalis, diuretics, sodium restriction, and rest. Therapy for congestive heart failure in infants and children is discussed in detail elsewhere in this text. Vasodilators may be helpful in severe congestive failure. Complicating arrhythmias are treated specifically as indicated by the electrocardiographic findings and the clinical course. Corticosteroids have not been found useful in dilated cardiomyopathy.

It has been suggested that endomyocardial biopsy assists in the diagnosis and classification of dilated cardiomyopathy, but its use is not generally indicated. The prognosis is usually poor, and death often ensues in days, weeks, or months.

Hypertrophic Cardiomyopathy. Hypertrophic cardiomyopathy is characterized pathophysiologically by a disarray of myocardial fibers, hypertrophy of the intraventricular septum, and some degree of left ventricular outflow tract obstruction produced by septal hypertrophy. This condition was originally termed idiopathic hypertrophic subaortic stenosis.

Treatment may modify the natural history of this disease to some extent but is primarily symptomatic. Since digitalis increases cardiac contractility, this drug may increase the outflow tract obstruction and therefore is generally contraindicated. If rapid atrial fibrillation occurs, the cautious use of digitalis may be necessary. It is recommended that beta-adrenergic stimulants be avoided. Beta-adrenergic blockade is the most common form of medical therapy, and propranolol is the drug most often used. Beta blockade may prevent the increase in outflow tract obstruction, and angina and dyspnea, if present, may respond to beta-blocking agents.

The development of congestive heart failure complicates therapy because of the relative contraindication of the use of digitalis. Other anticongestive measures such as diuretics may be useful.

The prognosis is variable, and sudden death may occur. The familial aspects of this disease are important in diagnosis, management, and family counseling.

A particular form of hypertrophic cardiomyopathy to be considered in pediatrics is that which may occur in infants of diabetic mothers. This cardiomyopathy is usually transient but may be asymptomatic. Some infants develop congestive heart failure, and anticongestive therapy in addition to treatment for metabolic problems may be required.

Restrictive Cardiomyopathy. The usual cause of restrictive cardiomyopathy is an infiltrative process. Ventricular filling is inhibited, and therefore restrictive cardiomyopathies are functionally similar to constrictive pericarditis with the impairment of ventricular filling the major hemodynamic abnormality.

There is no specific treatment for the restrictive process. Digitalis is potentially toxic in this condition. If significant conduction system disturbances result, pacemaker insertion may be necessary. Steroid therapy has been recommended for treating the restrictive cardiomyopathy associated with sarcoidosis. Endomyocardial biopsy may be particularly useful in establishing the pathologic basis of the restrictive cardiomyopathy.

PERICARDIAL DISEASES

The most common pericardial disease in pediatrics is acute pericarditis. The disease is often viral or idiopathic, and it may not be possible to differentiate between these two etiologies. The treatment of viral or idiopathic pericarditis is generally symptomatic. Moderate doses of acetylsalicylic acid (60–80 mg/kg/day) usually alleviate the discomfort. The efficacy of steroids has not been demonstrated.

The postpericardiotomy syndrome should be considered in children with findings suggestive of pericarditis following cardiac surgery. This condition may occur in the immediate postoperative period, or may present several weeks or months after surgery. Steroids have been used, but aspirin and bed rest are usually effective.

Bacterial or purulent pericarditis requires particular comment, since it is a life-threatening disease and prompt initiation of therapy is essential. If purulent pericarditis is suspected, a diagnostic pericardiocentesis should be done and therapy initiated if the diagnosis is confirmed. This disease may be primary as a complication of bacteremia or may be secondary to diseases such as empyema, pneumonia and other systemic infection. In infants, *Haemophilus influenzae* type B is the most likely cause; in older children, the etiology is often penicillin-resistant staphylococcus. Large doses of organism-specific antibiotics must be administered promptly. The length of therapy is dependent on the organism and clinical course but is usually three or more weeks. Tuberculous pericarditis is uncommon but must be considered in the differential diagnosis. Prompt therapy with appropriate antibiotics and open surgical pericardial drainage have improved the previously very high mortality in purulent pericarditis.

Trauma and iatrogenic injuries secondary to diagnostic or therapeutic instrumentation may produce hemopericardium and death may ensue rapidly if treatment is not provided. Prompt diagnosis, possible evacuation of the pericardial sac, and often transfusion are indicated in this emergency.

Constrictive pericarditis is very uncommon in pediatrics and is usually idiopathic but occasionally tuberculous. Treatment, if required, is usually surgical and involves removal of the pericardium.

Systemic Hypertension

DAVID GOLDRING, M.D.,
ALAN M. ROBSON, M.D.,
and JULIO V. SANTIAGO, M.D.

Hypertension is the major health problem in our country, because it has been estimated that approximately 20 to 25 million people have hypertension and that about 250,000 die each year from the complications of this disease. Traditionally, hypertension has been classified as either primary or essential when the cause is unknown and as secondary when it is associated with or a consequence of renal, endocrine, or congenital vascular disease. Even in secondary hypertension, the specific cause is incompletely understood. The above classification profoundly affects the decision and results of therapy. For example, treatment for primary hypertension is usually effective, but it must be emphasized that the therapy is symptomatic. By contrast, for some forms of secondary hypertension the treatment may be curative. One must also keep in mind that the decision to treat a hypertensive patient depends upon the level of blood pressure which justifies a diagnosis of hypertension. This level of blood pressure is arbitrary. For example the World Health Organization has recommended that 140/90 mm Hg be designated borderline hypertension and 160/95 mm Hg and higher as definite hypertension in adults. These values are inappropriate for infants and children, whose blood pressure is lower than that of the adult and increases progressively with growth. A reasonable working guideline might be as follows: The pediatric patients whose blood pressures are persistently between the 90th and 95th percentile for age and sex be considered as suspect and those individuals whose pressures are persistently above the 95th percentile for age and sex be classified as hypertensives. Suggested blood pressure levels which we have used to identify suspect hypertensives are shown in Table I.

PRIMARY HYPERTENSION

If the above arbitrary definitions of hypertension are used, the most common type in the pediatric population is primary hypertension. Dur-

Table 1. APPROXIMATE GUIDELINES FOR SUSPECT BLOOD PRESSURE VALUES

Supine Position—Lowest of 3 Readings Boys and Girls			
Age in years	3–5	6–9	10–14
Blood pressure mm Hg	>110/70	>120/75	>130/80

Seated Position—Average of Second and Third Readings			
	Girls		Boys
Age in years	14–18	14	15	16–18
Blood pressure mm Hg	>125/80	>130/75	>130/80	>135/85

ing a 5-year period, we measured the blood pressures in approximately 20,000 subjects, 14–18 years of age, in the St. Louis metropolitan area; one student was found with coarctation of the aorta, and one with hypertension due to hyperthyroidism, but approximately 1000 suspected primary hypertensives were found.

Although the cause is unknown, effective symptomatic therapy is available.

The decision to use pharmacologic therapy in asymptomatic primary hypertensive pediatric patients must be examined from a different perspective than that used for the adult. Therapy may be more effective in the young, early hypertensive, and it may be possible to arrest or even cure the disease in the pediatric patient; this has not been possible in the adult. On the negative side, the undesirable, sometimes serious side effects of all antihypertensive drugs are well known, so that the risk-benefit ratio must be very carefully considered. The drug therapy must be a lifetime commitment, and there is no information about what serious untoward effects these drugs may have upon a young, growing subject. Finally, in a 10-year follow-up of approximately 100 young primary hypertensives we found that in 30% the blood pressure spontaneously returned to normal levels. In the light of the above, we feel that the nonthreatening, safe, therapeutic regimen discussed below is the preferred course to follow in the young primary hypertensive.

Weight Reduction. It has been shown in studies that at least 50% of young primary hypertensives are obese. The pathogenesis of the hypertension with obesity in unknown. In recent studies of adult obese hypertensives, significant reduction in systolic and diastolic pressures was achieved by weight reduction. There are no reported similar studies in pediatric patients, but we would recommend this approach in view of the above experience with hypertensive adults. Patient compliance would be difficult. Expert guidance by the physician is important, and the effectiveness of a weight reduction

program would be enhanced by consultation with a nutritionist, a social worker, and in some instances a psychiatrist.

Exercise. Regimens of dynamic exercise have been shown to normalize blood pressure in some adult primary hypertensives. We have just completed a study on a group of 30 adolescent primary hypertensives who all experienced a drop in systolic and diastolic pressures during and after an exercise regimen of 6–8 months. The mechanism for lowering blood pressure with dynamic exercise is incompletely understood. It has been suggested that several months of dynamic exercising produces a relatively hypokinetic circulatory state, which is probably due to the negative inotropic effect of reduction in heart rate and to adaptations in the neuroendocrine system, which results in increased vagal tone and decreased release of norepinephrine and epinephrine.

The regimen we suggest to our young patients is summarized in the following instructions. Supervision and surveillance are provided by weekly visits to the physician. This helps with patient compliance in this dramatic change in their lifestyle.

ENDURANCE EXERCISE TRAINING

For endurance exercise training to be effective in helping to lower your blood pressure, a few simple guidelines must be followed:

1. The activity should exercise a large amount of your muscle mass. Exercises which meet this requirement are running, cycling, and swimming.

2. The activity must elevate your heart rate to at least approximately 160 beats per minute. This can be measured by taking your pulse for 6 seconds *immediately after exercise* and multiplying it by 10. The pulse can be felt either at the wrist or in the neck below the angle of the jaw. Your doctor can help you locate the pulse if needed.

3. The activity must continue for 30–45 minutes at least every other day but preferably 5 times per week. If you select running, you should build up your endurance so that you run approximately 3 to 5 miles a day 5 times per week. If you select bicycling, you should build up your endurance so that you ride 10 to 15 miles a day 5 times a week. If you select swimming, you should build up your endurance so that you swim 1 to 2 miles a day 5 times per week.

The tendency is to start out much too quickly which will elevate your heart rate too much and not allow you to continue for 40 minutes. The idea is to start slowly. Find the running, swimming, or cycling pace which results in a heart rate of approximately 160 beats/minute.

Eventually you will have to increase your pace as your fitness level begins to increase. At this point, it is still essential that you attain a heart rate of approximately 160 beats/minute.

There are no shortcuts to physical fitness. It requires a sincere and serious promise to stick with the program, but it offers a way to lower your blood pressure without taking medicine.

Isometric exercise such as hand-grip and certain forms of weight lifting are not recommended for the adult primary hypertensive who may have in addition either known or silent coronary artery disease. In the young primary hypertensive the incidence of coronary artery disease is very low, therefore, isometric exercise does not pose a risk. However, more studies are needed before these exercises should be recommended for the young primary hypertensive.

Diet Modification (Blood Lipids). Some years ago a number of investigators proposed that elevated blood lipids predisposed an individual to the development of atheromatous coronary artery disease. Elevated blood lipids as well as hypertension were thus considered risk factors. Reducing the intake of foods with a high cholesterol content and drug therapy such as clofibrate, colestipol, and nicotinic acid to lower the blood cholesterol has been recommended for adults with hypertension to protect them against the development of atheromatous coronary artery disease. This subject is still controversial for the adult subjects. Therefore, advising radical changes in the diet for infants and children with primary hypertension to reduce the risk of developing coronary artery disease in adulthood is not justified, because we do not know what serious harm may come to the young individual from this drastic modification of the diet.

Dietary Salt Restriction. There is considerable circumstantial evidence suggesting a link between a high dietary salt intake and hypertension in genetically predisposed individuals. The degree of salt restriction required to produce a significant reduction in blood pressure is unknown. It is believed by some that a diet containing 50 mEq of salt per day may be effective in reducing blood pressure. The degree of salt restriction would be unpalatable, and most children would not comply. We, therefore, suggest that mothers do not add salt to food in cooking and that they restrict food with high salt content.

Other Forms of Therapy. Smoking should be prohibited, and contraceptive drugs, steroids, amphetamines, and liberal use of nose drops should be discontinued. Behavior modification methods such as biofeedback, relaxation techniques, and psychotherapy are of questionable benefit.

An occasional patient might be considered a candidate for drug therapy as described below under renal hypertension; e.g., a young primary hypertensive who is obese and has a strong family history of hypertension who has not responded to nonpharmacologic therapy and whose pressure is progressively rising.

Unfortunately, the treatment of hypertension in the young will continue to be symptomatic and weakly effective until the pathogenesis of primary hypertension is better understood.

SECONDARY HYPERTENSION
Renal Disorders

Secondary hypertension most often is the consequence of a renal lesion. It may present as an acute event, sometimes requiring treatment as a medical emergency. Alternatively, it may represent a problem of long-term management. Since the approaches to these two situations are different and the drugs used also differ, each will be discussed separately.

Management of Acute Hypertension and Hypertensive Crises. Patients who fit into these categories have no previous history of hypertension or have an acute increase in blood pressure above their previous stable values. Typically, blood pressure levels are elevated well above the 95th percentiles for age. When such an increase is associated with symptoms or signs of an encephalopathy or heart failure, it must be treated as a medical emergency. However, it is important to remember that children are more susceptible to the changes of malignant hypertension at lower blood pressure levels than are adults. Thus, we consider any child who presents with a systolic pressure of 170 mm Hg or greater or a diastolic pressure of 120 mm Hg or greater to be at risk of major complications and to require urgent treatment. Such urgent treatment may be indicated at even lower blood pressure values in the neonate or infant. The only exception to this general rule would be the patient with coarctation presenting in childhood, without heart failure.

Causes of such acute severe elevations in blood pressure include acute poststreptococcal and other acute glomerulonephritides, hemolytic uremic syndrome, collagen vascular diseases, especially when affecting the renal vasculature, chronic pyelonephritis, segmental renal hypoplasia, infantile polycystic kidneys, and renovascular diseases. The initial approach to treatment is the same, regardless of the underlying etiology.

Sodium retention plays an important role in the genesis of the hypertension in many of these patients. Thus, attempting to decrease body sodium content by limiting sodium intake and by increasing urinary sodium losses with diuretics often represents an important adjunct to therapy with antihypertensive drugs. However, it is inappropriate to rely upon this approach alone to treat severe acute hypertension. These measures take too long, frequently days, to become effective.

Dietary sodium restriction alone can only prevent sodium retention from becoming worse, and the kidney typically responds poorly to diuretics in many of the renal diseases causing acute severe hypertension. The loop diuretics are the most potent. Our preference is to use furosemide 0.5 to 1.0 mg/kg given either orally or parenterally. On occasion we have used larger doses without problems. The thiazide diuretics are less effective.

The drug that we usually use first is hydralazine. It is a vasodilator which also increases cardiac output and has the advantage of not decreasing renal blood flow even when blood pressure is lowered. Side effects are those seen with vasodilators, namely flushing of the skin, headaches, tachycardia, and palpitations. They occur infrequently in children. The drug is well absorbed when given by mouth, and an effect typically is seen within 1 to 2 hours. The initial oral dose is 0.25 mg/kg and can be repeated every 4 to 6 hours. The total daily dose can be as high as 4.5 mg/kg/day. An effect from a dose of hydralazine of 0.15 mg/kg may be seen within a few minutes when given intravenously and within 15 to 30 minutes when given intramuscularly. Doses may be repeated within 30 to 90 minutes, but oral therapy should be implemented as soon as possible. The intravenous injection of hydralazine often is effective in reducing blood pressure in patients refractory to the drug given orally.

The combination of reserpine, 0.02 mg/kg per day to a maximum dose of 1 mg given intramuscularly every 12 hours, with hydralazine may be effective if hydralazine alone does not lower blood pressure satisfactorily. When reserpine is used, the dose of this drug is kept constant and the frequency of dosage of hydralazine is modified according to the patient's response. Some begin therapy with this combination of drugs. We avoid reserpine when possible because of its side effects, which include symptoms of depression in older children, drowsiness, nasal congestion, and stimulation of gastric secretion, which may result in peptic ulceration and bleeding from the gastrointestinal tract. It should not be used in patients in whom surgery is anticipated.

Patients who do not respond to the regimens outlined above should be treated next with diazoxide. The initial dose is 5 to 10 mg/kg given by rapid intravenous infusion over 1 to 2 minutes. A slower rate of administration usually is ineffective, because the drug is protein bound. The dose can be repeated 30 minutes later if there is no response. The length of action of the drug, typically, is from 4 to 24 hours, although an effect for 36 hours or longer may be seen. Side effects are rare, although nausea and hyperglycemia have been reported. Hypotension does not occur unless frequent repeated small doses of the drug are given, usually in combination with other antihypertensive drugs.

Sodium nitroprusside is an effective intravenous antihypertensive agent which we use in patients who do not respond to any of the above drugs. Its onset of effect is immediate, and the response lasts for as long as the drug is infused. To prepare it for use, 50 mg are diluted in 1 liter of 5% dextrose in water (50 μg/ml). The solution is infused at a rate of from 0.5 to 8.0 μg/kg/min. The rate of infusion is titrated according to the blood pressure response. The drug is not stable when exposed to sunlight so the bottle and infusion lines should be wrapped with aluminum foil throughout the infusion. Blood pressure should be monitored constantly throughout the infusion. Whenever possible the drug should not be administered for longer than 48 hours, especially in patients with renal failure, since the drug is metabolized to cyanide, which normally would be excreted by the kidney. If the drug has to be administered for 48 hours or longer, blood thiocyanate levels should be monitored after this period of time.

Very few patients do not respond to the preceding approach. Those who do not respond typically have hypertension in association with markedly elevated levels of plasma renin activity (PRA) and do respond to the angiotensin-converting enzyme inhibitor, captopril. The recommended starting dose is approximately 0.33 mg/kg three times a day. The drug is not stable in solution and should be given in tablet, or crushed-tablet, form. If response is poor, the dose is increased in stepwise fashion, usually at 24-hour intervals, until a satisfactory response is obtained. The total daily dose should not exceed 6 mg/kg. The effectiveness of the drug often can be potentiated by the use of furosemide (1 mg/kg/day in 2 divided doses) and propranolol* (1 mg/kg/day in 4 divided doses, increasing to a maximum of 5 mg/kg/day). We prefer, however, to use a single drug, rather than a combination of drugs, when possible. Few acute side effects have been observed with captopril. Long-term complications include proteinuria and a decrease in the white blood cell count. If either abnormality develops, the drug should be discontinued.

The preceding, sequential approach to therapy is designed to control acute hypertension and to reduce the risk of major complications developing from the elevated blood pressure. Once blood pressures have been reduced below the 95th percentile for age, the physician should consider whether there may be a surgically treatable cause

---

* Manufacturer's note: Data on the use of propranolol in the pediatric age group are too limited to permit adequate directions for use.

for the hypertension and, in those patients in whom hypertension is likely to be chronic, begin to introduce the appropriate drugs for long-term control of blood pressure.

Renovascular lesions are the most likely cause of secondary hypertension that can be controlled by surgery. They should be considered in any patient with very severe hypertension and in those with elevated PRA levels. Nowadays, such lesions can usually be demonstrated most satisfactorily after an intravenous injection of contrast agent and digital vascular imaging in centers where the appropriate equipment is available. This methodology avoids the much more invasive technique of renal arteriography. There has been considerable interest in the use of percutaneous transluminal angioplasty (PTLA) to treat patients with vascular stenoses, including those of the renal artery. This method appears to have limited value in children, since many of the renal artery lesions occur at the origin of the renal vessels and typically involve the abdominal aorta. There have been reports of successful treatment of mid-artery lesions in children using PTLA. It is not clear, however, whether such stenoses will return with time. Treatment of segmental lesions within the renal parenchyma can be particularly difficult. Successful selective embolization of a stenotic intrarenal artery in a child has been reported and would appear preferable to nephrectomy. In all cases, the surgical success depends on the experience of the surgeon in this kind of work.

Management of Chronic Hypertension. The major difficulty in managing hypertension on a long-term basis is patient compliance. It is self-evident that if a drug is to be effective it must be taken regularly. Compliance is less a problem in the younger child, since most mothers ensure that the physician's advice is followed closely. Most problems are experienced in teenage patients. Compliance can be improved if the drug regimen is simple, is free from side effects, and is relatively inexpensive. A suitable regimen must be supplemented by extensive education of the patient and the family about hypertension, about the prescribed drugs, and about the reasons for prescribing those drugs. It is sometimes very hard to convince asymptomatic patients that they need to take potent drugs, usually for the rest of their lives. Follow-up should be as convenient for the patient as possible.

Antihypertensive drugs can be considered in three basic groups: vasodilators, diuretics that reduce volume, and those that modify release, metabolism, or function of pressor systems such as the renin-angiotensin system. The same principles about determining whether hypertension is volume-or pressor-related and treating with a drug that has an appropriate action applies to children as well as to adults. Again, as in adults, if a drug from one major group is ineffective and a second drug is to be added, it is better to use a drug from a different group than from the same group. Thus, if a patient has a less than satisfactory response to a vasodilator and has a component of volume expansion, it is usually better to add a diuretic to the therapeutic regimen than another vasodilator. If secondary hyperreninism develops, the addition of a drug such as propranolol would be appropriate. However, such an approach often results in a confusing or cumbersome regimen that contributes to poor patient compliance. Thus, we prefer, whenever possible, to use maximum doses of a single drug rather than to use multiple drugs.

It is difficult to recommend specific regimens to treat hypertension. Each patient must have an approach individualized to his or her needs. Below we consider the major groups of drugs and our experience with them.

Vasodilator Drugs. Hydralazine may be used on a chronic as well as on an acute basis. Its effectiveness, however, is limited in most patients with secondary hypertension. Its major value in our clinic is to treat night-time hypertension in patients treated primarily with guanethidine. Dosage and side effects have already been outlined. The protracted use of hydralazine in high doses may result in a syndrome resembling sytemic lupus erythematosus (SLE). Typically, but not always, this reverses when hydralazine is discontinued. For this reason we do not like to use this drug in patients with SLE even though there is no evidence that hydralazine exacerbates SLE in patients on concomitant immunosuppressive therapy.

Minoxidil is a vasodilator that is a valuable addition to our armamentarium, since patients resistant to other drugs frequently respond to it. The recommended initial dose is 0.2 mg/kg as a single daily dose. This may be increased in increments of 50 to 100% every 2 or 3 days until blood pressure control is achieved. The effective dosage range usually is between 0.25 and 1.0 mg/kg/day with a recommended maximum daily dose of 50 mg. It is advised that a patient receive a beta-blocker such as propranolol before starting minoxidil. Since minoxidil induces fluid retention, which can be severe and result in pericardial effusions and tamponade, a diuretic such as furosemide should be used concurrently. The side effect that is most distressing to patients and their families is hypertrichosis. Many patients are unwilling to accept the severe overgrowth of hair over their face and forehead, and female patients dislike this growth on other parts of their bodies. Because of its side effects and the inability to use minoxidil as a single drug, we reserve this drug for patients who are resistant to other drugs.

Prazosin† has a direct effect on vascular smooth muscle and also has features of an alpha-adrenergic blocking agent. Therefore, reflex tachycardia typically is not a major complication when prazosin is used to lower blood pressure. The initial dose in older children is 1 mg 2 or 3 times a day. This may be increased slowly until an adequate response is obtained. Daily doses above 20 mg rarely increase the efficacy of the drug, although some patients may benefit from doses as high as 40 mg/day. There has been relatively little experience with this drug in younger children, and the size of the smallest capsules (1 mg) makes it difficult to provide a suitable starting dose for very small children. The effects of the drug are enhanced by simultaneous use of diuretics and beta-adrenergic blocking agents. Postural hypotension has been the most important side effect. Blood pressure should be monitored with the patient in the supine and in the upright positions. The patient should be alerted to the possibility of postural symptoms, and if they do occur, the patient should be advised to assume the recumbent position. Such side effects should alert the physician to the need to modify drug dosage. The major advantages of prazosin are the few side effects experienced with its use and the need for only twice-a-day dosage. However, in our experience, it is not as potent as other drugs. When used in large dosage, tachycardia and fluid retention may occur. Drugs that inhibit the transmembrane influx of calcium ions decrease peripheral vascular resistance and may be an effective adjunctive therapy. For example, nifedipine‡ may be started in an oral dose of approximately 0.5 mg/kg/day given in three individual doses. The dose can be later increased to 1 or 1.5 mg/kg/day.

Drugs Affecting Adrenergic Activity. Propranolol§ has been found to be an effective antihypertensive agent in children. It is thought to act as a beta-adrenergic blocking agent. Since the renin-angiotensin system is regulated in part by beta-adrenergic activity, it was thought originally that propranolol worked through this mechanism. More recent studies have indicated that other modes of action must be involved too. The drug is readily absorbed from the gastrointestinal tract. The initial dose should be between 0.5 and 1.0 mg/kg/day. Originally it was advised that the total dose should be divided into 4 doses a day; more recently, twice-daily doses have been found to be

effective. Doses can be increased on a daily or every-other-day basis until a suitable response occurs. Daily doses as high as 16 mg/kg/day have been used. The major complication has been the development of heart failure. The drug should not be used, therefore, in any patient with heart disease or pulmonary disease, especially if heart failure is present. We do not use propranolol as a drug of first choice when treating chronic hypertension, because we have been disappointed with it when used alone. However, it is a most useful adjunct to other antihypertensive agents.

Several other beta-adrenergic blocking agents have been developed. The one that offers definite advantages for children is nadolol,‖ since it is effective when taken once a day.

Guanethidine blocks sympathetic activity and has a prolonged serum half-life, which permits a single daily dose. This is a major advantage when treating hypertension in children. It works only when the patient assumes the upright position and therefore is of very limited value in neonates and infants. In children between the ages of 2 and 10 years we usually use a single daily dose of 5 mg to start. In older children this dose should be 10 mg/day. Effects are rarely seen for 3 or more days. Thereafter, the dose can be increased in increments of 5 or 10 mg/day at weekly intervals. Most patients respond to a dose of 25 mg/day or less, occasional patients require up to 50 mg/day. The major side effect is postural hypotension, typically when the patient arises in the morning or stands up abruptly. Sitting with legs over the edge of the bed for a few seconds before standing up or standing up slowly usually eliminates this side effect. Diarrhea is a side effect in a small minority of children. Fluid retention has been reported with the drug but has not been a problem in our experience. The drug should not be used in any patient receiving a monoamine oxidase (MAO) inhibitor. When monitoring the effectiveness of guanethidine, blood pressure should be taken with the patient in the supine and the upright positions as well as after exercise to determine its postural effect. One major disadvantage of the drug is that it has little effect when the patient is asleep. This can be rectified by having the patient propped up on pillows when asleep. Alternatively, a small dose of hydralazine can be added to the regimen in the evening. Recently we have found that some teenage male patients in whom blood pressure is controlled by guanethidine have discontinued this drug when they became sexually active because of its side effect on inhibiting ejaculation. We now

---

† Safety and efficacy of prazosin in children have not been established.

‡ This use of nifedipine is not listed in the manufacturer's directions.

§ Manufacturer's note: Data on the use of propranolol in the pediatric age group are too limited to permit adequate directions for use.

‖ Safety and effectiveness of nadolol in children have not been established.

warn teenage males about this problem and convert their control, usually to prazosin, if it appears that this side effect may pose a problem. Extensive experience with guanethidine has convinced me that this drug often is a most effective agent which can be used alone and requires only a single morning dose, helping to ensure compliance.

Methyldopa is a moderately potent antihypertensive agent that probably works by interfering with the production of the neurotransmitter norepinephrine. Its absorption is very variable, and it results in a positive direct Coombs' test in 20% of patients. The first two patients we treated with this drug developed hemolytic anemia. Although this is a rare occurrence, it limited our enthusiasm for the drug. Other patients complain of a sedative effect when starting methyldopa, an effect that may or may not lessen with time. Methyldopa has been reported to be effective in controlling hypertension in children, especially when taken with a diuretic to limit sodium and water retention, which is sometimes seen when the drug is taken alone. The recommended starting dose is 10 mg/kg/day taken in 3 divided doses. The dose can be increased stepwise every 3 to 5 days up to 40 mg/kg/day. The maximum recommended daily dose is 2 gm.

Other drugs in this group include reserpine and clonidine. Used on a long-term basis, reserpine produces drowsiness, symptoms of depression, and nasal stuffiness. It must be stopped several days in advance of any operation requiring a general anesthetic. Its routine use is not recommended, although it may have a role in some patients resistant to or unable to take other drugs. Clonidine is a much newer drug which acts on alpha-adrenergic receptors. It too may produce drowsiness. Other side effects include dryness of the mouth and rebound hypertension if the drug is stopped abruptly. We have had limited experience with the drug but have not found any advantage for it in comparison to guanethidine or prazosin.

Drugs Modifying Renin-Angiotensin System. Beta-adrenergic blocking agents such as propranolol interfere with renin release, and at least part of their action is through this mechanism. More recently, drugs have been developed that inhibit the enzyme responsible for the conversion of angiotensin I to angiotensin II, which is the pressor substance. The drug in this category which is absorbed when taken by mouth and which is now available by prescription is captopril. Recent observations suggest that it is effective by acting on both the renin-angiotensin and the kinin systems. Its use in acute hypertension has been detailed already. We have found it to be an extremely valuable agent in the management of chronic hypertension too, especially that which is renin-mediated. The initial dose is 1 mg/kg/day divided into three doses, and this is increased in stepwise manner, at 8-hour intervals if necessary, until effective blood pressure response is observed. The maximum dose should not exceed 6 mg/kg/day. The use of beta-adrenergic blocking agents and diuretics will often potentiate the effect of captopril, and all antihypertensive agents other than those in these two groups should be discontinued before captopril is used. We have been most pleased by the effectiveness of the drug and by patient acceptance. To date, we have not seen proteinuria or decreased WBC count, the two complications that require discontinuing the drug.

Drugs Acting on Volume. Hypervolemia may contribute to chronic hypertension in many patients, or fluid and sodium retention may occur secondary to the use of several of the vasodilator drugs. Thus, the use of diuretics has an important role in the management of hypertension.

The most frequently prescribed diuretics are the thiazides. Their effect in hypertension appears to be through their action to increase urinary losses of sodium and water. The drugs are well absorbed when taken by mouth and are relatively free of side effects. Potassium wasting with or without hypokalemia may occur with prolonged use. Hyperuricemia, a common complication of using thiazides in adults, is seen infrequently in children. Nor have hyperglycemia and hypercalcemia been reported as a complication of thiazide use in children. Hydrochlorothiazide will be used as an example of a typical thiazide. The starting dose is 2 mg/kg/day taken in two equally divided doses, the second one of which should be given no later than early afternoon to avoid nocturia. The dose may be doubled, but one should wait for at least 7 to 14 days before increasing the dose, since the maximum therapeutic response may take this long to develop. Unfortunately many children with secondary hypertension have a renal cause for their elevated blood pressure and therefore do not respond optimally to the thiazides.

Chlorthalidone is chemically unrelated to the thiazides but has very similar actions. Its major advantage is that it has a longer length of action and is effective when taken only once a day.

Furosemide acts on the ascending limb of the loop of Henle and thus is referred to as a loop diuretic. It and ethacrynic acid are the most potent diuretics known. Although furosemide has a short plasma half-life, it needs to be given only once a day, in the morning. The usual starting dose is 0.5 to 1 mg/kg/day. There has been little published experience to show that larger doses given for protracted periods of time in children are safe but to date we have not experienced any problems.

The major complication is potassium wasting, necessitating oral potassium supplements. Most effective potassium preparations are extremely unpalatable. We have found that the use of a salt substitute on foods is best tolerated by our patients. Caution in administering any potassium supplement must be exercised in any patient with renal insufficiency in case hyperkalemia develops. Concern has been expressed that furosemide may be ototoxic, but there is little evidence to support this concern when the drug is used as outlined above.

Spironolactone is a competitive inhibitor of aldosterone. When used in conjunction with a thiazide diuretic or furosemide, it potentiates the diuresis and may have a slight potassium-sparing effect. We sometimes use it for this purpose, but do not believe that it is an effective antihypertensive agent when used alone. The starting dose may be up to 3.3 mg/kg/day in single or divided doses. Effects from the drug may not be seen for 3 or more days, and maximum effectiveness may take up to 14 days to develop.

Triamterene is a nonsteroidal potassium-sparing diuretic. We do not use it, since most of our hypertensive patients have renal disease, and we are concerned about the potential of this drug to induce significant hyperkalemia.

Any patient in whom a diuretic is indicated should also receive a salt-restricted diet. It is not practical to restrict sodium intake to levels as low as 0.5 gm (20 meq) per day in nonhospitalized patients. We have found that usually the best one can accomplish is to restrict intake to around 35 to 50 meq/day. It is important to emphasize to parents that the higher the sodium intake, the greater will be the dose of diuretics needed. We do not recommend attempting to control chronic severe or moderately severe hypertension with dietary sodium restriction alone. It rarely works; if a benefit is seen, this usually is short lived, since most patients find that adhering to a low salt diet is extremely arduous.

Summary. The therapeutic regimen that is developed should be as simple and as free from side effects as possible. Preferably, a single drug should be used. Those that we use most are guanethidine and prazosin. We are now using captopril more often, especially in patients with renin-mediated hypertension. Minoxidil may prove effective in patients resistant to other drugs. When a second drug is needed, we use a diuretic and dietary sodium restriction if volume expansion or sodium retention appears to be an etiologic factor in the hypertension. A thiazide diuretic or chlorthalidone is used if a moderate diuresis is required; furosemide for a more vigorous diuresis. If secondary hyperreninemia appears to be responsible for a reduced effect of the primary antihypertensive drug, we add propranolol to the regimen, but have begun to use nadolol, because it is effective when taken once a day.

Endocrine Disorders

Since some children with hypertension caused by endocrine disorders can be cured with appropriate surgical or medical therapy, consideration should be given early in the course of diagnosis or therapy to the possibility that hypertension may have an endocrine cause in all hypertensive children. Some of the more important causes of endocrine hypertension are briefly outlined in Table 2.

Pheochromocytoma usually presents as sustained rather than intermittent hypertension. Pheochromocytomas may present as isolated cases or in association with Sipple's syndrome (medullary carcinoma of the thyroid and bilateral pheochromocytomas). High perioperative morbidity requires expert use of alpha- and beta-adrenergic blocking agents as well as careful monitoring of the hydration status. Surgical removal is the treatment of choice.

Two syndromes associated with congenital adrenal hyperplasia can cause hypertension in young children. They are caused by the accumulation of desoxycorticosterone (11-B-OH deficiency) or mineralocorticoids (17 α-OH deficiency) due to an increased secretion of ACTH secondary to deficient cortisol production.

Approximately 80% of children with Cushing's syndrome due to bilateral adrenal stimulation by ACTH or to an isolated adrenal tumor will be hypertensive. Treatment consists of surgical removal of the tumor responsible for excess cortisol or ACTH production.

The presence of a low plasma renin in a salt-repleted patient with hypertension should lead to a suspicion that the patient has a form of congenital adrenal hyperplasia or hyperaldosteronism. These disorders are often responsive to appropriate glucocorticoid or spironolactone therapy or to surgical removal of an aldosterone-producing tumor.

Systolic hypertension is sometimes a manifestation of hyperthyroidism, and treatment may either be surgical or medical, as noted in Table 2.

Congenital Vascular Disease

Coarctation of the Aorta. Coarctation of the aorta is a congenital malformation characterized by constriction of the aorta distal to the origin of the left subclavian artery. Characteristically, there is hypertension in the upper limbs and hypotension in the lower extremities. It is generally agreed that surgical correction be carried out in the infant

Table 2.   CAUSES OF ENDOCRINE HYPERTENSION

Endocrine Disorder	Clinical Presentation	Therapy
1. Pheochromocytoma	90% sustained hypertension	Alpha-adrenergic blockade (phenoxybenzamine, phentolamine)
	80% headache, 65% sweating	Beta-adrenergic blockade (propranolol)
	35% intermittent abdominal pain	Careful monitoring of hydration status intraoperatively
2. Congenital adrenal hyperplasias	Hypertension Rapid growth	Replacement glucocorticoids
(a) 11-B hydroxylase deficiency	Virilization in females Elevated 11-desoxycortisol and DOC	
(b) 17-α hydroxylase deficiency	Hypertension Hypokalemic alkalosis Ambiguous genitalia in males Delayed puberty in girls	Replacement glucocorticoids
3. Cushing's syndrome	Growth failure Signs of glucocorticoid excess	Surgical removal of adrenal or pituitary tumor
4. Hyperaldosteronism	Hypokalemia in sodium-repleted state Low renin, high aldosterone	Surgery (for isolated tumor) or spironolactone
5. Hyperthyroidism	Systolic hypertension, emotional lability, goiter, increased sweating, increased height for age, weakness, tremor, tachycardia, elevated T_4, T_3, FT_4, and RT_3U	Surgical excision of thyroid gland or medical treatment with propranolol, propylthiouracil, or methimazole (Tapazole).

who presents with congestive heart failure due to coarctation of the aorta, and a left-to-right shunt such as a patent ductus arteriosus or a ventricular or atrial septal defect. Thus, a volume overload is imposed upon a pressure-overloaded left ventricle. The critically ill infant in congestive heart failure should be started upon treatment for the heart failure. The baby should then be evaluated by cardiac catheterization and angiocardiography. If the diagnosis of coarctation of the aorta is verified, the baby should be operated upon. The time elapsed from admittance to operation should be 24–48 hours.

There is also general agreement that surgical correction is imperative in patients with isolated coarctation in the age range of 5 to 8 years when the aortic lumen has achieved approximately 50% of the cross-sectional area of the adult aorta. A second operation will therefore not be needed in adulthood, even if the anastomotic site does not grow with age. Most patients have generalized hypertension postoperatively, which spontaneously returns to normal values in 2 or 3 weeks in approximately 90% of patients. Although some authors have advocated antihypertensive therapy during this period, I have seen no evidence to support the reason for such treatment. Nor is there evidence to support the suggestion that antihypertensive drug treatment is of any value in the preoperative state. About 10% of patients have persistent generalized hypertension even if the aortic obstruction is completely relieved. The reason for this is unknown. It may be that these patients are destined to develop primary hypertension.

Hypotension

HERBERT S. HARNED, JR., M.D.

The pediatric practitioner must be able to assess rapidly the severity of hypotensive states. To recognize hypotension, he must be aware of the normal range of blood pressures in children of differing age groups and be knowledgeable about the proper cuff sizes, manometric techniques, and interpretations of Korotkoff and Doppler sounds and flush methods. Recognition of shock must be made from observing tachycardia, thready pulses, venous collapse, delayed capillary filling, pallor, coldness and moisture of the skin, obtunded consciousness, and oliguria. These findings indicate inadequate oxygenation and perfusion of vital organs and call for immediate action.

Although the various etiologies of severe hypotension with shock require certain specific therapies, especially with septic, anaphylactic, or neurogenic shock, certain general measures must be directed toward the rapid reversal of this life-threatening state.

Recent knowledge of the treatment of shock has been derived from experience in ICU settings. Treatments in this relatively ideal setting will be presented initially. From this perspective, the practitioner can extrapolate appropriate therapeutic measures and monitoring techniques which might apply in his particular circumstances. An organized approach is needed, with one person as the leader. The more assistants one can mobilize, the better the chance of reversal of a case of severe hypotension. At least four active physicians or knowledgeable ancillary intensivists are desired to handle a severe hypotensive episode.

Shock often is the precursor of cardiopulmonary arrest, and similar therapeutic measures are initiated to those needed for the latter condition. An approach using the initials VIP for "ventilation-infusion-pump" has set proper priorities.

First, immediate attention to ventilation is vital, with realization that the Trendelenburg position (head down) is often detrimental. Improving the state of ventilation, by ensuring a proper airway, administration of oxygen, and hyperventilating the patient to lower Pco_2 and combat detrimental acidosis, offers a direct treatment of the basic problem in shock, i.e., decreased cellular oxidation. In an ICU setting, the person most skilled in endotracheal intubation and ventilatory management should immediately be assigned to the task of evaluating the need for establishing an orotracheal airway.

Suctioning, use of an oral airway, passage of a nasogastric tube for gastric decompression, mouth-to-mouth insufflation, use of self-inflating and reservoir-type resuscitation bags, use of face masks, and use of 100% oxygen need to be applied as necessary if ventilation is inadequate. The decision concerning endotracheal intubation may be difficult, but this must be done if the severely compromised patient is not improved within minutes. Even though evaluation of ventilation is absolutely essential, severe respiratory depression often develops relatively late during a hypotensive episode and attention needs to be paid to other therapeutic measures.

If the heart rate falls below 40 and severe shock is apparent, external cardiac massage is indicated. Immediate ECG monitoring needs to be instituted and systematic blood pressure recordings taken. An arterial sample for Po_2, Pco_2, and pH determinations may be taken. Additional, more precise monitoring techniques are to be instituted and proper intravascular lines established for administering fluids and drugs. Lack of access for giving drugs limits immediate treatment to such nonsclerosing medications as epinephrine and atropine, which can be injected intramuscularly, lingually, or endotracheally as well as by stat IV injection. The stat doses of these medications are as follows: epinephrine (0.1 ml/kg/dose of a 1:10,000 solution or 10 μg/kg) and atropine sulfate (0.01–0.03 mg/kg/dose).

The first line to be placed is a venous line preferably, using the most propitious site. Soon after this is in place, a central venous pressure line must be established and, concurrently, an arterial catheter for manometric recording of intra-arterial pressures and periodic sampling for blood gases and electrolytes, especially valuable if the course is protracted. A 12 lead EKG and chest x-ray are done as soon as possible.

With the establishment of a venous line, the therapeutic options are greatly enhanced, for it is now possible to administer emergency medications optimally. Also, isotonic crystalloid solutions such as 0.9% NaCl solution or Ringer's lactate (20 ml/kg) or colloids such as 25% salt-poor albumin (1 gm/kg) diluted to 5% with isotonic saline preferably, plasma or whole blood (10 ml/kg) infused over 15 minutes can be administered as a CVP line is being placed. These infusions are given to combat the second major feature of shock, poor peripheral perfusion.

While fluids are being administered through the venous line, the CVP and arterial lines should become activated. With the CVP for guidance, one can ascertain rapidly whether there is a cardiogenic element in the shock state of the patient. The bolus of crystalloids or colloids, presumably already under way and to be repeated if necessary, can indicate the degree of myocardial failure while the CVP is raised. The bolus increases cardiac filling in all states where decreased circulating blood volume is the cause of decreased cardiac output. Periodic fluid challenges can be given, using 2–4 ml/kg infusions over 10 minutes and attempting to bring the blood pressure back to normal. The rate of change in the CVP as well as its absolute value should be assessed concurrently. If the infusions do not result in any improvement in the hypotension and peripheral perfusion, one must be very concerned about the cardiogenic nature of the shock state. The CVP indicates right ventricular filling pressures that may differ widely from those on the left side, which may be estimated better by placement of a pulmonary wedge pressure line. This latter procedure requires special expertise for use in infants especially and may be reserved for special conditions in which complex inotropic and vasoactive drugs are to be used.

In many cases, poor cardiac function may be a temporary condition caused by metabolic acidosis, hypoglycemia, hypocalcemia, or hyperkalemia, and these possible factors should be considered and appropriately treated. If peripheral perfusion has been poor, one can assume the presence of lactic acidosis from anaerobic glycolysis and give $NaHCO_3$ solution (1–2 mEq/kg IV). This $NaHCO_3$ therapy has several immediate favorable effects, including 1) improvement of cardiac contractility, 2) potentiation of the sympathetic-adrenal responses to shock and of the actions of administered sympathomimetic drugs, 3) reversal of local acidosis with improved vasoconstriction of small arterioles, and 4) amelioration of the myocardial effects of potassium toxicity if this exists. Administration of $NaHCO_3$ may need to be repeated if the state of shock remains profound and if blood gas determinations continue to show severe acidosis. Adequate ventilation must be maintained to eliminate excessive CO_2 with this bicarbonate loading. Also, $NaHCO_3$ solutions chemically neutralize sympathomimetic drugs and must never be given in the same line without proper measures to avoid such a deleterious reaction. $NaHCO_3$ solutions are sclerosing and should only be given through adequate intravascular lines, as is the case with calcium and glucose solutions. Use of glucose to supply needed substrate for myocardial metabolism is often forgotten in the melee of resuscitative efforts. If a blood Dextrostix determination shows less than 45 mg/dl, then 25% glucose (2 mg/kg IV) is given, followed by an infusion of 10% glucose.

All of the measures described above should have been completed within 20 minutes. In addition, after several bolus doses of epinephrine have been given at 5 minute intervals, selection of effective inotropic agents for use during the ensuing hours must be considered if a precarious state continues. Decisions as to the preferred agent can be complex and may require consultations with cardiologists and anesthesiologists.

As the most widely used treatment, a continuous epinephrine infusion, administered by an accurate infusion pump, has several advantages, including stimulation of cardiac rate and contractility and increase of peripheral vascular resistance with improved coronary flow. The infusion can be prepared rapidly by adding 5 ml of 1:1000 aqueous epinephrine to a 250 ml bottle of 5% dextrose to make up a solution of 20 μg/ml. The infusion is started at 0.1 μg/kg/min (or 6 μg/kg/hr) and increased to as much as 1.5 μg/kg/min. An infusion chart must be prepared and kept current by one member of the ICU team responsible for recording and calculating the drug dosages. Disadvantages of epinephrine include its tendency to cause tachycardia with increased myocardial O_2 consumption and its arrhythmogenic effects in severe hypoxic states.

Two new drugs are being used widely for the treatment of hypotension, but the nuances of their complex effects in infants and children are still being evaluated.

Dopamine (Inotropin)* infusions have proved to be useful in cases of hypotension of cardiogenic origin especially. This agent significantly enhances myocardial contractility, heart rate, automaticity, and atrioventricular conduction (beta-1 adrenergic effects), but additionally has unique "dopaminergic effects" that can be favorable. Vasodilatation occurs during low doses (2–5 μg/kg/min) in the renal, splanchnic, coronary, and cerebral vascular beds, a property especially useful in improving renal perfusion. In higher doses (10 μg/kg/min), needed to augment cardiac output, vasoconstriction occurs and peripheral resistance increases.

Dobutamine (Dobutrex)* also has properties that make it an effective agent in treating cardiogenic shock. This synthetic drug increases myocardial contraction without increasing the heart rate and produces peripheral vasodilatation in doses as high as 10 μg/kg/minute. Careful monitoring and liberal fluid infusions may be needed to maintain the blood pressure as systemic blood flow is improved. In infants below one year of age, its inability to increase heart rate may limit dobutamine's effectiveness.

These two agents have superseded other inotropic agents to a degree and appear to be relatively safe with proper monitoring. On the other hand, isoproterenol (Isuprel) has very strong beta-1 adrenergic effects, which may result in tachyarrhythmias, especially in children on digoxin therapy. Its strong systemic vasodilatory effects can also result in increased hypotension in the hypovolemic patient. However, isoproterenol is still the agent of choice in patients with bradyarrhythmias not responding to atropine.

Digoxin is a slower-acting inotropic agent that is not as potent as the sympathomimetic drugs. It is also a dangerous drug in acute hypotensive states and has well-established toxic properties. Its primary effectiveness is in conditions where prolonged action is desired, as in low cardiac output states from cardiac failure.

When vasoconstrictor effects are desired primarily, norepinephrine (levarterenol, Levophed) infusions, starting at 0.1 μg/kg/min with stepwise increased doses, or phenylephrine (Neo-Synephrine) infusions in the same dosage may be used. These drugs constrict the renal and mesenteric vessels so that their prolonged use causes progressive impairment of perfusion of these regions.

When left ventricular pump failure is the major factor in hypotension, outflow resistance can be decreased effectively by primary vasodilator therapy. Special attention must be paid to the intra-arterial pressures, which must be monitored closely to maintain a pressure adequate for coronary perfusion. The systolic pressure should be maintained not lower than 3/4 that expected for the child's age as a guideline for dosage of these powerful agents. Sodium nitroprusside (Nipride) infusions, starting at 1 μg/kg/min and increasing to as high as 10 μg/kg/min, are widely used, especially in adults with severe myocardial dysfunction. With prolonged high doses, one must beware of inducing thiocyanate toxicity manifested by vomiting, sweating, and muscle twitching or of cyanide poisoning causing intractable acidosis. It

---

* Safety and effectiveness for use in children have not been established.

is highly advisable to monitor the use of this agent by insertion of a Swan-Ganz catheter for continuous estimations of LV filling, as delineated by the pulmonary capillary wedge pressures. Passage of this flow-directed catheter is accomplished readily in the older child and adult but is often difficult to achieve in the young child without the assistance of a pediatric cardiologist or anesthesiologist. Fluoroscopic guidance may be needed, but the catheter can be located in the RV outflow tract by echocardiography. Combined use of dopamine or dobutamine and sodium nitroprusside has been effective, especially in severe pump failure, but obviously needs particularly careful monitoring. Nitroglycerin solutions are under investigation as a safer substitute for nitroprusside infusions when preload reduction is desired.

If bradycardia develops in association with hypotension, a stat dosage of atropine (0.01–0.03 mg/kg/IV) may be useful, but emergency placement of a transvenous pacemaker by a cardiologist may be necessary. Calcium, most reliably given in the form of $CaCl_2$ (0.2 ml/kg of a 100 mg/ml-10% solution), must be administered IV with the aim of strengthening cardiac contraction through another mechanism than that of beta-adrenergic stimulation. One must be aware that this agent should never be given in the same line as $NaHCO_3$ because calcium carbonate will be precipitated. Also, it should be given cautiously to digitalized patients, since these two drugs potentiate each other. It is also an extremely sclerosing material and should only be given through well-established intravenous lines.

Cardiac arrhythmias may cause pump failure and require specific diagnosis and treatment. A variety of causes for these disorders may be identified. Electrolyte imbalance, especially potassium deficiency or excess, acidosis, alkalosis, digitalis toxicity, hypoxia, fever, hypovolemia, presence of pericardial fluid, and irritation from CVP or pulmonary wedge pressure catheters are treatable. Primary arrhythmias, such as paroxysmal tachyarrhythmias, may also require selective therapies, such as the drug regimens and external cardioversion and defibrillation discussed elsewhere. Not to be forgotten is the occasional effectiveness of sharp blows to the chest of the older child in reversing known ventricular tachyarrhythmias, and the vagal stimulating maneuvers (facial immersion, carotid massage, induced gagging, etc.) in reversing supraventricular tachyarrhythmias.

The effects of shock on various organ systems must be weighed in the therapeutic plan, especially if hypotension is persistent. Damage to endothelial cells and alveolar epithelial cells in the lung (shock lung) may result in permeability edema and decreased surfactant production (adult respiratory distress syndrome). Adequate ventilation by en-

dotracheal intubation, use of pancuronium (Pavulon), 0.06–0.1 mg/kg/dose IV every 30–60 minutes and sedation (such as morphine 0.1–0.2 mg/kg/dose q 2–4 hours), appropriate supplemental O_2, proper airway pressure adjustments, and chest physiotherapy are often indicated. Furosemide (Lasix), 1 mg/kg, increasing to as high as 5 mg/kg/dose, and colloid therapy to raise oncotic pressure may be needed to handle these pulmonary complications of severe hypotension.

The renal blood flow and urinary output must be maintained if possible. Low dose dopamine* infusions, mannitol (0.5–1.0 gm/kg over 30 minutes every 4–6 hours), and furosemide are used to combat oliguric renal failure.

If paralytic ileus has occurred, the stomach contents need to be emptied by nasogastric tube. Stress ulcers and erosive gastritis may develop from mucosal ischemia. Antacids such as aluminum hydroxide (Maalox or Amphojel, 5–20 ml q 4 h po) are given to raise the gastric pH to 4.0.

Adequate nutrition must be maintained to provide liver substrates, as well as nutrition, for host defenses against infection. The catabolic effects of shock need special attention if the patient was nutritionally deficient before hypotension developed. Intravenous alimentation may be needed under these circumstances. Glucose therapy may result in increased glycogen synthesis with lipogenesis causing hepatomegaly and abnormal liver function. Infusions of glucose with insulin and potassium have favorably improved cell membrane function and can improve cardiac carbohydrate metabolism.

If treatment is prolonged, concerns will arise about infection from catheters which act as foreign bodies, and difficult decisions must be made concerning antibiotic therapy. Patients with severe hypotension have lowered resistance to infection from a variety of causes. At present, prevention or early treatment with antibiotics aimed at preventing bacteremia is the best therapeutic approach, but treatments to specifically stimulate host defense mechanisms and granulocyte transfusions may find wider use soon.

Special mention must be made of hypotension from sepsis, anaphylaxis, and neurogenic causes. Early in septic shock, increased vascular capacity with peripheral vasodilation produces a picture different from other forms of shock. The skin may be warm and flushed, blood pressure may be normal with wide pulse pressure, and the patient may be febrile, hyperventilating, and having chills. Alpha stimulators, such as epinephrine, norepinephrine, and phenylephrine, are usually ineffective. The preferred treatment as the condition

---

* Safety and effectiveness for use in children have not been established.

progresses to systemic vasoconstriction appears to be vigorous volume expansion initially and then use of an agent such as isoproterenol or nitroprusside. Concurrent antibiotic therapy, platelet concentrates, fresh plasma or blood, exchange transfusions, and steroids (dexamethasone, 5 mg/ kg, or methylprednisolone, 30 mg/kg IV in form of a bolus) must be considered in this shock state especially. The corticosteroid treatment may be repeated every 4–6 hours in the severely compromised patient but has not been shown to be effective after 3 days. Another controversial but promising agent is naloxone† (Narcan), an endorphin blocker (given in repeated doses of 0.01 mg/kg IV), which may counteract the deleterious cellular effects of these intrinsic substances. Naloxone is also an effective stimulator of central respiratory drive.

Disseminated intravenous coagulation, present as a major complication of sepsis, may exist to a degree in most severe nonseptic shock states. Treatment is directed against the associated conditions (hypotension, anoxemia, acidosis, and infection), but platelet and fresh frozen plasma transfusions are also indicated. Vitamin K (1–5 mg IM or IV) should also be administered. Heparin (100 units/kg/dose q 4 h or 10–25 units/kg/ hour as an IV infusion) is only advised where thromboses have been demonstrated.

Anaphylactic shock is to be expected in the office as well as hospital setting because of the variety of drugs now being administered and other allergens patients may contact. The practitioner must be aware of the variable nature and time of occurrence of this condition, the latter varying from minutes to hours after exposure. Usually, symptoms with parenteral drug administration will occur within 30 minutes, hopefully while the child is still under observation. The treatment is clear-cut—epinephrine should be given, 0.1 ml/kg IM or IV of a 1:10,000 dilution (or 10 μg/kg), as soon as the diagnosis has been made. Withdrawal of the offending antigen or isolation of its site of injection by a tourniquet should be accomplished. Prophylactic administration of diphenhydramine HCl (Benadryl), 0.05–1.5 mg/kg po or IV may be useful. Concern for maintaining an adequate airway, use of aminophylline for persistent bronchospasm, and general circulatory support with fluids and vasopressors have a role in severe cases of anaphylaxis, as they do in other forms of shock.

Many hypotensive episodes detailed above can be reversed readily. Gradual development of hypotension can often be reversed by crystalloid infusions, with the realization that these may leave the vascular compartments significantly within minutes, or with plasma infusions. Attention to

maintenance of the hematocrit at 35–40%, continuous monitoring of blood pressure, heart rate, ECG, and urinary output (by indwelling catheter), and arterial blood gas determinations are needed. In refractory cases, withdrawal of inotropic agents and decisions as to when respiratory support and monitoring may be discontinued require artful judgments, often involving empirical trials. At least, these decisions can be made deliberately and after discussions with colleagues with special expertise.

Simple syncope can present major problems in differential diagnosis, but can usually be identified by its postural nature resulting in inadequate cerebral perfusion and by its rapid recovery when the patient's head is brought to or below heart level. Other neurogenic causes of hypotension, such as head injury and seizures, require special measures detailed elsewhere.

The practitioner must tailor the idealized treatments possible in an ICU setting to his own practice with the realization that patients with severe hypotensive episodes will present under suboptimal conditions, often without warning. Since acute shock states require equipment and drugs similar to those needed for other forms of emergency such as primary respiratory arrest states, it would seem wise to establish a "crash cart" in the office with the drugs and equipment detailed in the early part of the above treatment plan for severe shock. The desired equipment, techniques for ventilation, placement of intravascular lines, and emergency drugs are detailed elegantly in the Textbook of Advanced Cardiac Life Support, available through the American and local Heart Associations. This should be required reading by the pediatrician and his support personnel. It would be most desirable for many pediatricians, especially those not familiar with intensive care as it is now practiced in most teaching centers, to participate in the Advanced Cardiac Life Support teaching programs and other similar programs at their hospitals. Organization of the office personnel so that each worker has a defined role in such emergencies is important, as is a thorough knowledge of the effectiveness of the local rescue squad and hospital emergency room. Decisions as to adequacy of equipment and drugs in the office can also be made by studying the equipment on the hospital crash carts, especially that in locations away from the ER and ICU areas.

Peripheral Vascular Disease

WARREN G. GUNTHEROTH, M.D.,
and D. EUGENE STRANDNESS JR., M.D.

The clinical appearance of obstructed blood flow is common to venous disorders, as well as peripheral arterial disease. Arterial disease may be simply

† This use of naloxone is not listed by the manufacturer.

vasospastic, particularly in children, and a thoughtful approach to diagnosis as well as to selection of treatment is important, since therapy may correctly vary from adjustment of clothing on the one extreme to amputation on the other.

PERIPHERAL ARTERIES

Vasoactive Disorders

Raynaud's Disease. Raynaud's phenomenon with no underlying disease is a vasospastic disorder of fingers and toes with a characteristic sequence of pallor, cyanosis, and rubor. Criteria for the diagnosis of Raynaud's disease are excitation of the vasospastic disorder by cold or emotion, bilaterality, absence of gangrene, and absence of an underlying primary disease.

Therapy of Raynaud's disease should be conditioned by its generally favorable prognosis. Surgical sympathectomy is rarely, if ever, indicated in the primary disorder. If the symptoms are bothersome, selection of a warm, dry climate may be helpful. Clothing selection should be directed toward conserving body heat rather than just covering the affected extremities; our studies show that cold applied directly to the affected extremity is less likely to produce vasospasm than is general body cooling. The clothing should not be tight-fitting; hard-finish, tightly woven material is essential to block wind, and bulky woolen clothing is necessary for insulation against cold. Stocking caps may be quite helpful in reducing vasoconstriction of the fingers. In adolescent girls, a program of increased physical exercise is probably beneficial. Biofeedback has been successful to some extent in increasing digital temperature and in aborting episodes of Raynaud's, or at least in reducing the severity of the attack. Medications may be required in more severe cases. The current drug of choice for adults in nifedipine, a calcium channel blocker. (Although this use of nifedipine is not included in the manufacturer's instructions, the use for blocking contractile response of smooth muscle is noted.) In adults, the dose is one 10-mg capsule three times daily; an appropriate basis for children is 0.2 mg/kg three times daily, although there has not been extensive usage in the pediatric age group. The side effects are largely those of vasodilatation, including lightheadedness, flushing, and headache.

When dealing with cold sensitivity, it is important to keep in mind that it may be secondary to some serious underlying problem such as one of the collagen disorders. Exhaustive workups, however, are not routinely indicated in a child with good health and mild vasospastic complaints. Although primary Raynaud's disease is a benign disorder, the secondary form may lead to digital artery occlusion, fingertip ulcers, and even gangrene.

The occlusion can be recognized by measurement of systolic pressures in the involved finger by either plethysmography or Doppler ultrasound. Finger pressures of less than 70 mm Hg, wrist-to-digit gradients of more than 30 mm Hg, and brachial-to-finger differences of greater than 40 mm Hg are consistent with occlusive disease in the hand or digits.

Chilblains (Pernio). Another disorder of cold sensitivity, chilblains involve itching, localized erythema, and sometimes blisters, occurring over the dorsum of the proximal phalanges of fingers and toes and over the heels and lower legs. It is said that this is a disorder of children in cool, damp climates, but, oddly, we have not seen this problem in Seattle. The disorder is more of a nuisance than a threat to life or limb. Treatment during the acute phase consists of antipruritic medications and a soothing ointment in a lanolin-petrolatum base. Management outlined under Raynaud's disease should be considered for the more persistent cases.

Acrocyanosis. This is probably more common than Raynaud's disease, but the overlap of acrocyanosis with the normal response to cold is greater than in Raynaud's. In acrocyanosis there is a more generalized response of the entire extremity in a glove or stocking pattern, and there is usually only unremitting cyanosis, without the pallor and rubor phases of Raynaud's. Ulcerations are rare, and therapy is rarely required except for cosmetic reasons. When required, therapy is the same as for Raynaud's disease.

Livedo Reticularis. Livedo reticularis and cutis marmorata are even milder peripheral vascular responses to cold, with netlike patterns of cyanosis in arms and legs. Therapy is not usually required, but the general comments pertaining to Raynaud's disease would apply to these conditions.

Erythromelalgia. Although the number of cases of erythromelalgia is smaller than that of Raynaud's disease, the symptoms are so much more debilitating that therapy must be considered briefly. Erythromelalgia presents as a peripheral hyperreaction to heat, the counterpart to reaction to cold in Raynaud's disease. The hot, swollen, and tender hands and feet are extraordinarily unpleasant and have led to suicide in a young adult in our hospital. Therapy should be directed toward physical factors as well as medication. Cooling of the body in general, as well as cool soaks to the affected extremities, bring some degree of relief. Ephedrine has been effective in some instances, at 0.5 mg/kg every 4 to 6 hours (average adult dose, 25 mg), preferably with a tranquilizer or a sedative.

Aspirin is definitely worth trying on a regular basis (every 4 hours), not only for its analgesic effects but also because there are indications that endogenous bradykinin may be involved.

Other authorities have suggested that erythromelalgia is a form of "peripheral migraine," and that release of serotonin is responsible. Accordingly, they have suggested antiserotonin medications, such as cyproheptadine. This use of cyproheptadine is not mentioned in the manufacturer's directive, however. For children, an average dose is 0.08 mg/kg (daily dose 0.25 mg/kg). It is available in a syrup containing 2 mg in 5 ml.

Causalgia. Although a deep wound with injury to a major nerve trunk leading to "major causalgia" is easily diagnosed, forms of minor causalgia often elude prompt and effective treatment by masquerading as primary vascular disorders. Unilateral vascular disorders, particularly when associated with exquisite tenderness, swelling, and abnormal perspiration, should suggest posttraumatic sympathetic dystrophy, a form of minor causalgia. The vascular disorder is most often vasospastic, but we have successfully treated a boy with a sympathetic dystrophy resembling unilateral erythromelalgia.

Therapy is the same regardless of the vascular disorder: paravertebral sympathetic blockade with injections of 1% lidocaine. If the diagnosis is correct, subjective relief is striking and will last for several hours. Permanent improvement will depend on vigorous physical therapy, beginning at once under the effect of the block, continuing for days or weeks, and usually requiring additional injections at intervals. It is imperative to interrupt the cycle of pain, disuse osteoporosis, and so forth; exercise of the affected limb is the essential therapy. The main function of sympathetic blockade is to permit relatively painless exercise of the limb. Sympathectomy is rarely indicated in the treatment.

Obstructive Disorders

Trauma. The immediate goal of therapy for traumatic interruption of arterial flow is to prevent loss of tissue and limb. Continuity of the arteries must be restored, spasm relieved, intraluminal clots removed and prevented, and tissue edema managed so that the arterial lumen is not compromised.

Maintenance or restoration of adequate circulating blood volume is of primary importance, not only for the preservation of life but also to permit intelligent assessment of the state of the local circulation. Although actual gangrene is rare in children, a nonoperative approach to vascular injury prolonged beyond 6 to 8 hours may lead to subsequent weakness and atrophy. Thus the ultimate function of the limb should govern the acute management, and early intervention by a skilled surgeon may be truly conservative. Arteriography may be helpful in locating the site and extent of obstruction, but the use of a transcutaneous Doppler flowmeter is less traumatic and may be repeated at will.

Proper surgical technique will include scrupulous débridement; end-to-end anastomosis if adequate vessel length is available to avoid tension, and autogenous vein graft replacement otherwise; complete removal of distal clots; relief of arterial spasm; fasciotomy to control complications of edema and hematoma; and possible anticoagulation with heparin (see under Thrombophlebitis).

An increasingly frequent source of arterial problems is medical cannulation. Poor technique, or overly long cannulation, may lead to embolic problems as well as occlusion. Left heart diagnostic studies via retrograde arterial catheterization have been found to produce leg shortening if the artery clots after the procedure. The instillation of heparin, 100 units/kg in the arterial catheter is helpful, and these patients should be followed closely for arterial pulses and long-term for leg growth.

Congenital Stenosis. Peripheral arterial stenosis rarely produces any definite signs or symptoms when it is congenital, reflecting the remarkable ability of youthful tissues to develop collateral circulation.

Arteritis. Inflammatory disease of arteries may occur locally or as part of a wide-spread disorder usually called polyarteritis. When smaller arteries are involved, a muscle biopsy is the only means of certain diagnosis. The most effective treatment is identification and removal of sensitizing drugs, infection, or toxin, and in severe generalized arteritis, the use of steroids. Major vessel arteritis that obstructs blood flow may require bypass grafting, depending upon the site and adequacy of collateral circulation.

Fistulas

Trauma. It is quite possible that the most frequent cause of this disorder in the pediatric age group is needle puncture of the femoral vein by physicians. The treatment is obviously surgical, with proper caution that closure of the fistulous connection does not compromise the arterial lumen.

Congenital. Abnormal communications between small arteries and veins, particularly if extensive, pose difficult problems. Because of the extensive and diffuse nature of the fistulas, it is rarely possible to treat by surgical removal. Since these patients often develop edema and incompetence of the superficial veins, it is necessary to treat the patient with gradient support stockings to prevent stasis changes.

PERIPHERAL VEINS

Thrombophlebitis

This is rarely a pediatric problem, but its occurrence is attended by considerable risk to life if treatment is not prompt and effective. The aggressiveness required in the therapeutic approach depends on the extent of the thrombophlebitis, whether it is progressing in spite of medical therapy and whether pulmonary embolism has occurred.

Massive deep thrombophlebitis (phlegmasia cerulea dolens) involves the entire limb with edema, severe pain, and cyanosis. The presence and quality of the pedal pulses depend on the systemic blood volume and pressure and the degree of edema. In some cases, there may be associated arterial spasm, which can reduce peripheral arterial flow as well. Thrombectomy should not be attempted unless there is a strong question of limb viability. Venous ligation or plication is performed just below the renal vein but is indicated only in those patients with pulmonary embolism that recurs while they are on adequate anticoagulant therapy. The use of fibrinolytic agents, such as streptokinase, to promote clot lysis and resorption is useful in adults with massive deep vein thrombophlebitis, but the problems with bleeding are substantial; there is inadequate experience in the pediatric age group to permit a recommendation of fibrinolytic therapy.

Venous thrombosis of the major deep veins is treated with bed rest, elevation, heat, and intravenous heparin. It is now recommended that heparin be given by continuous intravenous infusion to maintain either the whole blood clotting time at 2 to 2.5 times baseline values or the activated partial thromboplastin time at 50 to 80 seconds. An infusion pump is mandatory to avoid fluctuations in the rate of administration.

An oral anticoagulant, such as warfarin, is started when the status of the limb is satisfactory; the prothrombin time should be maintained at twice the normal control. While the duration of therapy has not been settled, it should be continued for a minimum of 3 months when major venous thrombosis has occurred. With pulmonary embolism, therapy should be continued for 3 to 6 months, or even longer if the patient remains at risk.

If there is any edema in the limb with ambulation, it must be controlled, preferably with tailored, pressure gradient stockings from the level of the foot to the upper thigh.

SMALL VESSEL DISORDERS

Frostbite. Rapid rewarming with moderately warm water (40 to 42°C) should be promptly initiated if the extremity is still frozen or cold.

However, for those situations in which the physician may be consulted by radio or telephone, and the patient is still remote from hospitalization, rewarming should not be undertaken unless all danger of refreezing is eliminated. The duration of rewarming required will depend on the depth to which the tissue is frozen; if there is through and through freezing, rewarming of the deeper layers may require over an hour.

The subsequent care requires fastidious hygiene of the injured extremity for a lengthy period; extirpation or amputation should be delayed, since surprising recovery is characteristic of frostbite injuries. Daily care should include gentle cleansing, avoidance of pressure or even light contact, bed rest, and analgesics until the acute inflammation has subsided. After that stage, physical therapy is essential to gradually restore full range of motion; whirlpool baths may aid in this.

Disseminated Intravascular Coagulation and Purpura Fulminans

RICHARD H. SILLS, M.D.

Disseminated intravascular coagulation (DIC) is an acquired failure of hemostasis triggered by an underlying disease process. The excessive intravascular clotting that precipitates DIC can be caused by a wide variety of disorders, including infections, respiratory distress syndrome, and malignant disease. A complex hemorrhagic disorder then develops as a result of depletion of platelets, depletion of factors II, V, and VIII and fibrinogen, and excessive formation of fibrin split products, which can inhibit fibrin polymerization as well as platelet function. A hemolytic anemia may also develop.

Success in managing DIC is most dependent on the ability to diagnose and treat the underlying disease. If the primary disorder is rapidly and successfully treated, the DIC will resolve without any specific hematologic therapy. Less frequently the primary disorder cannot be quickly managed and specific therapy for the DIC will need to be considered. Examples of this situation include malignant disease and giant hemangiomas. Most commonly, DIC represents a preterminal event, with death due to the primary illness and not the coagulopathy.

It is crucial to realize that no single therapy of DIC has been proved superior to any other. Furthermore, the only controlled study of the treatment of DIC demonstrated no significant improvement in survival or coagulation studies in neonates receiving specific hematologic therapy in comparison with those who only received treatment of their underlying disease. This serves to further emphasize the primary role of treatment of the underlying disorder.

Considering that no therapeutic modality has been proved superior to any other, including no hematologic therapy at all, routine therapy of DIC cannot be recommended except in a few clinical situations. These include potential or actual life-threatening hemorrhage, purpura fulminans or other clinically evident thromboses, and the need for emergency surgery. Laboratory abnormalities in the absence of potentially life-threatening bleeding should not generally be treated

Platelet and Blood Factor Replacement. Once a decision is made to intervene directly, the initial therapy should consist of replacement of consumed coagulation factors and platelets. Although theoretically this could add "fuel to the fire" and exacerbate the process, practically this has not occurred. The specific replacement therapy should be individualized based on the pattern of relative consumption of platelets, fibrinogen and factors II, V, and VIII. The source and dose of these factors, their minimal hemostatic levels, and the expected post-transfusion increments are noted in Table 1. Transfusions should be given to provide at least a minimal hemostatic level. If specific factor assays are not available, the safest approach is to give infusions of platelet concentrates and fresh frozen plasma in the doses indicated. Cryoprecipitate, which specifically concentrates fibrinogen and factor VIII, is given when these factors are more severely depleted. Subsequent tranfusions are based on the survival of the infused platelets and factors. This is determined by following the levels of platelets and factors every 3–6 hours depending on the severity of the DIC. If specific factor assays are not readily available the prothrombin time (PT) and the partial thromboplastin time (PTT) are adequate substitutes. The PT should be maintained under 1 to $1\frac{1}{2}$ times the control value while the PPT should be kept under $1\frac{1}{2}$ to 2 times the control. Transfusions are often required at least every 12 hours during the active phase of the disease.

Exchange Transfusion. Exchange transfusion is indicated if platelet and factor replacement using simple transfusions fails to control the DIC. Such failure may occur for 2 reasons. (1) There are limitations on the amount of fresh frozen plasma and/or cryoprecipitate that can be given without causing fluid overload and congestive heart failure. (2) Less frequently, simple transfusions may fail because of high levels of fibrin split products, which contribute to the coagulopathy by inhibiting both fibrin polymerization and platelet function. This situation can be identified by demonstrating evidence of an anticoagulant effect of fibrin split products using a modification of the PTT or PT. Regardless of the reason for failure of simple transfusion, exchange transfusion is more likely to succeed. Much larger amounts of platelets and factors can be provided, and inhibitory fibrin split products will be removed. A single or double volume exchange transfusion with fresh whole citrated blood or packed red cells reconstituted with fresh frozen plasma is generally used. Exchange transfusions are not used as initial therapy of DIC because of the potential risks of the procedure, including catheter-related and metabolic complications, vasomotor instability, and transfusion-related infections due to the greater amount of blood products required.

Heparin. The use of heparin in the treatment of hemorrhagic complications of DIC has fallen into disfavor. Theoretically it arrests the excessive intravascular thrombosis that is causing platelet and factor depletion. Practically there is little evidence that it is beneficial, and it can certainly exacerbate the bleeding diathesis. The use of heparin in hemorrhagic DIC is generally limited to patients with life-threatening bleeding who have failed to respond to both platelet and factor replacement as well as exchange transfusion. Exceptions include DIC secondary to acute promyelocytic or monocytic leukemia, which may respond well to anticoagulation with heparin.

The primary, widely accepted role for heparin

Table 1. TRANSFUSION THERAPY FOR DIC

Factor	Source	Minimal Hemostatic Level	Usual Dose	Expected Part-Transfusion Increment
Platelets	Platelet concentrates	30,000–50,000/mm^3	1 unit/5 kg	50,000–100,000/mm^3
Fibrinogen	Cryoprecipitate	100 mg/dl	1 bag/5 kg	150 mg%
Factor VIII	Cryoprecipitate	20–30%	1 bag/5 kg	40%
Factor V	Fresh frozen plasma	10–15%	10–15 cc/kg	15–22%
Factor II	Fresh frozen plasma	15–40%	10–15 cc/kg	10–15%*

* Volume will generally limit reaching a hemostatic level. Fortunately Factor II levels tend to be less severely affected by DIC than Factors V and VIII and fibrinogen.

in DIC is in treating thrombotic complications, including purpura fulminans and tissue ischemia due to septic shock or major vessel thrombosis. When the use of heparin is indicated, it is given intravenously in an initial bolus of 25–50 units/kg followed by a continuous infusion of 10–25 units/ kg/hr. The higher infusion rates are more likely to be necessary in treating purpura fulminans, but the actual dose of heparin must be individualized. This is best accomplished by measuring heparin levels, but these are often unavailable. The best alternative is to use the PTT to monitor heparin's anticoagulant effect while levels of fibrinogen, factor VIII, and platelets are used to monitor the severity of the DIC (since these measurements are unaffected by heparin). The PTT should ideally be maintained at 2 to $2\frac{1}{2}$ times the control, but the initial prolongation of the PTT due to the DIC itself will often confuse this regulation of heparin dosage.

If heparin therapy is successful, a response should be measurable in the first 24 hours. The fibrinogen and factor VIII levels should normalize within 24–48 hours, but the platelet count may not reach normal levels for 7–14 days. Therapy should be continued until the factor levels normalize, and in the case of purpura fulminans, for at least 2–3 weeks. Excessive heparin effect can be neutralized by giving 1 mg of protamine sulfate for each 100 units of heparin estimated to be present in the circulation, but this is rarely necessary. When treating purpura fulminans, replacement therapy with infusions of platelets, cryoprecipitate, and/or fresh frozen plasma may also be required.

Other Therapies. Other therapeutic modalities that have been used in the treatment of DIC include antifibrinolytic agents (aminocaproic acid), antiplatelet agents, dextrans, alpha adrenergic blocking agents, and antithrombin III concentrates. There is little evidence that they are efficacious, and their use cannot be generally recommended. Antifibrinolytic agents, specifically, are contraindicated in DIC.

Recurrent purpura fulminans in neonates is a rare disorder that is usually due to a homozygous deficiency of Protein C. In this situation, acute treatment of the purpura requires infusions of protein C using fresh frozen plasma or factor IX concentrates known to be rich in Protein C. Optimal long-term management of these patients has not yet been determined.

Acute Rheumatic Fever

SYLVIA P. GRIFFITHS, M.D.

Since there is no specific test for acute rheumatic fever, evaluation of the clinical picture and laboratory data, including electrocardiograms, is critical for diagnosis. This is not always clear, especially in children with arthritis alone. Hospitalization is advised in order to make close observations over a 24- to 48-hour period and eliminate other possible entities in the differential diagnosis. Because it is a poststreptococcal disease, the recommendation for long-term antibiotic prophylaxis against a rheumatic recurrence is pivotal. The crux of management, i.e., secondary prevention, imposes a significant responsiblity for accuracy of diagnosis on the physician as well as a formidable burden for compliance on the patient and family.

Once a diagnosis of acute rheumatic fever is made, penicillin should be administered in a dosage that eradicates group A beta hemolytic streptococci from the oropharynx regardless of whether the throat culture on admission is positive. A single intramuscular injection of 1.2 million units of long acting benzathine penicillin G (Bicillin) is preferred, unless there is a known hypersensitivity to this antibiotic, in which case erythromycin, 250 mg four times a day by mouth, is recommended for 10 days.

Today, in order of both frequency and time of appearance, the three major manifestations of acute rheumatic fever as originally outlined in the Jones' criteria are arthritis, carditis, and Sydenham's chorea. Whereas carditis may coexist with either arthritis or chorea, the latter two entities never present simultaneously because of the difference in their latent periods from antecedent streptococcal infection—short for arthritis (3 to 6 weeks) and long (up to 6 months) for chorea. Since rheumatic fever is a self-limited disease, whether a child develops one or more "manifestations" is not influenced by the anti-inflammatory effects of salicylates or steroids. Furthermore, suppressive therapy does not influence the eventual evolution of rheumatic heart disease. Guidelines for management other than streptococcal eradication will be discussed under the specific headings of manifestations below.

The incidence and severity of first attacks of acute rheumatic fever and recurrences in the 5 to 15 year age group have generally declined in the past 2 to 3 decades in the United States. It is noteworthy, however, that rheumatic fever has reappeared in New York City since 1982, with sporadic new cases including children who have come into the area from the Caribbean as well as Southeast Asia.

ARTHRITIS

Salicylates are invaluable for the relief of rheumatic joint inflammation associated with acute pain, erythema and swelling, and mild temperature elevation. Since multiple joints are usually involved, so-called polyarthritis, which predominantly affects the lower extremities (knees or ankles), involvement of a single joint by observation or history is not diagnostic. Hence, if on admission the arthritis is monarticular, rather than immediately start aspirin, it may be wise to use symptomatic treatment, such as acetaminophen (Tylenol) and codeine for pain, and allow time for involvement of a second joint to appear, which may indicate a more typical presentation for rheumatic fever. Also, auscultation of heart sounds and murmurs may be clarified with diminution of tachycardia associated with fever.

When a diagnosis of rheumatic polyarthritis is made, salicylates are usually given in the dosage of 75 to 100 mg/kg/day in divided doses every 4 hours for 1 week while on bed rest. If at the end of that time, the sedimentation rate is falling and auscultation reveals no significant murmurs, the salicylate dosage may be cut in half for the second week and ambulation started. If the patient remains symptom-free, he may be discharged at the end of the second week without aspirin and followed at weekly intervals on an outpatient basis. When the sedimentation rate is normal, probably within 4 to 6 weeks from the onset of arthritis, he may return to school on full activity.

In follow-up, particularly of boys, special attention should be given to the possible development of a high-pitched decrescendo aortic diastolic murmur in the third left intercostal space (Erb's point), which may be first audible 2 months following the onset of arthritis. The murmur of aortic valvulitis frequently develops later than that of mitral valvulitis, which usually presents within 2 weeks after the onset of arthritis.

CARDITIS

The medical management of carditis, particularly in the first attack of acute rheumatic fever, depends upon initial evaluation of its "severity," as does prognosis regarding the development of fixed rheumatic valvular heart disease.

The majority of patients have carditis of a "mild to moderate" severity, indicated by significant murmurs of mitral or aortic valvulitis. Certainly the most common presentation is that of "mild" carditis, with a grade 2–3/6 medium pitch pansystolic apical murmur of mitral involvement. Varying schedules of salicylates or steroids have no effect on outcome, judged by residual rheumatic heart disease, which in this particular group is estimated at 25% in follow-up 10 years later, presuming the absence of recurrence in this interval.

In contrast, the small number of patients with "severe" carditis have, in addition to murmurs of valvulitis, congestive heart failure secondary to profound myocarditis, or pericarditis. Such patients may have a fulminant course and die. For this group, in an attempt to save a life, steroids are employed to suppress the severe myocardial inflammation. The survivors, regardless of dosage schedules of steroids, with or without salicylates, will have 90 to 100% residual rheumatic heart disease.

Mild to Moderate Carditis. Salicylates are usually given at 75 to 100 mg/kg/day in divided doses for 1 to 2 weeks. If the clinical course shows improvement with decrease in sedimentation rate and stabilization of heart rate and murmurs, the dosage is cut in half, with anticipation of discharge between 3 and 4 weeks if home conditions are suitable. Outpatient observation is continued, with tapering of aspirin dosage, which would probably be discontinued by 6 weeks. Return to school and regular activity may be as early as 8 weeks after initial hospitalization. Participation in athletic activities is not permitted for at least 3 months.

Severe Carditis. The patient with congestive heart failure is usually critically ill and in need of special nursing care, often in an intensive care unit. The initial supportive cardiotonic regimen should include diuretics. For this, furosemide (Lasix) 1 mg/kg should be given as a single dose by mouth or intravenously, depending on the extent of pulmonary edema.

Digoxin may be cautiously added for the management of heart failure after 24 to 36 hours of suppression of myocarditis with prednisone. Because of the lowered threshold to toxicity in the presence of carditis, the initial digitalizing dose should not exceed one half of that usually administered for the age. Careful monitoring of digoxin blood levels and electrolyte levels is essential. Hypokalemia must be avoided as an additional problem conducive to digitalis intoxication.

The critical anti-inflammatory managment is provided by steroids as soon as possible. The prednisone dosage by mouth ranges from 40 to 60 mg a day, with anticipation of a 10- to 14-day course. Tapering may then be rapid, with the concurrent addition of salicylates at 75 to 100 mg/kg/day. The dosage and duration of both prednisone and aspirin must be strictly individualized according to clinical course and responsiveness. If prednisone is started without knowing the result of a tuberculin test or if there is any suspicion of tuberculosis contact, the patient should concomitantly receive a course of isoniazid.

Hospitalization frequently extends to 2 to 3 months. Limited activity at home may proceed with maintenance digoxin. The slow convalescence and return to school make a tutoring program invaluable so that the child does not fall behind academically. Athletic activities are usually restricted for 6 months.

CHOREA

This specific neurologic disorder of rheumatic fever ranges in presentation from mild clumsiness and slurred speech to thrashing and inability to ambulate. Symptoms may last from 6 weeks to 6 months, during which time the patient and his family may suffer considerable emotional distress in trying to handle the situation. Reassurance that recovery will occur without sequelae is critical.

The child should be protected from stressful activities and remain at home. Depending on the stage of the choreiform process, home tutoring should be arranged.

Mild sedation with diphenhydramine (Benadryl) is frequently helpful in alleviating some of the anxiety and restlessness and may be the only adjuvant necessary in addition to environmental control. If the movement disorder is more distressing, clonazepam (Clonopin) is prescribed to control the signs and permit satisfactory function. Should the severity of the chorea interfere with ambulation and self-help, haloperidol (Haldol) should be considered in consultation with a child neurologist.

PROPHYLAXIS AGAINST RECURRENCE OF RHEUMATIC FEVER

Continuous antimicrobial prophylaxis should be carried out in all children with a diagnosis of acute rheumatic fever, including chorea, in an effort to prevent subsequent attacks. Such a program should immediately be started 10 days after the initial treatment schedule to eradicate streptococcal infection, which may have been either a single intramuscular injection of benzathine penicillin G or a course of erythromycin.

The method of choice and the most effective protection in reducing the incidence of streptococcal infection and rheumatic recurrence is afforded by intramuscular injection of 1.2 million units of long-acting penicillin G (Bicillin) every 28 days. For the occasional patient who is sensitive to penicillin, it is suggested that oral sulfisoxazole* (Gantrisin), 0.5 gm, be given twice a day. Since prophylaxis is hard to maintain for long periods, whether parenteral or oral, its value and need for adherence should be constantly reinforced by regular contact with the prescribing physician.

Recommendation is made to families that prophylaxis for their child with a history of rheumatic fever be maintained until he is old enough to vote, or 18 years of age. If by then there is no auscultatory evidence of heart disease, mitral or aortic regurgitation, prophylaxis may be discontinued. However, if there is evidence of a significant murmur, then continued prophylaxis is urged "for a lifetime" or more realistically for approximately another 20 years through the period of parenting. The choice should remain that of either penicillin parenterally or Gantrisin by mouth.

---

* Sulfisoxazole is contraindicated in infants under 2 months of age.

PREVENTION OF BACTERIAL ENDOCARDITIS

For the child who has auscultatory evidence of rheumatic valvular heart disease, specific antimicrobial coverage should be initiated shortly before dental work involving gingival bleeding or operative procedures associated with the risk of development of endocarditis. This coverage should be in addition to the regular prophylactic program to prevent recurrence of rheumatic fever, which is inadequate for the prevention of bacterial endocarditis. The latter characteristically develops from invasion of organisms other than group A streptococci.

The indications for prophylaxis to prevent endocarditis and outlines of particular antibiotic schedules are periodically reviewed by the American Heart Association. The latest report, which is an update of 1977 recommendations, is published in Circulation, *70*:1123A–1127A, 1984.

Pediatric Cardiac Tumors

HERNAN SABIO, M.D.

Cardiac tumors are infrequent in adults and exceedingly rare in infants and children. Interest in cardiac tumors has paralleled the development of imaging procedures that are safe and reliable. The use of ultrasonographic techniques in the evaluation of suspected cardiac disease has led to earlier and possibly more frequent recognition of intracardiac tumors. Ultrasound also provides a noninvasive diagnostic modality, eliminating the potential risk of tumor embolization with catheterization.

Rhabdomyoma. The most frequent cardiac tumor in the pediatric age group is rhabdomyoma. Treatment consists of surgical resection as determined by the anatomic location of the mass or masses detected. Patients with tuberous sclerosis and documented cerebral involvement have survived successful surgical removal of rhabdomyomas. The ventricles are frequently involved by rhabdomyomas, leading to symptoms of outflow tract obstruction or recurrent arrhythmias. The success of surgical removal is largely dependent on the number of lesions present and their intracavitary or intramyocardial localization. However, even in the presence of multiple lesions, resection can be attempted with the combined use of profound hypothermia and cardiopulmonary bypass techniques. Because of the multiplicity of lesions observed in cardiac rhabdomyoma, it is suggested that sensitive two-dimensional ultrasound scanning be performed when an intracardiac mass is demonstrated or suspected in an infant. Although complete resection of each lesion should be attempted, selective excision of a major component of multiple lesions may result in the improvement of outflow tract obstruction. Mortality from cardiac rhabdomyoma is considerable, and an aggressive diagnostic and surgical approach is indicated.

Myxoma. Myxoma is the most common intracardiac tumor occurring in adult life. Although it is very infrequent in children, it merits discussion because of its potential curability. Definitive therapy consists of complete surgical resection, which is facilitated by cardioplegic arrest. The tumor usually is pedunculated and held by a stalk to the endocardium. The stalk and a full-thickness rim of normal tissue should be resected. Partial or incomplete resections should be avoided because of the risk of regrowth. The presence of a right atrial intracavitary mass should be further evaluated for evidence of direct tumor extension into the inferior vena cava. Inferior venocavography, sonography, or radionuclide imaging will more exactly define the extracardiac component of the tumor preoperatively. Tumors with inferior vena cava involvement can be resected in continuity with the right atrial component with the use of hypothermia and total circulatory arrest.

The postoperative management of infants and children with cardiac tumors should include periodic detailed ultrasonographic studies to identify recurrence or new tumor. Any persistent conduction abnormalities will also require appropriate therapy.

Fibromas. Fibromas are very rare tumors of the ventricular wall that occur predominantly during the first decade of life and especially during the first year of age. Treatment consists of surgical resection.

Rhabdomyosarcoma. Although rhabdomyosarcoma is the most uncommon primary cardiac tumor occurring in childhood, it is the most frequent histologically malignant cardiac neoplasm. It can form an intramural mass presenting with conduction abnormalities or an intracavitary mass with associated congestive heart failure. Unfortunately, there is usually mediastinal and extensive intramyocardial involvement as well as distant metastasis present at diagnosis and the therapeutic efforts then are palliative and directed at relieving critical intracavitary obstruction. Appropriate external-beam radiation therapy and chemotherapy utilizing drugs known to be effective in treating rhabdomyosarcoma, i.e., vincristine, cyclophosphamide, actinomycin D, and doxorubicin, can also add to the palliative effort. The potentiation of doxorubicin cardiotoxicity by radiation therapy should be considered in planning treatment. Other soft tissue sarcomas, including fibrosarcoma and angiosarcoma, can arise in the heart and have a similar clinical course.

Acute Leukemia. The most common noncardiac neoplasm to involve the heart is acute leukemia. This is usually clinically silent and responsive to systemic antileukemic therapy. Localized radiation therapy of pericardial leukemic implants can be used in the very unusual symptomatic case. Leukemic involvement of the heart is mostly observed as an autopsy finding with other evidence of extensive leukemic infiltration.

Metastatic Disease. Extra-cardiac malignant solid tumors can metastasize to the heart through venous or lymphatic channels or by direct intravascular extension. In several instances, osteosarcoma metastatic to the heart has been documented. Current advances in the control of localized osteosarcoma with the use of adjuvant and neoadjuvant chemotherapy suggest that a combined surgical-chemotherapeutic approach be considered when the metastatic foci are discrete and amenable to resection. A primary chemotherapeutic approach with subsequent re-evaluation of resectability should be reserved for cases with wide-spread metastatic disease. The most effective agents include doxorubicin, methotrexate in high doses with leucovorin rescue and combinations including cis-platinum, actinomycin D, bleomycin, cyclophosphamide, and vincristine.

Direct intravascular extension occurs most frequently from renal tumors. In most instances the tumor is a Wilms' tumor arising in the right kidney. In some instances hepatomegaly and edema of the lower extremities or ascites may be prominent. The presence of a heart murmur or other cardiac abnormalities in a child with a renal mass and the above findings should suggest direct intracardiac extension of Wilms' tumor. A complete resection should be attempted if other imaging procedures have not revealed evidence of metastatic disease. A combined thoracoabdominal approach with cardiopulmonary bypass and hypothermia has proved successful in the resection of these large intravascular tumors. Immediately after surgery, actinomycin D should be administered, and vincristine should be started approximately one week after surgery when adequate bowel function has been established. The tumor bed should be irradiated in contiguity, and the lung fields should also be irradiated. The addition of doxorubicin or cyclophosphamide to the treatment should be determined by the histologic type of Wilms' tumor. Follow-up evaluations should include abdominal and cardiac ultrasound studies as well as radiographic examination of the lungs for evidence of metastases.

6

Digestive Tract

Dental Caries

STUART D. JOSELL, D.M.D., M. Dent. Sci.

Dental caries is the most common dental problem found in children. In fact, it is the most common health problem in children. It is a disease of mineralized tissue and results from the interaction of three interdependent variables: a susceptible host (the teeth and saliva), a cariogenic diet, and pathogenic microorganisms. With time, these variables interact to initiate the caries process. Prevention and treatment of dental caries are aimed at disrupting the interactions of these variables.

Acids produced by microbial fermentation of sugar lead to the demineralization of tooth substance and the development of dental caries. One aspect of caries prevention involves making the teeth more resistant to acid breakdown. By incorporation of fluoride into enamel, especially during tooth development, the enamel can become more resistant to demineralization. Though fluoride can be incorporated into the teeth by topical application, it is most effective when it is administered systemically during the time of tooth development.

Community water fluoridation, at an optimal concentration of one part per million, is the main mechanism for systemic administration. At this concentration the incidence of caries can be reduced by 50–60%. If well water is used, it should be evaluated to determine if there is a need for fluoride supplementation.

It is necessary to use fluoride supplements in infants who are purely breast fed or fed prepared formula and when the water supply contains little or no fluoride. The American Academy of Pediatrics and the American Academy of Pediatric Dentistry recommend the following daily dosage of fluoride when there is 0.3 ppm of fluoride or less in the drinking water: 0.25 mg for infants less than 2 years of age, 0.50 mg for 2–3 year olds, and 1.00 mg for 3 year olds or older. When the fluoride content of drinking water is between 0.3 and 0.7 ppm, the daily dosage of fluoride is 0.25 mg for 2–3 year olds and 0.50 mg for 3 year olds and older. No supplementation is needed for infants less than 2 years old, and when the fluoride content of drinking water is over 0.7 ppm, fluoride supplementation is unnecessary for all age groups. The systemic use of fluoride during the years of dental development allows the formation of fluorapatite crystals instead of hydroxyapatite crystals in the tooth enamel. Fluorapatite is more resistant to acid demineralization than hydroxyapatite.

Topical application of fluoride through prescribed fluoride, professionally applied fluoride, over-the-counter mouth rinses, and dentifrices all have additional effects that reduce the incidence of caries. Dental sealants, plastic materials applied to teeth to smooth their fissured and pitted surfaces, also increase the host resistance to decay.

Prevention of caries must also incorporate nutritional and at-home oral hygiene information. Minimizing the consumption of fermentable sugars is important, but the frequency of carbohydrate ingestion and the physical form of the carbohydrates must also be considered. From the standpoint of preventive dentistry, an infant's diet should be high in iron and calcium and low in sugar. If a bottle is used at bedtimes, it should contain water and not cariogenic liquids; the bottle should be removed when the child falls asleep.

Oral hygiene, which disrupts the microbe-containing dental plaque, must be a parental responsibility in infants and toddlers. Daily parental assistance and supervision for plaque removal should continue for school-age children. Brushing, flossing, and oral irrigation (by rinsing or irrigation devices) must all be considered in an oral hygiene regimen. Early visits to the dentist, between 18 and 24 months of age, should be encouraged. If

171

discoloration or irregularities in the structure of the teeth are noted, referral to a dentist who readily treats children is advised.

Restoration of carious teeth is essential to the reestablishment of good oral health and prevention of future dental problems. The methods and materials for the treatment of decayed teeth may vary depending on the patient's age, dental status, behavioral maturity, and medical status. If caries goes untreated, it may extend to the dental pulp and cause a subsequent periapical infection. Though dental infections may cause acute problems, in some patients they may be asymptomatic and chronic in nature. These infections may be treated with pulp therapy or extraction with or without accompanying antibiotic therapy. Dental infections may severely compromise a child's health, especially when organic heart problems, anemias, diabetes, or immune deficiencies are present.

Dental caries is an entirely preventable problem. To optimally prevent and treat dental caries requires the cooperative action of child, parent, physician, and dentist.

Congenital Epulis of the Neonate

LAWRENCE A. FOX, D.D.S.

The congenital epulis of the neonate is a smooth, firm, benign tumor that arises on the anterior ridge of the alveolus. While it may be found on either the maxillary or mandibular ridges, it is most commonly found in the maxilla. It occurs 8–10 times more frequently in females. Lesions may be as small as 2–3 mm or as large as several centimeters. Because of their location in the oral cavity and the time of their occurrence, it is important to differentiate these lesions from the more common eruption cysts, which contain natal teeth. Since the tumors are lobular and pedunculated, they project into the mouth and restrict sucking and swallowing. For this reason, complete surgical excision of the lesion and its base is recommended. There have been no reports of either metastases or recurrence.

Diseases and Injuries of the Oral Region

HARVEY A. ZAREM, M.D.

CLEFT LIP

The primary problem with a congenital cleft of the lip is appearance. An infant can function effectively with a cleft lip; it is not a cause of a major difficulty in feeding or of a failure to thrive, and cleft lip is not associated with otitis media as is a cleft palate. Although some plastic surgeons repair the cleft lip in the newborn, the majority of craniofacial teams in the United States prefer to close the cleft lip at approximately age 3 months, when an infant better tolerates general anesthesia with less risk than does the newborn. There is no contraindication to postponing an operative repair of the lip if there are extenuating circumstances. A bilateral cleft lip presents problems of obtaining a satisfactory aesthetic result in later years and a bilateral cleft involving the alveolus will require extensive orthodontic management. The columella of the nose is usually extremely short, the alae of the nose are flared, and the midportion of the lip is attenuated. Although techniques have evolved over the last 10 years that permit a greatly improved repair of the bilateral cleft lip, the family must be alerted to the fact that it will take a number of therapeutic efforts over an extended period of time to obtain an optimal result. The teenage child with unilateral or bilateral cleft lip is usually primarily concerned with the nasal deformity associated with these clefts. It is common for the child to undergo several operative procedures in the pre-school era as well as in the teens before achieving a satisfactory aesthetic result.

CLEFT PALATE

A cleft palate presents several problems in addition to that of the cleft lip. Some infants may feed readily despite a cleft of the palate, but many infants do have difficulty with suction and feeding. A long, soft lamb's nipple is often effective. When the mother has learned to feed the infant patiently, the infant will thrive. If an infant with a cleft palate fails to thrive, it is usually due to frustration on the part of the family over the difficulty of feeding, and it is unwise to attribute a failure to thrive to a cleft of the palate alone. Efforts to educate the family to feed the child and hospitalization with feeding by a trained nursing staff should be tried before assuming that a failure to thrive is due to the cleft palate.

Children with a cleft of the palate have an extremely high incidence of otitis media, even in the neonatal period. Many otologists have recommended that children with clefts of the palate undergo routine myringotomy with insertion of tubes to maintain patency of the drum and to reduce the incidence of otitis media with subsequent hearing loss. The family must be alerted to the incidence of otitis media to facilitate early diagnosis and early treatment with decongestants and antibiotics to minimize the long-term scarring and hearing loss.

The major problem associated with a cleft of the palate is difficulty in speech. Although most craniofacial teams in the United States continue to close the palate at approximately age 18 months, we have frequently chosen to repair the palate at age 1 year in order to accommodate the otologist's need to perform myringotomies. Rather than subject the child to two separate anesthesias, we prefer to combine the two. If the child is thriving, anesthesia and cleft palate repair at age 1 year has been successful, and it is becoming our preference. In addition, speech pathologists believe that early phonation and speech habits can be affected by the cleft palate before the age of 3 years, which was previously doubted. Speech pathologists therefore are enthusiastic about early palatal closure, if it is deemed safe. Effective closure with respect to the anatomy and the use of pharyngeal flaps as well as other adjunctive techniques of palatoplasty and pharyngoplasty have resulted in a significant improvement in the quality of speech of patients with clefts of the palate. Working with the family to encourage them to speak clearly and deliberately with the child to encourage effective speech habits has been a worthwhile effort. If the child does have inadequate closure of the soft palate to the pharynx (velopharyngeal incompetence), several measures are available. A prosthodontist may contribute with the production of a speech bulb that will mechanically aid in the closure of the space between the soft palate and the pharynx, but we prefer to think of this as a temporary measure when other medical problems such as serious cardiac disease preclude operative closure of the palate. When a significant speech defect exists that is not improved with judicious speech therapy following palatal repair, a pharnygeal flap or a pharyngoplasty has been effective in closing the defect and allowing adequate speech. Problems with the pharyngeal flap or pharyngoplasty have included inadequate size of the correction with resultant inadequate speech improvement, denasal speech, and mild nasal airway obstruction. These problems are usually amenable to additional surgical therapy.

Routine tonsillectomy and adenoidectomy should not be carried out in the child who has undergone cleft palate repair. Frequently the hypertrophic adenoids and tonsils aid in the occlusion of the velopharynx and thereby aid speech by minimizing velopharyngeal incompetence. Concern must also be applied to the child who has a submucous cleft. A submucous cleft (which can be recognized by the bifid uvula, the thin blue midline in the soft palate, and a lack of a nasal spine with notching of the posterior border of the hard palate in the midline) has adequate velopharyngeal closure until a tonsillectomy and adenoidectomy have been carried out. Prior to recommending such an operative procedure, it is necessary to ascertain that the soft palate is normal.

The child born with a unilateral cleft of the lip and palate may expect a normal life pattern in view of the high quality of surgical, orthodontic, otologic, and speech therapy that has evolved today. The child with a bilateral cleft lip and palate, however, presents with a significant number of developmental deformities that produce problems even with excellent dental and surgical care. The midportion of the upper jaw (premaxilla) is prominent in infancy, but hypoplasia of the maxilla and collapse of the maxilla with collapse of the dental arch are frequent accompaniments of the bilateral cleft lip and cleft palate. The adolescent who has had a bilateral cleft of the lip and palate is likely to struggle with deformities of the maxilla and nose and with scars associated with the extreme lip deformity. Although judicious operative repair and sophisticated orthodontia have greatly improved the outcome of these patients in adolescence, the family should be alerted to the significance of the deformity and given encouragement to work with the child in a positive fashion. Numerous orthodontic, orthognathic, and soft tissue procedures will be needed to accomplish a satisfactory aesthetic and functional result.

MACROGLOSSIA

The term macroglossia is applied to an enlarged tongue. Occasionally the diagnosis is made when in fact the problem is a small mandible. The initial and primary concern in macroglossia is the potential for airway obstruction, as in the Pierre Robin syndrome. The major etiologies of macroglossia in children are lymphangioma, hemangioma, and neurofibroma; primary macroglossia may be associated with hyperthyroidism, amyloidosis, and glycogen storage diseases. In a surgical practice lymphangioma seems to be the most common etiology of macroglossia in children presenting at age 4–6 years. Small superficial vesicles on the mucosa are characteristic. An open bite and drooling are strong indications for excision of a portion of the tongue.

PIERRE ROBIN SYNDROME

Robin originally described a syndrome that included cleft palate, macroglossia (large tongue), and micrognathia (retruded mandible). The major significance of the Pierre Robin syndrome is the risk of glossoptosis in which the child may asphyxiate by "swallowing his tongue." Approximately 50% of affected children have cleft palate. Respiratory difficulty occurs most commonly at the time of feeding and may be manifested shortly after birth or as late as $1\frac{1}{2}$–2 months. The primary anxiety on the part of the treating physician is whether one should be conservative and risk the possibility that one of these respiratory difficulties could be fatal or continue with the conservative approach to tide the child over the first few months of life. The respiratory difficulty usually decreases when the child is on his abdomen and in some instances when an attempt is made to feed the child in the prone position. When this is not feasible, either because of the severity of the deformity or because of the lack of cooperation on the part of the family, an operative procedure to secure the tongue forward has been quite successful in experienced hands. This procedure is temporary and may be reversed after the neonatal period when the danger of respiratory obstruction has passed. Many of the children with Pierre Robin syndrome ultimately have normal mandibular development with correction of the glossoptosis and attain a normal occlusal relationship.

UNUSUAL CLEFTS

Although the most common clefts by far on the face involve the upper lip and palate, numerous other clefts may occur and have been classified, from both the therapeutic and the embryologic standpoints. Notching and clefts of the lower lip, alveolus, and tongue; bifid tongue; median cleft of the upper lip; and extensive clefts involving the nose, medial canthus, and orbit are now well recognized.

TONGUE-TIE

A significant number of infants are born with a short frenulum extending from the tongue to the central incisor area of the mandible. The majority of these children are asymptomatic. If the child can protrude the tongue, as in licking a lollipop, the likelihood of tongue-tie affecting speech is minimal. In significant tongue-tie, however, it is appropriate to release the tongue surgically. "Snipping" the tongue-tie is usually inappropriate, since a definitive procedure with Z-plasty and extension of the length of the frenulum is necessary. When the band is extremely thin, simple "snipping" may be effective. In children in whom the indication for surgery is questionable, an experienced speech pathologist may be most helpful.

MACROSTOMIA

The diagnosis of macrostomia is occasionally missed because it is associated with underdevelopment of the mandible. The distance between the midline of the upper or lower lip and the oral commissure is greater on the affected side than on the normal side. It is commonly associated with the first and second branchial arch syndrome (hemifacial microsomia) with hypoplasia of the entire half of the face, including the ear, the temporal muscle, masseter muscle, parotid gland, zygoma, and mandible. The macrostomia can be corrected by Z-plasty. The management of jaw deformity and hemifacial hypoplasia is a complex issue and should be deferred until development of the jaw and eruption of the teeth occur.

JAW DEFORMITIES
Micrognathia

Micrognathia may occur separately or in association with other syndromes such as Pierre Robin syndrome or hemifacial microsomia (first and second branchial arch syndrome). A significant number of micrognathias occur as hereditary features and not necessarily as a feature of a specific syndrome. Unless extreme, jaw development deformities are usually not apparent until the child is 5–6 years of age. The child should be evaluated by an experienced orthodontist, who is most capable of assessing dental and jaw development. Treatment of the majority of the children who require operative correction is deferred until full dental eruption, usually at age 18 or older. Severe facial deformities due to extreme jaw abnormality are treated at varying ages, depending on dentition.

Macrognathia (protruded mandible or prognathism) is also a deformity that is not readily apparent until the child is 5–6 years of age. It is characterized by an obtuse angle between the ramus of the mandible and the body of the mandible, and often an open bite. As in micrognathia, the diagnosis, evaluation, and treatment are sophisticated, and the patient should be evaluated by an orthodontist.

Bony Overgrowth of Jaws

A number of disorders with overgrowth of either the maxilla or mandible are not common but present a problem of diagnosis and treatment. Overgrowth of the jaw may be the result of arteriovenous fistula, which is usually apparent by the increased prominence of the vessels, by a bruit in the external carotid and its branches to the involved area, and by the increased warmth of the soft tissues. The management of an arteriovenous fistula involving the mandible or maxilla is difficult. The disease is invariably progressive. Patients may have dramatic episodes of bleeding that require blood transfusions. Frequently it is necessary to ligate the external carotid artery to control the bleeding, but the ultimate treatment is radical excision of the involved parts. This decision is difficult, since the surgery and the deformity are extensive; however, once the diagnosis is established and the course of progression of the arteriovenous fistula and progressive risk of serious hemorrhages have been clarified, definitive treatment should be instituted.

In a number of patients with neurofibromatosis, either local or diffuse (as in von Recklinghausen's syndrome), the face is involved. Overgrowth of the soft tissues and bones on the involved side of the face is the consequence. There is increased bulk of maxilla or mandible with gingival hypertrophy and displacement of the teeth. Management is effected by excising the offending tissues and sculpturing the tissues to correct the deformity. To "cure" the disease would entail an extensive operative procedure with removal of many normal structures and is never advisable. The course of this disease depends on the progression and age of onset of symptoms. The earlier the age of onset and the more rapid the course in youth, the worse the prognosis. Hemifacial hypertrophy, with enlargement of all of the facial structures (including jaw and teeth) unilaterally, presents a similar picture but is without the soft tissue neurofibromata.

Fibrous dysplasia of the jaws is an unusual condition involving the mandible or maxilla, which is enlarged because of the fibrous and noncalcified tissue within the bone. The presence of this entity is often not evident until late childhood, but it is usually self-limited when the child reaches puberty and growth ceases. This disorder must be recognized to avoid a misdiagnosis and radical excision of tissues. Contouring bone to reduce the deformity can be done in order to tide the child over until puberty and skeletal maturation. In some instances the excess bone that had been excised will recur, and this must be appreciated by the family before operative management of children with fibrous dysplasia of the jaws is undertaken.

Orofacial dysostosis is a congenital anomaly expressed in the oral region by alveolar clefts, tongue clefts, cysts of the upper lip, and supernumerary teeth; it is associated with anomalies of the hand and mental retardation.

Infantile cortical hyperostosis (Caffey's disease) is a self-limiting disease of children seen with onset of fever, soft tissue swelling, and periosteal new bone formation of the mandible. It occurs most commonly in the neonatal period (2–4 months of age) and could be mistaken for osteomyelitis of the mandible. The clavicles are often involved, and the x-ray picture is one of increased density on the surface of the bone due to new bone formation with overlying brawny induration of the soft tissues. In the mild cases no treatment is necessary except to maintain the comfort of the patient, but in the severe cases treatment with corticosteroids is indicated. It is recommended that the steroid dosage be continued over several months because exacerbations have occurred with early withdrawal of steroids.

TRAUMA

The majority of injuries about the oral region are minor and do not necessitate hospitalization. For the occasional severe injury, the most immediate dangers are exsanguinating hemorrhage and airway obstruction owing to loss of control of the tongue or to the blood. Most bleeding can be stopped by direct pressure.

If a child has eaten solids or liquids within 4 hours prior to the injury, it is generally not wise to consider general anesthesia except in dire circumstances. Emptying time of the stomach is prolonged after injury, so that the time lapse following an injury is often not reliable for judging a safe period. The majority of injuries about the mouth and face can be repaired using local anesthesia if some sedation is given and if the manner of the treating physician and parents is calm. Once the area is anesthetized, the majority of children relax and even doze during the repair.

Anesthesia about the face is often accomplished either by direct infiltration of lidocaine (Xylocaine), 1% with epinephrine, 1:100,000, or by regional nerve blocks. The entire upper lip can be anesthetized by injecting the infraorbital nerves. These simple nerve blocks are effective, and once the area is anesthetized, the child is usually cooperative.

Prior to the development of antibiotics, surgeons were cautious of closing any wounds that had occurred 4 or more hours prior to treatment. Today it is appropriate to close all facial wounds that are not overly contaminated despite the fact that more than 4 hours may have elapsed from the time of injury to the time of treatment. In animal bites or severe contamination, the use of tetanus toxoid, antibiotics, and judicious closure initially or closure secondarily (within several days of the injury) are appropriate. It is rarely advisable to allow a wound of the face or oral region to heal secondarily because of the resulting scar deformity. If a wound were closed and the degree of contamination underestimated, daily examination would allow the treating surgeon to open the wound at the first sign of infection and prevent a serious consequence.

A major portion of wounds seen in children in the emergency room are puncture wounds of the lower lip from the incisors. This wound lacerates the mucosa, the lower lip musculature, and the skin. This "through-and-through" wound is best cleansed with saline irrigation after local anesthesia and closed primarily. Small wounds may be closed with sutures in the mucosa and in the skin, but large wounds that are through-and-through should be closed in layers to include fat and muscle. Nonabsorbable soft suture material (preferably silk) should be used in the mouth when it is feasible to remove the sutures postoperatively.

Absorbable sutures cause inflammation in the mouth, and synthetic sutures such as nylon are stiff and extremely uncomfortable to the sensitive mucosa of the mouth. Closure of the muscle may be accomplished by absorbable sutures (Dexon,

Vicryl, or catgut), and closure of the skin should be effected with nonabsorbable sutures, such as a nonreacting fine (6-0) nylon, which can be removed. In the rare instances in which it is felt that the sutures cannot be removed from the skin, absorbable synthetic sutures such as Dexon or Vicryl are acceptable but only as second choices to the nonreactive synthetic fine nylon. Sutures on the skin of the face should be placed very close to the edge of the wound to avoid suture marks. They should also be removed approximately 4–5 days following the injury. The wounds can be supported after suture removal with a porous adhesive tape such as Steri-strips or Clearon. These paper tape closures will remain on the skin for approximately 5–7 days if left dry.

When the laceration about the lip extends across the mucocutaneous juncture (the white line between the vermilion of the mucosa and the white skin), care must be taken to align the fragments of the juncture. This is best done with the aid of magnifying loupes by aligning the fine white "roll" that is apparent owing to the thick sebaceous glands at the juncture. A small malalignment is conspicuous. When there is a significant loss of mucosa, it is often advisable to excise the wound in a V fashion and close the wound primarily. When there has been a loss of mucosa, such as from a dog bite, it is necessary to consider rotating a mucosal flap from the adjacent lip mucosa, a mucosal graft, or occasionally a tongue flap. Injuries in which there is a significant loss of tissue of the lip are difficult and the reconstruction to restore mucosa, muscle, and skin is complex. Sometimes it is best to close the wounds in a simple fashion and to defer extensive reconstructive procedures. When the immediate treating physician is not adequately experienced, it is always wisest to do a simple wound closure.

In general, it is preferable for the patient to undergo definitive wound repair at the time of the initial injury. If one allows the wounds to heal initially without definitive repair, scarring must be corrected secondarily. There are often circumstances (such as associated injuries, lack of available facilities and personnel, and the general condition of the patient) that may dictate secondary procedures rather than extensive primary repair. Secondary procedures, which include mucosal flaps, cross-lip flaps, and tongue flaps, should only be undertaken by an experienced surgeon.

Lacerations of the tongue are usually a problem because of extensive bleeding. The bleeding can be controlled by large sutures. The suture material should be silk because it is soft and relatively nonreacting, but this must be done only in the child who will cooperate to allow removal of the sutures.

In all significant injuries of the mucosa of the mouth, including lips, gingiva, tongue, soft palate, and pharynx, several steps have resulted in diminished infection and improved results. The child should be kept on a clear liquid diet for a minimum of three days and preferably seven days. A clear liquid diet consists of transparent liquids without particles. This prevents food particles from entering the wound as a nidus for infection. It is difficult to convince the family of the child that this diet is compatible with health and well being.

After solid foods have been resumed, it is wise to rinse the mouth after each meal with plain water or a milk salt solution (a quart of warm water in which 1 teaspoon of table salt and 1 teaspoon of baking soda have been dissolved). Frequent washing of the mouth and irrigating of the wounds in this manner have resulted in excellent wound healing. The use of antibiotics in these wounds is variable. Most surgeons agree that the use of an antibiotic for 5 days is safe and has resulted in a diminished incidence of wound infection and inflammation.

In all significant lacerations about the mouth, the treating physician should be aware of possible injury to the parotid duct and facial nerve. Parotid duct injury, if not recognized, can result in parotid secretions into the tissues, or in a parotid fistula, which is difficult to manage and often requires secondary procedures. If, on the other hand, the injury to the parotid duct is recognized at the time of the trauma, repair of the duct is simple and effective and is best accomplished under general anesthesia in the young child.

Injuries to the facial musculature or to the facial nerve should be appreciated prior to treatment, especially prior to the administration of local anesthetics. The child should be asked to activate all of the facial muscles of expression, and asymmetry should be carefully noted. If the injury to the facial nerve occurs anterior to a vertical line through the lateral canthus of the eye, the likelihood of recovery of function without surgical repair of the nerve is excellent. However, if the injury occurs proximal to this line, which is proximal to the anterior border of the masseter muscle, it is wise to undertake a search and repair of the nerve. This must be done under general anesthesia with magnification and with microsurgical instruments.

Electrical burns of the mouth are unusual. They usually occur when a toddler places the juncture of an electrical appliance and of an extension cord in the mouth. The saliva acts as a conductor and causes an electrical burn. Severe electrical burns can result in a loss of major portions of the upper and lower lip and gingiva, and even injury to the tooth buds and mandible. Fortunately, the majority of these injuries involve only the lips and oral commissure. Electrical injuries to the midportion of the upper and lower lip usually heal without severe deformities.

The treatment of the electrical injury to the lip must be definitive. Immediately after the injury, the degree of trauma is usually not evident. The child should be given sedation, antibiotics, and the family must watch the child carefully. Late bleeding from the labial artery can be dramatic and, if it occurs, does so 5 to 7 days following injury. Parents are instructed to watch for bleeding and, if it occurs, to pinch the lip between the fingers and to bring the child to the emergency room immediately.

The majority of surgeons prefer to treat electrical burns with antibiotic therapy and to allow secondary healing. If a deformity occurs at a later date, reconstruction is undertaken electively. The primary reason that this has been a chosen course is that it is often difficult to determine the extent of loss of tissues in the early post-injury phase. About 3 weeks following the injury, the degree of tissue loss is usually evident. If a significant portion of the upper or lower lip at the commissure has been lost, restoration of the bulk of the lip using the tongue as the source of muscle and mucosa can be done as a tongue flap 3–4 weeks after injury. This procedure must be carefully executed, but it is effective in extensive electrical burn injuries of the oral commissure.

Salivary Gland Tumors

DOUGLAS W. BELL, M.D.

Hemangiomas are the most common cause of parotid swelling in the newborn. Eighty per cent are present at birth, with the remainder discovered within the next 6 to 12 months. These benign lesions are diffuse, soft masses in the preauricular area and angle of mandible area. There may be a rapid growth for the first 6 months, but there is also regression because of vessel occlusion. There may be some redness of the overlying skin, but as the tumor regresses, the color subsides. The mass may increase in size with crying or straining. Only in a few cases in which the tumor continues to expand is surgery indicated. This involves a superficial parotidectomy, with identification and preservation of the facial nerve, which courses through the gland.

Lymphangiomas are benign congenital lesions of lymph vessels. Over 90% occur in the cervical region, and many involve the parotid or submaxillary gland. These lesions do not undergo spontaneous regression. Thus, surgical dissection must be utilized to remove all the small cystic lesions. Otherwise, there is a notable recurrence rate, and multifocal lesions develop. Laser therapy may be used at times, and cryotherapy is helpful for intraoral lesions.

If the tumor mass develops later in childhood, the mass is usually firmer, more discrete, nontender, and of variable mobility. The most likely tumor is a benign mixed tumor containing both glandular and ductal elements. If such a mass persists, excisional biopsy with facial nerve protection is necessary.

Only 10% of these masses are malignant. Such tumors expand rapidly and may be fixed to other tissues or may be tender. If there is facial paralysis, the tumor is assumed to be malignant. The most common malignant tumors of the parotid gland are mucoepidermoid carcinomas and sarcomas (rhabdomyosarcomas and undifferentiated tumors). Total parotidectomy with facial nerve preserved may be sufficient. If the nerve must be partially excised, immediate grafting techniques are used. Chemotherapy has made great advances and may be used as primary therapy. Radiation therapy is also part of the "triple attack" on these aggressive tumors. The exact protocol is determined by the cell type, rate of growth, and extent of tumor.

Submaxillary gland tumors are usually the benign mixed type and occur in older children. More rapid growth would signal a likely malignant potential. In either case, total removal of the submaxillary gland with sparing of the lingual nerve is the best treatment. Any further chemotherapy or irradiation would be decided based on the tumor cell type.

Recurrent Acute Parotitis

EDWARD J. O'CONNELL, M.D.

Recurrent acute parotitis is an unusual and troublesome condition that affects persons from infancy to adulthood. The highest incidence is in children 5–10 years old. Management of the acute episode consists of symptomatic relief, reestablishment of salivary flow, and antibiotic therapy. Analgesia with aspirin or acetaminophen and heat applied to the affected gland are of benefit. The affected gland should be milked to encourage salivary flo⋯ ⋯⋯⋯ probing the Stensen du⋯ ⋯⋯nspissated muc⋯ ⋯ructed in massage⋯ ⋯raged to have the⋯ ⋯ewing gum.

Antibi⋯ ⋯ to be of defini⋯ ⋯atment with am⋯ ⋯divided doses) s⋯ ⋯ure and sensitivi⋯ ⋯ Stensen duct; this therapy should be given for 10 days. Typical oral flora (*Streptococcus viridans*, *Staphylococcus aureus*, and *Streptococcus pneumoniae*) usually grow on cultures, although anaerobic bacteria grew on cultures in two recent cases. If the patient is sensitive to penicillin, erythromycin (30–50 mg/kg every 6 hours to a maximum of 500 mg every 6 hours for 10 days) should be used. If inflammation has progressed after the first 24 hours of antibiotic therapy, additional therapy with a coagulase-resistant antistaphylococcal drug (dicloxacillin, 25 mg/kg every 24 hours in four divided doses) should be strongly considered.

The usual episode lasts 4–6 days. A follow-up examination 4–6 weeks after the first attack is recommended. At that time, the parotid gland should be carefully examined bimanually to rule out small, partially obstructing lesions.

Preventing further attacks is much less rewarding than treating an acute attack. The prophylactic use of antibiotics, autogenous vaccines, corticosteroids, and antihistamines has been of no benefit. Maintaining salivary flow by the use of sialagogues, such as chewing gum, and, in some cases, preprandial massage of the parotid gland has appeared to be of some benefit. If recurrences continue, sialography should be performed to rule out stenosis, stones, and obstruction. This procedure has also been reported to be of therapeutic value in some cases.

Because most children with recurrent parotitis have few episodes after adolescence, surgical therapy is seldom necessary. However, patients in late adolescence or older patients who have had many recurrences despite optimal medical management and who have proximal ductal dilatation or cyst formation may benefit from surgical intervention.

Thyroglossal Duct Cysts

DOUGLAS W. BELL, M.D.

Thyroglossal duct cysts are typically asymptomatic and may pose no problem other than a cosmetic change. The longer the cyst is present, the more likely it is to become infected secondarily from an upper respiratory infection.

In 10% of children in whom the cyst becomes infected, it enlarges, tenderness increases, and it may progress to an abscess. Antibiotics such as amoxicillin or a cephalosporin are usually sufficent with warm compresses. Needle aspiration may be necessary for better culture of the organism if the infection fails to respond to antibiotics. In the extreme case, this abscess ruptures at the skin surface and a draining sinus tract persists. Antibiotics and local dressing care are used to control the infection. Later, the entire sinus tract and the cyst are surgically removed.

Unless the midportion of the hyoid bone is excised, there is a 25% recurrence rate of the cyst. If the cyst is large and little or no thyroid tissue is palpable, it is wise to perform a thyroid scan preoperatively. This is to document the entire thyroid tissue and to avoid possibly removing all the patient's functioning thyroid. The postoperative course is benign, with some dysphagia present only for a few days and no change in speech articulation.

Branchial Arch Cysts and Sinuses

DOUGLAS W. BELL, M.D.

The typical branchial arch cyst is a smooth, round, nontender cyst along the anterior border of the sternocleidomastoid muscle at any point from the external auditory canal to the clavicle. The cyst may not be noted until it becomes infected—usually in late childhood or adolescence. Then it enlarges and is tender, and the skin become erythematous. Antibiotic therapy usually controls the infection, and the cyst subsides after resolution of the illness. If a sinus tract persists, then it is palpable as a fibrous cord extending along the muscle border. The tract may develop into a fistula, with intermittent drainage onto the neck skin. The treatment of these various cysts and sinuses is surgical excision of the entire tract. It must be traced back to its origin, and the communication with the ear canal or pharynx must be closed.

In evaluating second and third arch fistula tracts, a radiopaque dye is used to identify the entire tract. The internal ostia may be in the tonsil and require a tonsillectomy to solve the problem completely. Knowing the embryology and development, the physician can anticipate any important vessels and nerves that need to be carefully protected during surgery. Antibiotic therapy should precede any surgical treatment so that inflammation is minimized. The excision should be as complete as possible.

Disorders of the Esophagus

JOYCE D. GRYBOSKI, M.D.

CONGENITAL DISORDERS OF THE ESOPHAGUS

Congenital lesions of the esophagus are usually obvious shortly after birth and present either as respiratory distress or as dysphagia. All infants with suspected esophageal anomalies should be managed in a high-risk neonatal unit.

Esophageal Atresia and Tracheoesophageal

Fistula. These disorders are among the most grave neonatal emergencies, for they are often associated with prematurity and other serious congenital anomalies. There is often a history of polyhydramnios. Although the infant may appear normal at birth, he will exhibit difficulty in swallowing and respiratory distress as secretions fill the esophageal sac and overflow into the oropharynx. Pharyngeal suction will temporarily remove the mucus from mouth and oropharynx. A number 10 or 12 F catheter, passed through the nose or mouth, will meet an obstruction at 10–13 cm. A plain chest film will show the position of the catheter and a dilated upper esophageal pouch that is filled with air. An abdominal film will show gas in the stomach and small bowel, indicating a distal fistula. The absence of air in the stomach denotes either no fistula or a proximal fistula.

Therapy is aimed at preventing pulmonary complications and ensuring adequate nutrition. The infant should be kept in an isolette and given oxygen as needed. Those with distal fisulas should be maintained in a semi-Fowler position. Continuous low-pressure suction is applied through a sump tube passed into the proximal pouch. A decompression gastrostomy may be indicated to prevent reflux through the fistula and to provide a portal for feeding. Broad-spectrum antibiotic therapy is begun immediately, and surgical correction should not be attempted until respiratory distress from pneumonitis or the respiratory distress syndrome has subsided.

The type of surgical treatment depends upon the size and condition of the infant. The full-term neonate weighing more than 2.5 kg who has no other anomalies or respiratory distress is a candidate for immediate single-stage correction using a right thoracotomy. Infants between 1.8 and 2.5 kg who are otherwise well, and larger infants with mild or moderate anomalies or pneumonia, fare best with gastrostomy and medical therapy for several days before surgery. Small premature infants (weighing less than 1.8 kg) and those with severe pneumonia or cardiac disease require gastrostomy, ligation of the fistula, and parenteral or gastrostomy feeds for several weeks before a primary repair can be performed.

End-to-end anastomosis with division of the fistula was the standard procedure for years but was associated with a high incidence of postoperative stricture (up to 25%). End-to-side anastomosis has decreased the incidence of stricture to 7–9% and permits feeding within several days after operation. If there is a long distance between the esophageal ends and primary anastomosis cannot be performed without tension, several techniques have been used, for example, stretching and elongation of the upper sac, circular myotomies of the upper sac, and colon interposition.

A major complication of these repairs is anastomotic leak, which occurs during the second and seventh postoperative days in 20–30% of infants. The complication is of less consequence in extrapleural repairs than in transpleural ones, where it leads to empyema. Many leaks heal spontaneously while the infant is fed parenterally or through the gastrostomy. Empyema is treated by cervical esophagostomy, closure of the distal esophagus, and chest tube drainage. A later complication is gastroesophageal reflux and stricture. Strictures are treated by dilation, and some patients may require fundoplication. Swallowing difficulties may persist to some degree, for most patients have some decrease of peristaltic activity in the esophagus below the level of the anastomosis.

Tracheoesophageal Fistula without Esophageal Atresia: "H-Type Fistula." This anomaly accounts for only 4.2% of upper esophageal lesions. It is usually situated higher than the other lesions of esophageal atresia and fistula. Most fistulas can be repaired by a cervical approach, but lower ones require thoracotomy. Both the esophageal and tracheal ends of the divided fistula are closed, and a flap of mediastinum or muscle is interposed between the two organs.

Esophageal Duplications. Duplication cysts of the esophagus may present with cyanosis and dyspnea in the neonate or with recurrent pneumonitis or dysphagia in the older infant or child. Most cysts can be simply excised, but some have a separate blood supply that must be identified and tied off.

Vascular Rings and Aortic Arch Anomalies. These vascular anomalies arise from faulty development of the aortic arch system and cause compression of the esophagus or the trachea. Symptoms are wheezing or stridor initiated or aggravated by feeding and dysphagia. If symptoms are mild, surgery may be postponed until the infant is larger, at which time the anomalous artery may be divided and ligated.

Congenital Diverticulum of the Esophagus. Congenital diverticulum may be asymptomatic for years or may cause respiratory distress by tracheal compression in the neonate. Once diagnosed, it should be resected, since its presence will prolong feeding difficulties and increase the risk of regurgitation and aspiration.

Esophageal Web. In our experience esophageal web has been seen in association with two disorders, epidermolysis bullosa dystrophica and dyskeratosis congenita. The symptoms are intermittent dysphagia that is more marked for solids than for liquids and pain referred to the neck. Radiologic examination shows a discrete cervical web. Some patients with epidermolysis bullosa will note a sudden pop when eating and have spontaneous resolution of their symptoms. Otherwise, the web may be disrupted by gentle dilation.

Esophageal Stricture and Epidermolysis Bullosa. Esophageal strictures due to epidermolysis bullosa must be treated differently from those due to acid reflux or caustic ingestion. Epidermolysis bullosa, which is now believed to be caused by a genetically altered collagenase, affects the esophagus as well as the skin, and minor trauma is followed by blistering and scarring. Lesions are most marked in young children. It is difficult initially to determine how much of the esophageal narrowing is due to edema and bulla formation and how much is actually stricture. Patients may spend hours ingesting one pureed meal. The conventional treatment has been high-dose prednisone (1–2 mg/kg/day) for at least 3 weeks with gradual tapering thereafter. Recently, phenytoin* has been shown to reduce skin blistering and has been used successfully in treatment of esophageal lesions. If there is no response to therapy, gentle dilation with rubber bougies is helpful. Colon interposition is reserved for patients with long, unresponsive strictures.

CAUSTIC INJURIES TO THE ESOPHAGUS

Most severe esophageal injuries are caused by the ingestion of lye, Drano, and Liquid Plummer. Now that the concentration of caustic in these has been reduced from 30 to 10% and child-proof caps have been substituted, burns are less frequent. Concentrated sodium hydroxide produces deep burns through liquification necrosis of the esophageal mucosa and underlying tissue. Weaker solutions such as ammonia also cause burns, but they are less deep and do not lead to stricture formation. Acid ingestion is less frequent and affects only the superficial layers of the esophagus.

Immediate first-aid treatment at home is for the child to drink a glass of milk to dilute the caustic. Vomiting should not be induced. The mouth must be inspected for burns. Although only one-third of children with oral burns have esophageal lesions, it is conversely true that severe esophageal burns may be present in the absence of oral lesions. Because one cannot be certain that a child does not have esophageal lesions, all children—even those only suspected of caustic ingestion—should be hospitalized and observed for 48 hours. Intravenous fluids are administered, and a chest film is obtained to rule out mediastinitis. Some investigators prefer early esophagoscopy, but it is better postponed for 24–48 hours to avoid increasing early edema about the arytenoids and the precipitation of respiratory distress. Esophagoscopy is performed under general anesthesia; by 48 hours burned areas are covered by fibrin patches and

are easily recognizable. One should not attempt to pass the endoscope beyond the first burned area recognized.

If there are no visible lesions, treatment is discontinued and the child is fed and discharged. If burns are present, an oral broad-spectrum antibiotic is administered for 10 days in combination with corticosteroid therapy (prednisone, 1–2 mg/kg/day), which is continued for 3 weeks. Early dysphagia, within the first 48 hours, is caused by inflammatory edema and may be so severe as to obstruct the esophagus. Usually, however, patients can swallow relatively comfortably by 48–72 hours and may be offered clear liquids and subsequently advanced to a soft diet.

Complications that contraindicate steroid therapy are aspiration pneumonia and mediastinitis. These develop within the first 48 hours and are heralded by fever and general deterioration of the patient. It must be stressed that bacterial invasion of the mediastinum can occur without demonstrable perforation. These complications mandate intravenous antibiotic therapy and fluid maintenance.

Since the depth of the burn cannot be truly estimated, one cannot predict with accuracy which patient will or will not develop a stricture. In some centers, when the patient can tolerate liquids, he is given a surgical thread to swallow (with the proximal end taped to the cheek) so that it may later be used as a guide for bougies. Cineesophagograms should be obtained after several weeks and at several-month intervals for a year. Half of untreated patients with severe burns develop strictures, whereas only 4–13% of those treated with combined steroid-antibiotic programs do so.

MOTOR DISORDERS OF THE ESOPHAGUS

Achalasia. Achalasia is a neuromuscular disease of the esophagus in which there is failure of the lower esophageal sphincter (LES) to relax in response to swallowing. The entire esophagus above becomes progressively dilated and has little or no peristaltic activity. The disease is thought to be due to a congenital absence or degeneration of the ganglion cells of Auerbach's plexus.

The treatment of achalasia is either surgical myotomy or pneumatic dilation of the LES. In the very small infant, temporary relief is provided by simple bougienage, but definitive therapy will be required later. Pneumatic dilation is used successfully in adults, and recent studies in the pediatric literature attest to good results in children. More than half have recurrent symptoms and require surgical correction. The risk of perforation of the esophagus increases with each successive pneumatic dilation. Surgical myotomy is successful in 85–90% of patients. Modifications of the Heller myotomy are used, varying from short division of

---

* This use of phenytoin is not listed by the manufacturer.

the lower esophageal musculature with sparing of the gastroesophageal junction to extension for less than 1 to several centimeters onto the stomach. If the myotomy is extended onto the stomach, a fundoplication should be performed to protect against gastroesophageal reflux. The LES pressure is reduced, spasm is decreased, and there is a slight return to peristaltic activity. Lifelong surveillance of the esophagus is necessary, for the disease carries an increased risk of carcinoma of the esophagus.

Isosorbide dinitrate and nifedipine (a calcium antagonist) both decrease LES pressure and have provided symptomatic relief in adults with achalasia. Not yet approved for therapy, their effectiveness is simply to be noted at this time.

Lower Esophageal Ring. The lower esophageal or Schatzki ring causes intermittent dysphagia in older children and adults. It may also be an incidental radiologic finding unassociated with symptoms. Initial treatment consists of instructing the patient to eat slowly and chew carefully. If symptoms persist despite these measures, dilation with bougies or a Mosher bag is curative.

Esophageal Muscular Ring. The esophageal muscular ring causes symptoms similar to those seen with the lower esophageal ring, but they are noted at an earlier age. The ring lies in the lower esophagus but well above the squamocolumnar junction. It may be associated with the VACTERL anomalies, a series of mesodermal malformations including vertebral and rib anomalies, radial limb malformations, single umbilical artery, anal atresia, ventricular septal defect, and tracheoesophageal fistula.

Familial Dysautonomia. Esophageal dysfunction in the Riley-Day syndrome of familial dysautonomia results in dilation of the lower esophagus. The only treatment is symptomatic. In some patients, parenteral neostigmine eases the swallowing difficulties. Patients should sleep prone in a semi-elevated position to prevent aspiration. Some patients eventually require fundoplication or gastrostomy to prevent aspiration.

Other Diseases. Abnormalities in esophageal motor function occur in a number of neuromuscular disorders and collagen diseases, as well as in diabetes mellitus. Abnormal motility is also associated with intestinal pseudoobstruction. Transient motor disorders may follow vagotomy but improve after several months.

Gastroesophageal Reflux and Hiatus Hernia

JOYCE D. GRYBOSKI, M.D.

Gastroesophageal reflux (GER) may or may not be associated with hiatus hernia. The significance of an hiatus hernia lies not in its size, but in the degree of reflux which accompanies it. Reflux represents the flow of gastric contents into the esophagus. Most often showing an effortless flow of gastric contents from the mouth after feeding, in some young infants, it may be quite forceful and even resemble the vomiting of pyloric stenosis. In some instances reflux may not be associated with any visible manifestation and a young infant may cough after feedings or in his sleep, suffer periodic apneic spells or recurrent pneumonitis, or simply be irreconcilably irritable after feeds. Older children may complain of recurrent abdominal pain, often epigastric, right upper quadrant or substernal in nature.

The initial therapy for infants and children with GER is dietary and positional. Since a few infants with GER vomit because of a dietary protein allergy, a trial of hypoallergenic formula may be attempted. A detailed history and observation of feeding habits are essential. Since reflux is less when the stomach is not filled to capacity or expanded by air, small, frequent feedings are recommended. For infants these should number 6 to 8 per day, and care should be taken that caloric requirements are met. Typically, solids are retained better than liquids. Infant formula may be thickened to a gruel-like consistency using up to 1 tablespoon of cereal per ounce of formula. Older infants may also be offered solids 15–20 minutes before their bottles. Children should eat smaller, more frequent meals, 4 to 6 per day. In all age groups, acidic foods and juices are to be avoided, as are other substances (e.g., chocolate, caffeine) that lower pressure in the lower esophageal sphincter (LES). Although tomatoes are not acidic, they are consistently identified as causing pain and should be eaten with discretion.

The head of the bed or crib should be elevated approximately 8 inches to a 30–45° angle. Pillows under the head are inefficient since the child rolls off them during the night. Sleeping in the elevated, prone position has been shown to decrease acid reflux significantly. The infant is kept from turning over in his sleep by a canvas harness whose straps are secured through the top rungs of the crib. The infant seat, long considered the mainstay of reflux therapy, has fallen into disrepute since such positioning has recently been shown to increase rather than decrease reflux.

Parents must be warned that clinical recovery will probably not be evident for several weeks and that therapy must be continued for a minimum of 6 weeks. Weight gain may be noted within the first week. Up to 95% of infants respond to such treatment, and a general rule is that reflux decreases significantly by 6 months and is no longer a problem by 1 year of age.

Some infants continue to reflux even after these measures have been employed and may require continuous nasogastric feedings for weeks to months before they develop the ability to feed safely. A few of these babies have small gastric capacities, although not the rare anomaly of microgastria.

Because increases in intraabdominal and intragastric pressure increase reflux, children who become symptomatic during athletic activities such as weight lifting, swimming, diving, or jogging should refrain from these activities until symptoms have subsided. Those with body braces should remove the braces postprandially. There is a frequent association of hiatus hernia and obesity and a probable association of reflux and obesity. Therefore, weight reduction will in itself often alleviate symptoms in the chubby older child.

Medical Therapy

Antacids, by their buffering effects, coat and alkalinize the esophagus. Five to 20 ml are administered every 2 hours or midway between feeds. Most products contain magnesium hydroxide and may cause diarrhea. Those containing aluminum hydroxide, on the other hand, are constipating, and it may be necessary to alternate the two forms. Mylanta II has proved palatable and efficient. If there is evidence of bile reflux, aluminum hydroxide antacids should be used because of their bile acid–binding properties.

Sucralfate,* a basic aluminum salt of sucrose octasulfate, is a nonabsorbed chemical with a number of unique properties. It becomes viscous and adherent when exposed to acid, forms complexes with protein molecules that are resistant to pepsin proteolytic action, adsorbs pepsin and bile salts, and is a strong buffer against acid. Its adhesive properties make it particularly effective in binding to injured mucosa and provide a "protective barrier" effect not accomplished by simple antacids. There is no established dosage for children; the adult dosage is 1 gm four times daily on an empty stomach. It is best given 1 hour before meals and at bedtime.

Cimetidine, a histamine H_2 receptor antagonist, functions specifically to decrease gastric acidity. It is occasionally used for the treatment of esophagitis† but has not proven superior to antacids. A dose of 20–40 mg/kg/day, given with meals in four divided doses, is recommended for children. Drowsiness, gynecomastia, and decreased white blood cell counts are rare complications. The drug decreases the hepatic metabolism of warfarin anticoagulants, phenytoin, diazepam, propranolol, and theophylline, causing a more prolonged elevation of their levels in the blood. Ranitidine,‡ a second-generation histamine H_2 receptor antagonist, has no reported side effects to date and requires only a twice-daily dosage schedule. A dosage regimen in children has not yet been established.

Dicyclomine hydrochloride relieves smooth muscle spasms of the gastrointestinal tract and may be extremely helpful in the treatment of infants with GER who have a demonstrated antral spasm or pylorospasm. The dosage for infants is $\frac{1}{2}$ teaspoon, diluted with an equal volume of water, three times daily. Use of the drug in infants under 6 months of age is now contraindicated owing to serious anticholinergic side effects. Older children are given a 10-mg capsule or 1 teaspoon three times daily. Side effects are urinary hesitancy or retention, tachycardia, nervousness, drowsiness, nausea, and vomiting.

Agents that increase gastrointestinal motility have proved effective in the treatment of GER. Bethanechol§ has been evaluated in several studies. It increases lower esophageal motility through its cholinergic action, and although it does not decrease the immediate acid reflux frequency, it improves acid clearance from the esophagus. It has been reported to increases LES pressure. Given 3 mg/m²/dose every 8 hours, 89% of treated infants and children showed improvement. A recommended weight dose is 0.3–0.6 mg/kg/day, divided in q 6 to q 8 hr increments. The drug does not increase gastric emptying. Salivation, flushing, sweating, nausea, vomiting, and diarrhea are signs of overdose, and the drug should not be used in asthmatics or those with urinary retention. Metoclopramide(methoxy-2-chloro-5-procainamide) increases both LES pressure and gastric emptying. The dosage for children 6–14 years old is 2.5–5 mg metoclopramide base (0.5–1 ml); for those under 6, it is 0.1 mg/kg metoclopramide base. The drug is administered 30 minutes before meals and at bedtime. It should not be used in children with epilepsy or extrapyramidal disease, and we do not use the drug in children younger than 3 months of age. In the central nervous system the drug acts as a dopamine antagonist, causing oculogyric crisis, torticollis, tremors, and dysarthria. Agitation is a milder reaction. Diphenhydramine reverses the dystonia.

Since all the motility-stimulating drugs have rather serious side effects, their use is best reserved for treatment of infants and children with significant failure to thrive, respiratory symptoms, or esophagitis.

---

* Manufacturer's warning: Safety and efficacy of sucralfate in children have not been established.

† This use of cimetidine is not listed by the manufacturer.

‡ Manufacturer's warning: Safety and efficacy of ranitidine in children have not been established.

§ This use of bethanechol is not listed by the manufacturer.

Surgical Therapy

Surgical intervention is not considered until failure of medical therapy has been demonstrated. Antireflux measures must be continued for 6 weeks, and often little improvement is noted until the second or third week of treatment. Most children and infants will respond to this type of therapy. The highest failure rates occur in those with mental retardation and, particularly, in those with scoliosis.

As noted, hiatus hernia itself is not an indication for surgery. Indications are respiratory problems or apnea, malnutrition, esophagitis and stricture, Sandifer's syndrome, and intractible vomiting. The Nissen fundoplication is the most frequently used procedure; it carries a success rate between 85 and 95% and remains effective during growth of the child. Complications are not unusual; studies showing rates as low as 0.6% are not accurate over the long term. Indeed, large series note a 15–20% complication rate. Major complications are para-esophageal hiatus hernia, small bowel obstruction, malalignment of the fundal wrap, and disruption of the fundoplication. Others are gastric ulceration, gas-bloat syndrome, and postoperative dysphagia. Most complications arise within the first 2 postoperative years. The gas-bloat syndrome occurs when the wrap is too tight and the patient is unable to belch or vomit. Loosening of the wrap and initially fashioning it over a large-bore stent with concomitant pyloroplasty and even parietal cell vagotomy are recent modifications. A transient dumping syndrome, in which the children develop diaphoresis, palpitations, syncope, abdominal fullness, and diarrhea during or within 30 minutes after meals, is now being reported. Laboratory studies document hyperglycemia and reactive hypoglycemia. These patients tolerate unsweetened foods well.

Fundoplication is not curative in all patients, particularly in infants with recurrent pulmonary disease. Problems may persist because of associated esophageal motility disorders or pharyngoesophageal incoordination. Some infants have greatly increased oral secretions associated with feeding and may require continuous drip rather than bolus feeds. A few may require treatment with atropine.

Barrett's Esophagus

With the increasing use of endoscopy, Barrett's esophagus is being more frequently recognized. This lesion represents a response of the esophagus to reflux in which columnar epithelium replaces squamous epithelium that has been destroyed by acid reflux. This mucosa contains parietal cells and can secrete acid.

Treatment is the same as for GER. Since there is some evidence that Barrett's esophagus, if it persists, may predispose to the development of carcinoma, treatment should be aggressive.

Nausea and Vomiting

DAVID R. FLEISHER, M.D.

Nausea and vomiting are signals of something gone wrong and should never be treated without considering and reconsidering their causes. Management of most of the disorders consists of removing the causes of vomiting and/or correcting fluid and electrolyte deficits until vomiting subsides. Antiemetics are relatively contraindicated when vomiting is a key indicator of some life-threatening process, e.g., meningitis or adrenal insufficiency, or when they are likely to produce unwanted side effects without significant benefit, e.g., in midgut volvulus. Antiemetics are useful when the causes of vomiting are known and the vomiting is predictable and of limited duration, e.g., in acute gastroenteritis, cancer chemotherapy, or motion sickness.

Antiemetic Drugs

Antiemetic agents include antihistamines, dopamine antagonists, and a miscellaneous group. Antihistamines—e.g., promethazine, dimenhydrinate, and cyclizine—are effective against motion sickness, probably because of their anticholinergic properties. Dopamine antagonists include phenothiazines, and metoclopramide. They suppress the chemoreceptor trigger zone (CTZ) but are generally ineffective against motion sickness. Phenothiazines have both anticholinergic and extrapyramidal side effects. Therefore, Thorazine is preferable to Compazine because it is less likely to cause extrapyramidal reactions. A dysphoric state with feelings of unreality is a side effect of phenothiazines that may be as common as their anticholinergic and sedative side effects and should caution against too liberal a use of these agents as antiemetics or sedatives.

Metoclopramide (Reglan) has a phenothiazine-like action on the CTZ and also affects the motor activity of the upper gastrointestinal tract. It increases the strength of the lower esophageal sphincter mechanism and enhances propulsive motility of the stomach, duodenum, and small bowel without affecting secretion or the motility of the colon. This action is blocked by atropine, and metoclopramide loses its effectiveness when used with anticholinergic antispasmodics. Like phenothiazines, it may cause extrapyramidal reactions and lower the seizure threshold. Metoclopramide blocks the hypotensive effect of dopamine; it should be used cautiously in patients recently treated with adrenergic agents, mono-

Table 1. DRUGS USEFUL FOR CONTROL OF NAUSEA AND VOMITING

Drug	How Supplied	Principal Side Effects
Antihistamines		
Promethazine (Phenergan, Remsed)	Injection: 25 and 50 mg/ml	Drowsiness, atropine-like
Child: 0.5 mg/kg/dose q 12 h	Syrup: 6.25 mg/5 cc and 25 mg/5 cc	
Adult: 25 mg bid	Tablets: 12.5, 25, and 50 mg	
	Suppository: 12.5, 25, and 50 mg	
Dimenhydrinate (Dramamine)	Injection: 50 mg/ml	Drowsiness, atropine-like
Child: 1.25 mg/kg/dose PO or IM, qid	Liquid: 12.5 mg/4 ml	
Adult: 50–100 mg/dose PO or IM qid, 100 mg PR qid	Tablets: 50 mg	
	Suppository: 100 mg	
Cyclizine (Marezine)*	Injection: 50 mg/ml	Drowsiness, atropine-like
Child (6–10 yrs): 1 mg/kg/dose PO or IM tid	Tablets: 50 mg	
Adult: 50 mg q 4–6 h		
Dopamine Antagonists		
Chlorpromazine (Thorazine)	Injection: 25 mg/ml	Anticholinergic > extrapyramidal, sedation, dysphoria, orthostatic hypotension, lowered seizure threshold
Child: 0.5 mg/kg/dose IM q 6 h, 1 mg/kg/dose PR q 6 h	Syrup: 10 mg/5 cc	
Adult: 25–50 mg/dose IM or 100 mg PR q 6 h	Oral concentrate: 30 mg/cc	
	Tablets: 10, 25, 50, and 100 mg	
	Suppository: 25 and 100 mg	
Prochlorperazine (Compazine)	Injection: 5 mg/ml	Extrapyramidal > anticholinergic, sedation, dysphoria, orthostatic hypotension, lowered seizure threshold
Child (>10 kg): 0.05 mg/kg IM q 6 h or 0.1 mg/kg PR or PO q 6 h	Syrup: 5 mg/5 cc	
Adult: 5–10 mg/dose IM or PO q 6 h or 25 mg PR bid	Oral concentrate: 10 mg/cc	
	Suppository: 2.5, 5 & 25 mg	
Metoclopramide (Reglan)	Injection: 5 mg/ml	Extrapyramidal, restlessness, sedation, lowered seizure threshold
Child: 0.1 mg/kg/dose PO, IM, or IV q 6 h	Syrup: 5 mg/5 cc	
Adult: 10 mg PO, IM, or IV q 6 h	Tablets: 10 mg	
Miscellaneous		
Trimethobenzamide (Tigan)	Suppository: 100 and 200 mg	Phenothiazine-like
Child: 100 mg PR, qid		
Adult: 200 mg PR, qid		

* Manufacturer's warning: Safety and efficacy in children have not been established.

amine oxidase inhibitors, or tricyclic antidepressants. Domperidone is not yet available in the United States but shows promise as an antiemetic motility agent. Its effect on gastrointestinal motility is similar to that of metoclopramide, but it does not enter the central nervous system as readily and is therefore less likely to cause dystonic reactions.

The pharmacologic properties of trimethobenzamide (Tigan) are similar to those of phenothiazine; it acts on the CTZ, is not useful in labyrinthine disturbances, and may cause drowsiness, extrapyramidal reactions, and lowering of the seizure threshold.

Emetrol, a mixture of glucose, fructose, and orthophosphoric acid, is available without prescription. Its alleged but unproved efficacy is said to result from lessening of stomach motility caused by the presence of a hypertonic sugar solution in the stomach; it should be taken undiluted. A placebo effect may be its most important action.

Emetrol's chief virtue is its safety; it has no systemic pharmacologic action, and it won't suppress nausea and vomiting due to serious organic disease. Table 1 summarizes the dosages and side effects of some common antiemetic drugs.

Specific Entities

Motion Sickness. The combination of scopolamine and amphetamine is most potent for the prophylaxis and treatment of motion sickness but is rarely, if ever, indicated in pediatrics because of its side effects. The antihistamines promethazine (Phenergan, Remsed), dimenhydrinate (Dramamine), and cyclizine (Marezine), in descending order of potency, suffice. The first dose should be given prophylactically $\frac{1}{2}$–1 hour prior to embarkation; further doses should be administered as needed. Side effects are somnolence and atropine-like. These drugs are appropriate for management of vertigo, nausea, and vomiting in other disorders of labyrinthine function. Persistent vomiting may necessitate intravenous fluids and electrolyte replacement.

Acute Vomiting Illness. Suppression of nausea and vomiting may be helpful in the management of acute, self-limited gastroenteritis. Antihistamine drugs are less potent than dopamine antagonists. One dose of chlorpromazine intramuscularly or by rectal suppository may allow the patient to resume oral intake of fluids and antipyretics and get some needed sleep. The risk of Reye's syndrome and meningitis must be considered prior to the use of this potentially hepatotoxic, soporific agent, and the patient's course should be monitored closely with the differential diagnosis of vomiting in mind. Fluids such as ice chips, Pedialyte, and Infalite are preferable to hypertonic fluids or fluids containing fat when oral intake is resumed. Intravenous fluids are necessary for seriously dehydrated children and when attempts at oral rehydration fail.

Functional Vomiting Disorders. Three vomiting syndromes that occur in infancy may mimic organic disease; two of them produce organic complications. They are innocent vomiting, nervous vomiting, and infant rumination syndrome.

Innocent vomiting occurs in 20% of healthy infants. They may vomit a small amount or a projectile gush, but the vomitus usually does not contain bile or blood and there is no sign of pain, nausea, or other distress. The vomiting is not lessened when the patient is upright and does not occur more frequently when the patient is supine, in contradistinction to the vomiting of pathologic gastroesophageal reflux. It is not relieved by changing to a protein-hydrolysate formula, as would be expected were the vomiting due to milk or soy sensitivity. There is no weight lag. Vomiting subsides by or before 12 to 18 months of age. Innocent vomiting may be due to the limited volume the infant's esophagus can accommodate during physiologic gastroesophageal reflux or to retropulsion during antral systole or pylorospasm. Management consists of reassuring the parents and continued vigilance for signs of organic disease.

Nervous vomiting is a form of nonorganic failure to thrive. The vomiting is a visceral reaction to stress or excitement and typically occurs in an infant who is intensely receptive for and reactive to environmental stimuli. The mother is typically conscientious and attentive but emotionally and physically exhausted. The reciprocity characteristic of the normal mother-infant relationship breaks down, and a vicious circle occurs in which the mother's anxiety is intensified by the infant's vomiting and weight lag and the failure of conventional antiemetic measures. She becomes less able to soothe her infant, who, in turn, reacts to the increased tension with more vomiting, fussiness,

sleeplessness, muscular tension, and episodes of opisthotonos-like arching of his back. He becomes more difficult to hold and to feed. The mother is troubled by ambivalent feelings toward her infant and becomes less tolerant of the irritability and vomiting. The mechanism of nervous vomiting may be an extension of the pylorospasm or antral dysmotility that probably causes innocent vomiting.

The diagnosis of nervous vomiting, like that of most other forms of nonorganic failure to thrive, can be confirmed only by a response to effective management. This may require an unhurried hospitalization that allows time for the weight loss trend to stop. The baby's comfort should be maximized. He should be promptly soothed when fussy and fed an undiluted, nutritious formula on demand, to satiety, even though his vomiting continues. He should be shielded from excessive excitement, especially during feedings and rest periods, which should take place in a quiet, nonalerting atmosphere. Diagnostic procedures should be spaced so as to minimize concentrated stress. Since organic and functional disorders do not preclude each other, an unbiased assessment of each patient is necessary.

Information ruling out diseases of the digestive, urinary, and central nervous systems is needed as a basis for management. Beyond that, the number and intrusiveness of diagnostic studies performed must depend on the evidence of organic disease and, equally important, on the infant's weight, vomiting, and irritability as his comfort improves. Interviews with each parent during the hospitalization permit a deeper appreciation of less apparent sources of distress that impair their ability to sense and satisfy their infant's needs. A conference with both parents at discharge elicits their questions and feelings about what was learned during the hospitalization and enhances collaboration during follow-up until symptoms resolve.

Infant rumination syndrome is a rare but potentially lethal functional vomiting disorder. Rumination is a form of self-stimulation seen in infants over 3 months of age who are unsuccessful at evoking comfort and satisfaction from their mothers. The vomiting does not occur during sleep and is lessened when the infant is engaged in social interaction. It occurs while the baby is awake, quiet, and self-absorbed. There may be other self-stimulating behaviors, such as head rolling, hand sucking, or sound making. Management of infant rumination syndrome requires that the baby receive satisfaction from the mothering environment, thereby allowing the self-stimulation habit to subside. This is best provided by a nurse or nurses maternal enough to enjoy spending time holding, interacting with, and feeding the patient; empathic enough to sense his needs and states;

and observant enough to respond early to each episode of rumination by engaging him in reciprocal interaction. A response to such a "therapeutic trial of comfort" consists of reversal of weight loss, improved hydration, and a gradual lessening of vomiting. The patient's mother may react with mixed feelings as her infant improves while cared for by a parent substitute. Good rapport between physician and parent is vital. The parents' permission should be obtained before a special nurse is employed for the purposes of helping with the demanding tasks of infant care and data collection. The nurse's role is that of helper to the physician and the mother, not didactic teacher of superior mothering techniques. The mother's own mothering often improves as her fears for her baby's life subside and she herself feels respected and cared for.

Infant rumination and nervous vomiting differ in that rumination is self-stimulating behavior that occurs in the absence of maternal responsiveness, whereas nervous vomiting is an involuntary, visceral reaction to excessive stress or excitement. Rumination begins beyond three months of age, after the infant becomes developmentally capable of self-stimulation, whereas nervous vomiting may begin during the first month of life. The mothers of ruminators tend to be emotionally distant and there is a poverty of interaction with the infant. Mothers of nervous vomitors interact attentively but dyssynchronously with their babys' cues so that their responses heighten rather than lessen tension.

Adult-type rumination is rare in neuropsychiatrically normal children. It typically presents in a child who habitually brings up into his mouth food eaten during a meal 1–2 hours before. He chews and reswallows, losing none from his mouth. Adult-type rumination does not seem to cause esophagitis, weight loss, or distress to the child, although it may be very distressing to his parents. It is an otherwise harmless habit. Theoretically, it should be lessened by metoclopramide, but beware of using a potent pharmacologic agent in an escalating power struggle between a parent and a child unwilling to give up this habit.

Oral-defensive vomiting occurs in infants and children old enough to resist spoon feedings they do not want. Individuals of any age may vomit involuntarily as a reaction to food they "can't stomach" or food they might enjoy but for their feeling that eating it is an obligation they are powerless to resist. Management consists of discovering what motivates the parents to feed coercively, relieving their fears, and having a reflective discussion about how their efforts to get their child to eat might jeopardize rather than protect his nutritional well-being.

Contentious vomiting occurs during anger caused by someone the child knows loves and cares for him. The struggles about independence and control characteristic of the "terrible two's" trigger intense emotions. When a child vomits during conflict with his parents, he soon realizes that this accidental occurrence gives them pause. They may view screaming and kicking as "behavior" but vomiting as a symptom of illness. This reflexive vomiting tends to be conditioned and reinforced by the parents' response to it; at first, it's merely part of the autonomic events during the conflict, but soon it acquires purpose. Such vomiting may be a chief complaint of distressed parents concerned that their child may be sick, and worried, too, by a feared loss of control in setting limits for their young child. Management aims at reassuring them that the vomiting neither results from nor causes organic disease and discovering and helping to resolve the aspects of the power struggle that are unnecessary or might be better handled with more flexibility. The vomiting begins to disappear when it ceases to frighten or anger the parents.

Two kinds of consciously self-induced vomiting are encountered in older children and adolescents, *vomiting as an act of malingering* and *factitious vomiting*. Malingering is done to deceive parents or other authorities in order to gain something or to be relieved of some obligation. Vomiting as an act of malingering ceases as soon as the manipulative behavior stops working.

Factitious vomiting, exemplified by the bulimic patient, is quite different from malingering. There is a compulsion to vomit and increased anxiety if vomiting is interdicted. The patient may acknowledge the harmfulness of her vomiting, yet she persists because it is too difficult for her to stop. Management ultimately requires psychiatric efforts at uncovering and ameliorating the unconscious motives that fuel the compulsion to vomit. Until this succeeds, surveillance for potassium deficits, Mallory-Weiss tears, gastric perforation, and other injury is necessary.

Children with *the cyclic vomiting syndrome* usually experience their first episode between 2 and 9 years of age, although onset during adolescence is not uncommon. Episodes tend to be stereotyped and self-limited, typically begin during the night or on arising, and last 12 to 48 hours, although some have symptoms for as little as a few hours and others for as long as 10 days. Crampy diarrhea and/or mild fever and/or headache may occur during vomiting episodes. Attacks recur fairly regularly in two thirds of the patients and at irregular intervals in one third. Recurrences may be more often than weekly or less than yearly. The majority of patients can identify specific phenomena that trigger attacks, most commonly, noxious emotional experiences, non-noxious excitement such as birthdays and vacations, and colds or flus.

Cyclic vomiting is probably a manifestation of migraine diathesis. The diagnosis is made clinically since there are no laboratory or radiologic markers of this disorder.

There is no curative treatment for cyclic vomiting syndrome. Fortunately, it tends to remit in most patients during adolescence or early adulthood. Establishing the diagnosis is, in itself, therapeutic because it relieves the child and family of the fears caused by such dramatic, incapacitating symptoms. Patients with episodes lasting no more than 1 or 2 days seldom develop severe fluid or electrolyte deficits. Chlorpromazine is sedative and antiemetic and may be given intramuscularly or by suppository pending spontaneous resolution of the attack. If vomiting episodes recur with predictable regularity, antiemetic drugs may be used prophylactically, e.g., 1 Combid spansule at bedtime on the night prior to the expected attack. If acute anxiety seems to be a major precipitant, the occasional use of an anxiolytic agent might be beneficial. Psychotherapy for chronically anxious children is helpful if practicable. Intravenous fluids may be given on an in-patient or out-patient basis to prevent severe fluid and electrolyte deficits during episodes lasting more than a day or two.

Indolent nausea without vomiting, diminished food intake, or weight loss is a chief complaint of some older children and adolescents who are chronically anxious. This symptom is usually functional. Management is directed at the underlying emotional distress.

Constipation and Encopresis

MELVIN D. LEVINE, M.D.

Children are said to be constipated when defecation is inordinately difficult or when the event occurs too infrequently. Commonly the stools are hard and may be difficult to pass. While occasional periods of infrequent or difficult elimination are normal occurrences in childhood, *chronic* constipation can be a source of discomfort, inconvenience, and anguish. Longstanding retention of stool can lead to encopresis, in which a functional megacolon or megarectum develops secondary to obstipation, with resultant loss of control or fecal incontinence, commonly encountered in school children.

Most children with chronic constipation have no other organic pathology. However, in rare instances chronic constipation can be a sign of an anatomic, neurologic, or metabolic disorder. Possible are various forms of imperforate anus in the newborn, sometimes accompanied by vulvar or perineal fistulas. Atopic anus also can impair defecation. Myelomeningocele and other spinal cord defects commonly are associated with this disorder. Although relatively rare, Hirschsprung's disease (aganglionic megacolon) is probably the most widely publicized neurogenic cause of constipation. It is particularly unusual to diagnose Hirschsprung's disease in a school-age child. Metabolic causes include hypocalcemia and hypothyroidism. Certain medications can cause infrequent bowel movements or hard stools. One example is methylphenidate (Ritalin), commonly used to treat attention deficits.

If all of the above organic causes of constipation are ruled out, it is inappropriate to assume that the problem is "psychogenic." Most cases represent neither organic nor psychiatric illness, but rather, a dysfunction, a bad habit, or a constitutional tendency toward sluggish bowel performance. Dietary factors may aggravate the process, but are seldom the sole cause.

MANAGEMENT

Newborn and Infancy. It is during the early months of life that the clinician must be most vigilant to possible anatomical causes of constipation that may require surgical intervention. In particular, Hirschsprung's disease may present at this time, often with symptoms of intestinal obstruction or necrotizing enterocolitis. The treatment of choice following appropriate diagnostic work-up generally is a colostomy followed by a pull-through operation late in the first year of life.

The newborn and infancy period also is a common time for symptoms of constitutional constipation to emerge. Treatment should be as noninvasive as possible, in order to prevent the induction of an "anal stamp," a permanent psychological scar associated with the later development of encopresis. The physician should emphasize to parents that the condition is benign, making every effort to minimize their anxiety. Frequent anal manipulations, such as digital disimpaction and the use of suppositories, should be discouraged. In mild cases, parents should be reassured and no therapy instituted. However, if the infant is uncomfortable and is producing consistently hard stools, one can add dark Karo syrup to feedings. Approximately 1–2 teaspoons per feeding generally is adequate. As the baby's diet becomes increasingly diversified, the need for such intervention diminishes. In rare cases, a mild laxative, such as milk of magnesia, may be needed. If so, use as little as possible (starting with $\frac{1}{2}$ tsp a day).

Some infants have considerable discomfort on defecation. A mother may note that her baby constantly strains to have a bowel movement. In some instances, the infant is actually struggling *not to have one!* Such early evidence of voluntary withholding should be noted. Typically, the affected infant hyperextends his legs and clenches his fists while defecating. This may result from discomfort during bowel movements. The physician should ascertain that there are no problems in the perianal area causing painful defecation. The most common offender is chronic diaper dermatitis. Appropriate management of any such condition therefore is important in preventing habitual voluntary withholding.

The Toddler and Preschool Child. Training is the most critical event related to bowel function during this period. Some toddlers develop an aversion to defecation because of coercive or compulsively executed training. Improper training methods can result in constipation. For example, some children have difficulty defecating with their feet suspended in air. They can benefit from the use of telephone books or some other kinds of support while learning to use a toilet. Constipation related to training sometimes must be managed by postponing or modifying the training routine. Some toddlers and preschool children acquire an irrational fear of the toilet. Apprehension may center on the possibility of falling in or encountering "fish monsters" lurking in the bowl.

This can also be a time during which the manifestations of constitutional constipation seem to worsen. Treatment should remain nonaggressive, avoiding especially therapies that entail anal manipulation. Dietary alterations introducing high bulk foods (fruits, vegetables, bran-containing items) may be helpful. If this is ineffective, stool softeners should be given in small doses. Maltsupex is a palatable example. If this fails, small amounts of a mild laxative (such as Senokot granules, $\frac{1}{2}$ tsp a day) can be instituted.

The School Years. There are many reasons why schoolchildren manifest chronic constipation. The phenomenon may be part of a continuing history of stool retention and poor bowel function that began in infancy or the toddler years. Or school itself may be an etiologic or at least aggravating factor. Some youngsters are reluctant to use school bathrooms because they lack privacy. They postpone defecation until safe, in the privacy of home. Some youngsters seem unable to "afford" to do this. That is, although they decline to use the bathrooms at school, they lose the urge when they get home. Over time, these children become constipated, and many develop a functional megacolon. Other schoolchildren acquire constipation because of a frenetic lifestyle. They race to meet the school bus each morning and are tightly scheduled all day. Homework, play, and alluring television shows occupy them until bedtime, leaving little time for something as trivial and uninteresting as defecation. Such children make relatively few trips to the bathroom, and when they do their defecation is partial or incomplete because of their haste.

Other youngsters have significant attention deficits. These children are overactive, distractible, impulsive, and impersistent at tasks. They seldom finish anything they start, including defecation. They too ultimately develop chronic constipation.

An understanding of the pathophysiology of the schoolchild's bowel disorder can aid in counseling and management. Alterations in life style, provisions for more privacy of bathroom use in school, and various forms of behavior modification may be critical. In treating schoolchildren with chronic constipation, one should distinguish between those with the complication of incontinence (i.e., encopresis) and those who are fully continent.

SIMPLE CONSTIPATION (WITHOUT INCONTINENCE). Schoolchildren with uncomplicated constipation can be subdivided into those with overt symptoms and those with "occult stool retention." The latter group can be insidious and difficult to diagnose. Occult stool retention is one of the most common causes of recurrent abdominal pain. The diagnosis is often missed, since there may be no history of infrequent or hard stools. A plain supine x-ray of the abdomen in such instances reveals abundant retained feces, the removal of which often is associated with pain relief.

Most cases of uncomplicated chronic constipation can be alleviated by educating the child to use the toilet regularly and to remain in the bathroom long enough to achieve complete emptying. Laxatives such as senna (Senokot, 1 tablet a day) or danthron (Modane, 1 tablet a day) often are helpful. Treatment should be continued for 3–4 weeks. If symptoms persist, the child may benefit from the ongoing use of light mineral oil (1–2 tablespoons twice a day). In more severe or protracted cases, treatment may need to be more vigorous and long lasting. The regimen suggested for encopresis is recommended under these circumstances.

Encopresis. It is not unusual for schoolchildren with chronic constipation to develop encopresis. Varying degrees of severity are encountered, ranging from multiple large accidents per day to occasional bouts of incontinence or steady but slight leakage. Virtually all children with encopresis have at least intermittent constipation. Although emotional factors may complicate the picture, in most instances encopresis (like enuresis) is not caused by emotional factors. However, children who have suffered from this condition over a long period may become secondarily depressed, anxious, and socially withdrawn. Peer interactions, family harmony, self-esteem, and school performance can deteriorate as a result.

Most cases of encopresis ultimately resolve spontaneously; however, medical treatment can accelerate the cure and thereby diminish the suffering and psychological toll. Management of this condition can be divided into its component steps. The treatment is summarized in Table 1. The following is an elaboration on the steps involved:

1. DEMYSTIFICATION. The first step in treatment is education of the child and parents. The physician should explain normal colonic function, using drawings or diagrams. There can be discussion of the ways in which intestinal musculature propels stool, with consideration of the role of nerves within that musculature in providing signals indi-cating the need to defecate. It should be explained that some children go through a period when they do not completely empty their bowels. This results in the progressive accumulation of stool with the consequent chronic stretching of intestinal musculature and the loss of tone and strength. It also should be pointed out that the stretching results in diminished feedback from nerves, so that children fail to experience the urge or sensation of needing to move their bowels. A plain film of the child's abdomen can then be reviewed with the

Table 1.   TREATMENT OF ENCOPRESIS

Treatment Phase		Treatment Program	Comments
Initial Counseling		1. Education and "demystification" 2. Removal of blame 3. Establishment and explanation of treatment plan	Include drawings, review of colonic function, joint observation of x-rays
Initial Catharsis	Inpatient	1. High normal saline enemas (750 cc bid) 3–7 days 2. Biscodyl (Dulcolax) suppositories bid 3–7 days 3. Use of bathroom for 15 minutes after each meal	Patient admitted when: 1) retention is very severe 2) home compliance likely to be poor 3) parents prefer admission 4) parental administration of enemas is inadvisable psychologically

	At Home	1. In moderate to severe retention, 3–4 cycles as follows:
		  a. Day 1—hypophosphate enemas (Fleet's Adult) twice
		  b. Day 2—biscodyl (Dulcolax) suppositories twice
		  c. Day 3—biscodyl (Dulcolax) tablet once
		2. In mild retention, senna or danthron, one tablet daily for one to two weeks
			1) Dosages or frequency may need alteration if child experiences excessive discomfort
			2) Admission should be considered if there is inadequate yield

		Follow-up abdominal x-ray to confirm adequate catharsis	
Maintenance		1. Child sits on toilet twice a day at same times each day for 10 minutes each time 2. Light mineral oil (at least 2 tablespoons) twice a day for at least 6 months 3. Multiple vitamins, 2 a day, between mineral oil doses 4. High roughage diet 5. Use of an oral laxative (e.g., Senokot) for 1–2 mo daily in moderate or severe cases	1) A kitchen timer may be helpful 2) A chart with stars for sitting may be good for children under eight 3) Bathroom reading encouraged 4) Mineral oil may be put in juice or Coke or any other medium 5) Vitamins to compensate for alleged problems with absorption secondary to mineral oil 6) Diet should be applied, but not to the point of coercion

Follow-up		1. Visits every 4–10 weeks, depending on severity, need for support, compliance, and associated symptoms
		2. Telephone availability to adjust doses when needed
		3. In case of relapse:
		  a. check compliance
		  b. trial of oral laxative (e.g., Senokot) for 1–2 weeks
		  c. adjust dosage of mineral oil
		4. Counseling and/or referral for associated psychosocial and developmental issues
			1) Duration of treatment program may be as long as 2–3 years or as short as 6 months
			2) Signs of relapse:
			  a) excessive oil leakage
			  b) large caliber stools
			  c) abdominal pain
			  d) decreased frequency of defecation
			  e) soiling
			3) Physician should spend time alone with child
			4) In cases slow to respond, physician should sustain optimism: persistence cures almost all cases eventually

All dosages and frequencies are calculated for an average-sized 7-year-old child. Appropriate adjustments should be made for smaller or larger patients.

patient and parents. The physician can point out the accumulation of "rocks." It then is explained that the good thing about muscles is that they can be restored when they become weak. The treatment strategy is presented. It is pointed out that it is critical to begin treatment by establishing an entirely empty colon. After this, the goal will be to keep it as empty as possible over a period of months so that the stretching can stop and the bowel can gradually return to its normal caliber, with restoration of muscle tone and feeling. It is important to point out that many other youngsters have this problem. A unique aspect of encopresis is that it is rare for any child who has it to have heard of any other who is similarly afflicted. Much anxiety can be relieved through demystification and the revelation that this is not an unusual condition. It also is helpful to emphasize that the problem is nobody's fault and that having it does not mean that a child is crazy, lazy, or immoral.

2. INITIAL CATHARSIS. A complete clean out is critically important at the beginning of treatment. In most instances this can be performed on an outpatient basis. In severe cases or when there is a very disturbed parent-child relationship, an inpatient program can be instituted. The components of these are summarized in Table 1. Following the initial catharsis the child should have a follow-up plain x-ray of the abdomen to establish that a good cleanout has been achieved. If this shows little or no improvement, the initial catharsis may need to be prolonged. If one begins a maintenance program following an incomplete cleanout, exacerbations are much more likely to occur.

3. MAINTENANCE. After the initial catharsis the youngster should be put on a laxative (Senokot, 1–2 tablets per day) or danthrone (Modane, 1–2 tablets per day). A stool softener should also be used. Most common and effective is light mineral oil. An average dose is about 2 tablespoons twice a day (for an average 7–8 year old). The flavor can be disguised with juice or soft drink. Light mineral oil should never be used when the bowel is impacted, since the lubricant itself is likely to leak around blockages, with the subsequent passage of a gold-colored liquid, which can be disconcerting as it streams down the legs of a schoolchild. In fact, if at any point during treatment excessive leakage of mineral oil is reported, one can assume that the youngster is again becoming retentive. In most cases after about a month of maintenance therapy, the laxative can be tapered off or discontinued. The stool softener should be continued for at least 6 months.

4. RETRAINING. A critical part of the treatment is retraining and toilet utilization. The child should be told to visit the bathroom twice a day at the same times each day, preferably after breakfast and supper. A minimum of 10 minutes should be spent therein. The youngster is told that he can read or listen to the radio, but he should try to empty out his bowel completely each time. In children under eight, it sometimes is helpful to set up a system of rewards, using a star chart, suitably embellished for each visit (with extra credit given for success).

It should be emphasized to parents that it is inappropriate to punish a child for having an accident. However, refusal to take medication or resistance to sitting on the toilet should constitute offenses. The child is not to blame for messing, but is to blame for not trying to do something about it. Following an accident a child should be required to clean himself. Underwear should be disposed of properly, although the child should not be expected to wash it, which could be interpreted as punitive.

For the child who soils himself in school, some arrangements may need to be made to provide a change of clothing in the nurse's office. Some youngsters may require a third visit to the bathroom, one that takes place in school. A sufficiently private setting for this should be sought. Most children feel strongly that they do not want school personnel to know about their problem, but most are agreeable to having one schoolperson aware of it. Their greatest fear is that peers will discover this most important secret. Therefore, every effort must be made to sustain their privacy.

5. FOLLOW-UP AND MONITORING. Encopresis is a chronic condition. The pediatrician should establish a strong alliance with the youngster and see him regularly (the frequency depending upon the severity and chronicity of the problem). During return visits, the physician should examine the child's abdomen and talk about management while alone with the youngster. There can be joint discussions with parents. Medication needs to be "titrated." When exacerbations occur, laxative therapy should be increased or resumed. It is important that parents and the pediatrician be aware that in many cases several years are required for restoration of normal bowel function. Although this can be frustrating, persistence has its rewards. In severe treatment-resistant cases, the physician should periodically review the condition and consider the possibility of complicating psychosocial factors. Referral for a psychological or psychiatric evaluation may help, especially when the child seems to be noncompliant and unable to discuss the problem, or when there is evidence that serious family problems are interfering with management. Surgical consultation should be sought in treatment-resistant cases in which aganglionic megacolon is suspected. However, the latter is extremely rare among schoolchildren, whereas slowly responsive encopresis is a common condition.

Acute and Chronic Nonspecific Diarrhea Syndromes

DORSEY M. BASS, M.D.,
and W. ALLAN WALKER, M.D.

Diarrhea, defined as excessive loss of fluid and electrolytes in the stools, is one of the most frequent problems confronting the pediatrician in clinical practice. In developing countries diarrhea is the leading cause of death in young children and in the West it remains the second leading reason for "sick" out-patient pediatric visits and nonsurgical pediatric admissions. Although the differential diagnosis of diarrhea is extensive, a brief but complete history and physical exam can usually exclude serious specific causes.

ACUTE GASTROENTERITIS

This usually self-limited illness occurs most commonly during the winter months in children less than 3 years old. The most common cause is rotavirus. The two mainstays of therapy are to treat and prevent dehydration and to avoid excessive nutritional compromise.

In recent years a large number of studies have demonstrated the efficacy of oral electrolyte solutions as therapy for dehydration secondary to diarrhea of any cause. The solutions used in these studies have generally contained higher electrolyte concentrations than the older commercial products. The World Health Organization oral rehydration solution (WHO ORS) contains sodium at 90 mmol/l and glucose at 111 mmol/l, while the older commercial formulations contained less than half the sodium and more than twice the glucose concentration of the WHO ORS. Newer commercial formulations (e.g., Pedialyte, Infalyte) are patterned after the WHO ORS, which is based on better understanding of glucose/sodium–coupled water transport in the small intestine.

These commercial solutions or WHO ORS can be given ad libitum to infants and toddlers with the addition of one bottle of plain or flavored water for every two bottles of solution. Patients with more severe dehydration may benefit from more specific instructions or even supervised administration in the clinic or in hospital. Patients in shock, with persistent severe vomiting, and those who do no respond to oral therapy need intravenous fluids, but oral therapy should be substituted as soon as possible.

The prevention of excessive nutritional compromise is especially important in the infant with acute diarrhea. Prolonged bowel rest or hypocaloric clear liquid diets can lead to starvation stools, and the malnutrition-dehydration cycle can rapidly accelerate into intractable diarrhea of infancy. Gener-ally, some kind of feeding can be started as soon as rehydration is completed. As lactase deficiency is very common in this setting, small, frequent feedings of soy formula are often successful. In more severe cases or in very young infants, a hydrolyzed formula such as Pregestimil may be indicated. Stool output, pH, and reducing substances can serve as guidelines to advancing the feedings.

Antibiotics have no role in the treatment of acute diarrhea in the absence of documented bacterial infection. Likewise, antiemetics and antiperistaltic medications are more likely to cause toxicity than provide any real benefit. Kaolin compounds merely change the cosmetic appearance of the stools and may camouflage significant fluid losses.

CHRONIC NONSPECIFIC DIARRHEA

Chronic nonspecific diarrhea is a benign symptom complex seen in healthy toddlers with normal growth and development. It is probably the pediatric equivalent of irritable colon syndrome. Many cases remit spontaneously with toilet training, but others continue for years.

The mainstay of treatment is reassurance of the parents. The child's continuing good growth should be stressed by the doctor at every visit. High-residue, high-fiber diets or the use of psyllium compounds can provide some symptomatic relief.

Intractable Diarrhea of Infancy

JEREMIAH LEVINE, M.D.,
and W. ALLAN WALKER, M.D.

Intractable diarrhea of infancy is a syndrome defined as diarrhea occurring in the first 3 months of life that persists for longer than 2 weeks with negative cultures. Because the diarrhea occurs during a period of high caloric need, those children affected can quickly become severely ill. Although some of these infants have an underlying disease entity that accounts for their illness, the vast majority of patients have no predisposing factor. In addition to the immediate concerns with regard to dehydration and electrolyte imbalances, these children almost universally suffer from malnutrition and its consequences. These infants often have severe small bowel histologic abnormalities as well as secondary enzyme deficiencies. The nutritional deficiency that is invariably present will prevent intestinal regeneration and prolong the time to complete recovery; therefore, aggressive nutritional support is needed in all patients. Mortality rates have declined from 45% to 5–7%, largely owing to the proper use of total parenteral nutrition and nasogastric enteral feeds.

The choice between enteral and parenteral alimentation should be based on the patient's clinical status as well as biochemical parameters such as total protein and serum albumin. In infants who have only mild disease and are not malnourished, a trial of an elemental diet such as Pregestimil may be attempted after a day of clear liquids such as Pedialyte. In patients who are moderately ill, hospitalization is indicated. The first 24–48 hours should be devoted to correction of acidosis, dehydration, and electrolyte disorders while providing the child with a period of bowel rest. If the child has only mild malnutrition and improves with resolution of the diarrhea, an elemental diet may again be attempted, starting with bolus diluted formula (5 kcal/30 ml) that is gradually increased both in concentration and in volume over the next few days. Many infants will not tolerate rapid increases in the volume or concentration of the formula. It is therefore important to follow daily weight, stool volume and stool-reducing substances, and pH.

If an infant has any difficulty in advancing feeds, peripheral alimentation should be initiated. A 10% dextrose and 2% amino acid solution can be used at a rate that, along with enteral feeds, fulfills daily fluid requirements. A 10% Intralipid solution may also be given and can be slowly increased to give 1–4 gm/kg/day in additional calories. While the infant is on peripheral alimentation, the formula is initially increased in concentration. Once full-strength formula is tolerated, the volume is slowly increased and the IV fluids are tapered accordingly.

If the child has moderate malnutrition on admission, does not resolve the diarrhea during the period of bowel rest, or relapses when bolus enteral feeds are attempted, continuous nasogastric feeding should be initiated. Initially 0.5 ml/kg/hour of 5 kcal/30 ml Pregestimil may be given; gradually both the volume and the concentration can be increased. Peripheral intravenous fluids should again be reduced as the volume of the enteral feeds is increased. Some infants are not able to tolerate full-volume enteral feeds, and it may be necessary to increase the caloric density of the formula to 24–27 kcal/30 ml. This can be done by adding glucose polymers and medium-chain triglyceride oil to the formula as well as by concentrating the formula. In special circumstances, such as fluid restriction, formulas can be increased to greater than 30 kcal/30 ml. This is usually accomplished by concentrating the formula for an additional 3 kcal/30 ml, adding medium-chain triglycerides for another 3 kcal/30 ml, and adding glucose polymers (polycose) for the remainder.

Once continuous feeds are well tolerated, the peripheral alimentation may be stopped. It may be necessary to maintain the infant on nasogastric feeds for several weeks before bolus feeds are cautiously reintroduced. If continuous feeds are not tolerated, a therapeutic trial of cholestyramine* at a dosage of 4–8 gm/day may be helpful. Cholestyramine is a nonabsorbable quaternary exchange resin capable of binding bile acids and endotoxin. Side effects include hyperchloremic acidosis, and electrolytes should be followed closely. In addition, steatorrhea occurs secondary to the loss of bile salts. Aluminum hydroxide (Amphojel) also has bile salt–binding activity and reduces intestinal motility; it has also been used in infants with chronic diarrhea. The starting dose of 150 mg/kg/day in six divided doses may be increased slowly and the patient observed for a therapeutic response. Side effects include antacid bezoar, aluminum intoxication, and steatorrhea. Finally, loperamide† (1 mg/kg in 4 divided doses) has been reported to be of benefit in some patients with severe diarrhea. Side effects include ileus, and the drug should not be used in patients with infectious diarrhea or electrolyte imbalances.

In the child who is severely ill at presentation or who is not able to tolerate continuous enteral feeds, total parenteral nutrition should be started. Initially, peripheral alimentation with lipids can be used, but if adequate calories cannot be provided through this route a central venous catheter is required. Once this catheter is placed under sterile conditions into the internal jugular or subclavian vein, a solution containing 10% dextrose is gradually increased to a maximum of 20–25%. Amino acids (2–4%) are also added. Intralipid (10–20%) is also given daily over an 18–20 hour period to provide 1–4 gm/kg/day. Trace elements and vitamins should be added on a daily basis, and serum electrolytes, glucose, minerals, and triglycerides should be carefully monitored.

Central hyperalimentation may be needed for several weeks before enteral feeds can be tolerated. During this period, small-volume continuous feeds of dilute elemental formulas should be given, since enteric feedings have a trophic effect on the hypoplastic intestinal epithelium and have been shown to induce a more rapid return of disacharidases such as maltase and sucrase. Caloric requirements in these children with severe malnutrition may approach 200 kcal/kg. Although initially one should strive to deliver 100–120 kcal/kg, daily weights and weekly anthropometric measurements are essential guides to caloric needs in all these infants.

Once an elemental diet is tolerated with adequate weight gain, the baby may be discharged with close

---

* Manufacturer states that dosage for infants and children has not been established.

† Manufacturer's warning: Safety and efficacy for use in children under 12 years of age have not been established.

follow-up. Hypoallergenic feeds are gradually reintroduced, but milk protein and lactose should be avoided for at least 6 months. It is not unusual for severely affected children to require hospitalization for several months. Support for the family and adequate stimulation of the infant are also important during this slow process. Fortunately, with critical attention to the nutritional rehabilitation of these infants and with prevention of infection and electrolyte disturbances, the overall prognosis is quite good. Early reversal of the malnourished state is the most important factor contributing to a favorable outcome.

Irritable Bowel Syndrome

ROY PROUJANSKY, M.D.,
and W. ALLAN WALKER, M.D.

Irritable bowel syndrome refers to a common clinical entity characterized by recurrent abdominal pain which may frequently be associated with alternating constipation and diarrhea. Although many adult patients date the onset of their symptoms to childhood, the diagnosis is infrequently entertained by pediatricians.

An approach to therapy in irritable bowel syndrome is hampered by the lack of specific diagnostic criteria for this syndrome. The nonspecific nature of the symptoms of abdominal pain, diarrhea, and/or constipation generates a broad differential diagnosis. Therapeutic intervention is often delayed then because of the clinician's pursuit of other treatable causes for the patient's symptoms. Nevertheless, careful history, physical exam, and a few screening laboratory tests should lead either to a specific diagnosis of irritable bowel syndrome or suggest alternative pathophysiologic mechanisms for the patient's complaints.

The history and physical should be directed toward excluding any other organic pathology that may present with similar symptoms. The presence of anorexia, nausea, vomiting, weight loss, rectal bleeding, fever, or other constitutional symptoms should be sought. A long history of symptoms without documented evidence of detriment to the patient is supportive of a diagnosis of irritable bowel syndrome. The physical exam should include careful abdominal palpation and a rectal exam with stool guaiac testing to exclude anorectal pathology. A pelvic exam should be included in the evaluation of the adolescent female. A normal complete blood count with differential, sedimentation rate, urinalysis, and urine culture help to support the clinical impression. Stool examination for ova and parasites, and abdominal or pelvic ultrasound should be performed in selected patients. A lactose breath hydrogen test may help exclude lactose intolerance, which may present with a similar clinical picture. Barium contrast radiography or endoscopy rarely lead to a specific alternate diagnosis when the history, physical, and screening laboratory tests support a diagnosis of irritable bowel syndrome.

Once the diagnosis of irritable bowel syndrome has been established, a critical step has been made in terms of treatment. Reassurance that this is the problem and that serious underlying pathology does not exist will help relieve hidden anxieties that may be aggravating the patient's symptoms. Attempts should also be made to reduce other stresses in the patient's environment. If these can not be identified in the history, keeping a diary of symptoms may assist the patient, parents, and physician in determining sources of stress.

Dietary manipulations are of benefit in some patients but should be carefully supervised. Vigorous dietary restriction is inappropriate for the growing child or adolescent and is often ineffective. Specific foods that the patient identifies as being associated with symptoms should be avoided on a trial basis. Some patients will improve after elimination of caffeinated or carbonated beverages. Sugar-free products containing sorbitol may also be causative agents. An increase in dietary fiber may help to regularize stooling habits in the patient with constipation or loose stools.

Finally, regular follow-up is an essential component of treatment. New symptoms or findings may suggest an alternate diagnosis or intercurrent problem. Occasionally, patients may embark on a trial of home remedies that may be detrimental to the overall therapeutic plan.

Recurrent Abdominal Pain

JEFFREY A. BILLER, M.D.

Recurrent abdominal pain is a common complaint in childhood. As defined by Apley, the term refers to three or more discrete epsiodes of debilitating abdominal pain over at least a three-month period. Using this definition, recurrent abdominal pain is reported in as many as 12–30% of school-aged girls (peak age, 9–10 years) and 9–12% of school-aged boys. In only about 5–10% of these patients, however, is the pain found to have an underlying organic etiology, divided evenly between urogenital and gastrointestinal disorders.

A thorough history and physical examination are essential in helping to distinguish between organic and nonorganic disease. Details relating to the location (diffuse or localized), severity (incapacitating or mild), radiation of pain, time of occurrence (in school, nocturnal, weekdays versus weekends, during menstrual cycle), and relationship with meals and particular foods may be helpful. In our experience, pain that wakes up the patient from sleep is more consistent with an organic etiology. Associated symptoms, including weight loss, constipation, headache, and nausea and vomiting are nonspecific. A detailed review of systems and medical history may suggest a site of organic involvement. A high incidence of abdominal pain is found in parents of patients with pain with a functional etiology. Information regarding the ethnic background and history of migraine or seizures in the family may also provide some assistance in the diagnosis. A detailed social history is vital, with special emphasis on school performance (often requiring direct input of teachers) and parent and sibling interactions. Identification of stresses both at home (parent-parent interaction and parent-child interaction) and at school may point towards an underlying cause. On physical examination, the presence of normal growth and general well being and absence of signs of systemic or localized disease are consistent with a functional etiology. Most patients will localize their pain to the periumbilical area. The presence of localized right lower quadrant pain (consistent with appendicitis or inflammatory bowel disease) or epigastric tenderness (consistent with peptic related disease) may be more suggestive of an organic etiology.

Laboratory evaluation must be individualized for each patient given the information obtained during the history and physical examination. It is justified, however, to perform a few selected screening laboratory tests in all patients, even in those in whom no clear organic etiology is suspected. These would include a complete blood count, an erythrocyte sedimentation rate, urinalysis and culture, and stool guaiac. Further evaluation, including liver function tests, serum amylase, stool for ova and parasites, lactose breath hydrogen test, serum lead level, and radiographic studies should not become part of the routine screening evaluation in these patients. Invasive studies, including endoscopy, laparoscopy and laparotomy, should only be performed when there is clear direct evidence suggesting their usefulness. Such studies may be detrimental psychologically to many patients with nonorganic causes. Occasionally, observation of the patient in the hospital setting away from the stresses of family and school may be helpful in directing further evaluation.

Once an organic etiology is excluded, therapy must be directed toward understanding the inciting factors, stresses, and motivations for the abdominal pain. This is often not possible until all family members recognize, accept, and understand that the patient is indeed experiencing a real pain that happens not to have any underlying organic cause. Trust and open communication within the family and confidence in the pediatrician may allow the patient to focus away from the abdominal pain and more toward the underlying emotional issue. In some cases, the degree of emotional disturbance in the patient and family is so severe that more formal psychological evaluation and guidance are useful. Medications are rarely helpful in managing nonorganic abdominal pain.

Preoperative and Postoperative Care of Patients Undergoing Gastrointestinal Surgery

ROBERT T. SOPER, M.D.

PREOPERATIVE CARE

Preparing pediatric patients for operations on the gastrointestinal tract can be as simple as withholding oral fluids and food for a few hours or as complex as spending several days restoring deficits (fluids, electrolytes, blood components, vitamins, nutrition), decompressing the bowel, and administering enemas and antibiotics. The variables that dictate these extremes include the magnitude of the operation, its urgency, the segment of gastrointestinal tract to be surgically manipulated, and how ill the patient is. The ultimate aim of these preparations is to bring to the operating room a patient who is metabolically as normal as the urgency of the operation allows, with a gastrointestinal tract that can be surgically manipulated to the degree necessary to cure or ameliorate the problem being addressed. These ideals cannot always be fully achieved. This section deals only with the specifics of preoperative care as they relate to the gastrointestinal tract; the important elements of psychological care of the patient and general supportive measures are discussed elsewhere.

An empty stomach is a necessity for anyone undergoing general anesthesia. This is assured in the well patient undergoing an elective operation on the stomach or small intestine by allowing nothing to eat or drink for a certain time, usually 8 hours in the older child and adolescent and 4 hours in the newborn and infant. Elective operations on the colon often require more sophisticated preparation to empty it of stool and reduce its bacterial flora. Allowing only clear liquids by mouth for 3 days, administering oral laxatives (e.g., milk of magnesia) in appropriate doses, and giving warm saline enemas on the day preceding operation ensure an empty colon. Neomycin (0.1%) added to the enema water reduces the bacterial count in the bowel. Prophylactic broad-spectrum antibiotics given systemically from immediately before the operation until 24 hours afterward are justified when the operation involves opening the bowel.

Urgent or emergent operations on the gastrointestinal tract (e.g., in cases of intestinal obstruction, bowel perforation, or peritonitis) require more aggressive and expedient preparation of the patient. Nasogastric suction is required (to empty the stomach and decompress the small bowel) with the largest-bore tube the nose will easily accommodate. We prefer sump tubes of the Replogle, Ventrol-Levine, or Salem type. They are placed on constant suction and hand irrigated with a premeasured volume of saline every 2 hours to ensure that they remain open and functioning. A large-bore intravenous catheter is percutaneously passed to begin fluid resuscitation with electrolytes to repair deficits and replace the fluid retrieved by nasogastric suction. A urethral catheter is passed to empty the bladder and monitor urine output as a measure of the adequacy of fluid resuscitation. Almost without exception, no patient is taken to the operating room until an adequate urine output (1–1.5 cc/kg/hr) is established. Broad-spectrum antibiotics (cephalothin, gentamicin, clindamycin) are administered intravenously during resuscitation.

POSTOPERATIVE CARE

Effective decompression of the gastrointestinal tract is one of the cardinal features of care following operation upon the stomach or intestine. The most common way to achieve this is to maintain suction and periodic hand irrigation of the largest-bore sump-type (Replogle, Ventrol-Levine, or Salem) nasogastric tube the nose will comfortably accept. Correct placement is ascertained at operation, and the tube is taped into place by the anesthesiologist. The nasogastric tube may be augmented (or substituted for) by a percutaneous gastrostomy tube placed at operation if lengthy decompression is anticipated. In the patient with recurrent adhesive small bowel obstruction, a long tube may be left indwelling in the intestine to decompress and stent the bowel for 10–14 days; this tube is usually passed percutaneously and should be managed by the surgeon.

Bowel decompression is maintained until effective peristalsis returns, heralded by diminishing fluid yield from the tubes, passage of flatus or stool, and, in the stomach, a change in color of its return from bile-stained to clear gastric juice. This may take only 24 hours after a simple appendectomy or up to a week or two in more complex cases. In the greatly stressed youngster, we measure the pH of gastric fluid return and maintain it above 5.0 by instilling appropriate volumes of antacids through the tube, which is then clamped for ½ hour.

Delay in the return of effective peristalsis beyond the expected time suggests ileus, either mechanical or paralytic. This should prompt an appropriate diagnostic work-up carried out under the direction of the surgeon familiar with the details of the operation. Plain abdominal radiographs, enteroclysis studies, blood cultures, and investigations into abnormalities of fluids, electrolytes, and blood products may be necessary. Treatment is dictated by the diagnosis and may include repeat laparotomy.

Once effective peristalsis has resumed, the decompression tubes are usually removed. In reinstituting feedings, we prefer to offer the patient small, measured volumes of clear liquids every 2 hours during the waking part of the day. Intravenous fluids are continued at maintenance levels. If the clear liquids are well tolerated, they are offered ad libitum the following day, and the intravenous infusions are reduced proportionately. The next day intravenous fluids are discontinued and the diet is progressively advanced as tolerated. Care of wounds, dressings, and drains is managed by the surgical team, as are "situp" routines, respiratory therapy, urethral catheters, and antibiotic administration.

BOWEL OSTOMIES AND THEIR CARE

Small bowel stomas must be covered at all times by a small plastic collection bag that is glued to the skin immediately adjacent to the stoma. The high-volume, thin effluent can then be measured as needed, and its enzyme-rich material will be kept from contact with the skin. Small bowel fluid digests and irritates skin; collection bags will not adhere effectively to peristomal skin once it is inflamed. Most bags must be emptied several times a day, but a new bag must be applied only after leakage; one bag may last for several days. Skin irritation is a constant threat, triggered occasionally by an allergic reaction to the adherent or bag but much more commonly by poor care. Occasionally, a poorly constructed ileostomy contributes to a poorly fitting bag: too short a stomal nipple, fistulas at skin level, stricture, and so on. Surgical revision of the stoma is then in order. Irritated skin can usually be managed by custom-fitting a disk of Stomahesive, to which the bag is glued, to the peristomal skin; karaya powder absorbs moisture and protects the nooks and crannies to which a relatively stiff appliance cannot conform. In the extreme case, the patient can be nursed prone so that the effluent drips into a receptacle. A hair blower is positioned so that its warm, dry current of air blows across and quickly dries the peristomal skin. However, skin irritation is better prevented than treated, and there is no substitute for meticulous attention to detail in stomal care.

Colostomies are easier to care for than ileostomies and jejunostomies, mainly because further downstream in the bowel the effluent is thicker, smaller in volume, and less irritative to skin. Stomas of the right, transverse, and descending colon usually benefit from a snugly applied bag because of the fluid nature of the feces. The clear plastic bags now available allow the physician to confirm stomal viability visually and to measure the volume and character of the stool output. Feces emanating from a sigmoid colostomy, on the other hand, are firm and nonirritating enough not to require a bag, unless the parents feel this is easier to manage than simply letting the stool collect in a diaper worn over the area.

Parents of ostomy patients require careful instruction in the management of the stoma before the patient is discharged from hospital. We have printed instructions to help in the educational process, but there is no substitute for experience by the parents under the tutelage of a nurse who is especially skilled in ostomy care. This instruction is immensely helpful in preventing skin problems, imparting confidence and self-assurance to the parents, and fostering better acceptance of the stoma by the older patient. Local ostomy clubs should also be enlisted for the support they provide to these families.

Pylorospasm

GIULO J. BARBERO, M.D., and JOAN
DiPALMA, M.D.

Pylorospasm is a descriptive term signifying that the pylorus closes more intensely and suggests an abnormality in gastric motility and emptying. At best, pylorospasm is predominantly a clinical entity, in which no tests or studies can readily confirm a definitive diagnosis. There are two situations in which pylorospasm is suspected. First, pylorospasm is considered partially responsible for the vomiting and abdominal pain seen in peptic ulcer disease and duodenitis. In these cases, the inflammation and ulceration are documented by upper gastrointestinal radiography, endoscopy, and biopsy. Proper treatment of these disorders with a histamine antagonist and an antacid regime usually manages the accompanying pylorospasm. Another situation is that of the infant less than three months of age who presents with recurrent vomiting. Upper gastrointestinal radiography may demonstrate delayed gastric emptying. Investigations for gastroesophageal reflux, infection, and metabolic disease are negative. The impact of pylorospasm in infancy is generally not profound. It is usually more of a nuisance, the vomitus frequently soiling all surrounding clothing and furniture. Fortunately, the degree of vomiting does not produce significant caloric deprivation to impair growth in most cases. Nevertheless, growth of the infant

requires careful surveillance. Small frequent feeds may be warranted. Changes of formula composition are of little value. An antispasmodic such as Donnatal Elixir, 0.5 ml four times a day, or an atropine 1:1000 solution, one drop prior to each meal, may be helpful. Metochlopramide hydrochloride, 0.1 mg/kg/dose, has been tried with variable success. Dealing directly with parental fears and concerns is also an important component to management. Environmental factors in the etiology of this uncertain entity are unclear. However, in examining such issues nonjudgmentally and supportively with the parents, a positive therapeutic alliance can frequently occur. Usually, the vomiting symptoms are limited in time and are not protracted. There is little evidence of this entity becoming chronic, but its relationship to other gastrointestinal disorders that may occur later in life is still of some interest.

Pyloric Stenosis

GIULIO J. BARBERO, M.D., and JOAN
DiPALMA, M.D.

Pyloric stenosis is a diagnosis that is reached after careful clinical, laboratory, and, at times, radiologic investigation. Diagnosis is based on the development of forceful vomiting usually 1–3 weeks after birth. The vomiting progresses in intensity, often with small and less frequent stools. Gastric waves pass across from left to right of the upper abdomen. The palpation of a pyloric "olive" confirms the diagnosis. Ultrasound and/or x-ray of the upper gastrointestinal area shows a dilated stomach with intensive contractions, and a pyloric string sign indenting the antral lesser curvature of the stomach. Once the diagnosis of pyloric stenosis has been made, there are three major components to therapy. First, the infant must be given required restorative care. Second, the hypertrophied pyloric muscle must be corrected surgically. Finally, the patient must be supported while being allowed to reach an adequate oral intake.

Infants with pyloric stenosis can present with clinical and metabolic derangements of varying severity. Some infants show little abnormality, particularly in the early part of the clinical process. These infants require minimal intervention and can proceed to the second phase of therapy. Other infants, because of intense vomiting and a decreased caloric intake, can present with dehydration, hypoglycemia, abdominal distension, or growth failure. The vomiting leads to a hypochloremic, hypokalemic alkalosis. If the vomiting is mild, it may be corrected by oral feedings every 3 hours with a 0.5 normal saline solution with 5% glucose and some added KCl. More severe vomiting and dehydration require intravenous treatment with 0.25–0.5 normal saline with 5% glucose at a rate of 125–150 ml/kg/24 hours. After urination has been established, KC1 can be added at 2–3 mEq/kg/24 hours. With severe salt depletion, it may be necessary to increase the amount of sodium chloride by using a 0.75–1.0 normal saline solution. Serum electrolytes, as well as the infant's weight and hydration status should be monitored carefully. Most infants will demonstrate a good response 12–48 hours into fluid and electrolyte correction. Occasional patients who show signs of recurrent hypoglycemia and poor nutrition may require parenteral hyperalimentation for several days. Marked abdominal distension can be managed with gastric lavage and gastric decompression via nasogastric suction. Once the infant has achieved an improved physical and metabolic state, the next therapeutic phase can be instituted.

Surgical intervention by Ramstedt pyloromyotomy is the procedure of choice for correction of pyloric stenosis. In this procedure the hypertrophied pyloric and antral muscular layers are incised, leaving the mucosa intact. Two major complications that can arise are the incomplete division of the hypertrophied pyloric muscle and perforation of the duodenal mucosa. The latter is usually detected and repaired by the surgeon during the operative procedure. Both of these complications can become evident in the postoperative period. The procedure's mortality rate is less than 1%. General anesthesia is required in most cases, and the patient should not be fed orally 8 to 12 hours prior to surgery.

Careful observation is imperative in the postoperative period. If the pyloromyotomy has been uncomplicated, nasogastric suction can be discontinued four hours after surgery. Two to three ounces of Pedialyte or a 5% glucose solution can then be administered orally every 2–3 hours. Feedings can be advanced on the second day to breast milk or full-strength formula 2–3 oz every 2–3 hours. Infants should be feeding liberally by the third postoperative day. Intermittent vomiting may occur in the first few days post surgery. On rare occasion the emesis may be severe and require continued intravenous replacement therapy and nasogastric suction. If a perforation of the duodenal mucosa is suspected, feedings should be discontinued and nasogastric suction should be reinstituted for a 24-hour period. Oral feeds can then be resumed. If incomplete lysis of the hypertrophied pyloric muscle is suspected, it is best to stop feedings and start nasogastric suction and intravenous hyperalimentation. The infant will be able to feed orally in approximately one week. Repeat pyloromyotomy is rarely necessary. An upper GI series is of little value at this point. Radiologic evidence of the pyloric abnormality may

persist for months despite adequate surgical intervention.

With careful management during the preoperative and postoperative period, an excellent outcome can be expected from the surgical approach to pyloric stenosis.

Peptic Ulcers
PETER K. KOTTMEIER, M.D.

The present confusion concerning both operative and nonoperative treatment of gastroduodenal ulcers in infants and children is partially related to the assumption that all these ulcers are "peptic ulcers." A correct classification of gastroduodenal ulcers in children is important not only to identify the cause—if possible—but also to select the appropriate therapy. True "peptic ulcers" in childhood are similar to adult peptic ulcers. Another group of children have gastroduodenal ulcers that appear to be neither secondary to stress nor compatible with peptic ulcers. These are loosely grouped together as "acute primary ulcers."

Acute Primary Ulcers. In patients with mild to moderate bleeding, gastric lavage with saline and buffering with antacids or milk will suffice to stop bleeding in most instances. In infants, care should be taken not to induce hypothermia with iced gastric lavage. In acidotic infants, the gastric lavage solution should be either isotonic lactate or isotonic half saline and half bicarbonate to reduce, or at least not to increase, a metabolic acidosis. The administration of isotonic crystalloid solutions, blood, or colloid depends on the amount of blood loss. If the blood loss is significant, either whole blood or packed cells and volume expanders can be used as replacement. In most instances an over-replacement should be avoided, since this may reinitiate gastric bleeding that may have stopped prior to the overadministration of blood.

If the blood loss within 24 hours exceeds the patient's blood volume, or if massive recurrent bleeding occurs, surgery is usually indicated. Since there is no recurrence of the ulcer formation after successful therapy, the most conservative operative procedure necessary to stop the hemorrhage should be used, such as the simple oversewing of isolated ulcers or suture ligation of bleeders. In an occasional infant with diffuse gastric ulcerations, a resection may be necessary, however. The perforation in a patient with a primary acute ulcer is also usually treated successfully by simple closure with or without the use of an omental patch.

A unique type of neonatal ulcer leading to gastric perforations within several days after birth has also been called an acute primary ulcer. Aspiration of the intraperitoneal air will improve diaphragmatic excursion and therefore respiration. The isotonic hypovolemia should be corrected with an initial push of isotonic solutions. The peritonitis, although predominantly chemical at onset, should be covered with broad-spectrum antibiotics. The operative procedure consists of closure of the perforation. If the patient recovers uneventfully, oral feedings can usually be resumed after 5 to 7 days; there is no need for postoperative antacids or other medications.

Chronic Primary or Peptic Ulcers. These usually begin at school age and increase during the teenage years. They represent the childhood equivalent of the adult peptic ulcer. The primary therapy, usually successful, consists of antacids between meals and at bedtime. Either magnesium or aluminum hydroxide can be used. Magnesium hydroxide appears to be a more powerful buffer used to keep gastric pH higher than 4, but serum hypermagnesemia has been reported not only in patients with renal failure but also in neonates, with resulting cardiorespiratory depression. While this is a rare complication, its possibility should be kept in mind with prolonged administration. Sodium bicarbonate, even though a powerful buffer, is contraindicated in view of the resultant alkalosis. Cimetidine appears to be as effective in children (20–40 mg/kg in four divided doses) as in adults. There is no proof that special bland diets are of any help; gastric irritants should be avoided, however, including alcohol, aspirin, coffee, tea, and cola-containing drinks. Psychologic assistance in children with overlying anxiety problems may be useful. Diazepam (Valium) has been used successfully in children with stress ulcers who have underlying or associated anxiety problems.

As in the adult, there is no unanimity as to the "ideal" operative procedure for peptic ulcers in children. Many investigators emphasize that the natural course of the childhood peptic ulcer is more benign than that of the adult. They report the response to medical therapy to be prompt in most instances. If surgery is necessary, limited operations, such as vagotomy and pyloroplasty, are supposed to suffice. Other series, however, show equally convincingly that childhood peptic ulcers often extend into adulthood and are more difficult to treat in the child than in the adult. Based on increased experience in the adult with selective or highly selective vagotomy, with or without drainage procedure or limited resection, the present trend toward truncal vagotomy plus pyloroplasty in children may change.

The indications for surgery in children with peptic ulcers consist of massive or repeated hemorrhage, perforation, obstruction, and the difficult to define "intractability."

Secondary or Stress Ulcers. In certain groups of patients, such as children with burns or CNS lesions, prophylactic therapy has been shown to decrease significantly the incidence of stress ulcers. The early use of milk feedings, immediately after stabilization of burn patients, can reduce gastric acidity and provide needed calories. The stomach is emptied prior to the nasogastric tube feeding to prevent aspiration. Diazepam (Valium), given orally at 1 to 1.5 mg at 6-hour intervals initially, gradually increased as needed and tolerated, in burn patients, is thought not only to decrease anxiety in burned children, but also to reduce gastric acidity through a direct effect on the hypothalamus. The nonoperative therapy of stress ulcers is otherwise similar to that described in patients with acute erosive gastritis. In contrast to patients with AEG, in patients with bleeding ulcers arterial embolization can serve as either a temporizing or definitive procedure when the general condition prohibits even a limited operative intervention. Stress ulcers can occur in either stomach or duodenum or both areas simultaneously. The majority of bleeding or perforating stress ulcers requiring operative intervention, however, are located in the duodenum. Since there is no recurrence of the ulcer once the underlying stress has ceased, the most conservative operative procedure able to control either hemorrhage or perforation is preferred.

Zollinger-Ellison Syndrome. This syndrome, responsible for multiple duodenal or jejunal ulcers, does occur occasionally in childhood. Non-beta pancreatic islet cells are responsible for the increased gastrin output, leading to a high gastric acidity. The treatment is identical to that in adults: total gastrectomy with esophagojejunostomy.

Gastritis

PETER K. KOTTMEIER, M.D.

Infectious gastritis, viral or bacterial, is uncommon even in children with "gastroenteritis." Bacterial gastritis can occur, however, in children with massive sepsis, such as, for instance, in emphysematous gastritis, where the therapy is directed toward the underlying etiology. Chronic granulomatous disease also occasionally can involve duodenum and stomach. Therapy is supportive, with appropriate antibiotics. Surgery is rarely indicated.

Acute gastritis is most commonly seen after the ingestion of medication or other chemicals. The therapy for acute gastritis after aspirin ingestion consists of the correction of a possible associated coagulopathy, restriction or appropriate selection of oral intake, and the temporary use of gastric antacids. Alcohol-induced gastritis is also self-limiting after the discontinuation of alcoholic intake and symptomatic treatment. Gastritis due to the ingestion of corrosive agents is almost entirely limited to the ingestion of acid solution, such as hydrochloric acid. The attempt of buffering the ingested acid with alkaline solution is useless, since the corrosive effect of the acid is almost instantaneous. The stomach should be put at rest with nasogastric suction after careful insertion of a nasogastric tube to avoid perforation. Diffuse necrosis with perforation is the most likely complication, requiring prompt operative intervention. Gastritis due to lye or alkali ingestion is extremely rare. If it occurs, it is usually associated with esophageal burns and should be treated accordingly: proof of the burn via endoscopy, followed by the administration of steroids and antibiotics for approximately 3 weeks with re-examination.

Chronic gastritis can occur as a protein-losing, benign, hypertrophic gastropathy similar to Ménétrier's syndrome in the adult. It is occasionally associated with cyclic vomiting, viral infections, or eosinophilia, suggestive of a hypersensitivity reaction. Hypoproteinemia and anemia are present in most patients. Therapy consists of the correction of hypoproteinemia, either by infusion of protein or a high protein and low fat oral intake. In contrast to the adult Ménétrier's gastritis, it is usually self-limiting in children, responding promptly to supportive therapy. Bile gastritis, sometimes seen in adults after gastric operations, is rare in children. It can occur after gastrointestinal surgery such as bypass operations or duodenal obstruction. The gastritis due to the exposure of gastric mucosa to bile salts may respond to therapy with cholestyramine, antacids such as aluminum hydroxide, or bethanechol chloride (Urecholine) to stimulate gastric emptying, which is usually delayed. If this fails, a duodenogastric diversional operation is usually indicated to eliminate gastric bile stasis.

Acute Erosive Gastritis (AEG). Although the etiology of AEG is similar to that of stress ulcers, pathologic changes, therapy, and prognosis vary considerably. Stress ulcers are often confined to a single, predominantly duodenal site. Even multiple ulcers are limited to localized areas without the complete and diffuse gastric involvement seen in AEG. Since AEG often occurs in patients undergoing recognizable or anticipated stress, as in postoperative patients or patients with burns or CNS lesions, the therapy should be prophylactic in many instances. Although gastric acidity in children under stress is not necessarily increased, the breakdown of apical mucosal integrity allows back-perfusion of even normal acid, with subsequent gastritis and ulcerations. The breakdown of the mucosal integrity may be related to the diminution of energy source in the stressed patient; part of the therapy consists, therefore, of restoration or maintenance of an anabolic state in the stressed

patient, if necessary through parenteral hyperalimentation. To prevent back-perfusion of gastric acid, buffers, such as antacids, or histamine receptor blockers, such as cimetidine, are used individually or together.

In patients in whom AEG has occurred, often leading to life-endangering bleeding, the following therapeutic approaches can be used: nasogastric tube suction with intermittent iced saline irrigation until the stomach is cleared of blood clots, followed by the instillation of antacids on an hourly basis. An attempt should be made to keep the gastric pH at or over 4. This can be supported or accomplished by the use of cimetidine. Cimetidine, a histamine receptor blocker, reduces basal and stimulated gastric acid output. It is also assumed to protect mucosal blood flow during hypotension. There is some evidence to suggest that a continuous intravenous infusion of cimetidine is preferable to a bolus infusion or oral administration in patients with AEG. Again, an attempt should be made to keep the gastric pH at or over 4. If the pH cannot be stabilized, uncontrollable sepsis or multiple organ failure is usually present or developing, with an extremely poor prognosis.

Other attempts to control bleeding from AEG consist of the systemic or localized arterial infusion of vasopressors. Arterial embolization, occasionally effective in children with localized duodenal bleeding, is usually not indicated with AEG in view of the diffuse gastric involvement.

Failure of nonoperative therapy requires operative intervention. As in adults, there is no uniformity of opinion as to what operative procedure is the most suitable. In contrast to patients with localized stress ulcers, in whom the most conservative procedure is usually recommended, substantial gastric resection with truncal vagotomy may be necessary for children with massive AEG, not only to control bleeding but also to prevent a rebleeding.

Fortunately, the prophylactic use of either antacids or cimetidine to control the gastric pH has reduced markedly the number of patients requiring operative intervention.

Malformations of the Intestine

E. THOMAS BOLES, JR., M.D.

Most congenital malformations of the intestines become symptomatic because of intestinal obstruction; therefore, relief of the obstruction is the primary goal of therapy. A few result in bleeding or inflammation, and some are asymptomatic.

DUODENAL ATRESIA AND STENOSIS

The newborn with congenital duodenal obstruction requires appropriate preoperative correction of any fluid and electrolyte abnormalities that may have developed. Evident dehydration with or without electrolyte disturbances requires adequate replacement and correction preoperatively. One method is to administer an intravenous bolus of 10 ml/kg of isotonic fluid (e.g., Ringer's lactate) and follow this by fluid calculated at a rate of 125 mg/kg/24 of a hypotonic solution (e.g., 0.45 normal saline with addition of 30 mEq. of KCl/L). The response of the infant is essential in guiding fluid management with attention to urine output, urine osmolality or specific gravity, hematocrit, and physical examination, including vital signs, presence or absence of pulmonary rales, and peripheral edema. A more detailed review of appropriate intravenous replacement and maintenance therapy is found in the article on that subject. The stomach and duodenum should be emptied of fluid and air and decompression maintained. For a full-term infant a 10 F catheter may be passed into the stomach via the nose, the stomach aspirated, and the catheter attached to a source of low suction. Five small holes should be cut in the distal 5 cm of this catheter, and the most proximal hole should be above the diaphragm. Exact positioning of the catheter is important and may require an x-ray. Antibiotic therapy is unnecessary for the uncomplicated case.

The operation is most easily and safely performed under general endotracheal anesthesia with appropriate monitoring of pulse, heart sounds, blood pressure, and core temperature. Placement of the baby on a warming blanket, plastic drapes around the trunk, wrapping the extremities with sheet wadding, a cloth cap over the head, and the use of radiant heat lamps all are helpful in preventing hypothermia during the operation; the ambient temperature of the operating room should be at 75 to 80°F. Of course, intravenous fluid administration should be continued during the procedure.

A right upper quadrant transverse incision just above the umbilicus provides excellent exposure. It is not necessary and is undesirable to eviscerate the intestines. The right colon is mobilized and displaced to the left to expose the duodenum, and a Kocher maneuver is performed. This permits precise identification of the atretic or stenotic area. Gastrointestinal continuity is restored by duodenoduodenostomy. A very satisfactory technique is to make a transverse incision through the proximal duodenum and a vertical incision of the same length through the duodenum just distal to the obstruction, and to fashion the anastomosis with a single layer of interrupted 5–0 silk sutures. The possibility of a mucosal web originating proximal to the terminal end of the dilated proximal duodenum should be kept in mind. If such a web is missed and the anastomosis is done distal to its origin, obviously the obstruction will not be relieved. After the incision through the end of the proximal duodenum has been made, a hemostat can be passed through this opening into the stomach and out through a gastrotomy on the anterior wall of the stomach. Free passage ensures that a web is not present. If a web is present, it will reject passage of the hemostat. A gastrostomy tube is placed into the stomach and led out through a stab wound in the left epigastrium after the anastomosis has been completed.

Postoperatively the infant is returned to an isolette with appropriate humidity and temperature control. Intravenous water and electrolyte replacement is maintained. The nasogastric tube is removed the day following operation and the gastrostomy tube connected to a straight drain. Usually after 2 or 3 days the gastrotomy tube may be elevated and gastric residuals measured at 8-hour intervals. Usually the anastomosis opens up satisfactorily within 4 or 5 days and oral fluids may be started. The oral feedings are slowly increased to an amount sufficient for maintenance of adequate hydration, and then progressively changed to a low-curd formula. Occasionally the anastomosis fails to open sufficiently within a week, and under these circumstances total parenteral nutrition should be started and maintained until full enteral feedings are tolerated.

Relief of the duodenal obstruction is excellent, and mortality and morbidity are low in uncomplicated patients. However, associated anomalies including Down's syndrome, cardiac defects, esophageal atresia, and imperforate anus are common and often multiple; so the overall mortality of these babies is high.

MALROTATION AND VOLVULUS

Malrotation in an infant with intestinal obstruction is a surgical emergency because of the strong likelihood of associated volvulus. Often the diagnosis is made in the first few days of life, but in some the condition may not become apparent until later in infancy or in childhood.

Preoperative preparation depends on the status of the child. In the infant without peritoneal signs or indications of sepsis or hypovolemia, the preparation is similar to that for an infant with duodenal atresia except that antibiotics should be started preoperatively. Ampicillin and gentamicin are recommended. If the infant shows clinical or radiologic signs of volvulus, fluid resuscitation should be more vigorous and started with a "push" of 20 ml/kg. Metabolic acidosis is often present, and the addition of sodium bicarbonate in dosage appropriate to the intravenous regimen is required. In any event, resuscitation should be done promptly and vigorously, so that the infant can be brought to the operating room within an hour or two in satisfactory hemodynamic status.

Under general endotracheal anesthesia the abdomen is opened through a transverse incision as with duodenal atresia, except that the incision should be extended to the left with division of both rectus muscles. Volvulus is readily apparent, since only loops of small intestine are initially apparent and the colon cannot be seen. It is essential to eviscerate the small intestine. This will disclose the base of the mesentery and the volvulus itself. Reduction of the volvulus requires counterclockwise rotation of the small intestine one to three complete turns. After the volvulus has been corrected, and in the absence of devitalized gut, the usual anatomy found is an unattached right colon with a narrow mesenteric pedicle of the midgut. The ascending colon and the distal duodenum will be fused on their antimesenteric surfaces by a peritoneal band. This band is divided, and the ascending colon with its mesentery and the distal duodenum (often with some proximal jejunum) and its mesentery are carefully separated in a fashion analogous to opening the pages of a book. This results in displacement of the distal duodenum and proximal jejunum to the right and the proximal colon to the left. A catheter should be passed down the length of the duodenum to exclude a possible intrinsic mucosal web obstruction. This can be done by manipulating the nasogastric tube distally, or alternatively can be done through a gastrotomy. An incidental appendectomy is usually performed but a gastrostomy is unnecessary. Postoperatively, intestinal function returns to normal within 2 to 3 days. Antibiotics are discontinued 24 hours postoperatively if there is no evidence of intestinal vascular compromise.

If the intestine shows evidence of significant vascular compromise, management is more complex. It is helpful in the interim between detorsion of the volvulus and determining viability to return the midgut to the peritoneal cavity. If it is clear after an appropriate period of observation that a relatively short segment of intestine is devitalized, it should be resected. Depending on the status of the remainder of the gut and of the baby itself, either primary anastomosis or exteriorization with later anastomosis can be done. If a long segment or virtually all of the small intestines involved in the volvulus appear severely compromised, the abdomen is closed and a "second look" laparotomy performed 24 hours later. In some instances, at the second operation bowel that previously appeared gangrenous will be viable, and a limited resection will be possible that will permit the infant to have sufficient gut for normal function. Postoperatively these infants require close management of fluid, electrolyte, and blood volume status.

Results depend primarily on intestinal viability. In children without volvulus or with volvulus but no gangrenous intestine, the prognosis is excellent.

In the few with devitalization of the entire midgut, resection is not advisable and the outcome is uniformly fatal. In those in whom a limited resection can be done, results are good in terms of mortality but may involve considerable morbidity if a short-gut syndrome ensues.

JEJUNOILEAL ATRESIAS AND STENOSES

The basic principles of preoperative management have been previously outlined; and achievement of normal fluid and electrolyte status, nasogastric decompression, and maintenance of normal body temperature again deserve emphasis. Antibiotic therapy ordinarily is not necessary.

Laparotomy is performed through a transverse incision in the upper abdomen, and the exact anatomic situation is determined. The primary obstruction is easily found because of the marked discrepancy of intestinal caliber above and below the obstruction. The two ends may be separated, or may be in continuity with a diaphragm type atresia. Although most obstructions are solitary, occasionally multiple levels of obstruction are noted (15%). These are obvious when the intestinal segments are separated but not when distal diaphragmatic atresias occur. Therefore, the potency of the distal gut should be determined by injecting saline into the intestine just distal to the primary atresia and following this fluid down to the cecum.

The gut proximal to the atresia ordinarily ends in a bulbous dilatation. With high jejunal atresias this proximal bowel should be resected back to the ligament of Treitz. A short segment of intestine distal to the atresia is removed as well. Continuity is restored by a primary end-to-end anastomosis. A gastrostomy is routinely performed. When the atresia is in the distal ileum, the distal bulbous segment proximal to the atresia is resected and an end-to-side ileocecostomy constructed. Gastrostomy is not required in infants with distal obstructions.

For atresias in the midportion of the small gut there are two techniques, both of which work well in uncomplicated cases. An end-to-end anastomosis may be done after resection of the bulbous proximal segment and resection of a short segment of the distal gut. Alternatively, a Bishop-Koop technique may be used. Again, the bulbous proximal segment is resected and the end of the proximal segment is anastomosed to the side of the distal gut 3 or 4 cm distal to the proximal end. This proximal end is then opened and exteriorized as a vent. At a subsequent operation, this short span of distal gut is resected and closed.

The important points in postoperative management have been discussed previously. If function returns to the gut within a week and oral feedings can be initiated, there are usually few problems. If functional obstruction persists beyond this time, total parenteral alimentation should be started and continued until full enteral alimentation has been achieved.

In the past 25 years the success rate in infants with jejunoileal atresias has increased to over 90%. Such success is due to significant improvements in the techniques of surgical management and to the development of total parenteral nutrition.

COLONIC ATRESIA

Preoperative management parallels that for more proximal atresias. At laparotomy the dilated proximal colon is simply exteriorized as an end colostomy. This is easily managed postoperatively, and intestinal function permitting adequate oral feedings returns in a few days. A colostomy bag simplifies care of the colostomy, and the parents are instructed in the management of this appliance. Weeks or months later, when the baby is thriving, continuity is restored by an appropriate anastomosis, either a colocolostomy or an ileocolostomy. Mortality in such infants is close to zero, and morbidity is minimal.

Colonic atresia is occasionally associated with gastroschisis. In such an instance the blind proximal end is exteriorized and the gastroschisis managed either by primary closure or with the "silo" technique. Delayed anastomosis is done as with the uncomplicated case. Jejunoileal atresias occur very uncommonly with gastroschisis and are also managed with initial exteriorization. The prognosis of babies with the combination of gastroschisis and an atresia is nonetheless excellent.

MECONIUM ILEUS

This condition, invariably associated with cystic fibrosis, may be either uncomplicated or complicated, depending in all likelihood on whether an intrauterine segmental volvulus of small intestine has occurred. In the uncomplicated instance, the obstruction is an obturation type caused by inspissated meconium. The obstruction can often be cleared by a Gastrografin enema. Prior to such a procedure the infant should be managed as though a laparotomy were to be done; i.e., by correction of fluid and electrolyte abnormalities and nasogastric decompression plus systemic antibiotic administration. The enema procedure requires great care and should be done under fluoroscopic control with a surgeon in attendance. Because the enema fluid is hyperosmolar, the infant requires hypotonic fluid administration and careful monitoring during the procedure. When the Gastrografin reaches the dilated, air-containing small intestine, the procedure is discontinued. The loosened meconium usually begins to pass within 12 hours, with progressive relief of the obstruction. Complications occur rarely, particularly intestinal perforations, and, hence, the baby must be closely watched for such a possibility and follow-up x-rays taken.

If meconium does not begin to pass within 6 to 12 hours post enema, laparotomy should be done. Resection of the hugely dilated loop of small intestine is followed by a Bishop-Koop reconstruction. The distal segment can then be cleared of the obstructing concretions of meconium by instilling a dilute solution of pancreatic enzymes through the enterostomy vent. With either a successful enema procedure or a laparotomy, the preoperative measures are continued until relief of the obstruction is complete. Furthermore these babies, who are very vulnerable to respiratory infections, are nursed in isolettes using careful isolation techniques, and the appropriate prophylactic measures for cystic fibrosis are begun.

The complicated cases present with volvulus (sometimes complicated by perforation and meconium peritonitis), ileal or jejunal atresia, giant cystic meconium peritonitis, or a combination of these. Operation is required in all such infants, and the same preoperative measures as noted above are in order. At laparotomy the procedure is dictated by the pathology. If an atresia is found, the Bishop-Koop procedure as described in uncomplicated atresias works very well. With volvulus, resection of the devitalized segment and a double-barrel ostomy is advisable. Meconium peritonitis complicates the operation and may contribute to significant blood loss. Some type of ostomy, using either a double-barrel technique or the Bishop-Koop procedure, is safer than a primary anastomosis. Postoperatively these infants require particularly close attention to the problems of proper fluid and electrolyte balance, nutrition, and prevention of nosocomial infection.

DUPLICATIONS

Management of this very diverse group of lesions depends on their size and shape, and on the secondary problems resulting from their presence. The rare duodenal duplications are usually cystic. When proximally located, they often result in obstruction, with findings mimicking pyloric stenosis. At times they can be removed by stripping them away from the contiguous duodenal wall. If they are more distally located in the duodenum, the bile and pancreatic ducts may be immediately adjacent, and anastomosis of the common wall between duplication and duodenum is preferred.

Duplications in the small intestine may be either cystic or tubular, are located between the leaves of the mesentery, and share a common wall with the adjacent gut. The uncomplicated cystic and short tubular forms are resected along with the contiguous bowel, and continuity is restored with a primary anastomosis. If the duplication is complicated by volvulus or intussusception, resection is again done, but a double-barrel enterostomy may be wiser than primary anastomosis. Delayed secondary anastomosis is, of course, then necessary. In long tubular duplications, removal of the duplication with the contiguous intestine could result in the short-gut syndrome. In these, the mucosa of the duplication is removed by stripping it from its attachments to the muscularis. This can be done through a series of incisions through the seromuscular coat of the duplication, avoiding the mesenteric vessels. Complete mucosal stripping is important, since some or all of this mucosa may be gastric and hence responsible for intestinal bleeding. Leaving the seromuscular coat of these long duplications in situ does not appear to result in complications.

The rare hindgut duplication may involve the entire colon and rectum and the distal ileum. The mucosa of the duplication invariably is the same as that of the adjacent gut. These patients may be asymptomatic, with no obstruction or bleeding. In some the duplicated colons end in some form of imperforate anus (rectal atresia) malformation with obstruction. In others, the outer colon may end in a normal anus and the inner colon end in a rectovaginal or rectourethral fistula. In the former patients, a colostomy is required initially. In the latter, the two colons can be joined above the peritoneal reflection, and the mucosa leading to the rectovaginal or rectourethral fistula can be stripped out.

MECKEL'S DIVERTICULUM

This remnant of the omphalomesenteric duct usually is totally asymptomatic and requires no treatment, but may be responsible for profuse intestinal bleeding, intestinal obstruction, or discharge of intestinal contents from an umbilical sinus.

When symptomatic, rectal bleeding is most common. The bleeding may be profuse, with resulting shock. The mucosa of the diverticulum in these cases is gastric, and a resulting ulcer in adjacent ileal mucosa produces the hemorrhage. At laparotomy the problem is usually obvious, but occasionally the diverticulum may be folded against the adjacent mesentery and be missed at first glance. In most instances, the diverticulum can be simply excised at its base on the antimesenteric surface of the ileum. If the base is quite wide or there is marked inflammation and induration, resection of a short segment of ileum with the diverticulum and a primary anastomosis may be necessary.

Occasionally a Meckel's diverticulum acts as the leading point in an ileoileal or, more commonly, an ileocolic intussusception. This will become apparent at laparotomy when the intussusception is reduced, and under such circumstances the diverticulum should be removed. This may be done primarily in many. However, if the involved gut shows marked induration and congestion, it is wiser to do this at a later laparotomy.

If the omphalomesenteric duct remains attached to the umbilicus, with or without patency, it may be responsible for a volvulus. This will be apparent at laparotomy, and the duct should be removed in its entirety after the volvulus is properly managed.

Rarely the omphalomesenteric duct remains patent throughout its length and results in the discharge of small intestinal contents from the umbilical opening. At laparotomy the duct is resected and the openings in the gut and at the umbilicus closed.

Very rarely a Meckel's diverticulum becomes inflamed, resulting in a clinical situation indistinguishable from acute appendicitis. At laparotomy, invariably with the wrong preoperative diagnosis, the inflamed diverticulum is identified as the culprit and is removed.

Foreign Bodies in the Gastrointestinal Tract

E. THOMAS BOLES, JR., M.D.

A swallowed foreign body that fails to pass uneventfully through the alimentary tract is most likely to become arrested somewhere along the course of the esophagus. If the foreign body reaches the stomach, and this is usually the case, the odds of it becoming arrested in its further passage down the gastrointestinal tract are exceedingly small, probably less than one time in 20. Accordingly, in most instances periodic observation of the patient, who is usually an infant or toddler, is all that is required.

The type and particularly the shape of the ingested object are important determinants of the possibility of its becoming arrested. Because most of these foreign bodies are visible radiographically, abdominal x-rays should be taken routinely. If the object is not radiopaque, it may be outlined by a small barium meal, although rarely a foreign body such as a toothpick may be ingested without symptoms and without knowledge of the parents, only to cause an inflammatory intra-abdominal lesion later as a consequence of ulceration or perforation through the intestinal tract.

If the object is rounded and smooth (marbles, coins, small plastic toys, etc.) the child may be followed on an outpatient basis, since the foreign body will almost certainly pass through safely. Usually this occurs within 2 days, and the parents should be asked to check the stools of the child to ensure passage and rejoice in this event. Even open safety pins almost always negotiate the gastrointestinal tract uneventfully.

It is possible for long, thin, pointed foreign bodies to become impacted at the pylorus, C-loop of the duodenum, duodenojejunal junction, or terminal ileum. Straight pins, bobby pins, and segments of pencils fall into this category. Hat pins are particularly dangerous. Children who have swallowed objects of this type should be observed in the hospital, and the progress of the foreign body documented by abdominal x-rays at 12-hour intervals. If there is failure of progression over a period of 2 to 3 days or if worrisome symptoms develop, the object should be removed. In the stomach and duodenum extraction can sometimes be performed successfully with the use of a flexible fiberoptic gastroduodenoscope. Otherwise, laparotomy with gastrotomy or enterotomy is required. Another type of foreign body of recent concern is the small alkaline battery, which is potentially harmful because the casing is not biologically sealed and may release corrosive fluid. Management is similar to that for long, pointed foreign bodies. If the foreign body does become arrested, it may erode the mucosa and produce bleeding or it may perforate through the intestinal wall. In the latter event a localized, walled off inflammatory process usually results. When either of these events occurs, the foreign body should be removed.

Rarely a foreign body gains access to the intestinal tract through the rectum. In infants, most often this is a glass thermometer that escapes upward or is broken off. These require prompt removal, which may be possible by digital manipulation alone. If this is not easily accomplished, proctoscopy under general anesthesia should be performed. In older children, a bizarre assortment of foreign objects will at times be inserted into the rectum. Often these pass without incident, but if they are large or fragile (e.g., light bulb), their extraction may prove to be a challenging exercise. Protoscopy under anesthesia is ordinarily required.

Bezoars are masses of hair or vegetable fibers that form a cast in the stomach, sometimes extending down into the duodenum or even the upper jejunum. These are usually trichobezoars (hair balls) and occur most commonly in girls. Typically there is no history of eating hair, but clearly this is the mechanism. These patients are often asymptomatic, but symptoms that may develop include loss of appetite, intolerance of solid foods, vomiting, and abdominal pain. The child may show evidence of malnutrition and is often somewhat withdrawn or disturbed. The breath is characteristically fetid. A large, firm, movable mass is palpable in the upper abdomen. A barium swallow with fluoroscopy confirms the diagnosis by outlining the intragastric mass. Treatment is by gastrotomy, with removal of the bezoar, which forms a cast of the stomach. The small intestine should be traced down to the cecum to determine whether or not portions of the bezoar have separated from the main mass and have lodged downstream.

Intussusception

HARRY C. BISHOP, M.D.

Intussusception, the telescoping of bowel into itself, is a leading cause of acute intestinal obstruction in infants and is most common between the ages of 3 and 12 months. Ileocolic intussusception is the most common type and in over 90% of the cases it occurs without known cause. It usually occurs in a well infant, although there may be a preceding viral illness with gastrointestinal symptoms. It can occur in association with Henoch-Schönlein purpura, where a presumed hematoma of the bowel wall has acted as a lead point. In children over 2 years of age an inverted Meckel's diverticulum, a small intramural duplication, a polyp, or, very rarely, a lymphosarcoma of the ileum may be a lead point.

Characteristically, the patient has severe intermittent abdominal pain that recurs every 15 to 30 minutes. Between episodes of pain the infant or child is completely comfortable and may sleep. Occasionally, a small infant will present with lethargy and pallor rather than the more typical spasmodic pain, crying and flexing the legs on the abdomen. Vomiting usually occurs. Since the bowel mesentery is compressed between the intussusceptum (invaginated segment of bowel) and the intussuscipiens, venous obstruction occurs while the arteries are still pumping and this leads to edema and intraluminal bleeding and the typical currant jelly stool. As the intestine becomes more tightly incarcerated, the arterial supply is occluded, leading to less rectal bleeding and inevitably gangrene with associated signs of toxemia and complete intestinal obstruction. To avoid this potentially fatal result, early suspicion and confirmation of the diagnosis and reduction of the intussusception are essential. Examination of the abdomen will usually show soft distention and mild generalized tenderness. There may be a palpable "sausage-shaped" mass, most frequently along the transverse colon. Peristalsis is hyperactive initially and absent in the later stages of the disease. The intussusception may be felt on the rectal exam if it has gone the full route through the colon. Rectal exam may produce a current jelly stool appearing for the first time.

MANAGEMENT

All infants and children suspected of having intussusception should be hospitalized and under the care of a surgeon. Nasogastric suction is begun, as is intravenous replacement of fluid and elctrolyte losses, blood is crossmatched, and the operating room is alerted for a possible emergency operation. With the surgeon attending, the patient is moved to Radiology, where a barium enema confirms the diagnosis and hydrostatic reduction will be attempted. If the patient is septic, has signs of perforation with peritonitis, or is considered critically ill, he or she may be taken directly to surgery rather than the physician attempting hydrostatic reduction.

Barium Enema Reduction. Hydrostatic reduction is safe if properly performed. Most radiologists use a Foley catheter with the inflated balloon pulled down against the internal sphincter and the buttocks strapped tightly together. Thin barium is allowed to flow by gravity into the recutum, with the reservoir no higher than 3 feet above the table top. Manual manipulation through the intact abdomen is avoided. Steady hydrostatic pressure is exerted on the intussuscipiens, which is outlined by the barium column. Several attempts might be made, evacuating the barium between attempts. Intussusception usually reduces easily back to the cecal area but the last reduction through the ileocecal valve may be delayed. Some radiologists use glucagon or morphine, in an attempt to relax the bowel and the patient. It is vitally important for the reduction to be complete. Only if there is a free flow of barium into two or three loops of ileum can reduction be confirmed. If an intussusception has been reduced hydrostatically, the patient should remain in the hospital. He should be free of abdominal pain; his abdomen should be soft and free of a palpable mass, and he should pass stool and flatus in the early postreduction period. Careful observation is important to ensure complete reduction and rule out recurrence.

Unfortunately, the condition can start as an ileoileal intussusception, and then this whole mass prolapses through the ileocecal valve, producing a so-called ileoileocolic intussusception. This treacherous variation must be considered and the possibility eliminated by a free flow of barium high into the ileum, guaranteeing a reduction of the ileoileal segment as well. If there is any doubt about the completeness of the reduction, the child should be taken to surgery and the condition explored. Since the entrapped bowel is in danger of becoming gangrenous, early surgery is mandatory.

Indications for operation are (1) incomplete reduction of a known intussusception; (2) suspicion of a jejunojejunal or ileoileal intussusception with intestinal obstruction; and (3) perforation during the barium enema, which is rare if the proper safeguards are taken.

If operation is scheduled, antibiotics should be given preoperatively, assuming that the bowel has been damaged. Most surgeons use a right lower quadrant McBurney type incision, which can be enlarged if necessary. An intussusception should be milked out from the distal end proximally, with great care to avoid splitting the bowel wall. At no time should the bowel be pulled from the opposite end. Frequently the appendix will have invaginated into the intussusception and may be traumatized. Ileal mesenteric lymph nodes are frequently enlarged, and it is difficult to know whether these were there primarily or occurred as a result of the intussusception. If the bowel can be completely reduced, there is always edema of the lead point and the Peyer's patches may seem hypertrophied. The cyanotic bowel frequently will improve once the reduction has been accomplished, especially if covered with warm gauze sponges. Care is taken to look for a lesion leading to the intussusception, as mentioned above. Most surgeons feel appendectomy can be safely accomplished, and often it is wise to include an appendectomy, since the appendix has been damaged. If the intussusception is gangrenous or cannot be reduced manually, the bowel is resected and ordinarily a primary anastomosis is done. The bowel should be resected if perforation occurs during the attempted reduction, but a careful effort should be made to avoid this complication. Postoperatively these patients are continued on nasogastric suction, intravenous replacement and support, and antibiotics. They frequently have a low-grade fever that might last for 2 or 3 days, presumably from damage of the intestinal wall.

Recurrent Intussusception. If the symptoms of intussusception recur following hydrostatic reduction, one must suspect that the original reduction was incomplete or that an etiological lead point lesion is present. Therfore, surgical exploration is indicated for any recurrence. A rare patient will repeatedly intussuscept and require resection of the ileocecal area or suturing of the terminal ileum up along the ascending colon. A very rare individual might have a chronic intussusception without the acute symptoms, which may be discovered while investigating mild abdominal complaints. This possibility should be surgically explored.

Postoperative Intussusception. Jejunojejunal or ileoileal intussusception can occur during the early postoperative period following other unrelated operative procedures. It is frequently confused with paralytic ileus or obstruction due to adhesions and cannot be diagnosed by barium enema. Early surgical exploration is therefore indicated when this diagnosis is suspected.

Hirschsprung's Disease

WILLIAM K. SIEBER, M.D.

Hirschsprung's disease is a congenital anomaly characterized by partial to complete, acute or chronic low intestinal obstruction associated with absence of intramural ganglion cells in the distal alimentary tract.

When Hirschsprung's disease is suspected, prompt surgical consultation for diagnosis and treatment should be obtained. Nonsurgical treatment is ineffective. Cathartics and smooth muscle stimulants such as methacholine (Mecholyl) may be harmful, promoting fatal enterocolitis. Older children with moderate chronic constipation as the only symptom may respond to enemas administered daily or every second or third day. Since the rectum is inactive, impactions occur frequently and may require the use of detergent retention enemas, dioctyl sodium sulfosuccinate (Colace), one part in three parts of saline, followed by a cleansing enema in 12 hours. The dangers of rectal perforation and water intoxication from enemas are well documented. Enemas should be isotonic. Fecal impactions are avoided by preparations that tend to keep the stools soft, such as mineral oil or psyllium hydrophilic mucilloid (Metamucil).

In infancy, acute colonic (90%) or low small bowel obstruction (10% aganglionosis coli) requires emergency relief by enterostomy in the normally innervated intestine just proximal to the aganglionic intestine. Frozen-section control of the placement of the enterostomy requires the aid of a pathologist familiar with the histologic appearance of intramural ganglion cells in infants. The colostomy is done as a loop colostomy or as a divided colostomy with the proximal end brought up to function as a single lumen, the distal end being closed and returned to the peritoneal cavity. When the aganglionic segment is short and involves only the rectum, a right transverse loop colostomy is done. An emergency colostomy is indicated to prevent the development of enterocolitis, a frequently lethal complication in infancy. A colostomy is done preliminary to definitive surgical treatment in the newborn, in symptomatic infants up to 6 months of age, and in older patients with longstanding symptoms. Definitive surgical treatment is deferred until the infant is over 6 months of age or, in an older child, until general health improves and colonic impactions are completely removed. This usually takes 6 months.

Preparation for definitive surgery includes mechanical emptying of the colon with enemas, a clear liquid diet, bowel preparation with neomycin and erythromycin base, and digital dilatation of the anus.

Definitive surgical treatment involves the resection of the aganglionic intestine and reestablishment of the continuity of the alimentary tract. This is currently done by one of three abdominoperineal procedures—the Swenson, Duhamel, or Soave procedure.

The Swenson procedure is the original and time-tested standard procedure. In this operation, the aganglionic intestine is freed and removed to within 1.5 cm of the pectinate line anteriorly; the procedure includes a sphincterotomy of the internal anal sphincter posteriorly. The normally innervated intestine is then brought down and anastomosed to this remaining rectal stump.

In the Duhamel procedure, the aganglionic intestine is resected down to the rectum. The rectum is sutured closed but left in place. A retrorectal channel is developed, and the normally innervated intestine is pulled through this channel and through an incision in the posterior rectal wall 1 cm above the pectinate line. Half the circumference of the distal rectum is then anastomosed to the posterior half of the pulled-through colonic wall and is opposed to the posterior half of the retained rectum. Clamps are placed intraluminally to remove this common wall, or the wall may be divided by the anastomotic stapler, resulting in an anastomosis of the end of the colon to the posterior wall of rectum. Variations of the Duhamel procedure involve differences in the type of crushing clamp or suturing method used. When long segments of aganglionosis are present, the Martin procedure—in which a long side-to-side anastomosis of the pulled-through intestine and the distal aganglionic colon is done—is now preferred.

In the Soave procedure (the endorectal pull-through procedure), the mucosa is removed from the rectum down to the skin of the anus. Normally innervated intestine is then pulled through the resultant muscular cuff and anastomosed either directly, as in the Swenson procedure (Boley), or in delay fashion, as a two-stage procedure (Soave), to the anal skin.

The operative mortality associated with these procedures is negligible, and the initial result in all is very good. At present the personal experience of the operating surgeon should determine the best procedure for the individual patient. My preference is the one-stage endorectal (Boley) procedure preceded by a right transverse colostomy.

Enterocolitis may occur as a serious complication of Hirschsprung's disease. The sudden abdominal distention, disinterest in nursing, vomiting, and foul diarrhea result in high fever with dehydration and may cause death within 24–48 hours. When enterocolitis is suspected, intravenous fluids, gentle copious saline rectal irrigations, antibiotics, and gastric suction followed by decompression by colostomy may be lifesaving. Enterocolitis may first appear after a colostomy has been done for obstruction, or it may appear as long as 6–8 years after an uneventful definitive procedure. The Swenson procedure is more likely to be followed by enterocolitis than are the other procedures.

Short-segment Hirschsprung's disease, in which only the lower rectum is aganglionic, sometimes responds to transluminal rectal myectomy (actually an extension of full-thickness rectal biopsy). My experience with this procedure has been disappointing.

Ulcerative Colitis and Crohn's Disease

JEFFREY A. BILLER, M.D.

Inflammatory bowel disease is being recognized with increasing frequency in pediatric patients. Approximately 15% of all patients with ulcerative colitis and 30% of those with Crohn's disease have onset of symptoms before the age of 20, with the majority of these presenting during the adolescent years. Both disorders are associated with enormous medical and psychosocial problems, each of which must be treated individually to manage the disease effectively.

The clinical presentation of ulcerative colitis and Crohn's disease is similar. Most patients have complaints of abdominal pain and development of diarrhea. Approximately 50% of patients with Crohn's disease and almost 100% of patients with ulcerative colitis will present with hematochezia. Weight loss is common in both groups (approximately 60–80%); however, the magnitude of weight loss in patients with Crohn's disease is often significantly greater. In addition, the presence of growth failure is noted in as many as 35% of pediatric patients with Crohn's disease and 15% of those with ulcerative colitis. Fever, a common presenting sign, occurs in approximately 40% of patients. Extraintestinal manifestations, which may either precede or occur after the onset of gastrointestinal symptoms, include stomatitis, uveitis, clubbing, splenomegaly, liver disease (pericholangitis and sclerosing cholangitis), and dermatitis (erythema nodosum, pyoderma gangrenosum). Patients with Crohn's disease have a higher incidence of developing perianal disease (abscess, fistulae, and skin tags) than do those with ulcerative colitis.

The distribution of intestinal involvement of Crohn's disease is similar for adult and pediatric patients. Approximately 40% will have disease localized to the small bowel (half of whom have solely terminal ileal involvement), 50% will have ileo-colonic involvement, and 10% solely colonic involvement. At the time of presentation, 25% of pediatric patients with ulcerative colitis have disease restricted to the rectosigmoid and decending colon, 50% have disease extending to the transverse colon, and pancolitis is noted in the other 25%.

The goal of treatment of inflammatory bowel disease is to control the inflammatory process in order to reduce or eliminate symptoms, maintain long-term remission, and allow as normal a lifestyle as possible. Therapy must be individualized, based on the severity of the disease, its location, and the response to treatment.

THERAPY

Sulfasalazine. Sulfasalazine is very useful in the treatment of mild cases of ulcerative colitis and Crohn's disease when there is evidence of either ileocolonic or colonic involvement. It has been shown to decrease the frequency of recurrences in patients with colitis in remission. There is no clear evidence, however, that sulfasalazine is useful for the treatment of acute severe colitis. Sulfasalazine consists of 5-aminosalicylic acid linked by an azo-bond to sulfapyridine. This bond is cleaved by colonic bacteria, releasing both compounds. The 5-aminosalicylic acid is believed to be the active moiety, and indeed enemas of this compound are now being tested for use in the treatment of rectosigmoid disease. Side effects of the drug include headache, rash, nausea, vomiting, hepatotoxicity, hemolysis, and myelosuppression. Azoospermia has been noted in adults taking sulfasalazine; however, this effect has been shown to be reversible after discontinuing the drug. Rarely, exacerbation of symptoms has been noted with the use of sulfasalazine. The usual daily dose* is 50 mg/kg/day divided bid (maximum, 3–4 gm/day). Because of the possibility of an allergic reaction, the initial dose is often 10 mg/kg/day, increased over 1–2 weeks to the total daily dose. Because sulfasalazine can interfere with the absorption and utilization of folic acid, routine daily supplementation with folic acid (1 mg) is indicated.

Corticosteroids. Corticosteroids remain the most important and effective medications for the treatment of moderate and severe cases of both ulcerative colitis and Crohn's disease. There is no evidence that chronic low-dose therapy is effective in preventing recurrences. For the acute episode, doses of 1–2 mg/kg/day of prednisone orally (maximum, 60 mg/day), or its equivalent parenterally, are prescribed, usually given in one or two daily doses. Significant improvement is noted in most patients within the first 1–2 weeks of therapy. High-dose prednisone is often continued for approximately 1 month, then tapered by 5 mg every 1–2 weeks, depending on the clinical response. In patients with evidence of significant steroid side effects (cushingoid facies, hypertension, hyperglycemia, cataracts, osteoporosis), or when low-dose chronic prednisone is required to maintain remis-

---

* Sulfasalazine is contraindicated in infants under 2 years of age.

sion, alternate-day administration of steroids may be indicated. High-dose prednisone interferes with growth; however, it has been shown that significant growth can be achieved even with doses as high as 20–30 mg/day if optimal nutrition is achieved. For those patients with rectosigmoid involvement, treatment with steroid enemas or foam may be very helpful in reducing the need for systemic steroids, as well as in relieving tenesmus. Intravenous corticotropin (ACTH) in doses of 1–1.5 units/kg/day has in some cases promoted remission faster than the equivalent dose of prednisone, especially when the patient has not recently been treated with steroids.

Metronidazole. Metronidazole† has been shown to be an effective agent for the treatment of perianal Crohn's disease and may be helpful in the treatment of mild to moderate ileocolonic Crohn's disease as well as for the management of fistulae. Administration of 20 mg/kg/day (maximum, 1 gm) in three divided doses is suggested. Side effects, including paresthesias, metallic taste, nausea, vomiting, and neutropenia, have been noted and may limit the usefulness of metronidazole.

Antispasmodic Agents. In some patients with inflammatory bowel disease, diarrhea and cramping may be a source of considerable morbidity. The use of antispasmodic agents—including tincture of opium, in doses of 5–10 drops three times a day, or diphenoxylate hydrochloride with atropine sulfate (Lomotil), in doses of 2–5 mg three times a day—may be helpful. It must be noted, however, that the use of such agents has been associated with the development of toxic megacolon in patients with colitis. Although no causal relationship has been clearly shown, these drugs should not be used when the patient is experiencing severe cramping or when there is evidence of intestinal dilatation on x-ray. More recently, studies in adults have shown that loperamide (Imodium) may be as effective as other opiates in reducing cramping and diarrhea and has fewer neurologic side effects. Further experience is needed, however, before this drug can be routinely prescribed for children.

Immunosuppressive Agents. Immunosuppressive medications, such as 6-mercaptopurine and azathioprine, may be efficacious in managing patients dependent on high-dose corticosteroids, as well as in the treatment of patients with chronic recurrent fistulae related to Crohn's disease. Azathioprine in doses of 1–2 mg/kg/day divided bid has been used to treat such adolescents. The mean time for response in these patients is approximately 3 months; consequently, this agent has little value in the acute treatment of active disease. Azathioprine therapy for the purposes described remains investigational at present.

---

† This use of metronidazole is not listed by the manufacturer.

NUTRITION

At the time of diagnosis, most pediatric and adolescent patients with ulcerative colitis or Crohn's disease have a history of weight loss (in one study a mean of 9 kg and 12 kg, respectively). The underlying cause of this weight loss is multifactorial, but it does not seem to have an endocrinologic basis. Many of the patients have low caloric intake, in part related to anorexia, with increased symptoms of cramping and diarrhea associated with meals. Some may have altered taste secondary to zinc deficiency. Excessive weight loss may occur as a result of malabsorption and protein-losing enteropathy. Malabsorption is common in adolescents with Crohn's disease; 30% have steatorrhea, 20% have lactose intolerance and abnormal d-xylose absorption, and others have low serum folic acid, vitamin B_{12}, iron, and calcium levels. Nutritional requirements are greater in these patients because of fever, losses due to fistulae, and the need for rebuilding of body stores. A general nutritional evaluation, including anthropometrics, is helpful to document the degree of nutritional deficit.

Nutritional repletion may be achieved either voluntarily, with high-calorie supplements, or involuntarily, with nighttime nasogastric infusions or hyperalimentation. Some patients require initial hospitalization for hyperalimentation without oral intake to decrease their symptoms of cramping and diarrhea, as well as for treatment of cutaneous fistulae or severe perianal disease. Patients who receive no enteral nutrition for longer than a week should be maintained on central rather than peripheral hyperalimentation, since the latter does not supply the required calories. Although no higher incidence of lactose intolerance exists in patients with inflammatory bowel disease than in the general population, a lactose-free diet should be followed until a lactose breath hydrogen test can be performed. In patients with severe colitis or evidence of a stricture, a low-residue diet may also be helpful.

A delay in both skeletal and sexual maturation in patients with inflammatory bowel disease may be the most devastating sequela of the disease, especially in the adolescent patient who is extremely concerned about body image. It is vitally important to treat growth failure early, before significant fusion of the epiphyses of the bones occurs. We have had good success with vigorous alimentation—either enterally, with nighttime nasogastric infusions, or parenterally, initially in the hospital and subsequently at home—to ensure approximately 150% of ideal caloric intake.

SURGICAL THERAPY

The indications for intestinal resection in children and adolescents with inflammatory bowel disease are similar to those for adults and include the presence of massive hemorrhage, intestinal obstruction, intestinal perforation, intractable fistulae and perianal disease, and intraabdominal abscess. In addition, localized disease causing severe symptoms unresponsive to medical therapy also mandates surgery. Because of the high risk of recurrence after surgical resection, medical therapy should be tried first whenever possible. Elective surgery to reverse growth failure in the prepubertal patient should be attempted only in patients unresponsive to aggressive medical and nutritional managment in whom all areas of active disease can be resected. The results of surgical resection to reverse growth failure remain controversial. For patients with severe colitis—defined as anemia, fever, tachycardia, gastrointestinal bleeding, and hypoalbuminemia—who are unresponsive to medical therapy for longer than 2 weeks (on hyperalimentation and high-dose steroids), strong consideration must be given to performing a colectomy with an initial ileostomy. Since the advent of surgical pull-through procedures, fewer patients with ulcerative colitis will require permanent ileostomies.

EMOTIONAL SUPPORT

Inflammatory bowel disease and its complications place severe emotional stress on both the patient and his or her family. The difficulties of adolescence are magnified manyfold because of lingering symptoms of abdominal pain, diarrhea, growth failure, delayed sexual development, and medication side effects. For some patients, this burden is overwhelming. It is vitally important that an honest, trusting relationship develop between the patient and the physician.

Literature explaining the complications and treatment of inflammatory bowel disease is abundantly available and answers many of the questions families are most concerned about. Once a patient is diagnosed as having inflammatory bowel disease, we routinely seek the assistance of a social worker or psychologist, already part of our health care team, to give care on a regular basis, rather than having them first involved during a crisis situation. Both patient and parent support groups are available and, in our experience, are of great benefit. A team approach—with caregivers including pediatrician, gastroenterologist, nutritionist, surgeon, social worker, psychologist, and ostomy nurse—is important in managing the challenging chronic problems of the pediatric and adolescent patient with inflammatory bowel disease.

Necrotizing Enterocolitis

CHARLES R. BAUER, M.D.

Over the last decade, necrotizing enterocolitis (NEC) has become one of the major contributors to both mortality and long-term morbidity in the low birthweight infant. This disease brings particular devastation to the family and nursery staff because the infant has usually weathered most of the critical, life-threatening period of his illness and is already seen as on his way to recovery when NEC strikes.

The mortality in infants medically managed is as high as 20% and rises to 60% when surgical intervention is mandated. The prognosis for normal long-term growth and development in survivors of medically managed NEC is in the range of 80%. However, only one-third of surgical survivors of NEC have adequate growth and developmental outcomes.

Since prevention is not yet possible, minimizing risk is the ultimate goal. An acute index of suspicion and early, aggressive management of suspected or established disease are the only effective methods of halting progression. Although any infant may be at risk, attention centers on those infants with recognized risk factors, primary among which is bowel ischemia occurring during the first few days of life.

Conservative management of these at-risk infants in their neonatal recuperative period includes the slow and cautious introduction of enteral nutrition, adequate fluid support, and prompt, aggressive treatment of situations that may evoke or exacerbate bowel ischemia, such as hypoxemia, hypotension, dehydration, and thromboembolism.

The symptomatology of NEC is insidious and mimics the nonspecific signs of infection in the newborn. The initial signs may not even implicate the gastrointestinal tract as the source of the problem. The classic signs of abdominal distention, feeding intolerance, bilious vomiting and/or blood in the stool may only follow nonspecific indicators such as lethargy, irritability, temperature instability and apnea. However, once the clinical suspicion of NEC is aroused, treatment should be immediate and should not be delayed until diagnostic confirmation.

Medical Management

Each nursery should develop its own protocol for immediate implementation once NEC is suspected. The goal of medical management is to put the bowel at complete rest and to avoid central hypoxemia or hypoperfusion by assuring adequate respiratory and circulatory support and by treating any associated conditions that may lead to or exaggerate bowel ischemia. The diagnositc workup should proceed simultaneously.

The infant must be made NPO at the first sign of impending NEC. Abdominal decompression is critical and is accomplished by the insertion of a nasogastric tube. The use of a sump-type tube allows maximum depression while minimizing trauma. The tube is best inserted nasally so that it can be adequately anchored in place. Oral tubes are unstable and easily displaced so that esophageal and not gastric decompression results. The tube should be connected to intermittent suction to remove all gastric contents and secretions and provide complete rest to the bowel.

Adequate intravenous hydration must be simultaneously instituted to assure adequate circulatory support and electrolyte balance. Replacement of gastric secretions must be considered in calculating the fluid and electrolyte requirements because of its high electrolyte concentrations. Frequent measurements of serum osmolality and specific electrolyte levels are necessary to avoid dangerous imbalances.

The initiation of broad-spectrum antibiotic coverage is warranted because the nonspecific initial symptoms may herald sepsis. Also 30–40% of infants with documented NEC have positive blood cultures. The use of penicillin or ampicillin and an aminoglycoside to cover both gram-positive and gram-negative organisms is indicated. A septic work-up, including blood, urine, spinal fluid, stool and surface cultures, is initiated early so that antibiotic therapy can be appropriately adjusted when specific infecting agents are isolated. Cultures for anaerobic organisms are important and should be specified, but the addition of a third level of antibiotic coverage for anaerobes is not generally recommended at the present time.

The use of enteral antibiotics remains controversial. This practice arose following the surgical custom of using enteral antibiotics prior to acute bowel surgery to "sterilize" the bowel. Because of the bowel injury, it was felt that keeping the bacterial colony count low might be helpful, both in preventing progression of the NEC and perhaps in avoiding perforation. In addition, there might be theoretical advantages if the infant eventually did require surgical intervention. Several recent studies have failed to support these ideas and caution that the bowel may become populated with antibiotic-resistant microflora. In addition, the idea that aminoglycosides placed in the bowel are not absorbed, although true for the normal, intact bowel, is not true for the ischemic, mucosa-damaged bowel. Therefore, potentially toxic levels of aminoglycosides must be considered as a possible complication in these immature and unstable infants. The trend is definitely away from the additional use of enteral antibiotics. However, their use does continue, and the recommended dosage is 15 mg/kg/day of either gentamicin or kanamycin, placed down the nasogastric tube 3 or 4 times per day. After administration, the tube is clamped for 30 minutes to allow gastric emptying.

The duration of medical management depends on the results of the diagnostic work-up as well as on the clinical course of the infant. If the work-up is negative, that is, the radiographs do not demonstrate pneumatosis, and the cultures are negative, then therapy can be tailored to the infant's condition. If the symptoms have improved, therapy can be stopped in 3–7 days and feedings cautiously reinstituted. If, however, a specific diagnosis is confirmed other than NEC, such as sepsis, urinary tract infection, patent ductus arteriosus with congestive heart failure, and so on, then treatment for NEC can be modified and redesigned to treat that specific underlying problem.

When NEC is confirmed by demonstrating the presence of pneumatosis intestinalis or portal air, then the established protocol should be maintained for at least 10 to 14 days following the resolution of the pneumatosis. Individual clinical judgement will require extensions of treatment if grossly bloodly stools, apnea, positive blood cultures, or severe abdominal distention persists for prolonged periods. Because occult blood and reducing substances in the stool may persist for prolonged periods in resolving NEC, other signs of clinical well-being should be present before treatment is stopped or modified. This may at times require a full protocol for 21 to 28 days, or even longer in rare circumstances.

Usually nasograstric suction is discontinued first and with it enteral antibiotics if they had been prescribed. This usually occurs 7 days after the x-ray has become normal. Systemic antibiotics are discontinued 10–14 days after cultures have been negative. Refeeding must be initiated slowly and cautiously, using small amounts with diluted concentrations. One must expect a stormy refeeding course and be prepared for setbacks and slow progress. Signs of bowel dysfunction must be treated cautiously by allowing a longer time for repair by reinstituting support with parenteral alimentation. There should never be an urgency to re-establish oral feeding following a course of documented NEC.

The most common complication seen after successful medical management is stricture formation at the site of the original ischemic injury. This may occur acutely but most often occurs weeks after refeeding has been started and when the infant is already at home. Vomiting, distention, and acute intestinal obstruction occur and must be relieved surgically. The outcome is uniformly good, and the setback is only temporary. Chronic diarrhea is another possible problem, which may require multiple manipulations of formula and diet, but does eventually resolve with time.

Surgical Management

When medical therapy fails, surgical management is the remaining alternative. At present, the primary indication for surgery is perforation of the intestine. This diagnosis is a life-threatening emergency and requires immediate action. In the acute phase of NEC, abdominal radiographs should screen the abdomen for signs of free peritoneal air every 4 to 6 hours, or more often if clinical symptomology indicates the possibility of a perforation. A left lateral decubitus film, looking for free air over the liver, is the most desirable screening tool.

Often, the clinical condition of the infant with fulminant NEC is so poor that a prolonged definitive surgical procedure is not possible. In most cases, the extent of damage is quickly assessed and the perforation and areas of clearly nonviable bowel are resected. The remaining areas of involved bowel are often exteriorized for later more definitive surgery. The mortality during surgery and in the immediate postoperative period approaches 60% in many centers.

Much controversy presently revolves around surgical intervention in the infant in whom medical management is failing and perforation is not radiologically demonstrable. These infants have a continuing downhill course. Their abdomens become grossly distended, tight, shiny, erythematous, edematous, and exquisitely painful to touch. Their platelet counts fall and they may develop a bleeding diathesis. Their respiratory status is compromised by the tremendous intra-abdominal pressure, and they therefore often require intubation and ventilation. Their abdominal radiographs may show an airless abdomen or a fixed loop of bowel that does not move or change configuration over a period of days. The erythema of the abdominal wall often becomes quite prominent and extensive.

This course is felt to be compatible with a silent or walled off perforation and/or peritonitis. Whether surgical exploration is helpful here is the subject of the debate. Neonatologists argue that surgery is the only hope, as the infant has continued to deteriorate with the most aggressive medical management and that in spite of the high mortality surgery offers the only chance of survival. Surgeons argue that surgery realistically offers the infant no advantage and only added risk. They describe large areas of acutely ischemic bowel with no clear demarcation between viable and nonviable bowel tissue, thereby making treatment impossible. They further suggest that any time that can be gained by intense medical support will make eventual surgical intervention more productive. Paracentesis and peritoneal drains have been offered as temporizing procedures in these very complex cases. Previous experience demonstrates that early surgery is deleterious, but waiting too long may also often be fatal. Guidelines based on radiographic features of peritonitis and results of peritoneal taps and other diagnostic maneuvers are being studied to provide other indications, in addition to free air, that would signify the need for immediate surgical intervention.

The postoperative course is always prolonged and stormy. Every effort is made during surgery to remove the smallest amount of bowel possible and to preserve the ileocecal valve, so that ultimate recovery and reinstitution of enteral nutrition will be possible. The maintenance of these infants during this interval period, which often lasts months, is filled with hazards and complications. Intravenous access always eventually becomes a major problem; formula intolerance, diarrhea, dehydration, and infection are all potentially lethal complicatitons in these infants. Recurrent bouts of NEC and late strictures are reported. Even the majority of those who are eventually discharged have serious growth and development problems. Survivors of surgically managed NEC are a selective subset of the most critically ill infants requiring the most complicated care in neonatal intensive care units today.

Prevention

There are at present no preventive measures to definitively avoid the ravages of NEC. Recognizing those infants at greatest risk and avoiding additional stresses to an already potentially compromised bowel and following a slow and cautious feeding schedule during the recuperative period may be the best we have to offer. Recent reports suggest that NEC may be related to the bowel as respiratory distress syndrome is to the lung, that is, a manifestation of immaturity. If bowel development can be pharmacologically accelerated, either prenatally or postnatally, as has been attempted with some success in the lung, perhaps the effects of ischemia can be minimized or structural development enchanced to allow for a more mature response to the initial enteral feedings. This is an area of interesting current investigation and holds promise for the possible prevention of NEC.

Peritonitis

DANIEL L. MOLLITT, M.D.

The peritoneal cavity responds to injury or insult with the outpouring of fluid and inflammatory cells, cessation of normal bowel activity, and deposition of fibrin. This reaction, or peritonitis, is associated with evidence of systemic toxicity, significant clinical symptomatology, and marked fluid and electrolyte derangements. Recognition and initial [resuscitation] of peritonitis are paramount to the determination of specific etiology.

The initial therapy of diffuse peritonitis should consist of gastrointestinal decompression, fluid resuscitation, and correction of electrolyte abnormalities. A nasogastric tube and a secure large-bore intravenous line are placed, blood for hematocrit and serum chemistries is obtained, and normal saline or lactated Ringer's solution is administered. Glucose-containing solutions are avoided initially as the large volumes frequently necessary result in hyperglycemia, as well as obligate glycosuria with factitious urinary response and subsequent increased fluid loss. Similarly, colloid solutions, although transiently expanding the intravascular volume, ultimately result in increased fluid loss and should not be utilized for primary resuscitation. The initial fluid administration is bolus therapy, 10–20 cc/kg, until a response is obtained. Further therapy is then guided by the patient's clinical condition and urinary output (minimum, 1–2 cc/kg/hr). Placement of a central venous line and bladder catheterization are indicated in instances of severe hypovolemia. Only when resuscitation has begun and a response is obtained should efforts be turned toward the determination of a specific cause.

PRIMARY PERITONITIS

The peritoneum is remarkably resistant to infection, and the majority of cases of peritonitis involve predisposing factors or concomitant irritation or injury. In the absence of these, peritonitis is rare and is only occasionally encountered. If a primary intraabdominal process cannot be ruled out in the septic child with abdominal findings, peritoneal lavage with Gram staining, culture, and cell count is performed. The finding of bile, meconium, or gram-negative organisms is an indication for surgical exploration. Without evidence of an intraabdominal focus, broad-spectrum antibiotics such as a third-generation cephalosporin (e.g., cefotaxime, 100–200 mg/kg/day) and penicillinase-resistant penicillin (e.g., nafcillin, 50–100 mg/kg/day) are begun pending culture results. If enterococcus is suspected, ampicillin (100 mg/kg/day) should be substituted for the penicillin. The gastrointestinal tract is decompressed and placed at rest.

Yersinia enterocolitica has recently been recognized as one of the more common causes of "spontaneous peritonitis" outside of the neonatal period. The clinical findings may be indistinguishable from acute appendicitis. When the diagnosis can be made without surgery, trimethoprim-sulfamethoxazole is the therapy of choice.

Primary peritonitis is an important complication of the nephrotic syndrome and must be considered in these children who present with abdominal pain. Initial therapy should include both gram-positive and gram-negative coverage, and the second-generation cephalosporin cefoxitin (100 mg/kg/day) or the aminoglycoside gentamicin (7.5 mg/kg/day), plus penicillin (100,000–200,000 units/kg/day), will usually provide adequate coverage pending final culture results.

Chronic ambulatory peritoneal dialysis predisposes to primary peritonitis. In the absence of significant systemic toxicity, therapy is initiated by mechanical flushing of the peritoneal cavity by means of two to three rapid lavages. Antibiotics are then begun locally by adding antibiotic to the dialysate. A broad-spectrum agent such as cefazolin is utilized pending culture results. An initial loading dose of 500 mg/l of dialysate is followed by 250 mg/l for 10 days. The child with significant systemic signs should be hospitalized and treated parenterally. Infection or leak at the catheter site predisposes to peritonitis and should, following therapy, prompt catheter removal. Similarly, recurrent episodes may respond to catheter change.

INTESTINAL PERITONITIS

By far the most common cause of peritonitis in childhood is gastrointestinal disease or injury. In the neonate, necrotizing enterocolitis is the most frequent etiology. In the absence of surgical complications, therapy consists of physiologic support, correction of fluid and electrolyte abnormalities, gut rest, nutritional support, and broad-spectrum enteric antibiotic coverage. Following cultures, gentamicin (5–7.5 mg/kg/day), ampicillin (100 mg/kg/day), and clindamycin (40 mg/kg/day) are begun and continued for a minimum of 7 days. Indications for operative intervention include intestinal perforation, obstruction, and hemorrhage. Without obvious pneumoperitoneum, peritoneal lavage is indicated in any suspicious case or in the newborn whose condition continues to deteriorate despite seemingly adequate therapy.

Outside the newborn period, acute appendicitis is the most frequent cause of intestinal peritonitis in childhood. The sine qua non of diagnosis is right lower abdominal peritoneal irritation. In the face of this physical finding, appendectomy is indicated unless there is overwhelming evidence for an alternative diagnosis. In the child with accompanying high fever or dehydration, surgery should be delayed until adequate resuscitation has been performed. Enteric aerobic and anaerobic antibiotic coverage (e.g., cefoxitin, 100 mg/kg/day; or gentamicin, 7.5 mg/kg/day, ampicillin, 100 mg/kg/day, and clindamycin, 40 mg/kg/day) is employed perioperatively in nonperforated cases and for a minimum of 5 days when perforation has occurred.

Additional uncommon gastrointestinal causes of peritonitis in childhood include perforated ulcer or foreign body, closed loop obstruction, and neglected intussusception.

PELVIC PERITONITIS

Pelvic inflammatory disease (PID), the ascending infection of the female genital tract, can result in peritonitis and is increasingly encountered in childhood. It is now apparent that *Neisseria gonorrhoeae* is not the sole cause of PID. Other commonly encountered organisms include *Chlamydia trachomatis, Bacteroides,* anaerobic gram-positive cocci, and *Escherichia coli.*

Pelvic examination is indicated in any female with lower abdominal findings. If the diagnosis remains in doubt, pelvic ultrasonography is indicated. A serum pregnancy test should also be routinely done to rule out ectopic pregnancy. Initially therapy consists of broad-spectrum parenteral antimicrobials such as doxycycline (2–4 mg/kg/day) and clindamycin (40 mg/kg/day). The intravenous administration of antibiotics is continued until the patient has been afebrile for 48 hours and abdominal tenderness has resolved. Oral medications are then substituted, based upon culture results, and continued for 10–14 days. In the absence of anaerobes, doxycycline is used. When anaerobic cultures are positive, clindamycin is substituted. If PID cannot be reasonably differentiated from acute appendicitis, surgical exploration is indicated.

MISCELLANEOUS CAUSES OF PERITONITIS

Acute cholecystitis can occur in the child, particularly in the presence of hemolytic disease. Initial therapy consists of gastric decompression, fluid resuscitation, and antibiotics (cefazolin, 100 mg/kg/day). Failure of response is an indication for surgery. Pancreatitis can result in peritonitis and is usually posttraumatic in the child. Pancreatitis usually responds to gut rest and decompression. Ovarian torsion will present as pelvic peritonitis of acute onset. Treatment consists of surgical excision. Psoas abscess, acute discitis, sickle cell crisis, and ventriculoperitoneal shunt complications may also result in signs of peritoneal irritation in the child and should be considered in the appropriate settings.

Peritonitis

ANNE KOLBE, M.B., B.S. (HONS.), F.R.A.C.S.,
and J. ALEX HALLER, Jr., M.D.

Generalized peritonitis in children is a serious condition with an estimated mortality rate of 1 to 2% and substantial morbidity. However, careful initial assessment, appropriate resuscitation, timely surgical intervention, and diligent postoperative care can minimize the complications associated with this condition such that an excellent long-term result can be expected in the vast majority of children.

Peritonitis is inflammation of part or all of the parietal and visceral surfaces of the abdominal cavity. The causes of peritonitis in children are

Table 1.   CAUSES OF PERITONITIS IN CHILDREN

Common
    Acute appendicitis
    Pelvic inflammatory disease
    Ischemic intestinal obstruction
    Traumatic gastrointestinal perforation

Uncommon
    Postanastomotic gastrointestinal leak
    Necrotizing enterocolitis
    Pancreatitis
    Meconium peritonitis
    Primary Peritonitis
    Secondary Chronic ambulatory peritoneal dialysis
    Secondary Urine, bile, or chyle leak
    Tubercular peritonitis

numerous (Table 1), but the presentation, assessment, and management of a child with peritonitis are basically the same regardless of the etiology. To manage a child with peritonitis it is necessary to understand the basic anatomy and physiology of the peritoneum as well as pathophysiological changes that result from the inflammatory insult.

Initial Management

The initial management of a child with peritonitis involves seven basic steps.

1. Fluid Replacement. *All* children with peritonitis are dehydrated. The extracellular fluid volume may be depleted by as much as 10–15% of body weight. The aim of fluid resuscitation is to correct this extracellular fluid deficit rapidly, thus minimizing the risks of hypovolemia and allowing early operation on a stable child.

Ringer's lactate is an appropriate fluid to use, as it is a buffered solution with electrolyte concentrations that approximate extracellular fluid. Initially 20 cc/kg stat should be given followed by a continuous infusion at 2–3 times maintenance until homeostasis is restored, as judged by a clear sensorium, good peripheral perfusion, normal blood pressure, fall in pulse rate, an adequate central venous pressure, and a urine output greater than 2 cc/kg/hr. Then the IV fluids can be changed to dextrose 5% with $\frac{1}{2}$ normal saline with 20 mEq of KCl/liter at $1\frac{1}{2}$ times maintenance until operation.

2. Antibiotics. Antibiotics must be administered as soon as is practical after the diagnosis of peritonitis is made. The initial choice of antibiotics is empirical but is guided by the knowledge that peritonitis in children is almost always polymicrobial, involving aerobes and anaerobes. The usual organisms isolated from the peritoneal cavity are *Escherichia coli,* enterococcus, Enterobacteriaceae, and bacteroides. On this basis the first-line drugs of choice are the following: (a) gentamicin, 5–7.5 mg/kg/day, divided and given IV q 8 hr; ampicillin, 200 mg/kg/day, divided and given IV q 4–6 hr; and clindamycin, 20–40 mg/kg/day, divided and given IV q 6–8 hr. All of these drugs achieve the same levels in the peritoneal fluid as they do in the blood.

3. Nasogastric Decompression. A large-bore sump nasogastric tube must be placed and attached to low-pressure suction. The tube empties the stomach of gastric secretions and swallowed air, which prevents vomiting, reduces the risk of aspiration, and minimizes further respiratory compromise.

4. Sedation. Once the diagnosis is established, all children with peritonitis should be given some form of analgesia and sedation. Either meperidine, 1–1.5 mg/kg IV, or morphine 0.1–0.2 mg/kg IV can be used.

5. Fever Control. Fever results in an increase in insensible fluid loss with ongoing dehydration. High fevers in young children may precipitate febrile seizures. Acetaminophen is usually sufficient to lower the temperature below 38.5° C. In addition, the use of cold sponges, a cooling blanket, or an electric fan may be helpful. Aspirin should not be used, as it alters platelet aggregation and increases the risk of intra- and postoperative bleeding. Aspirin has also been implicated in the pathogenesis of Reye's syndrome.

6. Oxygen. Severely ill children with hypoxemia and acidemia should receive oxygen via a face mask. If ventilation is severely compromised, intubation and mechanical ventilation may be necessary.

7. Emotional Support. In caring for a child with peritonitis, as for any ill child, it is important to remember the emotional impact of the child's illness on both the patient and the parents. A few minutes spent gaining the child's confidence before the initial examination and a brief explanation of proposed management and procedures is invaluable. Also a discussion of the child's illness and management protocol with the parents helps alleviate some of their concerns. This in turn is reflected favorably in their child's behavior.

Surgical Management

Operative intervention should be carried out as soon as the initial resuscitative management is completed. The aims of surgery are (1) to confirm the clinical diagnosis, (2) to prevent continued peritoneal contamination by removal of its source, and (3) to remove all foreign material from the abdominal cavity.

At operation, peritoneal fluid is obtained for Gram's stain and culture. The responsible lesion is identified and appropriately managed by closure of the defect, resection, or exteriorization. The peritoneal cavity is carefully and copiously lavaged with warm normal saline to remove all pus, blood, and foreign material and to reduce the bacterial load. No benefit can be demonstrated by the

Table 2.   POSTOPERATIVE COMPLICATIONS

Wound
    Hematoma
    Infection
    Dehiscence

Pulmonary
    Atelectasis
    Pneumonia
    Aspiration
    Pulmonary embolus

Gastrointestinal
    Acute gastric dilatation
    Adynamic ileus
    Adhesive small bowel obstruction
    Intra-abdominal abscess
    Anastomotic leak
    Stress ulceration of gastroduodenum

Urinary
    Retention
    Infection

Venous
    Phlebitis

addition of antibiotics to the irrigant in patients already receiving systemic antibiotics. Intra-abdominal drains are used only if a well-formed abscess cavity is encountered. In uncomplicated generalized peritonitis, drains are of no benefit and may, in fact, induce local septic complications. In cases of gross peritoneal contamination, the practice of leaving the skin and subcutaneous layers of the wound open decreases the incidence of postoperative wound infection.

Postoperative Care. The postoperative care of children with peritonitis is aimed at supporting them through the recuperative process and minimizing postoperative complications (Table 2).

In the immediate postoperative period, intra-abdominal sequestration of fluid continues, and temperature and respiratory rate remain elevated, which increases insensible losses. Intravenous fluid is therefore initially administered at $1\frac{1}{2}$ times maintenance using dextrose 5% with $\frac{1}{2}$ normal saline with 20 mEq of KCl/liter. As the child's condition stabilizes, fluids can be changed to dextrose 5% with $\frac{1}{4}$ normal saline with 20 mEq of KCl/liter at a normal maintenance rate, which is continued until bowel activity returns and an oral feeding regimen is fully established. In severe, complicated cases of peritonitis it may take many days for the adynamic ileus to resolve. These children are markedly catabolic and will develop severe protein depletion unless intravenous hyperalimentation is initiated.

Nasogastric decompression is maintained until bowel activity returns. The volume of aspirate should be measured regularly and replaced intravenously with an equal volume of $\frac{1}{2}$ N/S with 10 mEq of KCl/liter.

As soon as a correctly positioned nasogastric

tube that is attached to suction has no significant aspirate the tube should be removed. Leaving a nasogastric tube off suction or clamped for a trial of "gastric emptying" or oral feeding makes no sense. Nasogastric tubes are uncomfortable for a child, they hamper coughing, and they are associated with a significant incidence of otitis media in young children.

Antibiotic coverage may be altered according to the results of the pre- and intraoperative cultures. They should be continued for at least 5 days or until there are no remaining signs of sepsis. These include a normal temperature for 48 hours and a white blood cell count and differential within normal limits. During antibiotic administration appropriate serum levels must be monitored, especially in patients with renal impairment.

Postoperatively close attention must be paid to respiratory care. The child should be encouraged to cough and take deep breaths on a regular basis. Young children will usually not do this on demand; however, they can often be coaxed to blow up a balloon or a plastic spirometer, which provides excellent pulmonary physiotherapy.

Adequate analgesia postoperatively is necessary to permit satisfactory pulmonary physiotherapy and to facilitate early mobilization. This is best achieved by using *small, frequent* intravenous doses of a narcotic agent. The dose must be tailored to provide adequate continuous comfort for the patient without excessive sedation.

Intra-abdominal abscesses and wound infection occur frequently after surgery for peritonitis. The wound must be regularly and carefully inspected. Continuing fever, ileus, and a persistently elevated white blood cell count strongly suggest the presence of an intra-abdominal abscess, which must be aggressively searched for by clinical and radiological means and, when found, operatively drained.

Primary peritonitis is a monomicrobial form of peritonitis that occurs principally in children with nephrotic syndrome or cirrhosis. The infecting organism is usually *Streptococcus pneumoniae, Haemophilus influenzae, Neisseria meningitidis,* or *Escherichia coli.* The treatment consists of antibiotics and supportive measures; and provided objective improvement occurs within 48 hours, operative intervention is unnecessary. Primary peritonitis is an uncommon condition that is clinically difficult to separate from secondary peritonitis that is due to a surgically correctable lesion. Practically, the diagnosis is most frequently made by laparotomy, but the prognosis is unaltered by this surgical intervention. For these reasons primary peritonitis is a diagnosis of exclusion and should not be made except in a child with a specific predisposing condition.

Nonhemolytic Unconjugated Hyperbilirubinemia

M. MICHAEL THALER, M.D.

Unconjugated bilirubin is toxic to the brain, particularly in newborns with low birth weight, hypoxia, acidosis, and hypoglycemia. Older children with inherited deficiency of bilirubin conjugation (Crigler-Najjar syndrome) are also at high risk.

Neonatal Hyperbilirubinemia

"Physiologic" jaundice occurs in 60% of term infants and over 80% of preterm infants during the first week after birth. The infant with this type of hyperbilirubinemia (<9 mg/dl) is not at risk from bilirubin encephalopathy (kernicterus) unless severely ill for other reasons (extreme immaturity, respiratory distress syndrome, sepsis, metabolic acidosis, hypoglycemia). Such newborns, and those with severe hemolytic jaundice due to blood group incompatibility or glucose-6-phosphate dehydrogenase deficiency, may develop bilirubin encephalopathy unless the serum bilirubin levels are reduced. The standard procedures available for treatment of pathologic hyperbilirubinemia are exchange blood transfusion and phototherapy.

Exchange transfusion is indicated in *any* infant with serum bilirubin approaching 20 mg/dl. Those with early signs of kernicterus should receive an exchange of blood at any serum bilirubin level. Kernicterus should be suspected in jaundiced neonates with lethargy, poor feeding, and absent Moro reflex.

Phototherapy may be used in conjunction with exchange blood transfusions to reduce the rate of pigment accumulation. Exposure to light in the blue range (420–470 nm) converts the pigment to excretable derivatives, thereby performing a function similar to conjugation of bilirubin. Indications for phototherapy vary, but generally every infant with serum bilirubin approaching 10 mg/dl is treated, with the goal of maintaining the circulatory pigment below this relatively safe level.

The complications encountered in the course of phototherapy include diarrhea, overheating, dehydration, and a dark discoloration of the skin (bronze baby) due to accumulation of brownish photoderivatives of bilirubin in the blood. Bronze babies often manifest elevated direct-reacting bilirubin levels and other signs of cholestatic liver disease.

When phototherapy is used without exchange transfusion in infants with hemolysis, anemia may develop. Hematocrits should be checked for several weeks in infants with ABO hemolytic disease, and simple blood transfusions should be used to prevent anemia.

Other rare disorders associated with severe hyperbilirubinemia are Crigler-Najjar syndrome, types I and II. Unconjugated serum bilirubin values in excess of 30 mg/dl are commonly observed in neonates with these defects of bilirubin glucuronyl transferase. While type II is responsive to treatment with phenobarbital (5 mg/kg/day), type I patients must remain on phototherapy for life, or receive a liver transplant.

"Breast Milk" Jaundice

Breast feeding is associated with hyperbilirubinemia in approximately 1 of 250 term infants. While serum bilirubin levels may rise to peak values of >25 mg/dl during the third week, this type of jaundice does not appear to be linked with kernicterus. The causes of breast milk jaundice are poorly understood. However, interruption of breast feeding for 3–4 days is followed by a rapid decline in serum bilirubin. Subsequent resumption of breast feeding is not followed by return of hyperbilirubinemia to previous levels.

Cirrhosis

M. MICHAEL THALER, M.D.

Causes of cirrhosis potentially amenable to therapy include galactosemia, cystic fibrosis, Wilson's disease, and total parenteral alimentation. Cirrhosis following neonatal hepatitis, biliary atresia, and toxic hepatitis is usually irreversible. The management of these patients is directed toward optimal nutrient intake and absorption for growth and tissue repair, and prevention of complications. Frequent evaluation of clinical status is important for early detection of complications and for maintenance of adequate nutrition in the presence of biliary insufficiency.

Nutrition

A protein-rich (1.5–2.0 gm protein per kg), low-fat, calcium-containing diet is usually well tolerated. Daily supplements of fat-soluble vitamins should include K (2–4 mg), E (up to 1000 I.U., or 50 I.U. by intramuscular injection every 1–2 weeks if intestinal absorption in inadequate), D₂ (up to 4000 I.U.), and A (5–15,000 I.U.).

Pruritus may be controlled with cholestyramine, up to 16 gm daily, or with phenobarbital, 3–5 mg/kg/day.

Complications

The three major complications of chronic liver disease are bleeding from esophageal varices, ascites, and hepatic coma. Portal hypertension is an important factor in all three.

Gastrointestinal Hemorrhage. Bleeding from varices in cirrhotic patients is complicated by impaired synthesis of coagulation factors, including fibrinogen, prothrombin, and factors V, VII, IX, and X. Other complicating factors include thrombocytopenia of hypersplenism, excessive reabsorption of ammonia from the breakdown of red cells in the intestine, hyponatremia, and hypokalemia. Timely correction of these abnormalities has a direct bearing on prevention of coma and on eventual survival.

Transfusions of fresh whole blood are preferably given to maintain blood volume, to insure adequate tissue perfusion, and to elevate levels of circulating coagulation factors and platelets. Fluid and electrolyte balance should be managed parenterally. This is also a convenient route for administration of vitamin B complex and K. Venous pressure should be measured frequently, and a catheter in the urinary bladder may be necessary for close surveillance of urinary output. Measures for prevention of hepatic coma should be instituted in all cases of gastrointestinal bleeding in the presence of severe hepatic decompensation. Cathartics and enemas are administered repeatedly to remove blood from the colon and thus eliminate the absorption of ammonia from this source. Liquid neomycin, 2 to 4 gm/24 hr, is given orally or by enema in an effort to suppress bacterial production of ammonia. Blood can also be aspirated from the stomach through a lavage tube.

A patient with advanced liver disease may bleed from sites other than esophageal varices. Because the treatment of hemorrhage from peptic ulcer, gastritis, or other lesions differs from the aggressive procedures employed in intractable esophageal bleeding, the site of bleeding should be located endoscopically as soon as the patient has been given transfusions. The diagnosis can be established with a high degree of accuracy under direct vision, especially if the varices continue to ooze blood.

When bleeding esophageal varices are demonstrated, the following measures are taken. Vasopressin (or posterior pituitary extract) is administered intravenously over a period of 10 minutes in doses of 10 to 20 units in 25 ml of saline to reduce portal venous pressure. If the response is positive, the treatment can be repeated at hourly intervals. When massive life-threatening bleeding continues, the use of a balloon tube (Sengstaken-Blakemore tube) may become necessary. There are great hazards involved in the use of the tube, especially the danger of massive pulmonary aspiration of vomitus, suffocation by improperly positioned balloon, and damage to the esophageal mucosa. Although bleeding from esophageal varices can be controlled in most cases with these measures, sclerosing injections or portal shunting may become necessary in many survivors.

Ascites. A combination of hypoalbuminemia, hyperaldosteronism, and renal failure associated with impairment of liver function may result in retention of sodium and total body water, whereas portal hypertension appears to be mainly responsible for the localization of excess fluid in the abdomen. Sudden ascites can be precipitated during the course of chronic liver disease by intercurrent infections, hemorrhage, or surgery. Acute ascites is often reversed by limiting daily dietary sodium to 500 mg. Children on this diet should receive an adequate caloric and protein intake.

"Chronic" ascites, which is a reflection of progressive liver decompensation and portal hypertension, gradually results in discomfort, dyspnea, and severe limitation of physical activity. In addition to dietary management, successful diuresis in these patients may be accomplished with the combinations of diuretic agents and inhibitors of sodium-potassium exchange.

Treatment is initiated in the hospital. A dietitian prescribes salt-depleted proteins and starches to augment caloric intake and to make the diet more palatable and adds vitamin supplements. In children with advanced cirrhosis, protein intake is limited to 1 gm/kg/day because of the danger of hepatic coma. The most useful diuretic is spironolactone, 3 mg/kg/day. Dosages may be decreased or increased according to the diuretic response. A mean 24-hour weight loss of up to 1 pound is considered satisfactory. Serum sodium and potassium levels should be determined daily, especially during the initial stages of therapy. Spironolactone usually obviates the need for potassium supplements. Chlorothiazide (30 mg/kg/day) in combinations with spironolactone up to 7 mg/kg/day often controls refractory ascites. Furosemide, 2 mg/kg/dose, is reserved for the most resistant cases.

Coma. Coma can be precipitated in a cirrhotic patient by infection, fluid imbalance, diuretic therapy, hemorrhage, and surgery. Appropriate respective measures include antibiotics, correction of over- or underhydration, removal of diuretics, prevention of hemorrhage and, obviously, avoidance of surgery. Current therapy of hepatic coma is based on efforts to diminish ammonia by eliminating protein intake during the comatose period and using poorly absorbed antibiotics, such as neomycin, kanamycin, or paromomycin, to control intestinal ammonia-producing bacteria. A daily oral dose of neomycin, 2 to 4 gm, is given during the acute periods; smaller doses may be required for maintenance. Lactulose, 60 gm/day in 3 doses, is also effective in control of ammonia. This nonabsorbable sugar acts as substrate for acid production by colonic flora, resulting in flux of ammonia from the circulation to the intestinal lumen. Other measures include control of renal ammonia by maintenance of normal potassium levels and avoidance of diuretics.

Patients with uncomplicated chronic liver disease usually recover when treated in this manner, but those with progressive liver disease usually do not. Liver transplantation may offer a chance for survival in such patients.

Tumors of the Liver

SHUNZABURO IWATSUKI, M.D.,
and THOMAS E. STARZL, M.D., Ph.D.

MALIGNANT TUMORS

Mass lesions of the liver diagnosed by radiologic studies should be considered malignant until proved otherwise. The most common malignant tumor in children is hepatoblastoma. Hepatocellular carcinoma is the second most common and usually occurs in older children. Sarcomas of the liver, such as rhabdomyosarcoma and angiosarcoma, are rare. None of these has a favorable outlook, but fibrolamellar hepatocellular carcinoma, which is common in older children and young adults, has a better prognosis than other types of liver malignancy.

The treatment for all malignant liver tumors is complete surgical excision by anatomic hepatic resection. Hepatic resections of more than the right or left lobe of the liver can be performed quite safely. For example, a large tumor occupying the right lobe and the medial segment of the left lobe can be resected by right hepatic trisegmentectomy, leaving only the left lateral segment of the left lobe (to the left of the falciform ligament); or a large tumor occupying the left lobe and anterior segment of the right lobe can be resected by left hepatic trisegmentectomy, leaving only the posterior segment of the right lobe. These extensive right and left hepatic trisegmentectomies can now be performed by experienced surgeons with less than a 5% operative mortality.

We have found that computed tomography is most useful to assess the extent of the tumor, but it can be often misleading, particularly when a large tumor distorts normal anatomic boundaries. If resectability is uncertain after extensive preoperative investigations, the patient should be referred to a surgeon who is experienced in major hepatic resections rather than submitted to exploratory celiotomy by someone who is unprepared to undertake a definitive procedure.

After curative hepatic resections, we often recommend that patients receive adjuvant chemotherapy for at least a year. We have been using combination chemotherapy with doxorubicin, dactinomycin, vincristine, cyclophosphamide, and often mitomycin. The value of this approach has not been validated in randomized trials, but the patients who have received adjuvant chemotherapy have seemed to live longer, tumor-free.

Liver transplantation is an ineffective cancer therapy at this time. We have treated 50 patients with various primary liver malignancies by orthotopic liver transplantation (total hepatectomy and liver replacement). Nearly all the patients who received liver replacement for the treatment of nonresectable large malignant tumors developed tumor recurrences, with the exception of those with fibrolamellar hepatomas. Fibrolamellar hepatocellular carcinoma seemed to carry a better prognosis after liver replacement, just as after partial liver resection. On the other hand, most of the patients who have received liver replacement primarily for other end-stage liver diseases, such as tyrosinemia and alpha$_1$-antitrypsin deficiency disease, and whose malignant liver tumors were small and incidental, survived tumor-free for several years.

The most common metastatic liver tumors in children are neuroblastoma and Wilms' tumor. Although chemotherapy and radiation therapy may be helpful in treating these metastatic tumors, the lesion should be excised whenever possible, particularly if it is localized to part of the liver. We have performed nearly 100 liver resections for metastatic liver tumors without any operative mortality.

BENIGN TUMORS

Most of the benign tumors of the liver are asymptomatic and are found incidentally during studies for other disorders or during abdominal operations.

Hemangiomas are the most common benign tumors of the liver. Giant cavernous hemangiomas should be treated by surgical excision, particularly if they are symptomatic. The majority of giant cavernous hemangiomas require lobectomies or trisegmentectomies of the liver, but some, which are located on the surface of the liver or which are pedunculated, can be enucleated along pseudocapsular margins without significant loss of normal liver tissue.

Infantile hemangioendotheliomas are most often seen in infants during the first 6 months of life and are distinct from cavernous hemangiomas. The lesions should be excised by anatomic hepatic resection whenever possible. If the patient's condition prohibits surgery, treatment with prednisone, diuretics, and digoxin can be used initially. Response to prednisone may allow surgery to be performed safely in 2 weeks. In extensive lesions, radiation to the liver may be used after pathologic diagnosis is confirmed by open liver biopsy. Favorable responses to steroids, radiation, and he-

patic artery ligation or embolization have been reported. The treatment should be vigorous, because complete regression and cure are possible.

Other benign tumors include adenoma, hamartoma, focal nodular hyperplasia, fibroma, and teratoma. Radiologic differentiation of these benign tumors from malignant tumors is unreliable. Pathologic confirmation of benign tumor is mandatory for each lesion. Large benign tumors should be treated by surgical excision, particularly if they are symptomatic. Adenoma has a tendency to rupture and cause life-threatening hemorrhage. Some adenomas cannot be easily differentiated from low-grade hepatocellular carcinoma by needle biopsies. If the diagnosis is uncertain, the lesion should be excised with an adequate margin without delay.

Portal Hypertension

SHEILA SHERLOCK, D.B.E., M.D.

Portal hypertension is nearly always due to obstruction to blood flow in the portal venous system. It can be divided into two main categories: presinusoidal, and sinusoidal or postsinusoidal. It is important to make the distinction. In the presinusoidal type of portal hypertension, hepatocellular function is intact, whereas in the second form it is defective, and liver cell failure is liable to be precipitated by hemorrhage. Treatment depends upon accurate localization of the site of obstruction and, if possible, knowledge of the cause.

Management Before and Between Hemorrhages. Apart from any treatment necessary for underlying cirrhosis, the child should be allowed to lead as normal a life as possible and attend ordinary school. Provided the spleen is not too large, games and physical education may be allowed. Particularly vigorous sports, such as football, must be forbidden. The child should not be allowed to become overly tired. The school principal should be informed of the situation, and the parents should not press the child to be too competitive in either work or play.

Note should be taken of fecal color and the parents told to report if it becomes black. Hemoglobin estimations should be done if the child appears anemic or passes black stools. Oral iron treatment is given as required. The cirrhotic child requires occasional estimations of the prothrombin time, and intramuscular vitamin K$_1$ (5 mg) may be useful from time to time.

Hemorrhage commonly follows an upper respiratory tract infection, and this should be avoided if possible and all necessary inoculations given. If infection develops, it should be taken seriously and broad-spectrum antibiotics given from the start. Drugs containing acetylsalicylic acid must be avoided. Cimetidine is given at the first indication of bleeding.

Undue attention should not be paid to the platelet and leukocyte counts. Although both may be low, the effects on the patient are not definite. Multiple infections are unusual. Low values should not indicate splenectomy.

Management of Hemorrhage. Endoscopy should be done, using a pediatric endoscope. If the technique has not been performed previously, an emergency percutaneous splenic venogram or selective mesenteric angiogram is performed.

If the patient is cirrhotic, hepatic precoma and coma may be precipitated by the hemorrhage. This should be anticipated by giving no protein by mouth, keeping the bowels moving freely, giving an enema if necessary, and prescribing oral neomycin, 15 mg/kg 4 times a day for 3 days. All types of sedation should be avoided. If the child has extrahepatic portal venous obstruction and normal hepatic function, there is virtually no danger of the development of hepatic precoma. The precoma regimen is therefore unnecessary, and sedation can be given as required. It is unusual for these patients to bleed before the age of 4.

Blood transfusion is usually necessary. In patients with extrahepatic portal obstruction, hemorrhages are likely to be multiple over years. The greatest possible care must be taken to preserve peripheral veins for further transfusions and to give absolutely compatible blood.

If liver cell function is adequate, the bleeding usually ceases spontaneously. If liver cell function is deficient and if the bleeding continues, I prefer to use vasopressin* (Pitressin) IV, although this route is not recommended by the manufacturer. This drug lowers portal venous pressure by constriction of the splanchnic arterial bed, causing an increase in resistance to the inflow of blood to the gut. It controls hemorrhage from esophageal varices by lowering portal venous pressure. A large dose, 1 unit per 3 kg of body weight, is given well diluted in 5 per cent dextrose intravenously in 10 minutes. Mean arterial pressure increases transiently, and portal pressure decreases for 45 minutes to 1 hour. Control of hemorrhage is shown by the disappearance of blood from gastric aspirates and by serial pulse and blood pressure readings. Abdominal colicky discomfort and evacuation of the bowels, together with facial pallor, are usual during the infusion. If these are absent, it may be questioned whether the vasopressin is pharmacologically active. Inert material is the most common cause of failure. Regular vasopressin injections

may be repeated in 4 hours if bleeding recurs, but efficacy decreases with continual use. The ultimate failure of vasopressin to control terminal hemorrhage reflects hepatocellular failure rather than improper method of treatment.

The value of vasopressin is its simplicity of use. In an emergency it can even be used in the home. The short duration is obviously unsatisfactory, and the side effects are unpleasant even if short-lived. However, this dosage is necessary to achieve an adequate reduction in portal pressure.

If vasopressin fails to produce the desired effect, the Sengstaken trilumen esophageal compression tube is used. A special small-sized tube is available for pediatric use. A rubber tube is inflated in the esophagus at a pressure of 20 to 30 mm Hg, slightly greater than that expected in the portal vein. Another balloon is inflated in the fundus of the stomach. The third lumen communicates with the stomach. The tube is passed relatively easily if the pharynx is well anesthetized. When the tube is in position, traction has to be exerted, and this causes difficulty. Too little traction means that the gastric balloon falls back into the stomach. Too much traction causes discomfort, with retching, and potentiates gastroesophageal ulceration.

The compression tubes are very successful in controlling bleeding from esophageal varices. They do, however, have many complications. They should not be left inflated longer than 24 hours. Their use should be part of a plan of management culminating either in sclerotherapy or surgery. Complications include obstruction of the pharynx with consequent asphyxia, aspiration pneumonia, and ulceration of pharynx, esophagus, and fundus of the stomach. The tube is not well tolerated by the patient. Skilled nursing is required while the tube is in position.

Emergency endoscopic sclerotherapy may be used after the acute bleeding is controlled. It is usually successful in stopping the hemorrhage but complications are frequent, especially with inexperienced endoscopists. Emergency surgery is rarely necessary. If bleeding does not cease or if it recurs and active intervention becomes essential, the best surgical method is probably esophageal transection. In patients having normal liver function, and in whom the splenic venogram or mesenteric angiogram has shown a portal or superior mesenteric vein of adequate caliber, a portacaval or mesocaval shunt may be performed. Emergency shunt surgery has a high mortality rate if the patient has cirrhosis and, if possible, should be avoided in this circumstance. Esophageal transection using the staple gun is occasionally necessary in children with extrahepatic portal vein destruction and exsanguinating bleeding.

Elective Surgery. Prophylactic surgery is not indicated. The patient must have bled from varices

---

* This use of vasopressn is not listed in the manufacturer's directive; 1 unit/3 kg may exceed manufacturer's recommended dosage.

before operation can be considered. The choice of procedure depends largely upon the state of the portal venous system as revealed by splenic venography or selective splanchnic angiography. If the portal vein is patent and of adequate caliber, end-to-side portacaval anastomosis is the most satisfactory procedure. In experienced hands this operation carries a low mortality rate (less than 5 per cent). Because of vein size, the operation can rarely be undertaken before the age of 10 years. It carries a small risk of shunt encephalopathy. In children this is particularly small, and in the presence of a normal liver, e.g., obstruction to the portal vein at the hilus of the liver, the changes are almost nonexistent. In the presence of cirrhosis, the possibility varies with the degree of underlying damage to the liver. The operation should not be performed in the presence of jaundice, ascites, or a past history of hepatic coma.

Splenorenal anastomosis may be considered in portal venous occlusion if the splenic vein is of adequate size. It is less efficient than a portacaval anastomosis, because the shunt is small and often occludes. The danger of post-shunt encephalopathy, however, is very small.

Superior mesenteric vein–inferior vena caval shunt is used to treat portal hypertension in patients who have occlusion of the portal and splenic veins, making neither available for anastomosis. The vena cava is transected just proximal to the junction of the two iliac veins, and the distal segment is ligated. The proximal segment is then anastomosed to the side of the intact superior mesenteric vein. Sometimes an intervening Dacron graft is used and the superior mesenteric vein and inferior vena cava so anastomosed side-to-side. Failures may be due to superior mesenteric vein thrombosis, and the mortality rate is about 10%.

Direct attacks on the varices and on various dangerous collaterals are numerous and rarely of lasting benefit. They include splenectomy, transection of the esophagus, partial and total gastrectomy, and partial esophagectomy. In general, they are not recommended. Patients with extrahepatic portal venous obstruction rarely die of exsanguinating hemorrhage. Conservative management usually helps them over the acute episode. Bleeding becomes more infrequent as time allows for the opening of collateral vessels to the renal and lumbar veins. Ultimately, portal pressure may decrease. This possibility may be lessened with repeated operations and removal or transection of such benign collaterals. The operative and postoperative mortality rates of the local operations on varices in a cirrhotic patient with borderline liver function are high, and the ultimate benefit doubtful.

Repeated endoscopic sclerotherapy may be used to obliterate esophageal varices. Three or four sessions at 1–3-week intervals are usually necessary. Unfortunately, the esophageal varices recur and gastric fundal varices are not treated.

Chronic Active Hepatitis

SHEILA SHERLOCK, D.B.E., M.D.

Chronic active hepatitis is diagnosed by the continuation for longer than 6 months of fluctuant hepatocellular jaundice with increased transaminase and gamma globulin levels.

If specific causes, such as Wilson's disease or hepatitis B infection, can be excluded, then immunosuppressive therapy, usually with prednisolone, must be considered. The indications for such treatment are not clear-cut, but if the serum transaminase levels are increased five times and gamma globulin levels are more than twice elevated, steroid therapy should be given. Liver biopsy findings of piecemeal necrosis with inflammation and bridging necrosis between portal zones and central areas are also indications. The initial dose is 0.4 mg/kg of prednisolone for 2 weeks. This is then reduced to a maintenance dose of 0.2 mg/kg.

Twenty per cent of patients fail to respond, deteriorate, develop hepatocellular failure, and die. In such patients a trial of higher doses of prednisolone (0.8 mg/kg) is worth considering. Prednisolone usually must be used for at least 6 months and usually for 2–7 years. Attempts are made to withdraw therapy when serum bilirubin, transaminase, and, if possible, gamma globulin levels are normal. Relapses follow discontinuation of treatment in about half of the patients, usually within 6 months of stopping, and necessitate reinstitution of the drug.

Retardation of growth may be a problem in those less than 10 years old. In these children, alternate day therapy with prednisolone, 0.4 mg/kg every other day, must be considered. This may minimize the effects of corticosteroids on growth. Alternatively, if complications such as facial mooning, obesity, growth retardation, or diabetes are a problem, then prednisolone (0.15 mg/kg) may be combined with azathioprine (1 mg/kg). Azathioprine alone gives less satisfactory results than when prednisolone is used.* Corticosteroid therapy is of particular value in preventing deaths during the first 2 years after diagnosis, when the disease is most active. Although most patients end with cirrhosis, a lesion which is irreversible, there are many examples in which the disease has become inactive and the patients have survived 10 to 20 years.

* This use of azathioprine is not mentioned in the manufacturer's directions.

Hepatitis B related active hepatitis is more indolent and treatment is not so urgent. If the patient is hepatitis e antigen positive, corticosteroids should on no account be given as they increase virus replication. Treatment with antiviral drugs such as interferons must be considered, but their position has not been established and they are not generally available. If the patient is hepatitis e antigen negative, a trial of prednisolone may be considered, but if clinical and biochemical improvement has not followed three months' therapy, it should be stopped.

Disorders of the Hepatobiliary Tree

SHUNZABURO IWATSUKI, M.D.,
and THOMAS E. STARZL, M.D., Ph.D.

Biliary Atresia, Biliary Hypoplasia, and Arteriohepatic Dysplasia (Alagilles Syndrome). Extrahepatic biliary atresia is responsible for approximately one-third of the cases of neonatal cholestatic jaundice. In 10% of biliary atresias, the lesion is either a distal atresia with patent proximal hepatic ducts or a cystic dilatation of ducts adjacent to the hilum of the liver. In these correctable forms of biliary atresia, reconstruction can be achieved by anastomosis of the patent extrahepatic bile duct or the gallbladder to a Roux-en-Y jejunostomy. Prognosis is excellent after biliary reconstruction.

In more common, noncorrectable forms of biliary atresia, there are no patent extrahepatic ducts, and the gallbladder is absent or rudimentary. For these lesions, hepatic portoenterostomy (Kasai operation) has been tried with varying degrees of success. Successful bile flow may be established in nearly all patients when the intrahepatic bile ducts at the hilum are greater than 150 μ in diameter but in only one-tenth of patients in whom such ducts are not demonstrable. In addition, the surgical success rate is related to the timing of operation. Success rates of 80–90% are reported if surgery is performed before 2 months of life, but the success rate falls to 20% after 3 months. It is deceptive to define success in terms of bile flow, since only 25% of patients are alive and free of jaundice 1–6 years after operation.

Cholangitis is a major problem after hepatic portoenterostomy. Prophylactic use of oral antibiotics, such as trimethoprim-sulfamethoxazole and cephradine, for a year has been advocated to suppress recurrent cholangitis. Various types of cutaneous enterostomy and complicated enteroenterostomy have been devised to reduce the risk of cholangitis, but none has been proved to be superior to a simple Roux-en-Y jejunostomy. Bleeding at or near the mucocutaneous junction is a common and serious complication of stomas that are left in place in the late stage of biliary atresia.

Revision of hepatic portoenterostomy should be limited to patients who became jaundice-free after an initial Kasai operation and who later develop recurrent jaundice due to obstruction or to a patient whose operation is judged to have been inadequate after review of previous medical records and pathology specimens.

Liver transplantation has become an alternative treatment of biliary atresia in the last several years. Before 1980, 1-year survival after liver transplantation for biliary atresia was 25% using conventional immunosuppressive therapy (azathioprine, prednisone, and antilymphocyte globulin). Since early 1980, 1-year survival has increased to 75%. Improvement has been due to better immunosuppression with cyclosporine and low doses of steroids. Five-year survival is projected at more than 50%.

Almost all recipients with biliary atresia have had earlier attempts at hepatic portoenterostomy. The 1-year survival rate of patients with biliary atresia is 20% less than that of patients with liver-based inborn metabolic errors, such as alpha$_1$-antitrypsin deficiency, tyrosinemia, and Wilson's disease. The previous hepatic portoenterostomy, which made the transplantation operation extremely difficult in many patients, has been responsible for the poorer outlook. Revisions and re-revisions of hepatic portoenterostomy, the placement of cutaneous enterostomy stomas, and the use of complicated enteric anastomoses other than simple Roux-en-Y jejunostomy are all adverse factors if liver transplantation is finally needed.

Although some authors advocate aggressive surgical therapy for biliary hypoplasia, hepatic portoenterostomy cannot be recommended. It is not only ineffective, but it also causes recurrent cholangitis. Arteriohepatic dysplasia (Alagilles syndrome) can be diagnosed by the characteristic features of broad forehead, deeply set and widely spread eyes, pointed chin, vertebral arch defects, pulmonary artery stenosis, and cholestatic jaundice due to a paucity of intralobular ducts. Both biliary hypoplasia and arteriohepatic dysplasia are good indications for liver transplantation.

Nutritional support is essential for children with these diseases to maintain their development. Vitamins, particularly A, D, and E, and calcium should be supplemented. Nutritional support consists of a diet high in proteins and low in fats. Formula with medium-chain triglycerides is now available.

Choledochal Cyst. In the past, choledochal cysts were drained by choledochocyst-duodenostomy or choledochocyst-jejunostomy in Roux-en-Y. The majority of patients so treated became relatively asymptomatic for a number of years after the internal drainage operation, but many developed delayed complications, such as recurrent cholangitis, formation of biliary calculi, and progressive hepatic fibrosis. The development of malignant disease within the choledochal cysts or elsewhere in the biliary duct system has been reported repeatedly. The incidence of this complication is approximately 5%.

As a consequence of these complications and their increasing recognition, more and more surgeons are advising partial or complete excision of the cysts with performance of a Roux-en-Y jejunal anastomosis to the relatively normal proximal end of the duct system. If a part of the cyst wall cannot be resected because of technical difficulties, the mucosa lining should be stripped.

Caroli's Disease. Congenital segmental dilatation of the intrahepatic biliary duct system is called Caroli's disease. This disease is occasionally associated with congenital hepatic fibrosis, cystic spongiosis of the renal medulla, and cystic disease of the pancreas.

The large intrahepatic ducts of both lobes of the liver are usually involved. If the right and left main intrahepatic ducts are dilated at the hilum, a large hepaticojejunostomy in Roux-en-Y will relieve bile stasis, thereby reducing the chance of cholangitis and stone formation. If many biliary stones have already formed, the tip of the jejunal Roux loop is brought up to the skin to create the jejunal stoma. Through this stoma, the retained stones can be removed postoperatively by endoscopic or radiologic maneuvers.

Rarely, the cystic dilations are confined to one lobe of the liver. Hepatic resection is indicated only in these unusual circumstances.

Cholecystitis and Cholelithiasis. Cholelithiasis in children is usually a complication of hemolytic diseases, such as hereditary spherocytosis, sickle cell disease, and thalassemia major. Adult types of cholesterol stones are occasionally seen in postpubertal children. Children with cholelithiasis should undergo elective cholecystectomy in the same way as adults. If the cholelithiasis is complicated by acute cholecystitis, the child should be treated with antibiotics first. If the signs of acute inflammation subside with antibiotic therapy, the cholecystectomy is performed electively during the same hospitalization, but if there is not a good response within 48–72 hours, emergency cholecystectomy is carried out.

Acalculous cholecystitis may occur in children during acute febrile illnesses, severe diarrhea, and postoperative convalescence, or it may follow major trauma and large burns. These patients are ordinarily treated by intensive antibiotic therapy and gastric suction. However, if gallbladder distension is progressive, cholecystectomy is performed. If recovery from the acute illness is complete, residual gallbladder disease is not apparent.

Pancreatic Diseases

KENNETH L. COX, M.D.

ACUTE PANCREATITIS

The general principles of treatment of acute pancreatitis are (1) to treat hypovolemia and electrolyte abnormalities, (2) to relieve pain, (3) to reduce pancreatic secretions, and (4) to remove the precipitating cause.

Correction of hypovolemia should begin immediately, utilizing a large-bore central venous catheter for fluid replacement and to monitor central venous pressure. Hypotension and low central venous pressure should be corrected as rapidly as possible with plasma, dextran, albumin, or whole blood. Shock is the main cause of death in acute pancreatitis. Shock is primarily a result of exudation of plasma into the retroperitoneal space and peripheral vasodilatation caused by increased kinin activity.

After hypovolemia has been corrected, the rate of intravenous infusions should be reduced so as to provide maintenance plus replacement of ongoing losses from nasogastric suctioning and exudation into the peritoneal and retroperitoneal spaces. Monitoring urine output and central venous pressure are mechanisms for assessing the adequacy of the fluid replacement. Major complications of treatment of severe acute pancreatitis are pulmonary edema and congestive heart failure; these usually occur 3 to 7 days after the onset of pancreatitis. Though in many cases the cause is unknown, in some cases fluid overload has occurred because of excessive fluid replacement. Thus, the amount of fluid replacement must be adjusted frequently for changes in intravascular volume.

Serum electrolytes, including calcium and magnesium, serum creatinine, and blood urea nitrogen determinations, will aid in selecting the appropriate electrolyte composition of intravenous solutions. Since between 2 and 17 per cent of patients with acute pancreatitis have renal failure, potassium should not be added to IV solutions until stable urine output has been established. In addition to maintenance sodium chloride and potassium chloride of 3 mEq/kg/24 hr and 2 mEq/kg/24 hr, respectively, losses from nasogastric suctioning should be replaced. Though 5 per cent dextrose solutions should be initiated, hyperglycemia and hypoglycemia occasionally seen in severe pancreatitis warrant careful monitoring of urinary reducing substances and blood glucose concentrations and changing the concentration of dextrose in the IV solution appropriately. Symptomatic hypocalcemia, i.e., tetany and seizures, should be treated with IV calcium gluconate, 0.1 to 0.2 gm/kg/dose (not over 2 gm) as a 10 per cent solution administered slowly and stopped for bradycardia. For asymptomatic hypocalcemia, replacement may be accomplished by adding 10 ml or more of 10 per cent calcium gluconate to each 500 ml of IV solution. In severe pancreatitis, serum electrolytes, including calcium, should be measured at least daily so that adjustments in the electrolyte composition of IV solutions can be made if necessary.

Pancreatic exocrine secretions are reduced by fasting the patient. Usually feeding should not be reinstituted until abdominal pain and ileus have resolved and serum amylase, urinary diastase, and the amylase-creatinine clearance ratio have returned to normal. If oral alimentation cannot be taken within 5 days, then parenteral nutrition should be given. Since carbohydrate is less of a stimulant to pancreatic exocrine secretion than are protein and fat, the initial diet should consist of carbohydrates only. If the carbohydrate diet is tolerated without worsening or exacerbating symptoms, then a low-fat and protein diet may be given. Again, the diet should be discontinued if symptoms should recur.

Nasogastric suctioning should be used to relieve nausea, vomiting, and abdominal pain. Since there is no evidence that gastric suctioning alters the clinical course of pancreatitis, it is not required in the treatment of mild-to-moderate pancreatitis. However, in severe pancreatitis or marked ileus, nasogastric suctioning should be used.

Relief of the severe abdominal pain associated with pancreatitis not only is important for patient comfort but also may reduce the cephalic phase of pancreatic secretion. Morphine sulfate should be avoided because it may worsen pancreatitis by causing sphincter of Oddi spasm. Meperidine hydrochloride (Demerol) may be administered IV or IM at 1 to 2 mg/kg every 3 to 4 hours for severe abdominal pain. If this does not reduce pain sufficiently, then the effect of Demerol can be potentiated by administering chlorpromazine (Thorazine) at 1 mg/kg IM simultaneously.

Other therapies for acute pancreatitis remain controversial. Prophylactic antibiotics have not been shown to be beneficial. Secondary infection of the pancreas, usually by streptococci, coliforms, or staphylococci, occurs in 2 to 5% of cases of pancreatitis. Identification of the infective organism(s) and the antibiotic sensitivities will allow selection of the appropriate antibiotics. If pancreatic abscess forms, surgical drainage is usually necessary. There is insufficient clinical evidence

that suppressors of pancreatic exocrine secretion, such as anticholinergic drugs, glucagon, somatostatin, calcitonin, and tranquilizers, and inhibitors of pancreatic enzymes, such as aprotinin (Trasylol)* and epsilon-amino-caproic acid (EACA), are useful in the management of acute pancreatitis.

Persistence of abdominal pain and of elevation of serum amylase levels for 2 or more weeks after the onset of acute pancreatitis suggests the formation of a pseudocyst. Ultrasonography is an effective method of identifying pseudocysts, differentiating pseudocysts from inflammatory masses, and monitoring the size of pseudocysts. Many pseudocysts spontaneously resolve in 4 to 12 weeks. If the pseudocyst persists for 6 or more weeks or is enlarging, surgical internal drainage of the cyst into the stomach or upper small intestine has been the treatment of choice. More recently, ultrasonography has been used to guide percutaneous needle aspiration of the cysts and to place catheters for external drainage. This technique may be particularly useful in patients who are poor operative candidates.

Pancreatic fistulas most often occur following pancreatic trauma or drainage of pseudocysts. Most fistulas will spontaneously close. Those that have a high output or interfere with providing adequate oral alimentation often require prolonged periods of fasting and total parenteral nutrition. Intravenous lipids can be given as a part of TPN therapy since they do not appear to stimulate pancreatic secretion. Rarely, surgical closure of the fistula is necessary.

Chronic and recurrent acute pancreatitis are rarely seen in children. Continued exposure to the precipitating cause, i.e., alcohol, cholelithiasis, child abuse, and so on, or familial pancreatitis must be considered. Hereditary pancreatitis is transmitted autosomal dominantly and is associated with lysinuria and cystinuria in some cases. Most cases of hereditary pancreatitis require total pancreatectomy for control of symptoms. Endoscopic retrograde cholangiopancreatography (ERCP) should be performed if etiology is unknown, since congenital papillary stenosis may be identified and treated by endoscopic papillotomy. ERCP may identify other obstructive abnormalities such as gallstones choledochal cysts, or duplication cysts that can be surgically corrected. Malabsorption due to pancreatic exocrine insufficiency and, rarely, diabetes mellitus requiring insulin therapy are sequelae of chronic pancreatitis. Malabsorption should be treated with oral pancreatic enzyme replacement therapy. Severe chronic abdominal

*Aprotinin is an investigational drug and may not be available in the United States.

pain may require prolonged fasting, using home parenteral nutrition or pancreatectomy.

PANCREATIC EXOCRINE INSUFFICIENCY

Cystic fibrosis, Shwachman-Diamond syndrome (pancreatic insufficiency and bone marrow hypoplasia), and chronic pancreatitis are main causes of pancreatic exocrine insufficiency in children.

Oral pancreatic enzyme extracts are the primary treatment, independent of the cause. The dose of pancreatic enzymes extract to be administered with meals depends upon the severity of pancreatic exocrine insufficiency, the patient's age, the fat content of the diet, and the type of enzyme preparation. In general, dietary fat restriction is not necessary, and approximately 8000 lipase NF units (one Cotazym capsule or one Viokase tablet) should digest at least 15 gm of dietary fat. Higher doses of enzymes may not improve digestion and may result in hyperuricemia. Ineffectivenss of oral pancreatic enzymes to completely correct malabsorption is in part due to the suboptimal pH of the stomach for enzyme activity. Reduction of gastric acidity with antacids or cimetidine or protection of preparations with enteric coating (Pancrease or Cotazyms) have been reported to improve enzyme activity.

Deficiency of fat-soluble vitamins D, A, K, and E may occur with severe malabsorption. Clinical manifestations from vitamin deficiencies are rarely seen. Occasionally, bleeding diathesis due to hypoprothrombinemia from vitamin K deficiency and hemolytic anemia from vitamin E deficiency will occur. Prevention of vitamin deficiencies is usually accomplished by reducing malabsorption with oral pancreatic enzymes and by administering a multiple vitamin preparation at twice the minimal daily requirements. Additional supplementation with water-miscible vitamin E, 50 to 100 U daily, and with vitamin K, 0.5 to 5 mg daily, should be given to those who have severe malabsorption or laboratory evidence of deficiency in these vitamins.

Advising patients and families of the appropriate diet for age and dose of oral pancreatic enzymes will usually allow normal growth and development without significant malabsorptive symptoms. Occasionally, additional calories in the form of dietary supplements will be desired, or limited fat restrictions in the diet, i.e., a 15 to 20% fat diet, will be necessary to control steatorrhea. Because elemental dietary supplements like medium-chain triglycerides and predigested protein are unpalatable, children will often refuse to take these preparations, especially for long periods of time. In these cases, nonelemental dietary supplements, such as Ensure, Sustacal, and Meritene, given with enzymes may be more acceptable.

ISOLATED PANCREATIC ENZYME DEFICIENCIES

Isolated pancreatic enzyme deficiencies are extremely rare. Diagnosis is made by pancreatic secretory studies revealing normal concentrations of pancreatic enzymes in duodenal aspirates except for the absence of a single enzyme.

Isolated lipase deficiency is an autosomal recessive disease that presents shortly after birth with oily diarrhea. Standard oral pancreatic enzyme preparations, as are used in cystic fibrosis, will correct the malabsorption.

Isolated amylase deficiency usually presents after 1 year of age. As starch becomes a larger part of the diet, watery diarrhea occurs. Analysis of the stool will reveal reducing substances (Clinitest positive at more than $\frac{1}{4}$%) and an acid pH of less than 6.0. The diagnosis can be confirmed with a starch loading test, i.e., failure of blood glucose to rise following ingestion of 50 gm of starch per square meter of body surface area. Treatment consists of starch elimination and supplementation with disaccharides.

Isolated trypsin or trypsinogen deficiency presents shortly after birth with diarrhea, anemia, hypoproteinemia, edema, and severe failure to thrive. Absence of trypsin or trypsinogen results in lack of proteolytic enzyme activity in duodenal secretions. Treatment consists of standard oral pancreatic enzyme preparations.

Isolated enterokinase deficiency is an autosomal recessive disease that will also present in the neonatal period with severe watery diarrhea, failure to thrive, anemia, hypoproteinemia, and edema. Enterokinase is produced in the brush border of the proximal small intestine. Since this enzyme is necessary for the activation of trypsin, duodenal aspirates lack proteolytic enzyme activity, which can be activated by adding enterokinase to the aspirate. Enterokinase can be assayed in the small intestinal biopsies. Standard oral pancreatic enzyme preparations are the required treatment.

CONGENITAL MALFORMATIONS

Annular pancreas is a ring of pancreatic tissue encircling the descending portion of the duodenum. Surgical intervention consists of a duodenoduodenostomy or duodenojejunostomy. The pancreas is left undivided so as to avoid formation of pancreatic fistulas. Pancreatic function is normal in these patients.

Approximately 2% of the population have ectopic pancreatic tissue. Ninety per cent of these occur in the stomach, duodenum, or jejunum. Occasionally, the ectopic pancreas will produce abdominal pain, gastrointestinal obstruction, bleeding, or intussusception. When these complications occur, the ectopic pancreatic tissue should be excised.

PANCREATIC TUMORS

Pancreatic tumors in children are very rare. Most are endocrine-secreting tumors, e.g., insulinoma, gastrinoma, VIPoma, and so on.

Ninety per cent of insulinomas are solitary tumors. Severe hypoglycemia often results in irreversible neurologic sequelae. Diazoxide, from 5 mg/kg/24 hr up to 20 mg/kg/24 hr, will usually prevent hypoglycemia. Most children who have insulinomas during the first year of life will have remission before 5 to 6 years of age. Thus, surgical resection is not usually necessary in these younger children if hypoglycemia is prevented by diazoxide. Earlier surgery is indicated in children with localized tumors seen after 1 year of age or who have hypoglycemia that is poorly controlled by diazoxide. Blind resections are often unsuccessful.

Twenty per cent of gastrinomas are solitary and benign. Gastrin secreted by the tumor stimulates gastric acid secretion, resulting in multiple gastric and duodenal ulcers and often diarrhea. Fasting serum gastrin levels may be only marginally elevated, but will be markedly elevated (> 400 pg/ml) following IV secretin injection or calcium infusion. In adults, cimetidine, an H_2-receptor antagonist, has been shown to be an effective drug for controlling symptoms caused by the gastric hyperacidity. Those whose symptoms are not controlled by cimetidine usually require a total gastrectomy. Since the tumors are usually multiple and difficult to localize, surgical resection is often impossible.

Fortunately, carcinoma of the pancreas rarely occurs in children. However, recent reports from Japan indicate an increasing incidence in pancreatic carcinomas in children. Since clinical manifestations usually do not appear until extensive metastasis has occurred, prognosis of pancreatic carcinoma is poor, with a mean survival of 6 to 9 months after diagnosis in adults. Pancreaticoduodenectomy is recommended for the rare patient who has a small, localized lesion. In those with inoperable disease, supportive therapy consists of providing adequate nutrition and analgesia.

Cystic Fibrosis

LUCILLE A. LESTER, M.D.,
and RICHARD M. ROTHBERG, M.D.

Cystic fibrosis is a multisystem disorder associated with generalized exocrine gland dysfunction. Optimum treatment of this disorder at any age can be provided only if its various manifestations and complications are recognized and the wide spectrum of disease severity is appreciated.

Once the diagnosis of cystic fibrosis is confirmed by two positive sweat tests (Cl > 60 meq/l in at least 100 mg of sweat), coordination of care with a designated cystic fibrosis center often facilitates development of an appropriate regimen. A conference should be held to familiarize the family with the disease process and its treatment, prognosis, and *genetic implications*. Arrangements should be made for instruction in chest physiotherapy, the use of inhalation therapy equipment, the child's special nutritional needs, and the need for vitamin and pancreatic enzyme supplementation.

Following the institution of a care regimen, close follow-up, initially at 2- to 4-week intervals, is required to re-evaluate therapy and answer questions. As the patient's condition stabilizes, less frequent visits are needed. Children who are doing well only need to be seen every 4 to 6 months. At each clinic visit, information should be elicited about frequency and character of cough, sputum production, exercise tolerance, appetite, and recent weight and height changes. Pulmonary function testing should be done when possible, and a minimum yearly chest x-ray examination and liver function tests should be obtained. Exacerbations of the chronic pulmonary disease may thus be detected early and treated in an outpatient setting with oral doses of antibiotics and intensification of the chest physiotherapy regimen. If the patient does not improve, admission to a hospital for parenteral antibiotic therapy, intensive pulmonary toilet, and nutritional support is indicated.

Prevention of complicating diseases is also important. Routine pediatric immunizations should be given to patients who are not acutely ill, even if cough is present. Yearly immunizations against influenza are recommended, but Pneumovax (pneumococcal vaccine, polyvalent, MSD) is not indicated.

PULMONARY THERAPY

For unknown reasons, there is marked heterogeneity in the severity of the pulmonary disease. Since the disease spectrum includes infants under 6 months of age who present in a severely compromised pulmonary status during an episode of bronchiolitis, often caused by respiratory syncytial virus, to adults with nearly normal pulmonary function and lifestyle, specifics of treatment must be individualized. Close supervision and continuity of care permit an anticipatory therapeutic approach. It is generally accepted that a team approach, together with improved antimicrobial agents and more aggressive management of pulmonary complications, has resulted in the recent prolongation of life expectancy.

Chest Physiotherapy. Chest physiotherapy is utilized to facilitate mobilization of the thick mucopurulent secretions from the tracheobronchial tree. In children who produce sputum, it is usually preceded by inhalation therapy. We routinely teach nine position segmental bronchial drainage techniques at the time of diagnosis, even if there is no evidence of pulmonary disease. The combination of percussion and vibration, together with deep breathing and cough maneuvers in the older child, is performed in each of nine positions, with the average treatment session requiring 20–30 minutes. In infants or children with early radiologic signs of bronchial obstruction or chronic cough, we initiate postural drainage once a day. Children 10 to 12 years of age and older should be instructed in how to perform the therapy themselves, and when the patient becomes self-sufficient, it may be helpful to add a mechanical percussor or vibrator to do some of the posterior positions effectively. In school-age children it is difficult to manage more than 2 sessions per day, but patients with severe bronchiectasis do benefit from three to four treatments per day.

Compliance with daily chest physiotherapy is often poor in the active, seemingly healthy youngster despite repeated attempts to reinforce need and benefits. Recently, along with other centers, we have been substituting or adding a regular program of aerobic exercise such as running, swimming, gymnastics, or tennis for 15–30 minutes every other day. Patients with moderate symptomatic involvement should undertake such an exercise program only with medical supervision. The patient's sense of well-being is often enhanced by such activity.

Aerosol Therapy. In patients who cough and produce sputum, whether it is expectorated or swallowed, the addition of aerosol inhalation therapy appears beneficial. This therapy delivers fluid to the lower respiratory tract in an attempt to thin the tenacious mucus and to facilitate its removal, especially during chest physiotherapy. It is also used to administer medications to the lower respiratory tract. Small compressor-driven, hand-held nebulizers can be used, but larger ultrasonic units deliver a greater volume of smaller particle-sized mist to the lower airway. They are more durable and, thus, more practical for long-term daily use.

To enhance the effectiveness of chest physical therapy, a bronchodilator followed by 15 to 20 minutes of a tussive mist is usually employed prior to postural drainage. We routinely add isoproterenol as a 0.05% solution (1 drop/10kg + 1) to 0.45% saline solution for nebulization treatments. The isoproterenol acts promptly, and its effect dissipates within 30–60 minutes. More recently, we have used a 5% solution of metaproterenol with good results. Mucolytic agents, such as N-acetyl-L-cysteine, may be beneficial in some patients. Since it often induces bronchospasm, it is usually given by aerosol with the bronchodilator. One to 4 ml of a 10–20% solution of N-acetyl-L-cysteine is administered over 10–15 minutes. In the severely ill patient who has been unable to mobilize secretions, the initial N-acetyl-L-cysteine may lead to sudden, rapid mobilization of secretions, which may compromise ventilation. Therefore, the patient should be closely monitored, and nasotracheal suction should be available during and after the administration of the first few doses.

The use of aerosolized antibiotics has been controversial, but a recent enthusiasm has developed for this treatment modality. Prospective, crossover, blinded studies are currently evaluating the effectiveness of different inhaled antibiotic regimens. The most frequently used drugs are the aminoglycosides alone or in combination with a semisynthetic penicillin. We have been administering tobramycin (parenteral solution; 80 mg/ml) by nebulization after chest physical therapy in selected patients. The major benefit of this therapy, observed in our patients with moderate to severe lung disease, is a significant reduction in the necessity for hospitalization. Patients on long-term inhalation therapy with aminoglycosides must be monitored for otoxicity, nephrotoxicity, and the development of drug-resistant strains of *Pseudomonas*.

Antibiotic Therapy. The progressive, destructive pulmonary disease of cystic fibrosis is initiated by infection in obstructed areas of the lung. Aerosol therapy and bronchial drainage aim to mobilize and remove tenacious secretions. Antibiotics are used to control the chronic infection. We feel strongly that antibiotics should not be used alone or in place of measures to mobilize secretions. Intermittent culturing of expectorated sputum (older children) or nasopharyngeal aspirates at the time of induced coughing (younger children) and determination of antibiotic sensitivity on all isolates of pathogens are the best guides to appropriate antibiotic therapy.

Staphylococcus aureus is usually the first organism to be cultured from the respiratory tract, and many feel that it is the initial and major pathogen in cystic fibrosis lung disease. However, *Pseudomonas aeruginosa*, especially the mucoid strains, almost invariably becomes the predominant organism in sputum. There is evidence that *S. aureus* remains a significant offender, despite the isolation of only *P. aeruginosa* in a given sputum specimen. Intermittently, patients who have harbored only *S. aureus* or *P. aeruginosa* may have *Hemophilus influenzae*, *Escherichia coli*, *Proteus mirabilis*, or *Klebsiella pneumoniae* grow from their sputum. When this occurs, treatment for these organisms should be considered. Patients who have received numerous courses of parenteral anti-*Pseudomonas* antibiotics may develop strains resistant to the aminoglycosides and/or semisynthetic penicillins. Also, multiple drug-resistant *Pseudomonas* strains, such as *Pseudomonas cepacia*, have recently emerged as major problems in some patients with cystic fibrosis.

Significant controversy still prevails over the question of the use of daily prophylactic oral antibiotic therapy. We strongly favor the use of intermittent courses of antibiotics to treat exacerbations of pulmonary symptoms in an effort to delay the early appearance of *P. aeruginosa* and the development of antibiotic-resistant strains. However, patients with severe pulmonary disease and compromised pulmonary physiology have been empirically found to do better with daily administration of oral antibiotics.

Choice and timing of antibiotic therapy may be difficult, since signs of infection are frequently lacking, making it hard to differentiate between colonization and low-grade infection. Abnormalities on chest auscultation and increasing obstructive disease demonstrated by pulmonary function tests are often the main indications of pulmonary exacerbations. Additionally, findings such as increased cough, significant nighttime cough, increased irritability, decreased activity, poor appetite, and weight loss may also be present. Patients with these findings or with symptoms of an upper respiratory tract infection should be treated with a 10- to 14-day course of an oral antibiotic that has significant anti-*S. aureus* activity. Trimethoprim-sulfamethoxazole is often the first drug we prescribe because it is well tolerated and has to be taken only twice a day. Dicloxacillin, cephalexin, cefaclor, and erythromycin are also frequently prescribed. Tetracycline, particularly doxycycline, is useful alone or in combination with dicloxacillin in patients 9 years of age and older. Chloramphenicol remains a frequently used and particularly efficacious drug because of its high biopenetrability and its action against *S. aureus* and *H. influenzae*. Using short courses limited to 2 to 3 weeks, we have as yet not had hematologic or ocular complications.

Patients with more advanced pulmonary disease who develop acute or chronic symptoms and patients who have failed to improve on an outpatient regimen of oral antibiotics and intensified chest physiotherapy require admission to the hospital for intravenous antibiotics. Patients with only *S. aureus* cultured from their sputum are usually treated with nafcillin alone or nafcillin and gentamicin. In patients with *P. aeruginosa*, we use a combination of a semisynthetic penicillin and an aminoglycoside given intravenously for 10 to 14 days. High doses of aminoglycosides are usually required, and it is often necessary to administer

them every 6 hours instead of every 8 hours to achieve levels of 6–9 μg/ml 30 minutes after infusion. Trough levels should be < 2 μg/ml. Some centers favor the addition of nafcillin in patients not improving on the double antibiotic regimen. After hospitalization, we frequently administer another 2 to 4 weeks of oral antibiotics. The recent interest in home administration of intravenous antibiotics is presently being evaluated. This has been successfully undertaken in selected families trained in administration of intravenous drugs or in those who have access to home care service companies to supply and maintain the intravenous lines. We have a limited experience with central venous lines or semipermanent peripheral venous access lines for chronic antibiotic administration at home. These catheters for chronic administration of antibiotics are an appropriate treatment approach for a select group of highly motivated patients and families. The intramuscular route is seldom used, since the patient's muscle mass is small and repeated painful injections are poorly tolerated for protracted periods of time.

Treatment of Allergy and Reactive Airway Disease Symptoms. Cystic fibrosis patients have an incidence of allergy equal to that in the general population. The symptoms are often difficult to distinguish from milder pulmonary symptoms of cystic fibrosis. Antihistamines may thicken and dry lower respiratory tract secretions but can be employed for short periods together with decongestants to relieve allergic rhinitis symptoms. Cystic fibrosis patients may develop hyperactive airway disease on an allergic basis. However, those with bronchiectasis may have clinically evident bronchospasm secondary to the chronic inflammation. If pulmonaray function testing demonstrates reversibility of obstruction, oral theophylline or beta-adrenergic agents may be helpful. In patients with cold- or exercise-induced bronchospasm, symptoms usually respond to a bronchodilator given 20 to 30 minutes before exposure to cold or exercise. These measures, along with treatment of pulmonary infection, are usually sufficient and we avoid the use of steroids to treat the hyperactive airway disease in patients with cystic fibrosis.

Bronchial Lavage. This modality has been recommended as an efficacious way to "clean out" large quantities of mucopurulent material. We feel it has little long-term efficacy, and the severely compromised patient may experience significant hypoxia during the procedure. For these reasons we no longer perform this procedure.

Expectorants. No systemic drug has proved useful in specifically clearing secretions from the lungs. Prolonged use of iodides may be helpful but is limited by the frequent development of goiters. We have not found oral expectorants useful and caution against the use of over-the-counter expectorants or cough preparations. These mixtures often contain antihistamines or cough suppressants, which are potentially detrimental.

PULMONARY COMPLICATIONS

Atelectasis. Lobar or segmental atelectasis is frequently encountered in infants and young children with cystic fibrosis. The right upper and middle lobes and the lingula are most commonly affected. Such atelectasis may be an unsuspected finding on a routine chest roentgenogram, but even in asymptomatic patients aggressive treatment with inhaled bronchodilators followed by chest physiotherapy is indicated. Antibiotics are used if atelectasis is noted during the course of an exacerbation and infection. Re-expansion may not occur despite intensive treatment given in the hospital. In such patients we have seen re-expansion after several weeks of continued vigorous bronchial drainage at home. Rigid bronchoscopy with or without lavage is usually without benefit. Removal of the obstruction using a flexible fiberoptic bronchoscope may result in re-expansion and could be attempted.

Hemoptysis. Blood-streaked sputum is common in cystic fibrosis patients with widespread bronchiectasis. It is usually related to increased bronchial infection, and antibiotics should be prescribed. If mild hemoptysis (< 30 ml) continues despite antibiotic treatment, hospitalization for parenteral antibiotics is indicated. Postural drainage may be stopped for the first 24 hours and is then gradually resumed. Vitamin K is administered if prothromin time is prolonged. Massive hemoptysis (500–700 ml/24 hr) may occur in older cystic fibrosis patients with more advanced disease. Bed rest, cessation of postural drainage, and blood replacement are urgent steps to be taken. Supportive treatment, including oxygen and parenteral antibiotics, should be instituted. If bleeding persists, an attempt to localize the site of bleeding by bronchoscopy can be tried. This should be followed by percutaneous angiography and embolization of the dilated bronchials on the affected side. Gelfoam and Ivalon (polyvinyl alcohol sponge) have both been used successfully. In patients who continue to have significant hemoptysis, elective embolization of the remaining bronchial arteries is suggested.

Pneumothorax. Spontaneous pneumothorax is a complication most often affecting adolescent and young adult cystic fibrosis patients who have extensive pulmonary involvement. If the pneumothorax is less than 10% of lung volume as determined by chest roentgenogram, and the patient is stable, he can be observed in the hospital. In larger pneumothoraces or in tension pneumothoraces, immediate insertion of a chest tube is mandatory.

Due to the high risk of recurrence, we do chemical pleurodesis after the lung has re-expanded. After appropriate sedation, tetracycline or quinacrine is inserted into the chest tube, and the patient's position is changed frequently to expose as much of the pleura as possible to the irritant medication. If pneumothorax recurs after chemical pleurodesis, open thoracotomy with parietal pleurectomy, oversewing of visible blebs, and visceral pleural abrasion are done. This procedure is tolerated even in severely compromised patients.

Cor Pulmonale. Cor pulmonale, strictly defined as right ventricular hypertrophy, can be detected using echocardiography in patients with mild to moderate pulmonary disease. This hypertrophy progresses slowly with advancing hypoxemia and is probably exacerbated by the increased hypoxemia experienced during exercise and sleep. Nighttime low-flow oxygen at home may delay progression of this cardiac abnormality. Fulminant right heart failure or acute cor pulmonale is a near-terminal event in patients with severe lung disease but often responds to treatment. Humidified oxygen at low flow rates should be administered to maintain the PaO_2 at about 50 torr without depressing the ventilatory drive. Furosemide, 1 mg/kg IV, produces rapid diuresis and can be repeated at 8- to 12-hour intervals. Moderate dietary salt restriction is reasonable in these patients, who may also be receiving intravenous antibiotics with high sodium concentrations. Digitalis is of questionable usefulness, though short-term improvement in ventricular function has been documented. Tolazoline was initially found to be useful for reducing pulmonary hypertension, but its effectiveness is short lived and its side effects undesirable. Newer drugs (hydralazine, nifedipine) with possible pulmonary vasodilating effects may be more promising for use in patients with severe pulmonary hypertension.

Aspergillosis. Aspergillus species are most often encountered incidently in sputum cultures from patients receiving antibiotics for chronic conditions. In this situation it is thought to represent colonization rather than infection. Invasive aspergillosis requiring antifungal treatment has rarely been documented in patients with cystic fibrosis. In contrast, a hypersensitivity pneumonitis (allergic bronchopulmonary aspergillosis) does occur in cystic fibrosis patients. This complication responds well to low-dose steroid therapy, but care should be taken to adjust the basic care regimen to prevent exacerbations of bacterial infection.

Pulmonary Osteoarthropathy. Digital clubbing is commonly observed but is usually only of cosmetic importance. Periostitis of the ends of long bones with new bone formation may be roentgenographically evident in older patients with painful swelling of the larger joints. Aspirin, acetominophen, and nonsteroidal anti-inflammatory agents such as ibuprofen are effective in relieving the pain and swelling that are exacerbated during active pulmonary infections.

Respiratory Failure. Although usually thought of only as the end result of the chronic progressive bronchiectasis, respiratory failure can be precipitated by acute pulmonary infection in patients with mild to moderate lung disease. Short-term mechanical ventilatory support may be employed for such a patient. In more chronically ill patients developing hypoxia (Pao_2 between 50–60 torr on room air), low-flow oxygen by nasal cannula is used. We begin its use during sleep only and extend its use to daytime activities as indicated. Oxygen concentrators or liquid oxygen systems are both convenient for home oxygen administration. This oxygen therapy significantly improves the patients' quality of life by allowing them to be more mobile and less fatigued and dyspneic, and they have decreased headaches and deep bone pain. Mechanical ventilatory assistance appears to be of little benefit for the severely compromised patient with end-stage lung disease. This decision should be completely discussed with family members before the need for ventilatory assistance is clinically obvious. Supportive care, including antibiotics, tranquilizers, chest physiotherapy, and chronic oxygen, is routinely given.

GASTROINTESTINAL THERAPY

Pancreatic Insufficiency. Clinically evident pancreatic insufficiency occurs in most patients with cystic fibrosis, though it may vary in age of presentation and severity. Infants or young children who present with a positive sweat test and frequent, large, foul-smelling stools and failure to thrive do not need a 72-hour fat balance study to document the pancreatic insufficiency. Such infants may be severely malnourished, and we provide them with readily absorbable nutrients by starting them immediately on special infant formulas containing hydrolyzed proteins and medium chain triglycerides (Pregestimil or Portagen) as well as pancreatic enzyme supplements. These formulas, which can be prepared in concentrations up to 27 cal/oz are used to supply the needed extra calories without increased volume. When the special formula is no longer tolerated (around 12 months of age), skim milk fortified with nonfat dry milk powder (20 cal/oz) or 2% milk is introduced, and the pancreatic enzyme dose is increased appropriately.

Pancreatic enzymes should be given with meals and snacks. Sufficient enzyme is given to normalize stool number and consistency and to achieve maximal growth. The newer preparations circumvent the problem of gastric acid inactivation by an enteric coating designed to release active enzyme in the duodenum; thus, fewer capsules are required per meal. Young infants, however, are best treated with powdered enzyme mixed with a few teaspoons of formula or strained food (1/2 to 2 capsules of pancrelipase [Cotazym] per feeding), as the enteric coating of the microspheres may be incompletely removed by the gastric acid in young infants. At age 12 months we change to the enteric-coated microsphere preparations (Pancrease or Cotazym-S). As the child grows and intake increases, enzyme dosage must be increased, and older infants and children may need from 1 to 5 or 6 capsules/meal. Symptoms of bloating, abdominal distention, crampy abdominal pain, and diarrhea, which suggest inadequate enzyme intake, often lessen in older children and adults.

Low fat diets were previously the dictum for all cystic fibrosis patients with pancreatic insufficiency. With the improved enzyme preparations and with the recognition of essential fatty acid deficiency (lineolic acid) in cystic fibrosis patients with treated pancreatic insufficiency, the recent trend has been toward no fat restriction in the diet. Patients may vary in their ability to tolerate certain dietary fats even with good enzyme replacement, and diets must be individualized. We aim for 150% of the recommended daily allowance for age of calories and protein. When regular meal intake does not provide adequate calories, or when requirements increase, such as during infection, high-calorie liquid supplements are prescribed. Polycose or medium chain triglycerides can also be added to regular foods as a source of readily utilizable calories. In hospitalized children who have *lost* weight and cannot maintain adequate calorie intake, we have found supplemental peripheral hyperalimentation to be an effective and safe way to provide 700 to 1500 extra calories/day over a 2-week period. Solutions of 10% glucose, 1–2 gm/kg/day of crystalline amino acids, 1–2 gm/kg/day of 10% Intralipid solution (except in severely hypoxic patients) may be administered by peripheral intravenous infusion. All our patients receive supplemental vitamins containing water-soluble or miscible forms of A, D, and E.

Meconium Ileus. Meconium ileus is a common cause of neonatal intestinal obstruction and occurs in 5–10% of all children with cystic fibrosis. Perforation and meconium peritonitis can occur, and this requires immediate surgical intervention. More typically, clinical signs of obstruction develop in the first 24 hours of life, and if cystic fibrosis is not suspected, surgical intervention is usually prompt. In cases in which cystic fibrosis is suspected and the baby is stable, diatrizoate (Gastrografin) enemas with pressure may flush the contrast media above the area of obstruction. In about 50% of these cases, enough fluid is drawn into the bowel lumen to flush out the inspissated meconium. Diatrizoate is very hypertonic and must be administered only after an intravenous line has been established for fluid and electrolyte replacement. After relief of the obstruction, attention must be directed to achieving adequate nutrition, either orally or with supplemental parenteral alimentation.

Meconium Ileus Equivalent: Intussusception. About 20% of the older cystic fibrosis patients develop episodic (often recurrent) accumulations of bowel contents in the distal ileum and ascending colon. This partial obstruction, often associated with inadequate pancreatic enzyme intake, may lead to intermittent abdominal pain and a decreased number of stools. Adjustment of pancreatic enzyme dosage and saline enemas are often all that is needed. If more complete obstruction develops, the patient should be admitted to the hospital and treated with saline enemas containing N-acetyl-L-cysteine (4–5% by volume). If this treatment is not effective, diatrizoate* enemas under fluroscopic control are done in an attempt to flush out the obstructing material. Surgery to relieve the obstruction is occasionally required. A similar clinical presentation may also be observed with intussusception. This occurs with an increased frequency in the infant with cystic fibrosis, and cystic fibrosis is one of the few causes of intussusception in older children and adults. The intussusception is usually ileocolic and may be suspected on a plain film of the abdomen. Reduction by barium enema should be tried, but if it is unsuccessful, surgical reduction is required.

Liver Disease. A small percentage of newborn infants with cystic fibrosis may have prolonged cholestatic jaundice. Frequent monitoring of the transaminases is important, especially in those infants requiring hyperalimentation. This problem usually resolves completely within 6 to 12 months. Prior to diagnosis, some older infants may develop fatty infiltration of the liver secondary to malnutrition. This resolves promptly with the institution of appropriate diet and pancreatic enzymes. At least 25% of the patients develop a focal biliary cirrhosis that is characteristic of cystic fibrosis. In most, this is manifested by increased alkaline phosphatase and elevations of the transaminases. About 20% of the patients with focal biliary cirrhosis progress to a more severe multinodular cirrhosis and portal hypertension. There is no specific treatment for the liver disease, and hepatic function usually remains adequate until late in the course. The complications are managed in the same way as in other types of liver disease. Ascites is treated with a low-salt diet and at times with diuretics.

---

* This use of diatrizoate (Gastrografin) is not listed in the manufacturer's directive.

Esophageal varices may lead to frequent chronic blood loss or massive hemorrhage. Vitamin K should be given to patients with prolongation of their prothrombin times, and salicylates should be avoided. Effective control of acute hemorrhage can be achieved with nasogastric intubation, cold saline lavage, and infusion of vasopressin. If hemorrhage continues, endoscopy may identify the bleeding site, and homeostasis may be achieved by sclerosis of this area. Severe hypersplenism may result from portal hypertension, and when this occurs in association with bleeding varices, splenectomy and a splenorenal shunt are effective treatment. Portacaval anastomosis has been avoided because of the frequency of postoperative hepatic encephalopathy.

Gallbladder Disease. Up to 40% of older patients with upper abdominal pain have been found to have gallstones by abdominal ultrasound or cholecystogram. Only an occasional patient has colic or pain typical of cholelithiasis and requires surgical treatment.

Pancreatitis. The 10–15% of patients without clinically significant pancreatic insufficiency at an early age often develop acute or recurrent pancreatitis as young adults. The symptoms often are mild and may be similar to those of cholelithiasis. Patients with severe symptoms and elevated amylase levels are best treated with nasogastric drainage, intravenous fluids, and analgesics.

Rectal Prolapse. In the untreated cystic fibrosis patient who has frequent loose stools, the rectal mucosa may prolapse at the time of defecation. Similarly, prolapse may occur in patients with known cystic fibrosis taking insufficient pancreatic enzymes to control steatorrhea. In either instance, the prolapse often can be spontaneously reduced by placing the patient in the knee-chest position. If not, the rectal mucosa may be replaced manually. Prolapse ceases as steatorrhea is controlled by pancreatic enzymes. Surgical treatment is rarely indicated.

Gastroesophageal Reflux. In some infants the finding of gastroesophageal reflux has been used to explain recurrent pulmonary infiltrates, thereby resulting in a delay in the diagnosis of cystic fibrosis. Appropriate diagnosis followed by treatment of the cystic fibrosis lung disease with chest physiotherapy and antibiotics usually decreases the severity of the cough and eliminates the need for antireflux measures. A small percentage of older patients have been found to have significant reflux with or without hiatal hernia. These symptoms usually improve with medical reflux management and measures to minimzie paroxysmal coughing. Bethanechol should be avoided in patients with symptomatic pulmonary disease.

MISCELLANEOUS PROBLEMS

Salt Depletion. During the warmer months, infants with cystic fibrosis may present with a characteristic hyponatremic, hypochloremic dehydration with alkalosis secondary to excessive losses of electrolytes in the sweat. Maintenance of adequate salt and fluid intake during hot weather may prevent the development of such problems. Intravenous fluid and electrolyte correction have been necessary in some infants. Older children and adults may develop a similar state of dehydration if they work or exercise vigorously in hot weather. This can be controlled by giving salt supplements (500-mg tablets once or twice daily) in addition to the liberal use of dietary salt.

Hyperglycemia. In older patients fibrosis of the pancreas may be severe, and encroachment on the pancreatic islets may occur, with resulting carbohydrate intolerance. In 3–5% of patients, polyuria, polydipsia, and weight loss occur, and insulin is required. Ketoacidosis rarely develops, but during periods of stress (infection) increased amounts of insulin may be required.

Otolaryngologic Complications. Young children with cystic fibrosis may develop chronic serous otitis media and persistent rhinitis. Ventilation with polyethylene tubes may be required if hearing loss develops. Sinus opacification is radiographically evident in over 90% of the patients but is rarely associated with fever, pain, and purulent drainage. If repeated courses of antibiotics and decongestants are ineffective in the symptomatic patient, surgical drainage may be required. Nasal polyps also occur in a very high percentage of patients with cystic fibrosis. When very large, the polyps can obstruct one or both nares. Beclomethasone nasal spray may result in temporary relief. Surgical removal is sometimes needed, and postoperative recurrence is common.

Surgery. When surgical therapy is indicated in patients with cystic fibrosis, careful attention to pulmonary toilet will reduce the risk. Five to 10 days of maximized pulmonary therapy, including antibiotics, is given in the hospital prior to surgery. Every effort to use local or spinal anesthesia should be made. If this is not possible, general anesthesia time should be kept to a minimum. After surgery, postural drainage and coughing, with support of surgical wounds, are reinstituted as soon as feasible. A common surgical problem in older patients is inguinal hernia. This presents a particularly difficult situation during the postoperative period. Coughing is indicated for the pulmonary disease but even with support of the wound may have a detrimental effect on the healing surgical reconstruction.

Reproductive Problems. Ninety-eight per cent of males with cystic fibrosis are infertile. This is due to azospermia resulting from obstruction of the vas deferens. Females with cystic fibrosis have a reduced fertility rate, possibly due to abnormal cervical mucus. Significant lung disease may make pregnancy an undesirable medical risk, and birth control measures should be advised appropriately. These problems should be discussed with the patients and alternatives (such as artificial insemination of the spouses of males with cystic fibrosis) should be offered on an individual basis.

Chronic Diarrhea and Malabsorption Syndromes

WALLACE A. GLEASON, M.D.,
and LARRY K. PICKERING, M.D.

Chronic diarrhea in children is caused by a myriad of disorders, which can be classified into one of several catagories based upon pathophysiologic mechanisms and clinical presentation. This classification allows children with chronic diarrhea to be evaluated in a logical, systematic manner. These catagories include inflammatory and infectious diarrhea, osmotic diarrhea, secretory diarrhea, malabsorption, abnormal motility, and other causes that are not easily classified (Table 1). The approach to children with chronic diarrhea begins with a thorough medical history, a physical examination, and knowledge of pathophysiologic mechanisms underlying each of these categories. This information can then be used to determine appropriate use of laboratory facilities and to guide therapy. Chronic diarrhea is defined as diarrhea lasting for more than 3 to 4 weeks.

INFLAMMATORY AND INFECTIOUS DIARRHEA

Many bacterial, viral, and parasitic organisms produce diarrhea in humans. Their virulence determines the type of intestinal involvement and resultant clinical manifestations. Virulence is determined by intestinal invasion, cytotoxin production, enterotoxin production, and intestinal adherence. Only organisms that invade the intestine or produce a cytotoxin result in inflammatory diarrhea. Organisms that invade intestinal epithelium include *Campylobacter jejuni, Shigella, Salmonella, Yersinia enterocolitica,* invasive *Escherichia coli,* and occasionally *Vibrio parahemolyticus.* These bacteria produce symptoms that include abrupt onset of fever and, if the colon is primarily involved, abdominal cramps, tenesmus, fecal urgency, and the passage of scant stools containing blood, mucus, and fecal leukocytes. Vomiting is not common. Cytotoxins produced by *Clostridium difficile,*

Table 1. CLASSIFICATION OF CHRONIC DIARRHEA OF CHILDHOOD

Inflammatory and Infectious*
    Postinfectious including invasive or cytotoxin-producing organisms such as *Salmonella, Shigella, Campylobacter, Yersinia enterocolitica, Vibrio parahemolyticus, Escherichia coli, Clostridium difficile,* and *Entamoeba histolytica*
    Postinfectious, noninflammatory organisms, including parasites (*Giardia lamblia*, cryptosporidium, and *Strongyloides stercoralis*) and viruses (rotavirus, Norwalk-like viruses, enteric adenovirus)
    Noninfectious
        radiation
        dietary protein–induced enterocolitis
        Crohn's disease
        ulcerative colitis
        Hirschsprung's disease
Osmotic
    Lactose malabsorption*
    Sucrose-isomaltose malabsorption
    Glucose-galactose malabsorption
    Ingestion of nonabsorbable carbohydrates
Secretory
    Enterotoxin-producing bacteria
    Functional tumors
    Intestinal bacterial overgrowth (cholerrheic enteropathy, stagnant loop syndrome)
    Familial chloridorrhea
Malabsorption
    Small intestinal disorders
        celiac disease*
        immune deficiencies
        intestinal lymphangiectasia
        eosinophilic gastroenteritis
        abetalipoproteinemia
        Wolman's disease
    Pancreatic insufficiency
        cystic fibrosis*
        Shwachman-Diamond syndrome
        chronic pancreatitis
Other Disorders
    Chronic nonspecific diarrhea or irritable colon syndrome*
    Intractable diarrhea of infancy
    Acrodermatitis enteropathica

* Most common causes

enterocytotoxic *E. coli*, possibly enteropathogenic *E. coli*, and *V. parahemolyticus* damage intestinal epithelial cells, resulting in diarrhea containing blood, mucus, and leukocytes. A specific diagnosis may be confirmed by recovery of the organism on stool culture. These agents do not usually cause weight loss and usually are not chronic.

Pseudomembranous or antimicrobial associated colitis (AAC) refers to the presence of pseudomembranes or multiple plaquelike lesions in the colon caused by administration of an antimicrobial agent, most commonly a penicillin, cephalosporin, or clindamycin. The specific agent is a toxin produced by an overgrowth of *Clostridium difficile*. It must be stressed that diarrhea is a common complication of antimicrobial therapy in children and AAC occurs rarely. Patients with AAC present with watery diarrhea that often contains blood and mucus. Diarrhea may be the only manifestation of

disease or may occur in association with nausea, vomiting, abdominal pain or cramps, fever, and leukocytosis. If not treated appropriately, patients may develop toxic megacolon, colonic perforation, shock, and death. Diagnosis of AAC in a patient with diarrhea is suggested by recent antimicrobial therapy, a positive fecal leukocyte stain, exclusion of other enteropathogens known to cause fecal leukocytosis, isolation of *C. difficile* and its toxin from stool, and identification of pseudomembranes during sigmoidoscopy with rectal biopsy.

Four parasites are known to cause diarrhea in various populations in the United States. *Entamoeba histolytica* produces an inflammatory type of diarrhea; *Giardia lamblia*, cryptosporidium and *Strongyloides stercoralis* cause diarrhea that is watery, that may be protracted, and that is associated with villus tip flattening or microvillus destruction.

Amebic colitis due to infection with *E. histolytica* is an important problem in tropical and subtropical areas. The highest incidence of infection with clinical symptoms occurs in the third through fifth decades of life, although persons of all ages are susceptible. The most common mode of spread in the United States is person-to-person, including sexual transmission. Contaminated food and water have been shown to transmit the disease. *E. histolytica* organisms adhere to the intestine by microfilament invasion and produce microabscesses, probably through production of enzymes and cytotoxins. The clinical patterns associated with amebiasis consist of intestinal involvement with gradual onset of colicky abdominal pain and frequent bowel movements, tenesmus, and little or no systemic involvement; amebic dysentery characterized by profuse diarrhea containing blood and mucus and the presence of systemic signs such as fever, dehydration, and electrolyte alterations; and hepatic amebiasis, which usually presents as abscess formation without gastrointestinal tract symptoms.

G. lamblia is a flagellated protozoan that is an important cause of acute diarrhea as well as a causative agent of recurrent and/or chronic diarrhea and malabsorption. Conditions that predispose to giardiasis include youth, hypogammaglobulinemia, secretory IgA deficiency, peptic ulcer disease, biliary tract disease, pancreatitis, and travel to hyperendemic areas. The parasite may exist in the trophozoite or cyst forms. Trophozoites are usually seen in duodenal aspirates and loose stools; cysts, which are the infectious forms, are found in formed stools.

Cryptosporidia attach to epithelial cells in the gastrointestinal tract. Diarrheal episodes due to this organism have been reported in immunocompromised hosts, particularly those with acquired immunodeficiency syndrome (AIDS), as well as immunologically normal patients, often after exposure to infected animals or attendance in a day care center. The clinical illness is often protracted and is manifest by symptoms that include nausea, low-grade fever, abdominal cramps, anorexia, and five to ten bowel movements per day.

S. stercoralis is a nematode that infects humans via the intestinal tract or through skin that comes in contact with soil containing the larvae. Approximately one third of people with strongyloidiasis are asymptomatic, and the remainder may have skin, pulmonary or, more frequently, gastrointestinal tract involvement. Epigastric abdominal pain occurs and is associated with diarrhea that contains mucus. Some patients may complain of nausea, vomiting, and weight loss with evidence of malabsorption. Eosinophilia and an urticarial rash are prominent features of infection.

Acute infectious diarrhea of viral origin is generally a self-limited disease characterized by various combinations of diarrhea, nausea, vomiting, abdominal cramps, headaches, myalgia, and low-grade fever. Bowel movements are watery and do not contain mucus or blood. Vomiting is the most common manifestation of this condition. Rotavirus, Norwalk-like agents, and enteric adenovirus are important causes of viral gastroenteritis; the specific relationship between other viral agents and diarrhea is unknown. Norwalk-like agents characteristically produce epidemics of illness in adults and children, whereas rotavirus is a more important cause of endemic illness in infants and young children. Enteric adenovirus has been reported to cause outbreaks of diarrhea as well as sporadic episodes in infants. Clinical illness generally lasts 5 to 8 days but in rare cases may last as long as 1 month. Although rotavirus characteristically produces a transient diarrhea, it may cause a severely dehydrating illness that necessitates hospitalization. Rotavirus and Norwalk virus cause diarrhea by selectively destroying absorptive cells (villus tip cells) in the mucosa, leaving secretory crypt cells intact.

Many conditions that are not of an infectious origin produce inflammatory diarrhea (see Table 1). Radiation enterocolitis usually begins months after a course of radiation therapy and results from microcirculatory changes associated with the radiation therapy. The area of intestine involved must be within the portal to which the radiation therapy was delivered. The diagnosis is suggested by history of radiation therapy and can be confirmed by finding characteristic histologic changes in the small arterioles in the submucosa on biopsy.

Enterocolitis induced by dietary protein is a cause of bloody diarrhea in infants, generally those less than 6 months of age, who are fed commercial formulas containing intact proteins. Symptoms include bloody diarrhea with inflammatory lesions of the intestine and usually a peripheral leukocytosis with a marked left shift. In addition to diarrhea, infants with this condition may have other symptoms, including vomiting, abdominal pain, and colic. The mechanism of disease may involve excessive intestinal uptake of antigenic macromolecules. These antigens then elicit an immune response manifesting itself as enterocolitis due to a Shwartzman-like reaction in the colonic mucosa. Increased macromolecular transport also may occur after an episode of infectious diarrhea. There is roughly a 20% incidence of sensitivity to both cow's milk protein and soy protein, and it is therefore not unusual to see patients who have enterocolitis in response to refeeding with either of these formulas. Although evidence of a primary immune mechanism of this disorder is lacking, it is frequently referred to as "cow's milk allergy," "soy protein allergy," or "milk colitis." The diagnosis is considered when clinical manifestations resolve after milk elimination and reoccur within 48 hours following a trial feeding of milk. Another approach to diagnosis is serial intestinal biopsies after a milk challenge. During milk feeding mucosal villous atrophy is present. This resolves on a milk-free diet. Owing to wide variations in pathogenesis and manifestations of this disease, abnormal findings on small bowel biopsy are neither specific nor consistently present. A large number of immunologic tests have been reported to be variably abnormal in this condition; however, these tests have poor sensitivity and specificity and no single simple test that is readily available has been accepted as a diagnostic aid. Clinical manifestations clear by 2 years of age and many of these infants will not develop enterocolitis when the offending protein is reintroduced. Management is by encouraging breast feeding or feeding formulas, such as Nutramigen or Pregestimil, in which the protein source is casein hydrolysate.

Inflammatory bowel disease includes Crohn's disease and ulcerative colitis. An exhaustive discussion of these disorders is beyond the scope of this review, but inflammatory bowel disease should be included in the differential diagnosis of enterocolitis in the older child or adolescent, although it occasionally occurs in infants and younger children. The initial clue to its presence is the chronicity or recurrence of inflammatory diarrhea without an alternative explanation.

Hirschsprung's disease (congenital aganglionic megacolon) results from failure of retrocaudal maturation of the autonomic nervous system in the intestine. This results in unopposed tonic constriction of the aganglionic distal intestinal segment, producing obstruction and subsequent dilatation of the proximal, normally innervated colon. The vast majority of patients present with lower intestinal obstruction as newborns. A small number of patients who escape detection as young infants can present with a severe enterocolitis. Gram-negative sepsis and septic shock frequently occur, and the mortality is extremely high. The diagnosis of Hirschsprung's disease is suggested by abdominal distention and constipation, particularly in the absence of hard stools in a young infant. Digital rectal examination reveals a tightly constricted rectal ampulla in contrast to a dilated rectal ampulla present in simple constipation. The diagnosis is further suggested by radiographic demonstration of the "transition zone" between the dilated, normal proximal intestine and the constricted, aganglionic distal segment and confirmed by demonstrating the absence of ganglion cells in the submucosal or myenteric plexus of the constricted segment by rectal biopsy. This "transition zone" most commonly occurs in the rectosigmoid area. Since radiographic findings may be obscured by cathartics and enemas, patients undergoing barium enema examinations should not be subjected to the usual preparation for such radiologic procedures.

OSMOTIC DIARRHEA

Osmotic diarrhea results from incomplete absorption of osmotically active nutrients. In infants and children, dietary carbohydrate is primarily responsible; this type of diarrhea should cease when oral feedings are stopped. A test for carbohydrate in stools becomes, therefore, a test for osmotic diarrhea in children. Congenital lactase deficiency is a condition in which an abnormal enzyme protein with either decreased enzymatic activity or decreased affinity for substrate results from a genetic mutation. This rare disorder produces severe watery diarrhea from the very first feeding. A more common problem is acquired lactase deficiency, of which there are primary and secondary forms. Acquired primary lactase deficiency results from a decrease in intestinal lactase activity with increasing age. The presence of large amounts of lactase in the intestinal mucosa of the young mammal is an adaptation of the intestine of the suckling animal to its diet. As lactose becomes a less important dietary carbohydrate with weaning, intestinal lactase levels begin to fall. This decrease in intestinal lactase appears to be predetermined, since continued lactose feeding is generally ineffective in inducing persistence of enzyme activity. Infants who are destined to become lactase deficient as adults begin losing intestinal lactase activity between 2 and 8 years of age. It is therefore important to recognize that primary acquired lactase deficiency is not a cause of osmotic diarrhea in infants but may be an important cause of osmotic diarrhea in older children and adults.

Acquired secondary lactase deficiency refers to a nonspecific decrease in intestinal lactase activity accompanying many diarrheal illnesses. Lactase is an enzyme found only in relatively mature, well developed enterocytes. If such enterocytes are shed and replaced by a population of less mature enterocytes, a net decrease in intestinal lactase activity results. Acquired secondary lactase deficiency due to this mechanism is a common, nonspecific phenomenon in infants and children following a bout of infectious diarrhea. Lactose intolerance, by whatever mechanism, is characterized by watery diarrhea resulting in dehydration and acidosis in the young child. It is treated by using one of the soy formulas, which are lactose free.

Other causes of carbohydrate malabsorption in infants include sucrose malabsorption resulting from a decrease in activity of the intestinal sucrase-isomaltase enzyme complex and familial glucose-galactose malabsorption. Sucrase-isomaltase deficiency is rare and is inherited as an autosomal recessive enzyme defect. It should be suspected in children who develop watery diarrhea following ingestion of sucrose. It can also be a nonspecific result of intestinal brush border damage. The fact that sucrose-isomaltose malabsorption occurs much less commonly than lactose malabsorption has led to the suggestion that brush border lactase activity is more easily damaged by the insult of diarrheal illness. Familial glucose-galactose malabsorption is a rare disorder in which there is an abnormality of active hexose transport. Since this is a generalized epithelial transport problem not limited to the small intestinal epithelium, these patients generally have glucosuria as well as monosaccharide malabsorption, and are thus identified by the presence of glucose in urine and stool.

Transient, nonspecific monosaccharide malabsorption may occur as a result of decreased transport of the monosaccharides across the intestinal mucosal brush border membrane. This frequently complicates the oral rehydration and refeeding of infants with diarrhea. It results from disturbances in both active and passive transport of monosaccharides, probably due to repopulation of the intestinal villus with cells having a less well developed brush border and, therefore, less surface area available for absorption and less mature active transport mechanisms. Monosaccharide malabsorption is identified by the presence of fecal reducing sugars in patients fed only monosaccharides, such as 5% glucose and water. This is a transient phenomenon and usually disappears within 1 to 2 days of intravenous fluid therapy.

Hexitols are the sugars used in dietetic products. The main hexitols, sorbitol and mannitol, are not metabolized in the intestine and are only passively absorbed. Their accumulation in the intestinal lumen produces an osmotic diarrhea. The symptoms seem to be dose related.

SECRETORY DIARRHEA

Unlike osmotic diarrhea, secretory diarrhea results from excessive secretion of fluid and electrolytes into the gastrointestinal tract. This excessive secretion overwhelms the capacity of the distal small bowel and colon to increase its absorption of fluid and electrolytes. Secretory diarrhea can be differentiated from osmotic diarrhea by its persistence after oral feedings are stopped. Patients frequently have such severe watery diarrhea that only a several-hour period of fasting is required to demonstrate that their stool output is unabated.

Secretory diarrhea is due to the uncontrolled production of compounds that stimulate intestinal secretion. Enterotoxins produced by various bacteria are one class of compounds causing secretory diarrhea. Enterotoxin-producing bacteria cause profuse watery diarrhea and abdominal pain with little fever. These bacteria usually involve the proximal small intestine, where they adhere to the gastrointestinal epithelium but do not produce structural damage. Stools are devoid of blood and leukocytes. Many different species of bacteria are able to make closely related enterotoxins that have a direct effect on the intestinal mucosa by stimulating tissue adenylate cyclase to increase intestinal cyclic AMP (cAMP) concentrations. Organisms that produce these enterotoxins include *V. cholerae, E. coli, C. jejuni, Aeromonas hydrophila,* and Salmonella. There are no reliable markers such as serotype or biotype for enterotoxigenicity; demonstration of the toxin itself is necessary to identify which organisms are enterotoxigenic. Similarly, heat-stable, low molecular weight guanylate cyclase–stimulating toxins of *E. coli* and *Y. enterocolitica* can produce secretory diarrhea. The enterotoxins produced in the food poisoning syndromes of *Bacillus cereus, Clostridium perfringens,* and *Staphylococcus aureus* are not related immunologically or mechanistically to each other, to heat-stabile toxin (ST), or to heat-labile toxin (LT), but they also cause secretory diarrhea.

Other causes of secretory diarrhea are tumors that produce hormones that stimulate gastric, pancreatic, biliary, or intestinal secretion. The most frequently reported tumor causing secretory diarrhea in childhood is ganglioneuroma, whose secretion of catecholamines or vasoactive intestinal polypeptide (VIP) is associated with secretory diarrhea. Secretory diarrhea is also a feature of Zollinger-Ellison syndrome, in which gastrin-stimulated gastric acid production causes watery diarrhea. Determination of urinary excretion of vanylmandelic acid (VMA) and catecholamines and serum levels of VIP and gastrin should be diagnostic.

Small bowel bacterial overgrowth can result in secretory diarrhea. It can have a variety of causes.

In most cases there is stasis of small intestinal contents, allowing bacterial overgrowth. Predisposing conditions include anatomic abnormalities such as strictures resulting from Crohn's disease and motility disorders such as intestinal pseudo-obstruction, abnormal motility due to gastroschisis, and postoperative areas of stasis such as intestinal blind loops. Other abnormalities that make conditions favorable for bacterial overgrowth are immune deficiency states, resection of the ileocecal valve, and malnutrition, particularly in the tropics, where malnourished children live in unsanitary conditions and ingest large numbers of bacteria.

Normally the luminal contents of the upper small intestine contain less than 10^4 bacteria per ml. Concentrations of greater than 10^7 bacteria per ml are clearly abnormal. Steatorrhea results from bacterial deconjugation of bile salts. Deconjugated bile salts are insoluble at the neutral pH of small bowel contents. They precipitate and cannot be reabsorbed. Depletion of the bile acid pool results in duodenal bile acid concentrations below the critical micellar concentration, which results in fat malabsorption. Vitamin B_{12} malabsorption is caused by bacterial utilization or conversion to inactive metabolites. Carbohydrate and protein malabsorption also are due in part to bacterial consumption, but the mechanisms are not completely understood. Serum folic acid may be increased, apparently as a result of synthesis of folic-acid–like compounds by the bacterial contaminants. Not all findings are present in all patients with bacterial overgrowth.

This diagnosis can be difficult to prove, since it requires demonstration of decreased levels of duodenal bile acids or, alternatively, intestinal bacterial overgrowth. Specific treatment is available using cholestyramine, a nonabsorbable anion binding resin that binds bile acids, preventing their precipitation and interaction with the colonic mucosa. Use of cholestyramine should be reserved for this condition and not used in all children with secretory diarrhea, since important complications, including hypernatremia, hyperchloremic acidosis, and intestinal obstruction, have been reported from its use.

Familial chloridorrhea is most prevalent in Finland but has been described in other areas of the world. It is inherited as an autosomal recessive trait. Chloride-bicarbonate transport in the distal ileum and colon is impaired, resulting in increased fecal chloride loss and osmotic diarrhea. Stool potassium and sodium are normal, but total losses are increased because of the large volume of stool that is passed. Infants are born prematurely with abdominal distention and diarrheal stools that resemble urine. Growth is poor and the infants are hypotonic. Fecal chloride increases and urine is acidic, despite the presence of metabolic alkalosis. This is one of the only causes of diarrhea that is associated with alkalosis. Growth and absence of renal lesions have been noted in patients treated with supplemental sodium chloride with added potassium chloride to maintain normal levels of electrolytes and a normal pH.

MALABSORPTION

Before considering malabsorption as a pathophysiologic mechanism of diarrhea, it is important to emphasize that the concepts of diarrhea and malabsorption are not identical. Children with malabsorption do not always have diarrhea and, conversely, most children with diarrhea do not have malabsorption. Although malabsorption generally produces increased fecal mass, this is not synonymous with diarrhea, since increased fecal mass may be physiologic, for example in response to a high fiber diet.

Malabsorption in children may be divided into that due to small intestinal disorders and that due to pancreatic insufficiency. Of the small intestinal disorders associated with malabsorption in infants and children, the most common is celiac disease (gluten-sensitive enteropathy, nontropical sprue). Children with celiac disease present with irritability, growth failure, and diarrhea, frequently in the last half of the first year of life. The basis of this disorder is thought to be hypersensitivity to the alcohol-soluble gliadin fraction of dietary gluten, a component of grain flours. It generally occurs after cereals are added to the diet, around six months of age, when the primary teeth begin to erupt and the child begins to develop the ability to ingest solid foods. Symptoms can frequently be traced to the introduction of gluten-containing foods such as teething biscuits, bread, or cookies. Gluten sensitivity may result from introduction of complex foods into the diet of an infant at an age when absorption of intact macromolecules occurs. Although circulating antibodies to dietary protein can be demonstrated commonly in young infants, there is no clear relationship between the development of such antibodies and digestive disorders such as celiac disease.

A familial tendency towards development of this disorder has long been known. It appears to be most common in families of northern European descent, most notably the Scotch and Irish. Celiac disease has a strong association with histocompatibility type HLA-B8, further suggesting a genetic influence on gluten sensitivity. This diagnosis can be confirmed by finding the characteristic histologic pattern of intestinal villus atrophy and chronic inflammation on suction biopsy of small intestinal mucosa. Treatment with stringent dietary gluten restriction should produce symptomatic improvement, normal growth, and resolution of the histologic abnormalities, although the response may be slow. The characteristic flat intestinal lesion of villous atrophy, crypt hyperplasia, and cellular inflammatory response also occurs in cow's milk intolerance, soy protein intolerance, immunodeficiency, tropical sprue, eosinophilic gastroenteritis, giardiasis, bacterial overgrowth and other causes of chronic diarrhea.

A celiac-like disease is frequently seen in children with humoral and combined immunodeficiency. The mechanism of malabsorption in these disorders is incompletely understood, but some children have a lesion in the small intestinal mucosa that is identical to that in celiac disease. Although some patients may manifest only transient gluten intolerance, long-term dietary avoidance of gluten containing foods such as wheat, rye, barley, and oats is critical to prevent recurrences of intractable diarrhea and growth failure.

Intestinal lymphangiectasia results from an abnormality in the lymphatic drainage of the intestine. Since the primary route of fat absorption is into intestinal lacteals and ultimately the thoracic duct, anything that increases pressure in the thoracic duct or impedes flow of lymph can lead to dilatation of the intestinal lacteals. Absorption of fat causes further dilatation and rupture, discharging lymphatic contents into the intestine. Children with this condition generally present with fat malabsorption and systemic consequences of loss of the constituents of lymph, including chylomicrons, proteins, and lymphocytes. A clue to diagnosis is lymphopenia, which can be so severe as to cause recurrent infections. These children generally have gastrointestinal protein loss and will have low levels of serum albumin, immunoglobulins, and other circulating proteins.

Although rare, there are two distinct syndromes of eosinophilic gastroenteritis that have been reported in children. The first is a relatively superficial eosinophilic infiltration of the stomach and proximal intestine that produces a malabsorption syndrome much like celiac disease. The second more closely resembles Crohn's disease in that the eosinophilic infiltration is deeper, producing thickening of the bowel wall and involving the more distal small intestine. Peripheral eosinophilia occurs in both, and both are thought to be due to hypersensitivity to dietary antigens. Both are variably responsive to dietary restriction and corticosteroid treatment.

Abetalipoproteinemia is a rare, autosomal recessive disease, characterized by an absence of low-density lipoproteins resulting in an inability to form normal chylomicrons and defective release and transport of triglycerides from the enterocyte. Patients present in the first year of life with diarrhea, abdominal distention, steatorrhea, failure to thrive, and acanthocytosis of erythrocytes.

Frequently, the initial clinical picture may be indistinguishable from that of other causes of steatorrhea, such as celiac disease or cystic fibrosis. As patients get older, gastrointestinal symptoms may improve, but ataxia, muscle weakness, nystagmus, and retinitis pigmentosa develop. Milder forms of the disease exist in which patients have hypolipoproteinemia.

Characteristic laboratory findings include decreased plasma cholesterol and triglyceride levels and acanthocytes on hematologic smear. Vitamin A, vitamin E, and carotene levels are low. Lipoprotein electrophoresis shows absent or decreased beta-lipoproteins, and small bowel biopsy shows enterocytes engorged with fat droplets.

Wolman's disease or primary familial xanthomatosis is a rare, autosomal recessive lipid storage disease secondary to lysosomal acid esterase deficiency; cholesterol esters and triglycerides accumulate in all organs. Patients develop diarrhea, hepatosplenomegaly, and failure to thrive. Abdominal radiographs may show adrenal calcifications, and bone marrow shows lipid-filled macrophages. There is no treatment, and patients generally die before 1 year of age.

Pancreatic insufficiency is a relatively common cause of diarrhea in infants and children. The most common cause of pancreatic insufficiency in childhood is cystic fibrosis. Eighty percent of children with cystic fibrosis have decreased output of pancreatic enzymes, water, and bicarbonate. A common presenting feature of cystic fibrosis is severe steatorrhea and hyperphagia in a child who also has recurrent pulmonary disease. Definitive diagnosis is made by measuring the sodium or chloride content of sweat. This is frequently done after pilocarpine stimulation by iontophoresis. These children frequently develop fat-soluble vitamin deficiencies. Cloudy corneas due to vitamin A deficiency and hemorrhage associated with hypoprothrombinemia due to vitamin K deficiency are further clues to the diagnosis.

The Shwachman-Diamond syndrome is a cause of pancreatic insufficiency in childhood. Bone marrow dysfunction, including neutropenia and thrombocytopenia, growth retardation, and peripheral dysostosis are less frequent clinical features. This condition is distinguished from cystic fibrosis in that these children have a normal amount of sodium and chloride in sweat. Steatorrhea also occurs in hypoparathyroidism, especially during periods of hypocalcemia. The malabsorption due to syndromes of pancreatic insufficiency is most commonly treated by replacement of pancreatic enzymes and dietary supplementation of fat soluble vitamins.

Pancreatic insufficiency develops sufficiently slowly in children with recurrent acute pancreatitis that it is an uncommon cause of malabsorption syndrome in children.

OTHER DISORDERS

The most common cause of diarrhea in the preschool age group is chronic nonspecific diarrhea or irritable colon of infancy. This disorder is characterized by recurrent, watery diarrhea occurring in children between 6 and 36 months of age. These children have no other symptoms nor do they have clinical or biochemical evidence of malabsorption. The key to distinguishing these children from children with malabsorption syndrome or any of the other causes of diarrhea is their normal growth and development and the complete absence of any other symptoms, even when diarrhea is present. The family history is positive for other manifestations of irritable colon syndrome in two thirds of patients, strongly suggesting that this disorder is a specific symptom complex of a familial tendency towards colonic hyperreactivity. It may be the childhood counterpart of the irritable bowel syndrome of adults. The diarrhea in this disorder results from rapid transit from ileum to rectum and is best treated by decreasing the stimuli for colonic contraction by limiting fluid intake to mealtime, decreasing intake of cold, hypertonic liquids, and discontinuing dietary fat restriction. The most important reason to identify children with chronic nonspecific diarrhea is not to prevent their diarrhea, which is generally benign, but to prevent potentially harmful dietary or pharmacologic manipulation based on the theory that these children suffer from another disorder such as malabsorption syndrome or food allergy.

Intractable diarrhea is a serious condition resulting in poor absorption of essential nutrients, malnutrition, and failure to thrive. It usually occurs in infants less than 3 months of age and may be life-threatening if effective intervention is not undertaken. The syndrome of chronic nonspecific diarrhea is distinguished from intractable diarrhea by lack of evidence of malabsorption, growth retardation or dehydration, and a later age of onset (over 6 months of age).

Another rare cause of chronic diarrhea is acrodermatitis enteropathica, which is a cause of chronic diarrhea associated with zinc deficiency. Patients have an abnormality of zinc transport in the intestine, possibly resulting from an absence or abnormality of zinc-binding ligands within the intestine. Human milk provides some protection because zinc-binding ligands are present in it. Formula-fed infants present early in life and breast-fed infants after weaning. Patients develop moist or scaling erythematous eruptions about the mouth, anus, and interdigital areas. Alopecia, dystrophic nails, photophobia, conjunctivitis, and glossitis also may be present. The rash may occur before or with the onset of diarrhea. Loss of taste sensation, anorexia, irritability, lethargy, and depression are associated symptoms. Diarrhea tends to be intermittent, and usually there is steatorrhea. A deficiency of essential fatty acids in the serum has been described, and addition of Intralipid intravenously can help.

Diagnosis is based on a low plasma zinc (<65–70μg/dl) in association with typical clinical findings. Blood samples should be collected appropriately, as contamination can occur from glassware or rubber stoppers, raising the measured zinc level. Some patients with typical findings have been reported to have normal serum zinc levels, and some of these have responded to oral zinc therapy. Oral therapy with zinc sulfate or zinc acetate is recommended. Zinc deficiency can also be secondary to other diseases causing malabsorption, including Crohn's disease and celiac disease. Secondary zinc deficiencies will also respond to appropriate zinc replacement. Doses should be individualized and serum levels monitored.

TREATMENT

Treatment of patients with chronic diarrhea consists of nonspecific therapy, including nutritional support, and specific therapy, which may be administered once the diagnosis has been established. In all patients with chronic diarrhea and/or malabsorption, every attempt should be made to provide oral feeding. Both gut villous morphology and disaccharidase activity improve faster when stimulated by early enteral feeding than with prolonged bowel rest and intravenous alimentation. Nonspecific therapy of children with chronic diarrhea and/or malabsorption with drugs has included the use of anticholinergics, bile salt–sequestering agents, pancreatic enzymes, prostaglandin inhibitors, nonspecific antidiarrheal compounds, and antibiotics. These compounds should not be used indiscriminately as therapy for children with diarrhea.

Once a diagnosis has been established (Table 2) then specific therapy can be administered. Table 3 shows therapy for patients with diarrhea due to agents or diseases associated with inflammatory or infectious diarrhea. The type of syndrome produced by Salmonella influences the selection and duration of antimicrobial therapy. Antibiotics should not be used in the treatment of persons who are nontyphoid Salmonella carriers or in the vast majority of patients with mild gastroenteritis. Exceptions occur when the disease appears to be evolving into one of the systemic syndromes and in patients with a disease or condition that impairs host resistance to infection, such as neonates and young infants and patients with hemoglobinopathies or malignancies. Antibiotics used for therapy of patients with various Salmonella syndromes

Table 2. INITIAL LABORATORY EVALUATION OF CHILDREN WITH CHRONIC DIARRHEA

Test	Abnormality	Category or Cause of Diarrhea to Consider
Stool		
Fecal leukocytes	present	inflammatory (Table 3)
Ova and parasite	present	infectious (Table 3)
Sudan stain	positive	malabsorption (Table 6)
Reducing substance	present	osmotic (Table 4)
Culture	enteropathogen isolated	inflammatory, secretory (Tables 3 and 5)
Rotazyme or Rotalex	positive	rotavirus
Blood		
CBC with differential	lymphopenia	malabsorption (Table 6)
Immunoglobulins	low	malabsorption (Table 6)
Albumin/globulin	low	malabsorption (Table 6)
Carotene	low	malabsorption (Table 6)
Other		
Urine	glycosuria	osmotic (Table 4)

include ampicillin, trimethoprim-sulfamethoxazole (TMP-SMX), and chloramphenicol. The treatment of choice of shigellosis is TMP-SMX because of the increasing frequency of ampicillin resistance among Shigella isolates. In children with known ampicillin-susceptible strains, ampicillin can be given. Amoxicillin is not as effective as ampicillin and should not be used. In patients with Campylobacter enteritis, erythromycin is the drug of choice. Therapy will reduce fecal excretion but may not alter the clinical course. Insufficient data exist to support the use of antimicrobial agents in diarrheal disease caused by V. parahemolyticus or Y. enterocolitica. The most important aspect of therapy in patients with AAC is discontinuation of the antimicrobial agent. If symptoms persist or worsen, then specific therapy with orally administered vancomycin or metronidazole is indicated.

In treating patients with amebiasis, iodoquinol is the best luminal amebicide and is effective against both cysts and trophozoites in the lumen of the gut. Invasive amebiasis of the intestine or liver necessitates the additional use of metronidazole. Furazolidone, metronidazole, and quinacrine are effective against Giardia. Although quinacrine is the least expensive, it is associated with the highest incidence of side effects. Treatment for cryptosporidiosis has generally been unsuccessful. Patients with intestinal Strongyloides should receive thiabendazole. Currently there are no antiviral

Table 3. INFLAMMATORY OR INFECTIOUS CHRONIC DIARRHEA IN CHILDHOOD

Categories	Usual Age of Onset	Diagnosis	Specific Treatment
Inflammatory or Cytotoxin			
Salmonella	any	fecal leukocytes present and stool culture positive	ampicillin or trimethoprim-sulfamethoxazole (TMP-SMX) or chloramphenicol
Shigella	6 months–6 yrs		TMP-SMX or ampicillin
Campylobacter	any		erythromycin
Yersinia	any		none
Vibrio parahemolyticus	any		none
Clostridium difficile	any		vancomycin or metronidazole
Amebiasis	adults	microscopic examination of stool or colonic biopsy; serology	iodoquinol and metronidazole
Noninflammatory–Protozoa			
Giardia lamblia	any	microscopic examination of stool	furazolidone or quinicrine or metronidazole
Cryptosporidium	any		none
Strongyloides	any		thiabendazole
Noninflammatory–Virus			
Rotavirus	6 months–2 yrs	commercially available rapid diagnostic test	none
Norwalk	any	research test	none
Adenovirus	infant	research test	none
Inflammatory and Noninfectious			
Radiation	any	history; intestinal biopsy	none
Dietary protein–induced enterocolitis	less than 6 months	dietary manipulation with or without intestinal biopsy	remove implicated protein from diet
Crohn's disease	10 yrs	radiographs; intestinal biopsy	sulfasalazine and/or corticosteroids for relapses
Ulcerative colitis	10 yrs	radiographs; intestinal biopsy	sulfasalazine and/or corticosteroids for relapses; occasionally surgery
Hirschsprung's disease	1 yr	radiographs; rectal biopsy	surgery

agents available for the therapy of patients with viral gastroenteritis.

Therapy of patients with inflammatory, noninfectious diarrhea is variable (Table 3). No specific treatment exists for colitis due to radiation. Dietary protein–induced enterocolitis should be treated by replacing the cow's milk formula with other proteins such as soy or protein hydrolysate. Unfortunately approximately 25% of those allergic to milk protein may develop allergy to soy protein.

Table 4. OSMOTIC DIARRHEA IN CHILDHOOD

Deficiency	Predominant Age (onset)	Diagnosis	Therapy
Lactase			
Congenital	newborn period	small intestinal biopsy and enzyme analysis	avoid lactose-containing foods
Acquired			
Primary	2–8 yrs	small intestinal biopsy and enzyme analysis	avoid lactose-containing foods
Secondary	Any	small intestinal biopsy and enzyme analysis	avoid lactose-containing foods
Sucrase-isomaltase	6 mos	small intestinal biopsy and enzyme analysis	avoid sucrose- and isomaltose-containing foods
Glucose-galactose malabsorption	1 mo	small intestinal biopsy and enzyme analysis	avoid galactose-containing foods
Ingestion of nonabsorbable carbohydrates (sorbitol, lactulose)	1 yr	history	avoid or decrease intake of causative agent or food

Table 5. SECRETORY DIARRHEA IN CHILDHOOD

Category	Predominant Age (onset)	Diagnosis	Therapy
Enterotoxin-producing bacteria	any	enterotoxin assay	antimicrobial therapy
Neural crest tumors	under 2 years	vanillylmandelic acid and catecholamine concentration in urine	surgery
Intestinal bacterial overgrowth (cholerrheic enteropathy, stagnant loop syndrome)	any	intestinal bile acid measurement	antimicrobial therapy; cholestyramine
Familial chloridorrhea	1 month	stool chloride measurements; alkalosis; acid urine	replacement of electrolytes

Milk allergy is ultimately outgrown by most children, and they usually can tolerate milk within a year of restriction.

The course of ulcerative colitis is variable in children in that 10% experience only one episode, 30% become asymptomatic and have occasional exacerbations, and the remainder have a chronic, relapsing form of disease. Goals of treatment are control of symptoms with sulfasalazine and/or steroids, maintenance of adequate nutrition and growth, and return to a relatively normal life. Methods for treating Crohn's disease are similar to those used for treating ulcerative colitis with the exception that Crohn's disease is not cured by surgical resection. Hirschsprung's disease is treated by surgical resection of the involved aspect of the colon.

Treatment of patients with osmotic diarrhea due to a specific carbohydrate intolerance consists of instituting a diet that is free of the implicated carbohydrate (Table 4).

Treatment of patients with secretory diarrhea is varied (Table 5). Therapy of patients with an enterotoxin-producing bacteria such as *V. cholerae* or *E. coli* includes administration of antimicrobial agents. Patients with a neural crest tumor can be cured of the associated diarrhea by complete surgical removal of the tumor. Therapy of patients with intestinal bacterial overgrowth includes operative correction of any predisposing condition, administration of an antibiotic such as TMP-SMX for temporary control, and possibly cholestyramine to bind bile salts. Treatment of familial chloridorrhea should be sodium chloride solutions with potassium chloride to maintain normal serum concentrations of electrolytes and pH.

Table 6. MALABSORPTION IN CHILDHOOD

Category	Predominant Age (onset)	Diagnosis*	Therapy
Small intestinal mucosal disorder			
Celiac disease (gluten enteropathy)	6 months to 2 years	low carotene (10 μg/dl); intestinal biopsy	avoid gluten
Immune defects (humoral and combined)	1–2 yrs	immune evaluation; intestinal biopsy	correct immune defect, if possible
Intestinal lymphangiectasia	first year	radiographs	reduce dietary long-chain fats
Eosinophilic gastroenteritis	any	intestinal biopsy	dietary restriction, corticosteroids
Abetalipoproteinemia	6–12 months	lipoprotein electrophoresis (hypocholesterolemia), acanthocytes on peripheral smear, duodenal biopsy	fat-soluble vitamins, limit intake of long-chain fat
Wolman's disease	3 months	bone marrow; liver biopsy	none
Pancreatic insufficiency			
Cystic fibrosis	6 months	sweat test	pancreatic enzyme replacement, vitamins, therapy of pulmonary infections
Shwachman-Diamond syndrome	2 years	radiographs; duodenal enzymes	pancreatic enzyme replacement, vitamins
Chronic pancreatitis (traumatic and hereditary)	any	duodenal enzymes	pancreatic enzyme replacement

* Carotene levels in blood generally are below 50 mg/dl in malabsorption syndromes and if low are an indication for performing a xylose challenge test.

Therapy of patients with malabsorption revolves around dietary manipulation (Table 6). The dietary treatment of celiac disease consists of permanent elimination of wheat, rye, barley, malt, and oats from the diet, since all of these cause mucosal damage. Patients with immune deficiencies should be carefully observed and treated for recurrent infections. Patients with IgG deficiency should receive immunoglobulin monthly. Patients with intestinal lymphangiectasia generally have a normal intestinal absorptive capacity except for long-chain fat assimilation. Reduction of dietary long-chain fats may reduce enteric protein loss. Patients with eosinophilic gastroenteritis may respond to dietary restriction and corticosteroid treatment. Patients with abetalipoproteinemia should receive fat-soluble vitamins and limit their intake of long-chain fat. There is no therapy for patients with Wolman's disease. Patients with cystic fibrosis, Shwachman-Diamond syndrome, and chronic pancreatitis require replacement of pancreatic enzymes and administration of fat-soluble vitamins.

Therapy of patients with intractable diarrhea involves providing adequate nutrition. Patients with acrodermatitis enteropathica should receive daily zinc supplements. If untreated, exacerbations become more frequent and severe and are often associated with psychiatric disturbances. The disease usually resolves at puberty.

Disorders of the Anus and Rectum

JOHN H. SEASHORE, M.D.

ANORECTAL MALFORMATIONS

Imperforate anus is a complex spectrum of malformations resulting from arrested development at any stage of embryogenesis of the hindgut. Clinically these anomalies can be divided into three main categories depending on the relationship of the rectum to the puborectalis muscle. In low anomalies the rectum has descended normally through the puborectalis muscle, there is no connection to the genitourinary tract, and meconium is usually discharged from an external perineal fistula. In intermediate anomalies the rectum is at or below the level of the puborectalis muscle but is often displaced anteriorly, and there may be a persistent connection to the genitourinary tract. In high anomalies the rectum ends above the puborectalis muscle, frequently as a fistula to the urinary tract or vagina. These distinctions are important in planning treatment and determining prognosis, since the puborectalis muscle is essential for continence.

Low Anorectal Malformations. Imperforate anal membrane is ruptured with a probe or small dilator, and the accompanying anal stenosis is treated by serial dilatations over several weeks until the anus accepts a 12-mm Hegar dilator without difficulty. Anal stenosis without an obstructing membrane may not be diagnosed until later in infancy and is also treated by serial dilatation. In anterior ectopic anus the anus is perfectly normal but is displaced anteriorly. These children have severe constipation and straining because of the sharp angulation of the anorectal canal. Generous doses of mineral oil usually relieve the symptoms, but if constipation persists a posterior anoplasty is indicated. Covered anus, with or without anocutaneous or anovestibular fistula, is treated by perineal anoplasty. A cruciate incision through the anal dimple opens directly into the rectum, which is sutured to the skin. The anus is dilated for several weeks postoperatively to prevent stricture.

Intermediate Anomalies. In ectopic perineal anus the anal dimple and external sphincter are in the normal position but the anal opening is located anteriorly in the perineum. The anus is stenotic and is treated initially by dilatation. At about 6 months of age an anal transposition is performed. The rectum is dissected from the surrounding soft tissues for several centimeters and then tunneled posteriorly and sutured to a cruciate incision in the anal dimple. The treatment of rectovestibular fistula in girls is the same, but special care is taken to avoid injury to the posterior vaginal wall. Boys who have the rare rectourethral fistula to the membranous urethra are treated by colostomy at birth. Sacroperineal reconstruction and division of the fistula are performed at 6 months.

High Anomalies. All high anomalies are treated by double-barreled transverse colostomy at birth. Barium studies through the distal limb of the colostomy are helpful to define the anatomy. At 6 months of age an abdominoperineal pull-through procedure is performed. Through an abdominal incision the rectum is mobilized and the rectourethral or rectovaginal fistula, if present, is divided. A tunnel is created between the urethra or vagina and the puborectalis muscle down to a cruciate incision at the normal anal location. The external sphincter may or may not be present. The rectum is pulled through the tunnel and sutured to the skin. Girls who have a single perineal orifice have a cloacal anomaly. There are many anatomic variations of cloacal anomalies, and reconstruction can be very complex. In general, one-stage rectal and vaginal pull-through is preferred. The urogenital sinus is preserved as a urethra. Reflux of urine through large fistulas into the colon or vagina may lead to persistent urinary tract infection or hyperchloremic acidosis; early definitive surgery or division of the fistula may be necessary.

Long-term follow-up of children with high anorectal malformations is essential. Toilet training is difficult, and complete continence by age 3 or 4 is the exception. Bowel control slowly improves with time, but many children do not achieve an optimal result until the teenage years. Habit toilet training, dietary modification, and stool softeners are often helpful. Many of these children have sensory and motor deficits that make it difficult for them to achieve continence, but it appears that they gradually become aware of alternative sensory pathways and develop the perineal muscles to aid in bowel control. Moral support and reassurance that painfully slow progress is the norm are essential. Coercive toilet training is discouraged. Ultimately about 80% of these children achieve normal or at least socially acceptable continence. Permanent colostomy may be the best solution for a few patients who have total failure of bowel control.

A renal ultrasound is performed prior to discharge in all children who have anorectal malformations to search for major structural abnormalities of the urinary tract. Further evaluation is indicated if there is evidence of urinary tract infection, neurogenic bladder, or other symptoms.

ANAL FISSURES

Fissures are treated by warm baths and liberal doses of mineral oil to soften and lubricate the stool. The dose of mineral oil ranges from 1–2 teaspoons a day in infants to 3–4 tablespoons a day in older children. For infants under 6 months of age, corn syrup or molasses extract accomplishes the same purpose and may be safer than mineral oil because of the risk of aspiration. The dose is adjusted to keep stools soft, but not to the point of oozing. Treatment is continued for a week or two after the fissure heals. Vigorous treatment of fissures is indicated, since inadequately treated anal fissure is a common cause of chronic constipation and encopresis.

PERIANAL AND PERIRECTAL ABSCESS AND FISTULA

Superficial abscesses are incised and drained in the office, but deep abscesses should be opened under general anesthesia to allow adequate drainage. Anal fistulas, manifested by persistent drainage or recurrent abscess, are unroofed. Proctoscopy is helpful to identify the internal end of the fistula, which is opened in continuity with the incision. This may require cutting the external sphincter, but most fistulas in children are superficial to the sphincter. The lining of the sinus tract is curetted and the wound is packed open. Com-

plete healing in 7–10 days is expected. Persistent perianal disease in an older child may be a manifestation of Crohn's disease.

RECTAL PROLAPSE

Rectal prolapse is most common in toddlers and is usually caused by straining to pass a large, hard stool that overstretches the sphincter. The lax sphincter then allows prolapse to occur even without straining, and this prevents the sphincter from regaining its normal tone. Thus treatment is directed toward preventing prolapse until tone is restored. Generous doses of mineral oil may be sufficient. Tight strapping of the buttocks with tape is also effective. Children who are toilet trained should use an appropriate-size potty chair to prevent spreading of the buttocks and to provide a firm platform for their feet. As long as the prolapse is easily reducible, persistence in these simple measures is indicated since they almost always work. If the condition is progressive or does not resolve, a variety of operations are available, but none is totally satisfactory.

TRAUMA

Most foreign bodies in the rectum pass spontaneously. The most common foreign body encountered in children is a broken rectal thermometer. More harm may be done by vigorous rectal examination or proctoscopy than by the foreign body itself. Careful observation and administration of mineral oil by mouth to facilitate passage are indicated. Large impacted foreign bodies should be removed; general anesthesia may be necessary to achieve adequate relaxation and dilatation of the anus.

Careful observation after any kind of rectal trauma is indicated, since initial examination may fail to reveal the full extent of the injury. The rectum is so short, especially in infants, that thermometers, sticks, and other pointed objects may cause intraperitoneal perforation. Unrecognized extraperitoneal perforations may also have serious consequences. The urinary tract and, in girls, the vagina may be involved. If a more serious injury is suspected, examination under general anesthesia is performed. If gross or microscopic hematuria is present, retrograde urethrography and voiding cystourethrography are performed preoperatively. Rectal perforations and lacerations are repaired as accurately as possible, and the perirectal space is drained. Most patients who have major rectal injuries require a temporary loop colostomy to divert the fecal stream while the wound heals. Urinary tract injuries are repaired, and suprapubic urinary drainage is established.

—7—
Blood

Anemia of Iron Deficiency, Blood Loss, Renal Disease, and Chronic Infection

JOHN N. LUKENS, M.D.

IRON DEFICIENCY ANEMIA

The treatment of iron deficiency requires replenishment of body iron and correction of the factor or factors responsible for the deficiency state. Patients compromised because of severe anemia may require blood transfusion to rapidly correct cardiac decompensation. Iron supplements are indicated for groups at high risk for developing nutritional iron deficiency.

Iron Replacement. Iron can be given orally, intramuscularly, or intravenously. *Oral iron* is the safest, least expensive form of treatment, and is as effective as parenterally administered iron. There is no indication for the intravenous infusion of iron in children.

The treatment of choice for iron replenishment is ferrous sulfate. Ferrous gluconate and ferrous fumarate, while as effective, are more expensive. Numerous other iron salts, with and without adjuvants, are marketed with claims of improved palatability, enhanced absorption, or fewer side effects. Most of these preparations are therapeutically inferior to ferrous sulfate and all are more expensive. Ascorbic acid is a popular additive because of its known potential to increase iron absorption. However, the amount of ascorbic acid added to most iron preparations is much less than that needed to significantly influence absorption. In addition, ascorbate potentiates the undesirable side effects of oral iron. Thus, an increase in the dose of iron achieves the same result at a lower cost. Enteric coated tablets and sustained release capsules should be avoided, as they ensure transit of iron beyond the site of maximal absorption.

Ferrous sulfate is marketed in a variety of concentrations and forms for use in children of different ages. A concentrated solution containing 15 mg elemental iron per 0.6 ml is administered by calibrated dropper to infants and small children. An elixir, intended for toddlers, contains 30 mg elemental iron per 5 ml. Tablets and capsules contain 60 mg elemental iron.

The elemental iron content of the ferrous salt is used for dosage calculation. For ferrous sulfate, the elemental iron content is 20% by weight. An optimal therapeutic response is obtained with 5 mg elemental iron/kg/day (ferrous sulfate, 25 mg/kg/day). The usual adult dose of 180 mg elemental iron/day should not be exceeded. Larger doses are more likely to produce gastrointestinal disturbances without effecting a more rapid recovery. The daily dose is divided into three portions and given with meals. While meals interfere somewhat with iron absorption, the reduction in absorption is more than offset by better tolerance and patient compliance. If there are apparent side effects despite this precaution, the dose of iron should be decreased by 50%. Speed in the repair of iron deficiency is rarely important.

Subjective improvement may be noted within a day or two after starting iron therapy: irritability is less prominent, spontaneous activity increases, pica is corrected, and appetite returns. A reticulocytosis, inversely proportional to the initial hemoglobin concentration, is noted within 3 to 5 days. Reticulocytes are maximal (5–10%) at 5–10 days. The rate of hemoglobin rise is a function of the magnitude of anemia. The more severe the anemia, the greater is the daily increment in hemoglobin concentration. Approximately 18 days after initiation of therapy, the hemoglobin reaches a level midway between the initial value and that which is normal. Irrespective of the severity of anemia, approximately 2 months are required to achieve a normal hemoglobin concentration. Full

243

doses of iron are continued for 2 months after correction of anemia in order to provide iron reserves. Suboptimal response to iron most commonly reflects failure of iron administration, inadequate dosage, or use of an iron preparation that is poorly absorbed. Less frequently, a coexistent infection compromises marrow response to iron or ongoing blood losses obscure an appropriate marrow response. Rarely, treatment failure is due to iron malabsorption.

Side effects of oral iron therapy are more frequently encountered in adults than in infants and children. Adverse symptoms potentially related to medicinal iron include constipation, diarrhea, heartburn, and abdominal cramps. Temporary staining of teeth by liquid preparations can be avoided by using a straw or by placing the iron directly on the back of the tongue with a dropper.

Iron tablets should be dispensed in bottles equipped with safety caps. Parents are instructed to ensure inaccessibility of the tablets to small children. Because of their relatively low iron concentration, liquid preparations pose little or no risk of accidental iron poisoning.

Parenteral iron therapy is painful, expensive (relative to oral therapy), and attended by a slight but measurable risk of hypersensitivity reaction. The rate of hemoglobin rise is no greater than with iron given by mouth. Nevertheless, the intramuscular injection of iron is indicated in the face of steadfast noncompliance, for situations in which ongoing iron losses exceed that which can be absorbed by the oral route, and for states of iron malabsorption. Most iron deficient patients with peptic ulcer disease and inflammatory bowel disease do not require parenteral iron.

The parenteral iron preparation with which there is greatest experience is iron dextran (Imferon). This is a complex ferric hydroxide with high molecular weight dextrans in a colloidal solution containing 50 mg elemental iron/ml. The total required dose is calculated as follows: dose (mg Fe) = weight (kg) × desired increment Hgb (gm/dl) × 2.5. An additional 10 mg iron/kg is given in order to ensure replenishment of stores. The calculated dose is given over several days so as not to exceed 2 ml/day. Care is taken to deliver the preparation deep into the upper outer quadrant of the buttock. The skin and subcutaneous tissue are retracted laterally prior to insertion of the needle in order to avoid staining the skin.

Blood Transfusion. Because the response to iron is prompt and predictable, blood transfusion is rarely indicated. It is reserved for children whose anemia is of such severity as to produce frank or impending cardiac decompensation. In this setting, sedimented red blood cells are given as a modified exchange transfusion. Patient blood is replaced with packed red cells in 10 to 20 ml increments. The volume of the exchange need not exceed 20 ml/kg.

Correction of Predisposing Factors. It is very important to identify and correct the factors responsible for the deficiency. Iron deficiency is properly viewed as the expression of a primary disturbance rather than as a complete diagnosis in itself. Curtailment of milk consumption is required for infants whose deficiency is nutritional. Substitution of an evaporated milk preparation or a nonmilk-based formula for cow's milk is necessary to arrest the occult blood loss of milk-induced enteropathy. Nutritional counseling is provided for those of high school and college age. Search for occult disease is necessary when dealing with unexplained iron deficiency.

Preventive Measures. The risk of iron deficiency in the first years of life can be minimized by adoption of simple feeding practices. These include encouragement of breast feeding, avoidance of unmodified whole cow's milk during the first year, inclusion of foods that promote iron absorption (fruit and fruit juices, meat, poultry), and avoidance of excessive weight gain. Iron supplements are required during the first year if the recommended daily requirement (2 mg iron/kg) is to be met. For infants receiving cow's milk formulas, this is conveniently provided by using an iron-fortified formula. A medicinal iron supplement (2 mg/kg/day) is indicated for infants receiving milk formulas not fortified with iron. Twice this amount is required by small preterm infants after 3 months of age. Breast-fed infants also require an iron supplement between 6 and 12 months of age despite the higher bioavailability of iron in human milk. The negative iron balance of breast-fed infants after 3 to 6 months of age is due in part to a progressive decline in the iron content of breast milk and in part to a decrease in breast milk consumption that follows introduction of solid foods.

BLOOD LOSS ANEMIA

The management of blood loss anemia is dictated by the volume and chronicity of bleeding. The needs of patients who have sustained massive acute hemorrhages are different from those of individuals who have experienced chronic or remote bleeding. With both acute and chronic blood loss, remedial measures directed at the cause for bleeding must be addressed once any emergency has been dealt with.

Acute Blood Loss. Not until 20% or more of the blood volume is lost do disturbances in circulatory dynamics occur. Consequently, no therapy is required for blood losses unattended by alterations in vital signs unless recurrence of bleeding is anticipated. With losses of 30 to 40%, all the symptoms and signs of shock are observed: peripheral perfusion is poor, the skin is moist and cool, the blood pressure and central venous pressure are low, and the heart rate is accelerated. These physical findings are of far greater value than is the hemoglobin concentration in assessing the need for therapy. Since several hours are required for plasma volume expansion, the magnitude of acute blood loss is not revealed by alterations in hemoglobin concentration just after the event.

The immediate need is expansion of the blood volume, best accomplished with the transfusion of whole blood. If the urgency of the situation obviates the delay inherent in obtaining properly cross-matched blood, plasma or a plasma protein solution may be infused until blood is available. Approximately 20 ml/kg of the most readily available product is given by rapid intravenous infusion. The need for subsequent infusions can best be assessed by monitoring the central venous pressure. The initial transfusion is followed by repeat infusions of 10 ml/kg until a measurable central venous pressure is obtained and peripheral circulation is restored. In the absence of a central venous line, response to therapy must be assessed by changes in the pulse rate and blood pressure, and by the response of both pulse and blood pressure to assumption of the upright position.

If massive volumes of blood are lost, the infused blood must be fresh in order to prevent a "washout" of platelets and factor VIII. In general, coagulopathy resulting from massive blood transfusion is encountered only if more than the estimated blood volume of the recipient is replaced in a 24 hour period.

Chronic or Remote Blood Loss. The signs and symptoms of chronic or remote blood loss are those of anemia rather than hypovolemia. Because blood loss imposes a drain on iron, the anemia characteristically has all the morphologic and biochemical hallmarks of iron deficiency.

Anemia is usually well compensated. Because volume overload is a potential problem, blood is not given unless there is cardiac decompensation. This is best managed with a small exchange transfusion (20 ml/kg). The use of sedimented red cells instead of whole blood facilitates rapid correction of anemia and permits creation of a volume deficit. Correction of the iron deficiency that almost always accompanies chronic blood loss follows the principles described in the section dealing with iron deficiency anemia.

ANEMIA OF RENAL DISEASE

The anemia associated with severe renal failure has multiple contributing factors. Red blood cell production is limited, in part because of decreased erythropoietin production by the kidneys and in part because of decreased stem cell responsiveness to erythropoietin; red cell survival is shortened; blood is lost into dialysis equipment; and folate availability may be limited by poor dietary intake and by loss to dialysis baths. Contaminants in hemodialysis fluids (copper, nitrates, chloramines) may also trigger hemolytic episodes. The most significant of these contributing factors is deficient erythropoietin production. Since erythropoietin is not available for clinical trials, treatment of the anemia is symptomatic rather than substantive.

The cornerstone of therapy is blood transfusion. The indication for transfusion is based on symptoms rather than on an arbitrary level of hemoglobin concentration. Most active children with renal disease tolerate moderately severe anemia remarkably well. This is due at least in part to enhancement of oxygen unloading secondary to increased red cell 2,3-diphosphoglycerate. Symptoms attributable to anemia are infrequently experienced until the hemoglobin drops below 7 to 8 gm/dl. Many children tolerate 5 gm/dl with impunity. When dictated by symptoms, blood is given as sedimented red cells (approximately 10 ml/kg). If symptoms are alleviated, transfusions are repeated when symptoms recur. In the absence of symptoms, the hemoglobin concentration is allowed to fall until it stabilizes at approximately 5 gm/dl.

Patients on chronic hemodialysis programs are at risk for iron deficiency because of loss of blood into the dialysis apparatus. Therapeutic amounts of iron are indicated for such individuals unless the iron requirement is satisfied by blood transfusions. Since folate is dialyzable, reserves of this essential nutrient are also readily exhausted. Folate-limited erythropoiesis is easily prevented by giving 1 mg folic acid (pteroylglutamic acid) daily.

When successful, renal transplantation effectively restores both the endocrine and exocrine functions of the kidney. Although reticulocytosis followed by an increase in hemoglobin concentration is observed, anemia is not fully abolished unless or until immunosuppressive measures can be curtailed.

ANEMIA OF CHRONIC INFECTION

A wide variety of chronic infectious, inflammatory, and malignant states are associated with a mild anemia having well defined morphologic, kinetic, and biochemical features. The anemia is mild and nonprogressive. Rarely is the hemoglobin concentration less than 8 to 10 gm/dl. The significance of the anemia is its disclosure of a primary disease. Therapeutic efforts should be focused on the underlying disease rather than on the anemia. If anemia is so severe as to justify blood transfusion, additional pathogenetic mechanisms should be sought. Coexistent iron deficiency is particularly common. Chronic gastrointestinal blood loss associated with inflammatory bowel disease or salicylate therapy given for rheumatoid arthritis regularly compounds the anemia of chronic disease. The contribution of iron deficiency is best determined by the extent to which anemia is corrected by a 6 to 8 week trial of therapeutic iron.

Aplastic Anemia

ROBERT L. BAEHNER, M.D.

Aplastic anemia occurs in two forms, acquired and congenital. Acquired forms may be either severe or mild, and prognosis and treatment strategies are based on the severity of the bone marrow aplasia. Assuming that there is no evidence of congenital aplastic anemia and when the condition is severe, a specific therapeutic protocol must be instituted.

1. Transfusion of blood products should be minimized to reduce the risk of alloimmunization. If possible, red cells transfused should be buffy coat–poor or frozen-thawed in an effort to reduce sensitization to leukocyte and platelet antigens. The hemoglobin level should be maintained above 7.0 gm%. Platelet concentrates (1 unit/13 lb) should be administered for control of active bleeding or prevention of spontaneous hemorrhage when the platelet count falls below 20,000/mm^3. In allosensitized patients, control of thrombocytopenic bleeding from the nose and mouth may be helped by administration of aminocaproic acid (Amicar) 100 mg/kg every 6 hours. Improvement in platelet transfusion outcome in otherwise chronic refractory cases may be achieved by plasmapheresis on a monthly basis. Granulocyte transfusions should be reserved for treatment of sepsis when the absolute granulocyte count falls below 500/mm^3.

2. HLA typing of patient and family should be done as soon as possible. HLA-matched unrelated donors and single donors are ideal for platelet and granulocyte transfusions in these patients. Until the HLA typing and mixed lymphocyte culture (MLC) results are available (approximately 1 week), transfusion of blood products from family members should not be done, since such transfusions usually preclude a successful bone marrow engraftment.

3. If an HLA-MLC compatible family member is identified (usually a sibling), arrangments should be made for bone marrow transplantation. Every major pediatric hematology center in the United States can help in the referral of such patients. The cost for the procedure is between $25,000 and $50,000, but cure rates now exceed 60%, compared with less than 20% if transplantation is not performed.

4. If no donor is available for bone marrow transplantation, antithymocyte globulin* (ATG), 15 mg/kg/day for 10 days, should be tried. In some series, the outcome is almost as good as in bone marrow transplantation. The toxic effects of ATG include fever, chills, skin rash, arthalgias, abdominal pain, and liver dysfunction. Prednisone (2 mg/kg/day) or an equivalent corticosteroid usually controls these toxic effects during ATG administration. Platelet levels should be maintained above 20,000/mm^3 with platelet transfusions.

5. Androgen therapy is ineffective for patients with severe forms of aplastic anemia. However, for milder forms of the disease, as well as for Fanconi's anemia, androgen therapy usually improves the condition. A rise in the reticulocyte count with a subsequent rise in the level of hemoglobin, occurs within 6–12 weeks in the responsive patient. Platelet and granulocyte levels are slower to respond to therapy. We have employed nandrolone decanoate, 1.0–1.5 mg/kg IM weekly or twice monthly, since liver dysfunction is rarer with this preparation. Oral androgen preparations include oxymetholone (dihydrotestosterone) 2.0–6.5 mg/kg/day, and methandrostenolone (Dianabol) 0.25–0.5 mg/kg/day. Other parenteral preparations include testosterone enanthate in oil, 4 mg/kg IM weekly. If there is no response in 4 months, androgen therapy should be discontinued. Liver function (SGOT, SGPT, bilirubin, alkaline phosphatase) should be monitored closely; abnormalities usually cease when the drug is stopped. Acne and any masculinizing effects occur within several weeks after the drug has been started. Most responsive patients can be weaned from the drug or given it intermittently to maintain hemoglobin levels above 9.0 gm%.

6. Corticosteroids, usually prednisone, 1 mg/kg/day, have been combined with androgen in patients receiving the drug longer than 4 months in an effort to retard the accelerated bone aging stimulated by androgens. Prednisone has also been used in an effort to reduce bleeding tendencies at the capillary level, but clear cut benefits are lacking. Patients with severe aplastic anemia who have no bone marrow donor and who are unresponsive to ATG should receive a trial of high-dose bolus methylprednisolone therapy (20 mg/kg/day for 1 week), since a few patients given this treatment have shown a favorable response.

7. A few recent reports indicate that cyclosporin, 4–12 mg/kg/day IM for several months, may be useful in cases refractory to ATG or high-dose methylprednisolone. Tremors, hirsutism, and serum creatinine increases usually occur, but these side effects are generally reversible.

---

* Investigational drug.

Megaloblastic Anemia

PHILIP LANZKOWSKY, M.D.

Megaloblastic anemias in children are relatively uncommon and usually are due to folate or vitamine B_{12} deficiency. Most cases are due to folate deficiency. The causes of folate deficiency include inadequate diet, decreased absorption, which may be congenital or acquired (malabsorption syndrome), drug-induced inhibition of dietary folate absorption (phenytoin, phenobarbital), increased folate utilization (growth, malignant disease, hemolytic anemias), and drug-induced inhibition of folate metabolism (methotrexate, pyrimethamine, trimethoprim). The causes of vitamin B_{12} deficiency include dietary insufficiency (rare), absence or abnormality of gastric intrinsic factor, abnormal absorption of the vitamin B_{12} intrinsic factor complex due to previous small intestinal surgery or lack of intestinal receptors (rare), and inherited abnormalities of vitamin B_{12} transport protein.

The metabolism of folic acid and vitamin B_{12} is interrelated, however, and this must be considered when therapy is instituted. Large doses of vitamin B_{12} may correct the hematologic problems due to folate deficiency. Conversely, large doses of folate may correct the hematologic disturbances due to lack of vitamin B_{12}. Folate, however, will not correct the neurologic problem associated with vitamin B_{12} deficiency, and large doses of folate should not be given until vitamin B_{12} deficiency has been excluded.

Successful treatment of patients with *folate deficiency* involves (1) correction of the folate deficiency; (2) amelioration of the underlying disorder, if possible; (3) improvement of the diet by increased folate intake; (4) follow-up evaluations at intervals to monitor the patient's clinical status.

In cases of suspected folate deficiency, a therapeutic trial can be instituted with 50 to 100 μg of folate per day orally. This dose produces a prompt reticulocytosis in cases of folate deficiency but is without effect in patients with vitamin B_{12} deficiency. An optimal response occurs in most patients with 100 to 200 μg folic acid daily. Nevertheless, it is usual to treat deficient patients with 0.5 mg to 1.0 mg daily orally. Commercially available preparations include a tablet (0.3 to 1.0 mg) and an elixir (1.0 mg/ml). To reduce the folate content would not significantly reduce the cost, and since pteroylmonoglutamic acid rarely produces side effects except in patients with vitamin B_{12} deficiency, there is little reason to reduce the dose. Further, a smaller oral dose might not always be effective in patients with folate malabsorption. In most patients, 5 mg of folic acid given orally daily for 7 to 14 days induces a maximal hematologic response and significant replenishment of body stores. This may be given orally, since even in those with severe malabsorption, sufficient folate is absorbed from this dose to replenish stores. Before folic acid is given (in these large doses) it is always necessary to ensure that vitamin B_{12} deficiency is not present.

The clinical and hematologic response to folic acid is prompt. Within 1 to 2 days the patient's appetite improves (often becoming voracious) and a sense of well-being returns, with increased energy and interest in surroundings. There is a fall in serum iron (often to low levels) in 24 to 48 hours, a rise in reticulocytes in 2 to 4 days reaching a peak at 4 to 7 days, followed by a return of hemoglobin levels to normal in 2 to 6 weeks. The leukocytes and platelets increase with the reticulocytes, the megaloblastic changes in the marrow diminish within 24 to 48 hours, but large myelocytes, metamyelocytes, and band forms may be present for several days.

The duration of therapy depends upon the underlying pathology, but usually folic acid is given for several months until a new population of red cells has been formed. It is often possible to correct the cause of the deficiency and prevent the deficiency recurring, e.g., by an improved diet, a gluten-free diet in celiac disease, or treatment of an inflammatory disease such as tuberculosis or Crohn's disease. In these cases, there is no need to continue folic acid for life. In other situations, however, it is advisable to give folic acid continually to prevent the deficiency recurring, e.g., chronic hemolytic anemia such as thalassemia or in patients with malabsorption who do not respond to a gluten-free diet.

Patients receiving drugs that are folic acid antagonists (methotrexate, pyrimethamine) occasionally develop megaloblastic anemia. Trimethoprim, a pyrimidine analogue, inhibits the enzyme that reduces dihydrofolate to tetrahydrofolate. In some cases folate deficiency can be severe especially in patients with marginal or depleted folate stores. In these cases the antagonism can be overcome by folinic acid, one 5 mg tablet daily.

In conditions in which there is a risk of developing B_{12} *deficiency*, e.g. total gastrectomy, ileal resection, prophylactic administration of vitamin B_{12} should be prescribed.

Patients with suspected vitamin B_{12} deficiency are given a therapeutic trial with 25 to 100 μg of vitamin B_{12}. This dose corrects the hematologic problem due to this vitamin deficiency but will not correct the defect in folate-deficient patients. The reticulocyte response to this therapy is similar to that noted in folate deficiency.

Optimal doses for children are not as well defined as those for adults. When the diagnosis is firmly established, several daily doses of 25 to 100 μg may be used to initiate therapy. Alternatively, in view of the ability of the body to store vitamin

B_{12} for long periods, maintenance therapy can be started with monthly intramuscular injections in doses between 200 μg and 1000 μg. Most cases of vitamin B_{12} deficiency require treatment throughout life.

Patients with defects affecting the intestinal absorption of vitamin B_{12}, either because of abnormalities of intrinsic factor or of ileal uptake, will respond to parenteral vitamin B_{12}. Such a therapeutic maneuver completely bypasses the defective step, and is the chief means by which these two groups of patients are managed currently.

Patients with complete transcobalamin II deficiency respond only to large amounts of B_{12} (1 mg intramuscularly twice or three times weekly). The exact mechanism of this response remains to be defined.

Patients with methylmalonic aciduria with defects in the synthesis of vitamin B_{12} coenzymes are likely to be benefited from massive doses of vitamin B_{12} (1 to 2 mg vitamin B_{12} parenterally daily). However, not all patients in this group are benefited by vitamin B_{12}.

In vitamin B_{12}–responsive megaloblastic anemia, the reticulocytes begin to increase on the third to fourth day, rise to a maximum on the sixth to eighth day, and fall gradually to normal on about the twentieth day. The height of the reticulocyte count is inversely proportional to the degree of anemia. Beginning bone marrow reversal from megaloblastic ro normoblastic cells is obvious within 6 hours and is completely normoblastic in 72 hours.

Prompt hematologic responses are also obtained with the use of oral folic acid. Folic acid, is, however, contraindicated, since it has no effect on neurologic manifestations and has been known to precipitate or accelerate their development. Indeed, megaloblastic anemia should never be treated before a serum folic acid or vitamin B_{12} assay has determined the precise cause so that correct treatment can be administered. Iron is occasionally required when a generally inadequate diet has been given that is deficient in this mineral.

The indications for red blood cell transfusions are infection or incipient heart failure. For unknown reasons the bone marrow frequently is refractory to hematinic therapy during infections. When transfusions are indicated, packed red blood cells should be given at a very slow rate (2 ml/kg/hr).

Hemolytic Anemia

CATHERINE S. MANNO, M.D.,
and FRANCES M. GILL, M.D.

Appropriate therapy for the hemolytic anemias can best be planned once the etiology of the hemolysis has been determined. The premature destruction of red cells in this diverse group of disorders is due to defects that are intrinsic (membrane defects, enzyme deficiencies, or hemoglobin disorders) or extrinsic to the cell. Hemolytic anemias can be congenital or acquired. Red cell destruction occurs in the intravascular space or in the reticuloendothelial system. Hemolysis results in reticulocytosis, elevation of the serum indirect bilirubin level, and a decrease in the serum haptoglobin level. Hemoglobinemia, hemoglobinuria, and an elevated serum lactic dehydrogenase level are characteristic of intravascular hemolysis.

Therapy depends upon the severity of the hemolysis as well as on the etiology. Since increased red cell production, with a consequent increase in nucleic acid production, occurs in all hemolytic disorders, folic acid requirements are increased. Supplementation with 1 mg folic acid daily meets the increased need.

Red cell transfusion therapy is necessary most often in the acute hemolytic anemias but may be necessary in chronic hemolytic states if the anemia suddenly worsens. This happens most frequently during aplastic crises when the bone marrow temporarily stops making red cells. In disorders with brisk hemolysis, the hemoglobin level will drop dramatically after only a few days of aplasia. If the hemoglobin level drops low enough to result in cardiovascular compromise, a small transfusion of red cells (usually 5 ml/kg of packed red blood cells) given carefully is necessary. One transfusion is usually sufficient.

In some of the disorders chronic hemolysis is severe enough to require regular transfusions with red cells. These should be given on a regular schedule to maintain a hemoglobin in the range of 10 to 12 gm/dl. Prior to the first transfusion, complete red cell antigen typing should be performed. Consideration should be given to immunizing transfusion candidates against hepatitis B. If chronic transfusions are necessary over a period of years, accumulation of excessive iron occurs. For patients who no longer need red cell transfusions, excessive iron is best removed by therapeutic phlebotomies. If the need for transfusions continues, iron chelation with deferoxamine therapy is used.

Splenectomy is indicated in some patients. Destruction of damaged and antibody-coated red cells occurs in the reticuloendothelial system, primarily in the spleen. Splenectomy stops hemolysis in hereditary spherocytosis and significantly lessens red cell destruction in some of the other disorders. However, splenectomy carries not only the operative risk but also the risk of postsplenectomy sepsis, primarily due to *S. pneumoniae* or *H. influenzae*. The risk of postsplenectomy sepsis is greater in patients with red cell disorders than in those undergoing splenectomy because of trauma. The risk appears to decrease with age at splenectomy, and elective splenectomy should be deferred until the child is at least 5 years old. Polyvalent pneumococcal vaccine should be given prior to surgery, and prophylactic penicillin (250 mg of penicillin V orally twice a day) should be used daily after surgery. Careful evaluation of fever is mandatory in any patient who has undergone splenectomy.

MEMBRANE DISORDERS

Hereditary Spherocytosis. Hereditary spherocytosis is the most common hemolytic anemia among Northern Europeans. Since the degree of hemolysis ranges from barely detectable to severe, therapy must be determined on an individual basis. Splenectomy is curative, preventing future aplastic crises and stopping further formation of pigment gallstones, but is not necessary for all patients. Children often feel better with folic acid supplementation. If the patient develops fatigue or increased pallor, the hemoglobin and reticulocyte levels should be determined to see if an aplastic crisis is occurring.

Some infants have increased hemolysis during the first year of life, with a hemoglobin level as low as 7 to 8 gm/dl. If the child is growing and developing normally, red cell transfusions are not necessary. The hemoglobin level usually rises to 9 gm/dl or more after the first year. Occasionally the hemolysis may be so severe as to require regular or frequent red cell transfusions. These patients will benefit from splenectomy, which should be postponed until the patient is at least 2 years of age.

Pigmented gallstones have been reported in 23% of patients with hereditary spherocytosis between the ages of 10 and 20 years. Despite the high incidence of gallstone formation, it is not known how many patients will develop cholecystitis. Although splenectomy will prevent future pigment gallstone formation, its performance solely for this purpose is controversial.

Hereditary Elliptocytosis. Hereditary elliptocytosis is less common than hereditary spherocytosis, and chronic hemolysis occurs in only about 12% of patients. As in hereditary spherocytosis, some infants have marked hemolysis, which usually lessens after the first year. Treatment is similar to that for hereditary spherocytosis. Although splenectomy is not curative, the severity of the anemia almost always decreases after the procedure. The risk of pigment gallstone formation continues, however.

Other Membrane Disorders. The other congenital hemolytic disorders are much rarer. The forms of hereditary stomatocytosis can be managed like hereditary spherocytosis. In hereditary pyropoikilocytosis hemolysis may be severe from birth, and the infants often require regular red cell transfusions. In these cases it has been our practice to support the patient with chronic transfusions until the age of 2 or 3 years, when splenectomy is

Table 1. AGENTS TO BE AVOIDED IN G-6-PD DEFICIENT PATIENTS

Acetanilid
Chloramphenicol
Chloroquine, pamaquine, primaquine, quinacrine
Fava beans
Methylene blue
Nalidixic acid
Naphthalene (moth balls)
Nitrofurantoin
Phenacetin
Phenylhydralazine
Sulfonamides (sulfanilamide, sulfacetamide, sulfapyridine)

performed. Although hemolysis persists thereafter, regular transfusions usually are no longer needed. The severity of anemia is variable in congenital dyserythropoietic anemia, type II (known by the acronym HEMPAS). Some patients require transfusions from birth and early splenectomy. Others may be managed as patients with hereditary spherocytosis are managed. In HEMPAS iron overload is very common, and the patient must be monitored carefully for this.

ENZYME DEFICIENCIES

Energy requirements of the erythrocyte are met by production of ATP through glycolysis. Hemolysis results if red cell metabolism is altered by a deficiency of any of several enzymes in the glycolytic pathway, including those of the hexose monophosphate shunt. Deficiencies that cause chronic hemolysis have been called the congenital nonspherocytic hemolytic anemias.

G-6-PD Deficiency. The most common enzyme deficiency is that of glucose-6-phosphate dehydrogenase (G-6-PD). The two most common forms of this X-linked recessive disorder are the African and Mediterranean (Gd and Gd Mediterranean, respectively). The African deficiency occurs in about 10% of American black males. Females are affected less frequently. Hemolysis is limited to acute episodes, beginning hours to days after oxidant stress to the red cells, and the patients are well between episodes. Hemolysis is usually precipitated by drug or chemical exposure but occasionally by infection (e.g., hepatitis) or a severe metabolic disorder (e.g., diabetic acidosis). Since young red cells do contain some enzyme activity, hemolysis is usually self-limited. Red cell transfusions may occasionally be necessary. Avoidance of the inciting agents (see Table 1) will prevent almost all episodes of hemolysis.

Hemolysis in Gd Mediterranean deficiency may be severe, and exposure to oxidants produces hemolysis that may be fatal in a matter of hours. Since even young red cells are enzyme deficient, all red cells are susceptible to hemolysis. Transfusions are necessary in severe episodes. Neonatal hemolysis with hyperbilirubinemia can occur in this form. Exchange transfusions may be necessary. Oxidant drugs should be avoided.

In rare forms of G-6-PD deficiency hemolysis is chronic, resulting in anemia and hyperbilirubinemia. Acute exacerbations may require red cell transfusions, and aplastic crises can occur. Response to splenectomy is unpredictable. Vitamin E administration was not found to be helpful.

Other Enzyme Deficiencies. Deficiency of pyruvate kinase results in chronic hemolysis. The clinical spectrum ranges from mild anemia to severe anemia that requires regular transfusions. Splenectomy generally reduces or eliminates the transfusion requirement but does not eliminate hemolysis. Patients previously requiring regular transfusions may need phlebotomy therapy to remove excessive iron. Other enzyme deficiencies have been described but are rare.

HEMOGLOBIN DISORDERS

Sickle cell disease and the thalassemic disorders are discussed elsewhere. Hereditary alterations in the primary structure of hemoglobin can result in instability of the hemoglobin tetramer. The most common unstable hemoglobin is hemoglobin Köln. The severity of hemolysis in the unstable hemoglobin disorders ranges from mild to severe. Most patients require only folic acid supplementation and avoidance of exposure to oxidant drugs, which can exacerbate hemolysis. Rarely, patients require chronic transfusion therapy. Splenectomy may be beneficial in patients with severe, chronic anemia and in those who develop hypersplenism.

AUTOIMMUNE HEMOLYTIC ANEMIA

In most children autoimmune hemolytic anemia is an acute, self-limited disease. The onset of the anemia is usually very rapid, with an acute fall in the hemoglobin level over hours to days. The Coombs' test result is positive in about 95% of the cases, establishing the diagnosis. In children the disease is usually idiopathic or associated with transient infections. The hemolysis is due either to warm-reacting antibodies or to cold-reacting agglutinins or hemolysins.

Most cases in childhood are caused by warm-reacting antibodies and respond to corticosteroid therapy. Treatment should be started immediately in an attempt to prevent worsening of the anemia. The standard dose of 2 mg/kg/day of prednisone in two divided doses is used initially. If the child is severely ill, the equivalent dose of intravenous corticosteroid, usually hydrocortisone, is given. Response, which may be evident within 1 to 2 days, is heralded by clearing of hemoglobinemia and hemoglobinuria and stabilization of the hemoglobin level. Corticosteroid therapy is continued at the full dose until the hemoglobin level reaches about 10 gm/dl. A slow taper over many weeks can then be started. Too rapid a taper may result in an acute exacerbation. Hemolysis usually stops within two weeks, but the Coombs' test may remain positive for several months. Most children have only one episode of autoimmune hemolytic anemia. The child who is markedly anemic and does not respond to the standard dose may benefit from a 5- to 7-day course of prednisone at 5 to 10 mg/kg/day. The dosage should be tapered after this short course.

Cold-reacting agglutinin disease is most frequently associated with infections, particularly those due to *Mycoplasma pneumoniae* and infectious mononucleosis. Hemolysis is usually mild and stops as the infection clears. Although most cases do not respond to prednisone, the disorder is usually so mild and transient that no other therapy is needed.

Red cell transfusions are not needed in most patients, even when the anemia is marked. The children should be placed at bed rest and observed carefully. If signs of hypoxia or congestive heart failure develop or the hemoglobin falls to extremely low levels, a packed red cell transfusion is necessary. When cold-reacting antibodies are present, the blood must be warmed to body temperature by passage through a blood warmer before transfusion. It is often impossible to find a unit of blood that is compatible by routine blood bank techniques. Every effort should be made to identify the autoantibody, if it has red cell antigen specificity, and to use blood that lacks the antigen. Although transfusion of incompatible blood may increase the rate of hemolysis, it is often necessary to use the most compatible unit of packed cells available. A slow infusion of 5 ml of the unit is given. The patient's plasma should then be checked to see if the level of hemoglobin in the plasma has increased. The human eye can see even small amounts of hemoglobin, and visual inspection of plasma in a spun hematocrit tube is usually satisfactory to detect increased amounts of free hemoglobin. If there is no increase after the test dose, the transfusion may procede slowly. One or two transfusions of 3 to 5 ml/kg each are usually sufficient to relieve symptoms. The hemoglobin level need not be raised to normal levels. If there is increased hemolysis, another unit should be tried with the same precautions.

Transfusions in the severely affected child may not produce a rise in the hemoglobin level. In these patients, a two-volume exchange transfusion or plasmapheresis with replacement by donor red cells is frequently effective in slowing hemolysis and obtaining a higher hemoglobin level. This may need to be repeated daily until the severe hemolysis abates. These forms of transfusion may also be beneficial to the child with severe hemolysis from cold-agglutinin or cold-hemolysin disease in whom prednisone is not effective.

Children who have slower onset of hemolysis or who have moderate anemia may report only fatigue. Prednisone therapy and bedrest until the hemoglobin level rises may be sufficient treatment. Patients who have a rapid fall of hemoglobin to very low levels may be gravely ill, requiring close observation and intensive care until their condition stabilizes. Patients with hemoglobinuria should receive intravenous hydration in an attempt to prevent renal tubular damage. Rarely, anuria results from the tubular damage, and the child will need temporary dialysis support.

The severely ill child with marked anemia who does not respond rapidly to prednisone may require other treatment. Although there is little experience to date, intravenous gamma globulin in the dosage schedule used to treat immune thrombocytopenic purpura (400 mg/kg/day for 5 consecutive days) may help. Treatment with immunosuppressive agents should be reserved for the child with refractory acute anemia or for those with chronic or relapsing disease. Splenectomy may also be of benefit but is rarely necessary in acute antoimmune hemolytic anemia.

Acute autoimmune hemolytic anemia is sometimes accompanied by thrombocytopenia and less frequently by neutropenia. These usually resolve as the hemolysis improves. However, since some deaths result from hemorrhage, severe thrombocytopenia with bleeding should be managed aggressively with plasmapheresis, intravenous gamma globulin, or splenectomy.

In some children the course of the disease is chronic, lasting for more than 5 months, or relapsing. These children more frequently have an underlying disorder, such as collagen-vascular disease or immunodeficiency, and more frequently have associated thrombocytopenia or neutropenia. Acute relapses often respond to prednisone therapy, particularly those in patients with systemic lupus erythematosus. Chronic autoimmune hemolytic anemia is a difficult disease best managed by hematologists experienced in this disorder.

Thalassemia

CAROL B. HYMAN, M.D.

SPECIFIC TREATMENT

No specific treatment of the thalassemias is available. Bone marrow transplantation, primarily for young infants, is being tried. However, even if the transplant procedure is successful, it must be considered investigational, as the long-term risks from preparatory chemotherapy and/or radiation are not known. We do know that under present day management, most patients can expect to live to at least the third or fourth decade. Also,

it can be anticipated that in the future drugs to increase hemoglobin synthesis and/or genetic engineering procedures will be effective in treating the basic abnormality.

SUPPORTIVE CARE

Transfusion Therapy.   Patients who cannot maintain a hemoglobin level of approximately 7 gm/dl should be on a regular transfusion program to prevent chronic hypoxemia and suppress ineffective erythropoiesis. A transfusion program to maintain the hemoglobin level at 10.5 gm/dl or greater will enable patients to feel well and carry out most age-appropriate activities. Young adults, especially those who are active, may feel better with a pretransfusion hemoglobin level of 12 to 13 gm/dl. This transfusion program will diminish or prevent development of the bony abnormalities usually associated with the thalassemias, decrease spleen size and, to a lesser extent, improve growth and development. Dietary iron absorption is also decreased. It should be noted that once patients have become accustomed to a high hemoglobin level, symptoms may occur if the level is allowed to drop. For this reason, and because fluctuation in hemoglobin level is not physiologic, our patients are transfused at 2- to 3-week intervals. In fact, some patients require less blood on a biweekly than a triweekly schedule. Frozen red cells or washed red cells less than a week old should be used, as unwashed cells may result in febrile reactions. Neocytes, the most recently produced red cells from a unit of blood, are being used at some centers. Given with partial exchange transfusion, the intertransfusion interval can be increased and total red cell requirement decreased by as much as one third. However, these procedures are costly and wasteful of blood, since only part of each unit is used. Caution should be observed with the rate of infusion of blood or other fluids in iron loaded patients to prevent fluid overload or heart failure. The older the patient, the less tolerant he or she will be of fluctuations in blood volume. Our patients receive each unit over 3 to 4 hours and wait at least 2 to 4 hours between units. Adults may require 12 to 24 hours between units.

Nonimmune patients should receive hepatitis-B vaccine.

Splenectomy. Splenectomy should be considered for correction of hypersplenism with a red cell transfusion requirement above expected (greater than 250 ml/kg/year), for leukopenia or thrombocytopenia, and for massive splenomegaly. Prior to determining whether the procedure should be done, the degree of hypersplenism and the risks of rupture from trauma or discomfort from spleen size should be weighed against the benefits of leaving the spleen in situ. The spleen's protective effect against severe overwhelming infection, especially from pneumococcus and *Haemophilus influenzae,* is well known. The role of the spleen as an innocuous storage site for excess iron is not well understood. The author feels it may offer a greater protective effect for the heart and other organs than has been previously appreciated, and this may be enough to counteract some of the risks of the higher transfusion requirement.

If splenectomy is necessary, consideration should be given to performing a partial splenectomy. At this time, partial splenectomy is not "standard procedure" for thalassemia, as data on its effectiveness are not available. If partial or complete splenectomy is planned, Pneumovax, a vaccine that provides partial immunity to some strains of pneumococci, should be given at least 2 weeks prior to the procedure. Patients and their parents should be educated about the risks of post-splenectomy infection, and this education should be reinforced repeatedly over the following years and for the lifetime of the patient. This education is more valuable than prophylactic antibiotics. However, prophylactic penicillin, 250 mg bid, should be prescribed and patients instructed to call WITHOUT DELAY if they develop fever of 101.5°F or above. Patients who live a distance from the medical center may be given a supply of ampicillin if they can be depended upon to call the physician and complete a course of therapy if needed.

Management of Chronic Iron Overload. Deferoxamine (DF), is the best iron chelating agent available for clinical use. Its effectiveness depends on dose, time in blood stream, total body iron, and the chelatable iron pool. DF is expensive and 20 mg/kg per day is the most cost effective dose, but higher doses increase iron excretion. DF must be given parenterally, as oral absorption is minimal. Daily intramuscular (IM) DF removes only one third of iron intake by transfusion, and subcutaneous (SQ) DF is inadequate to prevent continued iron accumulation. Therefore, we use a combined SQ-IV treatment program. SQ DF, 40–60 mg/kg over 8 to 10 hours, for 5 to 6 days per week is recommended. For SQ therapy, each 500 mg vial of DF is dissolved in 1.5 ml distilled water without preservative and the total volume increased to 7 ml, with distilled water or normal saline in a 10 ml syringe attached to a 25 G or a 27 G long tube butterfly needle. The needle is inserted in the thigh or lower abdominal wall, and the drug is administered by continuous infusion, using a mechanical pump. The maximum IV dose, 15 mg/kg per hour, is infused at the time of transfusion and, if possible for 24 hours post transfusion or for as many hours as pratical therafter, as it has been found that there is greater iron excretion after than during transfusion. If this is not possible, IV pulse therapy for approximately 48 hours at reg-

ular intervals should be considered to prevent continued iron accumulation, or in older patients to lower the total body iron load. For infants and young children too small to use the pump, IM DF can be used. Although there is no consensus of opinion, the author believes that chelation therapy should begin when the patient is as young as possible to prevent the chelatable iron from being transported to the heart or other parenchymal organs. With DF, iron is excreted in the urine, coloring it orange-red, and in the stool in variable amounts. Toxicity is minimal, and side effects include abdominal discomfort, mild diarrhea, itching at the injection site and, with rapid IV infusions, possible lowering of the blood pressure. Cataracts may occur but are very rare. Therfore, the patient should be seen by an ophthalmologist at 6-month intervals. To ensure the availability of chelatable iron, ascorbic acid, 50 mg, should be given after the daily dose of DF is started. Vitamin C without DF or in large doses is contraindicated, as it can increase iron toxicity, especially to the heart and, if given with meals, can increase food iron absorption.

Hearing should be monitored because sensorineural hearing loss has been reported, especially in young children on high-dose Desferal therapy.

Diet. Patients should be advised to avoid citrus and other high vitamin C containing foods with meals. Tea and cocoa are excellent mealtime beverages, as they interfere with dietary iron absorption. Vitamin E supplements are necessary to counteract the oxidant effects of iron. Infants should receive 100 units, young children 200 units, and older children and adults 400 units per day. Folic acid, 1 mg per day, should be given to all patients.

Iron overload patients should avoid all raw seafood because of the possibility of contamination with organisms, which can cause overwhelming sepsis.

COMPLICATIONS OF THALASSEMIA AND CHRONIC IRON OVERLOAD

Cardiac. The primary cause of death in thalassemia is cardiac disorders. Congestive heart failure, arrhythmias, and pericarditis should be aggressively treated, preferably by a cardiologist familiar with cardiac problems due to chronic iron overload.

Diabetes and Other Endocrine Abnormalities. These should be managed as indicated. Patients who do not go through puberty or develop secondary sex characteristics should be given replacement therapy. Hypoparathyroidism with low serum calcium levels may occur and require treatment with calcium supplements or 1,25 vitamin D or both.

Magnesium Depletion. Magnesium depletion is a frequent problem and may manifest with increased neuromuscular irritability or with cardiac arrhythmias, eyelid twitching, generalized muscle aches, neck pain, and changes in affect. Hypomagnesemia must be corrected, as it may significantly increase cardiac arrhythmias from chronic iron overload. The serum magnesium level should be observed at regular intervals beginning in early childhood and, if low, oral magnesium supplements given. If oral magnesium supplements are insufficient to maintain the serum magnesium level, intravenous infusions of magnesium sulfate may be required.

THALASSEMIA INTERMEDIA

This clinical term includes those patients with beta thalessemia who can maintain a hemoglobin level of 6 to 7 gm/dl or greater without regular transfusions. Each patient should be individually evaluated to determine if transfusion therapy and/ or splenectomy is indicated, as symptoms may be severe and crippling. The long term risks of chronic hypoxemia and erythroid hyperplasia with osteoporosis, bony deformities, energy wastage, retardation of growth and development, and marked splenomegaly must be weighed against the problems associated with a chronic transfusion program. Severe hemosiderosis, from increased oral iron absorption, can be a significant problem and requires diet modification, including folic acid and vitamin E supplements as outlined above, and sometimes chelation therapy. After considering the factors discussed above, splenectomy or partial splenectomy may be necessary.

THALASSEMIA TRAIT

The diagnosis of beta thalassemia trait (thalassemia minor) is important for three reasons: (1) to differentiate it from iron deficiency anemia and avoid the chronic use of hematinics. The exception is during pregnancy, when folic acid may prevent the hemoglobin from falling as low as would otherwise occur. (2) To reassure the affected individual that this is not a disease and will not cause illness or affect longevity. (3) For genetic counseling. Screening of family members who are potential parents should be carried out.

HEMOGLOBIN H DISEASE

This is a moderately severe form of alpha thalassemia and manifests as thalassemia intermedia, with a hemoglobin level of approximately 7 to 10 gm/dl. Symptoms are usually less severe than those of beta thalassemia intermedia, as ineffective erythropoiesis is less marked. Although these patients do not require regular transfusions, sporadic transfusions may be necessary. The red cells are susceptible to oxidant stress, so drugs such as sulfonamides, antimalarials, and high doses of salicylates should be avoided. Cholelithiasis, hypersplenism,

and hemosiderosis from increased absorption of dietary iron may be problems. Splenectomy or partial splenectomy should be considered (as discussed above) for correction of severe hypersplenism. Diet modification and vitamin E supplements as outlined are advisable.

Adverse Reactions to Blood Transfusion

IRA A. SHULMAN, M.D.

The transfusion of whole blood and blood components is usually a temporarily effective means of correcting red cell, white cell, platelet, and coagulation factor deficits. Unfortunately, there is a spectrum of adverse reactions associated with the administration of whole blood and blood components. These reactions may be immunologically or nonimmunologically mediated. Transfusion reactions may be mild or so severe that they jeopardize patients' lives.

It is imperative that transfusionists be aware of the signs and symptoms of transfusion reactions. Close clinical monitoring of patients receiving transfusions can result in early detection of adverse reactions and prevention of serious complications should a reaction occur. By discontinuing a transfusion at the onset of a reaction, and thus limiting the quantity of blood transfused, serious complications can often be avoided.

Transfusion reactions can be divided into two broad categories, acute and delayed. Acute reactions generally occur within twenty-four hours of a transfusion, while delayed reactions may occur days, weeks, or even months later. Approximately 3% of transfused patients experience an acute reaction and approximately 10% experience a delayed reaction. The most important acute transfusion reactions are as follows: hemolysis of transfused red cells, hemolysis of the recipient's red cells, nonhemolytic febrile reactions, urticarial allergic reactions, anaphylactic allergic reactions, congestive heart failure, noncardiogenic pulmonary edema, septic shock, arrhythmias, and citrate toxicity. The most important delayed reactions include the following: hemolysis of transfused red cells; alloimmunization to transfused red cells, white cells, and platelets; disease transmission; iron overload; and graft-vs.-host disease. It is important to remember that it is better to avoid a transfusion reaction than to treat one. Therefore, before any patient is transfused, the potential value of the blood transfusion should outweigh the risks to the patient.

HEMOLYSIS OF TRANSFUSED RED CELLS

Hemolysis of transfused red cells may be either immune or nonimmune mediated. Immune-mediated acute hemolytic transfusion reactions are most often due to ABO incompatible transfusions. These reactions occur when group A blood is transfused to a group O or group B recipient, when group B blood is transfused to a group O or group A recipient, or when group AB blood is transfused to a group O, group A, or group B recipient. Depending on their blood group, pediatric patients begin to produce anti-A and/or anti-B within the first year of life. Transplacental maternal anti-A and anti-B may be present at birth. It is the presence of these antibodies that can cause an acute hemolytic reaction if the wrong blood is transfused.

Almost all ABO incompatible transfusions are preventable. These reactions usually result from human error and complicate approximately 1 in every 25,000 units of blood transfused in the United States. They are rarely fatal unless more than 100 ml of ABO-incompatible packed red cells (or 200 ml whole blood) have been transfused to an adult. Smaller amounts transfused to pediatric patients may be fatal. Approximately 2 in every million units of blood transfused result in a fatal ABO mismatch. Hemolytic transfusion reactions may be accompanied by fever, chills, chest pain, hypotension, nausea, flushing, dyspnea, hemoglobinemia, hemoglobinuria, shock, generalized bleeding, oliguria, anuria, back pain, and pain at the infusion site. Some patients may complain of a feeling of impending doom. Although all of these symptoms probably will not be found in any individual patient, a common first symptom noted in conscious recipients is fever, which is frequently accompanied by chills. The severity of the patient's initial symptoms may forecast the severity of the ensuing clinical problems and is related to the amount of incompatible blood transfused. In unconscious or anesthetized patients the only manifestations of an acute hemolytic transfusion reaction may be unexplained bleeding at surgical and venipuncture sites due to disseminated intravascular coagulation (DIC), and/or unexplained hypotension.

The signs and symptoms seen with ABO-incompatible transfusions are triggered by immunologic events (antigen-antibody interaction and the activation of complement). This is followed by the release of vasoactive substances into the circulation, the activation of the clotting cascade, and reflex activation of sympathetic nervous system responses. Severe reactions may be associated with shock, DIC, and acute renal failure.

The investigation of an acute hemolytic reaction should begin with a check of the name and hospital number on the patient's wrist band against the same data on the identification tag of the donor blood. If these are not the same, the possibility of an ABO incompatible transfusion is great and the blood bank should be immediately notified. Not only is it important for the patient being transfused to have the diagnosis established quickly, but such identification errors resulting in ABO hemolytic reactions often involve two patients and it is imperative to determine if another patient is also in danger of receiving incompatible blood. An anticoagulated and a clotted sample of blood should be drawn from the patient and sent to the blood bank for investigation along with the remainder of the suspected unit of blood and all attached tubing. The blood bank laboratory can quickly rule out an acute intravascular hemolytc reaction by performing three "stat" tests. The first is a visual comparision of the patient's pretransfusion and post-transfusion blood samples for the presence of free hemoglobin or bilirubin, the second is a direct antiglobulin (Coombs') test performed on the post-transfusion sample, and the third is an ABO-Rh typing of the post-transfusion sample. If the visual inspection is properly performed, as little as ten ml of intravascularly hemolyzed blood can result in a positive test.

If ABO incompatible blood has been transfused, treatment depends on how much incompatible blood has been transfused. Usually, if a volume of incompatible blood less than 5% of the patient's estimated blood volume has been transfused, no specific therapy is necessary. Incompatible transfusions exceeding 5–10% may lead to hypotension, shock, DIC, and renal failure.

Vigorous treatment of hypotension and promotion of adequate renal blood flow are important. Renal failure may be secondary to shock, and if the shock can be prevented or adequately treated, renal failure may be avoided. Therapy should be directed at maintaining normal blood pressures and brisk urine flow. This may be accomplished with specific diuretic agents such as intravenous furosemide, which improves renal blood flow and produces diuresis, and the administration of fluids to help maintain the patient's blood pressure. These fluids may be either colloidal or crystalloid solutions.

Drugs that decrease renal blood flow are contraindicated. Dopamine dilates renal vasculature while at the same time increasing cardiac output. This drug may be useful in treating the acute phases of hemolytic transfusion reactions. Dopamine must be diluted and given intravenously, and the patient's urine flow, cardiac output, and blood pressure must be carefully monitored. The use of heparin to treat DIC is controversial, as heparin causes bleeding and may be contraindicated for patients who have undergone surgery. Heparin is probably only indicated when the reaction is due to an ABO mismatch and the patient has received more than 3 ml/kg body weight of incompatible blood. If heparin is administered, it probably needs to be administered only for as long as the stimulus for the DIC exists. Therefore, heparinization may only be required for 6–24 hours. Administration of platelet concentrates and cryoprecipitate (as a source of fibrinogen) might be necessary if bleeding due to DIC is life threatening. Patients should be monitored for evidence of acute renal failure. If acute tubular necrosis is suspected, an appropriate treatment regimen should be instituted.

Acute hemolytic tranfusion reactions are also due to incompatibility of other blood group antigens, although less often. Antibodies such as anti-Jk^a, anti-Kell, and anti-Fy^a have all been described to cause acute hemolytic transfusion reactions. Reactions of this sort may occur when a patient requires uncrossmatched blood (either group O Rh negative or group specific) in an emergency situation. Serologic incompatibility may not be discovered until the crossmatch has been completed. By that time the patient may have begun to experience a symptomatic reaction.

There are several nonimmune causes for acute hemolysis of transfused blood. These include osmotic lysis if incompatible crystalloid solutions are used to dilute blood (such as 5% dextrose in water), accidental freezing (which can occur when blood is stored in unmonitored ward or surgical refrigerators, accidental overheating by faulty blood warmers or microwave heating, and bacterial contamination. These problems are avoidable when proper protocols are followed.

HEMOLYSIS OF RECIPIENT RED CELLS

Transfusion of antibodies to red blood cells can result in acute hemolysis. Blood products such as platelet concentrates, fresh frozen plasma, cryoprecipitate, and clotting factor concentrates may contain anti-A or anti-B alloantibodies. For example, whenever a unit of group O platelets is transfused into a group A or group B recipient, 50 ml of incompatible plasma is transfused. With increasing dosage of incompatible plasma, the possibility of an acute hemolytic reaction due to transfused antibody increases. This may be of considerable importance when transfusing neonates and small children. Infants with *Clostridium*-associated necrotizing enterocolitis are at special risk for acute hemolytic transfusion reactions due to the transfusion of antibodies to red cells. Neuraminidase produced by *Clostridium* spp. can result in so called "T-activation" of the newborn's red cells. Although T-activation of the newborn's red cells would have no immediate detrimental effects, if the infant were transfused with plasma or whole blood containing anti-T, a hemolytic reaction could occur. Most normal adult plasma has some anti-T in it. Infants with necrotizing entercolitis should be tested for T-activation of their red cells. If T-activation is present, washed red cells should be given and plasma avoided when transfusions are necessary.

NONHEMOLYTIC FEBRILE TRANSFUSION REACTIONS

A nonhemolytic febrile transfusion reaction is defined by a temperature rise of 1° C or more in association with transfusion and without other explanation. These reactions are the most frequent acute adverse effects seen in blood recipients, complicating approximately 1% of blood transfusions. Most often these febrile episodes are due to the transfusion of white cells and/or platelets to which the recipient has antibodies. The fever may be mild to severe and may begin at any time from early in the transfusion to several hours after the transfusion has been completed. Unfortunately, hemolytic reactions to blood are also characterized by fever. Therefore, febrile reactions cannot be ignored and must be carefully evaluated. Only after a hemolytic reaction has been ruled out can the diagnosis of a nonhemolytic febrile reaction be established.

No specific therapy has been indicated for nonhemolytic febrile transfusion reactions, although antipyretics may be administered. Acetaminophen would seem to be superior to salicylates because the former drug does not affect platelet function. Patients who suffer repeated nonhemolytic febrile transfusion reactions might benefit from leukocyte-poor blood products if additional red cell or platelet transfusions are necessary. One can choose from an array of leukocyte-poor blood products. Red cell products can be made leukocyte poor by either centrifugation, filtration, washing, or freeze-thaw techniques. Plateletpheresis concentrates (prepared by cell separator devices) can be prepared so they contain a minimum amount of white cell contamination.

URTICARIAL ALLERGIC REACTIONS

Another common acute reaction is the urticarial allergic reaction characterized by erythema, hives, and itching and is probably due to allergy to soluble proteins in the donor plasma. Perhaps 1% of all transfusions are complicated by these reactions. If an urticarial allergic reaction occurs and is not associated with fever or other signs and symptoms of transfusion reactions, it is not necessary to discontinue the transfusion. Rather, the infusion may be temporarily interrupted and an antihistamine administered. Once the symptoms have subsided, the transfusion may be continued slowly. Patients who repeatedly suffer urticarial allergic reactions may be premedicated with antihistamine. The use of plasma-depleted blood products such as saline-washed or deglycerolized frozen red cells will also prevent urticarial allergic reactions; however, these blood products are costly.

BACTERIAL CONTAMINATION

Bacterial contamination of blood products is fortunately rare. Such contamination is more likely to affect products stored at room temperature such as platelets and blood products that are thawed in warm water baths that might be contaminated by bacteria. Refrigerated blood products, however, are not free of risk. Bacteria can get into the blood container during the donor phlebotomy, or during blood component preparation. Bacteria may also contaminate the blood container ports. When a blood product is contaminated with bacteria, transfusion of that product can result in a devastating septic transfusion reaction. The reaction is characterized by high fever, chills, shock, hemoglobinemia, hemoglobinuria, DIC, and renal failure. Treatment consists of intravenous antibiotic therapy combined with administration of vasopressor drugs such as dopamine. Corticosteroids may also be of benefit.

ANAPHYLACTIC TRANSFUSION REACTIONS

Anaphylactic transfusion reactions are rare. They are characterized by anaphylactic shock after the administration of only a few milliliters of blood. Patients may develop flushing, rash, chills, coughing, respiratory distress, vascular instability, abdominal cramping, vomiting, and diarrhea. They may lapse into unconsciousness. Other causes for acute analphylaxis, such as drug reactions, must be considered. Anaphylactic transfusion reactions typically are seen in patients with IgA deficiency who have formed anti-IgA antibodies. Approximately one in every 800 patients are IgA deficient but only a small percentage of IgA deficient individuals form anti-IgA. The treatment of such a reaction is to stop the blood transfusion, maintain a patent intravenous line, treat hypotension, and give epinephrine. Patients with anti-IgA must be transfused with blood products that lack IgA. Frozen-thawed blood may be used. If feasible, the patient's autologous blood should be stored for future use. If time permits, blood can be obtained from Rare Donor Files, where IgA deficient blood products are stored. Such files are maintained by the American Red Cross, The American Association of Blood Banks, the Irwin Memorial Blood Bank in San Francisco, and the Canadian Red Cross.

CIRCULATORY OVERLOAD

Increases in blood volume may be poorly tolerated if a patient has little or no cardiac reserve or an already expanded blood volume. Even small-volume blood transfusions may cause problems for very sick infants. Patients who are susceptible to develop circulatory overload may require very slow blood transfusions. However, no container of blood should "hang" for more than 4 hours (to minimize the risk of bacterial contamination). To administer blood very slowly and not exceed the recommended 4-hour duration per container of blood, the desired dose of blood should be divided into small aliquots so that no individual aliquot is allowed to hang in excess of 4 hours. The use of diuretics prior to and during transfusion may be useful. Under no circumstances should a diuretic be added to the blood container, as hemolysis might result. If circulatory overload does develop, the transfusion should be stopped, diuretics and oxygen should be administered, and the patient should be placed into a sitting position if possible. Phlebotomy and/or rotating tourniquets may be required.

NONCARDIOGENIC PULMONARY EDEMA

Noncardiogenic pulmonary edema is characterized by acute respiratory insufficiency without evidence of heart failure. Symptoms occur after infusions of small volumes of blood products insufficient to cause volume overload. This very rare reaction is due to the transfusion of antileukocyte antibodies present in donor plasma or due to the transfusion of white cell concentrates to patients with antileukocyte antibodies. Transfused leukoagglutinins react with recipient leukocytes to produce white cell aggregates that are trapped in the pulmonary microcirculation, whereas during transfusion of granulocyte concentrates, leukoagglutinins in the recipient aggregate the transfused leukocytes in the pulmonary microcirculation. If noncardiogenic pulmonary edema develops, the transfusion should be stopped immediately. Respiratory support should be provided. Intravenous corticosteroids may be beneficial.

ARRHYTHMIAS

The transfusion of ice cold blood via central catheters positioned close to the cardiac conduction system may precipitate cardiac arrhythmias. Pulling back on the catheter, reducing the rate of infusion, or using blood warmers may avoid this problem.

CITRATE TOXICITY

When large volumes of whole blood, plasma, or platelet concentrates are transfused in a very short period of time, citrate levels rise in the blood and serum calcium levels may drop. This problem may be managed by administering calcium solutions intravenously (i.e., during exchange transfusions). It is important not to give too much calcium because iatrogenic hypercalcemia may cause worse problems for the patient than transfusion-induced hypocalcemia.

ALLOIMMUNIZATION TO RED CELLS, WHITE CELLS, AND PLATELETS

As long as Rh-negative patients receive Rh-negative blood, the risk of forming red cell alloantibodies following blood transfusion is approximately 1–1.6% per unit of red cell component transfused. Antibodies such as anti-E and anti-Kell are among the most commonly formed alloantibodies following blood transfusion. With the initial appearance of these antibodies in the serum, few if any clinical symptoms are detectable because weeks to months pass before the antibodies are formed. By that time, most of the transfused red cells responsible for the initial immunization have been cleared from the circulation. When a clinically significant antibody is identified in a pediatric patient, the patient's family should be informed and ideally should be provided with a card or letter with this information. After the initial immunization, alloantibodies may diminish to undetectable levels. Once such an antibody has been identified in a patient, blood bearing the corresponding antigen should be avoided, even if the patient's serum appears to be negative for red cell antibodies. Sometimes the only clue that a patient previously formed a clinically significant antibody is the information provided by the patient or his family.

Alloimmunization can also occur to leukocyte or platelet antigens. Alloimmunization to leukocyte antigens may cause febrile transfusion reactions when the patient is subsequently transfused. Antiplatelet and antileukocyte antibodies may result in refractoriness to platelet transfusions.

DELAYED HEMOLYSIS OF TRANSFUSED RED CELLS

Symptomatic delayed hemolytic transfusion reactions result from an anamnestic immune response to transfused red cells bearing a blood group antigen that the recipient of the blood lacks. Typically, the immunizing stimulus is a previous blood transfusion or pregnancy. As previously stated, alloantibodies formed after the initial immunizing stimulus may diminish to undetectable levels in the patient's serum. Crossmatches may be compatible, yet within one to seven days following the transfusion of the "compatible" blood, an anamnestic immunologic response leads to rapidly increasing levels of unexpected antibodies that can mediate hemolysis of transfused red cells. These patients may present with fever and an unexplained drop in their hemoglobin. Only rarely does renal failure occur. Typically, no specific therapy is required, but monitoring the patient's urine output is suggested. Additional blood transfusions should be avoided unless absolutely necessary.

POST-TRANSFUSION HEPATITIS

Post-transfusion hepatitis is the most common serious complication of blood transfusion. It has been estimated that as many as 7–10% of blood recipients develop at least mild hepatitis following blood transfusion. Over 90% of these cases are so called "non-A non-B." Some patients develop chronic active hepatitis and even cirrhosis.

CYTOMEGALOVIRUS

Cytomegalovirus (CMV) can be transmitted by blood transfusion, and the resultant infections in term infants or children are usually manifested by asymptomatic seroconversion or a mild mononucleosis-like syndrome. The outcome of CMV infections in preterm infants is different in that they are more likely to develop symptomatic infections with respiratory difficulties, hepatosplenomegaly, gray pallor, and atypical lymphocytosis. Infants weighing less than 1250 grams whose mothers are CMV seronegative are at the highest risk for developing serious or fatal CMV infections should they receive more than 50 ml of blood from CMV seropositive donors. It has been recommended that these infants receive CMV seronegative blood. The American Association of Blood Banks states the following: "In geographic areas where post-transfusion cytomegalovirus (CMV) disease is a problem, components that contain formed elements should be selected or processed to reduce that risk to neonates weighing less than 1,250 grams at birth, when either the neonate or the mother is CMV-antibody negative or that information is unknown." Blood products that might reduce the risk of CMV disease transmission include blood drawn from CMV-seronegative blood donors, saline-washed packed red cells, certain types of filtered blood, and deglycerolized red cells.

MALARIA

Approximately three cases of post-transfusion malaria occur annually in the United States. As there is no exoerythrocytic stage following transfusion-induced malaria, the disease may be treated with therapy that kills the erythrocytic parasites.

SYPHILIS

Since the spirochete cannot survive at refrigerator temperature, only blood products stored at room temperature (platelets) or those transfused very promptly after donation have any risk of syphilis transmission.

TRANSFUSION–ASSOCIATED AIDS

At the time of this writing, 1.3% of AIDS cases have been attributed to blood transfusion; 111 cases of transfusion-associated AIDS (88%) have been diagnosed in the adult population, and 15 cases of transfusion-associated AIDS (12%) have been diagnosed in the pediatric group. As there is currently no cure for AIDS, prevention of its transmission is extremely important. Individuals likely to be carriers of the disease (homosexual or bisexual males, IV drug users, hemophiliacs, Haitian entrants, sexual partners of carriers) are encouraged not to be blood donors. In addition, soon all blood drawn within the United States will be tested for antibodies to HTLV-III.

GRAFT–VS.–HOST DISEASE

Graft-vs.-host disease may be seen in immunocompromised patients receiving cellular blood products. All cellular blood fractions, including erythrocytes, platelets, and granulocytes contain lymphocytes capable of causing graft-vs.-host disease. Moreover, storage of blood does not solve the problem, as lymphocytes capable of causing the disease can survive both liquid and frozen storage. A radiation dose of 1500 to 3000 rads will render 95% of the lymphocytes in a unit of blood, granulocyte concentrate, or platelet concentrate incapable of replication. The function of the platelets, granulocytes, or red cells is unaffected by this treatment. Irradiated blood products are available from regional blood centers, or blood products may be irradiated by the hospital transfusion service.

TRANSFUSION HEMOSIDEROSIS

When patients have received over 100 units of blood, iron deposition in such vital organs as the heart, liver, or endocrine organs may interfere with the function of these organs. Treatment is directed at reducing the patients overloaded iron stores. Administration of desferrioxamine, an iron-chelating agent, has shown promise for reducing body iron stores in such patients.

Sickle Cell Disease

ELLIOTT VICHINSKY, M.D.

Sickle cell disorders include sickle cell anemia (hemoglobin SS), hemoglobin sickle C disease (hemoglobin SC), and sickle-beta thalassemia (S-beta thal). In addition to chronic hemolytic anemia, unexpected acute medical complications and organ failure characterize the clinical courses of these diseases. In general, patients with hemoglobin sickle C disease and sickle-beta-thalassemia have a milder course than do patients with sickle cell anemia; however, a particular complication may be equally severe in all three disorders. Although there is no cure for sickle cell disease, a significant decrease in morbidity and mortality has been accomplished as a consequence of early diagnosis, parent and patient education, comprehensive medical care, and improved treatment of complications.

COMPREHENSIVE CARE

Comprehensive family counseling by well-informed medical staff may be the most important step in decreasing the morbidity of sickle cell disease in childhood. The optimal time for diagnosis is in the neonatal period. This allows time for family education before the child develops symptoms. Problems such as fever, infection, pain, and anemia should be repeatedly discussed with the parents. It is extremely helpful to plan ahead for communication and transportation needs that may arise during emergency situations. Plans to minimize the financial and psychological hardships of raising a child with sickle cell disease should be initiated early in the treatment program.

Comprehensive care should also include periodic assessment of growth and development, regular immunizations, visual screening, and dental care. After the age of 10, children with sickle cell disease should be examined annually by an ophthalmologist familiar with sickle cell retinopathy. Sickle cell disease patients have increased nutritional requirements and may need a high-calorie balanced diet with folic acid supplementation. The possibilities of delayed onset of puberty, short stature, and persistent primary enuresis must be discussed with the family.

Pain Crises

Adequate hydration, effective analgesia, and identification and treatment of any precipitating event are the essential components of a vaso-occlusive crisis treatment program. One must never assume that pain is due to a vaso-occlusive crisis without first excluding other possible causes. If fever is present, an aggressive search for its cause should be made. Painful, swollen extremities suggest the possibility of osteomyelitis or septic arthritis. Abdominal pain should not be attributed to sickle cell disease until other surgical and medical emergencies have been excluded.

Hydration. Hydration is necessary for the successful management of vaso-occlusive crises. Dehydration promotes sickling and frequently occurs because of the high incidence of hyposthenuria. During a vaso-occlusive crisis, reduced oral intake and increased insensible water loss further increase the likelihood of dehydration. Urinary specific gravity should not be relied upon as a measurement of hydration, because of the associated hyposthenuria. In mild painful crises, oral hydration is usually sufficient. Patients and families should be given specific guidelines for fluid intake, in terms of ounces of fluid per day necessary to ensure one-and-one-half times maintenance fluid hydration. Soft drinks, juices, and bouillon are recommended. When severe pain is present, parenteral hydration is usually necessary. The choice of the initial fluid giver is dictated by the patient's hydration and electrolyte status. In uncomplicated vaso-occlusive crises, a solution of 5% D5W and 25% normal saline is recommended. If cardiac status is normal, the older patient should receive 2500–3000 cc/m^2/day. In small children, 100 cc/kg/day is adequate. Parenteral hydration should be closely monitored to prevent iatrogenic congestive heart failure and electrolyte imbalance. Frequent physical examinations, daily weight measurements, and adequate intake and output measurements are essential.

Analgesia. The choice of analgesic therapy is based upon considerations of potency, duration of action, and side effects. Medication should be administered on a fixed time schedule, with an interval that does not exceed the duration of adequate analgesia. This approach improves the control of pain and decreases anxiety in the patient. One should be aware that the oral route of administration of a narcotic is always less than one-half as effective as the parenteral route. However, oral administration avoids the complications of parenteral therapy and is often adquate to treat mild to moderate pain. When narcotics are used, the physician should remember that side effects include respiratory depression, nausea, vomiting, hypotension, increased secretion of antidiuretic hormone, increased bladder tone, decreased seizure threshhold, and constipation. Nonnarcotic analgesics such as aspirin (10 mg/kg/dose q 4 hr) or acetaminophen (10 mg/kg/dose q 4 hr) are recommended for mild pain. Codeine (1 mg/kg/dose q 4 hr) is the preferred narcotic for outpatient pain management and should be added to acetaminophen or aspirin when nonnarcotic analgesics are ineffective. Moderate pain can usually be effectively managed with the use of intermediate-strength narcotic analgesics given orally. Meperidine (1.5 mg/kg/dose q 4 hr), oral oxycodone* (Percocet, $\frac{1}{2}$ to 3 tablets/dose q 4 hr), and oral hydromorphone† (Dilaudid, 0.04 mg/kg/dose q 4 hr) are commonly used for moderate pain. A maximum of 2–3 days' supply of narcotic analgesics should be dispensed, and daily contact should be maintained with the family during this period. Parenteral morphine (0.15 mg/kg/dose q 3–4 hr) or meperidine (1.5 mg/kg/dose q 2$\frac{1}{2}$–4 hr) is generally required for severe pain. Meperidine, while commonly used for severe pain, is associated with

an increased incidence of seizures and should be avoided in patients with renal or neurologic disease. Nonsteroidal anti-inflammatory drugs such as ibuprofen have a significant analgesic effect and may be helpful in some patients with chronic pain.

Inpatient Guidelines. Patients who require repeated parenteral doses of narcotics for pain relief should be admitted to the hospital. A hospital management plan should be developed by the patient's physician, written in the hospital record, and discussed with the patient and his or her family. Nurses should be encouraged to evaluate the patient's pain and record this information on a regular basis. Parenteral fluid should be administered, and fluid intake and urinary output should be monitored closely. Parenteral narcotics should be given at fixed intervals, not as needed. The medication treatment plan should be evaluated every 24 hours. When acute pain has diminished, the parenteral dose should be tapered, not the interval of administration. When the patient can tolerate a 50% decrease in the total parenteral dose, a switch to oral narcotics should be considered. These decisions should be made with the involvement of the patient and the nurses.

Adjunctive Therapy. Oxygen therapy is not of benefit in vaso-occlusive crises unless hypoxia is present. In the absence of hypoxia, oxygen therapy may induce reticulocytopenia. Sodium bicarbonate therapy does not improve the clinical course of painful crises and should be withheld unless acidosis exists. Diazepam and chlorpromazine do not potentiate the analgesic effects of narcotics and should be avoided. Behavior modification programs, relaxation therapy, self-hypnosis, and transcutaneous electric nerve stimulation may be helpful adjunctive therapies for selected patients. They do not, however, replace standard treatment methods.

HEMATOLOGIC CRISES

After early infancy, children with sickle cell anemia develop a chronic steady-state anemia with a hemoglobin usually between 6.5 and 8 gm/dl. Patients are usually asymptomatic as a consequence of the chronic hemolytic anemia, and transfusions are not required. However, life-threatening episodes of transient severe anemia may be superimposed upon the chronic hemolytic state. Most of these anemic events are due to either acute sequestration crises or aplastic crises.

The acute sequestration crisis generally occurs in infancy. It is the second most common cause of death in sickle cell anemia. This potentially life-threatening event is due to sudden intrasplenic pooling of massive amounts of blood, producing at times hypovolemia, shock, and severe anemia. This is a medical emergency requiring immediate treatment. Packed red blood cells (10 cc/kg) should

---

* Manufacturer's statement: Use in children is not recommended.

† Manufacturer's warning: Safety and effectiveness of hydromorphone in children have not been established.

be transfused as soon as possible. When indicated, plasma expanders can be given until red cells are available. If cardiorespiratory compromise exists, a partial exchange transfusion is the treatment of choice. Because of the repetitive nature of this life-threatening complication, splenectomy is recommended following a single severe sequestration crisis. Alternatively, a program of chronic transfusions can be employed in the very young. These transfusions will prevent future sequestration crises, but once the treatment is stopped, the risk of acute sequestration crisis returns.

The most common cause of a significant fall in the steady-state hemoglobin of a sickle cell disease patient is a transient reduction or cessation of erythropoiesis. This aplastic crisis is usually secondary to an intercurrent infection. Once the diagnosis is made, the patient's hemoglobin should be measured daily. If the hemoglobin falls to 5 gm/dl, or if cardiorespiratory distress develops, the patient should be transfused. In many cases, only a single packed red blood cell transfusion is required. If there is evidence of cardiorespiratory distress, a partial exhange transfusion should be performed.

INFECTION

Sickle cell disease patients have several immunodeficiencies that increase their risk of life-threatening bacterial infections. Infections due to *Streptococcus pneumoniae, Hemophilus influenzae, Neisseria meningitis, Mycoplasma pneumoniae, Staphylococcus aureus,* and *Salmonella* species are more common in these patients than in the general population. *Streptococcus pneumoniae* is the most common cause of death in the young child with sickle cell disease.

Prevention of Infection. The pneumococcal polysaccharide vaccine should be administered to all children with sickle cell disease. This vaccine is generally given to patients over 2 years of age because of the diminished antibody response in the younger child. However, there is no disadvantage to immunizing the patient at 1 year of age and again at 2 years of age. Booster immunizations should then be given every 4–5 years. Unfortunately, the vaccine is not completely effective, even for the strains included in the immunizations. Therefore, penicillin prophylaxis has been suggested for patients between 6 months and 3 years of age. While it has not yet been proved effective, prophylactic penicillin appears to be relatively safe. If one chooses to use prophylactic antibiotics, compliance must be closely monitored. Injectable penicillin (Bicillin, 600,000 U IM) monthly or oral penicillin (125 mg bid) can also be used.

Management of Fever. Fever in the young child with sickle cell disease should be considered a sign of sepsis until proved otherwise. All febrile patients under 5 years of age should be seen immediately and undergo a laboratory investigation. Antibiotics should be started before laboratory results are received. Most patients in this age group should be hospitalized until the initial cultures show no growth. The antibiotic initially given to the patient should be effective against pneumococcus as well as *Hemophilus influenzae.* Cephalosporins such as cefotaxime and cefuroxime are good choices. Mycoplasma pneumonia may cause severe problems in sickle cell disease patients. If suspected, erythromycin should be added to the treatment plan. Osteomyelitis, usually caused by *Staphylococcus aureus* or a *Salmonella* species, presents a diagnostic dilemma because it can be confused with bone infarct. In suspected cases, aggressive laboratory evaluation, including bacteriologic culture of bone aspirate, should be performed.

STROKES

Strokes occur in approximately 12% of patients with sickle cell anemia, and the recurrence rate is as high as 50%. Initial treatment should include close monitoring of the patient for development of increased intracranial pressure, seizures, and other progressive neurologic symptomatology. Partial exchange transfusion or a one-volume exchange transfusion should be done as soon as possible in order to lower the amount of hemoglobin S to 30% or less. Arteriography is usually not required and, if necessary, should be delayed until the exchange transfusion is completed. Following the initial transfusion, patients should be placed on a monthly transfusion regimen for a minimum of 3–5 years. The optimum duration of transfusion therapy is not known; periods longer than 3–5 years may be necessary. Patients should be started on iron chelation therapy with subcutaneous deferoxamine mesylate.

ACUTE CHEST SYNDROME

Acute chest syndrome is a common cause of morbidity and mortality in sickle cell disease patients. Except in very mild cases, all patients with acute chest syndrome should be admitted to the hospital. Analgesics, intravenous hydration, and antibiotics should be started. Oxygen is indicated when analysis of arterial blood gas demonstrates hypoxemia. Partial exchange transfusion should be considered if the PaO_2 is below 70 mm Hg.

PRIAPISM

Priapism occurs secondary to venous engorgement of the penis and is a common complication in male patients with sickle cell disease. This complication is extremely painful and can result in acute urinary retention, impotence, and serious psychological problems. Treatment should be given immediately, with intravenous hydration, adequate analgesia, and, if urinary output is compromised, insertion of a Foley catheter. An exchange transfusion to lower the percentage of sickle cells to 30% or less should be initiated. If there is no response within 24 hours following completion of transfusion therapy, surgical intervention may be necessary. A urologist should be consulted early in the clinical course. Follow-up counseling and evaluation for impotence are mandatory.

LEG ULCERS

After the age of 10 years, leg ulcers are increasingly common in patients with sickle cell disease. Initial treatment should include adequate nutrition. Zinc supplementation is viewed as important by some authorities. Carefully fitted shoes and supportive stockings are essential. The ulcer should be cleaned and debrided with wet to dry dressings frequently. Frequently it will heal with conservative treatment. If healing does not occur within a few months, an Unna boot should be added to this program. Patients with leg ulcers that remain recalcitrant after conservative therapy should be considered for a 6-month transfusion program. Occasionally skin grafting and long-term bedrest are necessary in order to heal a chronic ulcer completely.

CHOLELITHIASIS

Gallstones are found in at least 30% of children with sickle cell anemia. Patients who have gallstones can be asymptomatic or can have severe right upper quadrant pain, nausea, and vomiting. The treatment of the asymptomatic patient is controversial. Many physicians will not advise surgery unless the patient has characteristic abdominal pain. Some physicians recommend elective surgery on all patients because of the potential risk of severe acute cholecystitis. The most common approach to sickle cell patients with gallstones is to postpone elective surgery until the patient experiences significant right upper quadrant pain or chronic, vague abdominal symptoms. If acute cholecystitis occurs, it should be treated conservatively with antibiotics, hydration, and analgesia until the attack subsides. Elective cholecystectomy should be performed after the hemoglobin S has been brought below 30% and the patient is stable.

CONTRACEPTION AND PREGNANCY

Genetic counseling and information concerning contraception should be offered to all sexually active patients. Low-dose estrogen oral contraceptives are less desirable than barrier methods, but there is no evidence that sickle cell anemia patients are at greater risk for complications from oral contraceptives.

Pregnancy in women with sickle cell disease is associated with an increased risk to the mother and fetus. However, with close supervision and careful management, most women can have a successful pregnancy and a healthy baby. A pregnant sickle cell patient should be managed in a high-risk prenatal clinic. The role of transfusion therapy during pregnancy is controversial. When given, transfusions are usually begun in the third trimester.

Prenatal diagnosis of sickle cell disorders is readily available and should be offered to couples in conjunction with effective genetic counseling. Amniocentesis, if desired, should be performed in the first 17 weeks of gestation.

SURGERY

Surgery requiring general anesthesia in patients with sickle cell disease should be performed when the sickle hemoglobin is less than 30% and the hematocrit is between 30 and 35%. Minor surgery, without general anesthesia, does not require transfusion. For elective surgery, packed red cell transfusions may be given to maintain the hemoglobin at 11–12 gm/dl for 4 weeks prior to surgery. Higher hemoglobin counts may result in complications from hyperviscosity. For emergency surgery, a partial exchange transfusion is recommended. The preoperative administration of intravenous fluids to prevent dehydration is necessary. The patient should not be denied fluids by mouth as part of preoperative management unless intravenous fluids are being administered. Following surgery, careful attention is necessary to prevent hypoxemia, acidosis, and dehydration.

TRANSFUSIONS

As discussed, transfusions are used increasingly in the treatment of specific complications in sickle cell disease. This has resulted in an increased number of transfusion-related complications, such as transfusion reactions and alloimmunization. Certain steps can be taken to minimize these side effects. Washed packed red cells should be used in frequently transfused patients in order to decrease allergic transfusion reactions. All patients with a prior history of transfusion should be screened for alloantibodies. If a patient is to be repeatedly transfused, he or she should first have complete typing for common antigens and be transfused with blood that is matched for the major blood groups. In addition, the patient should carry a card identifying his or her red cell genotype and identified antibodies. Finally, the patient should be transfused only when absolutely necessary.

Leukopenia, Neutropenia, and Agranulocytosis

PHILIP A. PIZZO, M.D.

Children with low white blood cell counts share in common an increased risk of serious infection. The incidence of these infections is directly related to the depth and duration of the neutropenia and inversely related to the degree of preservation of other phagocytic host defenses. Neutropenias may be transient (such as those associated with drug-induced bone marrow suppression, viral infections, or immune medicated events) or prolonged in duration (such as those associated with congenital deficiencies of myelopoiesis or acquired bone marrow failure states). Less frequently, neutropenias can be cyclic and intermittent.

One of the major difficulties in the management of the neutropenic patient is the inability to distinguish a fever that portends a potentially life-threatening infection from a less serious complication. In our prospective assessment of 300 neutropenic children who developed fever, we were unable to ascertain any clinical or laboratory parameters that could distinguish a patient with a bacteremia from one whose cultures were entirely negative. Thus, when faced with a neutropenic child who has become febrile, a potentially life-threatening infection must be assumed until proved otherwise. For this reason, children with a neutrophil count of less than 500/mm³ who become febrile (we have defined fever as a single oral temperature elevation above 38.5°C or three oral temperatures above 38.0°C during a 24-hour period) require admission to the hospital for examination, a chest x-ray, urinalysis, cultures of throat and urine, and at least two preantibiotic blood cultures. The initial evaluation should be performed promptly and expeditiously, and as soon as possible after its completion (ideally with 2–3 hours after the onset of fever) the patient should be started on an empiric antimicrobial regimen.

The goal of empiric antibiotic therapy is to prevent rapid clinical deterioration and early mortality related to an undiagnosed and untreated bacterial infection. Because both gram-positive and gram-negative bacteria can cause such infections, it is imperative that the empiric antimicrobial regimen instituted effectively cover the predominant potential pathogens at a particular institution. In approximatley 10% of cases, bacteremias may be polymicrobial, which further underscores the need for effective broad-spectrum coverage. Indeed, perhaps more than any other aspect of managment, the practice of promptly instituting empiric broad-spectrum antimicrobial coverage when the granulocytopenic patient becomes febrile has accounted for a significant reduction in the incidence of fatal infectious complications. Until recently, it has been possible to achieve such broad-spectrum coverage only by the use of combination antimicrobial therapy. In most centers, this has included the combination of a first-generation cephalosporin or an antistaphylococcal penicillin with an aminoglycoside or an antipseudomonal carboxypenicillin. A variety of two- and three-drug combinations have been effectively utilized, and since no particular regimen has shown itself to be singularly effective, the choice of agents should be based upon the pattern of infection observed at a given treatment center. When an aminoglycoside is included in the drug regimen, it is imperative that serum levels be monitored within 24 hours after the start of therapy and then serially to assure that effective drug levels are being obtained and that potential oto- and nephrotoxicity is minimized.

During the last several years, a number of new beta-lactam antibiotics have been introduced, particularly the third-generation cephalosporins and the ureido- and piperazine penicillins. The third-generation cephalosporins are unique in having a very broad spectrum of activity that in some cases includes not only the enterobacteriaceae but also *Pseudomonas aeruginosa*, gram-positive isolates, and anaerobes. The extended-spectrum penicillins offer increased effectiveness against *P. aeruginosa*, *Klebsiella* sp., and a variety of anaerobes. The role that these new antibiotics will play in the granulocytopenic patient is still not fully defined. While a variety of combinations have already been introduced into the clinic, it remains to be established whether these agents, when used in combination, offer a significant advantage over more standard and less expensive combinations of antibiotics. On the other hand, the unique spectrum of some of the third-generation cephalosporins and carbapenems raises the possibility that one of these drugs might be used as monotherapy for the initial empiric managment of the febrile neutropenic patient. Studies addressing this possibility are in progress, but definitive results are not yet available.

It is also notable that the changing pattern of infection has led to the reintroduction of an older antibiotic, vancomycin. This drug is particularly effective in the treatment of infections by coagulase-negative staphylococci, methicillin-resistant *Staphylococcus aureus*, and the multiply resistant JK-corynebacteria. Indeed, vancomycin is increasingly used in centers where indwelling intravenous catheters are employed, and it should be considered for patients with indwelling catheters who develop new fevers.

MANAGEMENT OF NEUTROPENIC PATIENTS WITH DEFINED SITES OF INFECTION

Following the initial evaluation and institution of empiric antibiotic therapy, clinical and microbiological findings that clarify the etiology of the child's fever may become available. Under any circumstance, it is imperative that each patient be examined daily until the resolution of the granulocytopenic episode, since both evolving infections and the emergence of second or superinfections are not infrequent. Additions to or modifications of the initial empiric regimen are frequently necessary, particularly in patients who remain neutropenic for protracted periods. Some examples are considered in the following paragraphs.

Bacteremia. Positive blood cultures are surprisingly infrequent in the granulocytopenic patient with cancer, accounting for only 10–20% of the infectious complications. This low incidence may reflect the fact that patients are evaluated and treated early (the improved survival of these patients justifies this approach to managment). When the initial preantibiotic blood cultures are positive, it may be necessary to modify the antimicrobial regimen. When coagulase-negative staphylococci are isolated, the addition of vancomycin (40 mg/kg/day in 4 divided doses) is usually necessary, since these organisms are frequently resistant to beta-lactam antibiotics. While it has usually been felt to be necessary to remove a foreign body when a site of infection has been defined, nearly 90% of catheter-associated bacteremias (particularly with *Staphylococcus epidermidis*) can be effectively treated with antibiotics alone, without catheter removal. However, if the patient remains bacteremic after 48 hours of appropriate therapy, or if the infection recurs when the antibiotic course is completed (generally 10–14 days), catheter removal is necessary.

Another question that commonly arises when a gram-positive organism has been isolated is whether the spectrum of the antimicrobial regimen can be narrowed to control the pathogen specifically. Our results from a retrospective analysis suggested that patients remaining neutropenic for longer than a week had an increased risk of developing a subsequent infection with gram-negative bacteria when they were treated with a narrow-spectrum antibiotic (e.g., oxacillin, nafcillin). In our current prospective study, however, it appears that a narrow spectrum of therapy can be effective as long as the clinician is cognizant that second infections or superinfections might arise during the course of treatment.

The current standard of practice for treating gram-negative bacillary infections in granulocytopenic patients is to utilize a two-drug combination.

When such therapy is instituted early, current data suggest that nearly 90% of granulocytopenic patients will survive the episode. The duration of therapy is generally 10–14 days. However, if the patient remains neutropenic when treatment is completed (even though all sites of infection have cleared), recurrent infection may occur and the patient should be appropriately monitored. Should a residual focus of infection remain in the neutropenic patient, even at the completion of a standard 14-day trial of therapy, antibiotics should be continued until either the resolution of the granulocytopenia or the disappearance of all signs of infection.

In addition to antibiotics, adjunctive therapies are frequently considered in the neutropenic patient who has a positive blood culture. Foremost among these have been white blood cell transfusions. While this mode of therapy was popularly employed during the mid-1970's, current data suggest that leukocyte transfusions are largely ineffective in the supportive management of granulocytopenic patients, even when patients have a documented gram-negative bacteremia. Most probably this reflects the inability to transfuse adequate numbers of qualitatively normal neutrophils to overcome the quantitative impairment. At present, leukocyte transfusions seem best restricted to neonates with sepsis and, perhaps, to patients with chronic granulomatous disease. As an alternative to cell component therapy, recent consideration has been given to antibody replacement by passive immunization. Observations have suggested that patients receiving cytotoxic therapy may have decreased titers of antibody to the core glycolipid of the enterobacteriaceae. Recent studies have shown that the passive infusion of antisera with increased core glycolipid titers (so-called J5 antisera) may decrease mortality in patients with proven or putative sepsis. This is an area warranting further investigation.

Head and Neck Infections. The oral cavity is a frequent site of primary or secondary infection in the neutropenic patient. Aphthous ulcers frequently occur when the neutrophil count is lowered (e.g., in cyclic neutropenia). Drug-induced stomatotoxicity can result in ulcerations that become secondarily infected by endogenous oral bacteria, thus providing a nidus for local infection and a portal to systemic invasion. We have observed that approximately 20% of patients who receive antibiotics while neutropenic develop a marginal gingivitis characterized by a red periapical line of gingival necrosis. The addition of a specific antianaerobic antibiotic (e.g., clindamycin, 30 mg/kg/day in four divided doses) has appeared to improve this process and can result in the defervescence of the patient who had been febrile on standard antibiotic therapy.

Infection of the oral cavity with *Candida* sp. is common and is characterized by the presence of white mucosal plaques. The diagnosis can be confirmed by scraping and examining the material under wet mount for pseudohyphae and budding yeasts or by culture. Although many centers routinely utilize nystatin for both prophylaxis and therapy, our experience has been that this agent is relatively ineffective. Alternatively, clotrimazole oral troches can be effective. Ketoconazole has been shown to be effective for the oral thrush that occurs in patients with AIDS, but we have found that children with oral mucositis frequently have difficulty in swallowing the tablets. If the mucositis due to *Candida* becomes particularly severe, a short course of intravenous amphotericin B (0.1–0.5 mg/kg/day for 5 days) has the highest likelihood of success.

Gingivostomatitis can also be the result of infection with *Herpes simplex*, and a severe necrotizing mucositis may ensue. This infection can be treated with either parenteral acyclovir (750 mg/m^2/day in three divided doses) or vidarabine. In particularly high-risk groups (patients undergoing intensive chemotherapy or bone marrow transplantation), prophylactic administration of acyclovir may prevent herpetic gingivostomatitis.

While sinus infection in the neutropenic child might be due to aerobic or anaerobic bacteria, consideration should be given to the possibility that the process might be fungal (particularly *Aspergillus* or *Mucor*). Fungal sinusitis may result in the rhinocerebral syndrome with subsequent invasion of the cranial vault. Diagnosis requires histologic demonstration of invading hyphae, and treatment includes both surgical débridement and parenteral amphotericin B (0.5 mg/kg/day). These infections may require protracted courses of amphotericin, usually over 2 or more months. Patients developing the rhinocerebral syndrome should also be carefully monitored for the development of pulmonary aspergillosis, which worsens the clinical outlook.

It is also important to note that middle ear infections in the neutropenic child may be due to gram-negative bacteria as well as to the usual respiratory pathogens. Hence, we institute broad-spectrum antibiotic therapy for neutropenic children who develop otitis media, particularly if a specific diagnosis cannot be made by tympanocentesis.

Respiratory Tract Infections. The lung is the single most common site of infection in the granulocytopenic patient. Presumably, the majority of these infections are the result of aspiration, although they may also occur as part of a hematogenous infection. Indeed, when a gram-negative bacteremia occurs in concert with a pneumonitis, the prognosis is particularly ominous. It should be underscored that the usual signs and symptoms and even the radiographic manifestations of pneumonia may be muted in the granulocytopenic patient. It is, therefore, imperative to monitor serially and even to repeat chest radiographs in neutropenic patients who have persistent fever, since an infiltrate may not be apparent at the time of initial evaluation but may become evident later in the treatment course. A particular difficulty posed by pulmonary infections is their general inaccessibility to direct microbiological evaluation. Sputum is not a reliable diagnostic specimen and is rarely produced in children anyway. Because these patients are not infrequently thrombocytopenic as well, the performance of more direct diagnostic procedures is often fraught with danger.

For the child who presents with a localized pneumonic process and who is febrile and neutropenic, gram-negative pneumonia must be assumed although gram-positve bacteria, legionellae, mycoplasmas, viruses, and even drugs must also be considered. Our general policy is to start the neutropenic patient who has a localized pulmonary infiltrate on broad-spectrum antibiotics, following standard preantibiotic evaluation as outlined earlier. The patient is carefully monitored, and if improvement is observed within 48–72 hours after the initiation of antibiotics, a full course of therapy (at least 2 weeks) is administered. If, however, the patient has failed to improve or is deteriorating after an adequate 48–72 hour antibiotic trial, attempts to make a more specific diagnosis by bronchoscopy or open lung biopsy are then pursued.

Another perplexing problem is the finding of a new pulmonary infiltrate in the patient already on antibiotics. This is not an uncommon problem, since nearly one-third of all the pulmonary infiltrates we have observed in pediatric granulocytopenic patients during the last 10 years have occurred in this setting. In a recent analysis of this problem, we observed that when the infiltrate occurred together with a rise in the patient's granulocyte count, the outcome was nearly always favorable and the infiltrate probably reflected the "lighting up" of a prior site of infection by the recovering neutrophils. However, when the infiltrate occurred in a patient who was persistently granulocytopenic, and particularly when it progressed over 2–3 days, the most likely diagnosis was a fungal pneumonia (particularly *Aspergillus* or *Candida*). Ideally, it is preferable to establish a microbiological diagnosis in these patients so that the need for and duration of antifungal therapy can be clearly delineated. However, if the patient's clinical course prohibits the performance of an appropriate diagnostic procedure (such as an open lung biopsy), empiric antifungal therapy with amphotericin B should be promptly instituted.

Diffuse interstitial infiltrates are not unique to the granulocytopenic patient. When they occur in patients receiving immunosuppressive therapy, (particularly steroids), *Pneumocystis carinii* pneumonia should be considered. However, bacteria, fungi, and viruses can also present as interstitial infiltrates, raising the question of how aggressively the diagnosis should be pursued. Numerous investigations suggest that the open lung biopsy is the most reliable diagnostic technique, although not without hazard in the patient who is neutropenic and thrombocytopenic. Recent experience with bronchoalveolar lavage suggests that this procedure may have a role in the diagnostic repertoire, but futher evaluation is clearly necessary. Alternatively, a trial of antimicrobial therapy might be adequate. We observed in a recent randomized trial that empiric antibiotic therapy with trimethoprim-sulfamethoxazole and erythromycin was an effective alternative to an invasive diagnostic procedure in nonneutropenic cancer patients with diffuse pulmonary infiltrates, although improvement may not be observed for 4–5 days. It is not yet established whether similar recommendations can be drawn for neutropenic patients, but if empiric antimicrobial therapy is to be utilized in the neutropenic patient with diffuse infiltrates, it is important to include broad-spectrum antibiotics in addition to coverage for *Pneumocystis* and *Legionella*. Moreover, if the patient was already on antibiotic therapy at the time of onset of the pulmonary lesions, the addition of antifungal therapy appears warranted.

Cardiovascular Infections. Primary or secondary cardiovascular infections are surprisingly infrequent in the neutropenic child. While endocarditis has been described with gram-negative as well as gram-positive bacteria and fungi, this is a rare complication, even in patients who have had bacteremias and fungemias. Thus, unless there is evidence of persistent bacteremia in the patient on antibiotic therapy, we do not recommend protracted courses of antibiotics. Myocardial abscesses can occur with bacteria as well as fungi, and myocarditis may be a manifestation of toxoplasmosis in the compromised host.

Gastrointestinal Infections. The onset of retrosternal burning pain aggravated by swallowing in the patient who is already receiving broadspectrum antibiotics suggests the presence of esophagitis. While esophagitis can rarely be due to bacteria, it is more likely the result of infection with *Candida* or *Herpes simplex*. Since esophagoscopy can be associated with bleeding or a bacteremia in neutropenic patients, we prefer to establish a tentative diagnosis by looking for cobblestoning

with a barium swallow. If evident, we initiate either oral clotrimazole or a short course of amphotericin B, with the expectation that if the process is due to *Candida* sp. symptomatic improvement should be observed within 48 hours. If improvement does not occur, the addition of acyclovir or esophagoscopy and biopsy should be considered.

While the gastrointestinal tract is a major reservoir of potential pathogens, primary gastrointestinal sites of infection are less common in neutropenic patients. A syndrome worthy of note is typhlitis. Patients generally present with right lower quadrant abdominal pain and rebound, mimicking an acute abdomen or a perforated appendicitis. Patients are usually already receiving broad-spectrum antibiotics. Although it is possible that some patients may be treated with supportive care alone, several reports suggest that surgical intervention and removal of the necrotic cecum is essential for effective control.

Diarrhea in the neutropenic patient, particularly when there has been exposure to antibiotics or chemotherapeutic agents, may be due to *Clostridium difficile*. The diagnosis can be established by examining the stool for cytotoxins. The presence of toxin-associated diarrhea warrants the initiation of either oral vancomycin or metronidazole.

Hepatitis due to type B virus has decreased in recent years, but infection with non-A, non-B virus continues to be a problem for patients receiving cytotoxic therapy and blood transfusions. Using abdominal computed tomography scanning or ultracenography, we have recently observed a series of neutropenic patients who developed "bull's-eye" lesions in their livers; these have been shown by biopsy to be due to hepatic candidiasis. This process has required protracted courses of amphotericin B therapy. Indeed, our most recent experience suggests that the best response is likely to occur with the combination of amphotericin B and 5-fluorocytosine.

The incidence of perianal cellulitis in neutropenic patients has decreased during the last decade, perhaps because of the more aggressive and earlier used of antibiotics in these patients. While it is commonly assumed that the major cause of perianal cellulitis is gram-negative bacilli, our recent review of patients treated at the National Cancer Institute suggests that mixed infections (i.e., gram-negative rods and anaerobes) are most common. Whether patients developing evidence of perianal cellulitis should be managed conservatively or treated with surgical debridement remains controversial. We have observed that the early addition of a specific antianaerobic antibiotic (e.g., clindamycin or metronidazole) to standard gram-negative coverage when the patient first begins complaining of perianal tenderness may avoid the need for an invasive surgical procedure.

Genitourinary Tract. Except in patients with primary genitourinary malignancies or those who have indwelling catheters, infections of the genitourinary tract are infrequent, even in neutropenic cancer patients.

Rarely, the syndrome of bladder thrush may occur, hallmarked by the presence of *Candida* in urine cultures and cytoscopic evidence of superficial invasion. Treatment of this process generally requires the instillation of amphotericin B into the bladder on a daily basis.

Central Nervous System Infections. Surprisingly, bacterial meningitis remains uncommon in the neutropenic patient, even in patients with bacteremia. When evidence of meningitis is present, particularly in children with leukemia, careful examination of the cerebrospinal fluid for gram-positve rods should be made, since *Listeria monocytogenes* can be a noteworthy pathogen in this patient population.

UNEXPLAINED FEVER IN NEUTROPENIC PATIENTS

Nearly half the children who present with fever and neutropenia fail to have a clinically or microbiologically defined site of infection. Nonetheless, it is probable that many of these children have an occult site of infection and that the diagnosis has simply been masked by the early institution of empiric antimicrobial therapy. In the absence of overt infection, however, the duration of antibiotic treatment can be a real problem. We have found that patients can be stratified into low- and high-risk groups. Low-risk patients with unexplained fever have periods of neutropenia lasting a week or less. When the antibiotics are continued in these patients until the resolution of granulocytopenia and then are stopped, the patients appear to do quite well. On the other hand, high-risk patients have neutropenia for longer than a week. Stopping antibiotics in these patients while they remain neutropenic, particularly if they are also still febrile, appears to be associated with recrudescent infection and in some cases with clinical deterioration. Our studies suggest that patients with prolonged granulocytopenia who defervesce after the initiation of empiric antibiotic therapy should be treated for 2 weeks unless the granulocytopenia resolves before then. While stopping antibiotics at 2 weeks in the persistently neutropenic patient is still associated with recurrent fever in one-third of patients, careful and expectant observation can usually prevent serious sequelae. However, stopping antibiotics in patients who are persistently febrile and neutropenic is associated with serious sequelae in more than half. Simply continuing antibiotics alone is not a solution, since many of these patients develop evidence of invasive fungal disease. Therefore, our recommendation for pa-

tients with persistent fever and neutropenia is that they be continued on broad-spectrum antibiotics and that an antifungal agent be added until the eventual resolution of the granulocytopenia.

While these cases are challenging, it is clear that a high degree of success can be achieved in the management of infectious complications in granulocytopenic patients if treatment is started early and appropriate additions to and modifications of therapy are carefully employed.

Pediatric Hemostasis

ERIK L. YEO, M.D., *and* BRUCE FURIE, M.D.

Approach to Bleeding Disorders

Hemostasis is a host defense mechanism that requires a complex interaction between platelets, coagulation factors, and endothelial cells. Congenital or acquired abnormalities of these components can lead to minor bleeding tendencies or potentially life-threatening bleeding. The diagnosis of hemostatic disorders rests upon a thoughtful history and physical examination and ultimately depends upon laboratory testing to establish the nature of the defect. Treatment strategies are based upon the correction of the hemostatic abnormality.

The history should focus upon the type of bleeding: petechiae, ecchymoses, purpura; its anatomic sites; and its temporal relationship to an inciting event. The family history is especially important for determining sex-linked or dominant or recessive autosomal inheritance. The exposure to drugs or other therapies (e.g., aspirin, immunizations, or transfusions) or certain diseases (e.g., liver disease, leukemia, or infections) must be established. The best assessors of hemostatic function are not laboratory tests but hemostatic challenges, such as tooth extraction, circumcision, the cutting of the umbilical cord and major surgical procedures. These events should be carefully reviewed with consideration to any inappropriate bleeding above that expected, particularly if the surgical challenge led to a transfusion requirement. Conversely, the absence of bleeding after such a surgical challenge argues against a hereditary bleeding tendency.

Physical examination may give a clue as to the type of hemostatic defect. Petechiae, purpura, and mucosal bleeding from the gums, gastrointestinal tract, or bladder suggests a platelet defect or von Willebrand's disease. Bleeding characterized by hematomas and hemarthroses is more often associated with coagulation abnormalities. These problems occur with increasing frequency in children after the age of one, corresponding to a period of increased mobility and spontaneous minor trauma.

Laboratory Screening. The initial event in hemostasis is the formation of a platelet plug. The ability to form a platelet plug is assessed with a bleeding time and platelet count. Coagulation abnormalities are screened with the prothrombin time, partial thromboplastin time (PTT), thrombin time, and fibrinogen level. Additional tests and specific factor assays are available for a precise diagnosis. An abnormality with factor XIII will be missed with these studies and requires a specific clot solubility test. Similarly, alpha 2-anti-plasmin deficiency can be diagnosed only by measuring this protein directly. In spite of a negative laboratory *screen*, if the history is highly suggestive of a bleeding disorder, further intensive studies may well reveal a functional abnormality.

Platelet Abnormalities

Platelet defects may be qualitative (thrombocytopathy) or quantitative (thrombocytopenia) and are screened with a properly executed bleeding time, a platelet count, and review of blood smear.

The bleeding time, normally between about 3 to 9 min, is performed with a template device on the inner aspect of the forearm, longitudinally, with a blood pressure cuff at 30 mm Hg. This test is the single most reliable overall assessment of platelet contribution to hemostasis, but it is notoriously inconsistent in predicting which patients are at risk of bleeding at surgery. The bleeding time is also a measure of vascular integrity. Below a platelet count of 100,000/µl of functionally normal platelets, the bleeding time becomes proportionally prolonged in a linear fashion. If disproportionately prolonged, the bleeding time suggests a qualitative platelet abnormality.

Thrombocytopenia, defined as a platelet count of less than 150,000/µl, is the most common cause of bleeding. However, significant bleeding rarely occurs with a platelet count above 50,000. While a platelet estimate is possible from review of the blood smear, the platelet count should be determined directly. The blood smear is reviewed both to confirm this value and to look for helpful clues from the other blood elements as to the etiology of the thrombocytopenia.

A bone marrow biopsy and aspirate are necessary to differentiate these processes and to assess the marrow response to thrombocytopenia. A normal response of megakaryocytes to thrombocytopenia is to increase their numbers and size and release immature, larger platelets into the peripheral blood. Failure of this compensatory increase in megakaryocytes reflects ineffective thrombopoiesis. A primary marrow process such as infiltration, aplastic anemia, or leukemia can be determined only with a bone marrow biopsy.

Platelet antibody testing, while helpful if positive, is not always reliable for the diagnosis of immune thrombocytopenia. Assessment of drug-induced platelet destruction using such methods may be equally misleading.

Both hereditary and acquired qualitative platelet abnormalities, or thrombocytopathies, are defined by a prolonged bleeding time out of proportion to the platelet count. Acquired platelet disorders are most often associated with aspirin ingestion. Thrombocytopathies are further defined with more specific platelet function tests to establish a diagnosis.

Coagulation Abnormalities

The partial thromboplastin time (PTT) assesses the intrinsic pathway, including factor XII, prekallikrein, high molecular weight kininogen, factor XI, factor IX, and factor VIII, and the final common pathway, including factor X, factor V, prothrombin, and fibrinogen. A significant decrease in activity in one of these clotting factors will prolong the PTT compared to normal plasma. Mixing studies, in which the patient's plasma is mixed with normal plasma, will differentiate between a clotting factor deficiency and a circulating inhibitor of blood coagulation.

The prothrombin time is a measure of the extrinsic pathway, including factor VII, factor X, factor V, prothrombin, and fibrinogen. This assay is a sensitive measure of liver synthesis of the vitamin K–dependent blood clotting factors (prothrombin, factor VII, factor IX, factor X, protein S, and protein C) and will be prolonged in liver disease or vitamin K deficiency.

The thrombin time is a functional test of the conversion of fibrinogen to fibrin. It is prolonged with hypofibrinogenemia, dysfibrinogenemia, elevated fibrin(ogen) degradation products, and heparin. Levels of fibrinogen below 100 mg/dl may limit fibrin formation. Fibrin degradation products are elevated in liver disease and disseminated intravascular coagulation and in conjunction with fibrinolytic therapy.

Factor XIII is involved in polymerization and stabilization of the fibrin clot and is not assessed by the prothrombin time, PTT, or thrombin time. A clot solubility assay will result in solubilization of the clot in a factor XIII–deficient state.

Specific assays are available for each of the clotting factors, which are measured functionally by their coagulant activity.

Quantitative Platelet Disorders

Thrombocytopenia. Thrombocytopenia, the most common cause of bleeding, is due to decreased platelet production or destruction. The clinical approach to the diagnosis of thrombocytopenia includes a history, physical examination, platelet count, review of the blood smear, and coagulation tests. A bone marrow examination may prove necessary. The clinical presentation for severe thrombocytopenia includes petechiae, ecchymosis in sites of trauma, and mucosal bleeding, especially from the gums, nose, GI tract, and bladder. Stools should be checked for occult blood. Special note of the size and number of platelets on the peripheral blood smear should be made to confirm the automated platelet count.

A bone marrow biopsy and aspirate will assess the adequacy of the marrow response to the thrombocytopenia and will demonstrate whether or not a primary marrow process is the cause. In some circumstances, a trial transfusion of platelet concentrates, with subsequent platelet count determinations, will help to differentiate between peripheral destruction and ineffective production. The platelet count will rapidly fall within 1 or 2 hours if peripheral destruction is responsible for the thrombocytopenia. If there is simply ineffective production, the half-life of transfused platelets should be normal.

Pseudothrombocytopenia is a laboratory artefact due to the clumping of platelets in the presence of certain anticoagulants. This consideration may be eliminated by visualizing the blood smear and identifying giant platelets or aggregates before an extensive evaluation.

Disorders of Platelet Production. The disorders of ineffective platelet production include May Hegglin anomaly, Wiskott-Aldrich syndrome, a group of rare autosomal dominant syndromes, and vitamin B_{12} or folate deficiency. Thrombocytopenia may also be caused by absent or decreased megakaryocytes. In this group of hereditary or acquired disorders the bone marrow biopsy may be hypocellular, as in aplastic anemias, or hypercellular, as in leukemia or other infiltrating disorders. Congenital megakaryocytic hypoplasia is associated with Fanconi's syndrome, thrombocytopenia with absent radii (TAR), macrothrombocytopenia, congenital intrauterine rubella, and maternal ingestion of thiazides.

Aplastic Anemia. Aplastic anemia is a broad category of acquired disorders of marrow hypoplasia involving any or all of the cell lines in the bone marrow. It is seen with drugs (chloramphenicol, chemotherapy, and benzene), radiation, toxins, infections (hepatitis and other viruses), but it often occurs without obvious cause. In severe cases (granulocytes less than 500, platelets less than 20,0000 and reticulocytes less than 0.2%), it has a mortality rate of 80%. Patients with aplasia secondary to hepatitis (non-A, non-B) have a particularly grave prognosis, with the 1-year mortality rate approaching 90%. Bone marrow transplantation with a histocompatible sibling donor is the best form of treatment for severe cases, with a high engraftment rate and up to 75% survival at 2 years. Both chemotherapy and radiation therapy cause a predictable dose-dependent myelosuppression associated with thrombocytopenia. Blood component transfusions, including platelets, may be necessary to support these individuals through their nadir. Paroxysmal nocturnal hemoglobinuria, a rare disorder of a primary stem cell defect, may present with aplastic anemia or thrombocytopenia. Treatment of the thrombocytopenia in aplastic anemia involves platelet transfusions during periods of bleeding while waiting for either bone marrow recovery or a suitable transplant donor.

PLATELET TRANSFUSIONS. Most patients with the disorders reviewed above require platelet transfusion therapy. Platelets are harvested from a single unit of whole blood or by plateletpheresis. The platelets are concentrated in 50 cc of plasma and have a shelf life of 72 hours at room temperature. This shelf life has been extended to 5 days with newer methods of storage. With transfusions of ABO cross-matched random donor platelets one expects an incremental rise of the platelet count in the recipient of about 5,000–10,000 platelets/μl/unit. In the neonate, 10 ml of platelet concentrate per kg body weight is recommended. The platelet response is decreased in individuals with sepsis or fever. Platelet counts performed at 1, 12, and 24 hours allow a calculation of the survival of the transfused platelets and thus an approximation of subsequent needs. Surgical procedures can be carried out with a platelet count above 50,000/μl but optimally the platelet count should be above 80,000/μl. Preoperatively the bleeding time needs to be corrected with infusions of platelet concentrates to ensure adequate hemostasis. The platelet count must be followed closely postoperatively. If bleeding persists, a laboratory evaluation of hemostasis is indicated; this evaluation should include a bleeding time. If these studies are normal, a search for an anatomic bleeding site must be undertaken. Alloimmunization causes patients to become refractory to platelet transfusion. This problem routinely occurs within 2–6 weeks; a change to HLA-matched platelets will delay this phenomena. HLA-matched platelets are expensive and difficult to obtain. Furthermore, subsequent sensitization to HLA-matched platelets will decrease the chances of engraftment if transplantation is performed.

A controversial question is whether to transfuse platelets prophylactically or whether to use platelets only when bleeding occurs. Prophylactic transfusions are commonly given at or below 20,000 platelets/μl, when spontaneous hemorrhages become increasingly frequent. Prophylactic transfusions are recommended during periods of high risk for bleeding, particularly when severe thrombocytopenia is expected to occur over a short period.

Immune Thrombocytopenic Purpura. Immune

thrombocytopenic purpura (ITP) presents with the abrupt onset of petechiae, ecchymosis, and mucosal or major bleeding. It is often preceded by a viral illness. The thrombocytopenia is due to antiplatelet antibodies. The peripheral blood smear reveals sparse but large platelets, often in association with atypical lymphocytes and mild eosinophilia. The bone marrow reveals an increase in size and number of megakaryocytes with budding evident. A test for anti-platelet antibodies may be positive. The prognosis is excellent, with 55% having a normal platelet count at 4 weeks and 85% having one at 4 months. The spontaneous remission rate is high, leading to the controversy over the need for any therapy.

The risk of bleeding is greatest in the first few days to weeks of ITP. Depending upon the platelet count, the patient may be advised to curtail certain activities. Under no circumstances should patients with ITP take aspirin or any other nonsteroidal anti-inflammatory drug. These agents have an antiplatelet effect. The consideration to treat should be based not on the platelet count but on clinical grounds. If there are significant hemorrhagic manifestations, e.g., fundal bleed, GI bleeding, persistent hematuria, or massive ecchymosis, corticosteroids at 2 mg/kg/day should be used. The intent should be a short course of therapy, approximately 2–4 weeks in duration, with rapid tapering of steroids to avoid any morbidity associated with long-term therapy. Alternatively, IV gamma globulin in doses to raise the gamma globulin level to approximately twice normal has been successful, but its action is unpredictable. The onset of the gamma globulin effect is 3–6 days, and the effect is transient, lasting approximately 3 weeks. Azathioprine, an immunosuppressant agent widely used to treat ITP in older adults, has no place in the treatment of ITP in the pediatric age group. Similarly, there is no role for vincristine or vinblastine therapy in children. Danazol, an anabolic steroid with minimal masculinizing side effects, may have a role in the treatment of ITP but should be reserved for refractory cases and is considered an experimental agent.

In the event of rare CNS hemorrhage or other major uncontrolled bleeding, the platelet count must be raised as quickly as possible. An emergency splenectomy should be performed and, simultaneously, platelet transfusions and corticosteroids administered.

An elective splenectomy should be performed if the patient fails to respond to steroid therapy or if the maintenance of a suitable platelet count requires chronic steroid therapy. Prior to splenectomy, a pneumococcal and meningococcal immunization should be given. High-dose corticosteroids may be reinstituted for one month prior to surgery to optimize the platelet count at the time of the splenectomy. Platelet transfusions may be needed at the time of surgery if the platelet count is less than 20,000/µl or if there is intraoperative bleeding. Postoperatively, chronic prophylactic antibiotics (penicillin 250 mg PO daily) are required in the under 10 to 12 age range to minimize the risk of asplenic sepsis from pneumococcal or meningococcal infections. A response in 80% of patients is seen within 1 week. Two thirds of patients enter complete remission.

Splenectomized patients exist in a compensated state of ITP. Although the platelet count is normal or near normal, it may temporarily fall with a recurrent viral illness. If a relapse becomes chronic, an accessory spleen or splenosis must be ruled out with a liver-spleen scan. If either are present, the spleen or implants of splenic tissue must be removed surgically.

Secondary autoimmune thrombocytopenia occurs in lymphoreticular malignancies and autoimmune diseases such as systemic lupus erythematosus. The clinical picture of secondary immune thrombocytopenia is like that of chronic ITP but will remit with treatment of the underlying disease.

Drug-induced thrombocytopenia (heparin, gold, and sulfonamides) is suspected by the temporal association of thrombocytopenia and drug administration. The platelet count will return to normal with discontinuation of the drug. Steroids have not been demonstrated to hasten the normalization of the platelet count but may improve hemostasis if bleeding does occur.

Neonatal Thrombocytopenia. There are two syndromes of neonatal thrombocytopenia: (a) neonatal ITP and (b) isoimmune neonatal purpura. Neonatal immune thrombocytopenic purpura is seen in 50% of mothers with chronic ITP and in 15% of mothers with ITP in complete remission. This syndrome is due to the transplacental transfer of IgG antiplatelet antibodies. The risk to the fetus occurs during birthing and is directly related to the degree of thrombocytopenia and obstetrical trauma. Spontaneous remission occurs in the neonate 2–4 weeks post partum. Steroids may be used if the platelet count takes a precipitous fall or is less than 75,000/µl. The best predictor of neonatal ITP is not the maternal platelet count but the maternal IgG antiplatelet antibody level. If present, a cesarean section will avoid fetal trauma and bleeding.

Isoimmune neonatal purpura is analogous to erythroblastosis fetalis and is due to the fetal inheritance of a minor platelet antigen that the mother lacks. Bleeding may occur immediately post partum, with the typical presentation of thrombocytopenia. If severe and symptomatic, steroid treatment and/or maternal platelet transfusions are necessary.

Platelet Consumption. These disorders of increased platelet consumption may be isolated occurrences, as in thrombotic thrombocytopenic purpura (TTP) or hemolytic-uremic syndrome (HUS), or may occur in concert with activation of the coagulation cascade. Disseminated intravascular coagulation causes thrombocytopenia secondary to the activation of the coagulation cascade and consumption of the clotting proteins and platelets.

Thrombotic thrombocytopenic purpura is characterized by thrombocytopenia, microangiopathic hemolytic anemia, fever, transient neurologic symptoms, and renal abnormalities. The laboratory findings often demonstrate a platelet count of less than 10,000/μl, microangiopathic hemolysis, and normal PTT and prothrombin time. Fresh frozen plasma and/or plasmapheresis are used in conjunction with high-dose corticosteroids and antiplatelet agents such as ASA* and dipyridamole.*

Hemolytic-uremic syndrome is clinically and pathologically similar to thrombotic thrombocytopenic purpura. The major difference between these two syndromes is the marked renal failure associated with hypertension that characterizes the hemolytic-uremic syndrome. The mainstays of treatment include early and vigorous hemodialysis, transfusions with platelets if clinically required, and antihypertensive therapy. High-dose corticosteroids and antiplatelet agents are used, but heparin has not been demonstrated to be of benefit.

QUALITATIVE PLATELET DISORDERS

Patients with prolonged bleeding times and normal platelet counts have either primary defects in their platelets or a plasma defect that impairs platelet function. These congenital or acquired syndromes of defective platelet function have been recognized with increased frequency.

Hereditary Disorders. Bernard-Soulier syndrome is characterized by giant platelets that lack the von Willebrand factor receptor and fail to adhere to exposed subendothelium. Glanzmann's thrombasthenia is characterized by platelets that lack the fibrinogen receptor; these platelets fail to aggregate. Hereditary storage pool diseases, including Gray platelet syndrome, lack various internal granules. In release disorders, the normal mechanisms of granule release are impaired. Ehlers-Danlos syndrome presents in a similar manner owing to defective collagen and vascular fragility but the platelets may also be abnormal. These disorders may be associated with significant hemorrhagic problems and are treated with platelet transfusions for surgical procedures and serious bleeding episodes.

Acquired Disorders. Drugs are the most common cause of thrombocytopathies. Aspirin exposure is frequently the cause of platelet abnormalities, but platelet defects are also seen with other

---

* This use is not listed in the manufacturer's directive.

nonsteroidal anti-inflammatory agents, antihistamines, major tranquilizers, and heparin. Aspirin causes a slight but significant prolongation of the bleeding time in normal individuals without causing any bleeding problems. In about 10% of otherwise normal individuals, the bleeding time becomes markedly prolonged. This effect is exaggerated in patients with coagulopathies or thrombocytopenia, sometimes causing spontaneous hemorrhages. Aspirin and similar drugs that have an effect on platelet function should be avoided in these individuals. The effects on platelet function of these drugs disappear after they are discontinued. However, the aspirin effect on platelets is irreversible and lasts for the lifetime of the exposed circulating platelets, which is approximately 7 days.

Uremia causes a functional platelet disorder that is related to the accumulation of metabolic products. The prolonged bleeding time will correct with renal transplantation and peritoneal dialysis and less well with hemodialysis.

Hereditary Coagulation Disorders. The hereditary coagulation disorders are characterized by bleeding tendencies after trauma or during surgery or, in their more severe form, by spontaneous bleeding. Since mild bleeding problems are not uncommon to normal growth and development in the pediatric age group, a major issue is to identify the small numbers of children with a significant bleeding tendency and to sort them from their otherwise normal peers. On history, the points that need to be clarified are extraordinary posttraumatic or postsurgical bleeding. If blood transfusions were required, special note should be taken. The age of onset and the presence of a bleeding defect in other family members are also of importance in the initial evaluation. A history of spontaneous bleeding into muscle, skin, the retroperitoneum, or joints is suggestive of severe to moderate hemophilia.

If the index of suspicion is high that a bleeding defect exists, screening laboratory tests should be performed. As a minimum, these tests should include a prothrombin time, PTT, bleeding time, and platelet count. Specific factor assays that allow quantitation of the deficient clotting protein must also be performed. Hemophiliacs are classified on the basis of both their factor levels and clinical symptoms as severe (<1% of normal factor level), moderate (1–5%) or mild (5–25%).

GENERAL CONSIDERATIONS. The treatment of patients with severe congenital coagulation abnormalities is difficult and complex. Hemophilia is associated with severe physical, economic, and psychological hardships. Care involves a comprehensive interdisciplinary approach involving the blood bank, hematologist, coagulation laboratory, orthopedic surgeon, dentist, specialized nurses, physiotherapists, and social workers. This type of care is best carried out in a center that has considerable experience with these patients. Pain control and drug dependence are a major area of morbidity for severe and moderate hemophiliacs. The use of nonacetylated salicylates is very helpful in these situations. These agents, choline magnesium trisalicylate (Trilisate) and salicylsalicyclic acid (Disalcid), while remaining analgesics and anti-inflammatory agents, do not have the antiplatelet effect of aspirin. While analgesics such as major narcotics are necessary at times, the long-term use of these drugs must be avoided.

Hemophilia. Classic hemophilia A is an X-linked functional defect of Factor VIII. Christmas disease or hemophilia B is an X-linked functional deficiency in Factor IX. Both of these conditions are characterized by a normal prothrombin time, a prolonged PTT, and a normal bleeding time. They are further delineated with specific assays of the clotting activity and antigen level of factors VIII and IX. Hemophilia A has a functional deficiency of factor VIII, with normal or elevated levels of Factor VIII/VWF antigen. Hemophilia B has both functional and immunologic deficiencies of factor IX. Hemophilia A must be distinguished from von Willebrand's disease, in which a deficiency of Factor VIII is associated with a prolonged bleeding time and impaired platelet agglutination with ristocetin.

The clinical presentations of Factor VIII and Factor IX deficiency are identical and vary with the severity of this disease. Mild to moderate deficiencies are symptomatic only with trauma or surgery, while severe cases have recurrent spontaneous bleeds. Both the levels and clinical severity of these diseases remain constant within families. Manifestations of hemophilia occur at about 1 year of age or earlier. Bleeding involves the joints, muscles, renal tract, GI tract and mouth; intracranial bleeding is one of the most serious complications of hemophilia.

Joint disease is the single most important cause of chronic morbidity. Hemarthroses often involve the knees, elbows, ankles, and wrists. A severe bleed can be aborted with an appropriate infusion of Factor VIII for hemophilia A or Factor IX for hemophilia B. Management involves analgesics, often narcotics such as morphine, infusion therapy to raise the deficient factor level to 30–50% for several days, and immobilization of the joint with splints. In less severe bleeds, joint mobility is maintained and immobilization is avoided. Minor bleeds usually respond in 2 or 3 days. Hospitalization may be required with severe bleeds or failed outpatient therapy.

Chronic joint disease, the outcome of recurrent acute hemarthrosis in severe and moderate hemophiliacs, is characterized by flexion contractures, muscle atrophy, and joint abnormalities, the last of which is often complicated by recurrent small bleeds in the joint. Conservative management includes minimal analgesics, physiotherapy, corrective devices, splints, canes, and crutches. The involvement of an orthopedist skilled in hemophilia care is crucial.

Muscle bleeds and hematomas are frequent and disabling, presenting as painful, tender, expanding masses causing muscle spasm and flexion. They lead to compression of nerves and blood vessels, muscle necrosis, and fibrosis. Treatment is conservative, involving analgesics, immobilization, splints, and factor replacement until the symptoms resolve. Physiotherapy in combination with infusion therapy is required to regain strength and mobility. Hemophiliacs should never receive intramuscular injections.

Intracranial hemorrhage, fortunately a rare occurrence, is the most common cause of death. Because of the high mortality, all hemophiliacs who have sustained trauma to the head should be treated empirically to raise their factor levels to 60–100%. Hemophiliacs with severe headache, confusion, or irritability should be evaluated for intracranial hemorrhage until this diagnosis is formally eliminated from consideration. CT scan of the head is needed to rule out small bleeds, and decompressive surgery may be required.

Hematuria can be especially troublesome, occurring without specific pathology. All cases should be investigated to rule out obstruction, stones, and malignancy with an intravenous pyelogram. Paradoxically, obstruction from blood clots is not uncommon. Because of this, antifibrinolytic agents such as ϵ-aminocaproic acid should be avoided unless the problem is persistent and uncontrollable. Management of hematuria involves high fluid intake, analgesics, and antispasmodics. Infusion therapy of Factor VIII or Factor IX is usually employed, but is often ineffective. Steroids (0.5–1 mg/kg/day) in conjunction with the above may be helpful in some cases.

The earliest manifestations of oral complications of hemophilia often occur within the first year of life. These problems include persistent bleeds from split lips, torn frenulums and tooth eruptions. These complications can be managed conservatively, with patience and pressure. Fillings and minor procedures can be carried out with local anesthetics after factor infusion prior to the procedure. Extractions are usually performed in an inpatient setting after infusion therapy to obtain Factor VIII or Factor IX levels of 30–60%. An antifibrinolytic agent such as epsilon-aminocaproic acid, 2–4 gm every 4 hours for 10 days, can be used to prevent clot dissolution, but only reduces the amount of factor replacement required.

Surgical procedures are performed on an elective basis whenever possible. On the day prior to surgery, it is important to establish baseline Factor VIII or Factor IX levels, to confirm the absence of an inhibitor, and to evaluate the half-life of infused Factor VIII or Factor IX. In the event of emergency surgery or a major elective procedure, levels of the deficient factor should be maintained between 60 and 100% until wound healing is evident; then the dosage may be lowered until healing is complete.

Inhibitors of Factor VIII occur in 10% of severe hemophilia A and are due to alloantibodies to Factor VIII. An inhibitor assay should be performed regularly, since the appearance of an inhibitor abruptly alters the therapeutic strategies. Some inhibitors are not inducible and can be overcome with high doses of Factor VIII concentrate. Inducible inhibitors, if initially present at levels below 5 Bethesda Units, can be treated with large doses of Factor VIII replacement. Since the antibody amnestic response takes 3–6 days, significant levels of Factor VIII can be maintained until the inhibitor titer rises and reduces the half-life of circulating Factor VIII. Inhibitors in excess of 5 Bethesda Units cannot be treated with Factor VIII replacement. Therefore, any transfusion therapy should be held in reserve for life-threatening bleeding episodes. Minor bleeding episodes in hemophiliacs with inhibitors are treated conservatively with immobilization and analgesics. Immunosuppressives are generally not useful in preventing induction of the alloantibodies. With more significant bleeding complications, Factor IX concentrate, 25–50 units of Factor IX/kg, is used to bypass the inhibitor. However, this therapy may be associated with disseminated intravascular coagulation or thrombosis, and can also induce the antibody titer. Activated Factor IX concentrates (e.g., Autoplex) may be useful but are prohibitively expensive.

Prenatal diagnosis of hemophilia is now available with safe amniocentesis at 12–14 weeks to determine the sex of the fetus. If the fetus is male, an informed decision for a therapeutic abortion can be taken.

von Willebrand's Disease. This is a heterogeneous autosomal dominant disorder characterized by low levels of functional Factor VIII, low levels of von Willebrand's factor, a prolonged bleeding time, and impaired platelet agglutination to ristocetin. The most common type has a prolonged bleeding time and a Factor VIII coagulant activity and Factor VIII/VWF antigen of 10–40%. Cryoprecipitate and fresh frozen plasma induce the Factor VIII coagulant activity and correct the platelet defect.

FACTOR VIII REPLACEMENT THERAPY. At the present time, all products containing human Factor VIII or Factor IX are derived from human blood. Factor VIII concentrates are prepared commercially from large pools of fresh frozen plasma. As such, they carry a certain risk of hepatitis B and acquired immunodeficiency syndrome (AIDS). However, these concentrates can be prepared on an economical scale and provide stable Factor VIII with a prolonged shelf life. In contrast, cryoprecipitate and fresh frozen plasma come from a single donor and carry the risk of viral infection from that donor alone. In general, most hemophiliacs with a chronic infusion history continue to be treated with Factor VIII concentrates. The introduction of heat-treated Factor VIII has reduced, and hopefully eliminated, the risk of AIDS infection. Single-donor replacement therapy, in the form of cryoprecipitate, is reserved for the young pediatric age group, in particular children who have not been exposed to the Factor VIII concentrates. Because of cost considerations, the limited availability of plasma, and the potential toxicity of replacement therapy, the aim is the early treatment of bleeding episodes and not the prophylactic prevention of bleeding.

The baseline level of Factor VIII, the half-life of the infused factor VIII, the presence of a Factor VIII inhibitor, and the severity of the bleed must be factored in when calculating the replacement Factor VIII dose. The calculated Factor VIII dosage is the estimated plasma volume multiplied by the desired increment in factor level. The plasma volume is estimated as 40 ml of plasma per kg of body weight. One unit of Factor VIII is defined as the level (100%) of Factor VIII in 1 ml of normal plasma. Thus, in a 40-kg child with a Factor VIII level of 5%, 720 units of Factor VIII will raise the plasma Factor VIII level to 50%. Cryoprecipitate contains approximately 100 units of Factor VIII/bag and 250 mg of fibrinogen. Fresh frozen plasma has approximately 250 units of factor VIII/250 ml bag. The heat-treated Factor VIII concentrates are assayed for Factor VIII activity, and each bottle is marked with this assay amount. The frequency of Factor VIII replacement depends upon the half-life of the infused Factor VIII. The normal half-life of Factor VIII is 6 hours. Therefore, to maintain a relatively constant range of Factor VIII levels between infusions, one half of the initial Factor VIII dose is administered each Factor VIII half-time. Since these calculations offer rough approximations, Factor VIII recoveries should be directly measured by the assay of the plasma Factor VIII. Adjustments to dosage and the frequency of infusion can be then made on a rational, empiric basis.

The introduction of home infusion therapy has simplified the lives of hemophiliacs, decreased morbidity, and lowered the total cost of hemophilia care. Patients, or members of their family, are taught to administer intravenous Factor VIII upon recognition of a minor bleeding episode. Early therapy obviates long treatment delays in emergency rooms and often leads to rapid, satisfactory resolution of the bleeding disorder. This type of therapy should be reserved for patients with recurrent bleeding episodes. A basic requirement is a mature adult, such as the parent, who can recognize the indications for therapy and facilitate administration of the Factor VIII concentrate. Serious bleeds still require the attention of the hematologist.

Patients with mild hemophilia may respond to a vasopressin analog, DDAVP. The Factor VIII level will increase 4-fold in normal individuals as well as hemophiliacs after the infusion of 0.3 µg/kg of DDAVP intravenously. This increase may be sufficient to treat bleeding problems without plasma products. However, this strategy should be reserved for patients with Factor VIII levels in excess of 5%. Others should be tested in advance to monitor the effect of DDAVP on the Factor VIII level.

VON WILLEBRAND'S FACTOR. Fresh frozen plasma contains both Factor VIII and von Willebrand's factor and is adequate for replacement if there are no volume considerations. Single-donor cryoprecipitate is most effective in von Willebrand's disease and is the preferred plasma product therapy. Infusion therapy addresses either the low Factor VIII level or the prolonged bleeding time. To raise the Factor VIII level, one unit of cryoprecipitate is administered 24 hours prior to surgery. The factor VIII level should be subsequently measured and shown to be in an adequate range. More commonly, the bleeding time must be corrected by infusion of adequate amounts of von Willebrand's factor in cryoprecipitate. Approximately 0.15 bag per kg may be required every 8 to 12 hours.

DDAVP, a synthetic analog of the antidiuretic hormone, raises factor VIII and von Willebrand's factor approximately 4-fold. It can be used in type 1A (common variant) von Willebrand's disease. The response to 0.3 µg/kg of IV DDAVP is seen within 30 minutes. It appears to be as efficacious as cryoprecipitate in those individuals who respond.

FACTOR IX REPLACEMENT THERAPY. Factor IX concentrates contain the vitamin K–dependent proteins (prothrombin and factors VII, IX, and X) and are useful for the treatment of Factor IX deficiency and Factor VIII deficiency complicated by Factor VIII inhibitors. This therapy is effective but carries certain risks not characteristic of the Factor VIII concentrates. Besides hepatitis and AIDS, thrombosis and DIC are associated with replacement therapy with this concentrate. Since Factor IX rapidly equilibrates between the intravascular and extravascular space, the calculated dosage (as described for Factor VIII) must be doubled to estimate the plasma Factor IX level after infusion.

Complications of Factor IX concentrates include thrombosis and DIC. In general, the large quantities of Factor IX concentrate required for surgical procedures put these patients at a special risk for pulmonary embolism and deep venous thrombosis. Some hematologists use small doses of heparin concurrently with treatment with large quantities of Factor IX to minimize these risks. Hemolytic reactions in non–ABO cross-matched transfusions require the discontinuation of the product, recrossmatching, and assessment of the degree of hemolysis. Allergic manifestations are not uncommon and include acute febrile reactions, chills, rash, and hives. These complications can be reduced or eliminated by switching to an alternate commercial product. Chronic complications include acquired inhibitors to Factor IX, hepatitis, and AIDS. Acquired inhibitors preclude any therapy other than life-threatening bleeds. Fortunately, inhibitors occur in only about 5% of patients with Factor IX deficiency. Chronic, persistent hepatitis and a mild increase in serum transaminases are common. Acquired immunodeficiency states, so far a rare complication of transfusion therapy, is of significant concern. Tests for HTLV III (LAV) antibody are now available, and all transfusion products are being screened.

Deficiency of Contact Phase Proteins. Deficiency of any of three of the contact phase proteins, Factor XII, high molecular weight kininogen, and prekallikrein, causes a prolonged PTT but is not associated with any bleeding tendency. However, Factor XI deficiency may be associated with a mild bleeding disorder, particularly if the Factor XI level is less than 15%. Replacement with the infusion of fresh frozen plasma (15–20 ml/kg daily) is sufficient.

Deficiency of Vitamin K–Dependent Proteins. Factor VII and Factor X deficiencies are rare. Plasma infusions are indicated to treat bleeding episodes. Hypoprothrombinemia or dysprothrombinemia (mutant prothrombin) is not usually associated with a bleeding tendency because these disorders are usually heterozygous. The treatment of choice is fresh frozen plasma infusion.

Factor V Deficiency. Factor V deficiency presents with mild to moderate clinical bleeding. Levels of only 10–15% are needed for adequate hemostasis, and this is attained with fresh frozen plasma (15–20 ml/kg). Alternatively, platelet transfusions have been successfully used to manage serious bleeding episodes.

Fibrinogen Deficiency. Hypofibrinogenemia is associated with a minimal bleeding tendency. Bleeding complications are limited to trauma and surgical procedures. Serious bleeding problems are corrected with cryoprecipitate. Dysfibrinogenemia (mutant fibrinogen) may be mild or asymptomatic, but paradoxically some patients have a thrombotic tendency. These fibrinogen abnormalities are corrected with cryoprecipitate. Cryoprecipitate (2–4 bags) will raise the fibrinogen level to 50–100 mg/dl.

Factor XIII Deficiency. This rare disorder may have a mild to moderate bleeding tendency and is missed by the standard screening tests. Clinically these patients manifest with delayed bleeding, poor wound healing, and keloid scars. The specific test for diagnosis is the clot solubility test. Factor XIII levels of 5–10% are needed for adequate hemostasis. Because of the long half-life of Factor XIII, 1–2 units of fresh frozen plasma, or 2–3 ml of fresh plasma/kg monthly is sufficient for therapy.

ACQUIRED COAGULATION ABNORMALITIES

Liver Disease. Hemostatic abnormalities in hepatic disorders are due to decreased synthesis of certain coagulation factors and decreased clearance of activated enzymes. These problems are seen with hepatic parenchymal disease. Vitamin K deficiency is also a common cause of hemostatic problems associated with liver disease. The severity of chronic or acute hepatitis correlates best with a prolongation of the prothrombin time, which reflects the decrease in production of the vitamin K–dependent proteins. A trial of vitamin K either intravenously or subcutaneously to improve the prothrombin time will show benefit within a day if the problem is simple vitamin K deficiency. In severe liver disease the thrombin time becomes prolonged owing to a decrease in fibrinogen to less than 100 mg/dl. An increase in fibrin(ogen) degradation products due to decreased clearance interferes with fibrin polymerization. Successful management of severe liver disease is difficult because of the multiple hemostatic defects. If the prothrombin time is prolonged without evidence of bleeding, a trial of vitamin K (10 mg IV or SQ daily for 3–4 days) is suggested. If there is bleeding, therapy entails daily vitamin K injections as above, replacement therapy with fresh frozen plasma, and platelets to treat serious thrombocytopenia. Factor IX concentrates for replacement of the vitamin K–dependent blood clotting proteins are contraindicated because of the hazards of hepatitis and the induction of a hypercoagulable state.

Vitamin K Deficiency. Prothrombin, Factor VII, Factor IX, and Factor X require vitamin K in the post-translational step involving carboxylation of the glutamic acid residues in these proteins so they can bind to Ca^{++} and phospholipid surfaces. A deficiency of vitamin K is reflected in a prolonged prothrombin time and prolonged PTT. Vitamin K deficiency is associated with dietary deficiencies and malabsorption syndromes, anti-

biotic suppression of normal gut flora that synthesize vitamin K, obstructive jaundice and impaired enterohepatic circulation, and vitamin K antagonists of the coumarin class. Management will depend on bleeding manifestations and the urgency for correction of the coagulopathy. Therapy involves vitamin K, 5–15 mg IV; because of rare anaphylactoid reactions, a test dose should be given and epinephrine should be immediately available. Alternatively, 10 mg of vitamin K IM or 5 mg SQ daily may be used. Rapid correction of the hemostatic defects is accomplished with fresh frozen plasma, but this carries the risk of hepatitis. Therefore, plasma should be used only in acute bleeding emergencies. Coumadin that is accidentally ingested or taken in excess for therapy of thrombosis may be associated with clinically significant bleeding. Vitamin K, 25 mg IV, will correct the prothrombin time rapidly. Infusion of fresh frozen plasma, 15–20 ml/kg, should partially normalize the prothrombin time. Factor IX concentrates are contraindicated for replacement therapy.

Hemorrhagic Disease of the Newborn. Almost all newborns have a vitamin K deficiency at birth. In its most serious form, vitamin K deficiency can lead to serious bleeding in the first week of life. To prevent vitamin K deficiency in the newborn, vitamin K is routinely administered at birth during in-hospital deliveries. Prophylaxis entails 1 mg of vitamin K_1 IM or SQ. If clinically significant vitamin K deficiency is suspected, particularly in premature infants, vitamin K should be administered (0.5–1.0 mg IV or 1–2 mg PO). Alternatively, 15–20 ml/kg of fresh frozen plasma should be infused if there is clinical bleeding. Vitamin K is not sufficiently supplied by human milk.

Disseminated Intravascular Coagulation. Disseminated intravascular coagulation (DIC) is a disorder of regulation characterized by a hypercoagulable state. In its fulminant form, spontaneous bleeding from mucosa and venipuncture sites is observed. Its chronic form is manifested by thromboembolic complications. It is characterized by the activation of the coagulation pathways and consumption of clotting proteins, fibrinogen, and platelets with deposition of fibrin thrombi in the microvasculature. The diagnosis hinges upon the laboratory findings of a prolonged prothrombin time, PTT, and thrombin time with thrombocytopenia, elevated fibrin(ogen) degradation products, and decreased fibrinogen. On the blood smear, fragmented red blood cells are seen.

The management of severe DIC emphasizes the treatment of the underlying disorder. Suspected bacterial sepsis must be treated without delay with aggressive antibiotic therapy, for example. The patient must be assessed for the clinical severity of the disorder. If the patient is not actively bleeding, no special measures need be taken. Blood component replacement is necessary in the face of active bleeding. Packed red blood cells and fresh frozen plasma are used for volume expansion and partial correction of the coagulopathy. Platelet concentrates may be effective in relieving the severe thrombocytopenia. In the neonate, aggressive blood component therapy is facilitated by exchange transfusion. There is no role for heparin in patients with DIC characterized by a severe bleeding disorder. Only in the presence of thrombosis is there a clear indication for the use of heparin.

Circulating Anticoagulants. Circulating inhibitors of blood coagulation are acquired as complications of other diseases or, in the case of hemophilia, as the result of allosensitization to specific therapeutic proteins. In the pediatric age group, circulating inhibitors are most often associated with systemic lupus erythematosus. The classic lupus anticoagulant is not associated with a hemostatic defect. Indeed, the presence of a lupus anticoagulant is more often associated with thromboembolic disease. These inhibitors are immunoglobulins that bind to the phospholipid used in the PTT assay, causing a prolongation of the PTT. Alternatively, some anticoagulants may be directed against specific coagulation factors such as factor VIII, interfere with fibrin polymerization, or inhibit platelet function.

The clinical importance of a detected inhibitor cannot be ascertained by a laboratory test. Although many of these inhibitors may be considered laboratory curiosities, the risks of elective surgery must be weighed carefully in the face of such an inhibitor. In the hemophiliac, the inhibitor always plays an important role in dictating management strategies.

Acute Leukemia

DONALD PINKEL, M.D.

Acute leukemia is a curable disease. The cure rate depends not only on the species of acute leukemia and certain prognostic variables but also on the skill of treatment. For this reason, every child with acute leukemia should be referred to a pediatric hematology/oncology research and treatment center where the best-honed skills are available to the child.

Treatment of acute leukemia is continuously evolving, so that methods outlined here may be more or less obsolete when they are published. This is an additional reason for referral to a center where the latest and often yet unpublished information about treatment is known.

After initial evaluation of the child and planning

of treatment are completed in a research and treatment center, much of the week-to-week care of the child can be managed by the child's community pediatrician with periodic consultation and monitoring by the center.

Chemotherapy of acute leukemia varies with biologic species and prognostic variables. Supportive measures are similar for all types.

CHEMOTHERAPY OF ACUTE LYMPHOCYTIC LEUKEMIA

Prior to chemotherapy, all children are evaluated with regard to peripheral blood and bone marrow findings. This includes cytochemical staining, immunologic phenotyping, cytogenetic analysis with banding, and flow cytometry of the leukemic lymphoblasts and lymphocytes in the marrow specimens.

Children with common type acute leukemia (ALL) demonstrating hyperdiploidy with low initial white blood cell counts (less than 20,000) have the best prognosis with current chemotherapy. Those with pre-B ALL, null ALL, pseudodiploidy, or high initial white blood cell counts (more than 20,000) have less favorable outlooks. We provide similar drugs to all of these children, but we are inclined to give more intensive chemotherapy when the outlook is less favorable.

Children with thymic ALL are treated differently than those with common, pre-B, and null ALL. Prognosis is worse with white blood cell count levels over 100,000 and with pseudodiploidy. However, all receive the same chemotherapy program, with emphasis on the combination of cytosine arabinoside and cyclophosphamide.

Children with B-lymphoblastic ALL ("Burkitt cell" ALL) have the worst prognosis. Highly intensive chemotherapy is used with particular emphasis on cyclophosphamide, high-dose methotrexate, high-dose cytosine arabinoside, and intensive intrathecal chemotherapy.

Remission Induction. For common, pre-B, and null ALL, we administer prednisone, vincristine, and asparaginase in order to produce clinical and laboratory disappearance of leukemia and to allow regeneration of normal hematopoiesis. Most patients will experience a complete clinical and hematologic remission after 4 weeks of this treatment. For children with thymic ALL we add daunomycin as a fourth drug. Children with B-lymphoblastic ALL receive high-dose cyclophosphamide and cytosine arabinoside in addition to the three primary drugs.

Preventive Meningeal Chemotherapy. In order to destroy leukemia cells in the arachnoid meninges and thus prevent meningeal relapse, intrathecal chemotherapy is employed weekly during the first 6 weeks of treatment and periodically thereafter. I recommend 8-week intervals for 2 years for those with common, pre-B, and null ALL, 4-week intervals for 18 months for those with thymic ALL, and 2-week intervals for 6 months for those with B-lymphoblastic ALL. We use methotrexate 15 mg/m^2 (maximum dose 15 mg), hydrocortisone 15 mg/m^2 (maximum dose 15 mg), and cytosine arabinoside 30 mg/m^2 (maximum dose 30 mg), with all three drugs dissolved in one solution of preservative-free normal saline and administered within 3 days of preparation (see Table 1). The solution is injected through a millipore filter attached to the syringe in a volume of 10 ml/m^2 (maximum 10 ml) after an atraumatic tap and free gravity removal of 5 to 10 ml/m^2 of cerebrospinal fluid. The solution is allowed to reach room temperature before injection. The patient is maintained in a lateral position during administration and in a prone position without a pillow for a half hour afterward.

Continuation Chemotherapy. Once clinical and hematologic remission is achieved, children with common, pre-B, and null ALL receive mercapto-

Table 1. DRUGS USED IN CHILDREN WITH ACUTE LEUKEMIA*

Drug	Usual Dosage	Route	Principal Side Effects
Asparaginase	6000 units/m^2 three times weekly	IM	Hypersensitivity reactions, anaphylaxis, pancreatitis, coagulopathy, hyperglycemia, fatty liver, ketosis, azotemia, emesis, cerebral dysfunction, alopecia, immunosuppression
Azacytidine†	150 mg/m^2/day for 5 days by continuous infusion	IV	Hematosuppression, emesis, mucositis
Cyclophosphamide	(1) 100–150 mg/m^2 daily for 7 days	IV, Oral	Hematosuppression, immunosuppression, emesis, alopecia, hemorrhagic cystitis, inappropriate ADH secretion, bladder carcinoma, oligospermia, amenorrhea, permanent sterility, cardiac toxicity
	(2) 300–600 mg/m^2 once weekly	IV	
Cytosine arabinoside	(1) 100–200 mg/m^2 daily by continuous infusion for 3 to 10 days	IV, SC	Hematosuppression, immunosuppression, mucositis, fever, alopecia, emesis, diarrhea, conjunctivitis
	(2) 1 gm/m^2 by continuous 24-hour infusion	IV, SC	
	(3) 30–50 mg/m^2 (maximum 30–50 mg) once a week	Intrathecal	Headache, backache, emesis, arachnoiditis, seizure, encephalopathy, paraparesis
Daunorubicin	25–35 mg/m^2 once weekly or daily for 1 to 3 days (maximum total cumulative dosage = 300 mg/m^2)	IV	Hematosuppression, immunosuppression, mucosal ulcers, emesis, diarrhea, cardiomyopathy, aggravation of radiation reaction, alopecia, phlebitis, paravascular tissue necrosis
Etoposide (VP-16)	(1) 150–300 mg/m^2 once or twice weekly	IV	Hematosuppression, emesis, diarrhea, alopecia, hypotension, allergic reactions
	(2) 100 mg/m^2 daily for 5 days		
	(3) 200 mg/m^2 daily for 2 to 3 days		
Mercaptopurine	50–75 mg/m^2 daily	Oral	Hematosuppression, immunosuppression, hepatic dysfunction, alopecia, mucositis
Methotrexate	(1) 20–30 mg/m^2 once weekly	IM, Oral, IV	Mucosal ulceration, megaloblastosis, abdominal cramps and diarrhea, malabsorption, cerebral dysfunction, hematosuppression, immunosuppression, leukoencephalopathy, hepatic dysfunction, hepatic fibrosis, photosensitivity, alopecia, dermatitis, conjunctivitis, pneumonitis
	(2) 1 gm/m^2 by continuous 24-hour infusion followed by leucovorin rescue	IV	
Prednisone, prednisolone	40 mg/m^2 daily in two to three divided doses	Oral, IV	Hypertension, hyperglycemia, edema, polyphagia, potassium deficit, acne, obesity, behavior change, muscle atrophy, striae, immunosuppression, ketosis, cataracts
Teniposide (VM-26)‡	100–200 mg/m^2 once or twice weekly	IV	Hematosuppression, emesis, diarrhea, hypotension, allergic reactions
Thioguanine	40–60 mg/m^2 daily	Oral	Hematosuppression, immunosuppression, hepatic dysfunction, alopecia, mucositis
Vincristine	1.5 mg/m^2 weekly (maximum 2 mg)	IV	Peripheral neuropathy, constipation, inappropriate ADH secretion, alopecia, ineffective erythropoiesis, seizure, immunosuppression, paravascular tissue necrosis

* Special precautions are needed in the preparation and administration of antileukemic drugs. For example, parenteral injections and infusions must be prepared in a vertical laminar flow hood. Patients must meet certain criteria of renal, hepatic, and hematopoietic function. High-dose methotrexate requires concurrent hydration and alkalinization.

† Available from the National Cancer Institute.

‡ Investigational drug.

purine daily and methotrexate weekly for $2\frac{1}{2}$ to 3 years. It is important to monitor these patients closely, at least once every 2 weeks, with assessment for infection, nutrition, growth, compliance, emotional and social adjustment, and hematologic status. On the one hand, it is important to avoid life-threatening toxicity. On the other hand, it is necessary to assure that the child is receiving maximum tolerated dosage in order to have optimal benefit of the drugs. I adjust the dosage of mercaptopurine to keep the white blood cell count between 2000 and 3000/mm^3 with 700/mm^3 or more phagocytes (granulocytes + monocytes) and 700/mm^3 or more lymphocytes. I adjust the methotrexate dosage to maintain moderate macrocytosis of the red blood cells and hypersegmentation of the granulocytes while avoiding oral ulcerations, sruelike symptoms, or evidence of cerebral dysfunction. Methotrexate polyglutamate can be measured in the patient's red blood cells to monitor adequacy of dosage and compliance. For children with pre-B or null phenotypes, pseudodiploidy, or high initial white blood cell counts, additional chemotherapy is often used because of the higher risk of relapse. Although there is no proof of additional efficacy, high-dose intravenous methotrexate, 2-week courses of prednisone and vincristine, the combination of teniposide (VM-26)* and cytosine arabinoside, additional courses of intensive asparaginase therapy, and periodic administration of an anthracycline are among the additional measures sometimes tried.

For children with thymic ALL, periodic courses of cyclophosphamide and cytosine arabinoside are given during continuation chemotherapy. Many other measures are also used by some hematologists, such as those mentioned in the previous paragraph. For B-lymphoblastic ALL, highly intensive chemotherapy with multiple drugs, particularly cyclophosphamide, is used in attempts to prevent the usual course of early hematologic and central nervous system relapse.

Continuation chemotherapy is usually terminated after $2\frac{1}{2}$ to 3 years of continuous complete remission, provided that bone marrow, spinal fluid, and—in boys—testicular biopsy are free of leukemia.

CHEMOTHERAPY OF ACUTE NONLYMPHOCYTIC LEUKEMIA

Acute myelocytic and myelomonocytic leukemias are the most frequent varieties of acute nonlymphocytic leukemia in children. Acute histiocytic, promyelocytic, monocytic, erythrocytic, and megakaryocytic types are unusual. Clinical features, light and electron microscopy studies, cytochemical stains, and cytogenetics are used to classify the

leukemia and to assess prognosis. With modern chemotherapy, approximately 30% of children with acute myelocytic and acute myelomonocytic leukemias are experiencing long-term leukemia-free survival and possible cure.

Remission Induction. Conventional therapy consists of cytosine arabinoside by continuous infusion for 7 to 10 days and daunorubicin by daily injection for 3 days. This treatment results in a hazardous period of mucositis, granulocytopenia, and thrombocytopenia lasting about 2 weeks that is often followed by hematologic remission. For patients with persistent leukemia in the bone marrow after 3 weeks, the initial course of chemotherapy is repeated.

For acute promyelocytic leukemia, a low-dose heparin infusion is initiated prior to chemotherapy and continued for 7 to 10 days in an effort to control the consumptive coagulopathy characteristic of this type of leukemia. Fresh frozen plasma and fresh platelets are usually required also.

For acute monocytic and acute histiocytic leukemia, etoposide (VP-16), an epipodophyllotoxin, is a highly effective drug.

Preventive Meningeal Therapy. Triple-drug intrathecal chemotherapy is utilized as in acute lymphocytic leukemia. Generally, it is not started until remission is achieved. There is no established schedule, but I would recommend monthly administration for 18 months.

Continuation Chemotherapy. Various combinations and schedules are in use, and none can be recommended over another. In addition to daunorubicin and cytosine arabinoside, the drugs effective against acute nonlymphocytic leukemia include the purine analogs thioguanine and mercaptopurine, azacytidine,† and etoposide (VP-16). Methotrexate, prednisone, and vincristine also are used in some treatment protocols but with less evidence of efficacy.

Bone Marrow Transplantation. In many hematology centers, children with acute nonlymphocytic leukemia who have histocompatible siblings are treated by bone marrow ablation and transplantation shortly after achieving remission. This involves the immediate risks and long-term sequelae of total body irradiation and/or highly intensive chemotherapy, severe prolonged hematosuppression and immunosuppression, graft versus host disease, and intractable pneumonia. Autologous bone marrow transplantation and mismatched donor transplantation are under investigation.

SUPPORTIVE CARE

Evaluation. Since acute leukemia involves all tissues and organs and has profound influence on the life of the child and his family and friends,

---

* Teniposide (VM-26) is an investigational agent.

† Azacytidine is available from the National Cancer Institute.

extensive supportive care is required. The following studies are carried out routinely.

AT DIAGNOSIS. Complete blood cell count, differential, reticulocyte count; SMA-18 panel; prothrombin and partial thromboplastin times; urinalysis; chest roentgenogram; tuberculin skin test; serology for varicella-zoster and cytomegalo virus; hepatitis panel; bone marrow aspiration with differential count, special cytochemical stains, cell surface markers, cytogenetic analysis with banding, electron microscopy when indicated, flow cytometry; cerebrospinal fluid examination with cytospin preparation; dental evaluation and care; oral hygiene instruction; nutritional evaluation; neuropsychological assessment; social service evaluation.

DURING TREATMENT. Periodic blood cell counts, bone marrow examination, spinal fluid cytology, SMA-18 panel, urinalysis; growth charting and reassessments of nutrition and psychosocial status.

FOLLOWING TREATMENT. Periodic blood cell counts and bone marrow examinations; growth charting; psychosocial and vocational evaluation and counseling; endocrinological assessments by physical examinations and measurements of T_3, T_4, TSH, FSH, LH, and testosterone or estrogen levels.

Metabolic Disorders. Children with rapidly evolving leukemia, high initial white blood cell counts, and large masses of tumor are prone to have hyperuricemia initially or after treatment is started. Consequently, these children receive intravenous hydration with 2.5 to 3 liter/m^2/24 hours of 5% glucose and 0.25 normal saline, alkalinization with $NaHCO_3$, 1 gm/m^2 every 6 hours orally *or* 25–30 mEq/l of intravenous fluid, and allopurinol 100 mg/m^2 orally every 8 hours for the first 3 to 4 days of treatment. Urinary output, specific gravity, and pH are monitored to ensure appropriate pH and dilution.

Hyperkalemia, hypercalcemia or hypocalcemia, hyperphosphatemia, azotemia, and lactic acidemia are other metabolic disturbances seen in children with leukemia at diagnosis or relapse. They often require prompt corrective measures. Prednisone and/or asparaginase can cause hyperglycemia and ketosis to the point of demanding therapy with insulin, intravenous fluids, and sodium bicarbonate.

Infections. The hematosuppression and immunosuppression resulting from chemotherapy as well as the leukemia itself make children with leukemia highly susceptible to serious infections. Preventive measures include minimal hospitalization, scrupulous handwashing by physicians, nurses, and technologists, removal of infectious foci such as dental abscesses, and maintaining the absolute phagocyte count (granulocytes + monocytes) above 700/mm^3 and the absolute lymphocyte count above 700/mm^3. Co-trimoxazole, 5 mg/kg of trimethoprim and 25 mg/kg sulfamethoxazole in two divided doses daily is administered three times weekly to prevent *Pneumocystis carinii* pneumonia.

Fever in the child with leukemia is assumed to be the result of infection. Physical examination and blood cultures are generally followed by intravenous antibiotic therapy if the child has granulocytopenia. For the child in relapse, suspect organisms are staphylococcus, *Hemophilus influenzae*, and enteric bacteria, but fungal infections can appear after prolonged antibiotic treatment. *Staphylococcus epidermidis* is a threat to children with central venous lines.

Varicella-zoster can be a catastrophic infection in susceptible children with leukemia. Varicella-zoster vaccine and varicella-zoster immune globulin are useful preventive measures. Acyclovir (acycloguanosine) 500 mg/m^2 intravenously every 8 hours for 5 to 10 days is the treatment of choice.

Blood Component Support. Red blood cell transfusions, 10 ml/kg, are used to maintain hemoglobin levels above 7 gm/dl or higher if the patient has pneumonia or sepsis. The red cells are washed prior to transfusion. If the patient is severely immunosuppressed, the red cells are irradiated to avoid risk of graft versus host disease.

Platelet transfusions, 4 to 6 units/m^2, are administered for significant bleeding associated with platelet counts less than 30,000/mm^3. Platelets are irradiated when the patient is highly immunosuppressed.

Granulocytes obtained by single donor leukapheresis are used in some centers for patients with granulocytopenia and proven bacterial sepsis that fails to respond to several days of appropriate antibiotic therapy.

Psychosocial Support. Every child with leukemia needs his or her own personal physician to provide continuous comprehensive care, advocacy and counsel. The child needs to know the diagnosis and to be consulted as feasible along with parents about management decisions. Families need the help of nurses, social workers, and psychologists in learning how to cope with the numerous challenges of caring for the child with leukemia. However, the child's personal physician retains primary responsibility.

Home health service is an integral component of treatment. Home visits are important for social assessment, reinforcement of medication schedules, family instructions, and care of the dying child.

RELAPSE

Hematologic relapse of acute leukemia during combination chemotherapy usually signifies drug-resistant leukemia. Although second and third remissions can be induced, they tend to be brief. Patients with relapse while on therapy are considered for bone marrow ablation and transplantation if they have histocompatible donors. Autologous and mismatched donor transplantations are experimental possibilities.

Hematologic relapse 6 months or more after cessation of therapy may signify inadequate duration of treatment. Remission induction and continuation chemotherapy utilizing both previously administered and additional drugs often result in lengthy second remissions and sometimes cures.

Isolated meningeal relapse at any time can be effectively treated with intrathecal chemotherapy followed by craniospinal irradiation. Approximately one fourth of these patients become long-term survivors.

Clinically isolated testicular relapse is treated by testicular irradiation, modification of chemotherapy, and an additional 2 years of drug treatment. Prognosis is better when the relapse occurs after cessation of chemotherapy than during chemotherapy.

Neuroblastoma

JAMES FEUSNER, M.D.

Neuroblastoma is a tumor of the sympathetic nervous system. It is the fourth most frequent pediatric solid tumor overall, and the most common such tumor in young children. Its incidence is estimated at 9 per million children per year.

There are several features of this tumor (such as spontaneous regression or maturation) that favor survival, but in its disseminated form it has remained resistant to curative treatment. Unfortunately, in two thirds of children, the tumor is disseminated at diagnosis.

In order to better understand and treat this tumor, it is important to fully estimate the extent of disease at diagnosis. We routinely stage our patients according to the system of Evans (Table 1). The validity of this system has been amply confirmed in several large studies since its proposal in 1971. Patients with completely resected disease (stage I) have an excellent chance (>85%) for long-term survival. On the other hand, children older than 1 year with stage IV disease have a very poor prognosis (10% 2-year survival). Age is next most important in estimating prognosis. Survival for all infants is approximatley 74% as compared with 12% for children over 2 years of age at diagnosis. Other factors considered to indicate a more favorable prognosis include urinary vanillylmandelic acid (VMA) to homovanillic acid (HVA) ratio of >1, serum neuron specific enolase (NSE) of <100 mg/dl, serum ferritin of <150 mg/dl, thoracic or cervical site of primary tumor, and presence of some ganglionic differentiation in the primary tumor.

TREATMENT MODALITIES

Surgical. Surgery may involve biopsy only, radical attempts at complete excision of huge tumors, or "second look" operations attempting complete resection of tumors initially felt to be unresectable. Most recently the surgeon has been called upon to attempt "debulking" of tumors before bone marrow transplantation is performed.

There is no question of the vital role of surgery in stage I and II neuroblastoma. However, it has not been clearly demonstrated that primary tumor resection of the primary tumor has altered the ultimate outcome for children with stage III or IV neuroblastoma. The importance and timing of surgery before marrow transplantation remain to be determined in future studies.

Radiotherapy. Neuroblastoma is a radiosensitive but not often radiocurable disease. Most centers utilize radiotherapy for treatment of emergencies involving organ compromise (e.g., spinal cord compression), for palliation of pain, or as an adjunct in treating stage III patients. It clearly is not necessary for stage I patients and may not be necessary for many stage II patients.

Total body irradiation has been attempted as the primary treatment of advanced neuroblastoma. It has not improved upon the results of contemporary radiotherapy and chemotherapy protocols. Perhaps if it were utilized in higher dosage along with chemotherapy (as in current transplantation protocols), it might contribute to improved outcome.

Chemotherapy. In the last 15 years many chemotherapeutic agents have been used in the treatment of neuroblastoma. Those that have proven activity include vincristine, cytoxan, doxorubicin (Adriamycin), DTIC, nitrogen mustard, VM-26, cisplatin, and melphalan. Past studies have not demonstrated improved survival for patients of stage I or II treated with chemotherapy. In stage III and IV patients, the median disease-free survival *has* been improved but not the ultimate survival. Current emphasis is on using newer agents (e.g., melphalan) added to regimens of proven activity (e.g., vincristine, cytoxan, and DTIC). In addition, investigational agents are being utilized sooner in patients who have sustained relapses on standard therapy.

Bone Marrow Transplantation. In the last 5 years several centers have begun utilizing bone marrow transplantation in treating patients with relapsed neuroblastoma. The exact preparative regimens have varied, but most have included high-dose chemotherapy (VM-26, doxorubicin, Cytoxan, cisplatin, melphalan) followed by total body irradiation. Both allogeneic and autologous transplants have been attempted. Although it is still early, this treatment regimen appears to be providing some patients longer disease-free periods than would otherwise be expected. For example, D'Angio and colleagues reported 23 of 63 patients surviving following transplantation in a mixed group of advanced neuroblastoma patients in whom only an 11% 2-year survival would be expected with standard therapies (personal communication).

The largest pediatric oncology cooperative group in the United States (Children's Cancer Study Group) is planning a BMT treatment approach for all non-infants with newly diagnosed stage IV neuroblastoma.

Other. Several other more novel approaches to treatment are being investigated. One is based on the infrequent but well-known occurrence of maturation of neuroblastoma. Laboratory studies have shown that several drugs can induce maturation of neuroblastoma cell lines. Vitamin E and retinoic acid are two such agents being studied in certain patients who have recurrent disease.

Another approach stems from monoclonal antibody technology. Either chemotherapy (daunomycin) or radioisotopic therapy is being administered to some patients by coupling the treatment "agent" to monoclonal antibodies raised to neuroblastoma. The advantage of this therapy would be lessened toxicity to the patient, since the therapy would be directed primarily to the tumor(s) and not to normal tissue.

Although these approaches are based on sound observations, it is far too early at this time to predict how successful they will be in the clinic.

SPECIFIC THERAPY RECOMMENDATIONS

Stage I. These children require only a careful surgical resection. In several reported series 90–100% of these children survive. Even those who have not had a complete excision of their tumor almost always do well without further therapy.

Stage II. The same approach for stage I patients applies to most children with stage II disease. There is some controversy concerning the role of radiotherapy in children with residual disease following surgery. It is our opinion there has not been a clear demonstration of added benefit from use of radiation in this setting. Therefore, we do not use radiation routinely, only considering it if bulk disease remains after surgery, especially in children over 2 years of age.

Stage III. In some respects this stage is arbitrary; not many children fit in this category. According to Evans' original criteria, such children have had a 50–60% 2-year survival, with therapy consisting of surgery, radiation, and combination chemo-

therapy. Recently, the CCSG has re-examined this group of patients and redefined them.

Those children whose tumors crossed the midline of the body by invading tissue, in contrast to those in whom the tumor merely hung over the midline, had a much worse prognosis. Their outlook approximated that of stage IV patients, e.g., 15–20% survival. Because of this, we currently approach this type of patient like a stage IV patient (see the following). There are two exceptions: all children less than 1 year of age and those of 1–2 years with low levels of serum NSE at diagnosis both have better prognoses (CCSG preliminary data). In these latter two instances we still utilize standard radiotherapy for bulk disease following initial chemotherapy utilizing vincristine, Cytoxan, and DTIC in cycles every 3 weeks as follows: *Day 1:* Cytoxan (C) 750 mg/m^2 IV; DTIC (D) 250 mg/m^2 IV; *Days 2–5:* DTIC 250 mg/m^2 IV; *Day 5:* Vincristine (V) 1.5 mg/m^2 IV.

Stage IV. Because of the uniformly dismal outcome for these patients when using standard chemotherapy and irradiation, we explore the possibility of bone marrow transplantation (BMT) for these children. All children, along with their parents and siblings, are HLA-typed at diagnosis. Those patients who have an HLA and MLC matched donor are referred for transplantation after induction therapy with VCD (preceding schedule) alternated with melphalan (1.5 mg/kg IV every 3 weeks). Further "debulking" radiation therapy and/or surgery is attempted in those who have residual disease after 12 weeks of chemotherapy. The doses and fields for radiation must be coordinated very carefully with the transplant center, to avoid excess toxicity with the transplantation therapy.

Children who do not have an acceptable donor are considered candidates for an autologous BMT if their marrow is shown to be free of neuroblastoma. They undergo the same induction therapy as already described.

For those patients not having a bone marrow donor and not having marrow free of tumor, we continue the VCD/melphalan chemotherapy regimen as long as there is no progression of disease. In the event of disease progresssion, we utilize combinations of cisplatin, VM-26, doxorubicin, and Cytoxan plus radiotherapy. If these regimens fail, we encourage the use of investigational drugs to discover more effective agents to combat neuroblastoma.

Stage IV-S. Children with this stage of neuroblastoma (Table 1) have an excellent prognosis (80–90% 2-year survival) with minimal therapy. Unless there is a life-threatening problem with compression of a vital organ (e.g., respiratory compromise due to massive hepatomegaly), we

Table 1. STAGING CRITERIA FOR CHILDREN WITH NEUROBLASTOMA (SYSTEM OF EVANS)

Stage	Criteria
Stage I	Tumor confined to the organ or structure of origin
Stage II	Tumor extending in continuity beyond the organ or structure of origin but not crossing the midline Regional lymph nodes on the ipsilateral side may be involved
Stage III	Tumor extending and infiltrating beyond the midline Regional lymph nodes may be involved bilaterally
Stage IV	Remote disease involving the skeleton, organs, soft tissue, and distant lymph node groups
Stage IV-S	(Special category) Patients who would otherwise be Stage I or II but who have remote disease confined to liver, skin, or bone marrow and who have no radiographic evidence of bone metastases on complete skeletal survey or bone scan

take an expectant stance on treatment. Low-dose (400–600 R) radiation, delivered via lateral ports, may be utilized to decrease liver size, if needed. Otherwise, we provide full supportive care to allow time for these children to outgrow their tumors.

SUPPORTIVE CARE

As the therapy has intensified for neuroblastoma, so has the need for supportive care. This is a tumor that demands the expertise of a comprehensive pediatric facility. Chemotherapy and radiotherapy will produce nausea and vomiting, which deserve treatment with the newest antiemetics, singly or in combination. We usually start with metoclopramide (1 mg/kg IV) plus diphenhydramine (0.75 mg/kg IV). If these fail, we increase the doses, up to 2 mg/kg and 1–1.25 mg/kg, respectively.

Weight loss and poor nutritional state can occur during treatment or prior to it in some aggressive stage IV cases. There is a growing body of data suggesting that nutritional deficiencies may be harmful to these children by prolonging the myelosuppression following therapy or even possibly by affecting the patient's response to chemotherapy. We generally institute supplemental alimen-

tation when the patient has lost 5–10% of his initial lean mass.

Graft versus host disease (GVHD) has been reported in patients transfused with nonirradiated blood products. In fact, one of the earlier reports involved a neuroblastoma patient from our institution. It is our policy to irradiate (1500 R) *all* blood products given to patients with neuroblastoma. To our knowledge there has never been a case of graft versus host disease in a patient transfused with blood so irradiated.

Interstitial pneumonia due to *Pneumocystis carinii* is a well-known potential complication of immunosuppressive therapy. This complication can affect neuroblastoma patients as well. Therefore, it is our policy to use trimethoprim/sulfamethoxazole (Bactrim) prophylactically (5 mg/kg/d trimethoprim, 25 mg/kg/d sulfamethoxazole) in all patients.

Other infections are occurring more frequently than in the past, reflecting the greater degree and duration of myelo- and immunosuppression effected by new treatment regimens. The prompt institution of broad-spectrum intravenous antibiotics is mandatory in any child with fever (38.5°C or 101.3°F) and neutropenia (absolute granulocyte count of 500/μl). In addition, amphotericin B for presumed systemic fungal infection is often added in children who remain febrile for 4 to 7 days on antibiotics. We utilize granulocyte transfusions only in patients with proven sepsis or soft tissue infection who are severely neutropenic (absolute neutrophil count <200 μl) and not responding to appropriate antibiotic therapy.

A rare but recently emphasized potential complication is hypertension. Some children may present with serious systolic and diastolic hypertension, while others will manifest it during surgery or chemotherapy. This problem may be serious enough to warrant short-term use of alpha-adrenergic blocking agents.

Finally, the nature of neuroblastoma makes the child who is affected a classic example of the patient who needs comprehensive psychosocial support. There can be tremendous financial, social, and psychological stresses on the patient and family. The effective delivery of appropriate and thorough care to these children requires a multidisciplinary team approach that includes the skills of a social worker, child-life worker, psychiatrist, and compassionate physician.

8

Spleen and Lymphatic System

Postsplenectomy Syndrome

JERRY A. WINKELSTEIN, M.D.

Although the spleen was once considered to be of relatively little value to the host, in recent years there has been a growing appreciation that it plays a critical role in defense against infection. The spleen is composed of two distinct but interrelated immunologic compartments. Fixed phagocytes of the reticuloendothelial system line the sinusoids of the red pulp and are important in the clearance of hematogenously borne bacteria in the nonimmune host. Lymphoid tissue found in the follicles and periarteriolar sheaths of the white pulp apparently plays an important role in producing early antibody in response to particulate antigens in the blood.

Since 1952 when the first report on postsplenectomy sepsis appeared, it has become clear that the risk for developing sepsis after splenectomy is not the same for all patients, but rather is related to a number of different variables. The age of the patient at the time of splenectomy is one such variable; the younger the patient at the time of splenectomy, the greater the risk of sepsis. The interval since splenectomy is another important variable; the risk is greater in the first few years after splenectomy and diminishes somewhat thereafter. Finally, the reason for which the splenectomy was performed influences the risk considerably; the risk is greater if splenectomy was performed because of some underlying disease that involves the reticuloendothelial system or the immune system than if splenectomy was performed because of trauma. Thus, the risk of developing postsplenectomy sepsis is much greater for the 3-year-old child with histiocytosis within the first few years after splenectomy than it is for the 50 year-old adult who had a traumatic splenectomy 20 years previously. Nevertheless, although the risk varies, it is clear that *any* patient who is missing his/her spleen carries some risk for postsplenectomy sepsis.

One reason so much attention has been focused on patients with postsplenectomy syndrome is the nature of their infections. As one would expect, patients without a spleen do well when infections are confined to mucosal surfaces or soft tissues. If bacteria invade the blood, however, a fulminant sepsis may develop. The episode of sepsis is usually characterized by subtle early clinical findings, a rapidly progressive course, and a high rate of mortality, even when treated with appropriate antibiotics. Pneumococci are responsible in one-half to two-thirds of cases. Meningococci, *Escherichia coli*, *Hemophilus influenzae*, and *Streptococcus pyogenes* account for most of the additional cases.

The physician who cares for the asplenic patient must be concerned with both preventing blood-borne bacterial infections and treating the episodes of sepsis once they occur.

Indications for Splenectomy. Splenectomy should be performed only when clearly indicated and with the knowledge that any patient who has had a splenectomy will have some finite future risk for postsplenectomy sepsis.

Conservative Management of Splenic Trauma. Although traditional therapy for traumatic injury to the spleen has been splenectomy, in recent years more conservative management aimed at preserving the spleen has been advocated. If possible, lacerations of the spleen are repaired. In some instances, if repair is not possible, partial splenectomy with preservation of the vascular pedicle is performed. Only when repair or partial splenectomy is not possible is total splenectomy for trauma indicated.

282

Immunization. Patients without a spleen should receive polyvalent pneumococcal vaccine. The current vaccine contains the polysaccharide capsules from the 23 pneumococcal serotypes most commonly responsible for bacteremic disease. Unfortunately, like most polysaccharide antigens, the pneumococcal vaccine is poorly immunogenic in children under the age of 2, the very ones with the greatest age-related risk for postsplenectomy sepsis. Nevertheless, pneumococcal vaccine should be given to all asplenic individuals over the age of 2.

Prophylactic Antibiotics. The question of whether to use prophylactic antibiotics, such as penicillin, in asplenic patients is difficult to answer, since not all splenectomized patients have the same likelihood of developing sepsis and, therefore, the risk-benefit ratio of prophylactic antibiotics is not easy to establish for the group as a whole. In addition, there have been no controlled studies performed to assess the effectiveness of antibiotic prophylaxis in these patients. Finally, once antibiotics are initiated, it is difficult to know when to discontinue their use.

Most physicians would agree that prophylactic oral penicillin (200,000 units bid) or oral ampicillin (50 mg/kg/day) is indicated for all asplenic children under the age of 5 regardless of the indication for splenectomy or the interval since splenectomy. A case can also be made for penicillin prophylaxis (400,000 units bid) in older children through adolescence, especially those patients in whom the splenectomy was performed for an underlying disorder involving the reticuloendothelial system, the immune system, or a malignancy and especially in the first few years after splenectomy.

Patient and Family Education. Neither immunization, prophylactic antibiotics or both used together will guarantee protection from postsplenectomy sepsis. For example, even though the patient may have received the pneumococcal vaccine, he may be challenged with pneumococcal serotypes not contained in the vaccine or with other bacterial species, such as *H. influenzae*. Similarly, the patient may not respond normally to the vaccine because of the underlying hematologic or immunologic condition for which the splenectomy was performed. Finally, even though the patient may be on prophylactic antibiotics, the possibility of infection with resistant pneumococci or other bacterial species still exists.

Thus, one of the most important elements in the care of the asplenic host is to counsel the patient and his family as to the role of the spleen in host defense and the relative risk that the given patient will develop sepsis. Armed with that information and with the knowledge that postsplenectomy sepsis is rapidly progressive and has an extremely high mortality rate, both the patient and the physician will be in a better position to assess any febrile episode and initiate early and intensive antibiotic therapy.

Treatment of Suspected Sepsis. It is difficult to recommend specific conditions under which the asplenic host should be admitted to the hospital and treated for sepsis. Each patient's risk is different, response to immunization will vary, compliance with prophylactic antibiotic regimens may not be known, and clinical symptoms and signs will necessarily be highly individual. Nevertheless, if there is any question that the asplenic child may be in the early stages of bacterial sepsis, he should be promptly treated and admitted to the hospital. It is hoped that as rapid diagnostic tests for bacterial pathogens become more widely available, they will offer help in deciding when to treat for sepsis.

The treatment for sepsis in the asplenic host is generally the same as for any other patient with sepsis. Special consideration should be given to the kinds of organisms responsible for postsplenectomy sepsis and to the fulminant nature of the sepsis and the high incidence of disseminated intravascular coagulation.

Indications for Splenectomy

WILLIAM H. ZINKHAM, M.D.

Over the years thousands of splenectomies have been perfomed for a variety of reasons. From this vast experience several important facts have emerged. First, the mortality associated with the procedure is extremely low. Second, splenectomy has been and continues to be the only effective form of therapy for certain medical and surgical disorders. And third, the benefits of the procedure should outweigh the risks of the patient developing the postsplenectomy syndrome. Medical and surgical conditions for which splenectomy may be indicated are the following.

Congenital Spherocytic Hemolytic Anemia. This entity comprises a heterogenous group of disorders in which an abnormality of spectrin and possibly other membrane proteins causes selective sequestration of red cells in the spleen. The spectrum of clinical severity is quite broad. Splenectomy is indicated in children with severe anemia requiring frequent transfusions. Whether and when to do a splenectomy in children with mild to moderate anemia is less clear. Splenectomy prevents the formation of gallstones, aplastic and sequestrative crises, and the development of leg ulcers. However, the risks of splenectomy and the postsplenectomy syndrome may exceed those associated with these complications.

Other Hemolytic Disorders. A variety of inherited red cell membranopathies (e.g., elliptocytosis) and enzymopathies (e.g., involving pyruvate kinase or hexokinase) may be associated with severe hemolysis. The decision to do a splenectomy should be based on transfusion requirements, the affect of the anemia on growth and development, and the frequency of aplastic or sequestrative crises.

Immunohematologic Disorders. The majority of children with idiopathic thrombocytopenic purpura or autoimmune hemolytic anemia recover spontaneously. However, life-threatening situations may arise, including serious bleeding or severe, recurrent anemia. If the patient fails to respond or cannot tolerate the dose of medication necessary to maintain remission, splenectomy should be performed. Splenectomy, therefore, is indicated only after medical management fails. A rare exception to this rule is the child with idiopathic thrombocytopenic purpura who early in the course of the disease develops signs of an intracranial hemorrhage. Under these circumstances, an emergency splenectomy may be life-saving and may also prevent crippling neurologic disturbances.

Hypersplenism. This term is applied to a heterogenous group of disorders characterized by varying degrees of cytopenia in the peripheral blood, a large spleen, and normal bone marrow. The blood abnormalities may be corrected by splenectomy or a shunting procedure in patients with portal hypertension. Rarely is the degree of anemia, thrombocytopenia, or leukopenia of sufficient severity to justify a splenectomy. Two major candidates for splenectomy are transfusion-dependent patients who have developed red cell antibodies—e.g., children with Cooley's anemia—and patients with splenic gigantism.

Malignant Tumors of the Spleen. Laparotomy with splenectomy remains the standard procedure for defining abdominal and pelvic malignant disease in patients with Hodgkin's disease. Alternative approaches under review are, e.g., subtotal splenectomy for staging and irradiation of the spleen without splenectomy. Both procedures have inherent risks; the first may fail to define malignant cells, and splenic atrophy may occur after splenic irradiation.

Splenic Gigantism. In some patients the spleen is enormous, ocuppying a large portion of the abdominal cavity. An appropriate description of this clinical situation is "splenomegalopolis." Splenic gigantism may occur in children with lysosomal storage diseases (e.g., Gaucher's disease, sea-blue histocyte syndrome), thalassemia major, hemangiomas, lymphangiomas, cysts, and hamartomas. In these patients the movement of the diaphragm is compromised, there is postprandial abdominal discomfort, and the risk of splenic rupture is great. In addition, most of these con-ditions are associated with a moderate to marked degree of pancytopenia. Thus, splenectomy may be beneficial for a variety of reasons.

Traumatic Rupture of the Spleen. In the past traumatic rupture was a major indication for splenectomy. The risk of postsplenectomy infection in subjects splenectomized after trauma is relatively low. Even so, alternative forms of therapy should be considered: nonoperative management of splenic injury, suturing of lacerated surfaces, and subtotal splenectomy or hemisplenectomy.

Lymphangitis

MAX L. RAMENOFSKY, M.D.

Lymphangitis is an inflammation of the lymphatic channels due to a local spreading distal infection. This was referred to in the past as "blood poisoning." Clinically lymphangitis is manifested as painful red streaks starting distally and moving proximally from the site of an infection. Regional lymph nodes are also usually affected.

In children, erysipelas is the most common cause, although deep puncture wounds are often incriminated. The most common organism is the group A beta hemolytic streptococcus, and consequently any bacterial therapy is directed at eradicating this organism. Other occasionally involved organisms are staphylococcus and the gram-negative organisms.

Treatment. The infection at the site of entry must be cleaned, cultured, drained (if indicated), and appropriately dressed. Initial antimicrobial therapy is penicillin, and the route of administration is dictated by the severity of the illness. Usually, oral penicillin V, 250 mg every 6 hours, is adequate for the child under 10 years of age. For the older child, 500 mg every 6 hours is a reasonable dosage. The child who is septic and toxic and whose disease process is rapidly progressing should receive parenteral penicillin G, 100,000 u/kg/day. Should the child be allergic to penicillin, erythromycin, 50 mg/kg/day in four divided doses is effective therapy. Antibiotics should be continued for 10 days and the physician should be alert for complications of streptococcal infection. Should staphylococcus be the offending organism, dicloxacillin, 50 mg/kg/day in four divided doses orally, or penicillinase-resistant beta-lactam antibiotic, 100 mg/kg/day IV, for severe infections should be used.

Puncture wounds deserve special attention when they result in lymphangitis. The puncture may have resulted in the inoculation of *Clostridium tetani,* which in the unimmunized child may be catastrophic. The puncture should be opened in a sterile fashion, irrigated, and dressed. If tetanus prophylaxis is not adequate, tetanus toxoid, 0.5 ml, or tetanus immune globulin, 250 units IM, should be given.

Patients at special risk for the development of lymphangitis as well as lymphadenitis are those in whom there is an abnormality of the lymphatic drainage system, such as lymphedema. The group A beta hemolytic streptococcus is a common offending organism in this situation, although gram-negative organisms are more frequently cultured than in patients who do not have lymphedema. The appropriate antimicrobial drug should be started depending on the results of the culture. Oral penicillin V at doses described previously should be the drug of choice until the cultures return.

Lymph Node Infections

(Lymphadenitis)

MAX L. RAMENOFSKY, M.D.

Lymph node enlargement is common in childhood and adolescence but quite rare in the newborn. The most common cause of a mass in the neck during childhood is an enlarged lymph node, and it must be differentiated from other congenital cystic cervical masses such as branchial cleft cyst, thyroglossal duct cyst, and cystic hygroma. Infectious causes should be differentiated from noninfectious causes such as hyperplasia or neoplasia. Lymph node infections are either acute, developing over a period of 2 to 3 days, or chronic, developing over weeks to months.

Lymph nodes anywhere in the body provide drainage from other more peripheral areas. The location of the node(s) will give one an indication of where to look for the primary infection. The most common inflammatory lesion of a cervical lymph node is suppurative lymphadenitis, which is generally an acute process. The most common chronic cervical lymph node infections are atypical mycobacterial lymphadenitis, tuberculous lymphadenitis, and cat-scratch disease.

ACUTE SUPPURATIVE CERVICAL LYMPHADENITIS

Acute suppurative lymphadenitis is generally thought to be secondary to bacterial entry at some distal site. In the child it is most common from the first to the eighth year. Prior to the penicillin era, the most common offending organism was group A beta-hemolytic streptococcus. At present, the most common organism is *Staphyloccus aureus,* with streptococcus occupying the second position, and gram-negative organisms and anaerobes being found with increasing frequency.

There is a sudden onset of a rapidly growing painful, red swelling in the neck, 2 to 3 days after an upper respiratory infection. The patient may be febrile and appear toxic. A leukocytosis is usual, with a left shift. At this point, unless the mass is fluctuant, needle aspiration or drainage is not recommended. A diligent search for the primary organ of entry should be done. In cervical lymphadenitis, sites to be carefully examined are the ears, the pharynx for tonsillitis or pharyngitis, and the oral cavity, particularly for dental caries and dental abscess. Therapy is started with an antistaphylococcal drug such as dicloxacillin sodium, 25 mg/kg/day orally, or a parenteral beta-lactamase–resistant semi-synthetic penicillin, 100 mg/kg/day IV in four divided doses for 10 days. At these dosages both staphylococci and streptococci are adequately covered. The use of the antibiotics for greater than the prescribed interval is to be discouraged, as prolonged use often results in a chronic granulomatous lymphadenitis that will neither resolve nor fluctuate.

The lesions should be followed at frequent intervals and the antibiotics continued for 10 days. If, however, the lesion softens and becomes fluctuant, incision and drainage are mandatory and should be carried out following the principles of adequate drainage with optimal cosmesis. The incision should be along Langer's lines in the neck, with insertion of a soft rubber drain and a collecting dressing. At the time of drainage an adequate culture and Gram stain should be done to identify the offending organism. Anaerobic cultures should be included in the examination.The antibiotic may be discontinued twenty-four hours after a lesion has been drained unless there is evidence of a spreading cellulitis. The drain should be removed when there is adequate saucerization of the wound.

On occasion organisms other than staphylococci and streptococci have been identified. Of particular note is the plague-causing organism *Yersinia pestis.* Tularemia is another cause of cervical lymphadenitis but is usually associated with an eye infection or skin ulceration. The treatment for *Yersinia pestis* is streptomycin, 30 mg/kg/day, or chloramphenicol sodium succinate, 50 mg/kg/day IV, in four divided doses for 10 days if the child is less than 8 years of age. For older children, tetracycline, 25 to 50 mg/kg/day in four divided doses, is effective therapy. Occasionally the involved nodes from plague or tularemia require incision and drainage but these nodes should not be drained until after 24 hours of antibiotic therapy.

CHRONIC LYMPHADENITIS

Most patients with chronic lymphadenitis have enlarged, nontender, asymptomatic cervical masses.

Mycobacterial Lymphadenitis. Most cases of

mycobacterial cervical lymphadenitis are no longer due to *Mycobacterium tuberculosis* but to nontuberculous mycobacteria (MOTT, mycobacteria other than tuberculosis). Cervical lymphadenitis due to *M. tuberculosis* is usually an extension of a primary pulmonary infection and thus involves the supraclavicular nodes. Cervical lymphadenitis due to atypical mycobacteria is thought to be a primary infection gaining entrance through the pharynx or tonsils and thus involves higher cervical nodes such as the submandibular group.

The nodes of the child with tuberculous lymphadenitis are generally large, matted, and asymptomatic. Evidence of pulmonary tuberculosis is frequently found when the cervical lymphadenopathy is encountered but progress of the disease from lymphadenitis to pulmonary tuberculosis is rare. Central necrolysis of the involved nodes with the development of sinus tracts is uncommon but may occur if the nodes have not been aspirated or were incompletely excised at biopsy.

MOTT infection occurs in high cervical lymph nodes, generally the submandibular group. Very rarely will there be extranodal involvement and then only in the child who is immunosuppressed either primarily or secondarily. The involved nodes are usually large, matted, fixed, and nontender. The nodes of MOTT are likely to break down spontaneously and drain externally with the development of sinus tracts.

Diagnosis. The diagnosis of *M. tuberculosis* can be aided by identification of pulmonary tuberculosis on chest films. Skin testing will identify most children with mycobacterial infections. Most of these children have a positive skin test to PPD-S, first strength. In children having atypical mycobacterial lymphadenitis this is not so. Use of first strength PPD-S in MOTT infections will yield negative or questionable results in over half of children tested. Second strength PPD-S may confirm infection due to MOTT.

Treatment. The treatment of tuberculous lymphadenitis is antituberculous chemotherapy. Regardless of how the diagnosis is made, antituberculous chemotherapy should be instituted and continued for 2 years unless a rifampin containing regimen is utilized. In this situation, 9 months of therapy are usually adequate to eradicate the infection. Complete resolution of the disease is to be expected, including cutaneous sinus tracts. Chemotherapeutic agents for tuberculous lymphadenitis are isoniazid, 10 to 20 mg/kg/day up to 300 mg daily, and rifampin, 10 to 20 mg/kg/day up to 600 mg daily.

The treatment of lymphadenopathy due to atypical mycobacteria is complete excision of the involved nodes including culture. Antituberculous chemotherapy is neither indicated nor necessary.

The vast majority of these children are cured, if all the involved nodes are removed.

CAT-SCRATCH DISEASE

Although the etiology of cat-scratch disease has never been proven, the infectious agent is thought to be a bacillus of the *Chlamydia* genus, other members of which cause lymphogranuloma venereum and psittacosis. Cat-scratch disease is the most common cause of chronic, nonbacterial lymphadenopathy.

The disease is generally transmitted by the scratch of a kitten, but monkeys and dogs as well as a thorny plant have been implicated in transmission. The animal carrier is not affected by the disease nor does it react with the antigen of cat-scratch disease.

Patients, when closely questioned, give a history of a minor scratch by a kitten 2 to 4 weeks before the onset of the lymphadenopathy. The inoculation site generally reveals a papule or blister. The most common sites of lymphadenopathy, corresponding to a distal inoculation site, are, in order of decreasing frequency, axillary, cervical, preauricular, submandibular, and epitrochlear.

Diagnosis. The diagnosis can be confirmed by a positive reaction to a skin test antigen prepared from the purulent aspirate of an involved node. As the antigen is not commercially available and difficult to obtain, the appropriate history with the findings of a chronic lymphadenitis allows a presumptive diagnosis of cat-scratch disease. Occasionally the diagnosis can be suspected from stains on involved lymph nodes which reveal gram-variable organisms.

Treatment. There is no chemotherapy available for this disease. Excision of the involved node is generally curative, but on occasion aspiration will allow the node to heal. However, observation alone will see the gradual subsidence of symptoms in most cases. Culture and histologic evaluation of the aspirated or excised material will exclude other causes of chronic lymphadenopathy. Supportive care for such symptoms as headache, malaise, fever, and vomiting is indicated.

Cat-scratch disease is self-limited, and complete resolution is to be expected.

Lymphedema

LEWIS B. HOLMES, M.D.

In infants and children lymphedema either is present at birth or develops during childhood, usually in the teenage years. The most common congenital form is Milroy's disease, which is due to an autosomal dominant gene. Lymphedema with late onset includes one type that involves a recurrent lymphangitis that can be prevented by antibiotic prophylaxis and another type that is associated with other anomalies, such as an extra row of eyelashes (distichiasis) and a widened spinal canal. Both these types of late-onset lymphedema are hereditary, each being due to a different autosomal dominant gene.

For all types of lymphedema, efforts should be made to control the swelling. As the lymphedema primarily involves the legs, the swelling can be controlled with elastic stockings. Unfortunately, many commerically available stockings are not strong enough to prevent swelling. Without adequate support the redundant skin folds can become abraded and infected.

Surgical reduction of the swollen extremity has not produced satisfactory results. The primary defect of lymphatic hypoplasia is not amenable to surgical repair at this time. Treatment with diuretics is not recommended.

The appearance of the untreated lymphedematous leg, as well as the support stockings, requires a major social adjustment. The affected child will need assistance in learning to facilitate periodic mechanical drainage of the legs, while maintaining activity as close to normal as possible. The social difficulties produced by chronic lymphedema require sympathetic long-term psychological assistance, as with any chronic illness.

Lymphangioma

MICHAEL B. LEWIS, M.D.

Most lymphangiomas are present at birth, and almost all have manifested themselves within 2 years. A significant number clinically disappear (not truly involute), and if the situation allows, the lesion should be observed over 6–36 months. Lymphangiomas are best thought of as lymphatic malformations containing endothelium-lined lymphatic tissue in the form of capillary, cavernous, or large cystic channels. They can cause skeletal overgrowth and distortion, especially in the head and neck region. Malignant change has not been reported.

The treatment of persistent lymphangiomas is surgical removal. The degree to which this is possible (i.e., the prognosis) is determined by the location and extent of the lymphangioma and the involvement of important neural, vascular, and skeletal structures. The timing of surgery depends upon the degree of aesthetic and functional impairment.

The head and neck are the most common sites of presentation. More than 50% of lymphangiomas occur in the neck, often with extension into the contiguous regions, including the mouth, medias-tinum, and axilla. They may transiently enlarge in association with upper respiratory infections. Very large and extensive lesions in this area can cause obstructive airway problems requiring tracheotomy.

Macrocheilia and macroglossia can be due to the capillary form of lymphangioma, which intimately involves all the tissue layers. In these cases incomplete excision to debulk and recontour is indicated.

Cystic lymphangiomas (cystic hygromas) of the head, neck, axilla, and mediastinum can often be completely excised. Surgery, however, can be lengthy and difficult because of the need to identify and preserve important neural and vascular structures. Temporary improvement can be obtained in these cases by aspiration of large cysts.

When the lymphangioma is extensive, involves the head and neck, and is associated with skeletal overgrowth and distortion, multiple surgical procedures are usually required and complete removal impossible. Residual disfigurement is likely.

If the lymphangioma involves the breast area in a female, surgery should be delayed, if possible, until breast development is complete so as not to injure the breast bud.

Radiation therapy, sclerosing therapy, and steroids have no role in the management of lymphangiomas.

Malignant Lymphoma

LUCIUS F. SINKS, M.D.

The lymphomas represent several different disorders having in common a neoplastic process involving lymph nodes. Included in this group are Hodgkin's disease, non-Hodgkin's lymphoma, and Burkitt's lymphoma.

HODGKIN'S DISEASE

This disease is very effectively treated and cured. In early stage disease (Stage I) (see Table 1), over 90% of the patients are expected to be cured. The therapy is radiotherapy alone or in conjunction with combination chemotherapy. Even though the therapy is effective, a number of clinical research trials are underway to refine it to ensure minimal long-range side effects. When dealing with children and adolescents with this disease, long-range side effects are of prime consideration. Such effects include secondary oncogenesis, growth impairment, breast atrophy, immune suppression, and sterility.

Stage I and II Disease. Early stage disease is usually treated by radiotherapy alone, with so-called extended fields to a dose of 3500 rads, based on the fact that the patient undergoes a staging laparotomy with splenectomy and that one is con-

Table 1. ANN ARBOR STAGING FOR HODGKIN'S LYMPHOMA

Stage I: Involvement of single lymph node regions (I) or single extralymphatic sites (1^e).

Stage II: Involvement of two or more lymph node regions on one side of the diaphragm (II), or localized involvement of extralymphatic organs or sites and one or more nodal regions on the same side of the diaphragm (IIe).

Stage III: Involvement of lymph node regions on both sides of the diaphragm, which also may be accompanied by localized involvement of extralymphatic organs or sites (IIIe) or, for example, spleen (III^s) or both (III^{s,e}).

Stage IV: Diffuse or disseminated involvement of one or more extralymphatic organs or tissues, with or without lymph node involvement.

Each stage is subclassified into A or B according to the presence or absence of constitutional symptoms. These are unexplained fever of 38°C or more, night sweats, and unexplained weight loss of more than 10% body weight. Superscripts, after laparotomy, are applied to indicate sites of involvement, e.g., liver, spleen, lung, bone marrow, pleura, bone, and skin, respectively.

---

fident that no occult disease is located beneath the diaphragm. Such surgical staging procedures are avoided in children under the age of 5 because of the fear of life-threatening sepsis.

There currently exists a rational concept of radiation to *involved* fields only in combination with multiple drug chemotherapy in stage II disease. This has the advantage that the patient can be staged by nonsurgical means and offers the advantage of reduced size of the radiation field. This is particularly important in avoiding breast tissue atrophy in the prepubescent female. The administration of systemic chemotherapy thus ensures that occult disease below the diaphragm that has escaped detection by nonsurgical techniques will be adequately treated. This approach is comparable to extended field radiation; however, it will be several years before we can appreciate the relative long-range toxicities of the two different approaches.

Stage III and IV. In the patient with defined stage III disease, the current therapy best utilized in this age group is multiple drug chemotherapy followed by radiotherapy at 3500 rads directed to bulky disease only. Such therapy is very effective in controlling disease for prolonged periods of time. Fortunately, a smaller proportion of young children and adolescents present with advanced stage disease.

Staging. The surgical staging technique is less desirable in situations where systemic chemotherapy is utilized; however, when performed, it involves a splenectomy, periaortic lymph node biopsy, liver biopsy, bone marrow biopsy, and if radiation to the pelvic area is anticipated, an attempt at oophoropexy is made to remove the ovaries from the intended field.

Nonsurgical staging is undergoing technologic improvement as CT scans mature and replace older methods of radiologic procedures, such as lymphangiograms, which are extremely difficult to perform in young children and should only be attempted by skilled personnel.

Combination Chemotherapy. The original successful multiple drug chemotherapy of nitrogen mustard, prednisone, procarbazine and vincristine (MOPP) has paved the way for a number of other equally successful and, in some cases, less toxic combinations. One such is CVPP, which includes lomustine (CCNU), Velban, prednisone, and procarbazine. This combination has been equally effective and is less toxic. It also avoids the potential carcinogen nitrogen mustard. This has become of increasing concern as a number of adults who have been re-treated for relapsing Hodgkin's disease with MOPP and radiotherapy have developed acute leukemia.

Dose and Schedule
 CVPP Schedule

	Day 1	CCNU (75 mg/m² po) Velban (4 mg/m² IV) procarbazine (100 mg/m²/day po) prednisone (40 mg/m²/day po)
Course 1 4	Day 8	Velban (4 mg/m² IV)
	Day 14	last day of procarbazine and prednisone
	Wait 2 weeks then start Courses 2, 3, 5, 6	

	Day 1	CCNU (75 mg/m² po) Velban (4 mg/m² IV) start procarbazine (100 mg/m²/day po) × 2 weeks
Course 2 3 5 6	Day 8	Velban (4 mg/m² IV)
	Day 14	procarbazine (100 mg/m² po)—Last day
	Wait 2 weeks, then start Course 3 Wait 2 weeks, then start Course 4	

NON-HODGKIN'S LYMPHOMA

This disease in children and adolescents is usually a diffuse histiocytic or lymphocytic process involving lymph nodes; rarely is there a focal histologic pattern. In this age group the disorder is much more rapidly progressive than in older people and has a great tendency to involve the

Table 2. STAGING OF NODAL AND EXTRANODAL DISEASE IN NON-HODGKIN'S LYMPHOMA IN CHILDREN*

Nodal	Stage	Extranodal
One area.	I	One single site.
Two or more areas either above *or* below diaphragm	II	One site + regional node. Two sites + regional nodes either above *or* below diaphragm
Two or more areas above *and* below diaphragm	III	Two or more sites above *and* below diaphragm
All extensive intrathoracic		All extensive intrathoracic
All extensive intra-abdominal		All extensive intra-abdominal
Central nervous system and/or bone marrow involvement	IV	Central nervous system and/or bone marrow involvement

* Memorial Hospital Staging System

bone marrow, thus producing a leukemia-like picture.

The progressive and systemic nature of this disease dictates that the evaluation and staging of the patient be swift and that systemic therapy be administered.

Staging is controversial and does not influence the choice of therapy as it does in Hodgkin's disease. Radiation therapy plays a lesser role than it does in Hodgkin's and is usually limited to radiating bulky disease.

A number of combination chemotherapy schedules have been tested. The LSA_2-L_2 combination described by Wollner and associates at the Memorial Hospital for Cancer and Allied Diseases, New York, has gained wide acceptance, and although difficult to administer, has been successful. The most recent review demonstrates an 80% disease-free survival curve for such children, with a median of $7\frac{1}{2}$ years. This includes all stages of disease (Table 2).

LSA_2-L_2 Schema with Drug Doses

INDUCTION PHASE. On the first day 1200 mg/m^2 cyclophosphamide are given in a single push injection to reduce the bulk of the tumor. Radiation therapy to the major site of primary disease is started either on the same day or within the next 3 days. On day 3 or 4, a 28-day course is started. This consists of daily oral prednisone, 60 mg/m^2; weekly intravenous injections of vincristine, 1.5–2.25 mg/m^2; intrathecal methotrexate, 6.25 mg/m^2, between the first and second vincristine injections, and two consecutive doses of intravenous daunomycin, 60 mg/m^2 each, between the second and third vincristine injections.

After completion of this 28-day course and while the prednisone dose is being tapered, two more intrathecal injections of methotrexate are given, 2 to 3 days apart.

CONSOLIDATION PHASE. This phase starts within 1 week from the last dose of intrathecal methotrexate and consists of a combination of 15 doses of cytosine arabinoside, 150 mg/m^2, intravenously daily (Monday through Friday) and thioguanine given orally, 75 mg/m^2, 8 to 12 hours after the injection of cytosine arabinoside. If the white blood count remains adequate on the fifth day of cytosine arabinoside, the patient continues to receive the same dosage of thioguanine over the weekend. However, both drugs are discontinued temporarily if there is bone marrow depression; this usually occurs after the initial seventh to tenth doses of the combination and ordinarily recovers within 7 to 10 days. Hence, the patient may receive more than 15 doses of thioguanine orally but may receive only 15 doses of intravenous cytosine arabinoside. This first phase of the consolidation averages 30 to 35 days.

The second consolidation phase starts immediately after completion of the 15 doses of cytosine arabinoside and entails the administration of L-asparaginase intravenously, 6,000 u/m^2 daily for a total of 12 injections. Within 2 to 3 days after the last injection of L-asparaginase, two more intrathecal injections of methotrexate are given. These are followed within a few days by an intravenous injection of 1,3-bis(2-chloroethyl)-1-nitrosourea (BCNU), 60 mg/m^2, which completes the consolidation. The average duration of induction and consolidation is 125 to 132 days.

MAINTENANCE PHASE. Maintenance starts 1 to 2 weeks after the end of consolidation and comprises 5 cycles of 5 days each, with intervals of 7 to 10 days between cycles.

The first cycle starts with oral thioguanine, 300 mg/m^2, for 4 days, followed by intravenous cyclophosphamide, 600 mg/m^2 on the fifth day. The second cycle consists of oral hydroxyurea, 2400 mg/m^2/day for 4 days, followed on the fifth day by daunomycin, 45 mg/m^2 intravenously. In the third cycle, oral methotrexate, 10 mg/m^2/day, is given for 4 days, followed on the fifth day by intravenous BCNU, 60 mg/m^2. The fourth cycle consists of daily injections of cytosine arabinoside, 150 mg/m^2 for 4 days, followed by the intravenous injection of vincristine, 1.5 mg/m^2 on Day 5. The fifth cycle consists only of two intrathecal injections of methotrexate, 6.25 mg/m^2 2 to 3 days apart. The sequence of cycles, beginning with thioguanine, is restarted after a 7- to 10-day rest period. Each of these five-cycle courses of therapy usually takes from 55 to 65 days.

The initial therapy of non-Hodgkin's lymphoma requires very careful clinical observation, to avoid life-threatening complications secondary to acute tumor lysis, such as uric acid stones and hyperkalemia, and other problems, such as sepsis and bleeding. In these patients allopurinol should be started at the time of diagnosis and the serum potassium levels should be carefully monitored to avoid sudden cardiac arrest.

The incidence of central nervous system (CNS) involvement in this disorder is quite high in patients with bone marrow involvement and a leukemia-like picture. Under these conditions, the treatment may be modified to utilize prophylactic CNS measures such as cranial radiation. If CNS disease is detected during treatment by demonstration of blast cells in the cerebrospinal fluid, then effective therapy such as cranial radiation and intrathecal methotrexate must be used.

Non-Hodgkin's lymphoma involving the bowel, usually the terminal ileum, is one of the few instances where surgery plays an important role. These tumors and usually a segment of bowel should be resected and then the patient treated with chemotherapy. Radiation is sometimes necessary if bulky disease is left and is nonresectable.

Non-Hodgkin's lymphoma may in unusual circumstances present as a primary tumor of bone and is often confused with Ewing's sarcoma. Therapy should involve radiotherapy to the primary lesion with systemic chemotherapy.

Burkitt's Lymphoma

IAN MAGRATH, MB, MRCP, MRC Path.

Burkitt's lymphoma is a B-cell lymphoid neoplasm that has a growth fraction approaching 100% and an actual doubling time of 2–3 days. Although these characteristics are responsible for the extremely rapid progression of this tumor— and the early demise of the untreated patient— they are also important factors in its responsiveness to a wide variety of chemotherapeutic agents and doubtless contribute to its curability. Rare patients with Burkitt's lymphoma have achieved prolonged survival after surgical resection of localized disease (usually in the small bowel) without further treatment, but the majority of patients in this situation rapidly develop recurrent disease unless treated with chemotherapy. Similarly, in about two-thirds of patients with localized disease treated only by irradiation, relapse occurs within or outside the radiation field. On the other hand, over 90% of patients with localized disease can be cured by chemotherapy. Thus, surgery or radiation should never be used as the sole treatment modalities. It appears that in the majority of cases the disease is widely disseminated from the outset, and chemotherapy is therefore the primary treatment modality.

The rapid proliferation and high growth fraction of Burkitt's lymphoma, coupled with the high spontaneous cell loss rate, have an additional consequence—the predisposition to hyperuricemia and uric acid nephropathy. Further, because of the rapid response to treatment, there is an additional risk of potentially fatal renal and electrolyte disorders from rapid tumor-cell lysis within hours or days of the initiation of specific chemotherapy. Thus, Burkitt's lymphoma can provide a difficult challenge to the chemotherapist, yet at the same time it is one of the most gratifying of tumors to treat, since about 60% of all patients, and possibly more, when treated with appropriate chemotherapy, can be expected to achieve prolonged disease-free survival—which doubtless constitutes cure.

BURKITT'S LYMPHOMA AS A MEDICAL EMERGENCY

Burkitt's lymphoma should always be treated as a medical emergency because of the very rapid growth rate of this tumor. A number of acute conditions may occur as a consequence of the presence of tumor at specific sites—for example, intestinal obstruction (including intussusception), gastrointestinal hemorrhage, partial occlusion of the upper airway, raised intracranial pressure, hemodynamic disturbances resulting from massive serous effusions, and renal failure from uric acid nephropathy or mechanical obstruction. Even in the absence of these complications, inappropriate delay in the initiation of therapy may result in the development of an emergency owing to continued increase in tumor bulk. Since the most important prognostic factor appears to be tumor volume, the long-term prognosis of individual patients may also be worsened by significant delays. Thus, it is critically important to accomplish all diagnostic and staging investigations as quickly as possible. At the National Cancer Institute (NCI), we have attempted to initiate treatment within 48 hours of the patient's admission, and it is rare that longer delays are necessary.

Perhaps the most common complication resulting from massive tumor burden is renal failure. Eighty to 90 percent of patients present with intraabdominal disease, and in patients with large abdominal masses there is a high chance of ureteric obstruction. These patients are also at high risk for hyperuricemia due to massive tumor bulk— the most common cause of renal failure prior to treatment. Renal involvement is also frequent, although the extent of its contribution to the problem is not clear. Chemical and mechanical factors often combine to produce oliguric renal failure, which is exacerbated by dehydration from any cause, or by hypovolemia, which may be present in patients with large serous effusions. Patients with diffuse marrow involvement also appear to be at particularly high risk for the development of uric acid nephropathy, although whether this is due exclusively to the high tumor burden or also signifies a biochemical difference in the tumor cells is not known. Other metabolic problems, such as hypercalcemia and hypoglycemia, have been described but are very rare.

It is essential that biochemical abnormalities be corrected, or at least partially corrected, prior to the commencement of therapy. Rapid tumor-cell lysis will further compromise renal function, and if an adequate diuresis has not been established profound hyperkalemia will ensue, with a high probability of death from cardiac arrest. At best, posttreatment renal failure is much more likely to occur. In patients with significantly elevated serum uric acid levels, alkaline diuresis should be established as soon as possible (aiming for at least 125 ml/m^2/hr). Diuretic such as furosemide, if necessary combined with chlorothiazides, should be used in patients in whom the intravenous infusion of fluids is not sufficient to establish diuresis. Patients with large serous effusions are particularly difficult to manage in this regard, since a significant portion of infused fluids enters the "third space" and it may be difficult to maintain normovolemia. The infusion of albumin or plasma protein solutions prior to giving a diuretic may permit the establishment of a diuresis in such circumstances.

In the rare patient with inferior vena cava or iliac vein thrombosis secondary to compression by tumor, fluid managment may be even more difficult, and the risk of pulmonary embolus is also significant. We have preferred to insert an occlusive device such as a Hunter-Sessions balloon in the inferior vena cava below the renal veins to prevent pulmonary embolization in patients with venous occlusion because of the significant risk of gastrointestinal hemorrhage associated with tumor involvement of the bowel wall, which could be exacerbated by anticoagulants. Acute gastrointestinal bleeding may occur at any time within the first 2–3 weeks of therapy as a consequence of tumor necrosis. The handling of such complex hemodynamic problems is considerably facilitated by the monitoring of pulmonary wedge capillary pressures, which can be performed after the insertion of a Swan-Ganz catheter.

Close monitoring of urinary output is mandatory in all high-risk patients, and if a good diuresis cannot be established prior to chemotherapy, it may be necessary to commence hemodialysis immediately. In such patients we have been able to initiate specific treatment immediately after the completion of a period of hemodialysis (usually 4–6 hours initially), but it should be borne in mind that cyclophosphamide can be dialyzed, so that whenever possible several hours should pass after the administration of intravenous cyclophospha-

mide before another period of hemodialysis is commenced.

As soon as the serum uric acid level has reached a normal or near-normal value, chemotherapy should begin.

SURGICAL TUMOR BULK REDUCTION

In the United States about 25% of patients with Burkitt's lymphoma present with disease confined to the gastrointestinal tract, almost always in the right iliac fossa. In such patients the tumor is frequently amenable to complete resection, and when tumor resection is followed immediately (i.e., within a few days) by chemotherapy they have an anticipated long-term survival rate in excess of 90%. Thus, during the initial investigations of a patient it is always appropriate to consider whether surgical resection of all overt disease can be accomplished. The size of the tumor is not necessarily a determinant of its resectability. Ovarian tumors, for example, although often reaching a very large size, may be readily resected, whereas tumors involving the retroperitoneal structures cannot usually be completely removed. Although it can be argued that patients in whom all tumor can be resected would have had a better prognosis even without resection, since they usually have a smaller tumor burden (although this is not always the case), the clear relationship between prognosis and total tumor burden supports the policy of reducing the tumor mass to an absolute minimum whenever possible. Available evidence suggests, however, that unless the tumor bulk can be reduced by a factor of 10, surgical resection is probably of little benefit. Thus, there is no point in attempting partial resection. In some circumstances surgical resection may have the added benefits of preventing the possibility of gastrointestinal hemorrhage from tumor necrosis after the commencement of therapy and reducing the risk of renal complications arising from acute tumor-cell lysis.

The resection of localized extraabdominal tumor as a therapeutic stratagem is rarely an issue. Since the prognosis in such patients is known to be very good without surgery, and in many cases (particularly with head and neck tumors) mutilating surgery would be necessary, there seems to be no role for resection in such patients. A possible exception to this might be localized testicular tumor, in which drug penetration is an issue and resection is therefore probably preferable to chemotherapy alone. However, this form of presentation is almost unknown.

MANAGEMENT OF THE RAPID TUMOR-CELL LYSIS SYNDROME

Patients at high risk for rapid tumor-cell lysis syndrome invariably have large tumor burdens. Apart from the obvious findings upon clinical examination, this may be manifested by diffuse marrow involvement or by markedly elevated serum lactate dehydrogenase, elevated uric acid, or elevated serum lactic acid levels. In patients in whom a good diuresis (at least 125 cc/m^2/hr, and preferably more) has been established and in whom serum uric acid has returned to a level of 8 mg/100 ml or less, chemotherapy should be initiated without delay. Ideally, tumor-cell lysis should be controlled and spread halted over a period of several days. In practice, however, there is no sure way of accomplishing this, although it seems reasonable to spread initial chemotherapy over a few days. Methotrexate should be avoided at the initiation of therapy, since severe toxicity will ensue in the presence of renal failure, and serous effusions may provide a reservoir for the drug, with resultant prolonged methotrexate excretion.

Careful attention to fluid and electrolyte balance is essential. It is advisable to omit potassium from intravenous fluids at the commencement of therapy, since tumor-cell lysis can result in very rapid release of intracellular potassium. In the peritreatment period, intravenous potassium should be administered only in the presence of significant hypokalemia, i.e., a serum potassium level of less than 3.0 mEq/l. Although bicarbonate is administered as part of the treatment of hyperuricemia, care should be taken not to induce a severe systemic alkalosis that would take some time to correct. Phosphates are less soluble in an alkaline urine, so withholding bicarbonate shortly before the commencement of therapy is preferable, and a urine pH of about 7.0 during initial therapy is probably optimal. Urinary output must be monitored on an hourly basis, since if oliguria ensues, biochemical abnormalities will be rapidly compounded, leading to a significant risk of death from cardiac arrhythmia. Serum blood urea nitrogen (BUN), creatinine, electrolytes, calcium, and phosphate should be monitored every few hours in order to follow the progress of tumor lysis. In the presence of good urine flow hyperkalemia is almost unknown, and hemodialysis is usually necessary only in the event of oliguria unresponsive to diuretics or for symptomatic hypocalcemia. Elevated serum phosphate levels and lowered serum calcium levels are manifestations of tumor lysis, but intravenous solutions of calcium should rarely be given for fear of exceeding the calcium-phosphate solubility product and precipitating soft tissue calcification.

Increases in serum phosphate, BUN, and creatinine levels may be detected within the first 24 hours of therapy, and hyperkalemia may be observed within hours of the initiation of therapy in patients in whom an adequate diuresis has not been established. Patients in whom biochemical changes consistent with rapid tumor lysis have not been observed within 3 days will not develop a significant tumor-cell lysis syndrome.

The complexity of the tumor-cell lysis syndrome and the necessity for close monitoring of hemodynamic status, fluids, and electrolytes, as well as the potential for cardiac arrhythmias from hyperkalemia or hypocalcemia, are sufficient grounds for carrying out the initial chemotherapy of patients with large tumor burdens in an intensive care unit where careful biochemical, cardiac, and hemodynamic monitoring can be accomplished.

SPECIFIC CHEMOTHERAPY

A broad spectrum of agents are active in Burkitt's lymphoma, but among the most effective drugs are cyclophosphamide, methotrexate, vincristine, and probably Adriamycin. There is no doubt that combination chemotherapy is superior to single-agent therapy, and all of the most successful drug regimens include at least four or five drugs. In some centers epipodophyllotoxins, cytosine arabinoside (ara-C), and carmustine (BCNU) have been included in chemotherapeutic protocols, but the precise role of these individual agents and the optimal drug combination have not yet been determined.

At the NCI we have utilized a regimen containing a combination of cyclophosphamide (1200 mg/m^2), vincristine (1.4 mg/m^2), Adriamycin (40 mg/m^2), and prednisone (40 mg/m^2 daily for 5 days) followed 10 days later by an infusion of methotrexate over 42 hours, with immediate leucovorin rescue. A loading does of methotrexate—300 mg/m^2—is given in the first hour of the infusion and 60 mg/m^2 over each of the remaining 41 hours. Leucovorin, 48 mg/m^2, is given at the end of hour 42, then 12 mg/m^2 every 6 hours until the serum methotrexate level is below 5×10^{-8} M. In the first cycle of therapy only cyclophosphamide and methotrexate are given systemically. Cycles are repeated as soon as marrow recovery (defined as a granulocyte count of more than 1500/mm^3) has occurred, since short intervals between treatments are essential in managing this rapidly proliferating tumor. In this protocol we continue therapy for 15 cycles in patients with extensive disease, a designation that includes all patients except those with a single extraabdominal tumor site or a completely resected intraabdominal tumor. It is probable, however, that fewer cycles would be as effective. The interval between the cyclophosphamide-containing combination and methotrexate is increased to 14 days after the first six cycles of therapy. Prophylactic treatment, designed to prevent spread of disease to the central nervous system (CNS) and consisting of repeated doses of intrathecal ara-C and methotrexate, is given to all patients. Such intrathecal therapy may not be necessary for most patients with abdominal tumor that has been completely resected, but relapse confined to the CNS has occasionally been reported in such patients, and it is therefore prudent to provide some intrathecal therapy for this subgroup.

The NCI treatment protocol has resulted in prolonged disease-free survival in approximately 60% of patients and appears to be among the best reported regimens for the treatment of Burkitt's lymphoma. Patients with totally resected intra-abdominal tumors have a very good prognosis—in excess of 90%—while only about 25–30% of patients with diffuse marrow involvement are likely to achieve prolonged survival. Similarly, the majority of patients with CNS disease at presentation are likely to relapse, although a few such patients can achieve prolonged survival if given intensive systemic therapy combined with intrathecal treatment.

There are a number of unresolved questions regarding the specific therapy of Burkitt's lymphoma. Many of these, including the role of anthracyclines in combination therapy, the value of additional drugs, the optimal duration of therapy, and the role of radiation therapy in addition to systemic chemotherapy for localized disease, may be answered by currently ongoing clinical trials. Burkitt's lymphoma is, however, a rare disease, so that few trials have sufficient numbers of patients for differences found between treatment methods to achieve high levels of statistical significance. Nevertheless, the overall results in a number of recent clinical trials carried out in the United States and Europe indicate that with aggressive combination chemotherapy regimens, between 50 and 75% of all patients, and at least 90% of patients with limited disease, should achieve prolonged survival, which in this disease is synonymous with cure.

CENTRAL NERVOUS SYSTEM INVOLVEMENT

Involvement of the meninges and cranial nerves in Burkitt's lymphoma at the time of presentation is relatively rare in the United States and Europe. Paraplegia, a quite common presenting feature of patients in Africa, is also extremely uncommon outside that continent. Thus, there is essentially no possibility of establishing optimal treatment by means of classical clinical trials. There is no doubt, however, that the intrathecal administration of ara-C and methotrexate can result in cure of CNS involvement. At the NCI we have adopted regimens consisting of 2 or 3 days of ara-C followed by a single day of methotrexate intrathecally, both for the treatment of overt disease and for the prevention of CNS spread. With this approach, isolated CNS relapse as the first sign of recurrence has been quite uncommon (below 5%).

Although the delivery of intrathecal therapy via an Ommaya reservoir has a number of theoretical advantages, it has not been clearly established to be superior to the instillation of drugs into the lumbar sac in the treatment or prevention of CNS disease in Burkitt's lymphoma. Further, cranial or craniospinal irradiation does not have a defined role in either the treatment or the prevention of CNS disease. In fact, a trial of the value of craniospinal irradiation in preventing spread of Burkitt's lymphoma to the CNS that was carried out in East Africa did not show an advantage to this approach. Thus, cranial or craniospinal irradiation cannot be recommended as an appropriate means of CNS prophylaxis. Patients in whom intrathecally administered drugs have failed to prevent the development of CNS relapse are often treated with cranial vault or craniospinal irradiation, since few alternatives are available. Even in this situation, however, there is no evidence, other than anecdote, of its value. Similarly, patients with facial palsy or paraplegia are usually irradiated because of the high risk of permanent neurologic impairment in such patients. In such circumstances, because of the added toxicity with combined modality therapy, including significant impairment of marrow reserves in the case of irradiation of the spinal column, radiation should be considered only as an emergency measure and is best limited to a total dose of approximately 1500 rads.

Placement of an Ommaya reservoir for delivery of intraventricular methotrexate and ara-C in patients with CNS relapse after intensive intrathecal therapy is a reasonable approach (although of unproved value) because of the failure of the lumbar instillation of drugs to prevent CNS spread. More experimental approaches to the prevention or treatment of CNS disease in Burkitt's lymphoma include very high doses of intravenous methotrexate or ara-C. The value of such regimens is unknown at present.

HIGH-DOSE THERAPY IN RECURRENT BURKITT'S LYMPHOMA

In the United States and Europe, patients who develop recurrent systemic Burkitt's lymphoma have an extremely poor prognosis. Essentially all patients ultimately succumb from progressive disease if treated with conventional doses of drugs. However, the use of high-dose cyclophosphamide-containing regimens, particularly the BACT regimen consisting of BCNU, ara-C, cyclophosphamide (at four times the dose used in conventional treatment regimens), and 6-thioguanine, has clearly resulted in the survival of a proportion of patients—between 25 and 30%—with recurrent disease, and high-dose therapy must, therefore, be considered the treatment of choice for such patients. The BACT regimen has been administered without bone marrow reinfusion or transplantation, but intensive support of infectious complications is required, and there is a significant risk of fatal myocardial necrosis. A role for total-body irradiation has not been clearly demonstrated in high-dose regimens; therefore, treatment requiring allogeneic marrow transplantation should be considered experimental. A small number of patients with recurrent disease have, however, been successfully treated in this way. The risk of graft-versus-host disease with allogeneic marrow transplantation and the theoretical risk of the reinfusion of tumor cells with autologous cryopreserved marrow should be weighed in the balance when considering the optimal approach to the treatment of patients with relapse. Although monoclonal antibody "purging" of autologous marrow—i.e., the removal of cryptic Burkitt's lymphoma cells—may now be feasible, its value depends upon the efficacy of the treatment approach it is used with, and to date no regimen for the relapsed patient has been demonstrated to be superior to BACT.

FUTURE APPROACHES TO THERAPY

No form of immunotherapy has yet been shown to be of value in Burkitt's lymphoma. The in vivo use of monoclonal antibodies directed against B-cell antigens has the potential disadvantage that normal B-cells may also be destroyed. Such approaches should be reserved for patients in whom all reasonable chemotherapeutic approaches have failed. Interferon and other biological response modifiers have also not been evaluated in Burkitt's lymphoma.

Of considerable potential interest to the development of novel treatment approaches are the specific chromosomal translocations involving chromosome 8, the location of the *c-myc* oncogene, and one of the immunoglobulin gene loci on chromosome 14, 2, or 22. As more is learned about the molecular changes associated with these chromosomal translocations, it is not inconceivable that a means may be found whereby the consequences of the genetic abnormalities can be nullified. Although we are very far from such an approach at the present time, the possiblity that treatment directed toward the specific genetic abnormality may contribute to the management of Burkitt's lymphoma in the future is a real one. Because of the extremely high rate of cellular proliferation in this tumor, however, the difficult management problems encountered at the time of presentation in patients with extensive tumors will still exist, and it seems unlikely that circumvention of the genetic abnormality will be of value in inducing remission. If such an approach ever proves feasible, it is more likely to be used to prevent tumor regrowth after the induction of remission by cytotoxic drugs.

9

Endocrine System

Hypopituitarism

LOUIS E. UNDERWOOD, M.D.

Growth Hormone

In mid 1985 it was learned that 3 young adults who had received growth hormone (GH) therapy years earlier had died of degenerative neurologic disease. It is suspected that these individuals had contracted Creutzfeldt-Jakob disease (CJD), a "slow virus" infection affecting the gray matter of the brain. Because of concern that one or more batches of the National Hormone and Pituitary Program GH that these patients had received was contaminated with the pathogen for CJD, distribution of pituitary GH from all sources was discontinued. Approval of biosynthetic GH for the treatment of GH deficiency is anticipated at an early date. The dosage of GH most commonly used in the United States is 0.1 unit/kg body weight 3 times weekly. The growth response is a function of the log of the GH dose. While larger doses of GH are often desirable, their use is usually not possible because of the limited supplies currently available. GH has almost always been given intramuscularly, but recent studies indicate that subcutaneous injections are equally effective. GH-deficient children typically increase their growth rate from 3.5–4.0 cm/yr before treatment to 8.0–10.0 cm/yr during the first year of therapy. Young children usually respond better than adolescents; the obese respond better than the thin; and severely GH-deficient children respond better than those with partial deficiencies. As treatment is continued, the rapid growth that occurs early in therapy declines, so that after 2–4 years the growth velocity may be below average for age and developmental status.

If the growth response to GH therapy is inadequate, several possible causes should be considered. These include (a) incorrect diagnosis, (b) failure to administer the GH properly, (c) formation of growth-attenuating antibodies to GH, (d) development of hypothyroidism, and (e) intercurrent illness. The frequency with which GH antibodies develop during therapy depends on the GH preparation used. With high-quality preparations, it is as low as 5%. Such antibodies only rarely reach high enough concentrations to attenuate growth. If attenuation occurs, growth is usually restored by using another GH preparation.

Hypothyroidism

Most children with hypopituitarism are not clinically hypothyroid, but some may have serum thyroxine levels below the normal range. Modest doses of L-thyroxine (3 µg/kg) are given to children with subnormal serum thyroxine. Approximately 5–10% of patients receiving GH develop hypothyroidism. The cause of this phenomenon is unclear, but it may cause attenuation of the growth response to GH and should be treated by the administration of L-thyroxine.

Adrenal Insufficiency

Symptoms of hypoadrenalism are uncommon in children with hypopituitarism. Therefore, we usually do not prescribe glucocorticoids unless the patient has syncope, postural hypotension, attacks of hypoglycemia, or laboratory evidence of loss of pituitary-adrenal axis function as a result of pituitary-hypothalamic surgery (loss of function due to therapy) or x-ray therapy. Because excessive doses attenuate the growth response to GH, we administer glucocorticoids cautiously (approximately 10 mg/m^2 body surface area/day). Pharmacologic doses of glucocorticoids (approximately 50 mg/m^2) are given during periods of stress to any child with hypopituitarism who shows evidence of impaired pituitary-adrenal axis function (i.e., impaired response to metyrapone or to injections of ACTH).

Diabetes Insipidus

Deficiency of antidiuretic hormone is uncommon in children with idiopathic hypopituitarism but occurs frequently after pituitary-region surgery. It is effectively treated by administering desmopressin (DDAVP)* intranasally in a dosage of 0.05–0.1 ml one to two times daily. The dosage schedule of this agent must be individualized.

Gonadotropin Deficiency

Boys with prenatal-onset hypopituitarism may have micropenis (stretched penis <3 cm in length). This should be treated early in life, when it is easier to normalize penile size. We give 50 mg of testosterone enanthate intramuscularly and evaluate the response after 1 month. If results are not satisfactory, this treatment can be repeated 2 or 3 times.

In boys with hypopituitarism who fail to undergo puberty by 14 years of age we prefer long-acting testosterone enanthate intramuscularly. We begin treatment with 50 mg/month and gradually increase the dosage over several years to 300 mg every 3 weeks. Androgens usually augment the growth response to GH but often produce suboptimal growth of beard and sexual hair. Enlargement of the testes during therapy is taken as evidence of endogenous gonadotropin secretion, and testosterone therapy is discontinued.

In girls requiring estrogen replacement we begin conjugated estrogen (0.3–0.6 mg daily) or ethinyl estradiol (0.05 mg). After 9 to 12 months of continuous estrogen therapy, cycling with a progestational agent is begun.

Outcome

If GH treatment is begun in the first 2 to 3 years of life, an adult height within the normal range can be anticipated. Delays in diagnosis and suboptimal therapy will compromise the final adult height. Because of these, many patients treated in the past have not achieved heights above the 3rd percentile.

Delayed emotional development and problems in coping are common in GH-deficient children. These result from infantilization and low expectations on the part of those who come into contact with these children. Counseling of parents and affected patients is usually beneficial, and sometimes essential.

The Future. Biosynthetic methionyl hGH prepared by recombinant DNA techniques has been shown to be as effective as pituitary GH in the stimulation of growth of hypopituitary children. Once approved for sale, it will serve as the source of unlimited GH. Synthetic growth hormone re-

* Safety and efficacy of intranasal desmopressin have not been established in children under 3 months of age.

leasing factor (GRF) also holds promise as a treatment modality. Growth hormone releasing factor stimulates GH secretion in children with hypopituitarism in whom GH deficiency is due to a hypothalamic lesion. In preliminary studies GRF appears to stimulate growth in such children.

Short Stature

STEPHEN BURSTEIN, M.D., Ph.D.

Short stature is a nonspecific finding. It may represent the first manifestation of a serious disorder or it may be medically inconsequential. Whatever its etiology, short stature is of frequent parental concern because of its protean psychological, social, and economic implications; in extreme cases, it may impose physical limitations.

Unless there has been recent growth failure, it is usually unwarranted to pursue anything but a cursory evaluation of a child whose stature is above the 3rd percentile when corrected for parental heights. To attempt augmentation of height in such patients is meddlesome at best. The relationship of bone age, chronologic age, and height may be used with growth rate to categorize the causes of short stature. These variables may also be used to predict ultimate stature with fair accuracy using the tables of Bayley and Pinneau, which are found in the Greulich and Pyle atlas.

Medications Used to Augment Growth

The therapeutic modalities available for the augmentation of height in patients without an underlying endocrine, metabolic, or systemic disease include the administration of growth hormone and of sex steroids and their congeners, the anabolic steroids.

Growth Hormone Therapy. In April of 1985 the distribution of pituitary-extracted human growth hormone was temporarily halted by the National Hormone and Pituitary Program of the National Institutes of Health. It is suspected that several cases of Creutzfeldt-Jakob disease resulted from contamination of the hormone with the causative prion. Commercial suppliers were later requested to suspend shipment by the Food and Drug Administration. It is unlikely that pituitary-extracted human growth hormone will be available for clinical use for some time. The prospect of unlimited quantities of biosynthetic methionyl human growth hormone will alleviate the resultant shortage and remove the practical constraint that now restricts growth hormone therapy to clear-cut, documented growth hormone deficiency. Nonetheless, experience in its use for other than complete growth hormone deficiency is limited; its use in other conditions to augment height must be considered experimental. Administration of growth hormone for these purposes should be confined to those settings in which its effects can be assessed in carefully controlled clinical trials with informed parental consent as a part of a clinical research program approved by an institutional review board. It is not known whether ultimate stature is increased by its use in conditions other than growth hormone deficiency. While developments in this field are occurring rapidly, it is unlikely that the experimental nature of growth hormone therapy for these purposes will change within the next several years.

Doses of growth hormone used by most investigators range from the usual replacement dose of 0.08 IU/kg three times weekly to about 2.5 IU/kg on the same schedule, intramuscularly or subcutaneously. The lower replacement dose was dictated by the limited supply of hormone extracted from human pituitaries. With increased availability of the biosynthetic form, we can expect higher doses to be employed more commonly.

Although somatomedin-C levels tend to rise during growth hormone therapy, growth rate does not seem to correlate with the magnitude of this response, and it is doubtful that serial measurements of somatomedin-C during the course of growth hormone therapy contribute to the management of these patients.

There are a number of possible side effects of growth hormone therapy. These include the induction of growth hormone–neutralizing antibodies in about half the patients treated; they interfere with growth in about 1% of patients. There is concern that subcutaneous administration might increase the incidence of such antibodies. Patients also develop demonstrable insulin resistance and at higher doses some glucose intolerance. Hypothyroidism occasionally complicates the administration of growth hormone in patients with growth hormone deficiency; its pathogenesis is poorly understood, but it is possible that the administration of growth hormone to patients who are not growth hormone deficient might similarly induce hypothyroidism. Because of these possibilities, anti–growth hormone antibody titers, fasting glucose levels, and thyroid function should be assessed every three to six months. It is conceivable that coarse facies and other acromegalic findings might occur when high doses of growth hormone are employed.

Androgens and Anabolic Steroids. These medications should be used cautiously, especially in the prepubertal child. While growth rate may be augmented, it is controversial whether these agents can achieve increases in growth rate without at least commensurate advancement of skeletal maturation, and ultimate stature may be compromised. Therefore skeletal maturation should be assessed

twice yearly during their administration. It is prudent to allow the child to achieve a bone age of 10 before considering therapy with these agents. Parenteral therapy with repository testosterone enanthate or cypionate is probably more convenient and safe than therapy with the orally effective androgens. Low doses may be administered monthly, and there may be less danger of hepatic toxicity. Oxandrolone is an orally active anabolic steroid, an androgen analog, that is commonly used.

Doses of these agents depend on clinical circumstances. When used in prepubertal or early pubertal boys, lower doses should be employed to maximize growth: 50 mg/m^2 per month of depot testosterone or 0.1 mg/kg daily of oxandrolone will promote growth without undue virilization. When virilization is desired, the dose may be raised to 100 mg/m^2 per month; growth appears to be about the same on this as on the lower dose.

In the case of diagnosed male hypogonadism, two to three years of therapy at this dose will assure fulfillment of growth potential and pubertal progression without attainment of full sexual potency. If the diagnosis of hypogonadism is not established in boys with pubertal delay, androgen or anabolic steroid therapy should be administered for 6 months interspersed with 6-month periods of observation for diagnostic purposes. A fully virilizing dose of depot testosterone is 200 mg given every 2 weeks; orally active androgens and anabolic steroids do not appear to be fully virilizing.

Androgens and anabolic steroids should be used with circumspection in girls to avoid virilization. In short, hypogonadal girls, such as those with Turner's syndrome, a 6-month course of depot testosterone at 30 mg/m^2 per month after a bone age of 10 years is achieved promotes growth and pubic hair development without clitoral hypertrophy or undue bony maturation. Oxandrolone, 0.1 mg/kg daily, is also used for this purpose. Thereafter, estrogen therapy is instituted (see below).

Side effects are occasionally a problem. The more common include virilization in girls and prepubertal boys, hypercholesterolemia, sodium and water retention with edema, and hypercalcemia. In the case of the orally active agents, all of which are 17-alkylated, cholestatic jaundice has been reported occasionally and hepatocellular neoplasms and peliosis hepatatis rarely.

Estrogens. Estrogens also promote growth, but they are thought to give less skeletal growth for degree of skeletal maturation. They are never employed in males because they cause gynecomastia.

Short, hypogonadal girls with bone age greater than 10 years are usually treated for 6 months with low doses of androgens or anabolic steroids at first to maximize growth. An anabolic dose of repository estradiol cypionate with which to initiate estrogen therapy is 0.5 mg monthly. The orally active estrogen ethinyl estradiol, 5 μg orally daily for three weeks per month (there is no commercial preparation of ethinyl estradiol that provides such a low dose), may be employed instead. If pubertal progression is slow thereafter, these doses may be gradually raised. Girls who are hypogonadal will require cyclic estrogen and progestin therapy after the first year of estrogen therapy or when they begin to experience estrogen withdrawal bleeding. A fully feminizing dose is 3.0–5.0 mg of depot estradiol intramuscularly monthly used with cyclic progestin therapy. A 5-day course of medroxyprogesterone acetate 5 mg orally on the 15th to 19th days of the month induces progestin withdrawal bleeding 3 to 7 days later. About 30 to 50 μg of ethinyl estradiol orally three weeks per month with cyclic progestin therapy is approximately equivalent. After growth potential has been fulfilled, the patient may find cyclic low-dose birth control pills a more convenient therapy for maintaining feminization.

Side effects include thrombotic complications and hypertension. The lower doses possible with parenteral therapy may minimize their incidence.

The Therapy of Specific Causes of Short Stature

Attenuated Growth. Those children who are growing at a subnormal rate and have proportionate height and skeletal maturational retardation almost always have a diagnosable endocrine, metabolic, or systemic disease. Their growth retardation remits if they are promptly treated. Treatment of the endocrinopathies responsible for this growth pattern, including growth hormone deficiency, hypothyroidism, Cushing's syndrome, and hypogonadism, are discussed in other sections. There is no evidence that treatment with growth hormone or sex steroids can promote the growth of these children if their underlying disease continues to interfere with growth.

GROWTH FAILURE RELATED TO ABNORMALITIES OF GROWTH HORMONE SECRETION OR ACTION. There has been increasing recognition of a group of short children with incomplete growth hormone deficiency. These children may have partial growth hormone deficiency on the basis of a limited pituitary secretory reserve, or they may have abnormalities in the control of growth hormone secretion that result in altered and decreased release. The demonstration of these abnormalities requires frequent sampling of spontaneous, usually sleep-associated, growth hormone secretion. Replacement doses of growth hormone appear to ameliorate this situation.

Although bioactive growth hormone was pro-

posed early as the cause of attenuated growth in children who appear to be otherwise normal, there has been only one convincing demonstration of a patient with normal blood levels of a growth hormone molecule by radioimmunoassay who had decreased biological activity and an abnormal structure. This must be one of the rarer causes of attenuated growth.

Intrinsic Shortness. In its uncomplicated form, these small-bodied children are growing at a rate within the normal range and usually have skeletal maturation normal for their chronologic age. It is not yet clear whether treatment with growth hormone will increase the ultimate stature of such children. As time goes on, we can expect increasing doses of growth hormone to be employed in an attempt to promote the growth of such children. It appears likely that high doses of growth hormone might be effective in these children, but whether side effects supervene at an unacceptable rate will be critical.

GENETIC SHORT STATURE ON A FAMILIAL BASIS. A number of trials of growth hormone therapy in short children with no readily diagnosable pathology have included a few children who might belong to this diagnostic category. They appear to be relatively unresponsive to the usual replacement dose. Until appropriate clinical trials are conducted, it would be unwarranted to treat these children with growth hormone in other than a research setting. Furthermore, since these children mature at a normal rate unless they have some element of delayed growth, androgen or anabolic steroid therapy appears to offer little psychological benefit to them and might compromise their ultimate stature.

TURNER'S SYNDROME. High doses of growth hormone (on the order of 0.2 IU/kg three times weekly) increase the growth rate of girls with Turner's syndrome. Androgen therapy also increases their growth rate. The use of growth hormone and androgens in combination appears to be synergistic. Depot testosterone at a low dose for six months promotes growth without advancing bone age unduly; oxandrolone is also widely used. Whether either growth hormone or androgen treatment or their combination increases ultimate stature is controversial. Girls with Turner's syndrome require estrogen replacement therapy for feminization at an appropriate time. See Androgens and Anabolic Steroids and Estrogens above for specific recommendations.

POSTNATAL GROWTH RETARDATION FOLLOWING INTRAUTERINE GROWTH RETARDATION. This category includes a heterogeneous group of disorders, such as intrauterine infections, some genetic syndromes, and intrauterine undernutrition. Carefully controlled trials of growth hormone or androgens are still necessary in most of these conditions. Preliminary studies report variable responses to either treatment. Children with the Russell-Silver syndrome might respond to high doses of growth hormone or androgens, but height predictions for these children must be offered cautiously, since their retarded bone ages usually rapidly advance when they go into puberty at a normal time.

OTHER CAUSES. Children with Down's syndrome grow at a faster rate when treated with anabolic steroids, but their ultimate stature is probably not increased. Children with skeletal dysplasias might benefit from high-dose growth hormone therapy, but the question of whether ultimate stature will be increased is a real consideration for them. Of even greater concern in the case of children with achondroplasia is whether rapid or augmented growth will exacerbate the orthopedic and neurologic problems that frequently complicate their course.

Delayed Growth. CONSTITUTIONAL DELAY IN GROWTH AND DEVELOPMENT. Children with the pure form of this disorder have bone ages that are proportionately delayed compared with their height age. Both their growth and skeletal maturational retardation develop during infancy and early childhood, and the age of puberty is typically delayed in proportion to their skeletal maturational delay. Frequently there is a family history of such a growth pattern. This formal diagnosis appears to include a heterogeneous group of disorders, and it may include some children with incomplete forms of growth hormone or gonadotropin deficiency. Most of the studies of growth hormone therapy in apparently normal, short children with delayed bone ages, the so-called "normal variant short stature" syndrome, seem to include primarily children with constitutional delay in growth and development. Although about half of such children appear to respond to the usual replacement dose of growth hormone, it is not known whether their ultimate stature is increased. Use of growth hormone in these children at these or higher doses must still be considered experimental. Such children with good growth potential are best managed by reassurance, since ultimate outcome is usually excellent. When short stature or pubertal delay is psychologically damaging or persists after 14 years in boys and 13 years in girls (these ages are about 2 SD above the mean), a 6-month course of exogenous sex steroids may ameliorate social difficulties. The doses employed at first are low. See Androgens and Anabolic Steroids and Estrogens above for specific recommendations. Some authorities believe such a 6-month course may induce puberty; if puberty does not ensue, further evaluation for hypogonadism is indicated.

Tall Stature

NANCY J. CHAREST, M.D.,
and JUDSON J. VAN WYK, M.D.

Tall stature is generally considered an asset in our society, and most tall children accept their height without difficulty. Occasionally, however, an extremely tall girl is disturbed by her discrepant size and has visions of reaching adulthood with unacceptably tall stature. More commonly, however, it is not the girl who is disturbed but her mother, who is also tall. The mother remembers her adolescence as traumatic and would like to spare her daughter a similar painful experience.

It has been recognized for over 30 years that the administration of high doses of estrogen to these girls will cause immediate slowing of their growth rate and attenuate their adult stature. Much controversy, however, has surrounded the use of these potentially hazardous agents for the treatment of healthy girls for a condition that many would consider to be a problem of social adaptation to culturally determined norms. It is our policy not to consider treatment of a tall girl unless her height is predicted to be truly excessive (never less than 183 cm), and the child, her parents, and physician agree that the potential psychological benefit to the child outweighs the risks of treatment.

Indications for Treatment

The overwhelming majority of healthy tall children have familial tall stature. A thorough history and physical examination should rule out the rare disorders associated with tall stature—Marfan's syndrome, cerebral gigantism (Soto's syndrome), Beckwith-Wiedmann syndrome, sexual precocity, and virilizing disorders. Excessive production of pituitary growth hormone is more difficult to exclude, however, since some extremely tall children with no signs or symptoms of acromegaly exhibit a paradoxical increase in serum growth hormone after challenges with oral glucose or thyrotropin-releasing hormone. Such responses were previously thought to occur only in patients with growth hormone–secreting pituitary adenomas. In a 6-month trial Job et al. (J. Clin. Endocrinol. Metab. *58*:1022, 1984) found bromocryptine to be effective in reducing the adult height prediction in a small series of such children. Should further investigation confirm these results, tests of growth hormone dynamics should be routinely included in the workup of children with excessive stature. Furthermore, bromocryptine should be considered as an alternative to estrogen therapy for those girls found to have abnormal growth hormone responses but no demonstrable pituitary adenomas.

Because an accurate adult height prediction is critical to the decision for treatment, height should be meticulously measured against a wall-mounted stadiometer by an experienced observer. Bone age should be determined from either the Greulich and Pyle or the Tanner atlas. We make our height predictions from the Bayley and Pinneau tables found at the back of the Greulich and Pyle atlas, although others prefer to use the Roche-Wainer-Thissen or Tanner-Whitehouse 2 methods. Because these height predictions, which have a standard deviation of almost 4 centimeters at 9 years of age, become more accurate as the bone age advances, we reevaluate at 6-month intervals those girls who are interested in treatment but whose prediction is below our arbitrary limit of 183 centimeters (72 inches).

Contraindications to estrogen therapy are diabetes, extreme obesity, varicose veins, smoking, and hyperlipidemia. Fasting serum cholesterol and triglyceride levels should be measured to exclude the last.

Finally, since the ultimate indication for treatment is not the child's height prediction but its preceived emotional consequence, time should be devoted to the psychological and social assessment of the child and her parents. The family should understand the risks of estrogen therapy and have a realistic expectation for how much height reduction can be obtained. To facilitate a better understanding of the potential risks of estrogen therapy, we ask the parents to read the package insert found in all oral contraceptive products on the dangers of oral contraceptives. We also make sure they understand that the risks of some complications may be greater than those stated in the pamphlet because the doses used for tall stature are 5–10-fold higher than those used for contraception. Finally, we inform our patients that the FDA has not approved the use of estrogen for the treatment of tall stature.

Treatment

There is no single ideal time to start treatment. Psychological problems can develop in the young prepubertal girl from the rapid development of secondary sex characteristics, and numerous pelvic examinations are not readily accepted by the normal prepubertal girl whose peers show no sign of sexual maturation. The girl should be mature enough to understand the risks involved and participate in the decision to treat. On the other hand, the longer treatment is withheld from the growing child, the less effective estrogen becomes in reducing eventual height. In most girls, we feel the best compromise is to start treatment at a bone age of 11–12 years.

We use conjugated estrogens at a dose of 7.5 mg/day. After 3 months, 10 mg/day of medroxy-progesterone acetate is added for the last 10 days of each calendar month. Others perfer to use ethinyl estradiol 0.3 mg/day, with the addition of 5 mg of norethindrone for the last 10 days of each month.

The children are followed every six weeks for the first six months and then every three months. Particular emphasis is placed on blood pressure and height and weight measurements as well as breast and pelvic or bimanual rectal examinations. A Pap smear is performed annually, and the patient is advised to continue this practice after treatment is stopped. Bone age is determined every six months, and treatment is continued until the bone age reaches 15 years, when 99% of growth has taken place.

The endpoint of estrogen therapy is epiphysial fusion and not cessation of growth. Since the predominant growth-retarding effect of estrogen appears to be inhibition of somatomedin-C production, growth may stop while the epiphyses remain open. Unless treatment is continued until the epiphyses close, growth will resume when estrogen therapy is withdrawn.

Results

It can be anticipated that additional growth will take place after the initiation of treatment. In our experience 3–7 cm of growth occurs during therapy before the epiphyses fuse. The average duration of treatment is 2 years. Large studies of girls treated with similar doses of estrogen have shown a mean reduction in height of 3.5–7.3 cm. As expected, those girls treated before menarche had greater height reductions than those treated after the onset of menses. A few children have been treated with no apparent reduction in height.

Side Effects

Secondary sex characteristics develop rapidly with the initiation of high-dose estrogen therapy. Menses begin each month after the last day of progesterone administration and usually last for several days. Nausea, excessive vaginal secretions, weight gain, and mildly elevated blood pressure are frequent side effects of estrogen therapy. Suppression of the hypothalamic-pituitary-ovarian axis occurs, but menses usually resume spontaneously within 2 to 6 months after treatment is stopped. Several cases of ovarian cystadenoma and one case each of a breast intraductal papilloma and a fibroadenoma of the breast have been reported.

Thromboembolic events are the most serious potential complication of estrogen therapy. It is well documented that women of all ages taking oral contraceptives have an increased risk of all types of thromboembolic phenomena, including pulmonary embolism, myocardial infarction, and stroke. The risk appears to increase with higher estrogen dosages. It is impossible to calculate the risk of these complications in the population of tall girls receiving high-dose estrogen, however, because thromboembolism has a very low incidence at this age in the normal population, and relatively few young girls have been treated in this manner. One case of superficial venous thrombosis has been reported in a tall girl receiving high-dose estrogen.

Certainly the most feared complication of estrogen therapy is its association with malignancy of the breast, endometrium, or liver. Although there have been no reports of these malignancies in tall girls treated with high-dose estrogen, we advise our patients of the increased risk of hepatic adenomas in oral contraceptive users and of endometrial carcinoma in postmenopausal women taking estrogens. From our review of the literature, however, the increased threat of a catastrophic thromboembolic event poses a far greater real risk than the initiation of a malignant disease some time in the future.

Boys

In our experience tall boys rarely request treatment. Others have treated boys effectively with long-acting esters of testosterone. The major side effect is decreased testicular size, which returns to normal after treatment.

Thyroid Disease

THOMAS P. FOLEY, JR., M.D.

The management of pediatric thyroid diseases may vary considerably depending upon the age of the patient, the duration of the disease, and the specific diagnosis. Abnormalities of thyroid function during infancy require specific management, since thyroid physiology and metabolism are quite different in infants compared with older children and adults, and the diseases may cause specific permanent disabilities if not promptly recognized and properly treated.

Thyroid diseases usually present as an abnormality of function, the secretion of thyroid hormones (hypothyroidism or hyperthyroidism), as a structural alteration in the thyroid gland, such as an infiltrative mass or inflammatory process, or a combination of both (the toxic nodule). Satisfactory response to therapy is judged by improvements in clinical, biochemical, and anatomical assessments of the patient.

THYROID DISEASE IN INFANCY

Congenital Hypothyroidism

As a result of newborn screening programs to identify hypothyroidism in the neonate, most but not every infant with hypothyroidism will be de-

tected during the first month of age. Every infant with elevated thyroid-stimulating hormone (TSH) and low thyroxine (T_4) values on newborn screening, indicative of primary hypothyroidism, must be promptly evaluated so that therapy may be initiated without delay. Once the serum specimen for confirmatory tests is collected, therapy with sodium L-thyroxine (L-T_4) should be initiated.

A thyroid image (scan with ^{123}I-iodide or ^{99}Tc-technetium pertechnetate) is very important in establishing a definite diagnosis, but therapy should not be delayed for several days to obtain this test. Since TSH values are increased for 1 to 2 weeks after the initiation of L-T_4 therapy, the thyroid image can be performed up to 5 to 7 days after beginning treatment. The definitive diagnosis is important for parental counseling and long-term management. Infants with ectopic thyroid dysgenesis have a permanent, sporadically occurring disease that does not require additional studies at a later age. The hereditary nature of familial goiter (autosomal recessive mode of inheritance) should be explained to parents so that subsequent children can be evaluated at birth. Infants with congenital athyrosis may have transient disease caused by transplacentally acquired maternal blocking antibodies. Sometime after age 2 years the dose of L-T_4 should be decreased to 25 μg/day or discontinued for 2 weeks to determine if the neonatal disease is permanent or was transient and has resolved. An elevation of serum TSH values will be indicative of permanent hypothyroidism and the need for life-long therapy.

Oral therapy with sodium L-thyroxine is the treatment of choice for hypothyroidism during infancy and childhood. Since the peripheral tissues promptly convert L-T_4 to the metabolically active thyroid hormone, L-3,3′,5-triiodothyronine (L-T_3), it is not necessary to utilize other thyroid preparations containing T_3 for therapy. In fact, these preparations are often more expressive and may lead to confusion in the interpretation of thyroid function tests during therapy. Preparations of desiccated thyroid and thyroid extract have an additional disadvantage of variable potency and unpredictable T_4 and T_3 content.

Since one study in adults has suggested that L-T_4 is better absorbed if taken before a meal, we have advised that infants receive their medication at least $\frac{1}{2}$ hour before a feeding. The tablet(s) is crushed into a small volume of water or milk and fed to the infant by an eye dropper or spoon. Since approximately 50–75% of the oral dose is absorbed, the parenteral daily dose of sodium L-thyroxine should be adjusted accordingly for those infants in whom the oral route is contraindicated.

Therapy with L-T_4 should be initiated in a dose of 50 μg/day, not exceeding 14 μg/kg/day, and adjusted within the first week of therapy to ap-

**Table 1. GUIDELINES FOR REPLACEMENT THERAPY
FOR HYPOTHYROIDISM WITH ORAL SODIUM
L-THYROXINE**

Age	Sodium L-Thyroxine Dose	
	μg/kg/day	Range of Daily Dose
0–6 months	8–10	25–50 μg
6–12 months	6–8	50–75 μg
1–5 years	5–6	50–100 μg
6–12 years	4–5	75–125 μg
12 years–adult	2–3	100–200 μg

Higher or lower doses may be required in individual patients as determined by clinical response and thyroid function test results.

proximately 10 μg/kg/day. This regimen will replenish the depleted T_4 stores in serum and not induce hyperthyroidism. Small infants can be started on 10 μg/kg/day. It is rare for an infant to require less than 25 μg/day or more than 50 μg/day during the first 6 months of age. There is considerable individual patient variation in absorption and metabolic requirements for L-T_4 at any age, particularly during infancy. The clinician should follow the guidelines for the replacement dose of L-T_4 on the basis of body weight (Table 1) and adjust the dose according to serum T_4 and TSH values. These tests should be monitored at 1- to 3-month intervals depending upon the rapidity of normalization of the values and the clinical response of the infant. The T_4 value should be maintained in the upper two thirds of the range of normal for age, and the TSH suppressed below 10 μU/ml. In an occasional infant with an abnormal control of pituitary TSH suppression by T_4, the dose of L-T_4 would have to be increased to amounts that induce clinical thyrotoxicosis to suppress TSH values to normal. This should be avoided, since persistent hyperthyroidism in infancy is associated with deleterious side effects that include premature synostosis of the cranial sutures, osteoporosis, failure to thrive, and advancement in skeletal maturation.

Symptoms and signs of excessive L-T_4 therapy include fussiness, poor sleeping habits, excessive food and fluid intake with poor weight gain or weight loss, jitteriness, hyperdefecation with or without diarrhea, and diaphoresis. In patients in whom it is difficult to achieve the proper L-T_4 dose, a serum T_3 determination may be very useful; a value below 200 ng/dl (assuming normal thyroxine-binding proteins) should not be associated with hyperthyroidism except in infants with unrelated chronic disease. In the absence of increased binding proteins for T_4 and T_3, values exceeding 250 ng/dl usually require a reduction in the L-T_4 dose. A serum T_4 value between 10 and 14 μg/dl in the first year of life should be

associated with clinical euthyroidism, TSH value less than 10 μU/ml, and serum T_3 less than 200 ng/dl. Intermittent elevations of TSH suggest variable compliance or absorption; persistent elevations of TSH with T_4 values between 10 and 14 μg/dl usually indicate the abnormal TSH feedback defect.

Patients with clinical euthyroidism, normal growth in length and weight, normal development, and normal values for thyroid function tests for age do not require additional studies.

Transient primary hypothyroidism may occur as a result of iodine deficiency in iodine-deficient, nonsupplemented areas of the world or of maternal antithyroid drug therapy (iodides, propylthiouracil, methimazole, carbimazole), through the use of iodide-containing skin antiseptics and radiographic contrast dyes, and, infrequently, in immature infants. L-T_4 therapy is required for those infants with a low serum T_4 and elevated TSH in whom the incriminating condition has not terminated. Patients with thyroxine-binding globulin (TBG) deficiency and the low T_3, variable T_4 (euthyroid sick) syndrome do not need L-T_4 therapy.

Infants with hypothalamic-pituitary disease usually present with other clinical features, such as hypoglycemia, direct hyperbilirubinemia, midline central nervous system defects, and hypogenitalism. These infants require lower L-T_4 doses to maintain euthyroidism (25 μg/day), and often require additional hormonal therapy for ACTH, growth hormone, and antidiuretic hormone deficiencies.

Congenital Graves' Disease

Approximately one of every 70 women with a history of Graves' disease will deliver an infant who develops thyrotoxicosis during the first 2 months of life. The disease in the infant is usually transient, but infrequently the course is prolonged and recurrent. The disease in the mother may be active or inactive. The pathogenesis of the transient disease in the infant is believed to result from the transplacental passage of thyroid-stimulating immunoglobulins from mother to fetus. However, the infant may not present with thyromegaly and thyrotoxicosis at birth but may develop the clinical disease days to weeks later. The fetus is partially protected from hyperthyroidism by the transplacental passage of the maternal antithyroid drugs and the preferential conversion of T_4 to the metabolically inactive isomer of T_3 called reverse T_3.

The disease in the neonate may be mild and require only observation and serial monitoring of thyroid function, or may be severe and life-threatening. In addition to the supportive therapy of fluids, temperature control, adequate caloric intake, and digitalization for high output heart failure, the patient with moderate or severe thyrotoxicosis should be treated with antithyroid drugs and beta-adrenergic blockage. Iodides promptly block iodothyronine secretion from the gland and can be administered in a dose of 8 mg every 8 hours of Lugol's solution (5% iodine and 10% potassium iodide with 126 mg of iodine per ml). A thioamide, either propylthiouracil (5–10 mg/kg/day) or methimazole (0.5–1.0 mg/kg/day), in three or four divided doses, should be administered in severely affected infants.

The most serious complications of this disease are caused by the hyperadrenergic state induced by excessive iodothyronine secretion. Prompt and effective reversal of cardiovascular decompensation with exaggerated tachycardia can be achieved by treatment with beta-adrenergic blocking drugs, such as propranolol hydrochloride* using the recommended dose of 2mg/kg/day in 2 or 3 divided doses. Therapy should be continued until thyroid function has returned to normal, at which time the dose may be tapered and discontinued. Since the thioamides and iodides may cause a steady decrement in iodothyronine secretion, it is important to closely monitor the T_4 values and decrease the dose as the euthyroid state is achieved. Similarly, if there is minimal therapeutic response after 2 to 3 days of therapy, the dose of the thioamides and iodide can be increased 30 to 50%.

In severe congenital thyrotoxicosis, therapy with glucocorticoids would be indicated, since they are known to inhibit the secretion of thyroid hormone in Graves' disease. Prednisone, 2 mg/kg/day, in three divided doses for a maximum of 10 to 14 days may be beneficial.

Careful assessment of thyroid function during treatment is important to assure adequate but to avoid excessive therapy. Once the patient has been successfully tapered off medication, it is necessary to follow the patient for several months, since the disease may relapse after withdrawal of therapy.

THYROID DISEASE DURING CHILDHOOD AND ADOLESCENCE

Acquired Hypothyroidism

Beyond infancy, primary hypothyroidism presents as growth deceleration or thyromegaly. The management of the patient may differ depending upon the duration and severity of hypothyroidism. Growth retardation is caused by chronic deprivation of thyroid hormone secretion, whereas the duration of hypothyroidism presenting as thyromegaly will vary.

The association of hypothyroidism and permanent, irreversible impairment of the central nervous system occurs only during fetal life and the

first 2 years of postnatal life. Brain growth and maturation are virtually complete by 2 to 3 years of age, and the development of hypothyroidism after this age is not associated with mental retardation or neurologic sequelae. Therefore, the rapid achievement of euthyroidism is not as critical in the older child as in the infant. Whereas the neonate and infant are promptly treated with the full replacement dose of sodium L-thyroxine at diagnosis, this regimen is not essential for the child or adolescent; in fact, in children with chronic hypothyroidism, severe growth retardation, and myxedema, the initiation of full replacement dose of L-T_4 often causes the undesirable side effects seen in children with untreated thyrotoxicosis, including short attention span, insomnia and restless sleeping, irritability, restlessness, and some hair loss. For these children it is preferable to gradually restore euthyroidism over 4 to 8 weeks by initiating replacement therapy with 25 μg of L-T_4 for 2 weeks and increasing the dose by that amount at 2- to 4-week intervals until the desired dose for age (Table 1) is achieved. This regimen is not necessary for children with mild hypothyroidism or clinical symptoms of short duration. However, it is important to avoid excessive therapy and prudent to select the lower dose per kg body weight for age on the initiation of therapy.

Since patients with acquired hypothyroidism do not have an abnormality in the feedback control of TSH release, the adequacy of their replacement therapy can be monitored quite satisfactorily by the determination of serum T_4 and TSH concentrations at 1- or 2-month intervals until normal; thereafter, T_4 and TSH determinations need monitoring only at 1- or 2-year intervals if the patient is clinically euthyroid and exhibiting normal growth.

For the child with growth retardation and hypothyroidism, the bone age at diagnosis roughly estimates the onset of the disease. Within the first 2 years of therapy, one expects growth acceleration with catch-up growth into the normal percentile of growth for that child prior to the onset of hypothyroidism. If this growth pattern occurs, no further bone age determinations are necessary. An occasional adolescent with chronic hypothyroidism may demonstrate poor catch-up growth despite adequate therapy and the absence of other causes of growth retardation on evaluation. The reason for this unfortunate course is unknown.

Patients with hypothalamic or pituitary hypothyroidism usually require the lower dose of L-T_4 for age to achieve euthyroidism. It is important to determine the integrity of the hypothalamic-pituitary-adrenal axis so that therapy with hydrocortisone can be initiated simultaneously with L-T_4 therapy.

* Manufacturer's warning: Safety and efficacy for use in children have not been established.

Hyperthyroidism

Excessive production of T_4 and T_3 associated with symptoms and signs of thyrotoxicosis during childhood and adolescence is caused by Graves' disease in more than 90% of cases. The other causes include the early phase of toxic thyroiditis (Hashimoto's and subacute thyroiditis), hyperfunctioning thyroid adenoma(s), thyrotoxicosis factitia, and the very rare cases of TSH hypersecretion by pituitary adenoma or pituitary resistance to thyroid hormone. In the cases of the toxic adenoma and pituitary adenoma, surgical therapy directed to the specific cause of hyperthyroidism is curative. As for Graves' disease, a complex disorder of abnormal immune surveillance, therapy is aimed indirectly at the source of thyroid hormone hypersecretion, the thyroid gland, rather than the immune system or thyroid-stimulating immunoglobulin(s) secretion.

Although the diagnosis of Graves' disease generally is not difficult, therapy poses specific problems. There are three acceptable therapeutic modalities: (1) antithyroid drugs, propylthiouracil (PTU) and methimazole (MTZ) in the United States, (2) subtotal thyroidectomy, and (3) ablation with radioiodine (^{131}I-iodide). Each treatment is effective and has specific advantages and disadvantages. For the pediatric population, most treatment centers recommend antithyroid drugs as initial therapy. These drugs have the advantages of ease of acceptance by patient and parents, effective control of the disease in approximately 50% of patients within the first 2 years of therapy, and an association with permanent remission in some patients. The disadvantages include toxic drug reactions in approximately 5%, necessitating alternate therapy, chronic dependency on 2 to 3 times daily medication, and failure to induce permanent remission in as many as 50% of patients.

Subtotal thyroidectomy is the initial choice for therapy in some centers with expertise in pediatric thyroid surgery. The advantages include prompt, definitive therapy without need for chronic dependency on multiple-dose drug therapy. The disadvantages include (1) the need for L-thyroxine therapy to treat primary hypothyroidism in approximately 25% of patients within 20 years; (2) infrequent morbidity from recurrent laryngeal nerve palsy and permanent hypoparathyroidism, particularly in the hands of the occasional, inexperienced surgeon; (3) anterior cervical scar that may form keloid in susceptible patients, specifically blacks; and (4) a real, though exceedingly rare, surgical mortality. Surgical therapy in most clinics is reserved for those patients who for various reasons cannot take the antithyroid drugs. In an occasional patient the disease may relapse after surgical therapy.

Radioactive iodine ablative therapy is the treatment of choice for patients beyond the childbearing age and in patients who cannot tolerate the antithyroid drugs and are poor surgical candidates. A prevailing concern about the risks of ionized radiation exposure in children has dampened the enthusiasm for this effective mode of therapy. The advantages include the simplicity of treatment and usual lack of side effects during the early and late (decades) years of observation. The disadvantages include the high incidence (more than 50%) of permanent hypothyroidism, a relapse rate of approximately 10%, and the still uncertain potential deleterious side effects of ionizing radiation. The latter concern has yet to be definitively documented, although the numbers of children studied and the duration of therapy have been limited.

Severe thyrotoxicosis requires specific therapy in addition to the initiation of antithyroid drugs. Beta-adrenergic blockers (propranolol 10 mg tid) provide effective relief from the adrenergic hyperresponsiveness that causes the disturbing side effects of thyrotoxicosis. Usually this therapy is needed for only the first 2 to 3 weeks.

Initial doses for the thioamides (PTU and MTZ) in the adolescent range between 300 and 450 mg/day for PTU and between 30 and 45 mg/day for MTZ in three divided doses at 8-hour intervals. In children the total daily dose ranges between 150 and 200 mg/day for PTU and 15 and 20 mg/day for MTZ. Within 4 weeks the patient will experience an improvement in clinical symptoms, a decrement in serum iodothyronine (T_4 and T_3) concentrations, and an increase in the size of the thyroid gland. The last observation should not alter the decision to continue therapy at the initially prescribed dose. Once serum iodothyronine values are normal, there are two acceptable methods for maintenance therapy. The first requires continuation of full blocking doses of PTU or MTZ and initiation of a small, supplementary daily dose of L-T_4 (1 μg/kg/day) after the therapeutic effect has been documented by an elevation in serum TSH. This method assures an avoidance of persistent hypothyroidism while maintaining maximal antithyroid and, perhaps, an associated anti-immune, effect. The second requires a reduction by 30% to 50% of the dose of PTU or MTZ to maintain clinical and biochemical euthyroidism. Maintenance doses of PTU may be administered twice daily and MTZ once daily, since the latter has a longer half-life. Serum T_4 values are usually more helpful in monitoring control of the disease than serum T_3, but some patients are found to have low to normal T_4 values yet mildly elevated T_3 values. Usually therapy is continued for at least 1 year. If the disease remains controlled and the gland size decreases, therapy may be discontinued by tapering the dose of medication or performing a T_3 suppression test. The serum T_4 concentration should be reduced into the hypothyroid range when exogenous T_3 (Cytomel) is administered in a dose of 1 µg/kg/day in three divided doses for 3 weeks in normal subjects and patients with inactive Graves' disease. Sufficient experience in the use of serum values for thyroid-stimulating immuno-globulins, also known as thyrotropin (TSH) receptor antibodies, has not been reported in juvenile Graves' disease to warrant their determination to judge the activity of Graves' disease in individual patients.

There are specific toxic side effects of the thioamides that may occur at any time during the course of therapy but usually occur within the first few months. These include erythematous rashes, urticaria, agranulocytosis (usually presenting as persistent orolingual infections), arthralgia, arthritis, lymphadenopathy, lupuslike syndrome, and hepatitis. The occurrence of these symptoms demands an assessment of the neutrophil count and cessation of therapy. If the side effect is not severe, a trial on the other thioamide may be initiated under close observation, since cross-toxicity may occur.

For patients who are allergic to the thioamides, noncompliant with therapy, or nonresponsive to doses up to 600 mg/day of PTU (60 mg/day for MTZ), or require 4 or more years of treatment because of persistent thyromegaly or relapse, alternate therapy should be considered. Surgery should be selected when the expertise of an experienced pediatric thyroid surgeon is available. Radioiodine ablative therapy should be the second choice for treatment of the patient who is a poor surgical risk, has had relapse after previous thyroid surgery, or previously has formed disfiguring keloid scars at incision sites.

Inflammatory Thyroid Disease

Acute suppurative thyroiditis is a rare disease at any age. Although the patients are clinically and biochemically euthyroid, they appear quite ill with exquisite anterior cervical pain, erythema and tenderness, fever, diaphoresis, and tachycardia. The patient needs urgent therapy with antibiotics, fluids, antipyretics, and analgesics. Since thyroid abscess may develop within a few days, ultrasound examination of the thyroid needs to be performed on one or more occasions depending upon the clinical course. Once the acute infection process has subsided, special diagnostic studies to detect a persistent pyriform sinus tract or thyroglossal duct should be performed, since these lesions are the usual source of infection in acute thyroiditis.

Though uncommon during childhood and adolescence, subacute or granulomatous thyroiditis may present several days after symptoms of an upper respiratory infection. Usually the disease is self-limiting and requires no therapy. However, an occasional patient may have persistent pain and tenderness and experience symptomatic improvement from therapy with analgesics such as acetaminophen or aspirin. Glucocorticoids have not been shown to alter the course of this disease. There may be symptoms of toxic thyroiditis as a result of the release of T_4 and T_3 into the circulation in response to the presumed viral insult to the thyroid. Only rarely does this thyrotoxic phase of the disease require brief therapy with beta-adrenergic blocking drugs for symptomatic relief. Three to six months later the patient may develop mild, transient hypothyroidism that gradually resolves as the thyroid recovers. Rarely does the patient develop symptoms of hypothyroidism or permanent gland failure to necessitate L-T_4 treatment.

Chronic lymphocytic or autoimmune (Hashimoto's) thyroiditis is the most common pediatric thyroid disease. It usually presents as euthyroid goiter that does not progress to primary hypothyroidism or thyrotoxicosis. A few patients present with transient toxic thyroiditis and should be managed in the same manner as those with subacute thyroiditis. Approximately 10 to 15% of patients present with primary hypothyroidism, usually a permanent disease that requires continuous L-T_4 therapy (Table 1). Studies in adults suggest that even compensated primary hypothyroidism (elevated TSH and normal T_4) should be treated with L-T_4 doses sufficient to suppress TSH.

In general, L-T_4 therapy is not recommended for the patient with euthyroid goiter unless the appearance of the enlarged gland is quite disturbing to the patient, who should be advised that L-T_4 therapy usually will not reduce the size of the gland. Infrequently patients with autoimmune thyroid disease may develop other diseases found in association with the autoimmune polyglandular syndromes, such as Addison's disease, insulin-dependent diabetes mellitus, and pernicious anemia.

Thyroid Nodules

The child with a mass in the thyroid gland often presents difficult diagnostic and therapeutic problems. Whether the nodule requires surgical excision or not becomes the primary consideration at presentation. Patients in whom the remainder of the thyroid gland has the clinical features of autoimmune thyroiditis (firm, irregular, seedy, granular, asymmetric) and very positive thyroid antibody titers (antimicrosomal and/or antithyroglobulin titers in excess of 1:1000) should be either followed without therapy if serum TSH is normal or placed on L-T_4 if the serum TSH is elevated. These patients should not have surgical excision unless the nodule progressively enlarges on full replacement doses of L-T_4.

In the patient with an isolated thyroid nodule, the management will depend upon the results of thyroid function tests and thyroid anatomical studies that may include an ultrasound examination for thyroid cyst and a radioiodine or technetium image or scan for a hot (hyperfunctioning) or cold (hypofunctioning) nodule. The hyperfunctioning nodule should be surgically excised if the patient has clinical and biochemical (elevated serum T_3) hyperthyroidism or a nodule 3 cm or greater in diameter. The patient with a thyroid cyst may have the cyst aspirated and cytology performed on the aspirate. However, excision assures definitive histology and lack of recurrence.

A solitary, hypofunctioning, solid thyroid mass with normal thyroid function tests and negative thyroid antibodies should be excised to exclude the possibility of malignant thyroid disease. Following excision of a benign thyroid tumor, there is no evidence to suggest that the patient should be placed on L-T_4 therapy to prevent recurrence. Patients with malignant thyroid disease will require total thyroidectomy and, depending upon the histology of the tumor and presence of metastasis, ablative therapy with radioiodine.

The remaining patients with thyroid nodules, normal thyroid function, negative thyroid antibodies, and normal function on thyroid imaging may pose difficult management decisions. Surgery is indicated if there are symptoms and signs of thyroid carcinoma such as prior history of therapeutic head and neck radiation, a rapidly enlarging, hard mass, a family history of thyroid cancer, chronic cough or hoarseness, vocal cord paralysis, or fixation of the mass to adjacent cervical tissue. In the absence of these clinical features, the patient should be placed on suppressive doses of L-T_4 (3 μg/kg/day to suppress TSH to indetectable values) for 3 to 6 months. If the nodule enlarges on this therapy, surgical excision is indicated.

Parathyroid Disease

KEVIN E. HALBERT, M.D.,
and REGINALD C. TSANG, M.B.B.S.

Vitamin D and Metabolites

The mainstay of treatment for hypoparathyroidism and pseudohypoparathyroidism is vitamin D and its analogues. Ergocalciferol (vitamin D_2), which is of plant origin, traditionally has been the principal agent used. It has a prolonged onset of action, from 7 to 14 days after therapy has begun. Furthermore, because of a long half-life of 2 to 4 weeks, prolonged hypercalcemia (20 to 40 days) easily occurs if vitamin D intoxication occurs. Doses of ergocalciferol have ranged from 8,000 to 1,200,000 IU per day, with the usual range being 50,000 to 100,000 IU/day or 1,000 to 2,600 IU/kg/day. Individual responsiveness to ergocalciferol can be variable and can change after a period of prolonged control with a fixed dose. In addition, ergocalciferol has a very narrow therapuetic index, thus making undertreatment and intoxication real possibilities. Because of these problems ergocalciferol is no longer considered the primary agent for management of hypoparathyroidism or pseudohypoparathyroidism, and vitamin D analogues have moved to the forefront.

Dihydrotachysterol (DHT) is an alternative agent to ergocalciferol. This agent is an ultraviolet irradiation product of ergocalciferol and is marketed in a crystalline form. Because of its structural conformation it does not require 1α-hydroxylation by the kidney before it is biologically active. Its onset of action of 1 to 2 weeks is still relatively long. Usual doses range from 0.2 to 3.0 mg/day, or 8 to 22 μg/kg/day (1 mg DHT equals 120,000 IU of ergocalciferol). Because of its relatively long onset of action, dose adjustments should not be made more often than every 2 to 3 weeks.

25-Hydroxycholecalciferol (25-hydroxyvitamin D_3) is also effective in the management of hypoparathyroidism and pseudohypoparathyroidism. At high serum concentrations 25-hydroxycholecalciferol may have similar actions on intestine and bone as does 1,25-dihydroxycholecalciferol, the naturally occurring active vitamin D metabolite; i.e., 25-hydroxycholecalciferol will increase intestinal absorption of calcium and phosphate and increase mobilization of bone calcium and phosphate. Peak serum concentrations of 25-hydroxycholecalciferol are reached about 4 hours after an oral dose, and an onset of action is seen in less than one week after therapy is begun. Doses that have been effective in controlling the hypocalcemia of hypoparathyroidism and pseudohypoparathyroidism have ranged from 20 to 50 μg/day or 3 to 6 μg/kg/day.

Another vitamin D analogue that has recently become available is 1α-hydroxycholecalciferol (1α-hydroxyvitamin D_3). This agent requires 25-hydroxylation by the liver before becoming a biologically active form but avoids the necessity of 1α-hydroxylation by the kidney, which can be impaired with decreased serum parathyroid hormone concentration or hyperphosphatemia. Initial starting doses range from 0.5 to 1.0 μg/day, with maintenance requirements between 0.5 and 3.0 μg/day, or 0.03 to 0.08 μg/kg/day. The major advantages of 1α-hydroxycholecalciferol are rapid onset of action and short serum half-life, which allow for rapid resolution of hypercalcemia (usually within 1 to 5 days of discontinuation) when inadvertent intoxication occurs.

The metabolite that has the most utility in management of hypoparathyroidism and pseudohypoparathyroidism is 1,25-dihydroxycholecalciferol (1,25-dihydroxyvitamin D_3). This is the most active naturally occurring metabolite of vitamin D, being the product of 1α-hydroxylation of 25-hydroxycholecalciferol in the kidney. Once ingested, 1,25-dihydroxycholecalciferol requires no further biochemical conversions for bioactivity. Rapid onset of action enables rapid correction of hypocalcemia, usually within 1 to 4 days. Because of the serum half-life of less than 24 hours, discontinuation of the agent in the event of hypercalcemia during therapy results in return to normocalcemia in 1 to 2 days. Biologic activity, as manifest by continued increased intestinal calcium absorption, may persist for several days after 1,25-dihydroxycholecalciferol has been cleared from the blood. Therapy is usually begun at 0.25 μg/day (0.03 μg/kg/day) and increased daily by 0.25 μg in older children, or 0.015 μg/kg in infants, until normocalcemia is obtained. Usual maintenance doses range from 0.5 to 1.25 μg/day or 0.03 to 0.08 μg/kg/day.

Goals of Therapy

The main objective in treatment of hypoparathyroidism and pseudohypoparathyroidism is maintenance of normocalcemia and normophosphatemia with minimal complications. Whichever form of vitamin D is chosen for treatment, the initial dose should be at the low range of usual therapeutic efficacy and gradually increased while monitoring the serum calcium concentration carefully. For example, with 1,25-dihydroxycholecalciferol serum calcium concentration should be measured once or twice daily once therapy is begun. For the slower acting vitamin D metabolites serum calcium measurements need to be begun as one approaches the time of onset of action (e.g., since ergocalciferol has an onset of action of 7 to 14 days, serum calcium measurements need to begin near the end of the first week of therapy).

Increases in the doses of vitamin D metabolites should be made cautiously, taking into consideration the onset of action as well as half-life of the metabolites, each of which will affect the steady state. The target serum calcium concentration should be maintained in the 8.5 to 9.0 mg/dl range. Once stability has been obtained, serum calcium, magnesium, and phosphate values can be checked every 3 to 6 months. In addition, renal function should be assessed at least once every 6 to 12 months. Examination of serum concentrations of 1,25-dihydroxycholecalciferol have not proved to be of value, in that maintenance of normal serum concentrations are associated with a high incidence of hypercalcemia. Serum phosphate concentrations require much longer to correct than serum calcium concentration. Phosphate concentrations are usually corrected within 2 to 3 months after serum calcium concentrations are normalized. Larger doses of vitamin D may result in faster correction of serum phosphate concentration, but they also greatly increase the risk of vitamin D intoxication.

Dose requirements of vitamin D in pseudohypoparathyroidism tend to be lower than in hypoparathyroidism. Dose requirements for either hypoparathyroid condition also can change with time, even after years of stability on a single dose, resulting in either hypocalcemia or hypercalcemia. Thus, consistent long-term follow-up examinations are required. Finally, continuous anticonvulsant therapy can increase vitamin D metabolism, thus leading to increased maintenance vitamin D requirements.

Adjunctive Therapy. Although vitamin D is the primary agent in the management of these conditions, several adjunctive therapies have been utilized. The principal among these is oral calcium supplementation. Although not necessary in the patient who has a normal calcium intake, this can add a little additional margin of safety in the difficult-to-control patient. Usually 50 mg of elemental calcium per kg of body weight or 530 mg calcium gluconate per kg is given in 3 or 4 divided doses over the course of a day. Maximum doses are 1 gm and 10 gm, respectively, for elemental calcium and calcium gluconate. Doses greater than 75 mg of elemental calcium per kg of body weight or 750 mg of calcium gluconate per kg of body weight may result in diarrhea. Milk is not a desirable source of calcium supplementation because of its relatively high phosphate content.

A few patients resistant to vitamin D therapy will respond after magnesium supplementation. These individuals are usually hypomagnesemic (serum concentrations less than 1.5 mg/dl), and once this problem is corrected their condition becomes easier to control. Giving 7 to 15 mg of elemental magnesium or 70 to 150 mg magnesium sulfate per kg body weight per day is usually adequate therapy.

Chlorthalidone, a thiazide-like diuretic, plus sodium restriction has been suggested as a means of managing hypocalcemia secondary to hypoparathyroidism and pseudohypoparathyroidism without the use of vitamin D. It is thought to work by decreasing urinary calcium losses and contraction of extracellular water. There is no experience with the use of this regimen in children and it cannot be recommended as an alternative to standard therapy.

Complications of Therapy

There are principally two complications of vitamin D therapy: vitamin D intoxication with resultant hypercalcemia, and hypocalcemia that can progress to tetany. Vitamin D intoxication is characterized by weakness, fatigue, lassitude, headache, nausea, and vomiting. Polyuria and polydipsia are usually present. On laboratory examination an elevated serum calcium concentration and possibly elevation of serum blood urea nitrogen and creatinine concentrations will be noted. Treatment of this disorder requires the discontinuation of vitamin D and any calcium supplements, which may be the only necessary therapy when the faster acting vitamin D metabolites are used. Institution of a low calcium diet is advisable. Intravenous isotonic saline at 200–250 ml/kg/day should be given to increase urinary calcium losses. Furosemide diuretics 1 mg/kg three to four times daily should also be given to increase urinary losses of calcium. Careful evaluation of serum electrolyte concentrations is essential with furosemide therapy. Calcitonin (4–10 MRC units/kg every 3 to 4 hours IM with a maximal initial dose of 100 units) or prednisone (1 to 2 mg/kg/day) can also be given to lower serum calcium, but usually are not necessary. If either 1α-hydroxycholecalciferol or 1,25-dihydroxycholecalciferol is used, discontinuation of these agents will result in reduction of serum calcium concentration to normal levels in 1 to 5 days. On the other hand, when ergocalciferol is used, normocalcemia usually returns by 4 to 6 weeks; it is possible to have a 20-week period before normocalcemia is attained. If hypercalcemia is prolonged, nephrocalcinosis can develop, resulting in renal failure. Other areas of ectopic calcification may also be noted. One probable long-term sequela of moderately severe hypercalcemia is growth arrest. This can last for 6 months or more after the onset of hypercalcemia. The resulting deficit in height is sometimes not recovered once growth resumes.

Hypocalcemic tetany is readily corrected with 2 ml of 10% calcium gluconate per kg of body weight given via a slow intravenous infusion. While calcium is being given, the heart rate (via electrocardiographic monitoring) and blood pressure need to be measured. Rapid administration of calcium can result in cardiac arrhythmias or hypertension. After the acute episode of hypocalcemia is corrected, calcium should be continued at 50 to 70 mg of elemental calcium per kg of body weight per day to assure maintenance of normocalcemia. Until serum calcium concentrations are stabilized, serum calcium concentrations should be examined once or twice daily.

Hypocalcemia may occur during a febrile illness. The hypocalcemia may be effectively managed by temporarily increasing the dose of rapid acting vitamin D metabolites or calcium supplements. Parents and patients need to be aware of the association of fever and hypocalcemia and to seek medical care at the first sign of illness.

Associated Conditions

Chronic mucocutaneous candidiasis will be encountered in a small number of patients with hypoparathyroidism. Nystatin can be used to control the infections, but currently no satisfactory therapy is available for complete eradication.

Many patients with pseudohypoparathyroidism will also have associated hypothyroidism. This is usually mild but occasionally will require thyroid replacement. There are also patients with autoimmune hypoparathyroidism who have associated malabsorption and steatorrhea. As a result they may have difficulty absorbing fat-soluble vitamins, like vitamin D, and may seem resistant to therapy. Usually with large doses of vitamin D and oral calcium supplements these patients can be adequately managed. Occasionally patients will not respond until placed on a diet containing a significant proportion of fat as medium-chain triglycerides.

Disorders of the Adrenal Gland

MARIA I. NEW, M.D.,
LENORE S. LEVINE, M.D.,
and JEAN W. TEMECK, M.D.

It is prudent for every patient with adrenal insufficiency to wear a medic-alert bracelet, medallion, or card.

ADRENAL HYPERPLASIA DUE TO ENZYMATIC DEFICIENCY OF STEROIDOGENESIS

Classic (Congenital) (CAH). In the virilizing forms of this disorder (21-hydroxylase, 11β-hydroxylase deficiency, and 3β-hydroxysteroid dehydrogenase deficiency), females usually have clitoromegaly. If clitoromegaly is mild, the clitoris may become hidden by the labia majora as the child grows and is under treatment. However, most cases require surgery involving either removal (resection) of redundant erectile tissue with preservation of the sexually sensitive glans clitoris or clitoral recession. The procedure is usually done at the age of 1 year. A vaginoplasty may also be necessary and is generally performed during early adolescence.

Incomplete virilization occurs in males with cholesterol desmolase deficiency, 3β-hydroxysteroid dehydrogenase deficiency, and 17α-hydroxylase deficiency. The virilization may be so incomplete as to make the female sex assignment more appropriate. Surgery is performed to correct the genital abnormality to conform with the sex of assignment. Sex hormone replacement is necessary to induce and maintain secondary sex characteristics at puberty.

The glucocorticoid-deficient forms of this disorder (21-hydroxylase, 11β-hydroxylase, 3β-hydroxysteroid dehydrogenase, 17α-hydroxylase, and cholesterol desmolase deficiency) require cortisol replacement. This not only corrects the deficiency but also suppresses ACTH oversecretion. Therefore, excessive stimulation of the androgen pathway, and consequently further virilization, is prevented, allowing normal growth and puberty. Of the various forms of steroid treatment available, we employ hydrocortisone. The dose varies widely depending on the patient, but the average requirement is 20 to 25 mg/m^2/day in two or three divided doses.

The mineralocorticoid-deficient forms (salt-wasting 21-hydroxylase, 3β-hydroxysteroid dehydrogenase, cholesterol desmolase, 18-hydroxylase, and 18-dehydrogenase deficiency) require salt-retaining hormone replacement. Fludrocortisone (Florinef) is most commonly used, and the usual dose is 0.05 to 0.1 mg/day. It is also helpful in patients with simple virilizing 21-hydroxylase deficiency with high plasma renin activity (PRA), where the addition of salt-retaining steroids to the treatment regimen suppresses renin and may permit a decrease in the glucocorticoid dose. Sodium chloride tablets may be used for infants in a dose of 3 to 5 mEq/kg/day. There is a 17 mEq Na$^+$/tablet which may be divided into two to four equal parts, crushed, and added to the infant's formula.

Therapy should be regulated by clinical and biochemical parameters. Clinically, it is important to monitor the child's growth and pubertal development. Biochemically, sensitive measurements of control are serum 17-hydroxyprogesterone and Δ4-androstenedione. In females and prepubertal males, serum testosterone is also useful but not in newborn and pubertal males.

PRA is a helpful index of therapeutic control in virilizers as well as salt-wasters. PRA is closely correlated with the ACTH level, and normalization of PRA may result in decrease in ACTH. Also, normalization of PRA allows for improved statural growth. Monitoring of PRA is also helpful in those forms of CAH with mineralocorticoid excess (11β-hydroxylase and 17α-hydroxylase deficiency). In the mineralocorticoid-deficient forms, PRA is increased in poor control, and in the mineralocorticoid-excess forms, it is suppressed.

Follow-up visits should occur at 3 month intervals. In addition to monitoring the above parameters, a bone age should be obtained yearly.

Nonclassic 21-Hydroxylase Deficiency

SYMPTOMATIC (ACQUIRED OR LATE ONSET) DEFICIENCY. The nonclassic 21-hydroxylase deficiency form results from a milder defect in 21-hydroxylation than the classical congenital form. It may be symptomatic or asymptomatic.

Signs of excess androgen production in affected patients are not noted at birth, but at some time thereafter. Onset may not be until adulthood. Treatment consists of glucocorticoid replacement in lower or the same doses as in the classical congenital form.

ASYMPTOMATIC (CRYPTIC) 21-HYDROXYLASE DEFICIENCY. This is noted in family members of patients with classic CAH. In contrast to the patient with classic and nonclassic CAH, affected family members are asymptomatic. They may have one gene for a severe 21-hydroxylase deficiency and one gene for a mild deficiency, or two genes for the mild deficiency. No treatment is needed, as growth, puberty, and fertility are normal.

PRIMARY HYPERALDOSTERONISM

This condition is rarely seen in childhood. In children it is predominantly due to bilateral adrenal hyperplasia, as opposed to an aldosterone producing tumor. When a tumor is present, surgical removal, if feasible, is the treatment of choice. Response to surgery is less satisfactory in cases due to bilateral hyperplasia, and spironolactone is effective drug therapy. Spironolactone, an aldosterone antagonist, may also be used preoperatively in the surgical management of primary hyperaldosteronism due to a tumor. Amiloride* (Midamor), a potassium-sparing diuretic, is also effective. These agents may be used alone or in combination with diuretics, β-blockers, and vasodilators to control the hypertension.

DEXAMETHASONE-SUPPRESSIBLE HYPERALDOSTERONISM

This familial disorder is similar to primary hyperaldosteronism except that in the former the aldosterone hypersecretion is completely and rapidly suppressed with dexamethasone. The hypertension always remits in children given glucocorticoid therapy, though it does not always do so in adults despite aldosterone suppression. Thus, early diagnosis and treatment are essential to cure this form of hypertension. Adequacy of the glucocorticoid treatment can be monitored not only by blood pressure measurement but also by measurement of PRA, which is suppressed in the untreated state and rises to normal with effective treatment.

ACUTE ADRENAL INSUFFICIENCY— EMERGENCY TREATMENT

This is a medical emergency that requires prompt recognition and treatment. It may be precipitated in the hypofunctional adrenal cortical conditions (e.g., CAH, Addison's disease) when patients are not yet diagnosed or are noncompliant with therapy or are stressed. It may also occur with trauma and bacteremia and during surgery

---

* Manufacturer's warning: Safety and efficacy of amiloride in children have not been established.

in patients who are steroid dependent. There may be significant hyponatremia, hyperkalemia, hypoglycemia, and dehydration with shock. Therapy consists of volume expansion and steroid replacement:

Infuse normal saline in 5% dextrose at 1.5 to 2 times maintenance (i.e., 2250 to 3000 ml/m^2/day). Use plasma or Plasmanate at 10 to 20 ml/kg or normal saline at 20 ml/kg over 1 hour if patient is in shock.

Administer hydrocortisone sodium succinate (Solu-Cortef) in a stat dose of 2.0 mg/kg IV push or IM. One may estimate the emergency dose of hydrocortisone by IV bolus as follows: for an infant, give 25 mg; for a small child, 50 mg; a larger child or adolescent, 100–150 mg. After the emergency dose, use hydrocortisone at 100 mg/m^2/day as a continuous IV infusion or every 6 hours IM.

Give deoxycorticosterone acetate (DOCA) stat at 1–2 mg IM. A repeat dose is usually not needed more than once daily, but this should be determined by the patient's electrolytes. It should be remembered that large doses of glucocorticoids (hydrocortisone) have some mineralocorticoid action which, coupled with normal saline infusion, may make the use of DOCA unnecessary in the acute situation.

To treat hyponatremia, calculate the patient's sodium deficit as follows: (normal serum Na$^+$ − observed serum Na$^+$) × body weight (kg) × 0.6. Administer half of the total sodium deficit in the first 8 to 12 hours with IV fluids, in addition to maintenance sodium.

Resistant hyperkalemia may require a Kayexalate enema; rarely are other measures needed.

It is imperative not to overtreat the child. This may lead to sodium and fluid overload with resulting hypertension, hypernatremia, edema, congestive heart failure, and hypokalemia, with muscle weakness. Monitor the patient's clinical condition, weight, input/output, blood pressure, electrocardiogram, and serum electrolytes very closely.

As the patient recovers and is able to tolerate liquids, IV fluids and medications may be tapered over a few days, and when a single AM dose is reached, they may be discontinued. If a short-acting glucocorticoid such as hydrocortisone was used for less than 3 days, therapy may be discontinued without tapering. It is essential to search carefully for the cause of the adrenal insufficiency. If the problem was acute, no further treatment is necessary. If the problem is one of chronic insufficiency, then maintenance steroid replacement is required. The oral dose of hydrocortisone may vary from 12.5 to 25 mg/m^2/day in two or three divided doses, and fludrocortisone from 0.05 to 0.15 mg/day.

When a patient with chronic adrenal insufficiency is stressed, e.g., during a febrile illness or surgery, the oral dose of hydrocortisone must be doubled or tripled, depending on the degree of stress and the condition of the patient. If oral therapy is not tolerated, the drug must be given parenterally. The stress dose of parenteral hydrocortisone is 40 to 60 mg/m^2/day in three or four divided doses. If the stress is a febrile illness, the increase should be continued for the duration of the illness and then maintenance therapy resumed. If the stress is surgery, administer either IV or IM hydrocortisone in the above dose 24 hours prior to surgery. Continue the same on the day of surgery, but divide the total dose into three equal portions: one on call to the operating room, one as a continuous infusion during surgery, and one in the immediate (same-day) postoperative period. Thereafter, depending on the procedure and the patient's condition, continue the same stress dose of hydrocortisone for 3 to 5 postoperative days, at which time the maintenance regimen may be resumed.

For emergency surgery, administer hydrocortisone 50 mg IV or IM on call to the operating room for a small child, and 100 mg IV or IM for a larger child or adolescent, and continue the management outlined above during the operative and postoperative period.

If a patient has received glucocorticoids in the past year, it is prudent to follow the above protocol in times of major stress such as surgery.

PRIMARY ADRENAL INSUFFICIENCY (ADDISON'S DISEASE OR BILATERAL ADRENALECTOMY)—MAINTENANCE TREATMENT

This disorder requires replacement with glucocorticoid and mineralocorticoid hormones. The usual maintenance dose of hydrocortisone ranges from 12 to 20 mg/m^2/day in two or three divided doses, and fludrocortisone 0.05 to 0.1 mg/day.

Important parameters to monitor treatment include growth, blood pressure, serum electrolytes, and PRA. It is also important to concomitantly treat infection (e.g., tuberculosis or histoplasmosis), if this is the underlying etiology.

SECONDARY ADRENAL INSUFFICIENCY (ACTH DEFICIENCY)

In contrast to primary adrenal insufficiency, secondary adrenal insufficiency is characterized by deficient glucocorticoids but normal mineralocorticoid function. This occurs in steroid treated or hypophysectomized or hypopituitary conditions. Glucocorticoid replacement is the same as that described for primary adrenal insufficiency.

ACTH UNRESPONSIVENESS

Therapy is the same as for secondary adrenal insufficiency.

CUSHING'S SYNDROME

Treatment depends on the etiology. It may be iatrogenic or secondary to an adrenal tumor or result from excess ACTH secretion from either the pituitary or a nonpituitary source.

If it is due to an adrenal tumor, surgical resection, if possible, is the treatment of choice. When an autonomously functional unilateral adrenal adenoma is removed, as is usually the case, the remaining adrenal gland is often atrophic. Therefore, these patients should be supplemented with glucocorticoid therapy before, during, and after surgery until the remaining adrenal gland returns to normal, which may take many months, depending on the duration of pituitary-adrenal suppression. If bilateral tumors were present, then total adrenalectomy is indicated, and the patient must take lifelong glucocorticoid and mineralocorticoid treatment in the doses outlined for primary adrenal insufficiency.

If the cause is a nonresectable adrenal carcinoma, the following agents may be tried: o,p'-DDD (mitotane [Lysodren]), an adrenocorticolytic drug; metyrapone, an 11-hydroxylase inhibitor of cortisol production; cyproheptadine hydrochloride, a serotonin antagonist that suppresses ACTH; and aminoglutethimide, which blocks conversion of cholesterol to $\Delta 5$-pregnenolone in the adrenal cortex. However, these agents are not without side effects; there has been limited experience with them in children, and results are disappointing.

When the syndrome is secondary to a nonpituitary souce of ACTH, i.e., "the ectopic ACTH syndrome," treatment is that of the underlying disease.

Cushing's disease refers to bilateral adrenal hyperplasia resulting from excessive ACTH secretion by the pituitary. Several treatment options are available. Recent advances in surgical techniques include selective surgical removal of the pituitary microadenoma(s) via the transsphenoidal route. Postoperatively, the resulting pituitary insufficiency, primarily ACTH, is usually temporary, but replacement glucocorticoid therapy is needed until normal pituitary/adrenal function returns. Pituitary irradiation is another treatment option. Total bilateral adrenalectomy is outdated and has two major disadvantages: the need for lifelong steroid replacement therapy, and the postoperative risk of Nelson's syndrome.

VIRILIZING, FEMINIZING, AND NONFUNCTIONAL ADRENOCORTICAL TUMORS

Treatment is surgical removal in resectable cases. If the tumor is also cortisol-producing, then the patient requires glucocorticoid replacement until the remaining adrenal gland returns to normal.

Additional modes of therapy include radiation, drugs, and chemotherapy. O,p'-DDD (mitotane) destroys both normal and cancerous adrenal tissue. Therefore, it is important to initiate glucocorticoid replacement therapy when a response occurs (usually in several weeks). Mineralocorticoid replacement may also be necessary. Among the chemotherapeutic agents that have been used, alone or in combination, are alkylating agents such as cyclophosphamide, doxorubicin, and fluorouracil. Many others have been tried, but in the cases reported in the literature, there has been only limited success with these agents.

PHEOCHROMOCYTOMA

Pheochromocytoma generally arises from the adrenal medulla, but it may be found anywhere along the sympathetic chain. Definitive treatment consists of surgical excision. In children it may be bilateral, in which case bilateral adrenalectomy is necessary, as well as subsequent lifelong glucocorticoid and mineralocorticoid therapy. Three major complications may occur during surgery: severe hypertension, tachyarrhythmias, and hypotension. The first two result from excessive discharge of catecholamines during manipulation of the tumor, and the latter from catecholamine withdrawal and hypovolemic shock. Appropriate preoperative and operative management of the patient is crucial in preventing these complications. Preparation usually begins 1 to 3 weeks before surgery. To control catecholamine release, the patient is placed on α-blockers with or without β-adrenegic blocking agents. The most commonly used α-blocker is phenoxybenzamine hydrochloride (Dibenzyline). It is administered orally and, because of its long half-life, is given on an every 12 hour basis. The usual starting dose is 5 mg every 12 hours. However, the dose must be adjusted to the individual patient and this should occur in the hospital.

Phentolamine (Regitine) is equally effective but less satisfactory for prolonged use because of its short half-life. It is particularly useful, however, when these patients develop acute hypertension, such as during a diagnostic radiographic procedure or during surgery. The emergency dose of phentolamine is 1 mg intravenously or intramuscularly.

Additional preoperative therapy with β-adrenergic blocking agents is appropriate when α-blockade alone is not satisfactorily controlling the catecholamine excess or when tachyarrhythmias develop. β-blockers are myocardial depressants, and in patients with hypertensive cardiomyopathy, may precipitate congestive heart failure. Propranolol* (Inderal) is the most commonly used β-blocker.

---

* Manufacturer's warning: Safety and efficacy in children have not been established.

The usual dose is 5 to 10 mg orally every 6 to 8 hours, but again, the dose must be adjusted to the needs of the individual patient. The emergency dose for tachyarrhythmias is 1 mg administered IV over 1 minute.

Most recently, metyrosine (Demser) has been used in combination with adrenergic blockade when the latter alone is not sufficient treatment. Metyrosine is a tyrosine hydroxylase inhibitor that reduces the production of catecholamines. The usual starting dose is 5 to 10 mg/kg/day orally every 6 hours. Again, the dose must be adjusted to the needs of the individual patient.

There should be close intraoperative monitoring of these patients, including both central venous and arterial pressure. Also, during surgery it is essential to administer an adequate amount of intravenous fluid to prevent hypovolemic shock once the tumor is resected. Preoperative administration of phenoxybenzamine may also be helpful, as it permits intravascular volume expansion by its β-blocking capability.

Intraoperatively, hypertension can be controlled with either phentolamine or sodium nitroprusside IV. Supraventricular tachyarrhythmias can be treated with propranolol IV, and ventricular arrhythmias with lidocaine. It should be reiterated that hydrocortisone should be available, so that in cases of bilateral adrenalectomy a continuous IV infusion may be begun.

If hypertension persists for longer than 48 hours postsurgical removal, one must suspect a remaining tumor. In children, these tumors may be not only multiple but also extra-adrenal. This emphasizes the importance of complete abdominal exploration at surgery. It is important to document normal plasma and/or urinary catecholamines, as patients may be normotensive and asymptomatic postoperatively but may still have residual tumor.

It is wise to follow these patients and their families for many years, because these tumors may recur, and because of their association with conditions such as multiple endocrine adenomatosis, neurofibromatosis, and von Hippel-Lindau disease.

PREMATURE ADRENARCHE

This is a benign condition of isolated sexual hair growth (pubic, with or without axillary hair) in boys less than 9 and girls less than 8 years of age. The source of androgens is most likely the adrenal gland.

No treatment is indicated, but close follow-up is necessary to assess the patient's growth velocity and to note if additional signs of puberty appear. In this condition, the growth velocity is either normal or slightly accelerated. The bone age is usually slightly more advanced than the chronological age but compatible with the height age. On follow-up, these patients should show no other signs of virilization than the presence of sexual hair, and no other signs of puberty should appear. Baseline and follow-up serum androgens and 24-hour urinary 17-ketosteroids are elevated but remain in the early pubertal range. Serum 17OHP, gonadotropins, and the response to LHRH stimulation are all at prepubertal levels.

Endocrine Disorders of the Testis

JOHN S. PARKS, M.D., Ph.D.

PRENATAL DISORDERS OF THE TESTIS

Testicular dysgenesis, enzymatic deficiencies in testosterone production, and defects in the end-organ metabolism or recognition of testosterone impede differentiation of the external genitalia as well as later phallic growth. The combination of microphallus (stretched penile length less than 2.0 cm), hypospadias, and chordee deserves intensive investigation and careful consideration of sex assignment. The presence of a uterus by ultrasound examination, a chromatin-positive buccal smear, or a 46 XX karyotype identifies the child as a virilized genetic female who may need specific treatment for congenital adrenal hyperplasia. In the genetic male, normal testosterone levels after hCG stimulation, or during the physiological increase in testosterone at 2 to 4 months, suggest impaired conversion of testosterone to dihydrotestosterone or defective end-organ recognition of dihydrotestosterone. Males with the 5-α-reductase deficiency or partial androgen resistance respond poorly to testosterone treatment during infancy or at adolescence. Early recognition of these disorders should lead to a female sex assignment despite a 46 XY karyotype.

Isolated hypospadias and chordee usually reflect an embryopathy limited to the critical 8- to 12-week period of genital differentiation. In general, hypospadias with normal phallic size and bilaterally descended gonads does not require hormonal intervention and can be managed surgically.

Microphallus without hypospadias is most often due to deficient pituitary LH and FSH production during the second and third trimesters. Neonatal hypoglycemia should alert the physician to the likelihood of associated deficiencies of growth hormone, ACTH, and TSH. Treatment of microphallus during infancy is usually successful, resulting in phallic enlargement into the normal range without adverse side effects. Intramuscular injection of depot testosterone cypionate or testosterone enanthate, 25 mg every two weeks for a total of three doses, is generally adequate to cause the phallus to lengthen to greater than 5 cm and increase in width to greater than 1 cm. The optimum age for treatment is 2 to 4 months, when there is normally a surge in testosterone production. During this time, the infant responds to treatment with selective phallic growth without development of sexual hair, acne, or accelerated bone maturation. Later treatment may require higher testosterone doses, and there is a risk of inappropriate virilization.

The pediatrician should be aware that most instances of alleged microphallus in later childhood involve a phallus of normal size that is obscured by an abundance of fat. The phallus often disappears completely when the child stands and he may urinate by aiming his belly in the general direction of a toilet. Explanation and instruction are preferred alternatives to hormone treatment.

DEFICIENCY OF PUBERTAL DEVELOPMENT

Several types of male hypogonadism can be recognized in advance of the usual age of puberty. Examples of primary hypogonadism include surgically proven anorchia or testicular hypoplasia with increased LH and FSH levels. Boys with Kallmann's syndrome lack the sense of smell and have central hypogonadism. In these cases, one can begin treatment with small intramuscular doses of the long-acting testosterone cypionate or testosterone enanthate esters at around age 11. I use 50 mg/month as a starting dose and continue at this level for about a year. Clinical assessment of pubertal development and growth rate provides guidelines for adjusting dosage. The objective is to keep the boy in phase with his classmates. Increases to 100 mg and 200 mg per month are followed by an adult maintenance dose of 200 mg every two weeks. If treatment is started late, then one can start with 100 mg/month and advance dosage more rapidly to make up for lost time. Once sexual maturation is complete, with achievement of potency, deepening of voice, adequate beard growth, and cessation of growth in height, I raise the option of temporarily discontinuing treatment to let the young man determine whether the benefits of treatment are still worth the discomfort of the injections. Two common errors in the management of male hypogonadism are failure to increase testosterone dose to emulate the normal increments in testosterone production with advancing puberty and cessation of therapy before adult sexual development is attained.

The effects of testosterone treatment are generally beneficial, but some can be distressing if they are not mentioned in advance. It is common to have reddening and tenderness of the scrotum during early weeks of therapy. This reflects the fact that scrotal skin is a sensitive target organ for testosterone. Frequent and unanticipated erections are common, as they are during spontaneous puberty. Breast budding and tenderness occur but seldom progress to true gynecomastia. Salt and fluid retention can lead to noticeable edema and dictate a temporary decrease in testosterone dose. Hepatic toxicity is less common with the testosterone esters than with orally active androgens.

Methyl testosterone (17-α-methyltestosterone) and fluoxymesterone (the 9-α-fluoro-11-α-hydroxy derivative of methyl testosterone) have been given orally to promote pubertal development. Doses are 10 to 40 mg daily for methyltestosterone and 10 to 20 mg daily for fluoxymesterone. There are two reasons for preferring testosterone ester injections. The first is that the oral preparations are not as effective in producing complete sexual maturation. They are quite adequate for producing phallic growth, sexual hair, and a linear growth spurt but generally fail to produce adequate beard growth. The second concern involves reports of hepatic damage. Cholestatic jaundice is reversible on stopping treatment. Hepatic adenomas and hepatocellular carcinomas have been reported in patients receiving oral androgens for the induction of puberty as well as in patients treated for aplastic anemia.

The discussion to this point has involved hormone replacement as a substitute for testicular androgen production. In males with anorchia, testosterone treatment and implantation of testicular prostheses ensure a normal appearance and normal potency. In males with central (hypothalamic or pituitary) hypogonadism, there is also the issue of fertility. Prolonged treatment with hCG and FSH can promote testicular growth, androgen production, and maturation of germinal cells. However, current treatment protocols are too complicated and expensive for use as a means of inducing puberty at a normal age. The usual practice is to promote virilization with testosterone and treat infertility after other aspects of maturation are complete. In future years, it may be practical to administer luteinizing hormone–releasing hormone (LHRH) analogues intranasally or by pulsatile subcutaneous injection and achieve a more complete and physiological induction of puberty.

KLINEFELTER'S SYNDROME

Klinefelter's syndrome with a 47 XXY karyotype is one of the most common causes of male hypogonadism. The typical presentation is a male with sexual maturation in advance of the degree of testicular enlargement. Some males with this disorder produce subnormal quantities of testosterone and experience arrest of pubertal development. Measurement of serum testosterone will provide information about whether supplementation is needed.

CONSTITUTIONAL DELAY OF PUBERTAL DEVELOPMENT

Constitutional delay refers to a lag of two or more years beyond the mean in appearance and progression of signs of puberty. The term implies that pubertal changes will occur and lead to maturity, but at a later age. Systemic illnesses and acquired pituitary deficiency can produce a similar picture and can be confused with simple delay. The boy with delayed puberty is distressed by looking younger and being smaller than his classmates. Detection and explanation of subtle signs of puberty together with agreement to monitor progress, are helpful in allaying anxiety.

On occasion, delay of puberty is so severe or waiting is so painful that hormonal intervention merits discussion. I do not intervene until chronological age is at least 14 and bone age is at least 11. The aim is to provide enough short-time virilization to narrow the gap in physical maturity and at the same time prime the pump for advancement of endogenous puberty. If one begins before bone age 11, the prospect of sustained progress after stopping a course of treatment is small. However, a minority of boys with bone age less than 11 will continue through puberty on their own at an accelerated rate with rapid skeletal maturation and an adverse effect on adult height.

Intramuscular injections of long-acting testosterone cypionate or testosterone enanthate at 100 mg/month for 3 consecutive months will produce increases in linear growth rate and in muscle size together with appreciable phallic growth. If testicular volume increases during this time or over the next 3 months, then it is a sign that the boy's own pubertal mechanisms have been activated and no further treatment is indicated. Occasionally, a second 3-month course is required.

PRECOCIOUS PUBERTY

Extensive studies have shown that potent, long-acting analogs of luteinizing hormone–releasing hormone (LHRH) are effective in treating central precocious puberty. LHRH is normally secreted by the hypothalamus in a pulsatile manner, with a periodicity of 60 to 90 minutes. The LHRH agonists have a much longer half-life, and they provide continuous saturation of pituitary LHRH receptors when given by injection or by nasal insufflation once or twice a day. Under these circumstances, pituitary gonadotrophic cells as the source of LH and FSH are reversibly inactivated. Circulating LH, FSH, and testosterone decline to childhood levels. At the time of writing, these LHRH analogues are restricted to experimental use in the United States. A child must be referred to a center that is doing the research in order to be treated. We can anticipate that the drugs will be approved for use by prescription before the 13th edition of *Current Pediatric Therapy*. The reader is encouraged to consult a pediatric endocrinologist to learn the current status of this breakthrough in treatment of central precocious puberty.

Primary testicular autonomy does not respond to treatment with LHRH analogues. Medroxyprogesterone acetate (Depo-Provera) has been used in the treatment of central precocious puberty and it may have some marginal effect in this condition as well. It is given intramuscularly in a dose of 100 to 200 mg/month or by mouth in a dose of 10 mg two to four times per day. Effectiveness is monitored by lowering of serum testosterone and decrease in the rates of linear growth and bone age progression. The weak antiglucocorticoid action of the drug can cause both adrenal suppression and a cushingoid habitus. Concerns about long-term effects on gonads, chromosomes, and tumor development dictate caution in the use of medroxyprogesterone acetate.

The androgen antagonist cyproterone acetate has been used in other countries for treatment of central and primary testicular precocious puberty. It is effective when given orally in a dose of 70–150 mg/m²/day. The drug is distributed in the United States for treatment of metastatic cancer of the breast and prostate. It is not approved for use in children.

Male sexual precocity poses severe problems for the affected child and his family. Excess size, strength, and energy level make him stand out among his peers. Adults in his environment have difficulty reconciling his physical maturity with a behavior more in keeping with chronological age. Mothers often have difficulty in showing closeness by touching and hugging. The developmental burden of precocious puberty is much greater in males than in females. Prompt mental health evaluation and intervention are required.

Gynecomastia

WILLIAM W. CLEVELAND, M.D.

Breast enlargement in the male, gynecomastia, occurs in three groups, with different significance in each. Neonatal breast enlargement in the male infant is common and requires no diagnostic or therapeutic intervention.

Breast enlargement in the prepubertal boy is comparatively uncommon and deserves careful consideration. Investigation of exposure to estrogen or drugs is important. It should be recalled that certain adult vitamin preparations contain sex steroids. Clinical evaluation and hormonal measurements should be undertaken to exclude endogenous production of steroids by a tumor of either the adrenals or the gonads. Virilization due to sexual precocity may result in gynecomastia just as it does in normal adolescent development. Investigation ordinarily will not reveal any abnormality, however, and the condition will be considered idiopathic. No medical treatment is available. Although the condition spontaneously disappears, it may persist for many months or a few years. Tumors of the breast in prepubertal boys are very rare and have included carcinoma along with lipomas, neurofibromas, and hemangiomas. Surgical removal may be indicated if the patient manifests sufficent concern or if a tissue diagnosis appears warranted.

Gynecomastia occurs commonly in adolescent boys. In most there is coin-sized enlargement involving one or both breasts. In others obvious enlargement reaching diameters of 6 to 10 cm may be found. Significant gynecomastia occurs more commonly in males who are undergoing rapid pubertal development. The mechanism is not clearly understood but may reflect conversion of androgen to estrogen in a ratio that results in stimulation of mammary tissue. Adolescent breast enlargement may also occur in pathologic situations, including Klinefelter's syndrome; if the gonads are unusually small or abnormalities of mental development are present, a karyotype may be indicated. Measurement of testosterone, estrogen, and prolactin concentrations in serum will be helpful in excluding rare aberrations in hormonal function such as adrenal or gonadal tumors.

A particular problem is presented by the obese adolescent boy who has apparent breast enlargement. Differentiating mammary and adipose tissue by palpation may be difficult. In most instances the enlargement represents accumulation of adipose tissue in the area; this assumes importance in considering treatment.

No satisfactory medical treatment for gynecomastia has been established. Treatment with testosterone in an effort to bring about a more favorable androgen:estrogen ratio is not effective and is contraindicated. Clomiphene, a drug that has antiestrogenic action, has been used with equivocal results and its use at this time should be considered experimental. The only satisfactory treatment is surgical removal of mammary tissue. This relatively simple operation, involving a circumareolar incision, gives generally good results with minimal apparent scar. What are the indications for mammoplasty? Although breast enlargement tends to diminish with time, it may take months or years to disappear. Meanwhile many young men experience much embarassment from the condition, resulting in considerable alteration of lifestyle. Given the simplicity of the operation and its good results, it should be offered to patients with significant gynecomastia who are concerned to the point of being enthusiastic about treatment. Caution should be exercised, however, in management of the obese male with apparent breast enlargement, which is largely due to accumulation of adipose tissue in the area. In this case surgical treatment is more difficult and less apt to yield satisfactory results. Obviously the best approach in this instance would be to treat the obesity in order to achieve a reduction in the enlargement of the area, however difficult this may be.

Ambiguous Genitalia

R. MARSHALL PITTS, M.D.

When an infant is born with ambiguous genitalia, this problem should be handled as any other surgical emergency in the newborn. A decision concerning the choice of gender for the child must be decided immediately to avert psychological and social disaster, first for the family, and later for the child. If not settled promptly, this can be a problem for the child's life. A male with an abnormally small phallus that will not function sexually is destined for unhappiness. A satisfactory female can be constructed relatively easily with clitoral recession, vaginoplasty, breast implants, and estrogens at puberty. A genetic male can be raised as a happy female if "she" is considered female from early infancy. Children can be adopted. "Gender is learned."

A working decision concerning the best sex assignment for the child can be made on the first day of life. Buccal smear and fluorescent chromosome Y staining can be performed immediately. These determinations, together with careful examination of the anatomy, are sufficient for a working diagnosis, which is accurate enough to predict the most suitable sex assignment. Gonadal symmetry or asymmetry plus the chromatin mass determination enables the doctor to choose into which of the four major diagnostic categories the child fits.

In female pseudohermaphroditism, the chromatin study is positive, and the ambiguous genitalia are symmetrical. In male pseudohermaphroditism, the chromatin is negative, and the genitalia are symmetrical. True hermaphroditism, which is very rare, is usually associated with a chromatin-positive study and asymmetry. Infants with mixed gonadal dysgenesis are usually chromatin negative, with gonadal asymmetry. This is slightly oversimplified, but it is a useful guide for early decisions. These criteria were established by Patricia K. Donahoe, M.D., and W. Hardy Hendren, M.D., of Harvard Medical School, Boston, Massachusetts.

These criteria can guide the decisions regarding

the child's sex determination on the first day of life before karyotyping and steroid analyses are completed. The sex assignment should be decided on the basis of anatomy and what can be done surgically for the newborn, regardless of the chromosomal karyotype. Donahoe and Hendren advise, "Only those males with a phallus of adequate size should be considered for male rearing. Otherwise the baby should be reared as a female." Even though a working diagnosis can be made quickly, a careful, detailed diagnostic work-up is also necessary. The definitive diagnosis of the infant with an intersex problem is made from the following studies: (1) history, (2) physical examination, (3) buccal smear, (4) cytogenetics, (5) x-ray, (6) endoscopy, (7) biochemical studies, and (8) laparotomy with gonadal biopsy.

A history of drugs taken during pregnancy may indicate that drugs have masculinized a female or feminized a male infant. A history of habitual abortions suggests possible chromosomal problems. The unexplained death of a sibling or relative in the first few weeks of life may help establish the diagnosis of adrenogenital syndrome with salt loss.

A gonad in an inguinal hernia of a "female" infant may be a testis or ovotestis. A uterus in a newborn under the influence of maternal estrogens is large enough to be felt as a "pencil-like" structure by rectal examination. A mucous discharge from the "male genitalia" or urogenital sinus suggests the presence of a vagina.

The buccal smear preparation is made by scraping the inside of the cheek with a tongue blade to obtain the specimen. The cells from a female show chromatin masses or "Barr bodies" in over 20% of the nuclei (chromatin +). The cells from males show the chromatin masses in no more than 1–2% of the nuclei, if at all (chromatin −).

The infant's blood should be sent promptly for chromosomal study. The normal karyotype for the female is 46,XX; the normal for the male is 46,XY. Chromosomal abnormalities may be manifest as ambiguous genitalia in newborns with mixed gonadal dysgenesis and true hermaphroditism. Mixed gonadal dysgenesis, the second most common disorder of intersex, has sex chromosome mosaicism, which is most commonly 45,X/46,XY.

When a vagina is suspected but not obvious by inspection, x-ray studies of the genitalia may help establish the complete diagnosis. A blunt catheter tip is placed at the opening of the urogenital sinus to fill the urethra and vagina. The vagina is not always demonstrated by this method. Endoscopy may be required to see a vaginal opening missed by x-ray. Miniature endoscopes are available for use in newborn males and even small premature males. Obviously this study should be performed only by experienced pediatric endoscopists.

The following biochemical studies help establish the diagnosis of adrenogenital syndrome: 17 ketosteroids, 17 hydrocorticoids, and urinary pregnanetriol. These tests help make an accurate diagnosis, but require several days for results. The urinary gonadotropins and serum testosterone, steroids, and gonadotropins can be measured in some laboratories. Sex assignment should be decided by the anatomy of the infant, however, and what can be surgically done, rather than from a specific diagnosis by biochemical and other studies. Vaginal smears and urinary cytology provide quick information concerning the influence of estrogens.

Laparotomy and gonadal biopsy are not necessary to diagnose adrenogenital syndrome, but they are often necessary to make a diagnosis of other forms of ambiguous genitalia. The initial laparotomy should be for *diagnosis only* by inspection and biopsy. Other operations to alter the anatomy, remove gonads, and so forth should be done later.

Confusion is lessened by placing infants with ambiguous genitalia into four categories. The first two categories have gonadal symmetry, the result of an abnormal influence applied equally to both gonads.

Female Pseudohermaphroditism

The androgenized infant female with pseudohermaphroditism is chromatin positive with gonadal symmetry. Congenital adrenocortical hyperplasia is the classical example of this. This is the most common of the ambiguous genitalia aberrations, and the only one that is life-threatening.

Congenital adrenogenital hyperplasia is a hereditary recessive deficiency of cortisol synthesis that results in a compensatory overproduction of ACTH by the pituitary gland, which in turn causes an overproduction of androgen. The excess androgen masculinizes the female fetus. The diagnosis of congenital adrenocortical hyperplasia should be entertained in infants with bilateral "cryptorchism" and hypospadias, a small or abnormal phallus which is actually a clitoris, or in any neonate with vomiting and cardiovascular collapse in the first few weeks of life. One-half of the infants with this disease are male. Males are not easily recognized unless the problem is suspected by history of an affected sibling or relative. Males may have increased pigmentation of the genitalia.

The deficiencies of cortisol synthesis may be complete or incomplete. In the complete form diminished aldosterone may lead to excessive salt loss and a "salt loss" crisis. Lacking cortisol, the infant may become severely hypoglycemic. The infant may be hypertensive. Death may result unless treatment is immediate and maintained.

The diagnosis of adrenocortical hyperplasia is by laboratory tests. The infants have hyponatremia and hyperkalemia and may have hypoglycemia.

They have elevated levels of urinary ketosteroids and later pregnanetriol, and elevated serum levels of 17 hydroxyprogestrone. Laboratory tests may take several days. Treatment should be instituted on suspicion. EKG changes of hyperkalemia and hyponatremia in conjunction with the changes in the genitalia are sufficient for instituting immediate treatment with sodium and glucose in solution (but not potassium). Steroid therapy should also be given promptly.

A diagnostic laparotomy should not be necessary for diagnosis or treatment of adrenogenital syndrome, although diagnosis by inspection can be difficult sometimes because of the spectrum of abnormality of the external genitalia in females from mild clitoral enlargement to complete labial-scrotal fusion with severe clitoromegaly and urethral formation in the clitoral shaft. Prenatal masculinization or virilization can also occur from drugs during pregnancy or from certain androgen-producing adrenal or gonadal tumors.

The abnormal genitalia can always be successfully reconstructed for acceptable cosmetic appearance and sexual function. Clitoral recession should be done as soon as the infant is stabilized on steroid treatment, to lessen the parents' anguish. Vaginoplasty at the time of clitoral recession or clitorectomy helps prevent infection by preventing stagnation of urine and secretions in the distal "covered vagina." A skin flap from just anterior to the anus into the posterior vagina provides a wide posterior surface for the introitus. In a highly masculinized adrenogenital patient, the vagina may arise from the urethra above the voluntary urethral sphincter. This is detected by cystogram or endoscopy. In this case the more complicated Hendren vaginal "pull-through" repair is necessary. The vagina is pulled down behind the sphincter to avoid permanent incontinence, which would result from the simple marsupialization procedure.

Male Pseudohermaphroditism

The incompletely masculinized male with pseudohermaphroditism is chromatin negative with gonadal symmetry. This may be an inherited unresponsiveness or subresponsiveness of genital structures to testosterone. It may also result from prenatal ingestion of drugs that feminize, placental insufficiency of gonadotropin production, or failure of development or damage to gonads in utero. The classical presentation for male pseudohermaphroditism is the testicular feminization syndrome. These infants appear to have female external genitalia. They have inguinal hernias on occasion, which may contain a testis. Plasma testosterone and urinary gonadotropins are likely to be elevated. Gonadectomy should be done before puberty because of the high risk of malignancy after puberty. These individuals have a feminine appearance which can be augmented by gonadectomy and the administration of estrogens at puberty. Reifenstein's syndrome and dysgenetic male pseudohermaphroditism are included in this category. If the phallus is sufficiently large, some of these males can be treated with hypospadias repair, insertion of testicular prostheses, and hormonal therapy at an appropriate age. Gender assignment should be made on the basis of anatomy.

Mixed Gonadal Dysgenesis

Infants with mixed gonadal dysgenesis are usually chromatin negative with asymmetry of the external genitalia. This is the second most common problem of ambiguous genitalia. Internally the typical anatomy is a streak ovary on one side and a dysgenetic testis on the other. Other combinations, such as bilateral streak ovaries, a dysgenetic gonad on one side and tumor on the other, and other combinations are possible. The degree of virilization varies from female-appearing genitalia with an enlarged clitoris to male-appearing genitalia with hypospadias and scrotum containing a single gonad. These infants have sex chromosome mosaicism, which is most commonly 45,X/46,XY. They should be reared in the female role, since they would probably be inadequate males. The gonads should always be removed because of the high risk of malignancy, which increases over the years to about 75% of patients in their midtwenties. This high risk is probably the result of persistent unchecked pituitary gonadotropin stimulation of the abnormal gonads.

True Hermaphroditism

Infants with true hermaphroditism are usually chromatin positive with asymmetrical external genitalia. Diagnosis of this rare condition is established by finding well differentiated male and female gonadal tissue in the same individual. About 60% of these babies are a 46,XX karyotype.

Conclusion

Ambiguous genitalia is a bonafide emergency of the newborn. Although the congenital adrenogenital syndrome is the only actual life-threatening intersex problem, prompt decisions regarding the assignment of sex to an infant are very important psychologically to the family and infant. When there is any doubt that the patient can be an adequate male, the female gender should be selected. Even though the buccal smear is negative and the karyotype is male, a genetic male can function as a female and regard "herself" a female if reared as a female from early infancy. Anatomy, not genetic sex, must be the overriding factor in deciding which gender will best suit the infant.

10

Metabolic Disorders

Infants Born to Diabetic Mothers

NAOMI D. NEUFELD, M.D.

Advances in the obstetrical care of the pregnant diabetic patient, coupled with a greater understanding of the etiology of specific fetal disorders, have led to a significant reduction in both neonatal morbidity and mortality rates in infants of diabetic mothers (IDM). Nonetheless, the rates of perinatal morbidity are still significantly greater than in normal pregnancies; thus, the care of such infants is extremely critical. Care should begin in the prenatal period and, to be performed well, is best conducted in a tertiary medical center where the team approach of obstetrician, pediatrician, and specialist in diabetes is practiced.

The aims of prenatal care are (1) to strictly regulate diabetic control of the pregnant patient. Patients with poor diabetic control have a significantly higher incidence of fetal loss, and ketoacidosis in particular is associated with extremely high fetal losses. Better metabolic control has been shown to significantly reduce neonatal morbidity and mortality rates; and (2) to monitor continued viability and well-being of the fetus and allow prolongation of pregnancy to as near term as possible.

MATERNAL MANAGEMENT

Most authorities consider maternal hyperglycemia a major predisposing factor in the development of clinical complications in IDM. Since improvement of fetal outcome has been shown to occur with good metabolic control of maternal diabetes throughout pregnancy, diabetic patients should be seen on a weekly basis for supervision of dietary and insulin therapy. The aims are to maintain fasting blood glucose at 100 mg/dl and postprandial blood glucose at less than 140 mg/dl, and to prevent ketoacidosis. Insulin doses should be adjusted according to home urine test results for glucose and acetone, as well as the history of hypoglycemic episodes. Recent studies have suggested a role for home monitoring of blood glucose in pregnancy as an improvement in the care of these patients, leading to further reduction in perinatal morbidity rates. Rigorous diabetic management using a regimen of multiple insulin injections or continuous insulin infusion by portable pump has been shown to significantly reduce perinatal morbidity in diabetic pregnancy. It remains to be shown whether such management in the early stages of pregnancy would reduce the incidence of major congenital anomalies. Should diabetic control be difficult to achieve early in pregnancy, patients should be hospitalized for careful supervision.

FETAL WELL-BEING

Tests of fetal well-being in pregnancy should be performed routinely. Ultrasonography at 18 to 20 weeks will give a fairly accurate determination of fetal size, confirming the duration of pregnancy and ruling out the presence of gross fetal anomaly. Serial determinations may be performed to assess the rate of fetal growth. Urinary estriol, protein, and creatinine determinations should be performed at least weekly after 30 weeks' gestation. After 33 weeks' gestation, pregnant patients should have nonstress testing or oxytocin challenge tests for assessment of fetal and placental function. Patients with falling urinary estriol values, abnormal stress or nonstress testing, pre-eclampsia, or poor diabetic control should be admitted to the hospital immediately for close supervision.

Patients with uncomplicated pregnancies should be hospitalized at 36 to 37 weeks' gestation for further management. Alterations in insulin and dietary therapy during the hospital stay are made in accordance with the results of blood glucose determinations obtained two to four times daily. Prevention of hyperglycemia during the latter stage of pregnancy has been associated with a significant reduction in the incidence of fetal macrosomia and postnatal hypoglycemia. Use of techniques such as closed- or open-loop continuous insulin infusion devices during this period may further reduce the incidence of these problems. During that time, the daily urinary estriol determinations and weekly tests of fetal well-being mentioned above should be performed.

Prior to delivery, fetal lung maturation is assessed by amniocentesis, utilizing lecithin/sphingomyelin ratio (L/S) determinations or lung maturity profiles, which include measurement of phosphatidylglycerol and disaturated phosphatidylcholine. Since documented cases of the respiratory distress syndrome (RDS) have been shown to occur in IDM who have L/S ratios of 2:1, a ratio of 3.5:1 or greater may be necessary to assure good fetal outcome.

Timing of the delivery of the IDM should take into account the variables of maternal and fetal well-being described. Planning of the delivery should include the pediatrician, who is informed about the expected fetal status and who will be present in the delivery room to initiate resuscitation therapy as needed, as well as to identify other specific problems. The need for elected caesarean section for predetermined fetal macrosomia should be considered in order to avoid birth injury.

GENERAL NEONATAL MANAGEMENT

If maternal blood glucose values are normalized during pregnancy as described above, such infants should appear to require very little attention since the incidence of perinatal morbidity is reduced to normal. On the other hand, if normal blood glucose values are not documented during diabetic pregnancies, such infants should be monitored as outlined herein. Following delivery, essential information, including Apgar score, weight, sex, and any obvious congenital anomalies, should be carefully recorded by the nursing staff. A specimen of cord blood should be sent to the laboratory for glucose and pH determinations at that time. Infants are transferred to the stabilization nursery, where they are warmed and more carefully examined. Assessment of gestational age by Dubowitz criteria is recorded. Detailed examination of the heart, lung, kidneys, and extremities and the presence of obvious congenital anomalies and birth injuries, including Erb palsy, fractured clavicle, phrenic nerve injury, or intracranial hemorrhage, should be noted. Blood studies for initial determinations of glucose (using Dextrostix or BG Chemstrips), calcium, hematocrit, and bilirubin should be obtained according to the following schedule:

Glucose: 1, 2, 4, 6, 8, 12, 24, 36, 48 hrs of age
Calcium: 6, 12, 24, 48 hrs of age
Hematocrit: 2, 24 hrs of age
Bilirubin (total and direct): 24, 48 hrs of age

The incidence and severity of the specific problems seen in IDM are related directly to the severity of the maternal diabetes, as judged by the White criteria, as well as to the degree of prematurity at birth. Near-term infants with gestational diabetes have a reported incidence of perinatal morbidity of 25% or less. Infants delivered prior to 37 weeks of mothers with severe, long-standing diabetes have morbidity rates at birth approaching 60%. These infants in particular have a significantly greater incidence of serious complications, including major congenital malformations and hypocalcemia.

SPECIFIC PROBLEMS OF THE IDM

Hypoglycemia is defined as blood glucose value of less than 30 mg/dl in infants of any gestational age. This is the most common metabolic complication, occurring in as many as 56% of IDM. Most often it occurs between 1 and 1.5 hours of life. Oral feedings of glucose water should begin within 1 hour of life, and assessment of blood glucose should continue in association with feedings until stable. By 12 hours most infants are on formula with transfer to breast feedings as soon as possible, and supplemental feedings of glucose-water are given as necessary to prevent hypoglycemia.

For infants who are unable to feed well or whose hypoglycemia cannot be managed by oral feedings, treatment with intravenous glucose infusions at a rate of at least 6 mg/kg/min, or that rate which results in normal steady-state glucose levels, should be given. The use of hypertonic glucose in bolus doses should be avoided since, in the presence of persisting hyperinsulinemia, this may lead to rebound hypoglycemia. Treatment with glucagon, while recommended by some, is usually not necessary. In the usual case this is a transient phenomenon lasting no more than 24 to 48 hours. Persistence of hypoglycemia beyond 48 hours often necessitates glucocorticoid treatment. Persistence of hypoglycemia despite glucocorticoid therapy should prompt investigation for causes, such as beta-cell hyperplasia (nesidioblastosis) or islet cell tumor (see article on Hypoglycemia).

While the incidence of the *respiratory distress syndrome* has been reduced significantly because of a greater understanding of pathophysiology and improvement in prenatal care, this still remains a major form of neonatal morbidity in diabetic pregnancies. Treatment of RDS is discussed elsewhere in this book.

The peak incidence of *hypocalcemia* occurs within 48 hours of birth and is increased in the presence of other known causes of the disorder. Treatment is usually begun when calcium levels are less than 7 mg/dl. The treatment of choice is with calcium gluconate (10%) given either orally or intravenously. Acute symptomatic hypocalcemia is treated with 2 ml/kg of intravenous calcium gluconate given slowly (1 ml/min or less), with the careful monitoring of heart rate. (*Note:* calcium should not be added to intravenous solutions containing sodium bicarbonate since an insoluble precipitate, $CaCO_3$, will form). Oral supplementation can be continued with the addition of diluted calcium salts to formula at a dose of 0.5 to 1.0 gm/kg/24 hr.

To prevent further aggravation of hypocalcemia (neonatal tetany), feedings with only those formulas with low-phosphate loads should be provided. Breast milk is ideal, and nursing is beneficial for both the infant and the diabetic mother. Other specially prepared low-phosphate formulas such as PM 60/40 (Ca^{++}, 400 mg/l, P, 200 mg/l) can be used. Treatment is usually necessary for 4 to 5 days: during this time calcium levels should be monitored every 12 to 24 hours and supplemental calcium provided accordingly.

Persistence of hypocalcemia or its resistance to treatment should lead to a search for other causes. Hypocalcemia may occur in the presence of renal insufficiency, defective Vitamin D metabolism, or hypomagnesemia. Treatment of these disorders is described elsewhere in this book.

Hyperbilirubinemia is another problem commonly observed in the IDM, occurring in as many as 37% of infants in one series. The etiology of this disorder is unclear, although both polycythemia with increased hemolysis and hypoglycemia have been implicated. Treatment of the jaundiced infant is described elsewhere in this book.

POLYCYTHEMIA AND HYPERVISCOSITY SYNDROMES

The occurrence of elevated hematocrit (greater than 65% for a venous sample obtained within 2 hours of birth) is very common in IDM, although the exact incidence is not known. A direct relationship between the viscosity and venous blood hematocrit has been defined. The clinical findings in such infants are due to the increased viscosity of blood flow in the venous bed and include respiratory distress, cyanosis, jitteriness, jaundice, thrombocytopenia, necrotizing enterocolitis, and gangrene. Treatment, which is aimed at lowering the hematocrit to between 50 to 60% with exchange transfusion, is carefully detailed in the article on Hyperviscosity Syndromes.

Renal vein thrombosis, an unusual complication of polycythemia, is seen with a greater frequency than normal in IDM and is often associated with asphyxia and hypotension. Clinical manifestations include hematuria and renal enlargement. Treatment is conservative, based upon careful fluid and electrolyte management coupled with heparin

therapy. These are temporizing measures that permit observation for spontaneous resolution of the disorder. In rare instances, surgical intervention may be required.

The major cause of death in IDM in several recent studies was that associated with fatal *congenital anomalies* of various types, including severe cardiovascular defects, skeletal malformation such as sacral agenesis, and anencephaly-meningomyelocele. Careful management of maternal diabetes in the early stages of pregnancy has been suggested as the best means of lowering the incidence of these anomalies, which occur now in as many as 6% of all diabetic pregnancies. Treatment is dictated by the nature and severity of the particular lesion.

Diabetes Mellitus

JOSEPH I. WOLFSDORF, M.D.

The diverse needs of the child with diabetes can seldom be adequately met by a physician working in isolation. Therefore, whenever possible, care should be provided by a team consisting of health care professionals with complementary roles who are knowledgeable about the physical and emotional growth and development of children and experienced in the management of type I diabetes. The multidisciplinary team should include a pediatrician, a diabetes educator, a mental health professional, and a nutritionist, whose role is to provide nutrition education and assist with the details of individual meal planning. The members of the team should communicate with the important individuals in the child's life, for example, teacher, school nurse, school guidance counselor, and team coach. To provide optimal care for children with diabetes it is necessary to involve the entire family unit. The efforts of the diabetes team are aimed at ensuring that children and their families acquire the knowledge and skills necessary to cope successfully with this life-long disease. The diabetes treatment team provides not only medical and nutritional care for the child, but of equal importance, continuing diabetes education, family guidance, and psychological support.

EDUCATION

Patient education is the foundation of successful diabetes management. Few diseases demand so much day-to-day participation by the patient; consequently, the patient must possess extensive knowledge and understanding of all aspects of diabetes. Education involves more than just imparting facts and teaching skills; one of the most important aspects of a comprehensive patient education program is the promotion of desirable health beliefs and attitudes in the person who has to live with a chronic incurable disease. This applies particularly to adolescents with diabetes.

The educational curriculum for children must be concordant with each child's level of cognitive development, and in order to be meaningful, the process must be specifically adapted to the individual child. Parents should be fully involved, because delegating complete responsibility to the child is likely to have disastrous consequences. The educational program should be designed to gradually transfer the responsibility for diabetes care from the parents to the child so as not to impede the normal process of separation and attainment of independence that occurs during adolescence.

The process of educating the child and his family begins soon after the diagnosis has been made and evolves over a period of several years. The aim is to impart the fundamental knowledge and to teach the practical skills that enable the patient and his family to competently and confidently assume complete responsibility for self-care.

The grief reaction that follows the diagnosis of a serious disease leaves parents and patients too upset and anxious to assimilate an extensive body of largely abstract information; therefore, the initial educational goals should be limited. During the first several days the child and family should learn what diabetes is and how it is treated and acquire the survival skills necessary to care for the child at home and to permit his early return to school. During the next few weeks the child's metabolic status is stabilized and the basic aspects of diabetes care are consolidated by practical experience at home and frequent contact with the diabetes educator and physician. Once the grief reaction has subsided, the family is more ready to learn the sophisticated details of management necessary to achieve near-normal blood glucose levels and to cope with intercurrent illnesses and other variations in the child's daily routine. Many patients find it necessary and should be encouraged to periodically review and update their knowledge of diabetes self-care during the ensuing several years.

INSULIN

Replacement of insulin is the cornerstone of treatment of insulin-dependent diabetes. It is important to appreciate, however, that conventional insulin replacement therapy does not mimic normal insulin physiology. The healthy pancreas secretes insulin at a low basal rate upon which are superimposed bursts of increased insulin secretion that coincide with eating. Accordingly, insulin levels in the blood increase and decrease in concert with the rises and falls in blood glucose levels. Furthermore, insulin is secreted into the portal circulation, so that the liver, which is the chief site

of glucose disposal, is the target organ normally exposed to the highest concentration of insulin. In contrast, injection of insulin into the subcutaneous tissue results in absorption of insulin into the systemic circulation, so that the concentration of insulin to which the liver is exposed is reduced by dilution in the systemic circulation. Given these inherent limitations, conventional daily or twice daily insulin regimens can seldom restore normal carbohydrate metabolism. Even programs of intensive insulin therapy that include injections of quick-acting insulin (regular) before each meal cannot always restore the normal pattern, although the wide fluctuations in blood glucose concentration that typically occur with a single injection of intermediate-acting insulin or even two injections per day can be significantly improved.

Most children with total diabetes (patients without significant residual insulin secretion) can be satisfactorily controlled with a twice daily insulin regimen consisting of a mixture of rapid-acting (regular) and intermediate-acting (NPH or Lente) insulins drawn up into the same syringe and given before breakfast and again before the evening meal. The amount of rapid-acting insulin needed before breakfast is determined by the results of late morning and early afternoon blood glucose tests. Similarly, the decision to provide quick-acting insulin before supper is determined by the results of blood glucose tests at bedtime; if high at this time, regular insulin is added to the presupper dose of intermediate-acting insulin. When presupper regular insulin is not necessary, better glycemic control during the night and early morning and avoidance of nocturnal hypoglycemia are achieved when the intermediate-acting insulin is given at bedtime.

There is no way of predicting the precise dose of insulin that is necessary. Therefore, the insulin program must be empirically worked out for each patient. On an average, about 60 to 75% of the total daily dose is given before breakfast and approximately 25 to 40% before the evening meal. Usually about one third of each dose consists of quick-acting insulin; however, the optimal ratio of quick- to intermediate-acting insulin for each patient must be determined by trial and error based on the results of blood glucose monitoring. Shortly after starting insulin therapy, many children can be well-controlled using intermediate-acting insulin alone. Children's insulin requirements are not fixed; they change during growth and development. It is, therefore, necessary to periodically reevaluate and adjust each child's insulin regimen. Also, most children are considerably more active during the spring and summer months and usually require less insulin during this part of the year. The insulin dose should be changed by approximately 10% at any one time, and one should allow a minimum of three days to elapse after each change before further adjustments are made.

Whenever possible, regular insulin should be given at least 30 minutes before meals. This interval allows sufficient time for the quick-acting insulin to be absorbed; and when this is done, the rise in blood glucose after meals is significantly less than when the meal is eaten immediately after receiving the injection.

Early in the course of diabetes, some children achieve satisfactory glycemic control with a single daily injection of insulin. Persistent nocturnal hyperglycemia, manifested as nocturia or enuresis, or significant fasting hyperglycemia with or without ketonuria, usually signifies the need to give a second dose of intermediate-acting insulin, either before supper or at bedtime. If the morning dose of intermediate-acting insulin is substantially increased in an attempt to prolong its activity through the night and early morning hours, this may cause hypoglycemia or intense hunger and overeating during the period of maximum insulin activity, which is usually in the late afternoon and evening.

The technique of drawing up and injecting insulin should be taught to the patient when appropriate as well as to both parents. The average child of 12 or older can and should be encouraged to learn to give his own insulin injections. Although even younger children can also master this skill, they should not be coerced into giving their own shots. If a young child does wish to give his own injections, it is important to ensure that this always is done under close parental supervision. Young children should never be hurried into accepting full responsibility for their own injections until they are psychologically mature enough to fully appreciate the consequences of omitting insulin. Careful rotation of the injection sites (using the arms, thighs, buttocks, and anterior abdominal wall) prevents lipohypertrophy. Lipoatrophy is becoming less frequent with the use of highly purified insulin (pure pork or human).

The total daily insulin dose in prepubertal children is usually in the range of 0.5 to 1 unit/kg; in pubertal individuals, the usual range is 0.8 to 1.5 units/kg. Less insulin is needed during the phase of partial remission. When the dose of insulin exceeds the above ranges, one should consider the possibility that the patient may be receiving more insulin than is actually necessary and is experiencing intermittent hypoglycemia followed by rebound hyperglycemia; this is a well-recognized cause of unstable glycemic control.

During the remission period ("honeymoon"), the insulin requirement may decrease to a negligible amount, so that one may be tempted to eliminate it completely. Most physicians experienced in the care of diabetes in children insist that insulin should not be eliminated, even if only one or two units are given each day. The remission phase in children usually lasts a few weeks or at most a few months, and larger amounts of insulin will be required when it ends. Thus, by continuing to give insulin each day, one avoids fostering false hopes that the child no longer has diabetes or no longer requires insulin injections. Furthermore, it has been suggested that discontinuing insulin may lead to sensitization, which could cause an allergic response to occur upon restarting the insulin.

DIET THERAPY

Principles. When insulin is given subcutaneously, it is absorbed from the injection site in a more or less predictable fashion that depends on the type of insulin or combination of insulins used. Each type of insulin has a characteristic time of onset, peak effect, and total duration of action. The provision of food must be temporally related to these events. Consequently, meals have to be eaten regularly and timed so as to correspond to the profile of action of administered insulin.

The nutritional needs of children with diabetes do not differ from those of healthy children. They do not require special foods, nor do they need different amounts of vitamins or minerals. The total intake of calories must be sufficient to balance the daily expenditure of energy and satisfy the requirement for normal growth. This allowance has to be adjusted periodically to achieve an ideal body weight and to maintain a normal rate of physical growth and maturation. In the small minority of youngsters with type II (non–insulin-dependent) diabetes, most of whom are obese, the main objective of dietary therapy is to first lose weight and then to maintain a desirable body weight.

In contrast to healthy children in whom insulin secretion is regulated by the ingestion of food, the child with diabetes must match his food consumption to the time of action of injected insulin. Consequently, meals and snacks have to be eaten at the same times each day. Also, the total number of calories and the proportions of carbohydrate, protein, and fat in each meal and snack must be consistent from day to day. Because insulin is released continuously into the circulation from the subcutaneous injection site, there is a tendency to develop hypoglycemia if food is not eaten between the three main meals; hence, most children who are on a regimen of twice daily insulin injections have a snack between each meal and at bedtime. Adolescent patients may find that they can safely omit the midmorning snack but should nevertheless always have readily absorbable carbohydrate available if hypoglycemic symptoms do occur before lunch.

Dietary Fat. Individuals with diabetes are more

prone to develop atherosclerosis, and the current dietary recommendations are an attempt to reduce the risk of developing atherosclerosis. Fat should comprise no more than 30% of the total calories. Dietary cholesterol should be reduced and the amount of polyunsaturated fatty acids increased while the consumption of saturated fat is reduced by consuming less beef and pork and more lean meat, chicken, turkey, fish, low-fat milk, and vegetable proteins. The fat intake should provide a ratio of polyunsaturated to saturated fat of 1.2:1.0. The average ratio of polyunsaturated to saturated fat currently consumed in the United States is 0.3:1.0.

Fiber. Dietary fiber has recently become a subject of renewed interest because of its influence on the digestion, absorption, and metabolism of many nutrients. The inclusion of plant fiber in the diet may benefit patients with diabetes by diminishing the rise in blood glucose after meals. There is even a suggestion that certain plant fibers can reduce serum cholesterol levels. An increase in dietary fiber can be readily achieved by substituting unrefined or minimally processed foods, such as grains, legumes, and vegetables, for highly refined carbohydrates.

The clinical nutritionist or dietitian has the important task of educating the patient and family in the basic principles of nutrition and the application of these principles to the formulation of an individualized meal plan. The aim is to lay a foundation for a life-long change in eating habits. A single instructional session is totally inadequate; nutrition education, like all aspects of diabetes education, has to be an ongoing process, with periodic review of the meal plan and assessment of the child's and parents' levels of comprehension.

Exchange System. We use a method of meal planning based on the exchange system individualized to meet the ethnic, religious, and economic circumstances of each family and the food preferences of the individual child. The exchange system is based on six food groups: milk, fruit, vegetable, bread, meat, and fat. The foods listed in each of the six food groups contain approximately equivalent amounts of carbohydrate, protein, and fat. Each list also indicates the approximate amount of each food (portion size) either by weight or by volume. Thus, the meal plan is prescribed in terms of the number of exchanges from each food group that make up each meal and snack. This method ensures day-to-day consistency of total calories, protein, carbohydrate, and fat while allowing the patient to choose from a wide variety of foods.

EXERCISE

The effects of exercise on diabetes are complex. Exercise acutely lowers the blood glucose concentration to an extent that depends on the intensity and duration of the activity. Physical training increases tissue sensitivity to insulin, which can be demonstrated even in the resting state. It should be noted that acute vigorous exercise in a child with poorly controlled diabetes can actually cause blood glucose levels to increase further and stimulate ketoacid production. Therefore, if a child has marked hyperglycemia and ketonuria, strenuous physical activity should be discouraged until satisfactory control has been achieved by appropriate adjustments of insulin and diet. Exercising the limb into which insulin has been injected accelerates the rate of insulin absorption into the circulation and may contribute to the development of hypoglycemia. Therefore, if exercise is planned it may be possible to reduce this effect by injecting insulin into an area where its rate of absorption will not be accelerated by the effects of vigorous muscular contraction on regional blood flow. For example, if the child is expected to run a lot during the day, the morning insulin injection should be given into the subcutaneous tissue of the anterior abdominal wall. The reality, however, is that children's activities are often unplanned. Consequently, bursts of increased energy expenditure should be covered by providing extra snacks before, and, if the exercise is prolonged, during the activity. Sustained or prolonged intermittent physical activity, as occurs during the summer vacation, usually requires a reduction in insulin dose to avoid hypoglycemia.

Individuals who participate in organized sports are advised to adjust their dose of insulin in anticipation of sustained physical activity during a particular period of the day; e.g., reduction in the morning dose of NPH or Lente insulin for the youth who engages in an after-school sports program. The reduction in insulin dose is determined by trial and error.

Exercise may be a useful adjunct together with insulin and adherence to a meal plan in achieving good blood glucose control. It also has beneficial effects on mental health, cardiovascular function, and blood lipids; in addition, a program of regular exercise allows young people with diabetes more leeway with food, and enables them to occasionally have "forbidden" foods, which can be judiciously used as sources of quickly absorbed carbohydrate to combat hypoglycemic reactions.

MONITORING

Urine Testing. Although inexpensive and convenient for some patients, urine tests for glucose have many limitations. There is a poor correlation between simultaneous urine and blood glucose concentrations and at any given urine glucose concentration the corresponding blood glucose level can vary widely. Therefore, a single ("spot") urine glucose determination, even if obtained by the double-voided method, may not accurately reflect the concurrent level of blood glucose. This is due to many factors: variations in the renal threshold among different people and even in the same individual, the lag between secretion of urine and the time of testing, incomplete voiding, and the semiquantitative nature of the tests. Even with a normal renal threshold, a negative urine test cannot distinguish between a blood glucose level that is abnormally low from a normal or even slightly elevated level. Many parents worry when their child's urine contains no sugar, since they fear the possibility of a hypoglycemic reaction and, in the interest of safety, deliberately undertreat to ensure that there is always a little sugar in the urine. Much hypoglycemia is asymptomatic; and when the aim is to achieve continuously negative urine tests, frequent hypoglycemic episodes are likely to occur. Despite the drawbacks of testing urine for glucose, the urine should be tested for ketones whenever the blood glucose exceeds 250 mg/dl.

Blood Glucose. In the late 1970's various reagent strips were developed to enable the patient to measure blood glucose accurately on a single drop of blood. Given the limitations of urine tests, self-blood glucose monitoring at home (HBGM) would appear to be the obvious way to monitor glycemic control. It should be noted, however, that HBGM alone will not lead to better control. When performed frequently (4–6 times per day), however, in conjunction with intensive support, education, frequent adjustments in insulin doses, and diet, HBGM has been shown to improve glycemic control.

The patient should not come to view testing as a meaningless chore imposed by the physician. Effective use of HBGM requires knowledge of when to test and how to use the results. It is not necessary to perform blood glucose monitoring frequently every day unless the patient is going to adjust the dose of insulin and/or modify the diet in response to the test results. To guide the physician, a period of intensive testing before and 2 hours after meals and during the night (2–4 A.M.) for several days before each clinic visit is often enough to confirm satisfactory glycemic control or indicate where problems lie so that adjustments in the regimen can be made. Office visits with the physician without the results of monitoring may be helpful in solving other problems but are unlikely to improve glycemic control. Each patient and family must discover for themselves what program of monitoring is acceptable on a long-term basis.

HBGM in conjunction with urine tests for ketones has undoubtedly been a major boon in managing intercurrent illnesses at home and preventing ketoacidosis. It has been of great value to parents uncertain of the cause of their child's crankiness or unusual behavior. In general, children tolerate blood glucose testing well. Many teenagers find urine testing repugnant and if they are going to do any testing at all, prefer to test their blood. It should be recognized that patients can fabricate blood glucose results as readily as urine test results. The reagent strips maintain their color for many days and can be saved for review with the physician or nurse.

Glycosylated Hemoglobin (Hemoglobin A_1 or A_{1C}). Assessment of glycemic control by symptoms, home urine tests, or single clinic blood glucose measurements is unreliable. Diabetes in children is characterized by constantly fluctuating blood glucose levels over the course of a single day as well as from day to day. Because of this pattern of constant change, a single blood or urine glucose value has little or no value in accurately assessing a child's metabolic control over a period of several weeks or months. Glycosylated hemoglobin is formed when glucose is bound nonenzymatically to the N-terminal valine of the beta-chain of the hemoglobin molecule. This test of glycemic control has many advantages: it is objective, is independent of the patient's cooperation and the time of the last meal, and provides an integrated measure of the patient's blood glucose concentration during the previous two to three months. Values are linearly correlated with mean blood glucose concentrations measured by frequent self-monitoring during the preceding two to three months.

Relatively brief periods of poor glycemic control cause a disproportionate increase in glycosylated hemoglobin values. Therefore, if one wishes to use glycosylated hemoglobin measurements as an integrator of control during the preceding 6- to 8-week period, one should measure only stable glycosylated hemoglobin after prior removal of the labile fraction, which may account for up to 1–3% of the total. There are several methods of measuring glycosylated hemoglobin; therefore, when comparing results, it is advisable to use the same laboratory.

HYPOGLYCEMIA

Occasional episodes of hypoglycemia are virtually an inevitable consequence of insulin therapy. The aim of therapy should be to achieve the best glycemic control possible while minimizing both the frequency and severity of hypoglycemia. Patients and their families have to be taught to recognize hypoglycemia early and treat it efficiently. The well-controlled child with diabetes may experience mild symptoms of hypoglycemia almost daily, but if the symptoms are recognized early and promptly relieved by ingesting a suitable form of concentrated carbohydrate, the child's activity should be interrupted for no more than a few minutes.

The most common causes of hypoglycemia are bursts of physical activity without additional food, or meals that are delayed, omitted or incompletely consumed. Occasional severe reactions occur unexpectedly and inexplicably; one suspects that some of these are due to an error in the insulin dose, e.g., giving the morning dose in the evening or reversing the amounts of short-acting and intermediate-acting insulins. It should be noted that hypoglycemia after periods of sustained physical exercise may occur several hours after the activity has stopped. The child with diabetes who participates in prolonged physical activity should consume additional carbohydrate and protein before, as well as during, the exercise. It may also be necessary to reduce the dose of insulin. The precise amount of extra food and reduction in insulin dose has to be determined empirically for each individual and adjusted according to the duration and intensity of the exercise.

The symptoms of hypoglycemia are due to both increased adrenergic activity and impaired brain function. Enhanced activity of the adrenergic nervous system and increased catecholamine levels account for nervousness, pallor, tremulousness, palpitations, sweating, and hunger. Weakness, dizziness, headache, drowsiness, irritability, loss of coordination, convulsions, and coma are due to altered central nervous system function resulting from cerebral glucose deprivation.

If the patient is unable to perceive the onset of hypoglycemia for any reason, is too young to treat it himself, or has impaired counter-regulatory mechanisms, the physician should be cautious rather than zealous in attempting to achieve "tight" glycemic control. These circumstances place the child at a considerably greater risk of having hypoglycemia-induced seizures. All parents must learn how to use glucagon, which should be available at home to treat severe hypoglycemia when the child is unable to swallow or retain administered carbohydrate. All children with diabetes should carry with them sugar-containing candy (e.g., Life Savers or Charms) or a couple of packages of table sugar; a bracelet or necklace should be worn identifying the child as having diabetes mellitus.

Hypoglycemia itself can be a cause of poor glycemic control, since the counter-regulatory hormone responses to hypoglycemia stimulate hepatic glucose production and induce a state of relative insulin resistance, which persists for 12–24 hours or longer. This phenomenon, referred to as the Somogyi effect or rebound hyperglycemia, should be suspected in any child whose blood or urine glucose test results are high and who is receiving a relatively large dose of insulin (greater than 1.0–1.5 U/kg/day) and is gaining weight too rapidly. More frequent blood glucose monitoring, especially at times of anticipated peak insulin action and during the night (2–4 A.M.), usually helps to confirm that hypoglycemia is the cause of the hyperglycemia. Alternatively, one can empirically reduce the insulin dose; improved control is presumptive evidence that the patient was experiencing unrecognized episodes of hypoglycemia, which are especially likely to occur during the night.

ASSOCIATED DISORDERS

Autoimmune thyroid disease is commonly associated with type 1 diabetes. About one in every five white children and young adults with insulin-dependent diabetes mellitus (IDDM) have thyroid antimicrosomal antibodies (TMA) in their serum. The prevalence of TMA in black children with diabetes is lower. A goiter without any evidence of thyroid dysfunction may be the only clinical evidence of thyroiditis, however, either hyperthyroidism or hypothyroidism may develop. The latter occurs more commonly; therefore, it is important to carefully monitor the diabetic child's rate of linear growth with the aid of a growth chart and look for other signs of hypothyroidism. It has been recommended that all children with diabetes be screened for TMA; those found to have antibodies should have thyroid function tests performed annually. Because immediate family members are also at increased risk of developing autoimmune thyroid disease, examination of the neck for a goiter and screening for thyroiditis, especially in female relatives, has been recommended.

Adrenal autoantibodies have been found in nearly 2% of white children and young adults with IDDM; about 25% of those with antiadrenal antibodies have overt adrenal insufficiency. Patients with type 1 diabetes also have an increased risk of developing other autoimmune diseases such as atrophic gastritis and pernicious anemia; however, these disorders rarely appear in childhood. If antiadrenal antibodies are detected, the patient must be carefully followed for the possible development of adrenal insufficiency, which may first manifest as a progressive decrease in insulin requirement due to increased sensitivity to insulin.

PSYCHOLOGICAL ASPECTS

Diabetes management is not simply a matter of insulin administration, meal planning, and testing. It also involves a child's emotional and social development and the impact on the family of a chronic incurable disease in a child. The child's diabetes involves the whole family and frequently places a considerable strain on the family; some parents, perhaps already struggling with other issues, give up and leave the child to get on with diabetes care as best he can. This often results in dreadful glycemic control and numerous episodes of ketoacidosis.

The diagnosis of a chronic disease usually stirs emotions that are similar to those experienced by the bereaved: shock, disbelief, denial, anger, and depression. The emotional upheaval that follows the diagnosis may temporarily limit a family's ability to learn; therefore, the initial educational goals should be to teach survival skills.

The major psychological task of the adolescent is to develop increasing autonomy, and this often leads to turmoil. Growth towards independence is complicated for the teenager with diabetes for a variety of reasons. The need for closer medical intervention occurs at just the time that the teenager is striving for less dependence on adult guidance. Adolescence normally involves a struggle for self-identity and a temporary rejection of the values of parents or other authority figures. Diabetes care often becomes the battleground for this struggle. Some adolescents want to find out whether they really have diabetes; this may take the form of omitting insulin injections, overeating, or refusing to monitor. This is a period of rapid physical growth and sexual maturation, and both physical as well as psychological factors presumably lead to more erratic diabetes control during the adolescent years than during childhood. The teenager with diabetes, already vulnerable to feeling different, may wish to prove to his friends that "nothing is wrong"; this may lead to omitting insulin injections and eating haphazardly. Numerous emergency room visits due to recurrent episodes of ketoacidosis signal the need for intensive psychosocial intervention and support.

Caring for the young person with diabetes is not solely a medical problem. Emotional and behavioral issues inevitably arise and must be identified and dealt with. In this regard the mental health worker, psychiatric social worker, or clinical psychologist plays an extremely important role as a member of the diabetes treatment team.

DIABETIC KETOACIDOSIS

Initial Evaluation of the Patient. Carry out the following:

1. Rapidly perform a clinical examination to establish the diagnosis and determine the cause. Weigh the patient and measure either height or length.

2. Determine the level of blood glucose with a reagent strip method (e.g., Chemstrip bG) and plasma ketones (Acetest tablet method) at the bedside. Obtain a blood sample for the laboratory measurement of glucose, electrolytes, BUN, arterial pH, P_{CO_2}, P_{O_2}, hemoglobin, hematocrit, white blood cell count and differential, calcium, and phosphorous.

3. Perform a urinalysis and obtain appropriate specimens for culture (blood, urine, throat).

4. Perform an electrocardiogram for baseline evaluation of potassium status.

5. Record clinical and biochemical data on a flow sheet.

Supportive Measures. Treatment of ketoacidosis includes the following supportive measures:

1. To prevent the possibility of pulmonary aspiration, empty the stomach of its contents by continuous nasogastric suction in patients who are either unconscious or semiconscious.

2. Antibiotics should be given to febrile patients after the appropriate specimens have been obtained for culture.

3. Supplementary oxygen is given to patients who are cyanosed or have a Pa_{O_2} of less than 80 mm Hg.

4. Catheterization of the bladder is usually not necessary; bag collection or condom drainage suffices to permit an accurate assessment of urine output in most patients who are unable to void on demand.

Some of the details concerning the treatment of diabetic ketoacidosis are still controversial. However, a successful outcome is dependent upon meticulous monitoring of each patient's clinical and biochemical response to treatment and upon prompt adjustments in the treatment when necessary. The physician will be considerably aided in his task by maintaining an accurate flow chart that records the patient's clinical and laboratory data, the details of fluid and electrolyte therapy, administered insulin, and urine output. Ideally, the severely ill child with DKA should be treated in an intensive care unit or medical facility where intensive clinical and metabolic monitoring can be performed.

Fluid and Electrolyte Treatment. All patients with diabetic ketoacidosis are dehydrated; the average patient with severe diabetic ketoacidosis has lost approximately 10% of his body weight. Dehydration is accompanied by total body depletion of sodium, potassium, chloride, phosphate, and magnesium.

Prompt and adequate rehydration restores tissue perfusion and suppresses the elevated levels of stress hormones. The top priority of treatment is to start an intravenous infusion using a large-bore cannula inserted into the largest accessible vein and then infuse 20 cc/kg of isotonic saline (0.9% sodium choloride) in 60 minutes. If hypotension or shock persists, infuse an additional 20 cc/kg of isotonic saline over 60 minutes, or give an equivalent amount of colloid, e.g., fresh frozen plasma, or even fresh whole blood if available.

Once the circulation has been stabilized, switch to half-normal saline (0.45% sodium chloride) and aim to replace half the calculated fluid deficit in

Table 1. POTASSIUM REPLACEMENT IN DIABETIC KETOACIDOSIS

Serum Potassium	Infusate Potassium Concentration
<3 mEq/L	40–60 mEq/L
3–4	30
4–5	20
5–6	10
>6	0

8 hours. The remaining half is given over the subsequent 16 hours, so that hydration is completely restored within 24 hours.

When the blood glucose concentration falls to 250–300 mg/dl, 5% dextrose is added to the infusion fluid. In some instances, 10% dextrose may be necessary to avert hypoglycemia. Early in the course of therapy the continued osmotic diuresis may contribute significantly to ongoing fluid losses. The urine output should be replaced with half-normal saline. When the osmotic diuresis subsides, maintenance fluid is given at a rate of 1500–2000 ml/m^2/24 hr.

Potassium Replacement. Although the initial serum potassium level may be normal or even elevated, all patients with diabetic ketoacidosis are depleted in potassium (3–10 mEq/kg). Patients who initially have a low potassium level are the most severely depleted and should receive early (after the patient has voided and insulin has been given) and vigorous potassium replacement therapy. The administration of fluid and insulin may lead to a rapid decrease of the serum potassium with the attendant risk of cardiac arrhythmias. One should aim to keep the potassium level in the range of 4 to 5 mEq/L. If the laboratory has not reported the potassium level within an hour, potassium replacement should not be withheld if insulin therapy has already begun and the patient is urinating. Table 1 is a guide to initial potassium administration.

Use the electrocardiogram as a guide to therapy and follow the configuration of the T waves every 30–60 minutes on the lead that best shows them (usually standard lead II or V2). Flattening of the T wave, widening of the QT interval, and the appearance of U waves indicate hypokalemia. Tall, peaked, symmetrical T waves and shortening of the QT interval indicate hyperkalemia.

Half of the potassium is given as potassium chloride and the other half as potassium phosphate. This serves two purposes; it reduces the total amount of chloride administered and also partially replaces the phosphate deficit.

Insulin. We use low-dose insulin therapy because it is simple to adminster and is effective. Only regular (short-acting, soluble) insulin is used. Administer a bolus of regular insulin (0.1–0.25 U/kg) intravenously and follow this with a constant intravenous infusion at a rate of 0.1 U/kg/hr using an infusion pump. Frequent biochemical monitoring (blood glucose, bicarbonate, and pH) must be performed to evaluate the efficacy of insulin therapy. One rarely encounters a patient with severe insulin resistance who requires two or even three times the usual dose of insulin. If after an hour of therapy the glucose level has not decreased and the pH has increased, increase the insulin dose incrementally by 0.1 U/kg/hr until an effective dose is reached. When the blood glucose level reaches 250–300 mg/dl, continue to infuse insulin at a rate of 0.05–0.1 U/kg/hr until the pH and serum bicarbonate are normal. When the patient is ready to begin eating, subcutaneous insulin is given one hour before stopping the insulin infusion.

Bicarbonate. The weight of evidence now indicates that administration of sodium bicarbonate neither hastens resolution of the acidosis nor improves survival. Indeed, it may impair tissue oxygenation as a result of its effect on the oxygen-hemoglobin dissociation curve. We do not routinely give bicarbonate just because the pH is very low; however, one may still wish to give sodium bicarbonate to improve myocardial contractility and enhance peripheral vascular responsiveness to catecholamines in the patient who is in shock or has an unstable circulation. In these circumstances, sodium bicarbonate (1–2 mEq/kg or 40–80 mEq/m^2) is infused over 30 to 60 minutes.

Hypoglycemia

MARK A. SPERLING, M.D.

Hypoglycemia is not a disease; it is a concentration of blood glucose below the acceptable range for the age and size of the individual. In the neonate, clinically significant hypoglycemia is defined as two blood glucose values less than 30 mg/dl in full-term infants, or two blood glucose values less than 20 mg/dl in low birth weight infants (premature or small for gestational age). Beyond the newborn period, a blood glucose value less than 40 mg/dl is pathognomonic for hypoglycemia. These criteria are based on whole blood glucose measurements. Plasma or serum glucose values are 15 to 20 per cent higher than whole blood glucose values. Hence, when using plasma or serum, allowance must be made for higher values that are still compatible with a diagnosis of hypoglycemia. Thus, serum or plasma glucose values of 30 mg/dl or less in low birth weight infants, 40 mg/dl or less in full-term infants and 50 mg/dl or less beyond the newborn period should arouse suspicion of hypoglycemia and should be vigorously treated.

Obtain a rapid blood glucose assessment by Dextrostix or Chemstrips. Finding values below 40 mg/dl on this screening test should be immediately followed by obtaining a blood sample for blood glucose measurement by a formal laboratory procedure, as well as by saving 1 ml of serum for future measurement of hormones or substrates or both; this initial sample prior to treatment may be crucial to future diagnosis. As soon as this sample is obtained, glucose should be given intravenously; 0.5 gm/kg (2 ml of a 25 per cent solution at a rate of 1 ml/min) should abruptly terminate the symptoms. If symptoms persist, hypocalcemia, sepsis, intraventricular CNS hemorrhage, anoxia, or heart failure should be considered and treated appropriately when diagnosis is confirmed.

It is convenient to consider the treatment of hypoglycemia at three age groups: the immediate neonatal period, early infancy, and late infancy and childhood.

THE IMMEDIATE NEWBORN PERIOD
Transient Hypoglycemia in the Neonate

Symptomatic hypoglycemia in neonates varies from 1.3 to 3.0 per 1000 live births. Low birth weight infants are often vulnerable to hypoglycemia, which fortunately is usually transient, resolving spontaneously in 3 to 5 days. Milk feedings therefore should be introduced within 4 to 6 hours of delivery in these infants and glucose levels carefully monitored. When feedings are precluded because of respiratory distress or when feedings alone cannot maintain blood glucose concentrations above 40 mg/dl, intravenous blood glucose should be provided at a rate of 5 to 10 mg/kg/min for 24 to 36 hours. The amount of glucose provided may be limited by the 24-hour fluid requirement; the higher the 24-hour fluid requirement, the lower the glucose concentration that need be used. With a fluid requirement of 100 to 150 ml/kg/24 hr, 10 per cent glucose will provide calculated glucose needs; with 70 to 90 ml/kg/24 hr, 15 to 20 per cent glucose may be necessary to provide calculated glucose needs. Concentrations of glucose higher than 15 per cent promote thrombosis and tend to sclerose veins and should therefore be avoided if possible. When intravenous glucose is to be provided for 24 hours or more, the glucose should be made up to 0.2 N saline with KCl 20 meq/l so as to provide approximately 3 meq/kg of sodium and 2 meq/kg as potassium. Serum electrolytes, especially potassium levels, should be carefully monitored. When oral feedings are tolerated and blood glucose values are maintained above 30 to 40 mg/dl, the rate of intravenous glucose provided can be tapered by changing to 5 per cent glucose for 12 hours, then halving the rate of intravenous fluid provided for a further 12 to 24 hours before stopping the infusion. Hypertonic glucose infusion should *not* be discontinued abruptly, as this may provoke a rebound hypoglycemia.

If blood glucose remains less than 30 mg/dl despite provision of glucose at 10 to 12 mg/kg/min cortisone acetate should be given at a dose of 5 mg/kg/24 hr in three divided doses at 8-hour intervals. The intramuscular route ensures adequate absorption and provides a depot. Cortisone can be tapered when blood glucose is stable at over 30 mg/dl for 48 hours and stopped after 3 to 5 days of total treatment, depending on response. During treatment, glucose levels should be monitored at 4- to 6-hour intervals or more frequently if deemed necessary.

When the infant is large for gestational age, the most likely diagnosis is that of infant of a diabetic mother (IDM). Early feeding alone can sometimes maintain glucose over 40 mg/dl in these infants. However, treatment of these infants commonly requires provision of intravenous glucose for several days until hyperinsulinemia abates. In these infants, too rapid provision of glucose that results in hyperglycemia evokes prompt insulin release, which may result in rebound hypoglycemia. Thus, a vicious cycle may be established in which increasing amounts of glucose are required to maintain normal glucose concentrations. Provision of glucose at rates that do not exceed 6 to 10 mg/kg/min usually circumvent this problem, but the appropriate dose for each case must be individually adjusted. For similar reasons, bolus injections of glucagon at 0.05 mg/kg IM or IV should be avoided in infants of diabetic mothers. Although this will acutely raise blood glucose, glucagon injections commonly result in rebound hypoglycemia because, apart from its hyperglycemic effect, glucagon is a potent direct stimulus to insulin secretion. However, continuous intravenous infusion of physiologic amounts of glucagon may maintain blood glucose concentrations in infants of diabetic mothers. Dissolve 1 mg of glucagon in 1 ml of its supplied diluent and add 0.1 ml (100 µg) to 500 ml of the 10 per cent glucose solution. Infuse at a rate of 15 ml/hr. This will provide 1500 mg of glucose and 3 µg of glucagon per hour; for a 4-kg IDM this translates into approximately 6 mg/kg/min of glucose and 12.5 ng/kg/min of glucagon. Bolus injections of glucagon at 0.05 mg/kg IM or IV will be helpful in acutely raising blood glucose in low birth weight infants while starting the intravenous glucose infusion.

If, despite these measures, hypoglycemia persists beyond the first week of life, hyperinsulinemia, a hormone deficiency (ACTH, cortisol, or growth hormone), or an inborn error of metabolism should be suspected. These persistent hypoglycemias are particularly likely to result in permanent brain damage and must therefore be vigorously treated with intravenous glucose, glucocorticoids, or other measures as appropriate while definitive diagnostic investigations are awaited.

PERSISTENT HYPOGLYCEMIA OF EARLY INFANCY

Hyperinsulinemia

The majority of children with hyperinsulinemia that causes hypoglycemia are seen in infancy. Once organic hyperinsulism has been established through concurrent measurement of glucose and insulin, the differential diagnosis rests between nesidioblastosis, beta-cell hyperplasia and beta-cell adenoma. For practical purposes these three entities need not be distinguished clinically, and all must be treated in a similar fashion. An intravenous line providing glucose at 10 to 15 mg/kg/min must be established; because the use of hypertonic glucose solutions is anticipated and because treatment may be prolonged, a central venous line through the subclavian vein is most helpful. Occasionally, frequent feedings coupled with pharmacologic agents such as diazoxide can control hypoglycemia. Diazoxide is a thiazide derivative that inhibits insulin secretion. The initial dose should be 6 to 10 mg/kg/24 hr orally in 8- to 12-hour doses. It may be necessary to increase this dose to 10 to 15 mg/kg/24 hr. Diazoxide should not be discontinued suddenly after prolonged use. The side effects of this drug include salt retention, edema, hyperuricemia, hypertension, and hirsutism. A lowering of IgG levels also has been reported, as have anorexia and vomiting. These side effects and the therapeutic response are dose-related and all disappear upon withdrawal of the drug. Oral cortisone acetate at 5 mg/kg/24 hr or prednisone at 1 to 2 mg/kg/24 hr in two to three divided doses also may be helpful.

If hypoglycemia proves to be refractory to these measures, we strongly urge that surgery be undertaken and that subtotal resection of some 75 to 80 per cent of the pancreas be performed. Further resection of the remaining pancreas may occasionally be necessary if hypoglycemia recurs and cannot be controlled by medical measures such as the use of cortisone with diazoxide. When the diagnosis is established before 3 months of life, we strongly urge surgery as the initial approach to treatment. Too often, frequent feedings coupled with these pharmacologic agents neither maintain blood glucose concentrations nor adequately inhibit insulin release. Thus there is persistence of hypoglycemia with loss of precious time and the possibility of irreversible brain damage. If hypoglycemia first becomes manifest between 3 to 6 months of life, a therapeutic trial with medical approaches can be attempted for up to 2 to 4 weeks. Failure to maintain euglycemia without undesirable side effects from the drugs prompts the need for surgery.

Similarly, medical measures may be attempted for up to 1 month in infants who first present hypoglycemia after the age of 6 months. The same diagnostic and therapeutic approach is applied to patients with hyperinsulinemia and with the Beckwith-Wiedemann syndrome, characterized by macrosomia, microcephaly, macroglossia, visceromegaly, and omphalocele. Microcephaly and retarded brain development may occur independently of hypoglycemia in these patients, who also have a predilection for eventually developing tumors such as hepatoblastoma, retinoblastoma, and Wilms tumor.

Leucine-sensitive hypoglycemia is probably a variant of nesidioblastosis with some milder clinical features. Infants with these diseases manifest hypoglycemic episodes after milk feedings. An oral leucine load will provoke hypoglycemia in these infants, who can then be managed with a diet low in leucine but still adequate for growth. In infants, a variety of milk products (Similac, Enfamil, SMA-26) can be used and additional carbohydrate should be offered after feeds and before sleep. Diazoxide may be particularly helpful in these infants if there is a poor response to dietary measures alone. However, partial pancreatectomy may still be necessary in these children. When surgery can be avoided, there is a tendency for spontaneous improvement by the age of 5 to 7 years.

In these neonates with persistent and recurrent hypoglycemia, as well as in older infants and children, a glucagon tolerance test (0.05 mg/kg given IM or IV) is helpful in differentiating between hypoglycemia due to hyperinsulinism and hypoglycemia due to other causes. A brisk significant hyperglycemic response to glucagon implicates hyperinsulinism that has promoted abundant glycogen whereas nonresponse of glucose to glucagon suggests other causes.

Endocrine Deficiency

Hypoglycemia associated with endocrine deficiencies is usually due to adrenal insufficiency with or without associated growth hormone deficiency. Treatment of adrenal insufficiency consists of provision of cortisone at a dose of 15 to 20 mg/m^2/24 hr; mineralocorticoid may be required as well. During intercurrent illness, the dose of glucocorticoid should be doubled and provided via intramuscular administration if the patient is vomiting and not tolerating oral intake. With growth hormone deficiency, replacement treatment with human growth hormone at 1 to 2 units, three times a week, is indicated. Even if growth hormone deficiency is combined with ACTH deficiency, growth hormone treatment alone may suffice to prevent hypoglycemic episodes. A syndrome of severe hypoglycemia in the first hours of life associated with jaundice, hepatomegaly, midline abnormalities, and multiple pituitary hormone deficiencies, including growth hormone and ACTH, has been described; recognition of this syndrome and treatment with cortisone and growth hormone in doses outlined above can be lifesaving. Although isolated growth hormone deficiency may also result in hypoglycemic episodes in early life, there is a tendency for spontaneous amelioration of hypoglycemia in later years, even when growth hormone replacement is not given.

Epinephrine or glucagon deficiency could theoretically be responsible for hypoglycemia; both conditions appear to be extremely rare. Epinephrine deficiency, when diagnosed as the cause of hypoglycemia, can be treated acutely by injecting epinephrine, 0.03 ml of 1:1000 epinephrine per kg IM, not to exceed 0.3 ml (0.3 mg), and using ephedrine as an oral agent for long-term management. Dramatic response to long-acting glucagon administered by intramuscular injection has been reported in the one well-documented case of glucagon deficiency.

Inborn Errors of Metabolism

Hepatic Glycogen Storage Diseases. GLUCOSE-6-PHOSPHATASE DEFICIENCY (TYPE I GLYCOGEN STORAGE DISEASE). Glucose-6-phosphatase is the enzyme that hydrolyzes glucose-6-phosphate to free glucose in the final step of the glycogenolytic or gluconeogenic pathway; deficiency of this enzyme therefore must result in severe hypoglycemia from early infancy.

Recent advances have dramatically altered the poor prognosis for these children by demonstrating that many of their metabolic changes are secondary to hormonal changes induced by the chronic state of starvation. Accordingly, marked improvement can be achieved in these patients by frequent feedings on this schedule: *Daytime feedings* are given every 3 to 4 hours and consist of 60 to 70 per cent of the calories as carbohydrate low in fructose and galactose, 12 to 15 per cent of the calories as protein, and 15 to 25 per cent of the calories as fat. *At night*, a small nasogastric tube is passed and approximately one third of daily caloric requirements are continuously infused over the night-time 8 to 12 hours; Vivonex, which contains 89 per cent of the calories as glucose and glucose oligosaccharides, 1.8 per cent as safflower oil, and 9.2 per cent as crystalline amino acid, has proved to be particularly successful. This regimen can result in the maintenance of normal blood glucose concentrations and reversal of many of the metabolic abnormalities for a prolonged period, resulting in a marked acceleration of the growth rate.

Allopurinol, 100 mg on alternate days, may be necessary to reduce uric acid levels to the normal range; precise dose should be titrated to the serum uric acid.

AMYLO-1,6-GLUCOSIDASE DEFICIENCY (DEBRANCHER ENZYME DEFICIENCY; TYPE III GLYCOGEN STORAGE DISEASE). Spontaneous symptomatic hypoglycemia is much less common than in type I glycogen storage disease. However, during periods of caloric restriction, as occurs during intercurrent infections or vomiting, hypoglycemia and ketonuria may appear. Because gluconeogenic pathways are intact, frequent feeding of a high carbohydrate, high protein diet is effective unless the patient is vomiting. In severe cases, affected children also may have hepatomegaly, muscle weakness, myotonia, and growth retardation. When dietary therapy, in the form of a high protein, low carbohydrate, frequent feeding regimen, cannot avoid hypoglycemia, nocturnal continuous nasogastric infusion of Vivonex may be attempted.

LIVER PHOSPHORYLASE AND PHOSPHORYLASE KINASE DEFICIENCY (TYPES VI AND IX GLYCOGEN STORAGE DISEASE). Symptomatic hypoglycemia occurs only occasionally in these conditions and may be associated with hepatomegaly, excessive deposition of glycogen in the liver, and some growth retardation. A diet high in protein and reduced in carbohydrates usually prevents hypoglycemia.

GLYCOGEN SYNTHETASE DEFICIENCY. This is an extremely rare condition in which the liver lacks the enzymes necessary to deposit glycogen. Consequently, severe hypoglycemia will result with only short periods of fasting. Protein-rich feedings at frequent intervals may result in dramatic clinical improvement, including growth velocity. This condition mimics some of the features of ketotic hypoglycemia.

Enzyme Defects in Liver Carbohydrate Metabolism

Galactosemia (Galactose-1-Phosphate Uridyl Transferase Deficiency). Hypoglycemia in this condition is due to an acute impairment of glycogen breakdown by accumulating galactose-1-phosphate. Galactosemia should be considered in any newborn infant with failure to thrive, in whom vomiting, diarrhea, and hypoglycemia follow milk feedings. A presumptive diagnosis can be made by demonstrating a reducing sugar that is not glucose in the urine. Strict avoidance of lactose-containing milk, foods, or other products is essential to avoid long-term sequelae.

Fructose Intolerance (Fructose-1-Phosphate Aldolase Deficiency). This condition mimics the clinical findings described for galactosemia, including failure to thrive, vomiting, and hypoglycemia following ingestion of foods containing fructose. Again the urine contains a reducing sugar that is not glucose. Affected individuals often spontaneously learn to eliminate fructose from their diet. A fructose-free diet, avoiding sucrose, table sugars, sweets, and fruits, prevents all the symptoms.

Fructose-1,6-Diphosphatase Deficiency. The clinical features simulate those of type I glycogen storage disease, and treatment consists of a diet high in carbohydrates (56 per cent of calories as glucose, maltose, or lactose) but excluding fructose, which cannot be utilized, 12 per cent protein, and 32 per cent fat. This regimen has permitted normal growth and development. The continuous nocturnal provision of calories via the intragastric infusion system described for type I glycogen storage disease is also applicable to children with fructose-1,6-diphosphatase deficiency. Intravenous infusion of glucose is necessary to prevent hypoglycemia during intercurrent illness with vomiting when oral intake is curtailed.

Phosphoenolpyruvate Carboxykinase (PEPCK) Deficiency. Deficiency of this enzyme is associated with severe hypoglycemia during fasting. Avoidance of long periods of fasting through frequent feedings rich in carbohydrates should be helpful since glycogen synthesis and breakdown are intact. During intercurrent illness, intravenous glucose is necessary.

Other Enzyme Defects. Hypoglycemia is seen in several other inborn errors of metabolism. In maple syrup urine disease, symptomatic hypoglycemia is quite frequent and requires acute treatment with glucose. In addition, appropriate dietary therapy is necessary to reduce the intake of branched-chain amino acids (leucine, isoleucine, valine), the metabolism of which is defective in this condition. Some forms of this condition may respond to thiamine administration. Rare conditions in which hypoglycemia is encountered include methylmalonic aciduria, which occasionally responds to vitamin B_{12} treatment, and tyrosinosis, which mimics the clinical picture of neonatal hepatitis; in both conditions the treatment of acute hypoglycemia is by administration of glucose or carbohydrates.

LATE INFANCY AND CHILDHOOD

Ketotic Hypoglycemia. Ketotic hypoglycemia is the most common form of childhood hypoglycemia. In anticipation of the spontaneous resolution of this syndrome, treatment of ketotic hypoglycemia consists of frequent feedings of a high protein, high carbohydrate diet. During intercurrent illnesses, parents should test their child's urine for the presence of ketones, the appearance of which precedes the hypoglycemia by several hours. In the presence of ketonuria, liquids of high carbohydrate content should be offered to the child. If these cannot be tolerated, the child should be admitted to the hospital for intravenous glucose

administration or a short course of steroids. It must be emphasized that isolated hormone deficiency, especially that of cortisol or growth hormone, can mimic all the findings of ketotic hypoglycemia. Therefore, each child must be tested for the capacity to secrete appropriate amounts of cortisol or growth hormone or both.

Alcohol Intoxication. In children, the consumption of even small quantities of alcohol can precipitate hypoglycemia if alcohol intake follows caloric deprivation by several hours. Alcohol acutely impairs gluconeogenesis, and hypoglycemia results if glycogen stores are depleted by starvation or by pre-existing abnormalities in glycogen metabolism. The hypoglycemia responds promptly to intravenous glucose, which should always be given to a child at initial presentation of coma or seizure, after taking a blood sample for glucose determination. A careful history allows this diagnosis to be established and may avoid needless and expensive hospitalization and investigation. Hypoglycemia may also occur in aspirin overdose. In these and other conditions in which hypoglycemia occurs, glucose should be administered intravenously at an initial dose of 0.5 gm/kg followed by continuous infusion at a rate of 6 to 8 mg/kg/min until the hypoglycemia resolves.

Hormone Deficiency or Excess. Hypoglycemia can be caused by deficiencies of cortisol, growth hormone, or a combination of these factors as a result of hypopituitarism in older children. If insulin levels are markedly elevated, the possibility of deliberate administration of insulin to a nondiabetic should be considered. A serum C-peptide determination on the same sample will permit distinction between factitious insulin administration and endogenous insulinoma; in the former, C-peptide levels will be low, whereas in the latter, C-peptide levels will be high.

Acute hypoglycemia should always be considered a medical emergency. Once the initial blood sample is drawn for definitive glucose and hormone measurements and glucose given intravenously to elevate blood glucose, each case must be carefully assessed for its underlying cause, which can then be rationally treated; few cases now are classified as idiopathic.

Diabetes Insipidus

ROBERT A. RICHMAN, M.D.

NEUROGENIC DIABETES INSIPIDUS

The availability of DDAVP has greatly simplified the treatment of neurogenic diabetes insipidus. It has become the treatment of choice, replacing posterior pituitary extract, aqueous vasopressin, lysine vasopressin, vasopressin tannate in oil, and pharmacologic agents with antidiuretic properties, such as chlorpropamide, clofibrate, and carbamazepine. Some of the disadvantages of these agents include inconvenience and painful administration, allergic reactions, gastrointestinal upset, and short duration of action. DDAVP, on the other hand, is a highly specific agent and is long acting, easy to administer, and virtually devoid of side effects. It is many times more potent in effecting antidiuresis than the native hormone and possesses much less oxytocic and vasopressor activity. It is administered as an intranasal spray, using a soft plastic calibrated catheter called a rhinyle. The parent or older patient fills the catheter with the desired amount of DDAVP, inserts the tip of the catheter into the nose, and gently puffs on the other end. When administered correctly, the hormone is delivered to the nasal mucosa, with none running out the nose or down the nasopharynx.

The duration of action increases with the dosage. Parents are instructed in how to administer the drug and titrate the dosage until the antidiuresis persists for about 12 hours. If such a dose is given before breakfast and again 12 hours later, the child can both attend school without the inconvenience of developing polyuria and polydipsia during class and sleep through the night uninterrupted. To avoid chronic hyponatremia and reassess the duration of action, if the child has not had any spontaneous polyuria during the week, the drug should be withheld on a weekend morning until polyuria occurs. This has proven to be safe, effective, and satisfactory to the patients.

The dose of DDAVP,* in general, varies with the weight of the patient, but the intranasal route produces a great variability in the response to a given dose. We usually initiate therapy under close supervision with 0.05 ml (5 µg) and gradually increase the dose in 0.025-ml increments until 12 hours of antidiuresis occurs. Patients may require higher dosages or more frequent administration during upper respiratory infections. They should be cautioned against drinking excessively during periods of low urine output. When older patients are stabilized and parents are comfortable with the treatment regimen, it is only necessary to reevaluate the regimen every 6 months by measuring 24-hour urine output and the serum and urine osmolalities.

Unlike other vasopressin preparations, DDAVP can be used safely and effectively in young infants, even those with major cerebral abnormalities and possibly defective thirst mechanisms. In infants, the initial dosage should be 2 µg of DDAVP and gradually increased until antidiuresis persists for

about 12 hours. Since the volume of this dosage is only 0.02 ml, it cannot be accurately measured with the plastic catheter. The standard solution of DDAVP (0.1 mg/1.0 ml) is diluted 1:5 with normal saline, so that 2 µg is administered in 0.1 ml of diluted DDAVP. Then the dosage is titrated, using the diluted solution. The diluted solution should be discarded after one week.

The treatment of patients with diabetes insipidus receiving intravenous fluids presents a formidable challenge. The patient's own thirst mechanism, when intact, is a much better regulator of fluid homeostasis than any scheme that can be devised. Initially, a dose of DDAVP is given that lasts about 12 hours when administered intranasally. The injectable preparation (4 µg/ml) of DDAVP, which has recently been released, may be preferable in certain clinical situations. Administered subcutaneously or intravenously, it is about 10 times more potent than DDAVP given by the intranasal route and the dose is reduced accordingly. However, experience with this form of the drug is very limited in children. While the patient's urine output is low with high specific gravity, each hour the calculated insensible fluid losses plus the volume of urine output for the previous hour should be replaced with 5% dextrose and 75–150 meq/l of sodium chloride, depending upon the serum electrolyte concentrations. The next dose of DDAVP should be given as soon as the urine volume increases (above approximately 3 ml/kg/hr) and specific gravity falls below 1.010. If the patient has a prolonged period of high urine output with low specific gravity, the intravenous fluids need to be changed to 5% dextrose with 35 meq/l of sodium chloride until antidiuresis is re-established with DDAVP. The goal is to return the patient to oral fluids as quickly as the clinical condition permits.

In seven years of prescribing DDAVP, we have found that it has a wide margin of safety. Only two of 20 patients have had significant complications. One 20-year-old patient with panhypopituitarism and developmental delay had two seizures associated with hyponatremia while away from home. The second patient, who had inappropriate thirst as well as panhypopituitarism, became edematous from fluid overload. By simply withholding DDAVP for 24 hours, she diuresed and the problem was resolved. Subsequently, she has been treated every 12 hours with a dosage of DDAVP effective for only 6–8 hours.

NEPHROGENIC DIABETES INSIPIDUS

The treatment of nephrogenic diabetes insipidus is much more difficult than that described above. Because no treatment is available to eliminate the polyuria, polydipsia is essential for survival. The goals of therapy are to maintain fluid and electrolyte homeostasis while supplying adequate calories

---

* Manufacturer's warning: Safety and efficacy of DDAVP have not been established in children under 12 years of age (parenteral) or 3 months (intranasal) with diabetes insipidus.

for normal growth and development. By diluting proprietary formulas 25% to 50% with water to reduce the solute load and administering chlorothiazide (1 gm/m^2/day, divided into two or three doses), the serum osmolarity can be maintained within the normal range during infancy. Because of the reduction in calories consumed with this regimen, it may not permit normal weight gain, even with supplementation of the formula with dextrose-maltose or corn syrup. The addition of glucose polymers (Polycose, Ross Laboratories) has met with some initial success in one patient, but it remains to be seen whether normal weight gain will continue with long-term therapy. Older children maintain fluid balance by consuming large quantities of water.

Rickets

SUSAN M. SCOTT, M.D.

Rickets, a disease of the growing bones, came under control in the early 20th century with the discovery that vitamin D prevents this disease. It became a health problem once again with the advent of neonatal intensive care units. Defined as a decrease in the mineral/osteoid ratio of bone, rickets becomes evident in a prematurely delivered neonate only when good linear growth is not obtained. Only then do the poor mineral/osteoid ratios of infants born early in the third trimester of pregnancy and our inability to mimic intrauterine calcium to phosphorus (Ca/P) accretion rates become limiting factors in normal bony development. This usually becomes evident only after a premature infant is returned to a secondary care center for growth before discharge. Beyond the newborn period, rickets is usually linked to genetic causes (discussed later), although infants exposed to little sunlight and abnormal diets may present with nutritional rickets.

NEONATAL PERIOD

In premature infants being fed the newer generation, especially adapted formulas, inadequate Ca/P accretion leading to rickets is not a problem. There are, however, large numbers of premature infants who have as their sources of calories breast milk, full-term formulas, and/or TPN (total parental nutrition) for whom rickets is a potential disease. The pediatrician should strive for a goal of supplying 400 IU of vitamin D a day. Yet with the frequent combinations of different caloric sources used, it may be impossible to calculate the amounts of Ca/P being given. A few warnings will help at least to anticipate the infants who are at risk. Breast milk from mothers who have delivered low birth weight infants is inadequate in Ca/P for their infants. There are breast milk fortifiers (1 packet per 25 cc or 50 cc), which add calories, sodium, and Ca/P and can be used to compensate for the inadequacies of such breast milk. Soy formulas, which are not recommended for long-term use in premature infants, have decreased bioavailable Ca/P. TPN not particularly designed for premature infants may also be deficient in Ca/P. Finally, diuretics, such as furosemide, when used chronically in premature infants, may be a significant cause of urinary calcium loss.

Surveillance for signs of osteopenia or rickets includes bimonthly calcium (normal range 9–11 mg/dl) and phosphorus (5–10 mg/dl) measurements and alkaline phosphatase levels. This should begin when adequate calories and good linear growth have been established for several weeks. A normal range for alkaline phosphatase is more difficult to define, since active growth will increase alkaline phosphatase 3 to 5 times the normal adult values. Rising alkaline phosphatase over 2 or 3 measurements is probably an indication of inadequate Ca/P or vitamin D nutrition. If measurements are done only after good growth has been established, the normal increase in alkaline phosphatase will not be confusing. Vitamin D metabolites are not easy to measure or interpret, and x-rays are usually only helpful when an experienced neonatal radiologist is available.

The signs and symptoms of rickets, which include frontal bossing, rachitic rosary, and limb and rib deformities, as well as apathy, hypotonia and weakness, should alert the practitioner to potential rickets in an infant or child but should be anticipated and prevented in the premature infant. In infants who may become chronic lung patients, hypotonia and rib deformities leading to a worsening of their pulmonary status must be prevented, since the limb and rib deformities of rickets will take from months to years to correct.

VITAMIN D–DEPENDENT AND VITAMIN D–RESISTANT RICKETS

The genetic forms of rickets present as growth failure frequently because of an increasingly inadequate mineral:osteoid ratio, which slows linear growth outside of the newborn period. The two forms most frequently seen, vitamin D–dependent and vitamin D–resistant rickets, are both poorly descriptive names for these disorders. Vitamin D–dependent rickets (autosomal recessive), probably secondary to a deficiency of the 1α-hydroxylase enzyme for the production of 1,25-dihydroxyvitamin D (calcitriol), presents with tetany/convulsions and growth failure. It responds well to large doses of vitamin D (10,000–100,000 IU/day) or to 1–2 μg of calcitriol daily. Vitamin D–resistant rickets (also called X-linked hypophosphatemic rickets) is caused by a renal leak of phosphate of unclear etiology. This type of rickets causes growth failure, and although convulsions are uncommon and successful treatment of the rickets with vitamin D (10,000–50,000 IU/day) and oral phosphate (Neutra-Phos 450–600 ml/day) can be obtained, this therapy does not prevent short stature. As can be seen by the dosage ranges given and the real complication of hypercalcemia with overdosage, it is recommended that the care of these children be undertaken with the assistance of a pediatric endocrinologist.

RICKETS WITH ANTICONVULSANT THERAPY

This form of rickets, thought to be secondary to increased production of inactive vitamin D metabolites in the liver, is treated with 50–100 μg/day of 250H vitamin D.

RICKETS AND FANCONI'S SYNDROME AND RENAL TUBULAR ACIDOSIS

Although the causes of Fanconi's syndrome are multiple, phosphaturia and vitamin D deficiency are commonly associated findings. Replacement of phosphate, correction of acidosis and the addition of up to 25,000–50,000 IU of vitamin D are often required to treat the bone disease. Rickets associated with renal tubular acidosis usually responds to correction of the acidosis.

Tetany

SUSAN M. SCOTT, M.D.

The possible etiologies and therapies for tetany are dependent on the age of onset as well as on the ion involved (calcium, magnesium, or hydrogen). The end result is a hyperexcitable state of the peripheral and central nervous systems leading to muscular spasms and seizures.

NEONATAL PERIOD

Symptoms presenting within the first weeks of life are usually related to the hypocalcemia of prematurity, the various forms of hypoparathyroidism, or hypomagnesemia of a nutritional source.

Tetany is rarely seen or recognized in a premature infant but is readily treated with calcium gluconate, 200 mg/kg (2 ml/kg) given by intravenous injection at 1 ml/minute while observing the heart rate for signs of bradycardia. With the institution of feedings, this problem will resolve.

Hypoparathyroidism. The causes of hypoparathyroidism include a transient form of unknown etiology, maternal hyperparathyroidism, and a permanent, but usually incomplete, absence of parathyroid function in isolated disease or as a component of DiGeorge's syndrome. The net result of each cause is hypocalcemia with hyperphosphatemia. Treatment is with enrichment of calcium and/or decrease in phosporus in the diet, usually by the addition of calcium gluconate to the formula. This will continue usually for several days to months.

Transient Hypoparathyroidism. This hypocalcemia used to be described only in infants on cow's milk feedings because of its high phosphorus content. Since this is probably due to a relative dysfunction in PTH secretion, it can be seen with normal phosphorus load formulas. The result of PTH dysfunction is a retention of phosphorus that inhibits the production of 1,25-dihydroxy-vitamin D and thus decreases the absorption of calcium.

Maternal Hyperparathyroidism. A search for maternal disease must be considered when an infant presents with signs of hypoparathyroidism. Most patients with true hyperparathyroidism will have calcium concentrations within the normal ranges but consistently high-normal on repeat measurements. If maternal disease is found, the infant may require weeks of therapy, but parathyroid function will usually return to normal.

Congenital (Permanent) Hypoparathyroidism. This cause of hypocalcemia does not respond to calcium alone and requires large doses of vitamin D. In DiGeorge's syndrome, the low-set ears and cardiac anomalies, such as interrupted aortic arch, may be the presenting features. Also, immunologic abnormalities secondary to thymic aplasia or dysfunction will usually be more life threatening than the parathroid dysfunction leading to tetany.

For treatment in the neonate, the calcium gluconate preparation used for intravenous therapy can be given by mouth and will avoid the hyperosmolar insult of high concentrations of sucrose in the oral preparations, which will cause diarrhea in the dosages necessary for therapy.

Hypomagnesemic Tetany. The neonate with this cause of tetany will often have a mother with diabetes mellitus or with a poor diet, particularly as seen in alcoholism. Intramuscular injection of 50% solution of $MgSO_4$ in a dosage of 0.1–0.2 ml/kg will correct both the magnesium and the hypocalcemia that accompanies this disorder.

INFANCY AND CHILDHOOD

Tetany beginning outside of the neonatal period may be related to vitamin D disorders, primary hypomagnesemia of infancy, and alkalosis.

The vitamin D disorders described under rickets may have tetany associated with them. They are treated acutely with intravenous calcium (as above) and large doses of vitamin D (500,000 units over 24 hr).

Primary hypomagnesemia is usually secondary to an intestinal absorption abnormality and requires 500–2000 mg of magnesium per day in divided doses.

Tetany of alkalosis is usually due to hyperventilation and can be treated by rebreathing into a paper bag.

Idiopathic Hypercalcemia

F. BRUDER STAPLETON, M.D.

Hypercalcemia is defined as a total serum calcium concentration greater than 11.0 mg/dl. Severe idiopathic hypercalcemia may present in early infancy as a component of the Williams "elfin facies" syndrome.

In Williams syndrome, and in most instances of idiopathic hypercalcemia, increased gastrointestinal absorption of calcium appears to be responsible for elevation of the serum calcium concentration. Therefore, dietary calcium should be minimized and any source of exogenous vitamin D intake should be avoided. Frequently, corticosteroid therapy with prednisone (1–2 mg/kg/day) must also be given to reduce dietary calcium absorption. Due to the adverse effects of corticosteroids, chronic daily prednisone therapy should be avoided. A further reduction in gastrointestinal calcium absorption may be accomplished with cellulose phosphate (Calcibind, Mission Pharmaceutical, San Antonio, TX) at a dose of 10–15 gm/1.73 m^2/day administered with meals. Finally, increased bone resorption may contribute to hypercalcemia in some patients. Therapy with subcutaneous calcitonin at a dose of 1–5 units/kg/day may be beneficial. Since idiopathic hypercalcemia may be a "self-limited" condition, periodic attempts to discontinue therapy are warranted.

Neonatal hypercalcemia from parathyroid hyperplasia may occur in infants born to mothers with familial hypocalciuric hypercalcemia. Frequently, such infants are asymptomatic and no therapy is required; however, in selected infants, parathyroidectomy may be necessary.

Magnesium Deficiency

SE MO SUH, M.D., Ph.D.

Magnesium deficiency manifests with hypomagnesemia and clinical symptoms of neuromuscular irritability such as tremor, tetany, convulsions, cardiac arrhythmia, and mental disorientation. Frequently, hypocalcemia or hypokalemia, which are usually refractory to treatment with calcium or potassium unless magnesium therapy is added, may also occur. Normal ranges of serum magnesium levels in infants and children are 1.5–1.8 mEq/liter. Some of the clinical symptoms of magnesium deficiency may be manifest without obvious reduction in serum magnesium level but with tissue depletion of magnesium, particularly in patients with diminished renal glomerular filtration rate.

In acute episodes of hypomagnesemic tetany and convulsions, magnesium may be administered intravenously as 10% solution of $MgSO_4$ at the dose of 0.8 mEq of Mg per kg body weight (1.0 ml/kg of 10% $MgSO_4$) up to 20 ml. The infusion rate should not exceed 1.5 ml of 10% $MgSO_4$ per min. This may be followed by a continuous drip of Mg at the dose of 1 mEq/kg/day up to 40 mEq/day (10 ml of 50% $MgSO_4$) diluted in 5% dextrose or normal saline to make up less than 10% of $MgSO_4$

Table 1. MAGNESIUM SALT PREPARATIONS

	Amount of Salt to Make Up 100-ml Solution	Amount of Mg
Oral Solution		
Mg chloride	4 gm of $MgCl_2$ $6H_2O$	2 mEq/5 ml
Mg citrate	6 gm of $MgHC_6H_5O_7$ $5H_2O$	2 mEq/5 ml
Mg chloride and citrate	4 gm of $MgCl_2$ $6H_2O$ & 6 gm of $MgHC_6H_5O_7$ $5H_2O$	4 mEq/5 ml
Mg gluconate	4.2 gm of $MgC_{12}H_{24}O$	2 mEq/5 ml
Milk of Magnesia	7 gm of $Mg(OH)_2$ (in suspension)	12 mEq/5 ml
Tablet		
Mg hydroxide		13.8 mEq/400 mg
Mg gluconate		4.8 mEq/500 mg
Parenteral Solution		
Mg SO$_4$ 7H$_2$O	10%	0.8 mEq/ml
"	20%	1.6 mEq/ml
"	25%	2.0 mEq/ml
"	50%	4.0 mEq/ml

concentration for the first 24 hours. In severe convulsions, in addition to the initial intravenous dose, an equal dose of magnesium (0.8–1 mEq/kg) may be injected intramuscularly as 20% (0.5 ml/kg) or 25% MgSO$_4$ solution (0.5 ml/kg). The effect of a bolus dose of intravenous injection of magnesium takes place immediately and lasts about 30 minutes, whereas following intramuscular injection the onset of action occurs in about 1 hour and lasts about 3–4 hours. If an intravenous route is not readily available, intramuscular injection of MgSO$_4$ at the dose of 1 mEq/kg (0.5 ml/kg of 25% MgSO$_4$) may be repeated every 4–6 hours for the first 24 hours.

Parenteral administration of magnesium solution may be continued 3–5 more days in one half the dose of the first 24 hours; then the patient may be switched to oral therapy. Any form of magnesium salts shown on Table 1 may be used for this purpose. All magnesium salts in large doses tend to induce diarrhea. One should start with a smaller dose initially and increase gradually up to 2–3 mEq/kg/day in 3 to 4 doses.

Patients who waste magnesium in urine or stool require a larger dose, and patients with imparied renal glomerular filtration require as low as one-fourth the normal dose. Progress should be checked by repeated serum magnesium determinations.

Zinc Deficiency

PHILIP A. WALRAVENS, M.D.

The clinical findings and treatment of zinc deficiency depend on both the etiology and the degree of severity. In severe zinc deficiency, the prototype of which is an autosomal recessive disorder of zinc metabolism known as acrodermatitis enteropathica, skin lesions and gastrointestinal disturbances predominate and can be life threatening. In these patients, the oral provision of 30–50 mg of zinc daily causes rapid resolution of signs and symptoms and correction of biochemical abnormalities. These doses are sufficient to overcome the defect in intestinal zinc absorption that is characteristic of the disease. In young infants with acrodermatitis enteropathica, zinc should be started at a dose of 2–3 mg/kg/day and increased as needed to achieve clinical remission.

Severe zinc deficiency has also been reported in premature infants who were mainly breast-fed. While human milk is generally considered the best source of bioavailable zinc for term infants, in rapidly growing prematures the amounts of zinc present during later lactation may be insufficient to support anabolic needs. In such infants, zinc supplements at a dose of 1–2 mg/kg/24 hr will induce remission of clinical signs, and the supplementation needs to be continued for only a few weeks. This contrasts with subjects with acrodermatitis enteropathica, in whom treatment must be continued for life, with regular monitoring of zinc status, particularly in females of child-bearing age who are considering pregnancy.

The most frequent occurrence of severe acquired zinc deficiency is related to the practice of intravenous parenteral nutrition without zinc supplements. Currently, recommended intravenous maintenance doses are 100 μg/kg/day for full-term infants and 300 μg/kg/day for premature infants. Should signs of deficiency appear in infants receiving zinc-supplemented parenteral feeding, the principal cause is an important loss of gastrointestinal fluids from persistent diarrhea or ileostomies. The quantities of zinc required for replacement and treatment under such conditions are best determined by balance studies, although the intravenous administration of zinc, 300–500 μg/kg/24 hr, with concomitant monitoring of plasma zinc levels may suffice if accurate balance studies are not feasible.

At the other end of the spectrum, mild zinc deficiency is not uncommon in infants and young children who generally manifest decreased growth velocity and poor appetite. This mild deficiency can result from the poor bioavailability of zinc in some infant formulas or from inappropriate weaning or later feeding practices. Treatment consists of the oral provision of zinc, 1–2 mg/kg daily for two or three months. A parental report of increased appetite verified by an increase in growth velocity will generally be enough to confirm the diagnosis. Mild nutritional deficiency can at times be corrected through the generous provision of zinc-supplemented cereals and foods high in zinc, such as peanut butter, but the concomitant anorexia will often foil such attempts.

Secondary zinc deficiency has been reported in a variety of disease states that cause malabsorption or excessive fecal or urinary losses of zinc. Oral replacement can often be safely started with zinc at 1–2 mg/kg/day. The latter level is recommended in infants with protein-calorie malnutrition once feeding tolerance has been established.

Monitoring of zinc treatment is important and can be done through serial assay of plasma zinc levels, particularly in severe zinc deficiency states when high-dose replacement is used. Plasma copper or ceruloplasmin levels should also be monitored, as copper deficiency can occur with high-dose zinc treatment. A variety of soluble zinc salts are commercially available as supplements, although zinc sulfate and acetate are the most frequently used. As a rule of thumb, 5 mg of the sulfate corresponds to 1 mg of elemental zinc. Costlier chelated or amino acid–bound zinc preparations offer little advantage over the inorganic salts. Since foods have variable effects on zinc absorption, supplements should preferentially be given 1–2 hours before meals.

Hepatolenticular Degeneration

(Wilson's Disease)

OWEN M. RENNERT, M.D.

Wilson's disease may present in the pediatric patient without the classic clinical triad of Kayser-Fleischer corneal rings, hepatic cirrhosis, and neurologic dysfunction. Early diagnosis is paramount since effective treatment may prevent irreversible organ damage and progression of the disease. Symptoms occur as early as 4 years of age, though the second and third decades are the usual ages of onset. The mode of presentation is variable, but the hepatic form is most common in childhood. Presenting symptoms may include hand tremors, slurred speech, spasticity, decreased academic performance, and behavioral disturbances. Two neurologic variants have been identified: dystonic (predominantly seen in young patients) and pseudosclerotic; the dystonic variant appears to be less responsive to therapy.

It is important to stress the wide variability of expression of Wilson's disease. This extends to age of onset, mode of presentation, severity of organ system involvement, and response to therapy. The less common manifestations, such as renal, skeletal, hematologic, and psychiatric disturbances, may occur at any time during the disease course, and usually are preceded by hepatic or neurologic manifestations.

The liver is the *central* homeostatic organ for copper metabolism. Wilson's disease is characterized by a congenital inability to maintain normal copper homeostasis, with resultant accumulation in the liver and other viscera. Impaired secretion of copper via ceruloplasmin and diminished lysosomal biliary copper excretion are associated with saturation of hepatic binding capacity and subsequent release of copper into the circulation, leading to hemolytic crisis and diffusion into the central nervous system and kidneys, giving rise to the distinctive clinical manifestations.

Therapeutic Rationale

Excessive storage of copper in viscera leads to organ system failure because the organism is unable to mobilize, utilize, and detoxify this trace metal. The principles of therapy are based upon enhancing the mobilization and excretion of copper, limiting copper intake, and monitoring the function of copper-toxic target organs. Successful therapy requires early recognition and diagnosis.

Chemotherapy is the central approach for achieving negative copper balance in patients. Penicillamine is the most effective agent utilized in the treatment of these patients.

Therapy

Penicillamine. The dosage of penicillamine used in children is related to the age of the patient. Children under 10 years of age are treated with 0.5–0.75 gm/day—in adults the dose is 1.0–1.5 gm/day. Initial dosage may be calculated as 0.02 gm/kg/day, divided into 2–4 doses/day. *Treatment is lifelong.* Following initiation of therapy, cupruresis of 1000 to 5000 μg/24 hours may occur. Over a 4 to 6 month period, following initiation of therapy, the degree of cupruria gradually falls to approximately 1000 μg/24 hours. Because penicillamine inhibits pyridoxine-dependent enzymes, patients should be given daily supplements of 12.5 to 25.0 mg/day of vitamin B_6. In patients with far advanced neurologic disease L-dopa has been proposed as adjunctive therapy. Published data identify variable success of this therapeutic maneuver.

During the lifelong therapy, patients should be monitored regularly, not only for toxic side effects but also for assessment and maintenance of negative copper balance and clinical improvement. Improvement of symptomatology defines successful therapy, and demonstration on physical examination of symptom reversal usually postdates chemical laboratory evidence of betterment.

An adjunct to penicillamine therapy that has recently been proposed is the treatment of patients with orally administered zinc sulfate. Zinc sulfate is administered to patients at a dose of 100–300 mg given three times a day. This therapeutic maneuver is based on the following observations: (1) intake of supplemental zinc (zinc/copper ratio > 8:1 in diet) results in negative copper balance, (2) oral zinc therapy of patients with Wilson's disease leads to enhanced excretion of copper, and (3) oral zinc treatment results in induction of intestinal metallothionein, which in turn blocks absorption of copper. Since zinc therapy also competes with iron absorption, patients treated with zinc sulfate should be monitored for iron deficiency.

Patient evaluation includes regular assessment of serum copper and ceruloplasmin concentration, as well as 24-hour urinary copper excretion. Improvement of hepatic function is documented by measurement of prothrombin time, serum transaminases, and bilirubin determination. Renal function may be sequentially evaluated by measurement of serum BUN and creatinine; additionally, examination of the urine for the characteristic aminoaciduria and glycosuria seen as evidence of heavy metal intoxication (Fanconi's syndrome) is a valuable adjunct. Recent clinical studies have documented hypercalciuria as a component of the renal dysfunction seen in Wilson's disease.

Successful therapy can be confirmed by regular slit-lamp ophthalmoscopy to document disappearance or absence of the Kayser-Fleischer corneal rings, as well as absence of the "sunflower cataracts" seen in some untreated patients. Recent reports document the potential usefulness of computed tomography to evaluate central nervous system anatomy prior to and during therapy.

Hematologic manifestations occur as a consequence of the pathologic processes of Wilson's disease itself and also as a cytotoxicity of penicillamine therapy. The hemolytic crises seen have been ascribed to a variety of pathophysiologic mechanisms, including copper inhibition of erythrocyte glycolytic enzymes, direct erythrocyte membrane damage, and oxidative denaturation of hemoglobin. During hemolytic crises, patients show marked cupriuria and elevated serum copper concentrations. Thrombocytopenia and leukopenia have been reported to occur as a consequence of hypersplenism.

Thrombocytopenia may be an early sign of penicillamine cytotoxicity. Anemia or granulocytopenia may also occur. Regular evaluation of hematologic status is required. Anemia may develop during therapy as a consequence of red cell aplasia secondary to penicillamine toxicity. The toxic hematologic sequelae of penicillamine therapy are reversed by discontinuation of the drug. Early hypersensitivity reactions have occurred in one third of treated patients; however, these usually respond to gradual desensitization under steroid therapy, usually accomplished by a two week discontinuation of penicillamine. Subsequently, the patient is started on half the calculated penicillamine dose in addition to 20 mg/day of prednisone. The steroid therapy is continued for 2 weeks, then the penicillamine dosage is gradually increased. In certain instances penicillamine dosage may have to be reduced to 50 mg/day for 7 days, rather than the simple 50% reduction, and then gradually increased.

In the past decade clinical reports have identified undesirable side effects of penicillamine therapy. These toxicities are seen infrequently; however, the nature of the reactions is diverse. Descriptions in the literature include nephrotic syndrome, immunocomplex nephritis, immune system alterations (including lupus erythematosus-like syndrome, alterations in T-cell and B-cell function), lymphadenitis, dermatologic manifestations (including elastosis perforans serpiginosa, papular eruptions, and cutis hyperelastica), myasthenia-like syndrome, defects in retinal pigmentary epithelium, and Goodpasture's syndrome. These have remitted following discontinuation of penicillamine therapy.

Alternate chemotherapy is available for the pa-tient who develops toxic side reactions to penicillamine and who cannot be desensitized to this drug. The newly developed copper-chelator triene-2HCl (triethylene tetramine dihydrochloride)* has been shown to be a safe alternative for the treatment of Wilson's disease.

Other Considerations

To minimize copper deposition, dietary restriction of copper should be advocated. Foods high in copper that should be limited or excluded from the diet are liver, nuts, chocolate, cocoa, mushrooms, brain, shellfish, and broccoli. The average American ingests approximately 3.5 to 5.0 mg of copper per day; the patient with Wilson's disease should ingest no more than 1.5 mg per day.

Because of successful therapy of patients with Wilson's disease, it has become necessary to recognize the potential teratogenic action of penicillamine when used during the reproductive period. Penicillamine crosses the placental barrier. Considerations relating to its potential detrimental effect on the fetus are based upon three factors: (1) the drug's capacity to increase solubility of collagen and decrease intramolecular cross-linking, (2) its ability to chelate copper (and potentially other trace metals) and make it unavailable to the fetus, and (3) its structural antagonism to pyridoxine dependent enzymes. Thus, penicillamine dosage should be kept as low as possible when used in the pregnant woman.

Supportive therapy is directed at palliation and minimization of the handicaps that are a consequence of irreparable damage from copper toxicosis. These relate to treatment and rehabilitation of the neurologic sequelae and management of hepatic damage and cirrhosis. Treatment of the agitation and emotional instability has involved use of benzodiazepine and phenothiazine derivatives. Treatment of movement disorders has consisted of use of trihexyphenidyl and related drugs. In the past few years two patients have been treated with liver transplantation. This is consistent with the premise that the central metabolic defect of Wilson's disease is expressed in the liver. This therapeutic maneuver is reserved for the patient with irreversible cirrhosis as a consequence of copper toxicosis.

Hyperphenylalaninemias

STANLEY BERLOW, M.D.,
and VIRGINIA E. SCHUETT, M.S.

The hyperphenylalaninemias are a heterogenous group of autosomal recessive hereditary metabolic diseases that should be identified by newborn screening. Persistent hyperphenylalaninemia, without elevation of other plasma amino acids,

---

* Investigational drug, not commercially available in the United States.

**Table 1. CLASSIFICATIONS OF DEFECTS IN
PHENYLALANINE HYDROXYLASE**

	Phenylalanine Level (mg/dl)	Risk of Mental Retardation	Need for Treatment
Classical PKU	>20	High	All
Variant PKU	10–20	Low–Moderate	Most
Benign Hyperphenyl-alaninemia	<10	0	0

is most commonly secondary to a deficiency of phenylalanine hydroxylase. Multiple allelic mutations in the gene for phenylalanine hydroxylase (PH) and compound heterozygosity probably account for the range of decreased phenylalanine activity and the degree of hyperphenylalaninemia. For therapeutic purposes, Table 1 is an operational classification of these defects in phenylalanine hydroxylase: The incidence of these types of PH deficiency vary. In populations of North European ancestry about 1:10,000 newborn infants who are screened for PKU will require treatment, i.e., will have classical or variant PKU.

During the past 10 years, hyperphenylalaninemia secondary to dihydropteridine reductase deficiency and biopterin synthesis defects has been recognized. Much lower than that of phenylalanine hydroxylase deficiency, the exact incidence of these disorders is not known but has been estimated to be 1–3% of all hyperphenylalaninemic infants. Treatment for these 2 groups of conditions is quite different from hyperphenylalaninemia secondary to phenylalanine hydroxylase deficiency.

PHENYLALANINE HYDROXYLASE DEFICIENCY

Principles of Nutritional Management

Although other possible modes of treating phenylketonuria (PKU) have been suggested, there is currently no effective alternative to dietary manipulation.

Since phenylalanine is an essential amino acid, the primary goals of PKU therapy are to restrict dietary phenylalanine intake to the minimum required for growth and to avoid any excess that could compromise development. This balance of phenylalanine must be maintained, and at the same time an adequate intake of essential amino acids, protein, energy, and other nutrients must be assured. Needs of persons with PKU are presumed to be approximately the same as for normal individuals for all dietary components.

Following a decision to initiate diet therapy, whether the child has classic PKU or a variant form, the immediate goal is to lower the serum phenylalanine level to a therapeutic range as quickly as possible. Age at initial treatment is a strong predictor of the child's eventual I.Q.; infants treated within the first several weeks of life will have the best chance of achieving their expected intellectual potential.

Because of the variability in expression of the disease, the necessity for tailoring the diet to each infant's individual needs, the importance of frequent monitoring, and the ongoing need for family counseling, PKU can best be managed by experienced clinicians. In order for optimal therapy to be started immediately, prompt referral to one of over 100 specialized treatment centers in the United States should be made for any infant with an elevated blood phenylalanine level.*

A therapeutic range for serum phenylalanine levels is generally considered to be 2–8 mg/dl in young infants, and up to 10 mg/dl for older children. There is evidence from the National Collaborative Study of Children Treated for PKU (1967–1984) that loss of dietary control at young ages is related to a deficit in the intellectual performance of the PKU child compared with the performance of siblings or parents. Children who maintain good control have I.Q. and school achievement scores that are no different from those of their normal siblings. Maintaining blood phenylalanine levels of children with PKU in the normal range of 1–2 mg/dl can result in severe phenylalanine deficiency and lead to poor growth, dermatitis, brain damage, and death. Frequent monitoring of blood phenylalanine levels is essential to avoid a deficient or toxic intake of phenylalanine.

Phenylalanine constitutes approximately 3–5% of all protein, and it is not possible to design a diet based only on natural foods that is sufficiently limited in total phenylalanine yet nutritionally adequate. Formulas very low in, or free of, phenylalanine are available to substitute nutritionally for those foods that must be eliminated owing to their high protein/phenylalanine content (including milk, meat, fish, eggs, cheese, nuts, and legumes).

Formulas available in the United States now include Lofenalac† (a casein hydrolysate containing a small amount of phenylalanine), and Phenyl-Free,† PKU 1,‡ PKU 2 Maxamaid XP,§ and Maxamum XP§ (all synthetic amino acid preparations devoid of phenylalanine). Lofenalac and Phenyl-Free are currently the most commonly used formulas for infants and older children, respectively.

---

* Treatment Programs for PKU and Selected Other Metabolic Diseases in the United States: A Survey. DHHS Publication No. (HRSA) 83-5296, 1983.

† Mead Johnson Company, Nutritional Division, Evansville, Indiana 47721.

‡ Milupa Corporation, 397 Old Post Road, Darien, Conneticut 06820.

§ Scientific Hospital Supplies, Inc., P.O. Box 117, Gaithersburg, Maryland 20877.

They provide 80–90% or more of the child's requirement for protein, vitamins, and minerals and up to 75% or more of energy needs. PKU 1 (for infants) and PKU 2, Maxamaid XP, and Maxamum XP (for older children) are primarily protein supplements with added vitamins and minerals, with insignificant amounts of carbohydrate and fat. The amino acid pattern in PKU 1 corresponds more closely to that of human milk than Lofenalac. When prescribing PKU 1, PKU 2, Maxamaid XP, or Maxamum XP, great care must be taken to ensure that adequate calories are provided by low phenylalanine dietary sources of fat and carbohydrate. For young infants, fat in the form of corn oil and carbohydrate as dextrose, dextrimaltose, cornstarch, or preparations of glucose polymers (such as Polycose or Dietary Specialties Caloric Supplement) should be added directly to the formula powder.

Use of PKU 2, Maxamaid XP, or Maxamum XP for the older child allows flexibility in adjusting caloric intake for those who are gaining weight too rapidly; for children who dislike formula, protein, vitamin, and mineral needs can be met by a much smaller volume of with than either Lofenalac or Phenyl-Free.

All six formulas are expensive, costing from $1000–7000 per year depending on the child's age and consumption. Some states still provide formula free of charge. In many states they are available only through PKU treatment centers. When reconstituted with water, the formulas look much like regular milk or infant formula. These formulas have a very objectionable flavor for the unaccustomed, but for children begun on formula in infancy, acceptance is generally good to excellent given competent parental managment in the home.

Because any of the PKU formulas alone will not provide a child with adequate phenylalanine in infancy, natural protein is added to the formula as measured quantities of milk or infant formula. Solid foods are introduced at normal ages (4–6 months) and gradually substituted for the added milk or infant formula. Low phenylalanine foods are allowed in small weighed measured amounts, including fruits, vegetables, small cereal and grain products, and a variety of special low protein products. Phenylalanine-free foods such as carbonated beverages and popsicles are allowed as needed for energy and at parental discretion. Any food or drug containing the sweetener NutraSweet (aspartame) should be carefully avoided by children with PKU owing to the high phenylalanine content. There are cookbooks and food lists of phenylalanine content available to families from PKU treatment centers.

A PKU diet prescription will include recommendations for phenylalanine intake from foods, formula preparation instructions, and a minimum average formula intake. Formula is fed at the normal dilution (20 kcal/oz) during infancy, but is gradually concentrated to 30–45 kcal/oz as the child's protein and energy needs increase.

In recent years, partial breast-feeding of infants supplemented by PKU formula has been successfully carried out by a growing number of motivated mothers. Mature human breast milk is significantly lower in phenylalanine (mean 41 mg/dl) compared with infant formulas (mean 75 mg/dl) or cow's milk (159 mg/dl), and it may be used to provide the additional phenylalanine traditionally provided by milk or infant formula. Individual variability in breast milk phenylalanine content is great, however, and content decreases gradually with duration of lactation. Breast milk analysis for phenylalanine at intervals and more frequent analysis of the child's blood phenylalanine levels may be necessary. The infant's intake of phenylalanine can be estimated from the mother's breast milk phenylalanine content and by weighing the infant before and after feeding. Alternatively, a specified number of breast feeds may be prescribed. Usually 2–4 breast feeds are possible, with supplemental formula feeds. A guide to breast-feeding infants with PKU is available.

Serum phenylalanine levels in the newborn period are typically lowered to the therapeutic range within 2–7 days when formula without an added source of naural protein is fed. On such a phenylalanine-deficient regimen, the blood level will fall at a rate of approximately 7–9 mg/dl/24 hr. In the past, initial therapy has often been instituted in the hospital. More recently, many centers manage the neonate as an outpatient. This requires intensive parental education, counseling, and cooperation plus the utilization of frequent, mailed capillary blood samples for phenylalanine analysis.

After the serum phenylalanine level has dropped below 8 mg/dl, the infant's individual tolerance of phenylalanine must be established through weekly monitoring, in combination with diet intake records. Optimal dietary phenylalanine intake can sometimes be quickly determined, but in some infants this can take weeks or months of minor dietary phenylalanine adjustments. Individual phenylalanine needs are extremely variable, depending on factors such as residual enzyme activity, growth rate, and age.

Infants, including those with PKU, generally require phenylalanine at 60–90 mg/kg in the newborn period, with a rapid drop to less than 20 mg/kg by one year of age, and by late childhood to less than 10 mg/kg. Milk supplements and food intake must be frequently adjusted, especially during the first year of life, when growth is most rapid. As a toddler, the child with "classic" PKU will be able to consume no more than approximately 10%

of the average amount of phenylalanine consumed by normal children of the same age, and formula will continue to supply up to 90% of total nutritional needs. Children with a variant form of PKU may tolerate a somewhat more liberal diet.

Even with good parental management of the diet and appropriate recommendations from specialized health care professionals, many factors can adversely influence serum phenylalanine levels. Fluctuations in appetite or formula refusal, leading to inadequate energy, protein, or essential amino acid intake; physical trauma; and even minor illness can cause elevations in phenylalanine levels. Prompt attention to ear infections and other common childhood illnesses is essential to avoid prolonged high blood levels.

Despite the severe dietary restrictions and requirements of the diet, children with PKU fall within growth norms for age, suggesting that protein and energy intakes meet acceptable levels when the diet is properly managed. Further, vitamin and mineral supplements are unnecessary when formula consumption is adequate to meet protein needs. There are indications that for some trace minerals, intake or utilization of children on the diet may be lower than that of normal children, but the clinical significance of these findings has not been proved. No nutritional deficiencies have been documented in children on these formulas during the past 15 years.

Duration of Nutritional Management

In the past, the routine practice of most clinicians in the United States was to discontinue diet at early school age (5–8 years). In recent years, an increasing accumulation of follow-up data on children who discontinued diet at these ages has documented the risk of terminating diet. Problems reported post discontinuation, when blood phenylalanine levels typically range from 20–40 mg/dl, have included significant drops in I.Q., poor school performance, mood and behavior changes, EEG abnormalities, and eczema. Data from 119 children enrolled in the National Collaborative Study of Children Treated for PKU confirm that deficits in intellectual performance and on school achievement tests are more likely to occur in children whose levels are consistently above 15 mg/dl before the age of 8 years. Data on children beyond age 8 is incomplete. Levels somewhat lower than 15 mg/dl, especially if these occur early in life, may also place the child at greater risk.

A number of clinics have attempted to reinstitute diet, and significant improvement has been noted in some children. However, few patients have been able to achieve mean blood phenylalanine levels of 10 mg/dl or less, and many have not been able to tolerate returning to diet at all.

In a 1983 survey of diet termination practices, two-thirds of 90 clinics treating PKU recommended indefinite maintenance of diet, a growing trend both nationwide and worldwide. Experience with on-diet older children and teenagers points to the difficulty but also the feasibility of following a phenylalanine-restricted diet into adulthood.

Education

For the difficult PKU diet regimen to be successful, parents and the entire family (including grandparents) need to understand and accept restrictions and requirements of the diet. Ongoing counseling by an experienced team of professionals can help diminish chronic anxiety, the frequency of elevated blood phenylalanine levels, and behavior problems revolving around food and facilitate a positive family attitude toward indefinite diet maintenance.

Any amount of cheating on the diet can result in significant elevations of serum phenylalanine levels. It is crucial that the children themselves learn about their diets and gain self-control at an early age. Booklets designed to teach children as young as age 3 are available through treatment centers. By the teenage years, self-management is a goal that can be achieved by many.

DEFECTS IN THE METABOLISM OF TETRAHYDROBIOPTERIN

Tetrahydrobiopterin (BH_4) is the cofactor for the hydroxylation of phenylalanine, tyrosine, and tryptophan. Either a defect in the regeneration of BH_4, due to a deficiency of dihydropteridine reductase, or a biopterin synthesis defect will cause defective production of the neurotransmitters DOPA, serotonin, epinephrine, and norepinephrine. Thus, the defect in neural transmission must be the major focus of treatment in these disorders, although hyperphenylalaninemia is generally the first phenotypic marker that is recognized. All newborn infants with persistent hyperphenylalaninemia should be screened for these defects.[||] Total reported cases worldwide number about 50, and the majority are either dihydropteridine reductase deficiency or a biopterin synthesis defect.

The enzyme required in the first step in BH_4 synthesis from guanosine triposphate (GTP) has been identified. But the synthetic pathway consists of at least two other enzymes that have not been unequivocally defined. At present the remainder of the biopterin synthesis defects are a heterogeneous group, which have only been generically described as complete or partial ("leaky" mutants), transient (in the neonate), and "peripheral" which

---

[||] The following screen for defects in biopterin metabolism: Dr. Edwin Naylor, Department of Reproductive Genetics, Magee-Women's Hospital, Forbes Avenue and Hackett Street, Pittsburgh, PA 15213 (412-647-4168) and Dr. Reuben Matalon, Genetics Section, University of Illinois, 840 S. Wood Street, Chicago, IL 60612 (312-996-6714).

do not involve the brain. In the latter two conditions, therapy is probably not necessary.

Patients with a complete or partial biopterin synthesis defect have been treated with a low phenylalanine diet and neurotransmitter replacement (DOPA, 5-hydroxytryptophan, and a decarboxylase inhibitor), with BH_4 alone, or with a combination of BH_4 and neurotransmitter replacement. It is reasonable to begin BH_4 alone. Small doses of 2.5 mg/kg/day have been used and often lower phenylalanine blood levels without markedly increasing CSF neurotransmitter metabolite concentrations. Moderate (10 mg/kg/day) and high (20 mg/kg/day) doses of BH_4 have been employed with better clinical and CSF neurotransmitter response. Some patients do not respond even to high BH_4 doses and require neurotransmitter therapy. The doses that have been employed alone or in combination are DOPA, 5–10 mg/kg/day; 5-hydroxytryptophan, 2.5–10 mg/kg/day; and decarboxylase inhibitor, 1.0–2.5 mg/kg/day. Optimal management requires monitoring CSF neurotransmitter metabolities, since their determination in blood or urine may not accurately reflect CNS concentrations. However, this caveat is issued with the recognition of the need for more age-related data on major and minor neurotransmitter metabolites in the CSF.

The efficacy of treatment has been difficult to measure, since most patients have been identified because of severe neurologic manifestations. There is little doubt that some patients have been helped by therapy, which has by no means reversed all of the neurologic impairment. With earlier diagnosis based on neonatal screening for biopterin metabolic defects in all infants with hyperphenylaninemia, and treatment in the asymptomatic period, it is hoped that these poor results will be improved.

It is important to emphasize the limitations of neurotransmitter replacement which circumvents regulatory mechanisms. BH_4 is probably more physiologic but certainly more expensive. In addition, complications of DOPA therapy similar to those reported in the treatment of Parkinson's disease have been noted. On the other hand, experience with BH_4 is so limited that knowledge of its complications is meager.

In dihydropteridine reductase deficiency, it has been estimated that the theoretical requirement for BH_4 of about l gm/day for a 10 kg child would cost over $40,000 per year. This may explain why there are only a few—and conflicting—reports of short trials of BH_4 in this deficiency. In almost all of the reported cases to date, neurotransmitter replacement has been generally used in the doses described above. Higher doses occasionally have been employed, i.e., DOPA to 20 mg/kg/day, 5-hydroxytryptophan to 20 mg/kg/day, and carbi-

dopa to 4 mg/kg/day. Although the higher doses may be more effective at raising neurotransmitter metabolite levels in the CSF, they are also associated with an increased incidence of vomiting and dyskinesia. Neurotransmitter replacement therapy should be employed in conjunction with a low phenylalanine diet if blood phenylalanine levels are over 15 mg/dl. Finally, it has been demonstrated that patients with dihydropteridine reductase deficiency can become folate depleted and will respond to folinic acid administration.

MATERNAL PKU

Infants who are born to women with classic or variant PKU can suffer intrauterine growth retardation, microcephaly, congenital heart malformations, and mental retardation. For mothers with phenylalanine levels over 20 mg/dl, the risk of the maternal PKU syndrome is over 90%. In other hyperphenylalaninemic pregnancies, paucity of data precludes risk estimates. It has been estimated that by 1990, the incidence of mental retardation from untreated maternal PKU would equal the incidence of mental retardation secondary to PH deficiency were affected infants not identified in newborn screening and treated.

Counseling about maternal PKU should be included in parental interviews that discuss the genetics and course of the disease. Parents should be encouraged to discuss maternal PKU with their daughters during adolescence. The options of birth control, adoption, and dietary management should be introduced and reviewed in family counseling sessions.

Less than 50 case reports on the dietary managment of maternal PKU have appeared. At present it is considered that the best results will be obtained for women on diet prior to conception. This is a compelling reason for a young woman to remain on diet during the childbearing period in order to preserve her option to carry her own child. The published case reports on treatment of maternal PKU cannot substitute for a controlled study and a national collaborative study has been established. This research effort will employ a low phenylalanine regime adapted for pregnancy, frequent plasma phenylalanine and amino acid measurement, nutritional analysis, and routine ultrasound examinations.

Amino Acid Disorders

SEYMOUR PACKMAN, M.D.

Inborn errors of amino acid catabolism or anabolism are single gene disorders most often inherited as autosomal recessive traits. The diseases are the result of defective processing, disposition, or

Table 1. MODES OF THERAPY

1. Replacement of product
2. Antagonists
3. Restriction of precursor
4. Vitamins

transport of amino acids or of small molecules derived therefrom. This definition reflects the pioneering concepts introduced by Sir Archibald Garrod in 1908. Garrod postulated that metabolic disorders were inherited biochemical blocks in normal metabolic pathways. In this construct, reaction steps in a given intracellular metabolic sequence—as well as transport of metabolites across morphologic barriers—are mediated by proteins and are genetically determined. Inherited disorders of the sequence may exist when there is an insufficient quantity of, or aberrant structure and function of, the proteins mediating the various steps.

Although individually rare, the aggregate incidence of inborn errors of amino acid metabolism is relatively high and may be significantly greater than 1/2000 newborns. Given the burden of amino acid disorders, it is not surprising that recent emphasis has been on treatment and on prevention of morbidity and mortality; many such conditions may now be viewed as treatable disorders. Successful therapeutic protocols have been based on an understanding of fundamental pathophysiology and disease mechanisms and have particularly benefited from refinements in nutritional manipulations. The thrust of this article is to develop and review general principles of treatment that can serve as a framework in specific encounters among the myriad of amino acid disorders.

MODES OF THERAPY

Specific approaches to therapy can be directly derived from considerations of potential sources of toxicity. For example, if conversion of an amino acid to a product is inadequate, the resultant dearth of product may cause disease manifestations. Alternatively, a block in a reaction step may result in an intracellular or extracellular accumulation of an amino acid, which compound may be toxic and cause disease. Further, accumulation of a given amino acid may result in increased flux through an otherwise minor pathway, raising to toxic concentrations an otherwise minor metabolite. Similar consequences obtain if the block is at a transport step. Such considerations can be used to derive modes of therapy applicable in a wide range of aminoacidopathies (Table 1).

In some instances, the therapeutic exigency is the replacement of a product that is not being synthesized. Examples include provision of neuroactive agents in disorders of biopterin metabo-

lism (cf. the article on Hyperphenylalaninemias) and the administration of arginine in certain of the disorders of the urea cycle.

In other instances, it may be possible to provide an antagonist to eliminate or otherwise detoxify offending accumulated metabolites. An example is the use of penicillamine to increase the solubility of urinary cystine, thereby preventing urolithiasis in children with cystinuria. Glycine supplementation in isovaleric acidemia can promote the formation of rapidly excreted isovalerylglycine, a nontoxic conjugate of isovaleric acid. In this connection, carnitine administration has been shown to favor the formation (and excretion) of acetyl- and other acylcarnitines, thereby decreasing ketosis in a number of organic acidemias. Finally, the urea cycle disorders are prototypes for quite innovative treatment approaches exploiting alternative reaction pathways for the removal of endogenously produced precursor nitrogen. The administration of phenylactate and benzoate, with the resultant formation and excretion of phenyl-acetylglutamine and hippuric acid, respectively, serves very effectively to reduce the frequency and severity of hyperammonemic episodes in these disorders.

Treatment in amino acid disorders can often be directed toward a reduction in the concentration of a precursor of a defective reaction step. This approach is valid whether toxicity is due directly to a proximately accumulating reactant or to derivatives thereof, and it currently constitutes a major component of our therapeutic efforts in such diseases. Such reduction in concentration may be achieved by dietary restriction of specific precursors (e.g., restriction of the amount of a particular amino acid ingested by a child) or by general restriction of protein intake. Examples are legion, with amelioration and even prevention of toxicity in a number of inborn errors of amino acid metabolism. The success of this kind of nutritional intervention is the basis for the widespread establishment of newborn screening programs for phenylketonuria, maple syrup urine disease, and other disorders of amino acid metabolism.

It is important to recognize that even in well-characterized entities amenable to nutritional manipulation, residual or relative intellectual impairment may be observed—even when properly maintained treatment begins presymptomatically or very early. Nutritional restrictions in such instances may well be deleterious in ways that are not completely understood. Residual deficits may also be due to an incomplete understanding of disease mechanisms or to possible prenatal damage not addressed even with presymptomatic postnatal intervention. Therefore, in discussions of prognosis with families, optimism may often be communicated, but it should be tempered with an honest assessment of the uncertainties extant in these therapeutic endeavors.

Vitamin-responsive or vitamin-dependent disease constitutes a category of amino acid disorder in which treatment has been especially successful. Such disorders respond to vitamins administered in pharmacologic doses (up to 1000 times the recommended daily allowance) or by a nonphysiologic route. The basis for such successful therapeutic responses is the notion that vitamins have specific chemical roles and perform such roles bound to enzymes. For example, normal catalysis in a given reaction step may require the presence and precise covalent binding to the enzyme of a cofactor (coenzyme) such as pyridoxine, cobalamin, or biotin. Failure to achieve such linkage of coenzyme to the enzyme protein (apoenzyme) will produce manifestations interpreted clinically as a disorder of that reaction step.

Vitamins are themselves small molecules and must be absorbed, transported to and into cells, reach the appropriate cell compartment, and perhaps be converted to other chemical forms prior to attachment to the apoenzyme protein. The processing of vitamins as small molecules is, therefore, not unlike that of metabolites such as amino acids. There is a possibility of specificity at each processing step, with mediation of that step by a specific protein. One can anticipate that an inborn error of metabolism may affect one of these steps for a given vitamin or may affect an apoenzyme protein so that the cofactor is poorly bound. In either instance, the end result is defective catalysis by the vitamin-dependent enzyme.

If there is residual activity of a protein mediating a reaction in vitamin processing or transport, there exists the possibility of overcoming the block by achieving a very high concentration of the vitamin at the intracellular reaction site. For example, in the instance of the interconversion of a vitamin from one chemical form to the final coenzyme form, the presentation to a reaction system of very high concentrations of precursor vitamin may result in the formation of enough product (i.e., the coenzyme form of the vitamin) to yield a physiologically satisfactory result. In clinical practice, this is done by administering pharmacologic doses of the specific vitamin.

Examples of vitamin-responsive aminoacidopathies include the cobalamin-responsive methylmalonic acidemias, thiamine-responsive maple syrup urine disease, pyridoxine-responsive homocystinuria, and the biotin-responsive multiple carboxylase deficiencies. In all such disorders, it is important to emphasize the requirement of pharmacologic doses of the cofactor necessary to produce a therapeutic response. Further, whether or not the precise defect in the reaction mechanism is known, it is desirable to demonstrate a reproducible improvement in specifically aberrant clinical chemistries, so as to identify patients who are candidates for such therapeutic approaches. The ultimate designation of responsiveness must of course be derived from observations of clinical efficacy of therapy.

The responsiveness of an aminoacidopathy to pharmacologic doses of water-soluble vitamins has been applied in the prenatal treatment of an affected fetus in the instances of cobalamin-responsive methylmalonic acidemia and biotin-responsive multiple carboxylase deficiency. Since complications from the use of high doses of water-soluble vitamins are relatively infrequent, one may be optimistic in anticipating few adverse effects in the application of such strategies. Nevertheless, caution must still be exercised, as the consequences of longer-term usage in children and in pregnancy have not been completely delineated.

When vitamins are used, we wish to emphasize that they are administered as pharmacologic agents—drugs—to treat specifically responsive aminoacidopathies. Even in those disorders in which the precise biochemical defect may not have been elucidated, cofactor administration is based on reasonable and focused hypotheses concerning underlying etiologies. Such administration is in sharp contrast to the use of "megavitamin" supplements in a random fashion in entities for which a response has not been documented or in patients with ill-defined dysfunctions presenting no clinically valid justifications for therapeutic trials. Indiscriminate use of vitamins in pharmacologic doses—as "megavitamin" supplements—is noted here in order to firmly decry such practice as an invalid approach to patient care.

ACUTE ENCEPHALOPATHY

The success of any of the treatment modalities used in aminoacidopathies is clearly a function of time—the longer the neurologic derangement persists before treatment, the poorer the prognosis. Accordingly, special attention should be given to the management of the patient presenting with acute and severe neurologic dysfunction. Two large subgroups—disorders of branched-chain amino acid catabolism and disorders of the urea cycle—account for a majority of disorders of amino acid metabolism presenting with acute symptoms in the neonate or infant. In such children, a number of additional considerations must supplement the specific therapies discussed above.

In aminoacidopathies presenting acutely, acidosis or alkalosis is commonly observed. Correction of acid-base status is essential and of immediate importance. Appropriate adjustments in electrolyte balance and hydration should, of course, be performed.

Selective avoidance of a particular amino acid

or protein is most crucial. Avoidance of protein should be widely employed for a short time in any child who presents with significant acute neurologic dysfuntion, especially since a clinical response to protein elimination may also be of diagnostic help. Cessation of protein feedings for a few days is harmless, whereas continuation of dietary protein in a child with an aminoacidopathy is often lethal. It is of major importance when instituting nutritional restrictions that attention be directed to total caloric intake. Maintenance of an adequate caloric intake (often utilizing glucose, glucose polymers, and lipid preparations) is essential for prevention of tissue catabolism and must be achieved by parenteral or oral routes of administration.

Exchange transfusion or peritoneal dialysis can contribute to improvement in some disorders of amino acid metabolism, including maple syrup urine disease and hyperammonemic states. In addition, in a child who is gravely ill and whose course has been one of inexorable decline, it is not inappropriate to administer a battery of rationally chosen cofactors in the hope that the baby's biochemical lesion will respond to one of the vitamins.

GENETIC COUNSELING

Treatment of heritable amino acid disorders involves considerations beyond the acute phase of the illness and even beyond the progress of the proband. Because of the importance of genetic counseling to the family, the physician has an obligation to try to arrive at a diagnosis, however grave the prognosis in the proband. Identification of a specific entity will enable counseling of families about their recurrence risks. Most aminoacidopathies are inherited as autosomal recessive traits, and such families are faced with a recurrence risk of one in four. In cases of X-linked ornithine transcarbamylase deficiency the counseling is more complex, and attention must be given to differential risks in males versus females.

Many of the conditions in question can be diagnosed prenatally, thereby offering families the option of pregnancy termination. Furthermore, the successful prenatal treatment of vitamin B_{12}-responsive methylmalonic acidemia and of biotin-responsive multiple carboxylase deficiency augurs an increasing focus on this unique kind of therapeutic opportunity in amino acid disorders.

GENE THERAPY

Advances in recombinant DNA technology and in our understanding of genetic regulation make it reasonable to anticipate even more specifically directed manipulations in aminoacidopathies, namely, correction of a defect by gene transfer. As of this writing, transfer and expression of defined human genetic material has been reported in cell cultures and animal systems. Such work,

while clearly investigational, is providing the basis for and the promise of gene replacement therapy in these disorders.

Hyperlipoproteinemia
PETER O. KWITEROVICH, JR., M.D.

The diagnosis and treatment of inherited disorders of plasma lipid and lipoprotein metabolism are important in order to prevent their two major complications, namely, atherosclerosis and pancreatitis. The hyperlipoproteinemias may be broadly classified into disorders of the major cholesterol-carrying lipoproteins, low density (beta) lipoproteins (LDL), or of those associated with increases in one or more of the triglyceride-rich lipoproteins, namely, chylomicrons, very low density (prebeta) lipoproteins (VLDL), and the remnants of their metabolism, chylomicron remnants and intermediate density lipoproteins (IDL). In certain children at risk for atherosclerosis, hyperlipoproteinemia may not be present; such children may have a very low level of high density (alpha) lipoproteins (HDL).

Dietary Management

For most children with hyperlipoproteinemia, the unified dietary approach currently developed by the Nutrition Committee of the American Heart Association can be used. This diet is used for disorders of both LDL cholesterol and triglyceride metabolism. It is divided into three phases of progressive stringency (Table 1). Many children will need a phase 2 diet to effect a significant lowering of their hyperlipidemia. In those with a disorder of LDL metabolism, a lowering of 10–15% in plasma total and LDL cholesterol level is often observed. For the hypertriglyceridemics, such a diet, often combined with suitable reduction in weight, often lowers and maintains the triglyceride level in the normal range.

Table 1. UNIFIED APPROACH TO DIETARY TREATMENT OF HYPERLIPOPROTEINEMIA

Nutrients as Percentage of Total Calories*	Phase 1	Phase 2	Phase 3
Fat	30–35%	<30%	20–25%
Saturated fat	<10%	8%	6%
Polyunsaturated fat	10%	10%	8%
Monounsaturated fat	10–12%	10%	8%
P/S	1.2–1.4	1.1–1.5	1.1–1.5
Cholesterol (mg/day)	<300	<200	100
Carbohydrate	45–50%	50%	55–60%
Protein	20%	20%	20%

* Approximate averages are provided; the percentage of nutrient intake will vary depending on the total daily caloric intake (e.g., 1200–2300 calories/day).

The principles of the diet include a reduction in total fat, which will decrease both chylomicrons (and their remnants) and LDL cholesterol (Table 1). The decrease in the percentage of calories as saturated fat will lower LDL cholesterol, and a reduction in dietary cholesterol and calorie control will lower VLDL, IDL, and LDL cholesterol. Restrictions of simple sugars (with an increase in complex carbohydrates) will decrease VLDL cholesterol. The major reductions include meat, dairy products, and eggs. Skim or 1% milk is substituted for whole milk, low fat cheeses are recommended, and only one to two eggs per week are permitted. Commercially baked goods and desserts, chocolate, fatty snacks, and fast foods are eliminated. Lean meat, fish, and poultry in limited amounts (3–5 oz/day) are recommended. This unified dietary approach to treatment of hyperlipidemia may be obtained in a booklet from from the American Heart Association, National Headquarters, Dallas, Texas.

For the unusual child with severe hypertriglyceridemia associated with increased chylomicrons, a more stringent restriction in dietary fat (at least phase 3) will be necessary. Medium chain triglycerides, which go directly to the liver via the portal vein and do not require chylomicron formation for absorption, can be used as an oil substitute, at up to 15% of the total caloric intake.

For the child with hypoalphalipoproteinemia, a phase 1 diet is recommended. Reduction to ideal body weight, regular aerobic exercise, and cessation of cigarette smoking may raise the HDL cholesterol level 5 to 10 mg/dl.

Drug Treatment

Familial Hypercholesterolemia. The majority of pediatric patients with hyperlipoproteinemia can be managed by diet alone. The primary need for therapy with drugs in the pediatric age group will be the child with heterozygous familial hypercholesterolemia. The drug of choice is a bile acid sequestrant, either cholestyramine (Questran) or colestipol (Colestid). These anion exchange resins bind bile acids in the intestine and prevent their reabsorption, and the complex is eliminated in the feces. Such an interruption of the enterohepatic circulation perturbs cholesterol metabolism in the liver. More hepatic cholesterol is converted to bile acid, prompting an increase in the production of LDL receptors, which mediate the uptake and catabolism of LDL from blood.

The decision to use a bile acid sequestrant must be individualized. We usually reserve the use of these agents for children at least 10 years of age who also have a family history of premature coronary atherosclerosis and who have not lowered their total and LDL cholesterol levels into the normal range with diet. The medication is dis-

Table 2. DOSAGE SCHEDULE FOR TREATMENT OF FAMILIAL HYPERCHOLESTEROLEMIC CHILDREN AND YOUNG ADULTS WITH A BILE SEQUESTRANT

| | Postdietary Plasma Levels | |
Daily Doses of Bile Sequestrant	Total Cholesterol (mg/dl)	Low Density Lipoprotein Cholesterol (mg/dl)
1	<245	<195
2	245–300	195–235
3	301–345	236–280
4	>345	>280

pensed either in a packet (cholestyramine 9 gm, 4 gm active ingredient; colestipol, 5 gm active ingredient), or in bulk form (1 scoop equals 1 packet). The dose-response relationship for children and young adults with familial hypercholesterolemia (FH) is summarized in Table 2. In general, heterozygous FH children will require a lower dose of bile acid sequestrant to lower their total and LDL cholesterol levels into the normal range than will adults. The dry powder must be mixed in a liquid, such as water or orange juice, before ingestion. The medicine is most effective when given just before, during , or after a meal. The primary side effects include constipation, abdominal bloating, and a feeling of fullness. Rarely, steatorrhea has been observed when the medicine is given in very high doses (6 packets or more/day). Potential side effects include malabsorption of fat-soluble vitamins and folic acid. A multivitamin containing vitamins, minerals, iron, and folic acid can be given when the child is being treated with the resin. Often, low plasma serum levels of folate will be observed during therapy, but it is rare for the folate content of the erythrocytes to be affected; consequently, anemia due to folic acid deficiency rarely occurs. The medication can also intefere with the absorption of other medicines, particularly digoxin, warfarin, and thyroxine, and consequently should be given at a time when other medications are not given.

Other medications have been used to lower the LDL cholesterol level in FH heterozygotes. These include D-thyroxine (Choloxin), in a dose of 0.05 mg/kg up to a maximum of 4 mg/day, and para-aminosalicylic acid. Such therapy is not routinely recommended for the pediatric age group.

The rare FH homozygote requires therapy with diet, bile sequestrant (6 to 8 packets/day) and nicotinic acid (up to 3 gm/day), but more aggressive measures such as plasmapheresis, portacaval shunt, and liver transplantation will usually be required. Partial ileal bypass is not effective in the FH homozygote.

Hypertriglyceridemia. Almost all hypertriglyceridemias are very responsive to weight reduction and diet (Table 1) and will not require the use of drug therapy in pediatric age group. In the rare patient with dysbetalipoproteinemia (type III hyperlipoproteinemia), clofibrate (Atromid-S),* 1–2 gm/day, is most effective.

Summary

In summary, the diagnosis and treatment of hyperlipoproteinemia in the pediatric age group is an important part of the traditional preventive approach taken by pediatricians. The recent results of the Lipid Research Clinics Coronary Primary Prevention Trial indicate that the treatment of patients with elevated LDL cholesterol levels is associated with significant reduction in morbidity and mortality from coronary artery disease. Such data, combined with the growing literature on the expression of hyperlipoproteinemia in children, the tendency of the hyperlipoproteinemias to persist into adulthood, and the strong association with coronary atherosclerosis, provide a strong rationale for appropriate diagnosis and treatment of these conditions. Finally, the rare child with profound hypertriglyceridemia needs to be treated to prevent life-threatening pancreatitis.

Galactosemias

MIRA IRONS, M.D.,
and HARVEY L. LEVY, M.D.

Of the three inborn errors of galactose metabolism, galactosemia is the best known and the most frequent and produces the most severe clinical consequences. It is due to a deficiency of galactose-1-phosphate uridyl transferase, an enzyme that catalyzes the second step of galactose degradation.

The elimination of lactose (galactose) from the diet is associated with the rapid reversal of clinical symptomatology, especially if begun within the first four or five days of life. The children treated earlier do better intellectually, although some have visual perceptual difficulties, speech defects, and problems with social adjustment despite early treatment. If the infant survives but remains untreated, the disease results in mental retardation, cataracts, and cirrhosis.

Dietary Therapy

The main form of therapy for infants and children with galactosemia is the elimination of lactose by removing milk and milk products from the diet. This is accomplished in infancy by the use of soybean formulas or Nutramigen, a casein

---

* Manufacturer's warning: Safety and efficacy for use in children have not been established.

---

hydrolysate. Older children should remain on milk-free diets with the addition of vitamins and calcium. The guidance of a nutritionist should be sought, since milk solid is a common additive to many foods and lactose is a common filler in medicinal tablets and capsules; thus, close attention to product labels is required. Patients and their families also require nutritional guidance to ensure that the diet is adequate for normal growth. Compliance with the diet is monitored by measuring erythrocyte or whole blood galactose-1-phosphate and urinary galactose. Even well-treated galactosemic patients have detectable erythrocyte galactose-1-phosphate and it is believed that this is formed endogenously from UDP-glucose. This endogenously produced galactose-1-phosphate may exert some toxic effects, most notably on the brain and ovary.

Prenatal Diagnosis

Prenatal diagnosis of galactosemia is available through midtrimester amniocentesis. Transferase measurement in cultured amniotic fluid cells can provide definitive fetal diagnosis. Mothers at risk are often placed on lactose-free diets with calcium supplementation during pregnancy on the premise that this decreases the galactose load to the fetus and thereby eliminates the complications of this disease. Cord blood determination, however, has revealed increased levels of galactose-1-phosphate in galactosemic infants even of mothers who strictly adhered to the diet. Consequently, it appears that the galactosemic fetus as well as the galactosemic infant and child can endogenously produce galactose-1-phosphate.

Other Complications

As already noted, even the early, well-treated child with galactosemia may develop learning disabilities, speech and language difficulties, and behavioral problems. Another recently described and potentially very distressing complication is that of ovarian failure in galactosemic females. This ovarian failure is hypergonadotrophic and varies in severity. It appears to be independent of early treatment and seems to affect most galactosemic girls. Current research is underway in various laboratories to determine the cause of these complications.

GALACTOKINASE DEFICIENCY

A second disorder of galactose metabolism is due to a deficiency of galactokinase, an enzyme that catalyzes the first step in the galactose metabolic pathway. This is also inherited in an autosomal recessive manner. In this disorder, galactose accumulates in blood and urine and galactitol accumulates in urine and ocular lenses, but galactose-1-phosphate is not formed. The only clinical complication is the development of cataracts early in life. Dietary restriction of lactose as described for galactosemia prevents the cataracts in these individuals.

Disorders of Porphyrin, Purine, and Pyrimidine Metabolism

PHILIP ROSENTHAL, M.D.,
and M. MICHAEL THALER, M.D.

THE PORPHYRIAS

The porphyrias are a group of disorders characterized by defects in heme synthesis resulting in excessive accumulation of heme precursors in the tissues. Most fatalities are caused by delays in diagnosis and treatment. Awareness of the clinical patterns associated with these disorders and investigation of family members of patients with porphyria will accelerate the diagnostic process and may prevent unnecessary surgery. Appropriate therapy will bring about relief from acute attacks and ensure a favorable long-term outcome.

Congenital Erythropoietic Porphyria (Günther's Disease). For this, one of the rarest inborn errors of metabolism, treatment includes avoidance of sunlight, screening window light, use of special light bulbs, protective clothing, avoidance of minor trauma to the skin, barrier skin creams, and appropriate topical and systemic antibiotics. Photosensitivity in some patients has been reduced with beta-carotene (30 to 150 mg/24 hr orally). Beta-carotene capsules may be opened and contents mixed in orange or tomato juice to aid administration in children. Recently, canthaxanthin (4,4-diketo-beta-carotene) has been utilized in doses of 25 to 100 mg/24 hr with good results. Instead of a yellow hue from beta-carotene, canthaxanthin causes a brownish discoloration of the palms and a pleasant suntanned appearance to the face.

Blood transfusions frequently are necessary to treat the hemolytic anemia. Splenectomy may reduce transfusion requirements and decrease formation of porphyrins responsible for photosensitivity. However, the increased risks of sepsis in children susceptible to repeated skin infections should be considered in the decision for splenectomy.

Erythrodontia, a pinkish-brown discoloration of teeth due to porphyrin deposition, may be improved cosmetically with dental crowns. Patients with such crowns should receive careful dental surveillance, since gingivitis may develop, forcing removal of the crowns.

Congenital Erythropoietic Protoporphyria. Congenital erythropoietic protoporphyria occurs more commonly than erythropoietic porphyria. Treatment consists of avoidance of sunlight by screening window light and by using special wavelength light bulbs (not in the 400 nm range), protective clothing, and barrier skin creams. Oral administration of beta-carotene at a dose of 30 to 150 mg/24 hr, maintaining serum carotene concentrations above 500 µg/dl over a period of months, has been found to dampen photosensitivity. Hemolytic anemia is a rare complication that may require splenectomy. Formation of porphyrin gallstones has been reported, which has been treated by cholecystectomy.

Acute Intermittent Porphyria (Swedish Type). Treatment of acute attacks includes provision of 450 to 600 gm of glucose/24 hr, infused through a central vein as 10 to 15% solution in water. Pain is treated effectively with chlorpromazine or chloral hydrate. Hyponatremia secondary to inappropriate secretion of antidiuretic hormone (ADH) often develops during an acute attack and should be managed with fluid restriction. Careful replacement of the sodium deficit with hypertonic saline may be necessary. Severe hypertension is an occasional complication and should be treated as primary malignant hypertension. Paralysis of intercostal muscles with respiratory insufficiency may develop in patients with acute intermittent porphyria in the acute phase. Paresis is often reversible with aggressive management in an intensive care unit. Treatment includes tracheal intubation or tracheostomy and mechanical respiratory support with frequent blood gas monitoring.

A recently introduced therapeutic strategy intended to reduce porphyrin production by means of IV-administered hemin for injection* appears to be extremely effective. An IV line running normal saline is used to inject hemin as a bolus over a period of 15 minutes at a dose of 1–4 mg/kg body weight. The tubing is then flushed with normal saline (0.9% NaCl). Hemin for injection administration may be repeated with 12- to 24-hour intervals depending on response, but no more than 6mg/kg in any 24-hour period.

Propranolol,† administered orally or IV to adults with acute intermittent porphyria, has been reported to exert a beneficial effect on acute attacks. The IV regimen consists of 1 mg propranolol every 1 to 2 hours initially, increasing each dose to a maximum of 40 mg if necessary.

Intravenous administration of the carbohydrate

---

* Hematin is available as Panhematin from Abbott Laboratories, which produces it by license under the FDA Orphan Products Development Program. It is obtainable only by direct request from Abbott Laboratories at 312-937-5558 during working hours or at 312-937-7970 at other times.

† This use is not listed in the manufacturer's official directive.

levulose‡ has also been reported to reduce the severity of acute attacks in adults.

In patients whose attacks may be precipitated by menstruation, the use of ovulatory suppressants, androgens, oophorectomy, and oral contraceptives may be indicated.

Porphyria Variegata (Congenital Cutaneous Hepatic Porphyria, South African Type, Mixed Porphyria). Treatment consists of protection from sunlight (see Congenital Erythropoietic Porphyria) and careful avoidance of even trivial trauma. Cholestyramine (note: dosage of cholestyramine resin for infants and children has not been established), 12 gm daily, has proved useful in the management of cutaneous manifestations. The resin binds porphyrins in the intestinal tract, thus preventing their reabsorption. Fat-soluble vitamins (such as vitamins A, D, and K) should be supplemented in patients treated with cholestyramine.

Porphyria Cutanea Tarda. For porphyrias of this type, treatment should be nonaggressive since the disease is not life-threatening. Dermatologic manifestations should be managed as previously described (see Congenital Erythropoietic Porphyria). When ingestion of toxic chemicals is discovered and discontinued, complete recovery often follows within a few months.

Other modes of therapy include attempts to increase porphyrin excretion by alkalinization of the urine and administration of cholestyramine. The antimalarial agent chloroquine forms complexes with uroporphyrin in the liver, which are readily excreted in urine. However, this form of treatment is potentially dangerous and should be avoided in most cases.

Vitamin E (alpha-tocopherol acetate), 400 IU daily, increased to 1600 IU daily, administered for several months has reduced the dermatologic complications in limited trials with adult patients.

Hereditary Coproporphyria. Treatment of hereditary coproporphyria is as described for acute intermittent porphyria.

DISORDERS OF PURINE AND PYRIMIDINE METABOLISM

Hyperuricemia. Hyperuricemia is rare in childhood. While gout is the major complication of hyperuricemia in adults, formation of urate renal stones is the most frequently observed manifestation of hyperuricemia in children.

Two categories of drugs are used in treatment: those for control of hyperuricemia and those for acute attacks of gout. Since hyperuricemia is rare in childhood, agents currently employed in treatment of hyperuricemia with or without gout have not been adequately evaluated in children. Rec-

‡ Investigational procedure.

ommended doses are the usual adult doses, unless specifically noted as designed for children.

The rapid cell turnover and breakdown of nucleic acids in neoplastic diseases such as leukemia and lymphoma induce hyperuricemia, which may lead to clinical complications, especially in the course of chemotherapy or radiation therapy. As mentioned, the major complication of hyperuricemia in childhood is formation of uric acid stones in the urinary tract. The xanthine oxidase inhibitor allopurinol (hydroxypyrazolo pyrimidine) is indicated in children with hyperuricemia due to malignancy. To ensure maximal inhibition of xanthine oxidase, treatment with allopurinol at 10 to 20 mg/kg/24 hr should be initiated several days prior to chemotherapy. When pretreatment is not possible, allopurinol in doses ranging from 120 to 500 mg/day is used concomitantly with cytotoxic agents. The actual dose of allopurinol is adjusted to body weight, monitored with determinations of serum uric acid, and reduced when renal function is impaired. Side effects of allopurinol include nausea and diarrhea, hepatotoxic manifestations, and skin rashes. Hepatic microsomal enzymes may be partially inactivated by allopurinol, resulting in prolongation of the effective half-life of other drugs metabolized by the liver. When the antileukemic agents mercaptopurine and azathioprine are used in conjunction with allopurinol, their usual doses must be reduced by two thirds to three fourths. Allopurinol and ampicillin should not be administered concomitantly because of an increased risk of serious skin rashes.

An abundant fluid intake and alkalinization of the urine to increase solubility of uric acid are important adjuncts in the treatment of hyperuricemia. This can be accomplished by the use of oral sodium bicarbonate (2 to 6 gm/24 hr) or sodium citrate (20 to 60 ml/24 hr). If renal stone formation occurs in association with diminished renal function, peritoneal dialysis or hemodialysis may be used to remove excess uric acid.

Dietary manipulation includes elimination of purine-rich foods such as organ meats (liver, sweetbreads, kidney), anchovies, sardines, wild game, meat extracts, and meat concentrates (gravies).

Acute attacks of gout are usually treated with colchicine administered orally (0.5 to 0.6 mg once hourly) until objective improvement is obtained. The drug must be discontinued when gastrointestinal complications of colchicine develop (cramping, diarrhea, nausea, vomiting). The maximum daily dose of colchicine is preferably administered IV (1 to 3 mg total dose, based on body size and weight, diluted in 20 ml normal saline) to minimize the gastrointestinal side effects. Colchicine is contraindicated in patients with leukopenia or substantial renal or hepatic disease. The drug must be injected slowly, with care taken not to infiltrate. In addition to gastrointestinal toxicity, side effects include granulocytopenia, alopecia, aplastic anemia, and respiratory depression.

The prostaglandin inhibitor indomethacin§ is also effective in acute gouty arthritis at 50 mg orally every 8 hours, continued until symptomatic relief is obtained. The dose should be rapidly tapered after resolution of inflammatory signs. Side effects include anorexia, nausea, abdominal pain, bleeding peptic ulcers, headaches, dizziness, mental confusion, depression, and convulsions. Bone marrow depression has also been described.

Phenylbutazone and its analog oxyphenbutazone (contraindicated in children under 14 years of age) are potent anti-inflammatory agents useful in the treatment of gout. Usual adult dosage for acute gout is 400 mg initially, followed by 100 mg every 4 hours until inflammation subsides, usually within 4 days. The smallest dose possible should be utilized. In general, 600 mg in 4 divided doses during the first 24 hours of an acute attack is sufficient in adults. Gastrointestinal toxicity is similar to that of indomethacin (see above). Other significant side effects are aplastic anemia and salt retention.

Naproxen, ibuprofen, fenoprofen, and piroxicam have been utilized with moderate success in adults to treat acute attacks of gout but have not been evaluated in children.

Lesch-Nyhan Syndrome. Severe deficiency of hypoxanthine-guanine phosphoribosyl transferase in this disorder causes marked uric acid overproduction associated with choreoathetosis, mental retardation, and self-mutilation. Hyperuricosuria and urate gravel or stone formation are treated with allopurinol‖ until the serum urate level and urinary urate excretion return to normal. Dosages must be individually titrated, but usually range from 100 to 300 mg daily in divided doses. Prevention of urate stones may be accomplished with increased fluid intake, which stimulates increased renal output of uric acid.

Treatment with allopurinol cannot reverse the neurologic manifestations of Lesch-Nyhan syndrome. Physical restraints (elbow splints and hand bandages) may be used to control self-mutilating behavior of patients. Lip biting may require extraction of teeth, but permanent teeth should be spared, since lip biting usually diminishes with age. Nondestructive behavior should be rewarded when possible, but attempts at self-injury should not be punished. This approach is based on reports which suggest that positive reinforcement is preferable to punishment in controlling self-destructive behavior in children with Lesch-Nyhan syndrome.

Recently, 5-hydroxytryptophan**, a precursor of serotonin, in a dose of 8 mg/kg/24 hr in four equal increments, in conjunction with the peripheral decarboxylase inhibitor carbidopa (safety in children not established), 1 to 10 mg/kg/24 hr in two to four equal portions, has been shown to reduce athetoid movement significantly and to produce a sedative effect without improvement in mood or self-multilation. Unfortunately, tolerance may develop within 1 month, with permanent loss of efficacy upon retreatment.

Xanthinuria. Xanthine accumulates owing to deficiency of xanthine oxidase, the enzyme that converts xanthine to uric acid. Uric acid levels are low in serum and urine, and xanthine stones form in the urinary tract. Treatment consists of reducing the intake of foods with a high purine content such as organ meats, anchovies, sardines, wild game, meat extracts, and meat concentrates (gravies). Fluid intake should be increased and the urine alkalinized to facilitate renal excretion of xanthine. These measures should be carefully monitored, since continuous alkalinization of urine may induce formation of calcium stones and may enhance susceptibility to infection with organisms that thrive in an alkaline environment. Once formed, xanthine stones may require surgical removal.

Orotic Aciduria. Hereditary orotic aciduria is due to a deficiency of two enzymes, orotidylic pyrophosphorylase and orotidylic decarboxylase. Mixtures of cytidylic and uridylic acid have been reported to produce remissions, but have not been well tolerated. Treatment with uridine, the nucleoside of uracil, in divided doses of 150 mg/kg/24 hr is readily tolerated, and has resulted in hematologic improvement and diminished urinary orotic acid excretion. A copious intake of fluids assists in dilution of orotic acid in urine and may diminish precipitation of orotic acid crystals.

Lysosomal Storage Diseases

ARTHUR L. BEAUDET, M.D.

The lysosomal storage diseases are due to the genetic deficiency or dysfunction of one or more lysosomal enzymes. This group of disorders includes the lipid storage diseases, the mucopolysaccharidoses, the mucolipidoses, glycoprotein storage diseases, and type II glycogen storage disease (Table 1). The pattern of organ involvement depends on the usual site of degradation of the

---

§ Manufacturer's Warning: Safe use in children has not been established.

‖ Manufacturer's Warning: Safe use in children has not been established.

** Investigational drug.

Table 1. LYSOSOMAL STORAGE DISEASES

G_{M1} gangliosidosis	Sialidosis
G_{M2} gangliosidosis, Tay-Sachs	Aspartylglycosaminuria
	Hurler, MPS IH*
G_{M2} gangliosidosis, Sandhoff	Scheie, MPS IS
Krabbe leukodystrophy	Hunter, MPS II
Metachromatic leukodystrophy	Sanfilippo A, MPS IIIA
	Sanfilippo B, MPS IIIB
Niemann-Pick disease	Sanfilippo C, MPS IIIC
Gaucher disease	Sanfilippo D, MPS IIID
Fabry disease	Morquio, MPS IV
Wolman disease	Maroteaux-Lamy, MPS VI
Cholesteryl ester storage disease	β-Glucuronidase deficiency, MSP VII
Farber lipogranulomatosis	Multiple sulfatase deficiency
Pompe disease, glycogenosis type II	Mucolipidosis II, I-cell disease
Acid phosphatase deficiency	Mucolipidosis III
Fucosidosis	Mucolipidosis IV
Mannosidosis	

* MPS, mucopolysaccharidosis.

accumulating macromolecules. Almost all the disorders are autosomal recessive defects, although a few are X-linked. Although these diseases are heterogeneous and often have infantile, juvenile, and adult forms associated with the same enzyme defect, the disorders regularly exhibit a progressive course. An enzyme-specific diagnosis is a prerequisite for optimal management.

Medical management of patients with these diseases is largely symptomatic and supportive, but a few specific forms of intervention are important. Hypersplenism develops frequently in adult Gaucher disease, and splenectomy is indicated for correction of significant hematologic abnormalities. The Morquio phenotype is associated with odontoid hypoplasia with instability at the atlantoaxial joint. This joint should be evaluated carefully, even in the absence of symptoms. Prophylactic cervical fusion is indicated during the first decade if instability is significant, since acute and chronic cervical cord damage is likely. Judicious use of corrective orthopedic procedures is appropriate, particularly for the mucopolysaccharidoses such as mild Hunter, Morquio, and Maroteaux-Lamy diseases in which intellectual impairment is minimal or absent. Careful cardiac and opthalmologic follow-up also is needed for the mucopolysaccharidoses and related diseases when these organs are involved.

Myringotomy and polyethylene tubes to prevent recurrent ear infections are very important in the mucopolysaccharidoses, mucolipidoses, and similar phenotypes such as mannosidosis. Hearing can be preserved in intellectually normal patients, and recurrent episodes of fever, irritability, and family stress can be avoided in profoundly impaired children.

Fabry disease has a progressive renal impairment, and renal transplantation and dialysis should be considered according to usual criteria. Renal involvement is usually severe enough to require such intervention in hemizygous males but not in heterozygous females. Painful neuropathy occurs in males and females with Fabry disease, and symptomatic relief often can be obtained with Dilantin in usual therapeutic dosage.

Cardiac and respiratory failure occur in type II glycogen storage disease and are managed symptomatically as for any cardiac and skeletal myopathy. Many of the disorders cause intellectual impairment, and special educational and training support is indicated. At times the possibility of progressive dementia exists, but the child should be given the usual special educational support, since prognosis is never certain.

Unfortunately, many children with these diseases experience progressive and ultimately severe neurologic impairment. Proper emotional and social support for the family is very important. Some of these diseases are most tragic and burdensome for families. The family should be encouraged early to explore local resources for institutional care. This can be of value in the event of family illness and can allow the family vacation time. Eventual long-term institutional care should be at the discretion of the family. Assistance can be provided with some medical problems. Seizures occur in many of the disorders and can be treated routinely. Constipation is frequent and can be managed with stool softeners, laxatives, and enemas in a usual manner. Feeding is progressively difficult and may require blenderized or liquid diets. Behavioral abnormalities, which include emotional outbursts, crying out as if in pain, and failure to sleep at night, are extremely burdensome for the family. Sedative medications may assist a family in managing a child at home, but erratic responses to drugs are not unusual in the face of brain damage. Behavioral difficulties are particularly severe in the Sanfilippo mucopolysaccharidoses but occur with other juvenile disorders. Major tranquilizers such as Mellaril,* in doses up to 3 mg/kg/24 hr may be quite helpful. Finally, there may be many difficult ethical decisions late in the course of these patients. When endless hours are required to feed the patient, tube feeding or gastrostomy may be necessary. Institution of these methods of nutritional support should be discussed with the family as they may prolong the life of a helpless child, a result that may or may not be desired by the family. The family should be involved in deciding when to hospitalize and how to manage pneumonias in terminally ill children.

Specific correction of the enzyme defects in these diseases is a subject of active research. While

---

* Manufacturer's precaution: Mellaril is not recommended for children under 2 years of age.

prenatal diagnosis and other reproductive options can prevent the disease in subsequent siblings, these diseases will continue to occur within families unless heterozygote screening, as applied to Tay-Sachs disease, can be extended to other disorders. For the present, effective therapy is a major need. Enzyme replacement is one research modality. Enzyme activity can be delivered to some organs, such as the liver and spleen. There might be cause for optimism that certain non-CNS manifestations could be treatable by enzyme infusion. To be effective in treating CNS damage, enzyme replacement must overcome the additional obstacle of the blood-brain barrier. At present, enzyme replacement is not of proven effectiveness and is not standard therapy in any lyosomal storage disease. Recent reports have revived interest in bone marrow transplantation or amnion implantation as modes of therapy. Carefully planned research trials are appropriate and are in progress. Some families may wish to explore the opportunities for their children to participate in human studies, but at present there is no proof of effective treatment or prevention of central nervous system symptoms. A variety of physical and biochemical methods for targeting enzyme to affected tissues and for overcoming the blood-brain barrier are being explored. The hope of replacing the defective gene itself is still quite uncertain, although considerably more realistic than at the time of the last edition of this book. Numerous cDNAs and genomic DNAs for genes encoding lysosomal enzymes are being cloned. Strategies for gene therapy are being formulated, and human trials are expected soon. Lysosomal storage diseases are attractive candidate disorders, since alternative treatment is so limited. On the other hand, there are potential drawbacks, such as the possible need to target genetic material to the central nervous system. Considerable obstacles still remain, and the feasibility of such therapy remains in question.

The final aspect of management of the lysosomal storage diseases is concerned with the family and prevention of future cases. The first step is complete genetic counseling, including a discussion of the risk of the disease, the burden of the disease, and reproductive options. In autosomal recessive conditions, the major risk is for subsequent pregnancies of the parents of the propositus. Occasionally a sibling of the mother will marry a sibling of the father, creating a high-risk situation. Genetic counseling must be extended to maternal relatives in the case of X-linked diseases. Heterozygote detection is feasible for most of the diseases in question and can be offered to aunts, uncles, and unaffected siblings of the patients with autosomal recessive disorders. For reliable heterozygote detection, however, a laboratory should have substantial experience in assaying normal controls and obligate heterozygotes. Samples from the obligate heterozygote parents of the propositus should be assayed simultaneously to assist in family-specific interpretation of unusual laboratory data which may result from rare alleles (mutant forms of the gene) in a family. Heterozygote testing of relatives is most important in disorders in which the carrier frequency is great, such as for Gaucher or Tay-Sachs disease in the Ashkenazi Jewish population. Mass screening for heterozygotes has been applied for the prevention of Tay-Sachs disease but has not been used significantly for other lysosomal storage diseases to date.

As part of the genetic counseling process, contraception, sterilization, adoption, and artificial insemination should be discussed as alternative methods for reducing the risk of disease. Prenatal diagnosis has been accomplished or presumably could be carried out for almost all the lysosomal storage diseases. The enzyme defects routinely are demonstrable in cultured fibroblasts and amniotic fluid cells. The newer diagnostic procedure of chorionic villus biopsy is proving reliable for most or all lysosomal storage diseases. This earlier prenatal test is attractive to many families with these high genetic risks. The vast majority of biochemical prenatal diagnoses in the last decade has involved the lysosomal storage diseases, with Tay-Sachs disease, type II glycogen storage disease, Krabbe leukodystrophy, metachromatic leukodystrophy, and Hurler disease among the most frequently tested.

11

Connective Tissue

Collagen Vascular Disease

EARL J. BREWER, JR., M.D.

Treatment of chronic rheumatic disease requires a cooperative effort by the pediatrician, pediatric rheumatologist, nurse educator, physical therapist, medical social worker, occupational therapist, ophthalmologist, and orthopedist, as well as the periodic help of consultant services such as cardiology, psychology, nutrition, nephrology, and school and vocational rehabilitation counselors. A basic goal is preparing the child or teenager to be a functioning member of society. Careful attention is required to assure an orderly transition to the adult responsibilities of employment and self-care.

The biggest medical problems center on control of inflammation leading to arthritis, tendinitis, fasciitis, muscular disuse atrophy and resultant weakness, and extraarticular complications (involving the eye, heart, kidney, and central nervous system). Thus, the main therapeutic goal is to reduce inflammation, which is responsible for pain, swelling, warmth, tenderness, and loss of motion in joints and other tissues. Inflammation of organs such as the kidney presents special problems of therapy.

Steppingstones to the successful management of these chronic illnesses include an initial and long-range management plan, parent and patient education and counseling, physical and occupational therapy, good health and nutritional training, specific drug therapy, orthopedic consultation, and periodic eye examination.

JUVENILE RHEUMATOID ARTHRITIS

Children and teenagers with systemic, pauciarticular, or polyarticular juvenile rheumatoid arthritis (JRA) have an excellent prognosis in that mortality is only 2–4% in the United States. At least 75% of these children grow up to lead normal lives with no crippling. Patients with nonarticular systemic complications such as pericarditis have the greatest risk of mortality. Iritis occurs most frequently in patients with pauciarticular JRA.

The milder the joint inflammation, the less therapy is necessary. In general, the greater the number of joints involved, the more likely the patient is to have progressive erosive arthritis; however, patients with only one or two inflamed joints can have severe erosive arthritis.

The therapeutic response of a specific joint or joints is unrelated to the type of JRA. There are no apparent differences among patients with the various types of JRA in adverse reactions to the different antirheumatic drugs.

The general therapeutic goals already discussed are essential to proper care. Virtually all aspects of treatment are directed toward reduction of inflammation and improvement of function and motion.

Drug Therapy

Drug therapy is an integral part of the overall management of JRA. So many antirheumatic agents are now available that it is useful to group them for discussion purposes. The nonsteroidal antiinflammatory drugs (NSAIDs) (aspirin, tolmetin sodium, ibuprofen, naproxen, and others) are antipyretic, analgesic, and antiinflammatory in action. The mechanism is at least partly due to inhibition of prostaglandin synthesis and its effect on the immune system. The pediatrician needs a detailed knowledge of these drugs, because several of them will become widely used for many inflammatory illnesses as well as for more effective fever control in children and teenagers. Slower acting antirheumatic drugs (SAARDs) (gold, D-penicillamine, and hydroxychloroquine) are added to the NSAID when two or three of the latter have been ineffective. SAARDs are also added when limitation of motion or contracture occurs. Perhaps 25% of JRA patients require SAARD therapy. These

353

agents take several months to have a clinical effect by reducing inactivity stiffness and joint swelling and improving joint motion. Corticosteroid medication is reserved for severe or life-threatening situations such as severe pericarditis or iritis. Patients who have incapacitating disease are given steroids for short periods to reduce pain and swelling sufficiently to allow more rapid mobilization. Cytotoxic drugs such as methotrexate, cyclophosphamide, and azathioprine are reserved for patients with extremely severe disease in clinical research situations.

NSAIDs. The NSAIDs currently marketed in the United States, including aspirin, are listed in Table 1. All these drugs act in a similar manner, and none is clearly superior. The three main useful effects are analgesic, antipyretic, and antiinflammatory. The relief of pain is perhaps the most striking attribute of the NSAIDs; this can occur in a matter of hours or days but is more often measured in weeks. Elimination or marked reduction of fever has been an important factor in reducing the need for steroids in patients with systemic JRA. This effect usually occurs in hours. The antiinflammatory effect, recognized by reductions in swelling, pain on motion, tenderness, and limitation of motion of involved joints, does not occur as quickly as the analgesic and antipyretic actions. Pediatric Rheumatology Collaborative Study Group (PRCSG) NSAID data reveal that the antiinflammatory effects occur on the average in 30–37 days. In patients who have not responded favorably (defined as 25% improvement) by 2 weeks, there remains a 50% probability that they will do so by 12 weeks; at 4 weeks the chance of response is still 25%; and at 8 weeks the probability decreases to 10%. It is useful to note that at 12 weeks 20% of the patients had just responded.

Twelve-month studies reveal that about 70% of patients improve, compared with only 50% at 12 weeks of therapy. Thus, these medications should not be stopped too quickly, even if they seem ineffective for several weeks. At least 1 month's trial seems reasonable.

The physician caring for a patient with JRA needs to know whether it is useful to try several NSAIDs. Our studies of PRCSG data reveal that 50% of patients who experience no relief with the first NSAID will improve when it is stopped and another is tried. An average of three or four NSAIDs may be tried before a drug that is both effective and safe for a given patient is found. Some physicians give two NSAIDs at the same time; one may help pain only and the second reduce swelling in a more satisfactory manner. Another method that is effective at times is to add a second NSAID to enhance the partial effect produced by the first drug.

Toxicity of a drug must always be balanced against its effectiveness. The removal rate of patients because of adverse reactions is about 5% with NSAIDs other than aspirin, for which it is 11–15%. The usual reactions are gastrointestinal (nausea, abdominal pain, or diarrhea), renal (hematuria or proteinuria), hematologic (anemia, leukopenia, or thrombocytopenia), and occasional tinnitus or blurred vision. Aspirin differs from the other NSAIDs in that up to 10% of patients must be removed when liver enzyme tests show levels several times greater than normal. One must remember that on rare occasions the NSAIDs can cause peptic ulcer, severe renal toxicity such as interstitial nephritis, liver toxicity, and severe allergic reactions.

Cross-toxicity is a continuing worry to the physician. Patients with JRA who develop a toxicity to

Table 1. NONSTEROIDAL ANTIINFLAMMATORY DRUGS

Name	Trade Name	Dosage (mg/kg/day)	Doses/Day	FDA Approved	PRCSG Study
Aspirin	Same	80	3–4	Yes	Yes
Indomethacin Group					
Tolmetin sodium	Tolectin	20–50*	3–4	Yes	Yes
Indomethacin	Indocin	1–2.5	3–4	No	No
Sulindac	Clinoril	?	2	No	No
Propionic Acid Group					
Naproxen	Naprosyn	10–20	2	No	No
Ibuprofen	Rufen Motrin	30–40	3–4	No	Yes
Fenoprofen	Nalfon	1200–1800/m^2	3–4	No	Yes
Other					
Meclofenamate sodium	Meclomen	4–7.5	3–4	No	Yes
Piroxicam	Feldene	?	1	No	No
Diflunisal	Dolobid	10–20	2	No	No
Phenylbutazone	Butazolidin	3–6	2–4	No	No

* Manufacturer's warning: Doses higher than 30 mg/kg/day have not been studied in children and, therefore, are not recommended.

one NSAID have a 50% chance of developing a significant toxicity to a second NSAID. Even more important is that one patient in four develops a similar toxicity (e.g., 25% of patients who experienced nausea with the first drug will have the same reaction to the second drug).

Why are there so many NSAIDs? As stated, 50% of children will respond to a different NSAID when the first one has failed or has lost its effectiveness. Formulation changes can sometimes reduce side effects; for example, substituting a pyrrole ring for an indole ring made tolmetin sodium sufficiently different from indomethacin to reduce such side effects as severe headhache. Patient compliance is much better if the medication is taken only one or two rather than four times per day. The development of longer half-life drugs such as naproxen (14 hours) and piroxicam (40 hours), requiring only once- or twice-daily dosing, has proved useful. Many children and teenagers prefer liquid preparations, and ibuprofen syrup will be welcomed when it is marketed. A few drugs, such as phenylbutazone and indomethacin, are thought to be more effective for certain kinds of arthritis, such as juvenile ankylosing spondylitis. Also, in some situations an NSAID will be effective for a number of months and then cease to help (this is called tachyphylaxis), requiring substitution of another NSAID.

The last matter to be discussed relates to Food and Drug Administration (FDA) approval and whether the physician on the front line of care can prescribe these useful drugs in children. At this time only two NSAIDs (aspirin and tolmetin) are approved for use in children by the FDA. As every practicing pediatrician knows, only about 30% of the drugs listed in the *Physician's Desk Reference* are officially approved for use in children, and it would be difficult to care for children if the others were avoided completely. It is essential to study these drugs, however, and one guideline is to restrict use to those drugs that have been studied adequately and the results published in a peer-review journal. Using that guideline, aspirin, tolmetin, ibuprofen, naproxen, fenoprofen, meclofenamate sodium, and indomethacin have all been studied, at least for dosage and safety, and the results published.

Aspirin has been until now the standard therapy for adult and pediatric arthritis patients. At a dosage of 80 mg/kg/day in divided doses, effective control of fever, joint swelling, pain, limitation of motion, myalgia, and morning stiffness can be expected in about 50% of children and teenagers. Adverse reactions, however, are more frequent with aspirin than with other NSAIDs; in patients studied by the PRCSG, the removal rate for adverse reactions to aspirin (usually increased liver enzymes and gastrointestinal problems) is 11–15%, compared with less than 5% for other NSAIDs (for which the complications are usually hematuria, proteinuria, or gastrointestinal problems). A problem peculiar to aspirin is the formation of caries in the chewing areas of the teeth, where material from chewed-up baby aspirin tablets tends to pack. There is also the issue of Reye's syndrome and its possible relationship to aspirin administration and an accompanying respiratory infection. In many parts of the country aspirin can no longer be given to the majority of children because of the adverse publicity and warnings issued by various governmental agencies regarding Reye's syndrome.

In spite of these criticisms of aspirin, none of the other NSAIDs has shown greater effectiveness, and the cost of aspirin is a fraction of that of the newer agents. In our center aspirin is tried first for at least a month unless fever control is a primary goal (then a week is sufficient). The next NSAIDs, in the usual order tried, are: Tolectin, Naprosyn, Rufen or Motrin (also sold over the counter as Advil and Nuprin), Nalfon, Dolobid, and Meclomen.

SAARDs. When NSAID therapy does not help sufficiently, the patient's disease is progressing, or limitation of motion with or without contractures occurs, a slower acting antirheumatic drug such as gold, D-penicillamine, or hydroxychloroquine is added to the NSAID being taken by the patient. These drugs are not considered antiinflammatory but do affect the immune system, at least in vitro. SAARDs must be given for several months before clinical effect is noted. Reduced morning stiffness and generally feeling better occur first, at about 2 months. At 4–6 months reduction of joint swelling and improved motion are seen. Parents and patients both report better mobility and less pain. As with the NSAIDs, about 50–60% of children will improve 25% or more. Such measures of disease activity as erythrocyte sedimentation rate and rheumatoid factor are reduced to normal, at least in some patients.

Injectable gold (Myochrysine or Solganal) or oral gold (Ridaura)* is the best SAARD to use initially. The dosage of injectable gold is 1 mg/kg/week IM for 20 weeks, followed by a reduction to every other week or monthly depending on response. The dosage of auranofin (Ridaura) is 0.15–0.2 mg/kg/day orally for an indefinite period. Response occurs with both drugs at about the same time; Ridaura may act a little faster. If the patient has not responded by 6 months, the medication should be stopped. If the patient does respond, gold therapy may be continued indefinitely.

Adverse reactions sufficient to discontinue gold therapy occur in about 10% of patients and usually

---

* Not yet approved for use in children. Studies are being completed.

consist of hematuria, proteinuria, anemia, neutropenia, and rash. The toxicity removal rate in fact was less than that for aspirin in at least two controlled studies in children. Severe reactions do occur, as they do with NSAIDs, and must be considered when weighing the risk/benefit ratio for a given patient. Nephrotic syndrome due to interstitial nephritis, hepatitis, exfoliative dermatitis, and severe allergic reactions are examples. The "nitritoid reaction," consisting of lightheadedness and weakness, is unusual; it occurs with the use of Myochrysine and is eliminated by changing to Solganal.

D-Penicillamine† is a chelating agent that has been found to possess antirheumatic properties. The dosage is 10 mg/kg/day in a single dose; it must be taken for at least 6 months before efficacy can be established. Studies in adults have clearly shown this agent to be more efficacious than placebo; however, a recent controlled and blinded study in children (USA-USSR PRCSG study) has shown a 60% improvement not only in patients on NSAID and D-penicillamine but in patients on NSAID and placebo.

Toxicity data reveal the usual problems with hematuria, proteinuria, anemia, neutropenia, and occasional thrombocytopenia. A rare patient can develop myasthenia gravis (usually reversible) or nephrotic syndrome.

Hydroxychloroquine is an antimalarial drug that has been widely used in the USSR and at a few centers in the United States. The dosage is 6–8 mg/kg/day orally to a maximum of 300 mg/day. Selected patients have seemed to respond dramatically to the compound, but recent PRCSG studies found that the results, improvement (defined as 25% or better) in 60% of patients, were no better than those obtained with NSAID and placebo in a 1-year controlled, randomized, blinded trial. Response is measured in months rather than weeks. A trial of 6 months is necessary to ascertain effectiveness.

Toxicity is minimal using the dosages described. Dosages greater than 10 mg/kg/day have resulted in visual acuity loss due to retinal toxicity. Alopecia, allergic reactions, and the usual abnormalities relating to the kidney, liver, and bone marrow occur in only a few patients.

Cytotoxic Drugs. Cytotoxic drugs such as cyclophosphamide,‡ azathioprine, chlorambucil, and methotrexate‡ are reserved for those patients who have severe debilitating disease and have responded poorly or not at all to more standard therapy with NSAIDs and SAARDs. The response

rate in severely involved adult patients with rheumatoid arthritis who received methotrexate was almost 70%, as opposed to only 20% in patients given placebos. A trial, funded by grants from the FDA to the PRCSG, to study the effectiveness of methotrexate in severely involved patients with JRA is now under way. In general, the serious adverse reactions that sharply limit the usage of cytotoxic drugs are malignancy and reduced fertility. Selected agents such as cyclophosphamide can cause painful, long-lasting hemorrhagic cystitis. In the past, fibrosis of the liver and lung limited the use of methotrexate; however, this finding is apparently not as serious as had been assumed.

The dosage of cyclophosphamide or azathioprine§ should rarely exceed 1–2 mg/kg/day. The dosage of methotrexate being tested is 5 and 10 mg/m²/week given 1 day per week. The dosage must not exceed 15 mg.

Physical and Occupational Therapy

A cornerstone of treatment is physical therapy. The main purpose of drug therapy is to relieve pain enough to allow strengthening and increase of muscular endurance along with improvement of motion. Exercises, which are taught by the physical therapist to the patient and parent, must be done daily. Moist heat is the best modality and the most economical. It is best administered by warm baths, usually taken in the morning to reduce morning stiffness. At times a waterbed is useful to reduce severe inactivity stiffness. The best single exercise, which is also fun for the patient, is swimming on a regular basis. Contact sports must be avoided, for obvious reasons, unless the patient's disease is very mild.

The real key to a successful physical therapy program is consistent follow-up of patients. There should be a definite plan for improvement, and continuing encouragement should be offered.

Orthopedic Care

The orthopedist is a necessary member of the care team, providing advice regarding splints and other orthotic devices to straighten contractures or rest a body part during periods of severe inflammation. Soft tissue release and later joint replacements in severely involved patients have allowed the orthopedist to make a major contribution to better care.

Ophthalmologic Care

A major concern in the treatment of JRA is the occurrence of inflammation of the eye, usually including iritis and occasionally papillitis, scleritis, myositis, choroiditis, or lens opacities. Frequent

---

† The efficacy of D-penicillamine in juvenile rheumatoid arthritis has not been established.

‡ This use of methotrexate and cyclophosphamide is not listed by the manufacturer.

§ The use of azathioprine in children for the treatment of rheumatoid arthritis is not listed by the manufacturer.

eye examinations by the ophthalmologist are essential to adequate care. Most patients are asymptomatic and are diagnosed at routine follow-up examination. Iritis is associated with pauciarticular JRA, but it does occur with the other types. Frequency of exams differs with the center giving care, but in general every 6–12 months is adequate except in cases of active iritis.

Treatment consists of local corticosteroid eyedrops, usually in conjunction with a cycloplegic. More severe problems require oral corticosteroid medication. Rarely, a patient with rapidly progressing iritis or retinitis requires cytotoxic drugs. The results of treatment are gratifying; usually fewer than 10% of patients lose significant visual acuity.

School, Family, and Social Problems

The most important contribution the physician can make to the care of the child or teenager with JRA is to establish rapport with the patient and parent so that there is early recognition of school, family, or social problems. A particular problem vexing parents and patients is the refusal of most schools to provide special adaptive physical education and to help with the physical limitation problems.

Great stresses are placed on the parents and siblings of children with long-term chronic illness. The physician, aided by the medical social worker and the parents, can do many things to minimize the natural stress of the disease. The social problems of children with any chronic illness are remarkably similar, having to do with restriction of a normal lifestyle. Great skill is necessary to be of service.

SYSTEMIC LUPUS ERYTHEMATOSUS

The spectrum of disease of systemic lupus erythematosus (SLE) is so broad that treatment must be individualized to fit the complication or manifestation exhibited. The mortality rate has been reduced dramatically, to about 10–15%, since steroid and other therapies have become available. Patients with mild disease should be treated with symptomatic therapies only; for example, patients with mild joint pain, malaise, and a mild skin rash should receive an NSAID at most. Patients with central nervous system problems or pulmonary or other systemic manifestations should be treated with oral corticosteroids (up to 1–2 mg/kg/day).

Children with SLE who have definite, diffuse proliferative glomerulonephritis should be treated with oral steroids in the dosage just specified. There is considerable controversy regarding whether pulse steroid therapy, in addition to daily or alternate-day administration of steroids and/or cytotoxic drugs, is beneficial to patients with SLE nephritis or other complications. Some recent reports indicate that using two cytotoxic agents at the same time improves survival. There are data to support the necessity of treating SLE nephritis with combined therapy in spite of the known risks. A particular problem is the child with a normal urinary sediment, elevated antinuclear antibody, and a low C3, C4, or Ch50. Many rheumatologists feel that a renal biopsy is necessary in this situation to document serious renal disease in the absence of abnormal urinary sediment.

Intravenous pulse corticosteroid dosage is generally 30 mg/kg/dose (1 gm maximum), given for a 1-hour period daily or every other day on three to six occasions, followed by oral steroids given daily or every other day at full or reduced dosage. There is evidence that the pulse therapy improves morbidity more quickly but does not alter long-term renal function. The initial hope was that pulse therapy would reduce adverse reactions while producing comparable therapeutic results. Unfortunately, patients usually require continuing daily or every-other-day steroid to maintain partial remission of disease.

Pulse cytotoxic therapy has not been studied sufficiently to establish its proper role in the treatment of SLE. Recent reports of combined usage of two cytotoxic drugs in adults seem to show better survival rates than when these drugs are used alone. Dosages are given in the JRA section.

Plasmapheresis or apheresis is controversial as an alternative mode of treatment in severely involved patients with SLE nephritis. The procedure involves removal and replacement of plasma or removal of predominantly lymphocytes from the blood. The exchange rate for plasma is usually 40 ml/kg/exchange, with 6 to 18 exchanges being given per treatment course. The interval of time varies, but the exchanges are given daily in groups of three with a several-day rest in between to allow the veins time to recover. In critical situations plasmapheresis can be life saving; in general, however, the expense and risk are usually too high to justify the procedure.

SLE patients with mild disease and cutaneous vasculitis can benefit from hydroxychloroquine therapy (6–8 mg/kg/day). Improvement takes several weeks to several months.

DERMATOMYOSITIS

The therapy of dermatomyositis is directed toward improving the strength of involved muscles. Physical therapy will not accomplish this goal. Corticosteroids (e.g., prednisone) at a dosage of 1–2 mg/kg/day are necessary until the patient can perform basic functions, including rising from the floor with or without help, climbing stairs, eating and drinking without help, and performing usual toilet functions. The muscle enzymes return to normal before the muscle function improves significantly. Many months often elapse before the steroid can be given only every other day. This may be accomplished by reducing the dosage on an every-other-day basis until no steroid is given on the alternate day. Subsequent reduction depends on whether a flare of muscular pain or weakness occurs at a certain level of oral steroid. When a flare occurs after a dosage reduction, many months may pass before partial remission occurs again, even on a much higher dose of prednisone.

There are a few reports of pulse steroid therapy, given in the manner described for treatment of SLE, that found a more rapid improvement of muscular strength and pain. Severely ill patients whose profound weakness even involves the muscles of respiration obtain relief with cytotoxic drugs at times. The dosage is the same as outlined earlier. Plasma exchange or apheresis can be helpful in life-threatening situations, particularly in those patients with weakness of the muscles of respiration. For patients with mild disease, particularly those whose chief symptom is arthralgia or mild myalgia, NSAID is the treatment of choice. Duration of therapy varies from months to years for all medications. The most common adverse reactions to steroids in children are excessive weight gain, hypertension, and growth failure. Compression fractures are worrisome but do not occur as often as the 10% reported in adults.

JUVENILE ANKYLOSING SPONDYLITIS

The therapy for juvenile ankylosing spondylitis (JAS) is basically the same as that for JRA, with a few exceptions. Closer attention must be paid to physical therapy and strengthening the back muscles and muscles of respiration. Classical teaching is that aspirin does not help the pain of JAS. Indomethacin and phenylbutazone seem to help more, and indeed many patients note marked relief with these two drugs only. More recently, such drugs as tolmetin and naproxen have also been found to help. Gold therapy is not well known to be useful, but there is at least one study showing its efficacy in patients with adult ankylosing spondylitis. Occasionally a teenager requires one NSAID to relieve peripheral articular pain and swelling and another for the lower lumbar arthritis. Dosages of drugs are as described in the section on JRA.

Acute iritis occurs in JAS; the rules and findings discussed for JRA iritis are applicable here.

SCLERODERMA

Scleroderma varies in expression from mild skin manifestations (morphea), to linear lesions causing severe destruction of soft tissues and muscles, to systemic sclerosis affecting key organs of the body. In general, children have more destructive disease of the limbs than organ involvement such as pul-

monary fibrosis or nephritis. Unfortunately, there is no definite treatment. NSAIDs help inflammation and pain in joints and muscles. Corticosteroids are useful during episodes of acute inflammation. D-Penicillamine has been reported to help some patients, and cyclophosphamide has been reported to help scleroderma nephritis and possibly other complications. However, neither drug has been validated for use in these conditions.

HENOCH-SCHÖNLEIN (ANAPHYLACTOID) PURPURA

The arthritis and purpuric vasculitis of this condition are self-limited, usually resolving within a few weeks, and treatment is symptomatic. NSAIDs are useful for arthralgias, myalgias, and arthritis. There is controversy concerning proper therapy of gastrointestinal vasculitis, but steroids given in the dosages previously discussed are necessary for periods of a few days to a few months. Many physicians do not feel that steroids have a place in the treatment of glomerulonephritis associated with Henoch-Schönlein purpura. The outcome is usually so favorable with no steroid therapy that risky treatments must be weighed against potential advantages.

OTHER COLLAGEN VASCULAR DISEASES

Mixed connective tissue disease is so similar to SLE that the treatment concepts are virtually the same. Polyarteritis nodosa is a rare arteritis that usually requires aggressive steroid and cytotoxic therapy. Reiter's disease is often, but not always, self-limited in children and teenagers. Treatment is symptomatic and is usually limited to administration of NSAIDs.

Eosinophilic Fasciitis

NICHOLAS A. PATRONE, M.D.

Most patients with eosinophilic fasciitis respond dramatically to corticosteroids. The dose of prednisone is 20–60 mg/day (0.5 mg/kg/24 hr), tapered gradually over 3–6 months to an every-other-day dosage. Length of treatment varies; there are no guidelines for total duration of therapy, but lack of response within 3 months should lead to discontinuation of corticosteroid therapy. Delays in diagnosis may lead to irreversible flexion contractures, but a response may occur with the institution of steroid therapy. The long-term natural history of eosinophilic fasciitis is unknown. Although most patients with this disease improve, flexion contractures and skin changes may remain for years after the onset of symptoms. Progression to systemic disease such as scleroderma is unusual. Physical therapy may be indicated for severe flexion contractures and muscle atrophy secondary to disuse.

12

Genitourinary Tract

Renal Hypoplasia and Dysplasia

WALLACE W. McCRORY, M.D.

RENAL HYPOPLASIA

Unilateral hypoplasia is usually undetected until urologic evaluation for urinary tract infection or hypertension demonstrates a unilateral "small kidney." These kidneys are considered to be prone to infection, lithiasis, and vascular disease, which occasionally leads to systemic hypertension. If none of these findings is present, no treatment is indicated. When it can be shown by selective renal vein renin determination that increased renin is produced by the small kidney, there is a greater than 90% chance that nephrectomy will cure associated hypertension.

If the presenting problem is infection and reflux is present in association with a unilateral small kidney, therapy is determined by several factors: the patient's age, the grade of reflux, the efficacy of suppressive anitbacterial therapy, and the amount of renal function contributed by the kidney. Nephroureterectomy may be appropriate if the degree of function provided by the small kidney is minimal (less than 10% of total function).

If hypertension is present and selective renal vein renin determinations lateralize hypersecretion to the affected kidney, surgery can be curative for the hypertension. With nonlateralizing main renal vein renin determinations, segmental renal vein renin determinations have been useful in discovering curable patients. Therapeutic failures have been related to bilaterality of the lesion, which is relatively common, and to mutliple areas of involvement.

Bilateral renal hypoplasia is a very serious problem and a cause of chronic renal failure in children. Patients should be managed from birth, if possible, on oral phosphate binders, vitamin D and calcium supplements, and sodium bicarbonate (see Chronic Renal Failure in this section). Slow but steady growth can sometimes occur even with markedly reduced renal function (i.e., a glomerular filtration rate less than 20% of normal). Renal transplantation is currently not routinely done until infants have achieved a weight of approximately 8 kg or more.

RENAL DYSPLASIA

Clinical forms of dysplasia include obstructive renal dysplasia, multicystic dysplasia, and aplastic dysplasia. The latter two are usually marked by nonfunctioning kidneys and are associated with ureteropelvic occlusions.

When unilateral dysplasia presents as a palpable flank mass in the newborn, treatment is usually surgical because of the theoretical danger of hypertension and infection. In the presence of a normal contralateral kidney the outlook is excellent.

Renal dysplasia associated with urinary tract obstruction requires relief of the obstruction. The functional capacity of dysplastic kidneys is usually subnormal. Function may improve with surgical relief of the associated obstructive uropathy, but this cannot be appreciated until relief of the obstruction is accomplished, since obstruction itself impairs renal function by hydrostatic back-pressure and urinary tract infection. Congenital lower urinary outlet obstruction (posterior urethral valves, urethral atresia) resulting in bladder enlargement, bilateral hydronephrosis, and hydroureter can also be associated with renal dysplasia. In such cases the long-term prognosis depends on the degree of renal parenchymal malformation, which, if severe, progresses to uremia in spite of successful relief of urinary tract obstruction. Lateral nephrostomies or loop ureterostomies should be established as early as feasible in these cases to maximize the actual functional potential of the kidneys. If there is significant renal reserve, an improvement in renal function can be seen as early as 1–2 weeks after relief of the urinary outflow obstruction.

Bilateral multicystic dysplasia is a lethal malformation associated with oligohydramnios, oliguria, and Potter's facies. There is no treatment of value.

Hydronephrosis and Disorders of the Ureter

EVAN J. KASS, M.D.

"Idiopathic hydronephrosis" is a descriptive term indicating the presence of an enlarged pelvicalyceal system. "Hydroureter," similarly, indicates the presence of a dilated ureter. Until recently, the mere observation of such upper urinary tract dilatation on an excretory urogram was often sufficient evidence to diagnose obstruction and justify corrective surgery. However, considerable evidence now demonstrates that not all dilatation of the upper urinary system is the result of an obstruction, and in such cases progressive loss of renal function is not inevitable. Nonobstructive dilatation may occur as an isolated condition unassociated with any underlying abnormality or in association with prune-belly syndrome, diabetes insipidus, or vesicoureteral reflux. The goal of any evaluation protocol is to determine whether an obstructive lesion is present, determine the location of this obstruction, and assess renal function. Only with all of this information can one decide on the appropriate course of management.

The magnitude of the pelvicalyceal dilatation is not a reliable guide to the presence of obstruction, since similar degrees of enlargement may be observed in both obstructed and unobstructed systems. Although the presence of abdominal pain, hematuria, or urinary tract infection may prompt the initial urologic evaluation, the presence or absence of such symptoms is not an absolute determinant of urinary obstruction. In addition, hydronephrosis is frequently detected incidentally during an evaluation for enuresis or cardiac defects; and more recently, with the use of antenatal ultrasound, the diagnosis of in-utero hydronephrosis is being made with ever-increasing frequency. Therefore, it is imperative that every child with urinary tract dilatation be objectively evaluated to determine the functional significance of this observed upper tract dilatation. Only then can a rational decision be made as to the best plan of management.

In obstruction the intrapelvic pressure is directly related to the urine flow rate and duration of the diuresis as well as the degree of obstruction. The loss of renal function is proportional to the magnitude and the duration of this rise in intrapelvic pressure. In a complete obstruction for more than one week, permanent deterioration of glomerular and tubular function will take place. However, congenital obstruction is rarely complete and the elasticity of the collecting system often serves to cushion the nephron from the full effect of the elevated intrapelvic pressure. Because the intrapelvic pressure remains within the normal physiologic range except when the diuretic load exceeds the transport capacity of the obstructed system, it is not unusual in chronic obstruction for the glomerular filtration rate to be preserved for a long period of time. Systems that are dilated but not obstructed do not demonstrate this rise in intrapelvic pressure, even under maximal diuresis, and therefore are not at risk for progressive renal damage.

This underlying physiologic difference between obstructed and unobstructed systems can be employed to discriminate between true obstruction and nonobstructive dilatation. The pressure perfusion study described by Whitaker is based upon the concept that an unobstructed urinary system is unable to transport urine at a rate of 10 cc/min without a concomitant elevation of intrapelvic hydrostatic pressure. Only an unobstructed system is capable of transporting fluid at this rate without a concomitant pressure rise. The major advantage of this study is that the perfusion medium is introduced directly into the renal pelvis via a percutaneous catheter; therefore, impaired renal function is not a limiting factor. However, since percutaneous puncture of the renal collecting system is required, the study is invasive and frequently requires sedation or general anesthesia.

The diuretic-augmented renal scan is a noninvasive isotope study capable of providing objective criteria for diagnosing urinary obstruction. Interpretation is based upon the concept that prolonged retention of the radionuclide in the dilated, unobstructed collecting system is the result of a reservoir effect. When urine flow is increased by diuretic administration, the urine containing the tracer rapidly leaves the unobstructed collecting system and is replaced by tracer-free urine. In the presence of obstruction the radionuclide leaves the system slowly, even with diuretic stimulation. With the aid of a gamma camera microcomputer system, the tracer activity within the dilated collecting system can be accurately counted and the time required for half the tracer to leave the collecting system measured. When this half-time is less than 15 minutes, no obstruction is present, and when the half-time is over 20 minutes, obstruction is thought to be present. With a half-time between 15 and 20 minutes, or when renal function is significantly compromised, this study is not reliable and other means of assessing urinary obstruction must be employed.

Both the pressure perfusion study and the diuretic augmented renal scan have an accuracy of greater than 90%. Frequently, both studies will be required to completely evaluate a dilated collecting system. At the present time, there is no single study or test that reliably diagnoses obstruction or excludes its presence with 100% accuracy.

The standard excretory urogram, even when combined with retrograde pyelography or ultrasonography, is not a reliable indicator of urinary obstruction. These studies merely depict the anatomy of the collecting system. When hydronephrosis is detected, a diuretic renal scan should be obtained to provide baseline information concerning individual renal function as well as an objective evaluation of obstruction. When the diuretic scan does not adequately define the situation, a pressure perfusion study may be required.

When objective evidence confirms the presence of urinary tract obstruction, surgical correction should be carried out promptly. Nonoperative management is indicated only for those children who show no objective evidence of obstruction; however, until long-term information is available as to the ultimate fate of the child with a dilated, unobstructed system, periodic renal scans are recommended to insure that asymptomatic renal damage does not occur.

The ureteropelvic junction is the most common site of upper urinary tract obstruction in infants and children. Ureteropelvic junction obstruction requires prompt surgical correction. The most commonly performed surgical procedure is a dismembered Anderson-Hynes pyeloplasty. In this procedure, the abnormal ureteropelvic junction is excised and the normal ureter spatulated and reanastomosed to the renal pelvis. It is not uncommon to find aberrant blood vessels or bands causing angulation of the ureteropelvic junction. Management of these extrinsic abnormalities alone rarely relieves the obstruction, since virtually all children with congenital ureteropelvic junction obstruction have an intrinsic ureteral abnormality responsible for the obstruction.

The second most common site of upper urinary tract obstruction is the ureterovesical junction. In all children with such dilatation a voiding cystourethrogram should be obtained to exclude vesicoureteral reflux and infravesical obstruction. Dilatation of the pelvicalyceal system is a common finding in children with vesicoureteral reflux and can also be seen in children with posterior urethral valves or neuropathic bladder dysfunction. In infants, significant transient ureteropelvic dilatation can be seen following a severe urinary tract infec-

tion that resolves with appropriate antimicrobial therapy.

The treatment of primary ureterovesical junction obstruction includes excision of the abnormal ureteral segment and reimplantation of the ureter into the bladder. Since the ureter that is to be reimplanted may be considerably dilated, it is often necessary to tailor it so that a proper ratio of ureteral diameter to submucosal tunnel length can be achieved. The abnormality responsible for a ureterovesical junction obstruction is an intrinsic abnormality of the muscle itself, similar to that seen in a ureteropelvic junction obstruction. Although this entity has been termed "obstructive megaureter," it does not share the aganglionic abnormality associated with congenital megacolon.

The majority of obstructed kidneys are salvageable, and nephrectomy is rarely necessary. In the past the criteria for nephrectomy have been subjective; however, a poorly visualizing kidney on an excretory urogram, or a kidney providing less than 10% of the total renal function on a renal scan, may still be salvageable. The final decision for nephrectomy should always be made at surgery. Since there is little risk to attempted salvage of a hydronephrotic kidney, nephrectomy should be reserved for obviously hopeless cases.

Long-term follow-up of renal function is required in all children with obstructive uropathy since delayed deterioration has been described in these individuals even when they appear to have maintained stable renal function for years. The diuretic-augmented renal scan provides an objective measure of individual renal function and drainage and, when compared with preoperative studies, gives invaluable information as to the success of corrective surgery.

The prenatal diagnosis of hydronephrosis is being made with ever-increasing frequency. Antenatal intervention strategies for the management of such hydronephrosis are currently being experimented with at some centers; however, extreme caution must be advised about general adoption of these techniques. At this time no objective criteria exist for defining upper urinary tract obstruction in utero, nor are there any data to suggest that in utero decompression of an obstructed kidney is superior to postnatal intervention. Until these data become available, the primary role of prenatal sonography will be to identify those infants with an abnormality who will benefit from early postnatal evaluation of their hydronephrosis. Following delivery, a prompt, thorough evaluation should be carried out, and those individuals found to have obstruction can be appropriately managed before complications occur, thereby maximizing the preservation of renal function. Individuals who do not meet the objective criteria for urinary obstruction do not require surgery but should be monitored for evidence of progressive hydronephrosis or loss of renal function.

Malignant Tumors of the Kidney

GEORGE T. KLAUBER, M.D.

Wilms' tumor or nephroblastoma is the most common malignant tumor of the kidney and urinary tract in children, accounting for approximately 95% of all such cancers. Survival rates have improved dramatically in the past 25 years, resulting in "cures" for the majority of affected children. This is due largely to the advent of chemotherapy plus the evolution of referral centers. Collaborative studies, such as the National Wilms' Tumor Study (NWTS), have shared group experience for a tumor that occurs approximately 500 times per year in the USA.

The diagnosis should be suspected in any child with an abdominal mass, hypertension, or hematuria. Radiologic studies, including computed tomography and ultrasound, if available, should be performed as soon as possible. Surgery should follow within 48–72 hours. Prognosis and specific therapy are dependent on accurate surgical staging and histology. Severe anemia, cachexia, or hypertension may need to be corrected or stabilized prior to surgery. Five to 10% of children are misdiagnosed preoperatively so that preoperative chemotherapy should be withheld.

Surgery

Excellent surgical exposure can be obtained with the child supine by elevating the tumor-bearing side. A large transverse incision is made from the tip of the twelfth rib across the midline. Both rectus muscles can be divided but frequently the contralateral rectus can be retracted laterally after incision of the sheath. This exposure allows access to both renal pedicles, vena cava, liver, spleen, and para-aortic lymph nodes from diaphragm to aortic bifurcation. Very large tumors can be biopsied and shrinkage induced with chemotherapy and radiation, thus making subsequent complete excision feasible. The contralateral kidney should be exposed, if complete ipsilateral excision appears possible, by opening Gerota's fascia and palpating both surfaces. Ligation of the renal artery followed by the vein should be attempted prior to mobilization of the tumor, and tumor spillage by rupture should be avoided. The adrenal gland can usually be spared, unless tumor occupies the upper pole of the kidney. Regional lymph nodes must be sampled for staging purposes, but radical lymphadenectomies are not necessary. En bloc resection of adjacent organs involved with tumor can be performed in some cases; otherwise maximal debulking is indicated, followed by tagging of residual tumor with surgical clips to delineate extent. If available, nonmetallic clips should be used to avoid interference with later CT scanning.

Prognostic Factors. NWTS I and II have clearly demonstrated three major prognostic factors in Wilms tumor. They are presence or absence of favorable (FH) or unfavorable histology (UH), hematogenous metastases, and lymph node involvement. Lesser factors are age, tumor size, intravascular extension beyond the kidney, operative tumor spillage, and direct abdominal extension of tumor. Histology appears to be the single most important prognostic factor, with anaplasia, rhabdoid tumors, and clear cell carcinomas constituting the unfavorable variants (12%). Tumors demonstrating any differentiation, FH, have a much better prognosis than tumors with UH.

Staging of the Wilms' Tumor (NWTS III)

Stage I: Tumor confined to kidney and completely excised

Stage II: Tumor extends beyond kidney but is completely excised

Stage III: Residual nonhematogenous tumor confined to the abdomen

Stage IV: Deposits beyond stage III, including hematogenous metastases

Stage V: Bilateral renal involvement (approximately 7%)

Treatment Protocols for NWTS III

Treatment is based on histology and stage, following results of NWTS I and II. All children should undergo preliminary surgery, and by stage, the following:

Stage I (FH): No radiation therapy. Randomized actinomycin D (AMD) and vincristine (VCR) for 10 weeks or 6 months.

Stage II (FH): Doubly randomized either to receive or not to receive 2000 rads radiation plus more intensive AMD plus VCR or triple therapy (TT)—AMD, VCR, and doxorubicin.

Stage III (FH): Chemotherapy identical to stage II but radiotherapy is randomized to 1000 or 2000 rads.

UH of any stage plus all Stage IV: All receive radiation therapy and are randomized to receive TT or quadruple therapy (TT plus cyclophosphamide).

Survival Rate (NWTS). The survival rate for FH is 90%, versus 54% for UH at two years. Relapse-free survival rate is 82.6% for patients without metastases at presentation versus 54% with positive nodes. Survival for synchronous bilateral Wilms' tumor is 87% and for metachronous ipsilateral involvement is only 40%. Thus, treatment for bilateral Wilms' tumor should be directed toward preservation of as much normal kidney function as possible, avoiding high doses of irradiation.

Other Tumors

Infants under 6 months of age constitute a special group of patients. The vast majority have mesoblastic nephromas, which should be treated by nephrectomy alone. Chemotherapy is potentially lethal in infancy and should be reserved only for those children with bilateral UH disease and for the rare rhabdoid tumors and sarcomas.

Renal angiomyolipomas can occur in up to 80% of patients with tuberous sclerosis. They are usually benign, although occasional malignant transformation can occur; they are almost invariably bilateral, so that nephrectomy should be avoided when possible. Rupture can cause retroperitoneal hemorrhage, which should be managed with transfusion and/or embolization of bleeding vessels whenever possible. Renal cell carcinomas are exceedingly rare in childhood. Complete surgical removal by means of a radical nephrectomy is the treatment of choice. Transitional cell tumors of the renal pelvis are also exceedingly rare and should be treated by nephroureterectomy. Fibro-epithelial polyps are not malignant and should be treated by local excision.

Glomerulonephritis

ALFRED J. FISH, M.D.,
and LAURIE S. FOUSER, M.D.

A child presenting with glomerulonephritis may have symptoms of hypertension and renal insufficiency with abnormal findings on urinalysis and electrolyte and acid-base imbalances. After the initial work-up and investigation of the patient it is usually several days before all laboratory data are available and it can be determined whether acute or chronic glomerulonephritis is present.

POSTINFECTIOUS GLOMERULONEPHRITIS

Postinfectious glomerulonephritis in childhood is usually an acute event with an excellent prognosis. Treatment is directed toward management of the consequences of acute glomerular injury with a reduction in glomerular blood flow and glomerular filtration.

Hospitalization. Patients with acute postinfectious glomerulonephritis, when presenting with edema and gross hematuria, are assessed for significant oliguria and hypertension. If these are not present, and if fluid and electrolyte balance is normal, hospitalization is not indicated. Children managed on an outpatient basis are observed carefully at home for oliguria, puffiness, and weight gain and are seen at regular intervals in the office or clinic to be checked for the development of hypertension or electrolyte imbalance.

Fluid Overload. Children with acute loss of glomerular filtration capacity become oliguric and develop edema and hypervolemia. Fluid restriction (to 300 ml/m^2) is begun if hypervolemia is present, and sodium intake is reduced. Diuretic therapy is usually helpful if significant edema and fluid overload are present. In most patients there is a response to hydrochlorothiazide, 1–2 mg/kg/day. Responsiveness to diuretics depends upon the degree of glomerular capillary injury; in some patients the use of furosemide, 1–5 mg/kg/day IV or orally, will be more effective. In rare instances, when complete anuria with severe fluid overload is associated with pulmonary edema and congestive heart failure, peritoneal dialysis or hemodialysis may be needed.

In some patients the development of edema is secondary to heavy proteinuria with hypoalbuminemia, decreased colloidal osmotic pressure, and hypovolemia. Management of these problems is outlined in Nephrotic Syndrome, later in this section.

Otherwise, it is important to monitor fluid balance carefully, with daily assessment of weight, total intake, and output. When ongoing oliguria is a problem, fluid intake should be restricted to the urinary output plus 300 ml/m^2, which replaces insensible losses. Fluids low in sodium and potassium are judiciously administered.

Electrolyte and Acid-Base Abnormalities. Children with severe forms of postinfectious glomerulonephritis may develop electrolyte imbalances due to the loss of glomerular filtration. In addition to the difficulties with water balance already described, hyperkalemia, acidosis, hypocalcemia, and hyperphosphatemia may be present.

Hyperkalemia is a serious complication of postinfectious glomerulonephritis, carrying the risk of cardiac electrical disturbances. Frequently hyperkalemia is associated with acidosis, intracellular shifts of retained hydrogen ions, and subsequent movement of potassium out of the intracellular compartment. Moderately stable degrees of hyperkalemia (5.0–6.0 mEq/l) are not associated with electrocardiogram abnormalities and are managed with potassium restriction and hydrochlorothiazide or furosemide, as outlined, to enhance urinary potassium excretion. However, serum potassium levels higher than 6.0 mEq/l indicate treatment with oral or rectal doses of sodium polystyrene sulfonate, 1.0 gm/kg in 20% sorbitol; this may be repeated every 2–3 hours until the hyperkalemia is controlled. The management of patients with electrocardiogram T-wave changes or with severe hyperkalemia exceeding 7.0 mEq/l should include the following: 10% calcium gluconate in a dose of 100–200 mg/kg IV given slowly over 10–15 minutes, which will temporarily diminish the cardiac effects of hyperkalemia, and 25% dextrose in water, 5 ml/kg (1.25 gm/kg) IV given over 30 minutes, followed by crystalline insulin 0.1–0.2 unit/kg. Simultaneous correction of acidosis using sodium bicarbonate, 2–3 mEq/kg IV, will enhance return of potassium to the intracellular pool.

Acidosis is more completely corrected using the formula of 0.6 × body weight (kg) × base deficit = mEq of sodium bicarbonate required. Ongoing administration of oral sodium bicarbonate, 1–2 mEq/kg/day, may be needed to maintain acid-base balance. If hypertension, dilutional hyponatremia, and fluid overload are evident, there may be limits to the amount of sodium-containing salts that can be administered.

Hypocalcemia and *hyperphosphatemia* may be encountered in acute glomerulonephritis. Hypocalcemia may result in tetany and convulsions, complications that may be precipitated by the correction of acidosis as previously outlined. Hypocalcemia is managed with 10% calcium gluconate in a dose of 100–200 mg/kg IV given over 3–4 hours, followed by elemental oral calcium, 10–20 mg/kg/day. Hyperphosphatemia is treated by restriction of phosphorus intake and the administration of aluminum hydroxide orally in a dose of 50–150 mg/kg/day.

Hypertension. Hypertension is a frequent and potentially serious complication of acute glomerulonephritis. Its etiology in this illness is probably related to both vasoconstriction and expanded intravascular volume from reduced glomerular filtration. Activation of the renin-angiotensin system may be affected as well. The goal of therapy is to prevent hypertensive encephalopathy with its sequelae and to avoid overtaxing a cardiovascular system already stressed by an expanded blood volume.

Severe blood pressure elevation in glomerulonephritis may lead to drowsiness, headache, stupor, palsy, or seizure and constitutes a medical emergency. Diazoxide,* a potent vasodilator, is given in a dose of 2–5 mg/kg as an intravenous bolus in a peripheral vein; it usually takes effect within minutes, with a duration of 4–36 hours. This dose is repeated if there is no response within 20 minutes. Furosemide, 0.5–1.0 mg/kg/dose IV, is given concurrently with diazoxide in patients with increased intravascular volume and edema. Both diazoxide and furosemide may be repeated at these doses in 4–6 hours if severe blood pressure elevations recur, although multiple doses of diazoxide may be associated with hyperglycemia. The rare patient with persistent severe hypertension who fails to respond to these measures can be stabilized with a continuous intravenous infusion of nitroprusside, beginning at 0.5 µg/kg/min and increasing gradually, as needed, to 2.0 µg/kg/min. This therapy requires very close monitoring of vital signs, as well as measurement of thiocyanate levels to avoid central nervous system (CNS) and bone marrow toxicity. The symptoms of hypertensive encephalopathy usually subside once blood pressures have been controlled, although diazepam or phenytoin may be needed acutely for seizures. The use of reserpine and alpha-methyldopa is discouraged in this clinical setting, since these agents may produce CNS depression that obscures the assessment of neurologic status in a patient at risk for encephalopathy.

Moderately severe, but non-life-threatening, blood pressure elevations are stabilized with hydralazine, 0.4–0.8 mg/kg/dose IM or IV, and furosemide IV as often as every 6–8 hours. Mild and moderate hypertension are managed with 2 mEq/kg sodium restriction and oral diuretic therapy (hydrochlorothiazide, 1–2 mg/kg/day in two divided doses if the glomerular filtration rate [GFR] is greater than 50% of normal; furosemide, 1–2 mg/kg/dose every 6–12 hours if the GFR is less than 50% of normal), with addition of hydralazine or propranolol if necessary. Propranolol† is instituted at 1 mg/kg/day in two divided oral doses and is increased by 0.5 mg/kg every 1–2 days until hypertension is controlled. Hydralazine is initiated at 0.75 mg/kg/day in three divided oral doses and can be increased, as necessary, up to 7.5 mg/kg/day (maximum, 200 mg/day). Use of propranolol is discouraged in patients with asthma, heart failure, or diabetes mellitus, and children on this drug are observed for bradycardia. Hydralazine may provoke a reflex tachycardia that can be effectively controlled with the addition of a beta-adrenergic blocking agent such as propranolol. The use of these medications is seldom required for long, since in the majority of cases of postinfectious glomerulonephritis hypertension is transient and resolves during the first week after presentation.

Supportive Care. *Nutrition* is an important consideration during the recovery from renal insufficiency in acute glomerulonephritis. Anorexia; dietary restriction of sodium, potassium, and phosphorus; and the ingestion of unpalatable medication contribute to inadequate total caloric intake. Although protein restriction is usually recommended, an intake of at least 2 gm/kg/24 hours should be offered as the renal insufficiency begins to improve.

Antibiotics (penicillin or erythromycin) are given to treat streptococcal pharyngitis, although they

---

* Manufacturer's precaution: Safety of diazoxide in children is not established.

† Safety and efficacy for use of propranolol have not been established.

will not alter the established course of the glomerulonephritis. Antibiotics are recommended to prevent the transmission of nephritogenic streptococci to other family members.

Dialysis, either peritoneal dialysis or hemodialysis, is recommended if severe oliguria is present in association with pulmonary edema, cardiac failure, hypervolemia, or hypertension that do not respond to the measures described. Similarly, severe hyperkalemia, acidosis, hyponatremia or hypernatremia, seizures, and stupor due to uremia are indications for dialysis.

Follow-up over the coming weeks will allow discontinuation of diuretics and antihypertensive agents when the blood pressure is consistently normal and the edema, oliguria, and uremia have resolved. If, after a period of convalescence (about 12 weeks), the serum complement (C3) level has not returned to normal, the glomerular filtration rate remains low, or severe proteinuria is present, a renal biopsy is indicated.

CHRONIC GLOMERULONEPHRITIS

Chronic glomerulonephritis may be a primary disease of the kidney, but it may also develop secondary to systemic disorders. Most primary forms of glomerulonephritis have a variable clinical course, and management is directed toward the avoidance of complications. In some instances, treatment of the systemic illness has a significant effect on the outcome of children with secondary types of glomerulonephritis.

Supportive Care. *Hypertension* accompanies most cases of chronic glomerulonephritis. The initial approach employs sodium restriction and diuretics (hydrochlorothiazide or furosemide) and, if necessary, propranolol in the doses previously outlined. Serum electrolyte levels are monitored in patients taking thiazides or furosemide since the kaliuresis that occurs with these diuretics may lead to hypokalemia. Thiazides may also cause hypercalcemia or hyperuricemia.

In more severe cases, drugs with different mechanisms of action are sequentially added to the above regimen until hypertension is controlled. Hydralazine, in the doses described, is usually the first drug to be added, followed by the alpha-adrenergic blocker prazosin,‡ 0.1–0.5 mg/dose, according to age and size, given two or three times daily. The first dose of prazosin may result in sudden loss of consciousness, so the patient should be observed carefully. When the combination of hydralazine and prazosin is insufficient to control hypertension, they are replaced by minoxidil, beginning at 0.1 mg/kg/dose (maximum initial dose, 2.5 mg) given every 12 hours. Since minoxidil is a potent vasodilator, reflex tachycardia and marked sodium and water retention may occur if propranolol and furosemide are not used adjunctively. Hypertrichosis is also seen with chronic minoxidil therapy. An alternative approach in patients refractory to a combination of diuretic and propranolol is the use of the angiotensin I–converting enzyme inhibitor captopril,§ starting with 0.5 mg/kg/dose every 6–8 hours and increasing gradually to 2.0 mg/kg/dose if necessary. Sudden hypotension may occur after the first dose in rare cases, so the patient should be observed closely. White blood cell counts are monitored during captopril therapy, and the drug dosage should be reduced or discontinued if mild or severe neutropenia occurs.

Edema due to nephrotic syndrome is managed with sodium restriction, hydrochlorothiazide (2 mg/kg/day), and spironolactone (2–3 mg/kg/day). For more severe edema, furosemide (2–5 mg/kg/day) is used. Attention to serum potassium levels is important, and supplemental dietary potassium, up to 2 mEq/kg/day, may be required.

The need for *nutrition* to sustain adequate growth in children is balanced against the recommendation of protein restriction to diminish the rate of progression of renal insufficiency. Protein intakes of high biologic value, 2–3 gm/kg, are required for growing children. Attention to the consequences of renal osteodystrophy involves the use of supplementary oral calcium, phosphate binders, and vitamin D analogues (dihydrotachysterol and 1,25 cholecalciferol). Either aluminum hydroxide or calcium carbonate (beginning with 1 gm/m²/day of elemental calcium PO) is used as a phosphate binder. Calcium carbonate therapy offers the benefits of simultaneous calcium supplementation and avoidance of aluminum toxicity but carries the risk of producing hypercalcemia as doses are increased to reduce hyperphosphatemia. Use of the vitamin D compounds is outlined in Chronic Renal Failure in this section.

Primary Glomerulonephritis. Type I *membranoproliferative glomerulonephritis* (MPGN) is a variably progressive form of glomerulonephritis. Some investigators have advocated the use of alternate-day steroids in these patients; however, we do not recommend this approach. Type II MPGN, or dense deposit disease, is also unresponsive to specific therapy and has a high rate of recurrence in the transplanted kidney.

Idiopathic membranous glomerulopathy is frequently associated with heavy proteinuria. Treatment of edema and nephrotic syndrome is managed with diuretics and spironolactone, as described. There is no convincing evidence to support the use of

---

‡ Manufacturer's warning: Safety of prazosin in children has not been established.

§ Manufacturer's warning: Safety and efficacy of captopril have not been established.

steroids or immunosuppressive agents in this disorder.

Diffuse crescentic glomerulonephritis may be idiopathic or associated with various etiologies. When this lesion develops secondary to circulating antiglomerular basement membrane antibodies, immunosuppression (prednisone and azathioprine or cyclophosphamide) and plasmapheresis are recommended. When it is part of a systemic vasculitic process (e.g., periarteritis, Wegener's granulomatosis), similar treatment strategies are used.

Secondary Glomerulonephritis. *Systemic lupus erythematosus* (SLE) frequently has associated renal involvement with variable degrees of glomerular injury. Long-term survival studies in SLE have shown that prognosis is closely tied to the extent of renal disease. In mild cases of mesangial lupus nephritis we use prednisone, 2 mg/kg/day in divided doses (maximum, 100 mg/day), to achieve immune suppression, which usually results in the disappearance of circulating antibodies to native DNA and the return of serum complement levels to normal. These parameters, as well as renal function and urinary protein excretion, should be carefully watched; patients are maintained on alternate day prednisone, 2 mg/kg as a single morning dose. In instances of focal or diffuse proliferative lupus nephritis we use the same regimen of prednisone therapy with the addition of azathioprine,‖ 2–3 mg/kg/day; the latter is continued over several years until the serologic parameters of SLE are controlled, along with reduction of proteinuria and restoration of renal function to normal. In certain selected patients who have a relentless progressive course in SLE, we have also added cyclophosphamide for immunosuppression.

Steroids used on a long-term basis have produced many recognized complications, including cushingoid facies, hirsutism, hypertension, infection, avascular necrosis, and osteoporosis. Similarly, immunosuppressive agents may reduce host defense mechanisms and result in bacterial infections (abscesses, sepsis) and opportunistic infections with fungal, parasitic (*Pneumocystis carinii*), and viral (herpes zoster) agents.

Anaphylactoid purpura nephritis occurs in approximately one-half of children with Henoch-Schönlein purpura. In the majority of patients, renal involvement is mild and does not require specific treatment. Children with severe glomerular injury who have loss of renal function and heavy proteinuria are at risk of permanent renal injury. In these instances we use a combination of prednisone and azathioprine,‖ as outlined in SLE.

Glomerulonephritis can also occur with *bacterial endocarditis, infection, sepsis, and infected ventriculoar-*

‖ This use of azathioprine is not listed in the manufacturer's directive.

terial shunts. These patients have continued chronic infection of bacterial origin. The chronic release of bacterial antigen is the source of antigen(s) resulting in immune complex injury of the glomerulus. Treatment with surgery and antibiotics to eliminate the offending microorganisms has a marked effect in ameliorating the glomerular injury.

The Nephrotic Syndrome

MELANIE S. KIM, M.D.,
and WARREN E. GRUPE, M.D.

The nephrotic syndrome, a clinical composite of massive proteinuria, hypoalbuminemia, hyperlipidemia, and edema, is the most common presentation of glomerular injury in children, with a prevalence of 16 children per 100,000 population. Whether classified as primary, when the syndrome is restricted to glomerular injury, or as secondary, when it is part of a systemic illness, two questions face the physician at the time of diagnosis; the probability of a complete response to corticosteroids and the value of a renal biopsy to therapeutic decisions. Almost 95% of pediatric patients between 1 and 10 years of age whose disease presents in the absence of hematuria, hypertension, or renal insufficiency with normal serum C3 complement levels and a renal clearance of IgG that is less than 10% of the renal clearance of transferrin (referred to as the selective protein index) will have complete resolution of proteinuria with therapy. Therefore, it is common practice to initiate a therapeutic course of corticosteroids without further morphologic definition in this group, who represent approximately 60% of children with primary nephrotic syndrome.

Initial renal biopsy, on the other hand, is reserved for those patients who present with gross hematuria, low serum levels of C3, diminished renal function, or hypertension. A biopsy is indicated later in those who fail to respond to an initial 8-week course of corticosteroids or whose protracted course might suggest the initiation of cytotoxic drug therapy.

Corticosteroid Therapy

Dosage programs vary among nephrologists even though none has been shown to be more efficacious than another. Initial intensive therapy with divided doses of oral prednisone, 1–2 mg/kg/day or 60 mg/M^2/day (maximum dose 60–80 mg) is maintained until the urine has been protein free for 2 weeks, at which point the steroid dosage is quickly reduced and finally discontinued over an additional 1–3 weeks. Using this therapy, 85% of patients will resolve their proteinuria within 4 weeks while less than 5% will require more than 8 weeks of daily steroids. Equivalent amounts of other corticosteroid preparations usually have similar efficacy.

Relapses occur in 80% of all patients in whom proteinuria initially disappears. Surveillance is maintained in the home by the patient or the family with reagent dipsticks to maintain a daily record of urine protein tests. If proteinuria recurs and persists for 7–10 consecutive days, daily oral doses of prednisone are reinstituted prior to the appearance of edema. Once the urine has been protein free for 2 weeks, an additional 3 or 4 weeks of maintenance therapy is provided at 3 mg/kg (maximum 80 mg) given as a single morning dose every other day. The prednisone is once more gradually reduced over a 4–6-week period, aiming for a total therapy course of 3 months.

Frequent Relapses or Steroid Dependency. "Frequent" relapses are defined as 3 or more relapses within a year; "steroid dependency" is defined as present in those patients who relapse as corticosteroid therapy is tapered or within two weeks of its discontinuation. Although cytotoxic drugs have been advocated in these patients, the demonstration of frequent relapses or steroid dependency is not in and of itself an indication for the use of such drugs. Many children experience a reduction in steroid toxicity, with prolonged periods of protein free urine and normal growth, when maintenance alternate-day therapy is continued for several months with a single morning dose varying between 0.5 mg/kg and 1 mg/kg. Cytotoxic agents should be contemplated only if relapses continue to occur, despite maintenance therapy, or if the degree of corticosteroid toxicity becomes dangerous to the patient.

Corticosteroid Resistance. Proteinuria persists in less than 5% of the patients with minimal change disease after 12 weeks of prednisone therapy. Approximately half will experience a resolution of proteinuria following the addition of an alkylating agent. An additional 3–5% may develop resistance after months to years of steroid responsiveness. In such patients, when minimal change disease is proved histologically, remission is more frequently achieved with one of the alkylating agents; subsequent relapses may then be steroid responsive again.

Occasional children have been noted in whom prednisone actually aggravates the proteinuria; this is demonstrated by the paradoxical appearance of protein in the urine during alternate-day prednisone therapy. In others with minimal change nephrotic syndrome, active, though subtle, infection may be responsible for steroid resistance; particularly common in children is a symptomatic

urinary tract infection. Extracorporeal ultrafiltration has been used for severe steroid and diuretic-resistance edema. Although some of these children may regain their ability to respond to steroids and/or diuretics, this treatment seems more effective when a modest reduction in renal function is already present, although it has been successful in patients with normal renal function. Other than potentially modifying the patient's response to other diuretics, ultrafiltration has no particular effect on proteinuria.

Cytotoxic Drugs

When prolonged high-dose steroid therapy cannot be avoided, when steroid toxicity is physiologically significant, or when steroid responsiveness is incomplete, cytotoxic drugs have been used successfully. The alkylating agents, cyclophosphamide and chlorambucil, have demonstrated effectiveness in controlled trials.

Cyclophosphamide. When given together with glucocorticoids, cyclophosphamide will either eliminate or reduce the frequency of relapses completely in 80–90% of frequently relapsing patients. Cyclophosphamide is given at a dose of 2–3 mg/kg/day, together with alternate-day steroid therapy for 6–8 weeks. Dosages less than 2 mg/kg/day generally do not alter the relapse rate, while dosages above 5 mg/kg/day are accompanied by unacceptable acute side effects. Steroid-dependent patients, treated below the age of 8 years or treated within two years of the onset of disease, do not have as sustained a reduction in the number of relapses. Second courses of cyclophosphamide can be as effective as the first. Seventy-five percent remain in remission at one year, while in 44% remission is sustained without further therapy for 4 years. Acute toxicity is dose related and includes bone marrow suppression, cystitis, gastrointestinal irritation, alopecia, and infections. Long-term problems include chromosomal damage, neoplasm, lung fibrosis, ovarian fibrosis, sterility, amenorrhea and menopausal symptoms. Most of the immediate complications are reversible or avoidable. The cumulative threshold dose for azoospermia appears to be between 150 and 250 mg/kg, although gonadal toxicity need not be permanent.

Chlorambucil. Chlorambucil has been effective in both controlled and uncontrolled studies when given together with corticosteroids. Chlorambucil is given at a dose of 0.2 mg/kg/day for no longer than 8–10 weeks. Cumulative doses above 11–14 mg/kg offer no advantage to the patient and clearly increase both acute and delayed toxicity. Although all studies support the value of chlorambucil in the frequently relapsing patient, two studies disagree about the effectiveness of the drug in the steroid-dependent person. Patients who are younger than 6 years of age, have had their disease for less than 3 years, or were treated for less than 7 weeks seem to have a diminished response to treatment. Ninety-six percent remain in remission at one year, and 84% at three years. Acute toxicity with chlorambucil is dose related and includes leukopenia, infections, focal seizures, and gastrointestinal irritation. Long-term effects include oligospermia, azoospermia, ovarian fibrosis, amenorrhea, and leukemia. Oligospermia has been noted at 60 days with cumulative doses of 6 mg/kg and at 45 days with cumulative doses of 9 mg/kg. Azoospermia occurs in all patients at a total cumulative dose above 18–25 mg/kg, which is twice the current recommendation. Most patients with gonadal toxicity have been treated for longer than 4 months. Gonadal toxicity need not be permanent.

Recommendations about the relative merits of chlorambucil and cyclophosphamide are controversial. The drugs share many characteristics and, in at least one study, had similar effectiveness. Response to both drugs appears to be dependent on dose, duration of therapy, age, and the duration of disease.

General Support

Activity. The overall philosophy of care encourages these patients to live as normally as possible. Children can remain remarkably active during this period with no clear evidence that restriction of general activity affects the outcome of this disease.

Diet. Nutrient intake should continue at a normal level for the child's age. Appetite is decreased in these patients; therefore a palatable diet that provides at least the recommended daily allowance of calories and protein for height-age should be encouraged. Salt restriction in the form of no added salt at the table and excluding foods with very high salt content is advised when marked edema is present and during prednisone therapy. However, salt restriction must be adjusted to the child's appetite and should never limit nutrient intake. Water restriction is less important if attention to sodium intake is maintained; however, restrictions should not be placed on any patient who is hypovolemic or who has increased nitrogen retention. There is no evidence that excessive protein intake is beneficial or alters the outcome of this disease.

Immunization. There is little information on whether immunizations can precipitate a relapse or whether a protective antibody response can be induced during active nephrosis. The influence of steroid therapy on developing a protective response is also unknown. Therefore it seems prudent to defer routine immunizations until the patient's urine has been protein free for 6–12 months.

Pneumococcal vaccine has been recommended for all patients with nephrotic syndrome. However, pneumococcal sepsis and peritonitis can still occur despite prior immunizations; hence, protection cannot be fully assured.

Edema. Treatment for anasarca is indicated in the presence of respiratory difficulty, skin breakdown, hyponatremia, hypotension, or nitrogen retention. Control of edema is mandatory in preparation for a renal biopsy or any other surgical procedure. Use of diuretics, particularly loop diuretics, in the absence of volume expanders, can be hazardous, and administration to children should be carried out carefully. These agents may produce severe volume contraction, which predisposes the nephrotic patient to hypokalemia, hyponatremia, alkalosis, renal failure, and vascular thrombosis. Hydrochlorothiazide in an oral dose of 2–5 mg/kg/day in two divided doses might be effective in a few patients. In more resistant cases, furosemide, 1–2 mg/kg/dose every 6–8 hours can be used. Spironolactone (3 mg/kg/day) alone is ineffective but can be added to loop diuretics for its potassium-sparing effects.

In the severely edematous patient in whom prompt control is essential, the intravenous administration of salt-poor albumin, 0.5–1.0 gm/kg/day, in conjunction with 1 mg/kg intravenous furosemide, is the most effective. This can be repeated every 8 to 24 hours until dry weight is achieved.

Complications

Infection. An increased susceptibility to infection is present in children with nephrotic syndrome, which is further aggravated by immunosuppression. Common infections include peritonitis, pneumonia, cellulitis, bronchitis, urinary tract infection, and septic arthritis. *Streptococcus pneumoniae* is the most prevalent organism, but the gram-negative organisms *Escherichia coli*, *Haemophilus influenzae*, and *Pseudomonas aeruginosa* remain common. Appropriate cultures should be obtained and antibiotic coverage for both gram-negative and gram-positive organisms should be started until the organism is identified and sensitivities determined. Prophylactic antibiotics have not been shown to be of benefit and may in fact confuse the clinical picture. Infection remains the leading cause of death in nephrosis; therefore prompt recognition and treatment remain crucial in the care of these patients.

Vascular Thrombosis. The nephrotic syndrome is a hypercoagulable state. Although unusual, arterial and venous thrombosis can occur in nonresponding nephrotic patients as well as in patients undergoing massive diuresis due to corticosteroid therapy or diuretics. The efficacy of anticoagulant therapy in these patients has not been carefully assessed, however.

Growth Impairment. Linear growth retardation is common in nephrotic children. The major cause is protracted corticosteroid therapy, although the effects of malnutrition, anasarca, hypoproteinemia, infection, and altered bone mineral metabolism cannot be discarded. To minimize growth impairment, unnecessarily prolonged courses of daily steroids in particular are avoided while efforts to maintain adequate nutrition are encouraged.

Steroid Toxicity. Side effects include a cushingoid appearance, large weight gain, increased appetite, skin striae, hypertension, gastrointestinal bleeding, cataracts, severe infection, seizures, diabetes, and electrolyte abnormalities.

Persistent Hyperlipidemia. Persistent hyperlipidemia in the steroid-resistant child represents an unknown risk. Although severe coronary artery disease can exist in the nephrotic adult, it is not clear whether it is intensified by the renal lesion; the prevalence of early atherosclerotic disease in nephrotic children is not clearly greater than expected in other patients of similar age. Although no long-term experience with lipid-lowering drugs has been accumulated in children, clofibrate may have a higher complication rate in the nephrotic adult, possibly due to the large unbound fraction of the drug.

Prognosis

Important to management decisions is the fact that childhood nephrosis is a self-limiting disease whose ultimate outcome, with rare exception, is favorable.

For children who respond completely to steroid therapy, the tendency towards relapse decreases with time. Nevertheless, the persistence of the disease is evident; half the children still experience relapses even after 5 years of disease and 20% still have recurrences after 10 years. Only an occasional child who is initially steroid responsive will ever become steroid resistant. Rarely, relapses after many years of a proteinuria free state can appear. Despite persistence of episodes of steroid-responsive proteinuria, even multiple episodes, progression to chronic renal insufficiency is minimal.

Renal Venous Thrombosis

ADRIAN SPITZER, M.D.

Renal venous thrombosis (RVT) has been observed in a variety of clinical settings such as dehydration and hemoconcentration; following trauma to the renal veins, renal biopsy, and renal transplantation; secondary to external compression of renal veins by tumors or other masses; and in association with ingestion of contraceptive agents, sickle cell anemia, and the nephrotic syndrome. RVT can be divided into two broad categories according to its cause: (1) primary thrombosis of renal veins in the presence of a hypercoagulable state, and (2) renal vein thrombosis consequent to impaired renal blood flow. Most of the cases reported fall within the first category.

RENAL VENOUS THROMBOSIS OF INFANCY

Management of RVT of infancy includes correction of the predisposing conditions, maintenance of fluid and electrolyte homeostasis, and, in certain instances, anticoagulant or surgical therapy. Patients with severe impairment in renal function associated with fluid overload and electrolyte and acid-base abnormalities can benefit from hemodialysis or peritoneal dialysis.

The use of anticoagulants, advocated by some authors, has never been subjected to appropriate testing. This therapeutic step should not be taken lightly, because the risk of bleeding complications is high among patients with renal insufficiency. The only clear indication for anticoagulation therapy is the development of pulmonary emboli (a rare occurrence among infants and children) and life-threatening disseminated intravascular coagulation. Heparin is given intravenously, as a constant infusion, in a dosage of 25 U/kg/hr, following an intial loading dose of 50 U/kg. The administration of heparin is then adjusted to maintain the activated partial thromboplastin time at 10–15 seconds above baseline. Heparin should be continued for 5 days or until the platelet count returns to normal or there is significant improvement in renal function. The platelet count and the clotting factors should continue to be monitored and heparin should be reinstated if evidence of consumption coagulopathy reappears.

Nephrectomy performed during the acute stage of the disease not only is unnecessary but can be harmful. Removal of the kidney may be undertaken several months later, particularly if hypertension intervenes. Other complications—such as defects in the renal tubular transport of glucose, phosphate, or amino acids; impairment in urinary concentrating ability; and type 4 renal tubular acidosis—may occur, but they are usually amenable to medical therapy. When severe or inadequately treated, they may result in rickets and growth failure. Hypertension remains the most common consequence of RVT.

RENAL VENOUS THROMBOSIS OF CHILDHOOD

RVT is seldom encountered among children beyond infancy. When it does occur it is most often associated with the nephrotic syndrome (NS), particularly secondary to membranous nephropathy. The prevailing opinion is that RVT is a consequence rather than the cause of NS and that its development is favored by a state of hypercoagulability present in patients with NS.

The thrombotic process of childhood, unlike that in RVT of infancy, starts in the main renal vein and spreads towards the periphery. Patients with established thrombosis should probably be anticoagulated with warfarin because heparin may be inefficient in nephrotics. Treatment should be continued for 6 months or until the severe nephrotic state subsides. Thrombectomy appears to offer few benefits over anticoagulation therapy.

Chronic Renal Failure

AILEEN B. SEDMAN, M.D.

The incidence of chronic renal failure (CRF) in children under 16 years of age in North America is estimated at 1.5/million total population/year. Many cases are not reported because the affected infants have fatal complications early in life.

The major causes of CRF in childhood include congenital urinary tract malformations (dysplasia, hypoplasia, obstruction), approximately 36%; glomerulopathy/glomerulonephritis, 37%; hereditary diseases (polycystic kidney, Alport's syndrome, cystinosis, nephronophthisis, oxalosis), 13%; systemic disease (including lupus), 9%; vascular disease, 2%; and miscellaneous disorders (including Wilms' tumor), approximately 3%.

A decade ago, the outlook for children with CRF was dismal except for those who received a successful transplant before severe retardation of growth and development occurred. Although hemodialysis had been widely used in adults by the mid-1970's and helped these patients to lead relatively normal lives, in small children the procedure was fraught with difficulties, including limited access, poor tolerance of rapid fluid shifts, poor psychologic tolerance of painful procedures and constant institutional care, and very severe growth retardation secondary to all of the above. In the late 1970's continuous ambulatory peritoneal dialysis was found to be an adequate method of therapy for children, providing for constant treatment that resulted in a more evenly controlled, albeit still abnormal, internal milieu. Also, peritoneal dialysis could be performed painlessly by families at home, allowing for a much more normal psychologic development of the child, with school attendance often being possible. Transplant procedures have also become more technically successful, and new immunosuppression regimens have increased 5-year patient survival rates post transplant to 95% and 5-year kidney survival rates

to approximately 70%. Because of these factors, meticulous management of children with CRF before renal replacement therapy is necessary has become crucial to maintain normal growth and development during the early stages of the disease.

The complications of renal insufficiency may begin to occur when the glomerular filtration rate (GFR) falls below 30–50% of normal, depending on the disease that initiated the process. The child may become anorexic or acidotic, and there may be a slowing of growth velocity. Bone histology has been shown to be abnormal in these early stages. There is evidence that intervention at this point with specified nutrition, involving adjustments in intake of calories, protein, calcium, phosphorus, and alkali, may prevent early growth failure. There is also evidence that control of protein intake may alter the progression of the insufficiency, although this is obviously dependent on the ongoing insult to the kidney. When GFR reaches 15–25% of normal, major complications begin to occur; renal replacement therapy (dialysis or transplant) becomes necessary when the GFR is approximately 8% of normal. During these later stages, anemia, renal osteodystrophy, growth failure, and encephalopathy are frequently noted. The goal of medical management of CRF, then, is to provide therapies in such a way that growth, schooling, and individuation of the child are supported and severe complications are avoided.

CLINICAL MANIFESTATIONS
Nutrition

A decrease in caloric intake is nearly universal in children with renal failure and may be of great importance in growth failure of children with CRF. Attempts should be made to monitor the intake of these children in such a way that, when inadequate intake occurs, dietary counseling can intervene to provide appropriate supplementation. Excessive protein intake has been implicated in causing a more rapid decline in GFR, and protein should be individually prescribed according to the child's need (e.g., a child who is nephrotic may need more protein than a child who is not). The general requirement for the growing child is 1.5–2 gm/kg/day of high-quality protein. Uremia is associated with insulin resistance and hypertriglyceridemia, and diets containing excessive saturated fat should be avoided. Exercise has been shown to lower insulin values and triglyceride levels and should be encouraged in the child with renal failure.

If dietary intake is inadequate in a child with CRF, there may be concurrent vitamin deficiency that can cause signs and symptoms indistinguishable from uremic symptoms (neuropathy, cardiomyopathy, etc.). Fat-soluble vitamins can accumulate in patients with renal failure, and vitamins A, E, and K are not supplemented beyond normal dietary intake. Vitamin D is supplemented in the form of 1,25-dihydroxy vitamin D (see Renal Osteodystrophy). Water-soluble vitamins should be given daily if the diet is inadequate. The most commonly available form is Berocca, which can be taken as a tablet.

Sodium, Potassium, and Water

Sodium, potassium, and water requirements in the child with renal failure are dependent on the volume and quality of urine produced. Children with CRF may not conserve sodium adequately and may have a tubular defect with aldosterone resistance leading to hyponatremia and hyperkalemia. Sudden strict water and sodium restrictions should be avoided. Intake and output volumes should be monitored to estimate approximate needs. Often children with dysplasia have polyuria with exacerbation of their uremia if water is restricted or if vomiting and diarrhea occur. All children with CRF who are unable to maintain normal oral intake or who have gastrointestinal losses must be monitored for fluid and electrolyte imbalances, which can be life threatening. Since the renal diluting and concentrating mechanism is often absent, the urine output dictates the intake necessary to maintain euvolemia. Fluid intake should be calculated as insensible loss plus the child's daily urine output. Intravenous support is often necessary in a child with CRF who has vomiting, diarrhea, or an illness that restricts intake.

Acidosis

Decreased net acid excretion may accompany a decline in renal function, and correction of acidosis with supplemental alkali is required. Electrolytes with total bicarbonate should be monitored whenever renal insufficiency is noted. Alkali should be administered to maintain the total bicarbonate content of the serum at 22–25 mEq/L. Alkali therapy is available as soda bicarbonate tablets or as Bicitra (1 mEq of sodium citrate/ml), which is then converted to bicarbonate, 1 mEq.

Renal Osteodystrophy

Calcium and phosphorus imbalances, with subsequent hyperparathyroidism and renal osteodystrophy, may begin to occur when the GFR is 20–40% of normal. We now recommend that children begin a phosphorus-restricted diet early in the course of renal failure by avoiding cow's milk and excessive intake of meat. A number of low-phosphate formulas that can be used as milk substitutes provide good quality protein without high phosphorus (Ross PM 60/40 and Wyeth S29 formulas are available). If hyperphosphatemia continues to be a problem, calcium carbonate can be used as a phosphate binder; the dose should be titrated to avoid hypercalcemia and gastrointestinal symptoms. Aluminum phosphate binders have been shown to cause aluminum loading when used chronically in children with CRF, leading to osteomalacia, anemia, and encephalopathy. Aluminum-containing antacids are used only for very short periods to treat severe hyperphosphatemia. When hyperphosphatemia becomes a problem despite adequate dietary restriction and calcium carbonate use, dialysis or transplant should be considered. Appropriate vitamin D therapy should be instituted when biochemical values, including hypocalcemia and increased alkaline phosphatase, indicate ricketic disease. 1,25-dihydroxy vitamin D is extremely useful in preventing severe renal osteodystrophy. These drugs must be used cautiously, as severe hypercalcemia can occur and in turn can cause more rapid deterioration of renal function. Two drugs are used to treat the vitamin D deficiency of renal insufficiency—dihydrotachysterol, 0.125–0.75 mg/day (Hytakerol); or 1,25-dihydroxy vitamin D (Rocaltrol, 0.125–2 μgm/day). The serum calcium level is monitored weekly when the doses of these drugs are being changed and monthly after the dose is regulated. It is allowed to rise to 11, and the alkaline phosphatase level is monitored until it is within the normal range. Vitamin D therapy is then maintained to adapt to the child's growth.

Anemia

Anemia is common in patients with renal insufficiency. Indices are usually normocytic and normochromic. If they are microcytic, iron deficiency or aluminum toxicity should be explored. Splenic sequestration of blood cells may exacerbate the anemia. Transfusions are given to maintain hematocrit in the 15–25% range, depending on how symptomatic the child is. Excessive blood transfusions should be avoided because of the potential for iron deposition and hemosiderosis. Ferritin levels are useful indicators of iron status.

Encephalopathy

Uremia can cause profound changes in the central nervous system. Both malnutrition and aluminum toxicity have been implicated in causing some of these effects, but it remains to be seen whether aggressive early medical management with nutritional therapy and avoidance of toxins such as aluminum can preserve normal neurologic function until transplant is accomplished. Children with renal failure should be monitored for their developmental status; if it is not normal, possible causes should be sought. Since many children with CRF have maintained normal intellectual function while supported on dialysis, it should not be assumed that any child with renal failure will be mentally retarded.

Hypertension

Hypertension in CRF may be due to salt and water retention or overproduction of renin by the diseased kidney. Plasma renin level determinations can help to differentiate the two if done with proper controls—that is, when the child is volume replete and is not on medications, such as diuretics or captopril, that can alter the renin status.

For children in whom hypervolemia is the problem, salt and water need to be restricted. Since thiazides are not efficacious in patients with renal failure, furosemide (1–5 mg/kg, two to four times daily) is given to increase the sodium and water loss, if a diuretic is necessary. The combination of a beta blocker and a vasodilator is used if further therapy is necessary (propranolol, 1–2 mg/kg, one to four times daily; hydralazine, 0.5–2 mg/kg, two to four times daily). If renin overproduction is the primary cause of hypertension, diuretics and hydralazine may make the hypertension worse by increasing renin production secondary to decreased renal perfusion. Captopril may be used in this situation, although it may cause hyperkalemia secondary to inhibition of aldosterone production or a decrease in GFR secondary to alteration in renal blood flow, especially in patients with renal vascular abnormalities. Captopril (0.1–0.4 mg/kg/dose in infants; 3.125–50 mg, two to four times daily, in children and adolescents) has also been associated with membranous nephropathy, proteinuria, and suppression of the bone marrow with neutropenia. The effect of captopril on hypertension may be profound, and it is our practice to start the drug only under hospital supervision. Minoxidil (0.1–1.4 mg/kg/day) is a potent vasodilator most commonly used after other drugs have failed; it may produce hirsutism. It should be used in combination with a diuretic and a beta blocker because it can cause fluid retention and tachycardia.

Cardiac Dysfunction

Cardiomegaly and congestive heart failure in patients with renal failure may be secondary to hypervolemia or hypertension, which should be treated aggressively. Pericardial effusion may occur in severe uremia and is an indication that dialysis should have been started sooner. Children who are severely anorexic may have vitamin deficiency; if cardiomegaly and peripheral neuropathy coexist, thiamine deficiency should be suspected. As discussed earlier, children with inadequate intake should be given water-soluble vitamin supplements.

INDICATIONS FOR DIALYSIS

The absolute indications for dialysis include: (1) electrolyte imbalance that is life threatening; (2) congestive heart failure secondary to volume overload, hypertension, or uremic cardiomyopathy, and (3) severe growth failure, secondary to renal osteodystrophy, anorexia, or acidosis, that is uncontrolled by conservative medical therapy.

In a child with progressive renal insufficiency, it is advantageous to plan for renal replacement therapy several months before it is necessary, preparing the family and the child when clearances are in the range of 15–20 cc/min/1.73 m². Obviously, some children do extremely well even when clearances are very low. This is the exception, however, and any child with CRF who shows growth and developmental delays should be evaluated early in the course of the disease to determine whether nutritional therapy or early dialysis would be helpful. Children with clearance below 10 cc/min/1.73 m² need replacement therapy imminently and should be monitored weekly until dialysis or transplant is accomplished.

Peritoneal Dialysis

AILEEN B. SEDMAN, M.D.

Peritoneal dialysis is a procedure that takes advantage of the semipermeable membrane of the peritoneum. This membrane allows for chemical and osmotic equilibrium between the peritoneal and extracellular spaces. Dialyzable substances diffuse through the walls of capillaries on the peritoneal surface. When fluid placed in the peritoneum mimics serum without containing urea, creatinine, phosphorus, and so forth, these substances can be removed by changing the fluid in the abdomen frequently enough to provide a constant gradient. Ultrafiltration of extracellular fluid is accomplished by adjusting the dialysate glucose concentration to provide osmotic stimulus for movement of water into the peritoneum. Peritoneal dialysis can be used acutely to treat renal failure, drug overdose (when the drug is dialyzable), and severe electrolyte or metabolic disturbances that cannot be handled conservatively. It should be recalled that hemodialysis is at least 10 times more efficient than peritoneal dialysis and may be necessary when a patient is severely catabolic or has had abdominal complications or when there is such poor perfusion to mesenteric vessels that diffusion cannot take place. But peritoneal dialysis has many advantages in children: the procedure does not involve rapid volume swings in the intravascular space, it allows for more controlled shifts of electrolytes and pH, and it removes middle molecules more efficiently than hemodialysis. Peritoneal dialysis has been used extensively for both acute and chronic dialysis in children.

ACUTE PERITONEAL DIALYSIS

Indications. The absolute indications for starting dialysis acutely are life-threatening electrolyte abnormalities and severe volume overload. In general, this situation usually occurs when the blood urea nitrogen (BUN) is greater than 100 mg/dl, the potassium is greater than 6 mEq/L, and the bicarbonate is less than 12 mEq/L. Severe hypocalcemia and hyperphosphatemia (< 7 mg/dl and > 15 mg/dl, respectively) can also necessitate dialysis but rarely occur without the other abnormalities. It should be remembered that a child who is anuric and catabolic or bleeding and needs emergent transfusion may move from safe electrolyte values to life-threatening values within hours, so dialysis should be started prophylactically.

Technique. Acute peritoneal catheters can be placed at the bedside with preoperative sedation and local anesthetic. In severely uremic children, morphine is our drug of choice for preoperative sedation as it can be easily reversed with naloxone. Many acute catheters and trays are available. We currently use an over-the-wire Cook acute peritoneal dialysis tray, which comes in both pediatric and adult sizes (C-PDSY-3 and C-PDSY-1, respectively).

After the child's bladder is emptied by urethral catheterization and he or she is sedated, an area approximately 2 cm below the umbilicus is anesthetized with 1% lidocaine. A plastic-sheathed, 18-gauge Intracath needle is inserted midline until a pop is felt passing through the linea and into the peritoneum. Often, at this time, proteinaceous ascitic fluid will return through the needle. The metal portion is discarded, and 10–20 cc/kg of dialysate fluid is allowed to flow into the abdomen through the plastic sheath to displace the gut from the area of the subsequent catheter insertion. The accompanying wire guide is passed through the plastic sheath with an estimation of length made to reach one of the colic gutters. The plastic sheath is slid off the wire, and the peritoneal catheter is passed over the wire, gently dilating the needle insertion hole with the tip of the catheter as it is passed. A small scalpel incision can be made at the insertion site if necessary. The wire is gently rotated and slid out of the catheter and discarded. An accompanying connecting tube is applied to the catheter, which accepts all dialysis tube delivery sets. The dialysis catheter is anchored either by suturing or taping to the skin the silicone disk that is attached to the catheter.

Dialysis is performed with the dialysate solutions warmed to body temperature. Typical dialysate contains 132 mEq/L of sodium, 0 mEq/L of potassium, 99 mEq/L of chloride, 35–45 mEq/L of lactate, 3.5 to 4 mEq/L of calcium, 1.5 mEq/L of magnesium, and 0 mg/L of phosphorus. Two concentrations of glucose are available—1.5% and 4.25% (15,000 mg/L and 42,500 mg/L, respectively)—with resulting osmolalities of approximately 347 and 500 mOsm/L (normal plasma osmolality is 275–290 mOsm/L). Potassium can be added to the dialysate when the serum potassium is below 4 mEq/L. The basic principle that any concentration of substance added to the dialysate must be compatible with what is safe in serum in the same concentration should always be kept in mind. The concentration of potassium in dialysate should, therefore, never be greater than 5 mEq/L. Potassium may be added as potassium chloride, potassium acetate, or potassium phosphate according to the patient's need for the particular anion. Patients with severe liver disease may be unable to metabolize the lactate in the dialysate, exacerbating their acidosis. Two approaches can be taken—giving bicarbonate as an intravenous infusion or replacing the lactate in the dialysate with 40 mEq/L of bicarbonate. The calcium must then be removed from the dialysate or precipitation will occur. The patient without calcium in the dialysate must receive it intravenously as a constant infusion.

The volume of dialysate instilled into the abdomen is approximately 30–50 cc/kg/pass. Patients with respiratory insufficiency may deteriorate with these large volumes and should be positioned with the head of the bed slightly elevated. Inflow and outflow are accomplished by gravity: fluid is run in over 5 minutes, allowed to "dwell" for 20 minutes, and drained for 5–10 minutes, accomplishing approximately one pass every half-hour. Longer dwell times of 1–2 hours can be used when the patient is euvolemic, but less free water will be removed. Antibiotics are not routinely added to the dialysate if the insertion procedure was sterile. If it was not, they can be added (dosage as listed in Table 1). Heparin is added to the dialysate at 500 units/L if there are small clots or fibrin in the dialysate.

The relative rates of diffusion of substances from the serum to the peritoneum are as follows: urea > potassium > chloride > sodium > creatinine > phosphate > uric acid > bicarbonate > calcium > magnesium. It can be expected to take 24 hours to lower a child's BUN by 50%. Hyperkalemia is usually rapidly controlled. Phosphorus levels are not easily controlled by dialysis alone, and phosphorus accumulation must be limited by decreasing the intake or avoiding the catabolic state. A rapid pH shift from acidemia to alkalemia will cause increased protein binding of ionized calcium and can lead to seizures and arrhythmias. This can be avoided by giving calcium supplementation and lowering the phosphorus to allow the serum calcium to return to normal.

Table 1.   RECOMMENDED DOSES OF
INTRAPERITONEAL ANTIBIOTICS IN THE
TREATMENT OF PERITONITIS IN CAPD PATIENTS

	Loading Dose*	Maintenance Dose*
First-line drugs		
Cephalothin	500	250
Tobramycin	1.7 (mg/kg/bag)	8
Second-line drugs		
Amphotericin	—	5
Ampicillin	500	50
Cloxacillin	1000	100
Ticarcillin	1000	100
Septra SMZ/TMP	400/80	25/5
Clindamycin	300	50
Amikacin	250	50
Penicillin	1,000,000 (units/L)	50,000 (units/L)
Vancomycin	1,000 mg or (10 mg/kg) (IV)	30

From Williams, P., Vas, S., Layne, S., et al.: The treatment of peritonitis in on CAPD: To lavage or not. Peritoneal Dialysis Bulletin 1:14, 1980, and Williams P: Loading doses of antibiotics for the treatment of peritonitis. Perit Dial Bull 1:45, 1981.

* Dose shown as mg/L dialysate unless otherwise indicated.

Complications. Complications of peritoneal dialysis are obstruction of the catheter, leaking around the catheter, and peritonitis. Outflow obstruction is often caused by mesenteric or bowel entanglement of the catheter. This can often be overcome by repositioning the patient, stimulating bowel activity with an enema, or irrigating the catheter in a sterile manner. Perforation of bowel, bladder, or blood vessel can also occur with insertion of the catheter. Small perforations can be handled by lavaging the abdomen with the dialysate. If there is a gut perforation, antibiotics should be added to cover the bacteria involved, as listed in Table 1. Moderate bleeding can simply be treated with blood replacement. If there is significant bleeding, the individual must be taken to the operating room for ligation of the vessel. Acute catheters must be used continuously to stay patent and prevent infection. If a child is to be dialyzed for more than 4–5 days or if he or she is very active (e.g., a toddler with hemolytic uremic syndrome), a chronic Silastic catheter should be placed in the operating room. A single-cuffed catheter with a small subcutaneous tunnel can be removed at the bedside when it is no longer necessary for therapy. Peritonitis is the most frequent and most serious complication of peritoneal dialysis. It is diagnosed by the onset of cloudy dialysate, abdominal pain, and fever. A 10-ml sample of dialysate is sent for cell count, Gram stain, and culture. Peritonitis is usually associated with a white blood cell count of greater than 100 mm^3, of which 50% or more are segmented neutrophils or bands. If cloudy dialysate, pain, and fever are obvious, immediate institution of rapid flushes and subsequent intraperitoneal antibiotics are necessary to prevent a rapid progression to catastrophic illness. Usually therapy is started empirically, with a cephalosporin and an aminoglycoside (dosages in Table 1), before the Gram stain results are known. Changes are made on the basis of the Gram stain and culture findings.

CHRONIC PERITONEAL DIALYSIS

Chronic peritoneal dialysis has gained wide acceptance as the method of choice for children who need long-term therapy because it is performed at home. Once the family has been trained, the acutal procedure is better tolerated psychologically by the children than is hemodialysis. With meticulous care and adequate nutrition growth on peritoneal dialysis seems possible. Hemodialysis is at least 10 times more efficient than peritoneal dialysis, but, because it is performed only 3–4 times weekly, it does not provide a stable internal milieu; furthermore, it usually requires in-center care during the procedure.

A chronic peritoneal dialysis catheter is usually placed in the operating room by the surgeon after partial omentectomy is performed. There are few statistics to support the choice of one catheter over another. In our center, for small children, we prefer the curled, single-cuff catheter (Quinton) with at least a 7-cm subcutaneous tunnel.

A number of different procedures are used to accomplish chronic peritoneal dialysis. The first and most popular is chronic ambulatory peritoneal dialysis (CAPD). The abdominal dialysis catheter is attached to tubing with an end spike that the patient (or parent) uses to enter a plastic dialysate bag in a sterile manner four to six times per day. The dialysate is run into the abdomen, and the collapsible bag is clamped, rolled up, and placed in a pocket or under an expandable belt. After the prescribed interval, the bag is unclamped and lowered, and the old dialysate is drained by gravity. The old bag is discarded and a new bag is spiked sterilely and allowed again to drain into the abdomen. Each "pass" procedure takes approximately 20–30 minutes, but because there are no machines involved and all the equipment is portable, it can be accomplished at school or while away from home. CAPD usually provides adequate clearance and ultrafiltration for older children and those with some urine output. For very small children who require large volume feedings or for those with anuria, four to six passes per day may not be enough for ultrafiltration and clearance. Also, constantly having dialysate in their abdomens may inhibit appetite and developmental tasks such as walking in some children. In these cases, continuous cycling peritoneal dialysis (CCPD) is considered. With this method, all cycling is done at night via a machine that does the passes automatically. In the usual routine, the parents sterilely put the child on the cycler at bedtime, and a pass is done every 1–2 hours over a period of 10–12 hours. The child is taken off the cycler in the morning, and a small amount of fluid is left in the abdomen. Thus, the child is up and around all day without the large amount of volume in the abdomen. Intermittent peritoneal dialysis (IPD) is the term used when the dialysis is done nonconsecutively. Initially, it was hoped that pertoneal dialysis could be done three to four times per week, as is hemodialysis; however, peritoneal dialysis is relatively inefficient and the advantages are lost when it is done less often than daily. Individual prescriptions for dialysis must be made with the goal that, when adequate nutrition is provided, dialysis will control the resulting volume and biochemical aberrations.

CAPD or CCPD is as effective as hemodialysis in controlling the biochemical and clinical manifestations of uremia and, as previously stated, may remove middle molecules more efficiently. Also, the more consistent therapy seems conducive to growth, better fluid control, and less anemia than hemodialysis. Most children on CAPD require only moderate fluid restriction. Since 1,25-dihydroxy vitamin D and water-soluble vitamins are lost at a high rate on peritoneal dialysis, water-soluble vitamins and one of the activated forms of vitamin D (Rocaltrol or Hytakerol; see the article on Chronic Renal Failure) must always be given. Protein is also lost in the dialysate at an approximate rate of 0.2 gm/kg/day, so total protein and albumin must be monitored along with the other biochemical parameters, with protein supplemented as necessary.

Adequate nutrition is a major problem for any child on dialysis. Although older children may eat well, many infants and toddlers will take in less than 50% of the recommended daily allowance. Dietary histories must be carefully followed, and supplementation with high-calorie, low-phosphorus foods is often necessary. Low-phosphorus formulas, such as Ross PM 60/40 or Wyeth S29, supplemented with corn oil, carbohydrate, and protein fortifiers are often necessary to provide adequate nutrition. When the child is unable to take the necessary amount, tube feeding by nasogastric feeding at night or by gastrostomy is often considered. Obviously, dialysis is an extremely time-consuming and expensive therapy. Dialysis without adequate nutrition for any length of time is unacceptable. Chronic malnutrition can cause myopathy, neuropathy, developmental delay, and eventual death. Symptoms caused by malnutrition are often difficult to distinguish from symptoms of uremia.

The most important complication of chronic peritoneal dialysis is peritonitis, which occurs as often as one episode every 6–13 months. The diagnosis and treatment of peritonitis are discussed in the section on acute peritoneal dialysis. Exit site infection, cuff extrusion, and tunnel leakage are less frequent. All can usually be handled without catheter removal. Infection that is caused by *Pseudomonas* or fungus and does not clear quickly with appropriate antibiotics does require catheter removal; the child should be placed on hemodialysis for 2–4 weeks before a new catheter is implanted. Ventral and inguinal hernias along with hydrocele are also complications of large volumes of fluid being carried in the abdomen. Hernia repair is often required, but cycling at night while the patient is recumbent may be helpful if repair cannot be performed immediately.

Peritoneal dialysis, along with appropriate nutrition and medical supervision, can adequately support a growing child. However, the burden of the time-consuming procedures and dependence issues make it acceptable only for finite periods. A successful transplant is always the ultimate goal for any child with end-stage renal disease.

Hemodialysis

ANTONIA C. NOVELLO, M.D., M.P.H.

Pediatric nephrologists consider renal transplantation the optimal therapeutic modality for children with renal failure; i.e., a successful transplant provides the best opportunity for normal growth and development and for alleviating the psychological distress of chronic renal failure. However, prolonged dialysis may be needed in some children.

Dialysis is a technique for removing metabolites and toxins and for maintaining a satisfactory equilibrium of electrolytes and volume in patients with disordered excretory capabilities. Hemodialysis, simply stated, is a diffusive process in which blood comes into contact with a balanced salt solution (dialysate) across a semipermeable membrane and solutes pass across by diffusion along a concentration gradient, their rate of removal being determined by their physicochemical properties. Isotonic fluid removal is achieved by applying a hydrostatic pressure gradient on the membrane.

Hemodialysis has been performed in children since the early 1960's. The technique has been utilized in preparation for renal transplant while searching for a suitable donor, after a failed renal transplant, and for the treatment of life-threatening clinical complications. Nevertheless, there seems to be limited experience with long-term (longer than 5 years) hemodialysis in children. Despite this, the overall survival is good, with one report indicating a 5-year actuarial patient survival rate of 95%. Several other options for the treatment of children with chronic renal failure (CRF) have become available during the past decade, e.g., continuous ambulatory peritoneal dialysis (CAPD), continuous cycling peritoneal dialysis (CCPD), and chronic intermittent peritoneal dialysis (IPD).

The number of patients in the pediatric age group with end-stage renal disease (ESRD) reportedly varies from 1 to 3.5 per million population per year. Prior to the widespread availability of hemodialysis and the newer peritoneal dialysis techniques (CAPD, CCPD, and IPD), definite treatment was not initiated until severe uremic complications were apparent. Currently, hemodialysis is begun before severe symptomatology occurs. Absolute indications for dialysis are uncontrollable hypertension with hypertensive encephalopathy or congestive heart failure, congestive heart failure unresponsive to loop diuretics, pericarditis, peripheral neuropathy, renal osteodystrophy, and bone marrow depression with either severe anemia, leukopenia, or thrombocytopenia.

In most instances, symptoms arising from involvement of a single organ system predominate and dictate the need for dialysis. In the child without such absolute indications, the decision to institute dialysis should be based upon his or her ability to perform usual daily activities. In these cases, derangements in biochemical parameters can be useful indicators for starting dialysis: i.e., blood urea nitrogen (BUN) greater than 150 mg/dl, carbon dioxide content less than 12 mEq/L, potassium level greater than 6.0 mEq/L, falling hematocrit (less than 20%, necessitating transfusion in the face of hyperkalemia and volume overload), and severe hypocalcemia (calcium level less than 7.0 mg/dl). These biochemical abnormalities in combination with a glomerular filtration rate of less than 5 ml/min/1.73 m^2 indicate the imminent need for dialysis.

Two other situations may require emergency initiation of hemodialysis: accidental poisoning and acute renal failure. As alternatives, hemoperfusion and peritoneal dialysis, respectively, might be considered in such cases. Peritoneal dialysis is widely available and has the advantage of not requiring heparinization.

DIALYSIS PRESCRIPTION FOR CHILDREN
Vascular Access

Patients undergoing hemodialysis require a vascular access that permits high blood flow rates. Three types of access are commonly used: shunts, fistulas, and temporary access. The Thomas femoral shunt is the preferred access for children weighing less than 15 kg or younger than 5 years of age who require hemodialysis. With any type of vascular access, the goal is to use the largest

cannula that fits comfortably without compromising the intima of the vessel in which it is inserted. Disadvantages of the shunt include infections, clotting episodes, and, in some children, inhibition of normal activity and anxiety because of the presence of the external cannula. Ischemic damage to the leg where a groin shunt was placed has been reported as a rare complication.

In children with ESRD who will undergo long-term dialysis and whose weight is more than 15 kg, an arteriovenous fistula—a forearm vein anastomosed to a radial artery—is preferred. Fistulas differ from shunts in requiring "maturation." They must be constructed at least 3 weeks before utilization is anticipated. When the anastomosis provides insufficient blood flow, an alternate internal arteriovenous fistula can be created using either a bovine graft or synthetic material. More recently, microsurgical techniques in infants weighing less than 5 kg have been described. A detrimental effect, as with the use of shunts, is thrombosis. At times the high fistula flow demands an excessively high cardiac output, resulting in eventual systolic hypertension and heart failure.

For temporary vascular access, percutaneous catheters have been used via femoral, subclavian, or internal jugular veins, even in children weighing as little as 6 kg.

Dialyzers

Because of the low cardiac output and the small vascular volume of children, the extracorporeal volume of the dialyzers, blood flow rates, and blood lines must be kept to a minimum. The ideal is to fill both the dialyzer and blood tubing with less than 10% of the child's blood volume (10 cc/kg body weight). Hollow fiber dialyzers are preferable to flat or coil dialyzers, since their blood compartment is relatively small and rigid.

There are three types of dialyzers available today: parallel plate, hollow fiber, and coil. Children are usually dialyzed with parallel plate or hollow fiber dialyzers. The main consideration in choosing a dialyzer is its ultrafiltration coefficient and blood compartment volume. Pediatric dialyzers are generally designed for children in either the 10–20 kg (0.5–0.6 m^2) or the 20–40 kg (1.0 m^2) weight range. Children weighing more than 40 kg (1.3–1.6 m^2) can usually be treated using adult dialyzers. Children weighing less than 10 kg require a 0.25 m^2 dialyzer.

Delivery System

No special modifications of existing delivery systems are required for pediatric patients. The usual dialysate solution has the following composition: calcium, 3.5 mEq/L; potassium, 1.0 or 2.0 mEq/L; sodium, 135 mEq/L; chloride, 100 mEq/L; magnesium, 1.6 mEq/L; acetate, 38 mEq/L; and glucose, 0–250 mg/dl. If the child demonstrates intolerance (nausea, vomiting, hypotension) to acetate, as may occur with high-efficiency dialyzers, bicarbonate can be substituted for acetate in the bath. Likewise, the use of dialyzers with inappropriately high clearance values should be avoided in children. Several techniques, such as intravenous infusion of saline, human albumin, vasopressors, or mannitol, can be used to minimize ultrafiltration-induced hypotension. Separate filtration followed by isovolemic hemodialysis may also be employed. In order to minimize the need for these interventions, the ultrafiltration rate should be calculated to remove the desired quantity of fluid evenly during the course of dialysis.

Prescription

Many schemes have been proposed to determine the optimal frequency, duration, and clearance of dialysis in pediatric patients. The most commonly used method to determine the adequacy of dialysis is kinetic modeling. This technique employs urea as a marker of uremic toxicity and allows for the development of treatment options permitting maintenance of BUN within predetermined limits. The goal is to keep a time-averaged concentration of urea within the range of 60–70 mg/dl (predialysis BUN level or about 80–100 mg/dl and postdialysis level of about 20–30 mg/dl).

The dialysis index, which compares and relates dialyzer surface area × weekly hours of dialysis ÷ body surface area, has been formulated according to values derived from adult experiences. In most pediatric centers the initial prescriptions of dialyzer clearance and time schedule depend on the child's weight (surface area), fluid accumulation between dialysis treatments, and the predialysis level of BUN. In most centers dialysis is usually prescribed three times a week for periods ranging between 4 and 6 hours, utilizing standard priming and heparinization techniques described in the literature.

Ultrafiltration

During ultrafiltration, fluid removed from the plasma is replaced with fluid equilibrated from the expanded interstitial space. The degree of ultrafiltration varies according to the desired weight loss. Excessive ultrafiltration (greater than 3 kg for adolescents or 2 kg for younger children) is frequently necessary. This can cause hypotension, nausea, vomiting, headaches, and cramps. When hypoalbuminemia (less than 3 gm/dl) is present and ultrafiltration is required, the albumin level must be raised to improve tolerance of ultrafiltration. Although equilibration is rapid, at times signs of plasma volume depletion occur. In this event, separate ultrafiltration for 1 hour prior to the initiation of dialysis will aid in the removal of fluid without concomitant hypotension.

Nutrition and Diet in Dialyzed Children

Since growth failure and nutritional energy deficiencies are commonly recognized in dialyzed children with ESRD, an effort should be made to maximize the number of calories ingested. This is difficult, inasmuch as caloric intake must be kept high while sodium, potassium, phosphorus, protein, and fluids must be limited. Today, the goal is to strike a fair balance among these needs. The energy and protein content of the diet must be supplemented and not limited, and dietary restrictions must not produce nutrient deficiencies, even if this means a greater dialytic requirement. The goal is to provide 80–100% of the recommended daily allowance energy requirements for these children. Daily dietary recommendations are: calories, $2000/m^2$; protein, 1.5–2.5 gm/kg, or 3–4 gm/kg in small children (less than 10–16 kg); sodium, 40 mEq/m^2; potassium, 30 mEq/m^2; and fluids, 500 ml/m^2 plus an amount equal to urine volume. B complex vitamins and folic acid, 1 mg daily, are also supplemented. Phosphate-binding gels (preferably without aluminum), 1–3 capsules three times a day with meals, or calcium carbonate is given to reduce the serum phosphorus level.

In general, therefore, the dietary intake of dialyzed children should include a balanced energy intake and a protein intake of approximately 2 gm/kg/day.

COMPLICATIONS OF HEMODIALYSIS

Hypertension. Virtually all patients undergoing hemodialysis have periods of hypertension. The usual mechanism is volume expansion, which generally responds to dietary fluid and salt restriction. Ultrafiltration to dry weight also controls hypertension in more than 90% of patients. Occasional hypertension episodes are not controlled by dialysis, and these patients may require hypertensive medication. Occasionally, hypertensive medications are ineffective and bilateral nephrectomy is necessary for blood pressure control. This is rare, however, with the availability of captopril and minoxidil. Most of these cases are associated with high levels of renin. Postnephrectomy hypertension is mostly volume related. If hypertension persists after nephrectomy, it may be due to changes in peripheral resistance or to vasoactive substances produced outside the kidney. Despite all, blood pressure control during hemodialysis generally improves once the patient is well dialyzed.

Anemia. Children with CRF have a normochromic, normocytic anemia secondary to deficient erythropoiesis. When they undergo dialysis, this state is complicated by a continuing loss of blood, mostly in the dialyzer and because of frequent sampling for laboratory determinations. Increased hemolysis due to the mechanical trauma of the extracorporeal circulation is a minor additional factor. If the patient has undergone bilateral nephrectomy, the anemia worsens. Most children need transfusions to maintain the hematocrit level above 20%. Complications from frequent transfusion procedures include infection with hepatitis B antigen, tissue iron deposition, and sensitization to HLA antigens. If patients fail to respond to iron (e.g., adolescents with fused epiphyses), benefit may be obtained from nandrolone phenpropionate* (Durabolin), 50–100 mg IM every week for boys and every 2 weeks for girls. This is helpful in stimulating erythropoesis. This treatment should not be used in patients with unfused epiphyses.

Osteodystrophy. Chronic dialysis usually stabilizes existing renal osteodystrophy. Two types of lesions have been recognized by x-ray examination: rickets-like lesions (osteomalacia) and subperiosteal bone resorption (secondary hyperparathyroidism or osteitis fibrosa). Meticulous control of acidosis and calcium and phosphorus balance by pharmacologic agents or dietary maneuvers may alleviate these problems. Controlling secondary hyperparathyroidism prior to dialysis is also important. During dialysis, the dialysate calcium should be high (7.0 mg/dl) to allow the ionized calcium to be transferred to the patient. Parathyroid hyperplasia, however, rarely involutes with the use of a high calcium–containing dialysate alone. Vitamin D analogs and supplemental calcium result in a more dramatic response. Dihydrotachysterol, 0.2 or 0.4 mg daily, and supplemental calcium carbonate, 500–2000 mg daily, have been advocated. If hypocalcemia persists, 1,25 dihydroxycholecalciferol (Rocaltrol), 0.25 μgm once or twice daily, should be used instead.

Despite dietary restrictions, most children are also hyperphosphatemic, requiring aggressive therapy to maintain serum phosphorus between 4 and 5 mg/dl. This should be accomplished with phosphate-binding gels (not containing aluminum) or calcium carbonate. If by x-ray examination the lesions of hyperparathyroidism fail to show evidence of healing, or if they worsen despite correction of calcium and phosphorus parameters, parathyroid gland extirpation ($3\frac{1}{2}$) may be indicated. In the presence of rickets, however, parathyroidectomy is not beneficial. Chronic aluminum loading may cause rickets, as is evident on bone biopsy. Aluminum can be chelated by weekly infusions of desferrioxamine.

Cardiovascular Alterations. Left ventricular performance, as measured by systolic time inter-

vals, may be depressed by uremia; this effect has been reported on echocardiography. In children, hemodialysis results in improvement in left ventricular function. Pericarditis develops in 2–19% of patients on dialysis; in some, years after the initiation of dialysis and in others within the first 3 months. Echocardiography appears to be the most helpful method for assessment of patients with pericarditis. Major hemodynamic complications occur as a result of cardiac tamponade and constrictive pericarditis. In patients with dialysis-associated pericarditis, intensive dialysis alone (3–4 weeks) is usually curative. Heparin dosage in these individuals should be reduced and carefully monitored because hemorrhage may cause cardiac tamponade. Other treatment modalities are peritoneal dialysis, charcoal hemoperfusion, systemic or intrapericardial steroids, and pericardial stripping. Furthermore, hypertriglyceridemia is frequently found in children on dialysis. Hypercholesterolemia and an increased fraction of low-density lipoproteins can also occur.

Psychosocial Problems. In children, dialytic treatments are time consuming, medical complications are common, and loss of schooling is frequent, often leading to poor peer-group interactions. Associated complications are loss of self-esteem, social isolation, and lack of independence. The treatment goal is to allow patients as much responsibility as possible for their daily care; the ultimate goal is rehabilitation and community integration.

Seizures. In most instances a specific etiology cannot be identified, and thus the seizure is attributed to the disequilibrium syndrome. Patients with high BUN, especially those during their first or second dialysis treatment, are at greater risk. Disequilibrium is prevented by using a relatively high dialysate sodium concentration (140–145 mEq/L), by decreasing the efficiency of urea clearance to 1.0–1.5 ml/min/kg, or by infusing 25% mannitol, 1 gm/kg over the course of dialysis, in order to maintain extracellular fluid osmolality. In some cases prophylactic phenobarbital prior to and/or during dialysis has been advocated.

Hepatitis. Evidence supports the conclusion that infection with hepatitis B virus increases morbidity and mortality. The incidence of hepatitis in children treated with chronic hemodialysis is approximately 10%. Blood paramenters to be followed monthly as a precaution are serum glutamic oxalic transaminase (SGOT), serum glutamic pyruvic transaminase (SGPT), bilirubin, and hepatitis B antigen levels. Elevation of SGOT and SGPT in the absence of hepatitis B antigen may be due to hepatitis A or hepatitis non-A, non-B. Methods established to decrease the incidence of HB$_s$AG-positive hepatitis among patients and staff of hemodialysis units include the provision of gowns

---

* This use is not listed by the manufacturer.

and gloves, use of disposable equipment, routine screening for hepatitis B virus, dialysis of HB_sAg-positive patients in isolation, and possibly utilization of home dialysis. To contain or prevent an epidemic, hyperimmune serum may be given to ESRD patients and staff members recently exposed to hepatitis virus. Hepatitis B vaccine is also an effective prophylaxis. There is a significant incidence of "e" antigenemia in children with persistent hepatitis antigenemia, indicating infectivity of these patients.

Renal Transplantation

ANTONIA C. NOVELLO, M.D., M.P.H.

The annual incidence of chronic renal failure in children requiring dialysis or transplantation approaches three per million total population if adolescents older than 15 as well as infants are included. Since 1972, renal transplantation has been the preferred mode of treatment for the alleviation of End-Stage Renal Failure (ESRD) in children in the developed nations. A successful transplant results in physiologic and psychologic benefits unsurpassed by current modes of chronic dialysis.

Factors determining the actuarial survival of both patients and renal grafts include donor age, donor source, underlying renal disorder, age of the recipient, closeness of HLA match, pretransplant blood transfusions, prior history of transplantation, immunosuppressive therapy, and the experience of the transplant center. Although age need not necessarily be a factor when treatment of a child with ESRD is under consideration, conflicting data have emerged regarding the impact of donor age on the outcome following cadaveric kidney transplantation. Patient and graft survival rates are significantly higher in children 10 to 15 years of age compared with those 5 to 9 years old or those less than 5 years of age. Survival rates in infants less than 1 year of age is very low; the short-term outcome of cadaver donor transplantation in these infants has been dismal.

Although technical problems are not inherently different, kidneys obtained from infants and newborns may fail to function more commonly than kidneys from older children or adults. Discouraging results have been obtained when anencephalic donors have been used. Recent studies have shown different graft survival in donor groups less than 11 years old when compared with donor groups between 11 and 50 years old (52% and 57% respectively). Improved graft survival in children receiving adult grafts rather than a pediatric graft (69%, 52% respectively) has also been reported.

The outcome of renal transplantation in children, as in adults, improves dramatically if living related donor transplantation is utilized, both in young (less than 10 years old) and older (11 to 20 years old) children. Thus if a live related donor is available, transplantation is the best option, since the results of cadaver donor transplantation in young children (1 to 5 years) have been disappointing and are worse in children less than 1 year old. By contrast, since the outcome for age group of 1 to 5 years using a live related (parental) donor organ has been encouraging, this is an acceptable mode of therapy.

Criteria For Acceptability

1. *Age*: No limit is generally placed.

2. *Mental Status*: It is known that the uremic state depresses cognitive functioning, which may improve with a successful transplant. Noncompliance is a major problem in children with ESRD, as is psychological or emotional instability. Children with severe mental retardation or behavioral or psychiatric problems require far more involvement with the health care team along with appropriate psychoemotional support. If emotional needs are not met, transplant success may be limited. Transplantation should probably then be deferred until the patient's psychoemotional status is improved so that it would be reasonable to assume that the post-transplant therapeutic regime will be followed.

3. *Preexisting Malignancy*: Prior malignancy is a real risk factor because of the possibility of recurrence following transplantation. Recurrence of the tumor or distant metastases have been known to occur in children receiving an allograft within one year following treatment for Wilms' tumor (47%). No recurrence has been evident when transplantation has been delayed for more than one year. Thus transplantation in children with Wilms' tumor should be deferred for at least one year following treatment of the tumor.

4. *Generalized Infection*: If unrecognized, infections can disseminate when immunosuppression is started. Therefore, it is of importance to eradicate infection before transplantation is considered.

5. *Bladder Adequacy*: The presence of an abnormal bladder is not a contraindication for transplantation, an encouraging point for pediatric patients with ESRD, in at least one third of whom obstructive uropathy is present. These children often have scarred and contracted bladders related to previous corrective lower urinary tract or bladder surgery. Although post-transplant urologic complications and urinary tract infections occur with increased frequency, allograft function is not adversely affected, since graft survival rate in pediatric patients with previous urologic surgery is comparable to survival in children with normal

lower urinary tracts. If the bladder is unsuitable, an ileal or nonrefluxing colon conduit can be utilized. The allograft ureter may also be anastomosed to an existing cutaneous ureterostomy. When a diversionary procedure is not feasible in patients with neurogenic bladders, clean intermittent catheterization can be performed.

Potential for Recurrence of the Primary Disease

The primary renal disease may influence patient and graft survival. Although graft loss is low, potential involvement with a pathologic process similar to that which affected the recipient native kidney is important when considering renal transplantation. The principal diseases for which recurrence is reported are membranoproliferative glomerulonephritis (MPGN), focal glomerulosclerosis (FGS), hemolytic uremic syndrome (HUS), cystinosis, and oxalosis. In MPGN no observed relationships between recurrence of the histologic lesion and alteration of allograft function have been reported. In FGS immediate recurrence in an initial allograft indicates substantial risks for recurrence in subsequent allografts. Despite this potential for graft loss and the variable incidence of recurrence, children with FGS should not be excluded from transplantation. In children with HUS, clinical manifestations of the disease after transplant have rarely been reported. Thus, in patients with HUS, it seems prudent to delay transplantation until all clinical manifestations of the initial episode abate.

Donor Selection—Surgical Procedure and Histocompatibility

As with adults, allografts from living related donors fare better than cadaveric transplants. The 5-year graft survival rates range between 71 and 85% following live related donation, and between 39 and 65% following cadaver donation. The best graft survival rates are obtained when kidneys from monozygotic twins and HLA-identical siblings are used. Children appear to accept kidneys from adult donors as long as they are 2 years of age and at least 10 kg. Parental or sibling donor allografts can be used. Siblings, however, should have expressed willingness to donate and be of age. Kidneys from a pediatric cadaver donor are excellent sources of donation, since anatomic hypertrophy occurs weeks after transplant. In cases in which the allograft is too large, it might be necessary to place the kidney intraperitoneally, anastomosing it to the recipient's aorta and vena cava if it cannot be placed in its usual extraperitoneal iliac-fossa site.

Improved cadaver graft survival rates do occur with better HLA-A and B antigen matching. A 20% difference in survival rate at the end of 2 years for a two-haplotype match is evident when compared with three or four mismatches. It has been shown that survival rates for grafts improve when the donor and the recipient share two DR antigens. Currently, children receiving parental transplants have significantly higher allograft survival than when cadaver transplants well matched for HLA antigens are used.

Blood Transfusions and Allograft Survival

Donor-specific transfusions (DST) have gained acceptance in pediatric renal transplantation, since they appear to improve the graft survival in one haplotype–matched live related donor recipients with a reactive mixed lymphocyte culture. Data shows prolonged graft survival when recipients are treated with donor-specific blood (98% one-year graft survival rate). The major disadvantage of this procedure is the risk of the development of antibodies against donor histocompatibility antigens. This has been known to occur in 15–29% of children. The future of DST in pediatric renal transplantation depends on the lowering (perhaps as low as 10%) of the sensitization rate, which may be accomplished with azathioprine therapy immediately before or during DST. The mechanism by which these transfusions protect against rejection is unknown. However, graft survival in first nontransfused cadaver donor recipients is poor (20–40%). Graft survival rates are superior in multitransfused patients (more than 5 transfusions)—85% vs. 57% (less than 5 transfusions).

Cross Match

Preformed lymphocytotoxic antibodies against donor antigens, acquired from blood transfusions, are associated with hyperacute rejection of the allograft. A negative cross match (utilizing donor T lymphocytes and recipient serum) is essential prior to transplantation. The detection of DR antigens on B lymphocytes—a so-called positive B cell cross match–is not deleterious to the allograft.

Bilateral Nephrectomy

Bilateral nephrectomy is no longer considered a prerequisite for transplantation. Pretransplant nephrectomies are performed for renin-dependent hypertension unresponsive to newer antihypertensive medications (i.e., captopril, minoxidil), persistent massive proteinuria, and persistent pyelonephritis. Reports of decreased allograft survival rate following nephrectomy, plus the importance of erythropoietin production and vitamin D metabolism in residual kidney mass, point to the importance of preserving even minimally functioning renal parenchyma.

Splenectomy

Despite recent controlled studies indicating improved allograft survival in splenectomized recipients receiving antilymphoblast globulin (ALG),

**Table 1. DOSAGE OF IMMUNOSUPPRESSIVE DRUGS
FOR RENAL TRANSPLANTATION**

Dosage	Post-transplant Period
Prednisone	
3 mg/kg/24 hr	First 2 weeks, taper to —
2 mg/kg/24 hr	3rd week through 5th week
1 mg/kg/24 hr	6th week through 8th week
0.5 mg/kg/24 hr	3rd month through 5th month
*7.5 to 15 mg/day	6th month through 12th month
*15 to 30 mg/day	After first year
(alternate-day therapy)	
Azathioprine (Imuran)	
3 mg/kg/24 hr	Initially and maintained at that level unless:
0.5 to 1.0 mg/kg/24 hr if any of these conditions are present	oliguria, or leukopenia <4000 mm³, or hepatic dysfunction

* Depending upon adequate allograft function.

this procedure is not generally indicated in pediatric renal recipients. Risk of infection in splenectomized patients is considerable; thus, the risks outweigh the potential gains.

Retransplantation

At 5 years after transplantation the actuarial survival rate for the second and third allograft is similar to the first (±45%). The primary factor influencing allograft survival is recipient sensitization. The survival rate varies, from less than 5% in nonpresensitized patients to 5–50% in moderately presensitized patients and to greater than 50% in highly presensitized patients. Thus, although HLA-A, B and C antigen does not have a statistically significant effect on retransplant outcome, in the highly presensitized patient 3 or 4 HLA-A and B antigen–matched allografts should be utilized whenever feasible for retransplantation, since this appears to influence allograft survival.

Immunosuppression

Steroids and Azathioprine. The dosage and indications for corticosteroids and azathioprine in pediatric renal transplants, are shown in Table 1. Recently, a new immunosuppressive agent, cyclosporine A has been used in pediatric renal recipients. It appears that superior allograft survival can be attained with relatively low corticosteroid doses when cyclosporine A is concomitantly administered with steroids. Although results using cyclosporine A in adults are encouraging, results in children are variable. Cyclosporine A should be closely monitored in whole blood or serum. In some patients it may be difficult to achieve adequate cyclosporine A blood levels and concomitant optimal immunosuppression; in order to maintain

desired blood levels, children may require more cyclosporine A than adults, calculated on a mg/kg basis. Other investigators prefer kinetic analysis of cyclosporine A blood levels in order to achieve optimal dosage intervals. The major side effects are a transient nephrotoxicity that reverses with dose reduction (27–50% of children), moderate depression in glomerular filtration rate (this might be a limiting factor in the future use of cyclosporine A in children, since diminished glomerular filtration rate may result in growth retardation), recurrence of the hemolytic uremic syndrome in some recipients, neurotoxic side effects (grand mal seizures, hypomagnesemia), facial hirsutism, and worsened cushingoid appearance. Thus, at present, the role of cyclosporine A in pediatric renal transplantation needs further evaluation.

Alternate-Day Therapy (ADT). Because growth suppression is known to occur when the daily prednisone dose exceeds 8.5 mg/m², the concept of ADT was introduced in the field of pediatric renal transplantation. With ADT, growth velocity improves and side effects of steroids (without increased evidence of rejection) are known to diminish. The usual dose is $2\frac{1}{4}$ times the daily corticosteroid dose, given on alternate days. If graft function remains stable, the dose is then reduced to an equivalent of $1\frac{1}{2}$ to 2 times the previous daily dosage. With ADT, the incidence of hypertension has been found to diminish, growth significantly improves (40 to 55% higher in 1 year on ADT), and serum cholesterol values fall. Controlled studies have not found that ADT is associated with increased incidence of rejection or with greater loss of renal function, as compared with patients on daily steroids.

Rejection Episodes. High doses of corticosteroids are the current treatment of choice for acute rejection episodes (methylprednisolone up to 30 mg/kg IV daily for 3 days), whereas other studies have shown that 3–10 mg/kg of methylprednisolone daily IV for 3 days (i.e., "pulses"), can be effectively employed. The previous oral prednisone dose, prior to pulsing, is then continued. The pulse treatment is best administered only twice in 3-month spans since the risks (infection and steroid side effects) may outweigh the benefits. Pulse therapy does not seem to significantly improve allograft outcome, and it may predispose the patient to life-threatening infection.

Postoperative Medical Complications

Infection. Infection occurs with increasing frequency and can cause death in transplanted children. The offending agent is often viral (herpes group—cytomegalovirus, herpes virus hominis, and varicella zoster). It is imperative to differentiate the presence of infection from rejection in the early post-transplantation course, since immunosuppressant therapy must be reduced or discontinued so as to protect the patient. Moreover, lower doses of oral prednisone have been found to provide as efficient immunosuppression as that of high doses, with equivalent graft survival. Other offending infectious agents are bacterial (*Staphylococcus, Legionella*), fungal (*Candida, Nocardia*), and parasitic (*Pneumocystis*). In the latter, prophylactic use of trimethoprim sulfa significantly reduces its development. In data collected from 6 large centers, of 167 deaths, 56 (or 34%) were due to infection. Thus, survival of transplanted patients can be improved by reducing the mortality related to infection.

Hepatic Dysfunction. Liver impairment is mostly related to drug toxicity (cyclosporine A, azathioprine), cytomegalovirus, herpes virus hominis (HVH), hepatitis A, B, or non-A non-B, or viral hepatitis. Progressive liver dysfunction has not occurred in pediatric recipients with persistent antigenemia; thus, these children are acceptable transplant candidates.

Hypertension. Hypertension can occur under various circumstances, and may indicate acute or chronic rejection. Hypertension immediately after transplant is usually related to hypervolemia (complicated with acute tubular necrosis or minimal urinary output) or to the administration of corticosteroids, which increase renin substrate and sodium retention. If hypertension develops during the first 3 months after transplant, renal artery stenosis should be considered. Treatment should be tailored to the cause. Antihypertensive therapy achieving adequate control may curtail deteriorating allograft function. Angiography, followed by surgery, transluminal angioplasty, and captopril have been used in renal artery stenosis. Captopril should be cautiously used, since deleterious effects on graft function have been reported. Finally, in the hypertensive child unresponsive to medications after transplantation, embolization of native kidneys may be performed.

Corticosteroid Toxicity. Several signs of toxicity occur when high doses of steroid are administered. Posterior subcapsular lenticular opacities develop in 55% of patients who have functioning allografts for more than one year. Hyperlipidemia, with an abnormal lipoprotein electrophoretic pattern (Type II and IV), which correlates with corticosteroid dosage, has been reported in one half to two thirds of pediatric allograft recipients. Aseptic necrosis involving any bone, multiple bones, or localized to the femoral heads or femoral condyles may occur. The incidence varies from 6 to 21% of pediatric renal recipients, and at least one femoral head is involved. Pain, rather than x-ray findings, antedates the diagnostic confirmation. A correlation between steroid dosage and the development of necrosis cannot be documented; however, a decrement in its incidence has been apparent coincident with a reduction in steroid dosage, with concomitant treatment of renal osteodystrophy.

Although malignancies are known to occur in adult transplant patients, their incidence in pediatric allograft recipients is low (1.3%).

Growth and Development

Growth Potential. Children with a bone age greater than 12 years at transplantation grow minimally, if at all, after transplantation. However, newer data suggest that substantial growth may follow transplantation despite a bone age greater than 12 years. Growth at a bone age under 12 is excellent as long as sexual maturation is not completed, since this may advance bone age as much as 4 years in a single year. Sexual maturity results in progressive epiphyseal closure and a declining growth rate. Improved growth follows in children who receive a transplant before 7 years of age and whose daily steroid dose is low. Male recipients grow better and catch up in growth more readily, than female recipients, despite comparable graft function and corticosteroid dosage.

Allograft Function. Modest reduction in glomerular filtration rate (less than 60 ml/min/1.73 m²) and modest rises in serum creatinine (1.3 to 2.0 mg/dl) often result in marked deceleration in growth velocity. This degree of renal impairment may reduce somatomedin activity and diminish growth velocity.

Corticosteroid Dosage. The amount, mode of administration, and route used for administering corticosteroids appear to be important in terms of growth potential. Lower daily doses of oral prednisone (0.1–0.18 mg/kg/day) may optimize growth, and linear growth can be maximized by maintaining optimal allograft function. Alternate-day steroid therapy has been associated with improved growth velocity. However, not all authors have found a relationship between glomerular filtration rate, ADT dose and post-transplant growth. Although "catch up" growth rarely occurs, linear growth can be maximized by utilizing ADT and performing transplantation at a younger age.

Puberty

The changes associated with puberty proceed following a successful transplant. In female pubertal recipients, menses return within a year following transplant. In males, genital maturation lags significantly behind chronologic and bone age. The pituitary testicular axis has been found to be normal when good renal function is restored. Androgen production is decreased, possibly due to corticosteroid administration. Exogenous androgen therapy should be considered in those male recipients with marked pubertal delay so long as bone age is acceptable and epiphyses are not closed.

Long-Term Outcome

In pediatric living related transplantation, 5-year allograft survival rate ranges from 55 to 73%, and 10-year graft survival rate ranges between 55 and 74%. The outcome for cadaveric survival rate, however, is less satisfactory, ranging from 39 to 43% at 5 years and from 31 to 44% at 10 years. Despite adequate function for 5 years, indolent chronic rejection (due to immunologic attack) probably occurs in most pediatric recipients. The results of long-term kidney transplantation, therefore, are as dependent on the outcome of immune factors as they are on the experience of the physician and the transplant center. Similarly, considering the age at which children receive renal transplants, the possibility that more than one renal transplant will be needed in order to achieve prolonged survival is great.

Hemolytic-Uremic Syndrome

ANTONIA C. NOVELLO, M.D., M.P.H.

Hemolytic-uremic syndrome (HUS) is a disorder of infancy and childhood. The syndrome is seen principally in pre–school-aged children, affecting males and females with equal frequency. The central lesion seems to be vascular endothelial damage, especially to the kidneys, yet other organs and tissues (the liver, brain, heart, pancreatic islet cells, and muscles) may also be involved. New insights into the pathogenesis of HUS point toward an inherited or acquired perturbation in prostacyclin metabolism.

Failure to recognize the heterogeneous nature of HUS and to distinguish the different predisposing factors has made advances in therapy difficult. Although no specific treatment exists, many therapeutic strategies have been attempted: heparin and other anticoagulants, steroids, exchange transfusion, fresh plasma, plasmapheresis, splenectomy, antithrombin III, prostacyclin, streptokinase, urokinase, aspirin, and dipyridamole. The most important treatment, however, is vigorous supportive care.

The prognosis in HUS appears to be related to signs and symptoms present early in the course of the disease. The most influential are the presence of hypertension, the duration of oliguria, and the severity of the central nervous system (CNS) symptoms. Prognosis is better with early diagnosis and with rapid and appropriate management. The value of dialysis, the therapy of choice, in the face of renal insufficiency cannot be overestimated. Dialytic treatment should be performed during the oliguric phase. It is also currently used as an adjunct to therapy to maintain a reasonable level of nutrition in cases of prolonged oliguria.

The general picture in HUS is of a nonspecific infectious disease, with a moderate degree of fever, malaise, irritability, vomiting, and slight diarrhea. The stools are watery and contain mucus and clumps of filaments of coagulated blood. Melena is found in 60% of patients and hematemesis in 20%. Colicky abdominal pain, which at times has prompted surgical exploration before the diagnosis is apparent, is common. The diarrhea is usually not severe enough to cause dehydration. Bowel rest, stool cultures to detect enteric pathogens, and fluid and electrolyte replacement are all that is usually required. Other forms of therapy do not alter the course of the disease and at times might be frankly contraindicated.

The associated pallor, vomiting, rectal blood, and abdominal tenderness in HUS are sources of confusion that have led to unnecessary surgical explorations. The presence of subserosal extravasations of blood in the operating field has further confused the picture. No excision of colon is advocated since colonic recovery is complete. It is important to remember that colonic symptoms are potential early findings in the patient with HUS, occurring prior to the onset of thrombocytopenia and hemolytic anemia. Other minor associated findings, such as hepatosplenomegaly, hepatocellular involvement, and acute diabetes mellitus, have been described. These usually disappear when the acute phase of the disease abates.

HEMATOLOGIC INVOLVEMENT

Patients have evidence of an acute, Coombs'-negative hemolytic anemia with red blood cell fragmentation and thrombocytopenia. The high plasma hemoglobin level, hemoglobinuria, and depressed haptoglobin level are indicative of the intravascular nature of the hemolysis. The anemia can last for a time and might necessitate transfusion if the patient is symptomatic. The goal is to keep the hematocrit level above 16–18%.

In nearly every case of HUS there is marked thrombocytopenia, with a mean platelet count of 75,000/cu mm (range, 16,000–175,000/cu mm). The half-life of the platelets is diminished as the result of increased platelet consumption and decreased platelet production. In patients with severe clinical involvement, recovery from thrombocytopenia may be irregular.

Although coagulation abnormalities have been demonstrated, there is little rationale for anticoagulation therapy. Until recently, heparin had been the most commonly used agent. The action of antithrombin III (which neutralizes activated coagulation factors) is known to be accelerated by heparin. The intravenous administration of heparin in patients with HUS is known to further reduce the levels of antithrombin III. It has been shown that once heparin administration is stopped the antithrombin III concentration may be too low to neutralize activated clotting enzymes. However, at present the use of antithrombin III in an uncontrolled fashion is not indicated.

Streptokinase and urokinase have been used to activate plasminogens, which induce lysis of intravascular clots, but there is no convincing evidence that the mortality rate or the degree of residual renal functional impairment is reduced by this treatment. A single study suggests a late beneficial effect on proteinuria and hypertension. Although some reports suggest that dipyridamole is effective, others have shown that it fails to attenuate the clinical course. Corticosteroids, on the other hand, increase blood coagulability and tend to aggravate azotemia. They are contraindicated in the treatment of HUS. Thus, there is no evidence that intervention with the previously mentioned anticoagulants, including aspirin, has any effect on the short-term outcome of HUS. The long-term benefits of such therapy have not been determined.

Recently, vitamin E has been used in the treatment of HUS, and patients so treated have done well even in the presence of adverse prognostic features. Before such treatment is advocated, however, more controlled trials are needed.

RENAL INVOLVEMENT

Renal injury occurs along with anemia and other disease manifestations. Acute renal failure (ARF) is present in over 90% of patients. Prolonged oliguria can persist for an average of 2 weeks (range, 4–47 days) and often necessitates dialysis. All complications of acute renal insufficiency are found, including hypervolemia, cardiac failure, hyperkalemia, hyperuricemia, metabolic acidosis, hypocalcemia, and hypertension. Bilateral renal cortical necrosis develops in some patients. Since most fatalities are due to these complications, early diagnosis and careful managment are indicated.

The initial supportive measures for most children are those used in the management of ARF. In a few cases, a team well versed in intensive care and dialysis techniques is required. Children need close observation and specific therapy for anemia, bleeding, heart failure, and ARF. Fluid replacement may be required and must be calculated with great care. Severe anemia should be corrected by using small packed-cell transfusions. Urine output should be monitored; if it falls below 200 ml, a treatment plan appropriate for ARF should be initiated. Dialysis should be considered when intractable hypertension, cardiac failure, pulmonary edema, hyperkalemia, metabolic acidosis, uremic symptoms, or hyponatremia does not respond to conservative management.

Two other aspects of the management of ARF in pediatric patients with HUS deserve special attention: hypertension and nutritional support. HUS frequently renders the patient anorectic and thus catabolic. Healing and repair of the kidney require adequate caloric intake and energy metabolism. Thus, a minimum of 20–30 cal/kg/day as carbohydrate and/or lipid is needed to minimize tissue breakdown. As much as 60% of the usual daily requirement may be necessary to reduce endogenous urea nitrogen generation. If dialysis is initiated, these dietary and fluid and electrolyte restrictions can be relaxed. Arterial hypertension is found in one-third of patients and may be secondary to fluid overload (or more vascular with left ventricular failure), hypertensive encephalopathy, and signs of hypertensive vascular damage to the kidneys, i.e., malignant hypertension. Hypertension may also compromise recovery from HUS. If it does not respond to usual volume-depleting maneuvers, hyperreninemia is likely, requiring therapy with propranolol or captopril. Other initial supportive measures used in the acute phase of HUS do not differ from those utilized for severe cases of ARF and discussed in Warren Grupes' chapter on HUS in the eleventh edition.

NEUROLOGIC INVOLVEMENT

Nearly all patients manifest signs of involvement of the CNS. In about half the patients, these signs are mild, consisting of somnolence, irritability, jerking, and ataxia. However, generalized convulsions, focal neurologic signs, and deep coma may occur. Seizures in the patient with HUS should be treated with diazepam in the acute phase and with phenytoin for the longer term. Hypertensive encephalopathy, however, is managed with diazoxide and fluid balance in the acute stages and propranolol* or other chronic antihypertensive drugs over the long term.

PROGNOSIS

The immediate prognosis is dependent on the severity of ARF and the extent of injury to the CNS. More than 90% of patients with HUS recover following careful management of the renal complications. With early recognition and improved technology for the treatment of ARF, mortality has declined, although it remains between 10 and 20%. The incidence of progression to chronic renal failure appears to be under 6%. Residual mortality may well be related to the severity of the nonrenal involvement. The prognosis is poor with prolonged anuria, oliguria, malignant hypertension, and CNS involvement, in the absence of prodrome, when the patient is more than 5 years old,

---

* Safety and efficacy for the use of propranolol have not been established.

and in cases of recurrent disease. Persistent proteinuria, hypertension, or reduced creatinine clearance occur in 6–20% of cases. In a few patients bilateral renal cortical necrosis may necessitate prolonged dialysis and transplantation. Renal transplantation is successful in the majority of patients, despite rare recurrences of HUS.

Perinephric and Intranephric Abscess

FRED G. SMITH, JR., M.D.

The conventional therapeutic approach for intranephric and perinephric abscess includes both parenteral antibiotics and surgical drainage. Selected cases, especially small renal cortical abscesses (less than 3 cm), may be treated effectively with appropriate parenteral doses of antibiotics without surgical drainage. If the child is treated with antibiotics alone and is not improving within 3–5 days, surgical drainage should be performed. Successful antibiotic treatment is usually indicated by defervescence of the fever, leukocytosis, and a decrease in the size of the abscess, which is determined by ultrasound studies. Large renal abscesses, especially those in the corticomedullary area, and perinephric abscesses should be treated with both surgical drainage and parenteral antibiotics.

Since the spectrum of pathogens causing perinephric and intranephric abscesses includes both gram-negative rods and staphylococci, intravenous doses of methicillin (100–200 mg/kg/24 hr q 6 hr) and intravenous or intramuscular doses of gentamicin (3–7.5 mg/kg/24 hr q 8 hr) should be given until the organism and its sensitivities are determined.

When the child has a history of a hypersensitivity reaction to penicillin, vancomycin (40 mg/kg/24 hr q 6 hr) or a cephalosporin may be substituted for methicillin.

In general, antibiotics should be administered parenterally for 14 days; these are followed by oral doses of antibiotics for an additional 2–4 weeks, depending on the resolution of the abscess as determined by follow-up ultrasound studies.

Urinary Tract Infections

FRED G. SMITH, JR., M.D.

The presumptive diagnosis of urinary tract infection must be confirmed by a urine culture. The child who presents for the first time with symptoms of urinary tract infection (dysuria, frequency, or urgency) without fever may be treated with either oral sulfisoxazole* (150–200 mg/kg/24 hr four times a day), co-trimoxazole* (6–12 mg/kg/24 hr of trimethoprim and 30–60 mg/kg/24 hr of sulfamethoxazole twice daily), or ampicillin (50–100 mg/kg/24 hr four times a day). With the first infection, I prefer to use sulfisoxazole because of its low cost, palatability, and relative safety. Therapy should always be guided by organism susceptibility studies. At this time, it appears that roughly 20–30% of *Escherichia coli* commonly seen in urinary tract infections will be resistant to sulfonamides, tetracycline, ampicillin, and oral cephalosporins. These drugs are nevertheless very useful and may be tried for several episodes provided follow-up cultures are obtained following cessation of therapy. In addition, if there is a question about the initial response, a urine culture should be obtained after 2–3 days of treatment. Dip slide cultures (such as Uricult) are an accurate, sensitive, convenient, and inexpensive way to monitor infection. Therapy should be continued for 10–14 days. At present I feel that children should not be treated with a single-day dose of amoxicillin or sulfonamide.

The child with clinical evidence of urinary tract infection accompanied by fever or other signs of renal parenchymal involvement (flank pain, tenderness, vomiting, or other signs of toxicity) should be admitted to the hospital. Urine and blood cultures should be obtained and intravenous ampicillin should be given for a minimum of 48 hours (100–200 mg/kg/24 hr every 4–6 hr). Usually the child's signs, symptoms, and fever defervesce within 36 hours, and if the organism is sensitive to the antibiotic he or she can be discharged after 48 hours and oral therapy continued at home for an additional 10 days. Again, a culture should be performed 3–5 days after discontinuing therapy. I also repeat a urine culture (Uricult) at monthly intervals for 3 months and then at 3-month intervals for the next 6 months to identify children with asymptomatic bacteriuria.

ASYMPTOMATIC BACTERIURIA

Asymptomatic children discovered to have significant bacteriuria on a screening quantitative urine culture (greater than 100,000 colonies/ml) should be treated in a manner similar to children with uncomplicated symptomatic urinary tract infections. It has been shown that young school-aged girls with significant bacteriuria will go into long-term remission after each treatment. Since there is a high recurrence rate of infection in females (70–80%), follow-up cultures are also important in this group.

---

* Contraindicated in infants younger than 2 months of age.

URINARY TRACT INFECTIONS IN THE NEWBORN

All newborn infants with suspected or proved urinary tract infection should have blood and urine culture specimens obtained prior to the initiation of therapy. Urine for culture should be collected by a suprapubic bladder tap. Ampicillin (100–200 mg/kg/24 hr q 6 hr) plus kanamycin* (15–30 mg/kg/24 hr) or gentamicin (3–7.5 mg/kg/24 hr) should be given parenterally because septicemia may occur in association with urinary tract infection and antibiotic absorption after oral administration may be erratic in neonates. Therapy should be continued for 10–14 days and a repeat urine culture performed 5–7 days after discontinuing treatment.

All newborns with documented urinary tract infection should have an intravenous pyelogram (IVP) and voiding cystourethrogram (VCUG) studies. Ultrasound studies of the kidney also provide a rapid noninvasive method to determine whether obstruction is present. If obstruction is present, a urology consultation should be obtained.

FOLLOW-UP EVALUATION

There is some controversy regarding the radiologic evaluation of the female child following the successful treatment of the first uncomplicated urinary tract infection; however, most authorities agree that following a documented urinary tract infection in the male both an IVP and VCUG should be performed. Recently, it has been our policy to perform IVP and VCUG following the first infection in all female children, primarily because of the high recurrence rate (70–80%) and the prevalence of vesicoureteric reflux (35–50%). Radiologic evaluation is especially important in the female child under 5 years of age because of the higher incidence of renal scarring in this age group. If there are associated anomalies or if moderate to severe vesicoureteric reflux (greater than Grade II) is discovered, a urology consultation should be obtained.

RECURRENT URINARY TRACT INFECTIONS AND VESICOURETERIC REFLUX

There is a group of female children without congenital anomalies of the genitourinary tract or vesicoureteric reflux who have recurrent urinary tract infections. Even though these children have less risk of upper tract injury, we feel they should receive long-term antimicrobial suppression. It is our policy to treat this group of children with nitrofurantoin† (2.5 mg/kg), co-trimoxazole‡ (tri-

methoprim, 6 mg/kg; sulfamethoxazole, 30 mg/kg), or cephalexin (25 mg/kg) given as a single dose at bedtime after emptying the bladder. After suppressive therapy is discontinued, a urine culture should be obtained in 5–7 days, then monthly for 3 months and every 3 months for an additional 6 months.

Children with vesicoureteric reflux, especially those with high-grade reflux or intrarenal reflux, are at great risk for renal injury. Therefore, long-term antimicrobial prophylaxis should be maintained as outlined. It is well recognized that reflux ceases in a high percentage of children (70–80%) with Grade 1 to II reflux if they are maintained free of infection. However, children with reflux who continue to have urinary tract infections in spite of suppressive antimicrobial therapy should be seen by a urologist for consideration of ureteral reimplantation. Constant monitoring of compliance in the administration of the antibiotic is also exceedingly important.

COMPLICATED URINARY TRACT INFECTIONS

Children with urinary tract obstruction, indwelling catheters, neurogenic bladder, or nephrostomy tubes pose difficult problems and usually do not respond to antibiotic therapy unless the complication is corrected. These children are at high risk for progressive renal scarring from infection, hypertension, defects in concentrating capacity, and renal failure.

Urolithiasis

F. BRUDER STAPLETON, M.D.

The problem of urolithiasis is being recognized with increasing frequency during childhood. Often children are faced with a future of repeated stone episodes unless specific preventative measures are undertaken. Fortunately, fewer than 50% of children with urolithiasis present with renal colic, although pain may be disabling at times. When stone-related colic is present, aggressive analgesic therapy is mandated. All children with urolithiasis in our center have had either microscopic or macroscopic hematuria at the time of detection.

Determination of the pathogenesis may allow specific therapy to prevent recurrent urinary stones. Regardless of the etiology of stone formation, the medical management of any child with urolithiasis requires that he or she ingest a large volume of dilute fluids to maintain a hypotonic diuresis in order to prevent supersaturation of the urine with lithogenic salts. Patients should be instructed to drink a large glass at bedtime and once during the night. In addition to maintaining diu-

---

* The dosage of 30 mg/kg/day is higher than that recommended by the manufacturer.
† Manufacturer's warning: Nitrofurantoin is contraindicated in children under 1 month of age.
‡ Contraindicated in infants younger than 2 months of age.

resis, specific measures to reduce urine excretion of crystalloids or to increase the solubility of urinary constituents have been extremely successful in reducing stone formation in our pediatric population with urolithiasis.

In the southern United States, metabolic abnormalities account for approximately 60% of urinary calculi in children. Increased urinary calcium excretion (hypercalciuria) is now recognized to account for 70% of these metabolic stones. Hypercalciuria is defined as a urinary calcium excretion greater than 4 mg/kg/24 hours. Idiopathic hypercalciuria with normal serum calcium concentration may result from a renal tubular defect in calcium reabsorption (renal hypercalciuria) or from excessive gastrointestinal absorption of dietary calcium (absorptive hypercalciuria). In children with renal hypercalciuria, hydrochlorothiazide at a dose of 2 mg/kg/day reduces urinary calcium excretion to normal values and reduces stone activity. In addition, a low-sodium diet is recommended, since urinary calcium excretion is related to sodium excretion and extracellular fluid volume expansion increases calcium excretion. Dietary calcium restriction is not recommended in patients with renal hypercalciuria, as it may result in negative calcium balance. Absorptive hypercalciuria, on the other hand, may be managed with dietary calcium restriction alone, although hydrochlorothiazide therapy may also be necessary in some patients. Therapy with cellulose phosphate has been advocated for some adults with a form of absorptive hypercalciuria. Cellulose phosphate is expensive, may result in secondary hyperparathyroidism, and is not recommended for use in children. Secondary hypercalciuria resulting in urolithiasis may occur from conditions such as hyperparathyroidism, immobilization, and metabolic acidosis or from pharmacologic agents such as furosemide. Whenever possible, the underlying abnormality should be corrected; however, in some instances, hydrochlorothiazide may be helpful.

Primary hyperoxaluria is a severe metabolic disorder that leads not only to recurrent urolithiasis but also to renal failure early in life. Normal urinary oxalate excretion is less than 50 mg/24 hours/1.73m^2 body surface area. Urinary oxalate excretion may be reduced and crystal formation prevented by aggressive medical management. As in all types of urolithiasis, maintaining a high urine flow rate is important. Dietary oxalate intake should be restricted. Hydrochlorothiazide diuretics may be beneficial to reduce urinary calcium excretion as well as to increase urine flow rate. Pyridoxine, 200 mg/day for children under 20 kg and 500 mg/day for children over 20 kg, may reduce oxalate production. Oral phosphate therapy with sodium or potassium phosphate solutions decreases calcium oxalate crystallization. Phosphate may be given in increasing doses until either diarrhea occurs or serum phosphate exceeds 5 mg/dl. Magnesium gluconate is given in an initial dose of 65 mg twice daily for children under 10 kg, 125 mg twice daily for children 10–20 kg, and 250 mg twice daily for children over 20 kg. This dose should be gradually increased to two to four times the initial dose in order to increase urinary magnesium excretion and decrease calcium oxalate crystal formation.

Uric acid stones account for 5% of the cases of urolithiasis in children in our clinics. Total uric acid excretion varies with age in children but is normally less than 0.56 mg/100 ml of glomerular filtrate. Urate calculi may be the result of hyperuricemia or renal hyperuricosuria. When hyperuricemia is present, allopurinol therapy at a dose of 5–10 mg/kg/day is given to reduce serum uric acid levels. Certain factors are known to increase uric acid precipitation. These include a low urine pH and a high urinary concentration. Urinary alkalinization with either sodium bicarbonate or sodium citrate increases urate solubility and may dissolve uric acid stones. Sufficient alkali should be given to maintain a urine pH greater than 8.

Cystinuria is a rare autosomal recessive disorder characterized by increased urinary excretion of the dibasic amino acids, cystine, lysine, arginine, and ornithine. A small number of patients with cystinuria may present with calcium oxalate urinary calculi. Normal individuals excrete less than 60 mg of cystine/day/1.73 m^2 body surface area. The mainstay of medical management is high fluid intake to reduce the urinary cystine concentration below 200 mg/l. Urinary alkalinization is important in the management of cystinuria. Sufficient alkali should be given to maintain a urine pH greater than 8. Approximately 35% of children with cystinuria may be successfully managed with fluid and base therapy. The remainder will require D-penicillamine to complex cystine and reduce cystine stone formation. D-Penicillamine is associated with hematologic, hepatic, gastrointestinal, and renal toxicity.

In approximately 10% of children urolithiasis is a result of infection of the urinary tract. Antibiotics may be given to provide prophylaxis against urinary infection. Adult patients at high risk for infectious calculi have been successfully managed with urease inhibitors such as acetohydroxamic acid. Unfortunately, urease inhibitors are not yet approved for urolithiasis in children.

A thorough evaluation fails to uncover a diagnosis in 10–15% of children with urolithiasis. To prevent repeated calculus formation, a large fluid intake is indicated. When recurrent calculi occur, addition of hydrochlorothiazide at a dose of 2 mg/kg/day may be helpful.

When a calculus is present in the urinary tract,

management requires determination of the degree of obstruction with excretory urography or, occasionally, computerized tomography. Surgical therapy is indicated when colic persists or when diuresis fails to move stones and relieve obstruction. A number of innovative and less invasive urologic therapies have been developed to supplement traditional nephro- or ureterolithotomy. Some of these new procedures are percutaneous endouroscopy, direct chemolysis, electrohydrolytic lithotripsy, ultrasonic lithotripsy, and extracorporeal shock wave therapy. Most of these techniques have not been applied to children; however, percutaneous endouroscopy has been successful in older children. Lower ureteral or bladder stones may be removed by a cystoureteroscope.

Vesicoureteral Reflux

TERRY W. HENSLE, M.D.
and KEVIN A. BURBIGE, M.D.

The understanding and management of vesicoureteral reflux (VUR) continues to stir controversy, as evidenced by the ever expanding literature. The prevalence of silent VUR in the general population is probably on the order of 0.5%. However, it may be detected in up to 30% of children undergoing urologic evaluation for recurrent urinary tract infection and in up to 25% of their siblings. Infection, then, would seem to be the marker for identifying a population at risk.

Abnormalities of the normal passive valve mechanism of the ureterovesical junction that predispose the patient to VUR include a deficiency of the longitudinal muscle layer of the submucosal ureter (short tunnel), an ectopic insertion of the ureter into the bladder, and deficient muscular support of the submucosal ureter (paraureteral diverticulum). The ratio of submucosal tunnel length to ureteral diameter would seem to be the major determinant in preventing VUR. VUR is generally accepted as a primary lesion of the ureterovesical junction and is not due to obstruction at the bladder neck, as was once thought.

The diagnostic tools best suited for detecting VUR and determining its severity are the excretory urogram, the voiding cystourethrogram, and, to a much lesser extent, cystoscopy. The radionuclide cystogram is a very adequate means of following VUR once it has been identified on a standard voiding cystourethrogram. The radionuclide study can be done with much less radiation exposure but cannot be used to quantify VUR initially. Radiologic evaluation of the child with a history of urinary tract infection is best done when the urine is sterile after antibiotic treatment. The degree of VUR is characterized by a grading system (Table 1).

Table 1. VESICOURETERAL REFLUX GRADING SYSTEM

Grade I— VUR into the lower ureter only
Grade II— ureteral and pelvic filling without caliceal dilatation
Grade III—ureteral and pelvic filling with mild caliceal blunting
Grade IV—marked distention of pelvis, calices, and ureter
Grade V— massive VUR associated with severe hydronephrosis

The aim of treatment is preservation of renal parenchyma, maintenance of renal function, and elimination of urinary infection. Factors to be considered when planning treatment are the grade of VUR, chronicity of the symptoms, number and severity of infections, presence of anatomic urinary tract abnormalities, and the patient's ability to adhere to a treatment program.

MEDICAL MANAGEMENT

It has yet to be shown that sterile VUR in the absence of increased voiding pressures causes renal damage. Therefore, if medical management is chosen it is extremely important that a sterile urine be achieved and continuous antibiotic prophylaxis be maintained until the VUR has subsided. Children with less than Grade III VUR are usually managed medically, since there is about an 80% probability of spontaneous resolution. As somatic growth progresses, the submucosal ureter will lengthen and VUR will often cease.

During this period of waiting, a sulfamethoxazole/trimethoprim* combination (Bactrim, Septra) or nitrofurantoin (Furadantin)† is most commonly used for prophylaxis, at about half the usual therapeutic dose. In the elixir form these are well tolerated by most children, have a high concentration in the urine and vaginal epithelium, and do not significantly alter bowel flora. In following patients, a urine culture should be obtained every 4 to 8 weeks and can be done at home by a dip slide method. A CBC should be done routinely every 3 months in children suppressed with sulfamethoxazole/trimethoprim in order to detect early signs of bone marrow depression, which is infrequent but must be recognized.

An excretory urogram and voiding cystourethrogram (conventional or radionuclide) should be done once a year to monitor renal growth and persistence or absence of VUR. Adjunctive measures such as good perineal hygiene and a frequent voiding schedule may also help to prevent lower tract infection in the female child who is an infre-

---

*Manufacturer's warning: Not recommended for children less than 2 months of age.

†Manufacturer's warning: Not recommended for children less than 1 month of age.

quent voider. Repetitive cystoscopy, meatotomy, urethral dilatation, and internal urethrotomy should be avoided unless significant pathology can be demonstrated radiologically and on urodynamic evaluation.

SURGICAL TREATMENT

The major indications for antireflux surgery are the presence of a significant anatomic abnormality at the ureterovesical junction, recurrent urinary tract infection despite continuous antibiotic therapy, high grades of VUR, noncompliance with medical therapy, intolerance to antibiotics, and VUR after puberty in the female. Children with high grades of VUR and dilated ureters due to VUR (grades IV and V) have only a 40% probability of spontaneous cessation of their VUR. Surgical intervention is generally required earlier in this group than in children with a lesser degree of VUR.

The Cohen cross trigone and Politano-Leadbetter methods of ureteral reimplantation are the most reliable and most often performed antireflux procedures. Creation of an adequate submucosal tunnel can be accomplished by either procedure; the success rate is over 97% when done by surgeons with appropriate pediatric urologic experience.

Cystitis may occur in approximately 20% of children following antireflux surgery but pyelonephritis is rare. Postoperatively antibiotics are continued until a voiding cystourethrogram demonstrates a successful result with no further VUR. Excretory urograms are done prior to discharge from the hospital, and at 3 months, 1 year, and 3 years after surgery to assess renal growth. Interestingly, accelerated renal growth may be observed in some children after successful surgery.

The medical and surgical managements of VUR are not competitive, and there are clear indications for each. The goal is the same, to protect renal parenchyma and maintain renal function.

Neurogenic Bladder

KEVIN A. BURBIGE, M.D.
and TERRY W. HENSLE, M.D.

Neuropathic voiding dysfunction in childhood can be secondary to many different primary etiologies (Table 1); in general, however, myelomeningocele is the most common cause in children. Our treatment approach is based on the myelodysplastic child; however, the general principles are applicable to most forms of neurogenic bladder. Experience has proved that a coordinated multidisciplinary effort by the pediatrician, neurosurgeon, orthopedist, and urologist will provide the best overall care for the myelodysplastic child. Just

Table 1. VOIDING DYSFUNCTION IN CHILDREN

Neurological
    Myelomeningocele
    Sacral agenesis
    Spinal cord trauma
    Spinal cord tumors
    CNS tumors
    Spinal dysraphism
    CNS inflammation
Functional
    Enuresis
    Non-neurogenic neurogenic bladder
    Urinary tract infection
Anatomic
    Exstrophy
    Severe epispadias
    Posterior urethral valves
    Lower urinary tract trauma
    Urethral stricture

as critical is the presence of nursing and support personnel specifically skilled in the care of these patients. The goals of urologic treatment of the myelodysplastic child are basically three: preservation of renal function, control of urinary tract infection, and socially acceptable urinary continence.

The bony abnormality of myelomeningocele occurs most commonly in the lumbosacral region (80%) but the level of neurologic impairment may vary. A differential growth rate of the bony somites and developing vertebral arches in relation to the neural tube accounts for the apparent foreshortening of the spinal cord in the developing fetus with myelomeningocele. Nerves at or below the level of the bony defect are generally most affected, but owing to this differential growth rate, proximal nerve root damage may also occur. Most children with myelomeningocele will have a lower motor neuron lesion of the bladder (detrusor hyporeflexia), although an upper motor neuron lesion (detrusor hyperreflexia) is seen in almost 30%.

The urologic evaluation of the myelodysplastic child should begin in the neonatal period, and should include a urinalysis, urine culture, and renal function studies as well as an excretory urogram or renal ultrasonography. The vast majority of these babies will have normal renal function and normal appearing urinary tracts by either imaging technique. Careful follow-up at regular intervals will facilitate early detection of renal deterioration; therefore, repeat excretory urography or ultrasonography should be done at 6 months of age and then yearly until age 10 years, when follow-up should be individualized. A voiding cystourethrogram should be part of the evaluation if there is a history of urinary infection, and probably should be performed in all myelodysplastic children along with the annual upper tract studies in order to assess bladder configuration and emptying.

Urodynamic testing may provide important information relative to bladder management in the child with a neurogenic bladder. This testing should include measurement of intravesical pressure during filling and voiding (cystometrogram phase) as well as simultaneous measurement of urinary flow rate (uroflow) and electromyography of the external urinary sphincter. These studies combined with measurement of a urethral pressure profile constitute a full urodynamic evaluation. The goal of urodynamic testing is to identify neuromuscular abnormalities not readily definable by routine neurologic examination or standard radiographic evaluation.

Simply stated, the bladder has two primary functions, urine storage and urine emptying, and both can be adversely affected in myelodysplastic children. In order to facilitate urine emptying, several options are available. In some few infants and young children the Credé maneuver, manual expression of bladder urine by suprapubic pressure, may be effective. Credé, however, has inherent drawbacks, and if post-Credé residuals become elevated or if there are signs of upper tract deterioration, another method should be selected. Credé is definitely contraindicated in the presence of vesicoureteral reflux or if significant outlet resistance is present. Just as outmoded are medications such as bethanechol chloride (Urecholine), which have been used to facilitate bladder emptying and have proved to be of little benefit in the hyporeflexic bladder.

Clean intermittent catheterization is the single most important advance in bladder emptying and has largely altered the treatment of children with neuropathic voiding dysfunction secondary to myelomeningocle. The bladder is emptied at regular intervals by means of a small caliber catheter, using a clean but not sterile technique. Clean intermittent catheterization is a simple and straightforward procedure easily performed by the parent or child, and urine sterility can be monitored on a routine basis by an inexpensive home culture method.

In terms of urine storage, adjunctive pharmacologic therapy is usually required to facilitate continence, and the use of these drugs should be based on both clinical and urodynamic findings. If uninhibited bladder contractures (hyper-reflexia) are producing incontinence, an anticholinergic medicine (Pro-Banthine, Ditropan) may be helpful. When outlet resistance is low, an alpha adrenergic agent (Ornade, ephedrine) may increase outlet resistance. If continued incontinence is due to poor bladder emptying (overflow) or there is an upper tract dilatation, then clean intermittent catheterization is indicated in association with the use of these drugs. These medications, used alone or in combination with clean intermittent catheterization, will in most cases produce a reasonable degree of continence. Low dose prophylactic antibiotics are often added to the regimen; however, their use is not universally advocated. Procedures designed to lower bladder outlet resistance, such as transurethral resection of the bladder neck, sphincterotomy, and overdilatation of the urethra, should be avoided since they may damage whatever continence mechanism is present.

In general, urinary incontinence is no longer an absolute indication for permanent urinary diversion. In selected instances diversion by means of a nonrefluxing color or ileocecal conduit may be required if clean intermittent catheterization is not technically feasible or upper tract deterioration continues despite appropriate conservative therapy. Temporary urinary diversion may be a reasonable alternative in a very young infant until the age of expected continence, when clean intermittent catheterization can be instituted, and cutaneous vesicostomy is probably the best method for this temporary diversion.

In summary, the urologic care of the child with neuropathic bladder dysfunction requires a thorough evaluation including clinical, radiologic, and urodynamic modalities. Follow-up evaluation is lifelong and therapy is directed at the preservation of renal function, the control of urinary infection, and establishing socially acceptable urinary continence.

Exstrophy of the Bladder

STEPHEN A. KRAMER, M.D.,
and PANAYOTIS P. KELALIS, M.D.

Bladder exstrophy is essentially always associated with complete epispadias. Surgical reconstruction in both male and female patients requires a planned and multistaged approach. The primary goal of surgical reconstruction in patients with exstrophy is to achieve complete urinary continence. In males, the establishment of a straight penis of adequate length, which is functional for normal sexual intercourse, is equally important. Factors critical to the achievement of complete continence include age of the patient at the time of operation, bladder capacity, and maturation of the prostate at puberty in boys.

Neonatal bladder closure is the preferred treatment of choice. In children seen within the first 48 hours of life, the bladder can be closed primarily without groin flaps or iliac osteotomies. The presence of circulating maternal hormones allows the pelvis to be approximated anteriorly at this early age.

It is desirable to complete the repair of bladder exstrophy before school age. Essentially all patients with exstrophy have vesicoureteral reflux and will require antireflux surgery. This should be accomplished in combination with vesical neck reconstruction in an attempt to produce urinary continence. These procedures are usually performed at $2\frac{1}{2}$ to 3 years of age. Penile elongation with release of dorsal chordee is performed as a separate procedure around 4 years of age. Six to twelve months thereafter, a neourethra is constructed to advance the urinary meatus to the glans tip.

In females, urethroplasty, approximation of the bifid clitoris, and mons plasty are accomplished at the time of the anti-incontinence procedure. Vaginoplasty is deferred until puberty. In both boys and girls, rotational skin flaps are necessary to improve the cosmetic appearance and distribution of hair in the suprapubic area.

In patients seen after the first week of life, bilateral iliac osteotomy is often required to achieve satisfactory bladder closure. Alternatively, if the bladder is not satisfactory for primary closure because of its small size or fibrosis, a temporary urinary diversion should be performed. We prefer a nonrefluxing colon conduit or nonrefluxing ileocecal conduit to prevent the deleterious effects of long-term vesicoureteral reflux. Ureterosigmoidostomy is an excellent choice to avoid a urinary stoma, provided that there is no anal prolapse and that fecal control is normal. It is important to note that the incidence of adenocarcinoma of the colon at the site of the ureterosigmoid anastomosis ranges between 5% and 8% in patients followed long-term. A sigmoidosigmoidostomy (end-to-side) or ileocecal sigmoidostomy avoids the mixing of urine and feces and may prevent the development of colonic cancer.

In selected patients with small bladder capacities, the temporary cutaneous diversion can be "undiverted" using an ileocecal cystoplasty, cecocystoplasty, or colocystoplasty. Even in patients who have undergone prior cystectomy, bladder substitution procedures, particularly with the ileocecal segment, can be used to replace the bladder; urinary continence then often requires placement of an artificial genitourinary sphincter.

It is imperative to follow the integrity of the upper tracts closely, as any deterioration would indicate the need to abandon efforts at achieving continuity of the urinary tract in favor of an antirefluxing intestinal diversion.

Patent Urachus and Urachal Cysts

FRANK HINMAN, JR., M.D.

The urachus, important in embryonic life, usually degenerates into a 5-cm cord containing an almost completely obliterated lumen. "Almost" is the key to urologic disorders. Should the lumen remain intact, patent urachus results. This is a disorder of the neonate, in whom the bladder has yet to descend fully and the mature urachal cord has not been fully formed. Should the lumen persist in some parts of the cord, the lining may degenerate and become colonized with bacteria, forming an infected urachal cyst or opening to the bladder or umbilicus as a urachal sinus. These are diseases of the adult.

Treatment is excision through a vertical midline incision, with care to include the opening into the umbilicus, and closure of the bladder in two layers with postoperative maintenance of catheter drainage. The sites of infected cysts must be drained postoperatively.

Disorders of the Bladder and Prostate

JOHN W. DUCKETT, M.D.

MALIGNANT TUMORS

Uroepithelial Tumors. These tumors are universally of low grade and stage and rarely recur. They are rare in the second decade and even rarer in the first but have occurred as early as 5 years of age. They may be resected transurethrally, fulgurating the base. They require periodic endoscopic reevaluation for several years but then have a benign course.

Rhabdomyosarcoma. Genitourinary rhabdomyosarcomas comprise 27% of all rhabdomyosarcomas; the incidence is approximately 1.2/100,000 children/year. There is a 3:1 male to female predominance. Approximately one-third of pelvic rhabdomyosarcomas arise in the prostate and bladder, while another 25% arise in the uterus and vagina. The remainder arise from the pelvis and grow intraperitoneally as a mass lesion with no specific site of origin.

By far the most common cell type is *embryonal rhabdomyosarcoma*. The *botryoid sarcoma* is a subtype of embryonal rhabdomyosarcoma that lies submucosally with a papillary component. This is commonly found in the bladder. The *alveolar* type is more common in the older child and carries a poor prognosis. It is decidedly more rare than the embryonal type. The *pleomorphic* type is exceedingly rare in children.

In the past the prognosis for these tumors was most discouraging, and radical extirpation was the primary treatment. In recent years, there has been a more encouraging response to vincristine, actinomycin D, and cyclophosphamide treatment, and primary ablative surgery has taken a secondary role.

Currently a tissue diagnosis is made, and the patient is treated with chemotherapy for approximately 2 months. Response of the tumor is monitored. Radiation therapy is added later if the chemotherapeutic response is not satisfactory. Extirpative surgery is used as a last resort to control local tumor, but it is hoped that such surgery is performed before distant metastasis has occurred.

Under this regime, there is approximately a 75% tumor-free survival rate, with maintenance of the bladder or vagina in over 50% of cases.

BENIGN TUMORS

The two benign tumors of the bladder are *hemangiomas* and *neurofibromas*. They usually co-exist with similar tumors in adjacent organs and may be controlled with local excision if symptomatic but otherwise should be left alone.

Polyps of the urethra are seen as hamartomatous growths arising from the verumontanum. They may protrude down the urethra and cause symptoms of outlet obstruction. The polyps may, in addition, float freely into the bladder as a mass lesion. They may be excised with transurethral manipulation or removed through the bladder. Recurrence has not been reported.

Bladder Diverticula

Diverticula of the bladder are congenital anomalies. Most occur at the hiatus of the ureter and are called *periureteral diverticula*. These are most commonly associated with vesicoureteral reflux involving a weak musculature adjacent to the hiatus and a laterally placed orifice. Resolution of reflux in this situation is unlikely but has been reported.

Periureteral detrusor weakness is associated with uninhibited bladder contractions in children with an unstable bladder. These contractions frequently resolve when the bladder is more mature.

Other diverticula may occur in the posterior wall and up to the dome. These may be multiple and generally require excision. They are associated with infection and hematuria. If left until adulthood, they are prone to develop malignancy of a transitional cell type. Bladder diverticula are also associated with outlet obstructions such as posterior and anterior urethral valves.

POSTERIOR URETHRAL VALVES

This is the most common severe obstruction in males. Most instances of this disorder are now being detected in the neonatal period (up to 75%), and early diagnosis is even more likely as prenatal ultrasound becomes prevalent.

Bilateral hydronephrosis with distended bladder is the typical appearance on ultrasound. If the fetus does not demonstrate oligohydramnios, there are no indications for intervention in the prenatal period. In the face of oligohydramnios, poor renal development is likely and bilateral pulmonary hy-

poplasia will prevail. These fetuses have little chance of surviving. Intervention has been accomplished as early as 21 weeks of gestation without altering the ultimate course. There are currently no indications for prenatal drainage procedures or early delivery.

Babies with posterior urethral valves may have a very weak urinary stream with abdominal masses and, especially, an enlarged bladder. Urinary ascites may be the presenting problem with respiratory distress.

If the diagnosis is delayed, the babies present with azotemia, acidosis, and failure to thrive. Infection may occur, with rapid dehydration and deterioration. If the diagnosis is delayed for several weeks to months, failure to thrive, vomiting, irritability, and dehydration may develop.

A stabilization period follows diagnosis. This entails drainage of the bladder with either a suprapubic cystocath or a No. 8 feeding tube through the urethra, control of infection with parenteral antibiotics, correction of acidosis, and electrolyte stabilization.

The valves should be destroyed either by transurethral electrocautery using miniature instruments or by creating a temporary vesicostomy to divert the urine through a vent in the bladder. The vesicostomy decompresses the upper tracts quite nicely, and it is not necessary to do high ureterostomies in the majority of cases. At a later date, the valves can be ablated and the vesicostomy closed.

If there is still renal failure following either drainage of the bladder or relief of the obstruction in the urethra, it is appropriate to perform a renal biopsy and to bring out a high ureterostomy if there is evidence of inadequate decompression. This is a rare occurrence these days.

This child is then followed carefully with a "wait and see" program. Reimplanting ureters and correcting reflux have been shown to complicate the situation more than improve it. These procedures may be appropriate but are better done at a later date for very specific reasons.

The long-term prognosis with valve patients depends on how much damage was done to the kidneys in utero. If, at the time of diagnosis, the creatinine level drops to below 0.8 mg/dl, the prognosis is generally satisfactory. This represents about 50% of glomerular filtration rate corrected for age.

The long-term prognosis of patients with posterior urethral valves who sustained kidney damage in utero is discouraging despite optimal care in the neonatal period; in later life, a significant number will develop chronic renal failure, and need dialysis and transplant. The outcome for many of these children can be predicted at an early age, and the parents can be well prepared for what lies ahead.

There are other subtle and symptomatic problems associated with posterior urethral valves, such as wetting. This incontinence is not uncommon in the years prior to puberty, but after puberty prostatic growth appears to control it quite satisfactorily. Inadequate bladder emptying is occasionally a problem and may require intermittent catheterization or other means of improving voiding. Some children will carry a full bladder that obstructs the upper tracts and require double and triple voiding at least twice daily to empty their entire systems.

About 20% of patients have a functionless kidney that refluxes, requiring a nephrectomy. Bilateral reflux carries a worse prognosis than unilateral reflux or no reflux at all.

ANTERIOR URETHRAL VALVES

These are more appropriately called a diverticulum of the anterior urethra. This is a defect of the spongiosum that creates a valvelike lip of the diverticulum. The condition requires excision or transurethral ablation of the lip. Some of these children have severe upper tract changes.

Congenital Urethral Membrane. This is a variable obstruction in the membranous proximal bulb that acts as a diaphragmatic obstruction. It has an etiology different from that of posterior urethral valves. It may be considered a congenital urethral stricture, but this term should be abolished. Males with this condition have severe upper tract changes.

Prominent Urethral Folds. These are normal folds coming from the verumontanum that may be quite prominent in little boys. They are similar to urethral valves but do not form a fusion anteriorly with an obstructing web. They should not be considered obstructing.

Posterior Urethra Polyps. These hamartomatous benign tumors of the verumontanum may obstruct the outlet and may be removed transurethrally.

Megalourethra. This is a rare lesion most often associated with prune-belly syndrome. There are two types: The *scaphoid* type is a deficiency of the corpus spongiosum that allows ballooning of the urethra during voiding and may be repaired with techniques used for the correction of hypospadias. The *fusiform* type involves a deficiency of the corpora cavernosa, as well as the spongiosum, that results in an elongated flaccid penis with redundant skin. This is usually seen in severe forms of the prune-belly syndrome and may be repaired if the patient survives.

HYPOSPADIAS

This anomaly occurs in a wide spectrum of presentations. There are two basic problems: one is the lack of completion of the urethral folding up to the tip of the penis; the second is chordee, a bending of the penis due to a deficiency on the ventrum with a fibrous replacement. The more severe the defect, the more likely it is that chordee is present. Classification should be based on the location of the meatus after the chordee is released. Under these criteria, 75% of hypospadias is a subcoronal situation and can be managed with a simple meatal advancement and glanuloplasty (MAGPI). Another 10% occur on the penis and may be repaired with a more extensive extension of the urethra to the tip. The other 15% are penoscrotal and more proximal, and these require much more extensive reconstruction.

Management. There are numerous techniques available for repair of hypospadias. The most modern include the MAGPI technique used to correct the simple distal subcoronal meatus, which makes up 70–75% of hypospadias cases. For the more proximally placed urethra, a Mathieu technique may be used with a perimeatal based flap extending the urethra onto the glans. An onlay preputial island flap may be utilized for those without chordee, leaving a distal urethral strip. Finally, the more severe types may be managed with a transverse preputial island flap with vascularized tissue creating the neourethra. Free skin grafts have also been used for this purpose.

Complications. A complication rate of about 10–15% should be expected. Problems include urethral cutaneous fistulas and strictures that require secondary surgical techniques. Other complications are infections, diverticula, and residual chordee.

The currently accepted techniques are one-stage procedures that may be done with short hospital stays and even as outpatient procedures. The earlier age, 6–18 months, is the preferred time for surgery. Microscopic and optical magnification with fine, delicate instruments is currently used.

Other Disorders of the Urethra

Urethral Strictures. A midbulbar urethral stricture is most commonly associated with trauma due to instrumentation or a straddle injury. "Congenital urethral strictures" are not a specific entity. Urethral dilatation for such a diagnosis is inappropriate. A narrowing of the bulbar urethra should not be considered a congenital stricture; there is a common bulbar spasm during a voiding cystogram that gives the appearance of a stricture.

Meatal Stenosis (Males). A narrowed urethral meatus is very common in the circumcised male and does not require meatotomy. A tight web on the ventrum will deflect the urinary stream upward, and a meatotomy is indicated for improvement in stream direction. Very few meatal stenoses create significant obstruction. These are usually an inflammatory replacement of the meatus with balanitis xerotica obliterans.

Meatal Stenosis (Females). "Lyon's ring" is a collagenous area just inside the meatus that is the narrowest spot in the female urethra. For many years it was considered an obstructing problem, and dilatation and fracture were recommended. There are occasional meatal stenoses that require enlargement, but this condition is much rarer than was previously thought.

Prolapse of the Urethra. This occurs predominantly in black girls and causes irritation and bleeding. There is a circumferential eversion of urethral mucosa, which becomes inflamed and should be carefully excised. This condition rarely recurs. Differential diagnoses to be considered are ectopic ureterocele and sarcoma botryoides.

Accessory Urethra. Urethral duplications in boys are usually asymptomatic and appear on the dorsum as an epispadiac extra urethra. More complex channels may be present, and is necessary to excise the accessory channel to correct chordee or troublesome double voiding.

Undescended Testes

ROBERT PENNY, M.D.

During the seventh to ninth months of gestation the testes descend from the abdomen, where they develop, into the scrotum. The 2.2° C lower temperature there as compared with the temperature of the peritoneal cavity permits spermatogenesis. A mass of tissue containing smooth muscle that is attached to the lower pole of the testes, the gubernaculum, assists testicular descent in some poorly understood way. The role played by hormones in facilitating and/or initiating the descent of the testes is unclear. In their journey, the testes remain behind a peritoneal tube, the processus vaginalis. The processus vaginalis is a peritoneal outpocketing that retains a communication with the general peritoneal cavity which projects down through the various muscle and fascial planes before the testis enters the inguinal canal. Normally the upper part of the processus vaginalis atrophies and closes, but if it does not do so, the sac remains as a congenital indirect inguinal hernia; and the lower part of the processus vaginalis is pinched off to form the tunica vaginalis of the testis.

"Ectopic testis" is the term used to described a testis that has progressed normally through the inguinal canal and, after passing through the external inguinal ring, has become lodged in the superficial tissue of the abdominal wall or upper thigh or within the perineum. A hypothesis has been developed explaining ectopic testis on the grounds of encroachment of the developing body wall fascia into the gubernaculum. The incidence of ectopic testis is approximately 0.008%. Ectopic testes can always be easily placed surgically into the scrotal sac, because they all have spermatic cords of sufficient length to permit this. Surgery is indicated when the diagnosis of ectopic testis is established. Published data suggest a very poor prognosis regarding normal spermatogenesis in this disorder.

"Cryptorchidism" is the term used to describe the failure of the testis to descend normally through the inguinal canal. Descent of the testis may be arrested at any point along its normal path. This most often occurs at the external inguinal ring. The cause of undescended testis where mechanical factors are absent is unclear, but disturbance of the hypothalmo-pituitary testicular axis may play a role. At birth, in term infants the incidence of cryptorchidism is 3.4%, and in premature infants it is 30.3%. By one year of age in approximately 75% of the term and premature infants the cryptorchid testes will spontaneously descend. After the first year of age the incidence of cryptorchidism is approximately 0.8%. Finally, the incidence in the post-pubertal male is 0.3 to 0.4%. In about 50% of the patients, undescended testes are right sided, in 20% they are bilateral, and in 30% they are left sided. Inguinal hernias are frequently (57 to 93%) associated with cryptorchidism. These hernias are usually of anatomic rather than clinical importance.

In newborns who present with bilateral undescended testes, congenital adrenal hyperplasia in a female infant must be excluded. This may be done by utilizing ultrasonography to detect the presence or absense of a uterus. If a uterus is present, peripheral blood levels of testosterone and 17-hydroxyprogesterone should be determined to confirm a diagnosis of adrenal hyperplasia.

Usually patients with cryptorchid testes are brought to the physician because the parents have noticed a small scrotum and are concerned about future sexual development. Undescended testicles are rarely a cause of discomfort. Inspection shows that the entire scrotum, or one side of it, is smaller than normal and appears incompletely developed. A slight bulge along some part of the inguinal canal may be revealed by inspection. Most commonly, a gonad can be palpated at the external inguinal ring or along the inguinal canal. An attempt should be made to place the gonad in the scrotum by placing the finger tips at the upper lateral edge of the mass and pushing it obliquely downward toward the scrotum. If the maneuver results in the gonad being placed in the scrotum (as occurs with a retractable or migratory testis), it is at once clear that the testis will eventually lodge in the scrotum spontaneously and will not require medical or surgical therapy. It may be presumed that if gonads cannot be palpated anywhere, the testes are atrophied (bilateral anorchia) or else reside within the abdomen.

A diagnosis of undescended testis or testes should not be made from a single examination, and one should inquire of the parents whether the testis have ever been seen in the scrotum. Elevated serum gonadotropins (which occur with bilateral atrophy of the testes) and/or response to HCG administration (2000 IU per day for 4 days) with serial measurement of serum testosterone levels (an increase of 3- to 12-fold would not occur with bilateral testicular atrophy) will aid in distinguishing bilateral cryptorchidism from atrophied testes.

Orchidopexy is indicated in bilateral undescended testes to provide the best possible chance for fertility, in unilateral undescended testis for possible impaired testosterone secretion, and in both because of the propensity for neoplastic change. The risk of developing a tumor in a cryptorchid testis is 35 times that in the testis that descended normally into the scrotum. Ten per cent of all germinal cell tumors occur in testes that were undescended. Orchidopexy does not decrease the risk of developing a tumor. There is no consensus as to the optimal time for orchidopexy. Published data suggest orchidopexy at between 1 and 2 years of age or between 4 and 5 years of age. The first recommendation is based on a cross-sectional retrospective study indicating that sperm morphology, in adult subjects, was satisfactory in approximately 90% of those who had orchidopexy by 2 years of age, compared with approximately 40–60% in those who had orchidopexy by 5 years of age. The second recommendation is based on histologic, cellular kinetic, psychological, and clinical considerations. At this writing, the author recommends that the time chosen for the performance of orchidopexy be based on the availability of surgical expertise, since technical problems resulting from variation in spermatic cord length can require considerable skill. All subjects, notwithstanding the limited effectiveness of human chorionic gonadotropin (HCG) before 3 years of age, should have a trial of HCG therapy. HCG should be administered at 1500 IU/m^2 IM three times weekly for 3 weeks. Patients should be examined for testicular descent prior to each injection. If testicular descent occurs, though it may be transient, it can be predicted that at puberty permanent descent will occur, and surgery will not be necessary. This dosage schedule should not damage the testes, nor should undesirable androgenic effects occur. A biopsy should be obtained at the time of orchidopexy to evaluate the status of the testis and the possibility of carcinoma in situ. Published data suggest that the prognosis for fertility following orchidopexy in bilateral cryptorchidism is good.

For the unilateral cryptorchid testis, the data suggest that the prognosis for normal spermatogenesis is poor.

Circumcision and Disorders of the Penis and Testis

GEORGE T. KLAUBER, M.D.

PENIS

Circumcision and Penile Hygiene. An uncircumcised penis is a normal penis. Presence of a foreskin and the need for penile hygiene are not considered indications for circumcision and the procedure itself should not be considered "routine." If circumcision is requested for nonreligious reasons, adequate counseling should be a prerequisite; however, when parents strongly favor circumcision, their request should not be denied. Circumcision, if elected, should be performed during the neonatal period in order to obviate the need for general anesthesia.

Normal penile hygiene for the uncircumcised infant penis consists of gentle washing with soap and water. Retraction of the foreskin is not necessary and should be carried out only if it can be performed easily.

Preputial Adhesions. The foreskin is normally adherent to the glans penis in the infant. At birth, such adherence is close to the urethral meatus; gradual separation occurs with time and is usually complete by age 6 to 8 years. The foreskin should not be forcibly retracted in the infant or young child because separation invariably occurs naturally. Forcible retraction may result in splitting the foreskin, with subsequent phimotic scarring. Penile skin bridging is somewhat different; it occurs between the shaft and glans penis. It is a complication of circumcision consisting of epithelialized adhesions that may or may not cover trapped smegma. Sharp dissection under local or general anesthesia is usually required.

Phimosis and Paraphimosis. Phimosis is a narrowing of the foreskin preventing retraction over the glans penis. It is normal in infants and little boys and usually disappears as the child grows and the distal prepuce dilates. Occasionally the preputial opening is narrow enough to obstruct the urinary stream and cause ballooning of the foreskin with voiding. Severe phimosis can be relieved by the Heineke-Mikulicz procedure, dividing the constricting outer preputial skin vertically and suturing transversely. This is an acceptable alternative to a circumcision, which remains the more popular treatment for phimosis.

Paraphimosis occurs when the foreskin is somewhat narrow and after retraction cannot be brought back over the glans penis. Edema occurs secondary to lymphatic obstruction. Reduction of paraphimosis can usually be achieved manually by squeezing the edematous foreskin and rolling it upon itself. If this cannot be carried out, immediate circumcision is the optimum therapy.

Balanitis. Balanitis is an inflammation of the glans penis and the inner aspect of the prepuce in the uncircumcised male, often associated with phimosis. Topical antibiotic ointments will usually cure the acute episode, but occasionally parenteral broad-spectrum antibiotics may be required if severe cellulitis occurs. Circumcision or a dorsal relaxing incision in the foreskin to permit retraction should be considered if balanitis recurs.

Meatal Stenosis. The most common complication of circumcision, meatal stenosis usually presents as a delicate web of epithelium producing a partial obstruction across the inferior portion of the meatus. This causes dorsal deviation of the urinary stream. The web variety of meatal stenosis can be dilated in the office using a forceps and lidocaine (Xylocaine) jelly. Stenosis that does not reduce the caliber of the urinary stream does not require therapy. Surgical meatotomy is indicated only for a very small or scarred meatus associated with a poor urinary stream.

Hypospadias. This refers to ventral ectopia of the urethral meatus anywhere from the ventral glans penis to the perineum. Hypospadias, especially the coronal or glandular variety, can now usually be corrected in infancy. A minihypospadias repair is little more than a modified circumcision combined with an advancement urethral meatoplasty.

Most cases can be corrected by a one-stage operation that must include chordee excision, complete straightening of the penis, and construction of a neourethra, with the meatus as close as possible to the tip of the penis. Staged repairs are still preferred by some surgeons, especially by the occasional operator.

Boys recognize the importance of their genitalia at a very early age, and standing erect to void is an important skill in western society. Severe psychological disturbances are common in boys if definitive reconstruction is delayed beyond school age.

Epispadias. This very rare defect affects the dorsum of the penis. Surgical reconstruction is always indicated and should include penile and urethral lengthening plus bladder neck reconstruction when necessary.

Micropenis. By definition a micropenis should be more than two standard deviations smaller than the norm. Two distinct types can be recognized. Corpus cavernosus tissue is present in the more common variety, which is often associated with intracranial pathology. Endocrine evaluation

should be performed and therapy with topical or parenteral testosterone considered. A normal penis will never develop in boys with a micropenis that consists of skin and urethra alone and lacks corporeal tissue. In this event, a serious case can be made for amputation of the penis and female gender assignment.

Concealed Penis. This is a penis of normal size hidden within the suprapubic fat pad. It can occur naturally in some obese boys and requires no treatment. Retraction of the penis and circumferential cicatrix formation of the shaft skin over the glans occurs as a complication of neonatal circumcision. Surgical release of the glans is required; this can be performed as an office procedure in the neonate. A partially concealed penis, pseudomicropenis, also a complication of circumcision, is caused by excessive removal of penile shaft skin. If the condition is recognized immediately, the skin edges should be separated and the denuded penile shaft allowed to epithelialize. If recognized later in childhood, surgical correction may be necessary.

SPERMATIC CORD AND TESTES

Torsion. Acute painful swelling of the scrotum should always be considered a torsion of the spermatic cord or testis until proven otherwise, as should the painful groin swelling associated with ipsilateral undescended testis. Surgical treatment, which is always required for torsion, consists of bilateral trans-scrotal exploration and orchidopexy, except in infants or in the presence of primarily groin symptomatology, when an inguinal approach is preferred. Viability of the testicle depends upon prompt treatment. Surgery can be temporarily delayed if manual detorsion is successful; the contralateral testicle should always be anchored.

Torsion of the Appendix Testis. Scrotal exploration is mandatory if there is any doubt in the diagnosis. Symptoms usually subside spontaneously in approximately 1 week; however, boys are often less incapacitated by prompt surgical excision, which allows them to resume normal activities within 24 to 48 hours.

Epididymitis and Orchitis. Both conditions are rare in childhood; they must be differentiated from testicular torsion, and thus diagnosed with caution. Treatment for both consists of bed rest, scrotal elevation, and ice packs. A broad-spectrum antibiotic such as ampicillin for 10 to 14 days should be added in the treatment of epididymitis. Subsequently, investigative urographic studies should be performed. Steroid prophylaxis may be useful in mumps orchitis to preserve future spermatogenesis.

Trauma. If the trauma is severe and testicular rupture is suspected, scrotal exploration should be performed. A hematoma or hematocele can be evacuated and a ruptured tunica albuginea repaired.

Testis Tumors. In children, these tumors usually present as firm, painless scrotal masses that do not transilluminate. Surgery is always indicated unless the child has leukemia. Preoperative studies should include serum alpha fetoprotein, beta-subunit of human chorionic gonadotropin, carcinoembryonic antigen, testosterone, luteinizing hormone, and follicle-stimulating hormone estimations, as well as excretory urography, chest x-ray, and a metastatic series. Speckled calcification in the neonatal scrotum strongly suggests prenatal meconium peritonitis.

Seventy per cent of pediatric testicular tumors are of germinal origin, and 80% of these are malignant embryonal cell carcinomas. However, leukemia relapses presenting as testicular tumors are common.

Testis tumors should be explored through the groin. The spermatic cord is cross-clamped with vascular instruments before the testicular mass is examined. If there is any question about the diagnosis of malignancy, a frozen section is performed; otherwise, a radical orchiectomy is indicated. CT scanning should be performed to evaluate the retroperitoneal lymph nodes (RPLN). The role of RPLN remains controversial; if preoperative tumor markers are elevated and fail to return to normal levels, RPLN dissection is indicated; otherwise, evidence that this procedure improves survival is inconclusive. Cancer chemotherapy is indicated for most germ cell tumors except for the rare cases of seminomas, for which radiation therapy remains the treatment of choice. Intermittent courses of a combination of vincristine, actinomycin D, and cyclophosphamide (Cytoxan) have increased the long-term survival rate to more than 80%. Leukemia of the testicle does not require biopsy and should be treated aggressively with radiation and chemotherapy.

Hernias and Hydroceles

STEPHEN L. GANS, M.D.,
and EDWARD AUSTIN, M.D.

Herniorrhaphy is the most frequently performed operation in infants and children. This procedure has an excellent record and offers reasonable and ample protection from the more serious and hazardous complications of hernia incarceration and strangulation. These occurrences may result in damage to or destruction of small or large intestine, omentum, bladder, testes, ovaries, tubes, and even the uterus.

Therefore, when the diagnosis of inguinal hernia has been made, operation is advised regardless of age or symptoms. Controversy exists concerning timing and safety of early repair in premature or other ill neonates. In this group, the incidence of complications, incarceration, intestinal obstruction, and gonadal infarction is about double that in the general childhood population. In the hands of experienced surgeons, anesthesiologists, and neonatal support personnel, early repair prior to discharge from the hospital has resulted in reduced morbidity.

Aside from this special group, failure to thrive, acute illness, some temporary household or psychological problems, or exposure to a contagious disease may prompt delay in surgical correction. Under these circumstances, yarn and other trusses have been used, but they are troublesome to the mother, are frequently associated with severe underlying skin irritation or furunculosis, and cannot be depended upon to prevent incarceration. We do not recommend them.

If repair is to be postponed, the parents must be informed about the symptoms and signs of an incarcerated hernia, instructed in simple measures to reduce it, and warned to call for help if complete relief is not obtained within a reasonably short time (see Incarcerated Inguinal Hernia).

Hospitalization for uncomplicated herniorrhaphy is now a matter of only a few hours (outpatient surgery) or, at the most, one day. Small infants are fed up to a few hours before the induction of anesthesia in order to prevent dehydration, and appropriate preanesthetic medication is ordered by the anesthesiologist.

When hernias are present bilaterally, both sides are repaired at the same operation. However, when a hernia is apparent on only one side, should the other side be explored? After many years controversy still rages, and there are reasonable arguments on both sides. We suggest that the situation be resolved in the following manner. If the history reveals an early undescended testicle that "came down" or a transient hydrocele, or if examination demonstrates thickened cord structures or a "rub" sign, exploration of this side should be considered. The experience and skill of the operating surgeon and the anesthesiologist are important factors in the decision for or against further exploration.

Postoperatively, the patient is discharged from the hospital when fully recovered from the anesthesia and when food has been retained, usually in 2–4 hours. The following instructions for home care are given:

1. Sponge baths instead of tub baths should be given for 1 week.

2. Infants still in diapers should be changed more frequently than usual during the day and once or twice during the night.

3. For pain, if present, acetaminophen is usually sufficient.

4. There are no physical restrictions for infants and toddlers. Older children need be restricted only from heavy lifting and pushing, wrestling and fighting, bicycle riding, and athletics for a total of 3 weeks.

5. School-aged children may attend classes as soon as they are comfortable but are excused from physical education for the same 3-week period.

HYDROCELE

Most hydroceles do not require treatment in the first few months of life, and many of them disappear spontaneously. However, patients with hydroceles that fluctuate significantly in size during the course of the day or from time to time or increase greatly in size over several weeks have a patent processus vaginalis and will eventually come to surgery for repair of an associated hernia. Hydroceles that persist or develop after age 6 months to 1 year are almost invariably associated with hernias; they should be treated like hernias and for the same reasons.

The operative approach is always through the inguinal regions, and the hernia sac is ligated high and removed along with part of the hydrocele sac. Postoperative care is the same as for herniorrhaphy, but the parents should be told that occasionally temporary discoloration and swelling of the scrotum occur.

INCARCERATED INGUINAL HERNIA

Reasonable attempts should be made to reduce an incarcerated hernia in an infant. Emergency surgery for this condition is frequently difficult, and the morbidity, complications, and recurrence rate are significantly higher than with elective surgery. At home all measures to comfort and relax the patient should be tried; a warm bath may help. If this fails to reduce the hernia, a trip to the emergency room is indicated. Often the hernia will reduce during the ride to the hospital because of the relaxing effects of holding and motion.

Usually the physician can reduce the hernia by gentle, firm pressure while the baby sucks industriously on a pacifier dipped in granulated sugar. If this maneuver fails, sedative or narcotic medication is given (e.g., Demerol, 2 mg/kg IM). Reduction may be tried again when the patient is well relaxed by the medication. If these attempts do not result in reduction of the hernia, immediate surgery is indicated. Nasal gastric suction and intravenous fluids are started. At operation, incarcerated bowel should be examined carefully before it is returned to the peritoneal cavity. Ovaries or testes may appear badly traumatized or infarcted, but this is not necessarily an indication for resection. Return of the ovary to the abdomen and the testis to the scrotum is the rule. Postoperative care is much the same as for elective herniorrhaphy, except that the patient should not be discharged for at least 24 hours.

Whenever possible, successful nonoperative reduction should be followed by elective repair in 48–72 hours, when reactive edema and inflammation have subsided.

INGUINAL HERNIA IN GIRLS

In general, the same principles apply for girls as for boys, but certain special considerations warrant discussion. When the hernia is represented by a small, firm mass in the groin or labium, several possibilities exist. Most frequently it is an incarcerated ovary or tube. Occasionally it will be a sliding hernia with ovary, tube, or even a corner of the uterus making up part of the wall of the sac. Even when the infant or child appears to be a normal female in all other respects, the mass may be a testis (male pseudohermaphroditism or testicular feminization).

If the mass is quite tender and the patient is symptomatic, treatment is carried out without delay as in the boy with an incarcerated hernia. If the mass is not tender and the patient is asymptomatic, elective surgery should be scheduled at the earliest possible date. Meanwhile, tests may be carried out and a further history obtained to help rule gonadal abnormalities in or out.

When these investigations prove normal, the operative procedure follows the usual description. Simple hernia in a girl is repaired in the same way as in a boy. Sliding hernias require a special technique.

FEMORAL HERNIA

Femoral hernias are rare in infants and children. The same principles of treatment apply as in inguinal hernias.

Vulva and Vagina

LOUIS FRIEDLANDER, M.D.

CONGENITAL OR DEVELOPMENTAL DISORDERS

Developmental abnormalities presenting in the newborn period require early recognition, diagnosis, and institution of appropriate medical therapy. Virilization of the female fetus in utero may result in the development of ambiguous genitalia.

Early diagnosis of ambiguous genitalia will lead to a determination of the child's sexual identity and, in turn, guide parental child-rearing attitudes. Early gender identification will permit reconstructive surgery at the appropriate time to create female genitalia in an infant with a testis.

Isolated clitorimegaly, when present at birth, is often the result of prenatal exposure to virilizing steroids of maternal or fetal origin. This condition may require plastic repair. Clitoral recession, with preservation of innervation and anatomic configuration, can be deferred to 18 months of age. Clitorectomy is rarely, if ever, indicated.

ACQUIRED HORMONAL DISORDERS

The white vaginal discharge of the neonate, which results from maternal estrogen stimulation, subsides after several days.

Hormonal stimulation of the vulva and vagina, such as precocious development of pubic hair (adrenarche), clitorimegaly, estrogenization of the labia minora, or menstruation, should be investigated for signs of a systemic process. Exogenous sources of estrogen, such as ingestion of birth control pills, estrogen creams, autonomous ovarian or adrenal sources, or central nervous lesions, must be excluded.

Imperforate hymen is generally not identified until menarche, when the patient may present with amenorrhea, abdominal pain, and lower abdominal swelling (hematocolpos) with or without a bulging introitus. Occasionally it may be identified in the newborn period by a bulging of the introitus due to the accumulation of vaginal secretions from the estrogenized vagina. When a large amount of secretions collects (hydrocolpos), lower abdominal swelling appears. Excision of the membrane is necessary for drainage. Vaginal or other defects are rarely associated.

With a transverse vaginal septum, symptoms similar to those seen with imperforate hymen may occur at any level above the hymen. The septum is usually resected.

Adhesions of the labia (labial agglutination) are extremely common. They usually occur in young girls 6 months to 6 years of age. The exact etiology of these lesions is unknown, but they are generally associated with mild vulvitis. Occasionally the vaginal orifice is completely covered, causing poor drainage of vaginal secretions. Urinary drainage may also be impaired. In mild cases, no treatment is necessary because the labia will separate completely with estrogenization at puberty.

When vaginal or urinary drainage is not impaired, an estrogen-containing cream (Premarin) should be applied twice a day for 2 weeks and then at bedtime for another 1–2 weeks, until the labia are separated. The cream must be rubbed into the area of the adhesion while the labia are gently separated. Treatment should be continued with a bland ointment at bedtime after the labia have separated. Forceful separation is discouraged because it is traumatic for the child and may cause the adhesions to form again.

CONGENITAL ABSENCE OF THE VAGINA

Vaginal Agenesis. Ultrasonography and laparoscopy should be done early to determine whether the uterus may be a source of pain. When the uterus is absent, a functional coital canal is created. When it is present, symptoms of primary amenorrhea and cyclic, recurrent abdominal pain are relieved by drainage of the retained blood; normal flow is maintained thereafter by the reconstructed vagina. Normal menstrual function, fertility, and vaginal delivery have resulted when the condition is promptly diagnosed and surgically corrected.

Testicular Feminization Syndrome. Testicular feminization syndrome (total androgen insensitivity) may be mistaken for vaginal agenesis. Patients have a male karyotype (46,XY), with testes that may be palpated in the labia or groin, a normal-looking vulva, and a blind vaginal pouch so short that it may be difficult to distinguish from vaginal agenesis. The cervix and uterus are absent. Pubic hair may be scanty or absent, and breast development is poor. Plasma testosterone is normal.

Testes are prophylactically removed after puberty (to retain the female habitus) because of the high rate of malignant degeneration. The patient's ability to have normal sexual relations, without menses and childbearing, should be discussed. After surgery, cyclic conjugated estrogen therapy (Premarin, 0.625 mg/day on days 1–21 of each month) is given.

TUMORS OF THE VULVA AND VAGINA

Fortunately, genital tumors in the child are rare.

Benign Cysts. *Mesonephric duct cysts* (Gartner's duct cysts) are common, representing wolffian duct remnants arising from the anterolateral vaginal wall. They present as a translucent, unilocular swelling that may protrude through the vaginal introitus. *Paraurethral duct cysts* are found in the urethrovaginal wall and may compress the hymenal opening or urethra. If they are symptomatic, simple surgical unroofing and marsupialization is preferred to total excision. *Inclusion cysts* on the vulva and vagina are secondary to trauma. They are simple cysts, lined by squamous epithelium, that contain cheesy material. They are treated by simple excision. *Cysts of the canal of Nuck* represent proximal obliteration of the processus vaginalis. If they are large or disfiguring they should be excised. *Bartholin's gland cysts* are treated by marsupialization. *Labial papillomas* (skin tags) are small, benign polyps. Excisional biopsy is mandatory if the diagnosis is in doubt. *Hymenal cysts* seen in the newborn period usually shrink and disappear.

Hemangiomas are the most common tumors of the vulva. They are of either the capillary or the cavernous type and generally tend to regress in time. Their treatment depends on size, distortion of adjacent structures, rapidity of growth, and susceptibility to injury (trauma). Recently, excision or cryotherapy of these vascular masses has been replaced by treatment with the argon laser. This technique effectively destroys large vascular tumors and has gained acceptance because bleeding is readily controlled and minimal scarring results. Lipomas, papillomas, and leiomyomas may be kept under observation and excised when symptomatic.

A *hydradenoma*, a cystic tumor of the sweat glands, presents as an umbilicated subcutaneous tumor. It should be removed only if the diagnosis is uncertain.

Tumors arising from mesodermal tissues are the fibroma, lipoma, leiomyoma, lymphangioma, and hemangioma. Solid tumors are treated by local excision, while lymphangiomas and hemangiomas can be followed carefully.

Bleeding, ulceration, or distortion due to a large tumor mass is an indication for excision. Dysplastic epithelial changes of the vulvar skin, in the form of hypertrophic, atrophic, or mixed lesions, should be biopsied if the diagnosis is in doubt. Malignant precursors should be treated by local excision or laser techniques. Vulvectomy with lymph node dissection is reserved for the rare malignancies in the adolescent.

Urethral prolapse is often confused with neoplasm. It is treated by simple excision and suturing of the mucosal edges to the vestibular mucosa. Digital reduction should not be attempted because it is painful and recurrences are common.

Sarcoma Botryoides. This is the most common malignant tumor arising in the vagina during childhood and early adolescence. Complete vaginectomy and hysterectomy are indicated. When the tumor extends beyond the confines of the subepithelial tissue, exenterative procedures, possibly with excision of the vulva and rectum, may be required.

Adjunctive chemotherapy (combinations of actinomycin D, doxorubicin, vincristine, and cyclophosphamide) is effective in controlling these tumors. Radiation is often employed in the therapeutic regimen.

The preservation of ovarian function is determined by the extent of pelvic involvement of the malignant process. Vaginal reconstruction should be contemplated.

Diethylstilbestrol. In utero exposure to maternally administered diethylstilbestrol and related synthetic compounds (dienestrol and hexestrol), given to women from the 1940s to 1960s in an attempt to prevent fetal wastage, is associated with the development of vaginal adenosis and clear-cell adenocarcinoma in the vagina and cervix in young women.

Vaginal adenosis is the presence of glandular epithelium resembling that of the endocervix and associated with transverse cervical and vaginal ridges. It is almost always present if there is a vaginal clear-cell carcinoma. Treatment of clear-cell adenocarcinoma is aggressive, as the lesion is invasive. Early staging to determine the extent of spread will help in selecting the appropriate procedures. Vaginectomy, hysterectomy, extensive lymph node dissection, adjunctive chemotherapy, and radiation therapy may all be indicated.

INFECTIONS AND SKIN DISORDERS OF THE GENITALIA

Vulvovaginitis is a common gynecologic problem in childhood; it is strikingly different in the prepubertal child and in the adolescent. Usually there is a primary vulvitis with a secondary distal vaginitis; less often, there is a primary vaginitis, requiring more careful investigation, that might be due to a foreign body, trapped pinworms, gonorrhea, a specific bacterial infection, ectopic ureter, or a neoplasm. Management involves ruling out a specific cause of the vulvovaginitis other than poor hygiene; treating the specific cause, if there is one; reducing the inflammatory reaction and symptoms; and improving local hygiene.

Nonspecific Vulvovaginitis

For acute weeping pruritic dermatitis, give sitz baths in tepid water with colloidal oatmeal (Aveeno) or baking soda. Alternatively, wet compresses with Burow's solution (1:40) or saline may be applied at intervals of 3–4 hours. The skin is blotted dry, and a bland medication (e.g., Desitin or calamine shake lotion) is applied. Skin infections are treated systemically. Preventive care includes washing with nonmedicated, nonperfumed soap. The vulva is gently dried or exposed to dry air and dusted with cornstarch. After each bowel movement, the patient must wipe from back to front with soft, white, unperfumed toilet tissue. Loosely fitting white cotton undergarments are worn. Bubble baths and detergent washing of underpants should be avoided. Topical hydrocortisone or hydroxyzine hydrochloride (Atarax) may be given for itching. Bacterial infections of the vulva transmitted from extragenital primary sites (e.g., nasopharynx, intestine, skin) are treated according to the sensitivity of the offending organism. Topical estrogen cream or Premarin cream may be employed for 3–4 weeks for persistent or recurrent nonspecific vaginitis after negative vaginoscopy. Creation of a thickened vaginal wall and an acid vaginal pH usually results in a cure.

Nonspecific Vulvovaginitis Secondary to Foreign Bodies. This condition presents as a profuse purulent discharge, sometimes with blood, that lasts for weeks. The most common cause is toilet paper or stool and there is a high rate of recurrence. In adolescents, the cause is usually a retained tampon. Pelvic radiography is useful for diagnosis if the material is radiopaque. The extraneous object is removed using a cystoscope with a fiberoptic light source, and the vagina is irrigated with warm water.

Specific Vulvovaginitis

Diagnosis of specific vulvovaginitis requires close inspection, vaginoscopy, and a culture. Pathogens derived from other sites (e.g., pharynx, ear, skin) are treated with systemic antibiotics. The high or microperforate hymen may trap urine and mucus in the vagina, where it may become infected by stool bacteria and be a source of recurrent infection. Excision of some tissue is preferred to a simple incision.

Trichomonas Vulvovaginitis. The prepubertal child is given metronidazole (Flagyl), 125 mg three times daily for 5 days. In the adolescent female, 1.5–2 gm, given in a single dose, is effective in 90% of patients. This drug is contraindicated in the first trimester of pregnancy since its teratogenic potential is unknown. The sexual partner should be treated at the same time.

Monilia Vulvovaginitis. Effective antifungal agents include miconazole nitrate (Monistat) cream, one applicatorful intravaginally nightly for 7 days, or clotrimazole (Gyne-Lotrimin, Mycelex-G), one applicatorful intravaginally nightly for 7–14 days or one tablet intravaginally nightly for 7 days. For candidiasis in the child 1 year of age or younger, oral nystatin, 100,000–1,000,000 units orally four times a day for 7 days, can be used in combination with local nystatin cream or suppository every day. Treatment failure may indicate a coexisting pathogen, such as *Trichomonas*.

Gardnerella Vulvovaginitis. Formerly termed *Haemophilus vaginalis* vaginitis, this is the most common form of bacterial vaginitis. Metronidazole* (Flagyl), 500 mg twice daily for 7 days, is the treatment of choice. A single oral dose of 2 gm may be given. The sexual partner should be treated at the same time.

Pinworm Vulvovaginitis. Pinworm infestations are common in preschool and school-aged children. Treatment with mebendazole (Vermox)—one chewable 100-mg tablet taken once only, regardless of weight—will clear the condition. Treat all other members of the family.

Gonorrheal Vulvovaginitis. Acute gonorrhea in the child causes marked inflammation of the vagina with a profuse purulent discharge and a secondary vulvitis with edema and dysuria. In contrast, the adolescent with gonorrhea has an

endocervicitis. Infection may be acquired from sexual abuse or contact with an infected person, improperly sterilized thermometers, and clothing.

Gonorrheal vulvovaginitis is treated with penicillin G procaine, 100,000 U/kg IM in two injection sites (maximum, 4.8 million units), administered simultaneously with probenecid, 25 mg/kg orally (maximum, 1 gm). Alternatively, oral single-dose therapy with amoxicillin trihydrate, 50 mg/kg (maximum, 3.5 gm) with probenecid can be used. In the patient allergic to penicillin, tetracycline is effective, but a single dose is not sufficient. A course of oral tetracycline, 25 mg/kg initially (maximum, 1.5 gm), followed by 10 mg/kg four times daily for 4 days, is recommended. If organisms are resistant to penicillin (penicillinase-producing *Neisseria gonorrhoeae*) or if the child is allergic to penicillin, spectinomycin (Trobicin), 40 mg/kg IM, may be given in a single injection (maximum, 2 gm). Children with complicated infections such as peritonitis or arthritis should be hospitalized for the intravenous administration of aqueous crystalline penicillin G, 100,000 U/kg/24 hr for 7 days. When meningitis is present, the dose of penicillin is increased to 250,000 U/kg/24 hr for 10 days.

Condyloma Acuminata. A viral venereal infection (caused by the papovavirus or papillomavirus), condyloma acuminata produces multiple small warts on the vulva, vagina, and, sometimes, the cervix. Large growths may become secondarily infected. The incubation period is 6 weeks to 8 months. Podophyllin resin (20%) in tincture of benzoin, applied to the vulva with a cotton applicator and removed by washing after 4–6 hours, is used once weekly until the lesions are cleared. Normal skin should be protected with petrolatum jelly. This preparation is contraindicated in pregnancy because it is absorbed systemically. Extensive lesions may require electrodesiccation, cryotherapy, laser therapy, or surgical excision under anesthesia. Excisional biopsy to exclude neoplasm is warranted when the diagnosis is in doubt.

Herpes Vulvovaginitis. Local application of antiviral cream (acyclovir), four to six times daily for 7–10 days, is effective in shortening the course of the disease and limits the viral shedding period. Acyclovir may be given intravenously for severe infection. Oral use of this agent seems promising.

COMMON SKIN DISORDERS AFFECTING THE GENITALIA

Vulvovaginitis may be secondary to staphylococcal skin infections, seborrhea, psoriasis, or atopic dermatitis; in such cases, it is usually associated with lesions in other parts of the body. Treatment includes hydrocortisone cream or Burow's solution soaks if the lesions are exudative. Secondary infection is treated.

Diaper Rash. Acute diaper rash may be treated

---

* This use of metronidazole is not recommended by the manufacturer, but it is recommended by the Centers for Disease Control.

with wet compresses of water, saline, or Burow's solution. The dermatitis usually responds to a 1% hydrocortisone cream or lotion. Nystatin powder is applied to the skin when dry to treat monilial infection.

Lichen Sclerosus. In addition to the treatment outlined for nonspecific vulvovaginitis, a short course of topical corticosteroids, e.g., 0.025% fluocinolone acetonide (Synalar), followed by a course of 1% hydrocortisone ointment for a few more months, is useful in bringing the condition under control. Testosterone (2%) in petrolatum gel may be effective; then testosterone propionate can be given once weekly as maintenance therapy.

TRAUMA

Vulvar and perineal ecchymoses, with significant vaginal lacerations and bleeding, are common with blunt trauma and straddle injuries. There can be significant vaginal laceration and bleeding or a transvaginal injury to the bladder, rectum, or peritoneal cavity even in the absence of external damage. Cold compresses will stop the bleeding. Lacerations may need sutures. Examination under general anesthesia may be necessary, with measures then taken as needed to prevent distortion of anatomy and secondary sepsis and to restore subsequent sexual and reproductive function. When child abuse or sexual molestation is suspected, attention is focused on evidence of vaginal penetration, abrasions, lacerations, contusions with hematomas, and spasm of the pubococcygeal muscle; laboratory work to check for seminal products should be performed.

With healing, multiple hymenal scars, rounded hymenal remnants with a large vaginal opening, and laceration extending to the perineum will be evident, in addition to an odorous vaginal discharge. The extent of anal injury may vary from acute spasm to swelling of the anal verge with abrasions, bruises, and localized hematomas. With chronic abuse, complete or partial loss of sphincter control may be found along with thickening of the skin mucous membranes and skin tags.

Uterus, Tubes, and Ovaries

LOUIS FRIEDLANDER, M.D.

PRIMARY AMENORRHEA

Primary amenorrhea is defined as the absence of spontaneous menstruation within 2 years after the onset of secondary sex development or no spontaneous uterine bleeding by the age of 17 years. Classification is based on the presence or absence of breast development and the uterus.

Primary amenorrhea in patients with sponta-

neous breast development and a normal uterus may indicate a disturbance of the hypothalamic-pituitary-ovarian axis after the initiation of thelarche. Patients should have a careful breast examination to detect galactorrhea and a serum prolactin determination to rule out a prolactin-secreting pituitary adenoma.

Menstrual cycles can be brought about by the administration of medroxyprogesterone acetate (Provera), 10 mg orally for 5–10 days, or progesterone in oil, 100 mg IM every 6–12 weeks. The endometrium will become secretory and withdrawal bleeding will be initiated. Subsequently, conjugated estrogens (Premarin), 1.25 mg, is given on days 1–21 and Provera, 10 mg, on days 15–21. After another week with no treatment given, vaginal bleeding will occur; the same steroid regimen is repeated. This will effect full maturation of the secondary sexual characteristics. The dosage can be reduced by one-half after full maturation.

Delayed menarche in the normal healthy teenager with adequate estrogen and normal anatomy may be related to overweight, underweight (e.g., anorexia nervosa), stress, depression, or certain drugs (e.g., phenothiazine). Spontaneous periods will commence when these conditions are corrected. Rarely, pregnancy may occur without menarche.

Gonadal dysgenesis (Turner's syndrome) is characterized by the absence of breast development in patients with a normal vagina and a uterus that is capable of responding to exogenous hormones. Serum FSH is consistently elevated. The presence of a Y chromosome, as in a mosaic karyotype such as 45, XO/46, XY, puts the patient at risk for the development of a gonadoblastoma in the streak gonad. Long-term gynecologic follow-up, peritoneoscopy or pelvic ultrasonography, or prophylactic surgical removal of the streaks is indicated.

Conjugated estrogen (Premarin), 0.3 mg once daily, is introduced around the age of 14 or 15 years and continued for approximately 1 year or until linear growth appears to be leveling off. The dosage is then increased to 0.625 mg, given on days 1–21 of each month, with 10 mg of medroxyprogesterone (Provera) added on days 15–21 to effect cyclic withdrawal bleeding.

Increasing the dosage of Premarin to 1.25–2.5 mg on days 1–21 for 6 months may improve breast development and may occasionally be required for normal menstruation. The use of weak androgens, such as oxandrolone, to stimulate growth is now under evaluation. Doses of 0.07–0.25 mg/kg/day during late childhood or early adolescence may result in a significant increase in growth velocity during the first year of treatment and a slight advancement in bone age over height age in the majority of patients.

Hypogonadotropic hypogonadism is due to congenital absence of the hypothalamic centers responsible for the secretion of luteinizing hormone–releasing hormone in patients without breast development and a palpable uterus. Reproduction is often possible if these women are given exogenous gonadotropins. Conjugated estrogen, 0.625 mg daily, is given to induce breast development. Ovulation may be induced by the sequential administration of intramuscular follicle-stimulating hormone (Pergonal), a human chorionic gonadotropin, when the patient wants to become pregnant. Hyperprolactinemic hypogonadism without a radiologically demonstrable pituitary tumor should be treated by the administration of the dopamine agonist bromocriptine (Parlodel), 7.5 mg daily for 6 months.

All patients with the testicular feminization syndrome, or androgen insensitivity, should have the gonads surgically removed once full height and breast development are attained because of the high incidence of malignancy (dysgerminoma). Detailed counseling is important before surgery. The physician should stress the patient's femininity and her ability to have normal sexual relations, but she must accept that she cannot have menses or bear children. Postoperatively, the patient should be placed on 0.625 mg of conjugated estrogen replacement for the first 25 days of each month to prevent osteoporosis and to preserve breast development. Since the uterus is absent, progestins are not indicated in these patients.

SECONDARY AMENORRHEA

The two most common causes of secondary amenorrhea in the adolescent are pregnancy and stress. Illnesses with fever, emotional upsets, weight changes, and involvement in competitive athletics or ballet may be associated with secondary amenorrhea of 6 months' duration or longer. Menses frequently returns during intervals of forced rest owing to injury and in patients who acquire chronic disease, e.g., chronic renal failure. Work-up on patients with secondary amenorrhea includes a pregnancy test and a progesterone challenge test. Provera, 10 mg by mouth twice daily for 5 days, or progesterone in oil, 50–100 mg IM, is given to induce withdrawal bleeding. When this occurs, the patient is normal.

The absence of withdrawal bleeding following this treatment indicates disorders such as polycystic ovary syndrome, ovarian tumors, thyroid disease, and diabetes mellitus. Patients with elevated protein levels with or without galactorrhea and without a radiologically demonstrable pituitary tumor should be treated by the administration of bromocriptine (Parlodel), 7.5 mg daily for 6 months. Neoplasms may be resected or treated with radiation or a similar dose of Parlodel.

Types of ovarian failure that cause amenorrhea include loss of ovarian function secondary to infection, hemorrhage, and a compromised blood supply, e.g., due to ovarian torsion. Another cause is polycystic ovarian disease (Stein-Leventhal syndrome), manifested by hirsutism, obesity, and infertility. The amenorrhea is treated with intermittent administration of progestin, the infertility with clomiphene citrate (Clomid), and the hirsutism with oral contraceptive steroids.

DYSFUNCTIONAL UTERINE BLEEDING (Menorrhagia, Metrorrhagia)

Dysfunctional uterine bleeding is due to chronic anovulation, usually secondary to faulty hypothalamic-pituitary-ovarian interactions, and is characterized by painless uterine bleeding of irregular duration, interval, and quantity. Treatment is dependent on the severity of the bleeding once diagnostic procedures are established that it is dysfunctional and not of organic origin. Patients who experience single episodes of mild to moderate flow and who have stable hematocrit or hemoglobin levels should be observed carefully. Normal periods are generally resumed after a month or two.

Moderate to severe bleeding, with a decrease in the patient's hematocrit and hemoglobin levels, usually requires hormonal therapy. Medroxyprogesterone acetate (Provera), 10 mg for 5 days each month, is usually sufficient to reverse the histologic pattern. Flow will cease by the third to fifth day. This dosage pattern is resumed on day 14 after the withdrawal flow and continued for 3–6 months. To control the acute episode of bleeding, as well as to reduce the frequency of recurrences, oral administration of conjugated estrogens, 2.5 mg four times a day, is usually effective. The bleeding will stop or be markedly reduced within 2–3 days. Treatment should then be continued for 21 days, with Provera, 10 mg/day, added for the last 5 days. The dosage of estrogen should be doubled if bleeding persists. Ferrous sulfate, 300 mg three times a day for 2–3 months, may be required to control anemia.

For heavy or prolonged bleeding, the initial use of an oral contraceptive such as Ortho-Novum (Norinyl), 2 mg, or Ovral for 21 days is useful. If bleeding continues the medication should be given twice a day. Bleeding is generally controlled within a few days. The patient should then be given cyclic medroxyprogesterone for 3–6 months.

Treatment of severe dysfunctional bleeding with a heavy prolonged flow, and a drop in hemoglobin to below 8 gm%, and clinical signs of acute blood loss requires hospitalization. Whole blood transfusions are given, as is estrogen-progesterone therapy: Ortho-Novum (Norinyl), 2 mg, is given every 4 hours until bleeding slows or stops and then once a day for 21 days. Alternatively, Enovid (norethynodrel, 10 mg, plus mestranol, 0.15 mg), may be used; 10 mg·is given orally initially, and the dose is then increased by daily increments of 5 mg until bleeding is markedly reduced or stopped. If hormonal treatment fails to control bleeding within 24–36 hours, the possibility of pelvic pathology should be excluded by dilatation and curettage under anesthesia. The patient is then maintained on the initial steroid therapy and given iron and folic acid supplements.

DYSMENORRHEA

Prostaglandin inhibitors are the drugs of choice if the pain is severe, and treatment is begun 1–2 days before the expected menses. Ibuprofen (Motrin), 400 mg every 4–6 hours, or mefenamic acid (Ponstel) or naproxen (Naprosyn), 250 mg every 6–8 hours, may be used. Aspirin may be tried for mild to moderate cramps in dosages of 300–600 mg every 4 hours. It should be avoided in patients with known or suspected ulcer disease, gastrointestinal bleeding, or clotting disorders and in those with allergies or aspirin-induced asthma.

If pain is not controlled by these measures, ovulation suppression with low-dose oral contraceptives is effective. This reduces the amount of menstrual flow and substantially relieves the cramping. Norinyl 1 + 50, 1 + 35 (Ortho-Novum 1/50, 1/35) Loestrin 1.5/30 or Ovral is useful and is used for 3 months unless contraception is required. If severe cramps persist despite hormone therapy, a thorough physical examination, including laparoscopy, is indicated to exclude organic causes such as endometriosis, disease-associated congenital malformations, and obstruction of the upper female genital tract, any of which can present with dysmenorrhea and requires careful gynecologic evaluation. Congenital scoliosis and urologic abnormalities require early evaluation of the female genital tract to exclude associated abnormalities.

GONORRHEA, PELVIC INFLAMMATORY DISEASE, AND SYPHILIS

Gonococcal Cervicitis. The preferred treatment for asymptomatic infections is aqueous procaine penicillin G, 4.8 million units IM, divided into two doses and injected into two different sites at one visit, with probenecid, 1 gm, given orally. Alternatives to this treatment are the following:

1. Ampicillin, 3.5 gm; or amoxicillin, 3 gm orally, and probenecid, 1 gm orally.

2. Tetracycline,* 500 mg orally four times a day for 5 days.

3. Doxycycline, 100 mg orally two times a day for 5 days.

With the emergence of penicillinase-producing *Neisseria gonorrhoeae*, which is resistant to the standard forms of therapy, new drugs have become available. These include spectinomycin, 2 gm IM in a single dose, or cefoxitin, 2 gm IM and probenecid, 1 gm orally. These drugs are also useful in penicillin-allergic patients and for treating gonococcal infections in pregnant women. Concurrent chlamydial infection will respond to tetracycline, 500 mg qid over 10–14 days. Erythromycin, 500 mg four times a day for a similar period, is a useful alternative. Cervical and rectal cultures repeated in 7–14 days will detect treatment failures. These patients should be given spectinomycin, but most positive follow-up cultures are probably the result of reinfection. All contacts of the patient, regardless of symptoms, should be cultured and treated at the same visit.

Gonococcal pharyngitis and gonoccocal proctitis require more vigorous therapy. Initial penicillin therapy is followed by either ampicillin, 500 mg orally four times a day for the next 5 days, or aqueous procaine penicillin, 2.4 million units IM daily for the next 4 days. Spectinomycin,† 4 gm IM, or tetracycline, 500 mg orally four times a day for 5 days, is indicated for patients allergic to penicillin.

Pelvic Inflammatory Disease. Ambulatory therapy, reserved for patients with mild symptoms who have no peritoneal signs, is less desirable than treatment given in the hospital because patient compliance is often poor or erratic and adequate coverage for polymicrobial infection is not provided, so there is often a higher incidence of residual tubal damage, infertility, and chronic pelvic pain.

The following four regimens may be employed for the outpatient treatment of salpingitis:

1. Aqueous procaine penicillin, 4.8 million units in two divided doses, with probenecid, 1 gm PO approximately 30 minutes prior to the penicillin injections. This therapy is usually followed by ampicillin or amoxicillin, 500 mg PO qid for 10 days.

2. Ampicillin, 3.5 gm PO; or amoxicillin, 3 gm PO, followed by ampicillin, 500 mg PO qid for 10 days.

3. Tetracycline, 500 mg PO qid for 10 days, or doxycycline, 200 mg PO to start and then 100 mg bid for 10 days if the patient is not pregnant.

4. Cefoxitin, 2 gm IM followed by cephradine (Anspor, Velosef), 500 mg PO qid for 10 days.

Patients should be reevaluated 48–72 hours after the initiation of antibiotic therapy, and those who are not responding favorably should be hospital-

---

* Use of tetracycline in children under 8 years of age can cause discoloration of permanent teeth.

† Safety of spectinomycin in infants and children has not been established.

ized for intravenous therapy. Sexual partners should receive appropriate treatment.

In-patient hospital treatment is advised for all but mild cases of pelvic inflammatory disease so that intravenous therapy can be given for at least 4 days or for at least 48 hours after the fever resolves. This practice is aimed at preservation of tubal function, which will prevent infertility and chronic pelvic pain. The available regimens are as follows:

1. Cefoxitin, 2 gm IV every 6 hours, plus doxycycline, 100 mg every 12 hours. Follow with oral doxycycline, 100 mg bid for 10–14 days after discharge. This regimen covers gonorrheal and chlamydial infections but is inadequate against certain anaerobes.

2. Clindamycin, 600 mg IV every 6 hours, plus aminoglycoside, 2 mg/kg initially followed by 1.5 mg/kg every 8 hours. Follow with oral clindamycin, 450 mg qid for 10–14 days after discharge. This regimen provides added coverage against anaerobes and facultative gram-negative rods. Serum creatinine and aminoglycoside levels must be monitored to prevent nephrotoxicity. Further, the patient should be watched for ototoxicity.

3. Metronidazole, 1 gm IV every 12 hours, plus doxycycline, 100 mg every 12 hours. Follow with oral metronidazole, 1 gm bid, and oral doxycycline, 100 mg bid for 10–14 days after discharge. Because they decrease menstrual blood flow, oral contraceptives protect against salpingitis in 50% of cases. Applies to barrier methods (diaphragm or condom). Alternative antibiotic therapy includes cefamandole, 8–12 gm IV in four divided doses (covers penicillinase-producing *N. gonorrhoeae* plus many gram-negative organisms), or moxalactam, 1–2 gm every 8 hours. Treatment is usually continued for 10 days.

Syphilis. See the article on syphilis.

ECTOPIC PREGNANCY

The sharp rise in the incidence of tubal pregnancies is attributed to the increase in venereal infection seen with pelvic inflammatory disease, induced abortions, and IUDs. Ectopic pregnancy should be suspected in adolescents with abdominal pain, vaginal bleeding, and menstrual irregularities (not always amenorrhea). The goals of treatment are preservation of the patient's life and her fertility; the latter has been made possible by advances in tubal microsurgery. When the uterus is left intact, term pregnancy is possible thanks to recent advances in techniques of in vitro fertilization and embryo transfer.

TUMORS OF THE UTERUS, TUBES, AND OVARIES

The ovary is the most common site for neoplasms occurring in adolescents, and ovarian tumors comprise 1–2% of all tumors in childhood. Thirty percent of all ovarian tumors in childhood and adolescence are cystic teratomas or dermoids. The majority of nonneoplastic lesions are cysts. These are considered a variation of the normal physiologic process. Dermoid cysts are detected on routine pelvic examination and can be diagnosed by X-ray or ultrasonography through the identification of calcification, tooth formation, or a particular fat-halo sign. Treatment is surgical excision, with preservation of ovarian tissue if possible. Follicular cysts comprise the bulk of nonneoplastic ovarian enlargements; forming from the unruptured follicle or corpus luteum, they enlarge and resemble cystic tumors of the ovary (cystadenoma). These may be identified by ultrasonography and laparoscopy. Small follicular cysts that cause no symptoms should not be removed or punctured. Those larger than 6 cm that have a solid component and cause menstrual irregularities may be treated with contraceptive pills to suppress the hypothalamic-ovarian axis. If these cysts do not resolve within 3 months, they may be aspirated at laparoscopy. In the absence of pain or bleeding, large luteal cysts may be treated with oral contraceptives and observed for further development. Laparoscopy or laparotomy is indicated if bleeding, torsion, or rupture occurs.

Neoplasms of the fallopian tubes are exceedingly rare.

Benign uterine tumors are uncommon in childhood. Excision of myomas depends on their size, location, and symptoms. Malignant uterine neoplasms, primarily adenocarcinoma and sarcoma, are extremely rare in pediatric patients. They require aggressive radical surgery and radiation therapy.

Lesions of the cervix, including polyps, papillomas, condylomas, and endometriomas, may present with bleeding and discharge. Early biopsy is important to establish the histologic diagnosis and treatment.

A papillary or polypoid vaginal or cervical tumor with or without vaginal bleeding or discharge requires excisional biopsy to exclude sarcoma botryoides. Reexamination at frequent intervals for several years is indicated even if the initial biopsy findings are negative.

Carcinoma of the Cervix

Cervical Dysplasia and Carcinoma in Situ. An increase in the incidence of cervical dysplasia progressing to carcinoma in situ has been reported in adolescent girls, probably related to excessive sexual activity at an early age, exposure to multiple sex partners, herpes type II vaginitis and other sexually transmitted diseases, and pelvic inflammatory disease. All high-risk patients, regardless of their age, should have a Papanicolaou smear every 6 months and should be referred to a gynecologist for appropriate treatment, which includes excisional biopsy, cryosurgery, or carbon dioxide laser treatment for diffuse ectocervical disease and 5-fluorouracil chemotherapy for diffuse vaginal disease. The treatment for severe disease is irradiation or surgery (conization or hysterectomy). Early detection and treatment results in a high cure rate, up to 90%.

Ovarian Tumors

The most common malignant tumor in childhood is the so-called immature teratoma. The prognosis is excellent following adequate excision if the tumor is localized. Dysgerminoma is the second most common malignant ovarian tumor in children. These are of low-grade malignancy and are often bilateral.

Surgical removal is indicated when an ovarian tumor is discovered in a patient of any age. The growth may be investigated by ultrasonography, laparoscopy, exploratory laparotomy, and frozen sections. Adjunctive radiation therapy, combined with chemotherapy, may be required. If possible, a fragment of an ovary should be preserved to induce a feminine habitus and induce normal growth and menarche.

If all ovarian tissue must be excised, substitute hormonal therapy is begun when the child is 8–9 years of age. Small doses of estrogen—e.g., 0.625 mg of conjugated estrogen or 0.02 mg of ethinyl estradiol—are administered orally.

13

Bones and Joints

Craniofacial Malformations

IAN T. JACKSON, M.D.

The treatment of craniofacial deformity is becoming better established in terms of what operation to perform and when to carry out corrective surgery. However, there are still areas of conflicting opinion, and it is not always possible to make hard and fast rules. The approach is multidisciplinary at the time of the initial assessment; the surgery is performed by the plastic surgeon and the neurosurgeon; occasionally an oral surgeon will be involved.

In some cases, total correction of the deformity can be achieved by initial repositioning of the skeletal component, followed by rearrangement of the soft tissue. In other conditions, however, a multistaged approach is necessary.

Bony defects, both those resulting from the deformity and those created by osteotomy, are reconstructed with bone. Usually this is accomplished using a free bone graft, but occasionally vascularized bone is employed. Mircrovascular techniques are now being used more frequently for reconstruction of soft tissue deficiencies. When indicated, soft tissue and bone can be replaced in this manner as a composite free tissue transfer.

Even in treating fairly standard, straightforward deformities (e.g., those of Crouzon's disease), it is usual that one major procedure is followed by one or two fairly minor ones in order to obtain the best possible end result. Recent advances in treatment include early correction of craniosynostosis, the use of skull as the primary bone graft site, the use of "mini" bone plates for stabilization in some situations, and—perhaps most important of all—a very considerable decrease in operating time.

CRANIOSYNOSTOSIS

All degrees of craniosynostosis, even the most minor, cause a rise in intracranial pressure. This may or may not be significant in terms of mental retardation, but high pressure levels may result in progressive papilledema, optic atrophy, and blindness. The advised timing of suture release is at age 3 months. This allows the normal rapid brain growth during the first year to help improve the result of the osteotomy. There is good correction of the frontosupraorbital deformities associated with craniosynostosis, and it is hoped that in the long term the facial deformity that can result from coronal and basal craniosynostosis can be minimized. This, however, remains to be proved.

Scaphocephaly. A wide strip of cranium is removed in the region of the fused sagittal suture. In the past, silicone was used to line the edges of the craniotomy; however, this procedure has become less popular since it seems ineffectual in preventing refusion of the cranium. In extreme cases of scaphocephaly, vertical osteotomies anteriorly and posteriorly, running in a coronal direction, can be carried out; the lateral bone plates are then outfractured, the line of fracture being in the temporoparietal area. In some cases there is posterolateral rotation of the supraorbital rims, and in this situation the sagittal osteotomy is continued down to the glabellar area. A coronal craniotomy is performed behind the coronal sutures. The supraorbital rims and lateral orbital walls are mobilized as described for the correction of bicoronal craniosynostosis. This segment is split vertically in the midline. The two large frontal bone plates and supraorbital rims are derotated to improve the appearance of the forehead and the orbits. This frontal segment is wired to the glabellar area and to the lateral orbital walls but has no posterolateral fixation.

Trigonocephaly. Correction is similar to that described for the anterior portion of the severe scaphocephaly. The frontal bone flap is removed, as are the supraorbital rims, both split in the midline. If the anterior cranial fossa is of adequate width (which is rather unusual in this condition), the frontal bone plates and the supraorbital rims can be rotated anteriorly by removing a wedge of bone based anteriorly along the central osteotomies; this flattens the forehead and supraorbital regions. In severe trigonocephalies, the two frontal bone plates and the supraorbital rims are left unsecured in the midline and are spread apart to widen the anterior cranial fossa. Fixation is to the lateral orbital rims and to the glabellar area. The two frontal bone flaps are wired to the supraorbital rims. This loose arrangement allows the expanding brain to remold the frontosupraorbital region. The bony gaps in the cranium are spontaneously filled with bone formed by the dura.

Plagiocephaly. A frontal bone flap is removed, and the involved supraorbital rim is removed. The latter is shaped with bone-contouring forceps until it matches the contralateral side; it is then advanced by a lateral rotation to achieve symmetry and is fixed with wires at the lateral orbital rim and in the midline. If the zygomatic area is flattened, this is included in the osteotomy. The craniotomy is continued down along the sphenozygomatic suture to the inferior orbital fissure. The frontal bone flap is now rotated 180 degrees, and the former *posterior* border is wired to the supraorbital rim. The flattened front area is transferred to the opposite side but now lies within the hairline. In this way, symmetry is restored to the fronto-orbital region. There is no posterior fixation, again following the pressure of the developing brain to hold the fronto-orbital region in the correct position.

Bicoronal Craniosynostosis. This may or may not be associated with retrusion of the midface. To correct the condition, a frontal craniotomy is performed and the supraorbital area is freed by osteotomies laterally, across the orbital roof, anterior to the cribriform plate, and in the root of the nose. The supraorbital rims are advanced as a single unit and fixed to the nasal bones and to the lateral orbital walls. The oxycephalic skull anteriorly is reconstructed either by rotating it 180 degrees or by recontouring as seems appropriate. The bone flap is wired to the supraorbital rim; again, no posterior fixation is used in order to allow expansion of the brain to carry the fronto-supraorbital area forward. The amount of advancement required is that which will position the ridges 1–1.5 cm anterior to the cornea.

CRANIOFACIAL DYSOSTOSIS (CROUZON'S SYNDROME) AND ACROCEPHALOSYNDACTYLY (APERT'S SYNDROME)

The frontosupraorbital deformities in these conditions are corrected at an early stage by the method described. Gross exorbitism is improved by the early surgery. The retrusion of the midface should be left until there is a strong reason for correcting it (e.g., peer or parental pressure or the danger of corneal exposure). The longer this can be postponed the better, as the dentition is increasingly able to cope with the fixation appliances required in the postoperative phase.

At the time of correction of the midface deformity, a LeFort III osteotomy is carried out. In this procedure the approach is subcranial, but a coronal flap is used. Osteotomies are carried out at the root of the nose, the nasal septum, the medial orbital walls, the floor of the orbit, the lateral orbital walls, and then behind the maxillary tuberosities to separate them from the pterygoid plates. In this way, the maxilla can be separated from the skull base and moved forward and, if indicated, downward as required.

In some cases, because of the lateral rotational deformity of the maxilla caused by a slight hypertelorism (telorbitism), a central wedge based upward is taken out of the nasal bone area and a midline split of the palate is performed. This allows the maxilla to be rotated medially in order to level off the occlusion. In patients with a vertical shortness of the maxilla in the midline, a LeFort I operation is selected, and the horizontal maxillary osteotomies are performed through a buccal sulcus incision. The dentoalveolar segment of the maxilla is placed in correct occlusion with the mandible. This may be done at the same time as the LeFort III procedure or at a later date. In older patients, exactly the same procedures are carried out; however, in some cases these may have to be varied, since often some kind of limited cranial release has been performed in the past. Therefore, combinations of intracranial and extracranial procedures may be necessary when larger amounts of the orbit are to be moved forward. In selected cases, the frontosupraorbital advancement will be performed with the LeFort III osteotomy.

Maxillary fixation is established by bone grafting the defects created by the osteotomies. Frequently "mini" bone plates are used in the lateral wall and temporal region to establish rigid fixation. This can also be done on the zygomatic arch. The correct position of the maxilla is obtained using an acrylic wafer containing impressions of the ideal occlusion, which has been determined in the laboratory from dental models. Intermaxillary fixation is maintained for 6–8 weeks.

HYPERTELORISM

This term is bandied about with little thought. *Hypertelorism* (telorbitism) indicates that the *orbits* are displaced laterally. *Telecanthus*, which may be either of bony origin or of soft tissue origin, indicates that the *medial canthi* are displaced laterally. These two conditions tend to be lumped together into the category of hypertelorism, and therefore the wrong operation may be carried out. For example, frontonasoencephaloceles, extensive mucoceles, and some minor midface clefting syndromes produce bony telecanthus but not hypertelorism. Careful examination in these cases shows the lateral orbital walls to be in the correct position; thus a relatively minor procedure is indicated. This is frequently referred to as "mild to moderate hypertelorism."

Telecanthus. The position of the lateral orbital walls determines whether an extensive orbital shift is necessary. In patients with bony telecanthus or small degrees of hypertelorism, the correction can usually be subcranial, using a coronal flap approach, although frequently the cranium is entered because of the low position of the dura in the cribriform plate area. This is not an operation for practitioners inexperienced in this kind of surgery. The central segment of bone is removed, judging the size so as to leave a small segment of nasal bone laterally without disrupting the nasolacrimal apparatus. As this segment of bone is removed, the nasal mucosa is dissected very carefully so as not to damage it. The contents of the ethmoid sinuses are removed. The nasal septum may be resected from this extramucosal approach. Osteotomies are then made vertically far back on the medial wall of the orbit; horizontal osteotomies run out to the supraorbital rim and to the inferior orbital rim. If the anterior cranial fossa is entered, small dural tears can occur; if this happens, they should be carefully repaired. In the older patient, if there is a large frontal sinus, its lateral wall is actually freed and moved toward the medial wall, making the whole procedure much safer.

The orbital segments are mobilized, brought together, and wired in the midline; the medial canthal ligaments are identified and wired into position (transnasal canthopexy). A skull bone graft is used to build up the nasal bridge line. Bone grafts are not required in the orbit. In some cases with a low-lying cribriform plate, particularly those associated with frontonasal encephalocele, an intracranial approach may be used to remove the encephalocele and to make the operation much safer.

Hypertelorism. When the total orbital bulk has to be moved, a combined intracranial and extracranial approach is used. Again, the central segment is removed with careful preservation of the nasal mucosa. The septum is removed by an extramucosal approach, and the ethmoid sinuses are totally resected. An osteotomy is made above the supraorbital rim, down the lateral wall of the orbit, and across the front of the maxilla under the infraorbital nerve. The intraorbital osteotomy is made circumferentially, far back in the orbit. The orbital blocks are mobilized, brought together in the midline, and wired in position. Skull bone

grafts are used to build up the dorsum of the nose and to fill in any lateral defects in the temporal area. Transnasal medial canthopexy and lateral canthopexies are performed.

Usually only a coronal approach is necessary; however, there may occasionally be some difficulty gaining access to the floor of the orbit and the front of the maxilla. If this is the case, a conjunctival incision is used. This is made deep in the inferior fornix and allows good exposure to the floor of the orbit and to the anterior aspect of the maxilla. If the nasal mucosa is broached it should be very carefully repaired, since there is always the danger of infection ascending into the extradural space. If this risk exists in any craniofacial correction, a galeal frontalis flap is used. This can be a long flap and is very vascular. It is based inferiorly on the supraorbital and supratrochlear vessels, then swung down to close off any openings into the nasopharynx, thus protecting the extradural space. Dural tears can be repaired with pericranium, fascia, or freeze-dried dura.

The timing of hypertelorism correction is dependent on the position of developing tooth buds; one must wait until there is enough room between the infraorbital rim and the tooth buds to perform the transverse osteotomy. Therefore, the correction is frequently delayed until around age 5, and many patients are much older.

HEMIFACIAL MICROSOMIA (LATERAL FACIAL DYSPLASIA)

The severity and extent of this condition are variable; frequently the cranium, orbit, maxilla, and mandible are involved.

If there is cranio-orbital involvement, this can be corrected at any time either by onlay bone grafts or by osteotomies; a coronal flap approach is used. Often the zygomatic arch is missing, and in order to widen the involved side of the face, the zygomatic arch is reconstructed or augmented using vascularized cranial bone. This is taken from the temporal area. The blood supply is from the temporal muscle and its overlying fascia; thus, the bone is pedicled on these structures. The bone flap is swung down and fixed in position with wire. Any onlay bone grafting of the orbit or the maxilla is performed with skull bone grafts. Correction of the enophthalmos involves advancement of the orbital contents and bone grafting deep in the orbit. If there is an associated macrostomia, this is corrected; any auricular tags are removed.

Should there be significant absence of the ascending ramus of the mandible, this can be reestablished at the age of 5 or 6 years with a costochondral graft. However, vascularized iliac crest is being used more and more, with microvascular anastomosis of the deep circumflex iliac vessels to the facial vessels. If soft tissue bulk is required, it is supplied by the muscles surrounding the graft. If skin is necessary, an ellipse of skin overlying the crest is added to the reconstruction.

In the older child with a mild to moderate deformity, a functional orthodontic appliance is used to guide growth and development of the mandible and maxilla and to realign the teeth. At a later date a mandibular reconstruction, which usually involves a bilateral sagittal split and bone grafting to the deficient side, is carried out together with a LeFort I osteotomy. In this way, tilt of the occlusal plane is corrected.

In adolescents and adults with severe deformities, the microvascular approach and the osteotomies described are used. Ear reconstruction is performed after the bony correction has been carried out. Costal cartilage is used to establish an ear skeleton; this is then elevated from the side of the head at a second stage, some 6 months later. No attempt is made to establish hearing in the unilateral case.

Bilateral cases of lateral facial dysplasia occasionally occur and are treated as outlined. An attempt may be made to establish hearing if it is totally absent.

TREACHER COLLINS SYNDROME (MANDIBULOFACIAL DYSOSTOSIS)

If there is a cleft palate, it is closed between 6 and 12 months of age. The recent tendency has been to do this earlier and earlier; thus, 6 months is the usual timing. Correction of the skeletal deformity is being performed earlier than in the past, often within the first year of life and certainly before age 5.

The first procedure, using a coronal flap approach, consists of:

1. Osteotomy of the supraorbital rims—an ellipse of rim is removed laterally and is shifted up and wired to the frontal area to form a new, more prominent supralateral rim.

2. Skull bone grafting to the inferolateral portion of the internal aspect of the orbit. (Steps 1 and 2 change the orbital axis and thus alter the position of the eye.)

3. Reconstruction of the zygomatic arch and lateral orbital wall with a full thickness vascularized skull graft based on temporalis muscle and temporalis fascia.

4. Skull bone grafts to the anterior aspect of the maxilla.

5. Reconstruction of the coloboma of the lower lid with a full thickness island flap of upper lid with a lateral skin pedicle.

6. Reposition of the lateral canthus.

Additional bone grafts may be required at a later date, and extensive and prolonged orthodontic treatment is usually necessary. Correction of the manibular and maxillary deformities is deferred until closer to adolescence. The ear deformities are managed as for hemifacial microsomia, and a similar approach is adopted for the hearing problems.

Disorders of the Spine and Shoulder Girdle

LAWRENCE I. KARLIN, M.D.

The treatment of skeletal disorders of the spine and shoulder girdle is best approached by an initial classification into acquired and congenital problems. Congenital disorders occur at a crucial time in the embryonal differentiation of the individual. As several systems may be at a critical stage in development at the same time, associated multisystem anomalies are frequent, e.g., spinal and genitourinary disorders. Often, one lesion of life-threatening consequence may initially be overshadowed by a less serious, but more visible, deformity.

Acquired disorders are either structural or functional. The latter will be an apparent deformity that is easily corrected when the causative factor is treated. An increased lumbar lordosis may merely be a compensatory posture caused by the structurally increased thoracic kyphosis of Scheuermann's disease. Structural deformities of variable etiology may initially appear quite similar. Spinal curvatures have a tremendous number of causative factors, including fractures, collagen disease, and neurologic and muscular impairments. Careful diagnosis is obviously indicated, as the treatment of identical deformities with different etiologies will be quite dissimilar.

DISORDERS OF THE SPINE

C1–C2 Instability. Atlantoaxial instability results from anomalies of the upper cervical spine or lesions of the supportive structures. It has been identified in children with Down's syndrome, Klippel-Feil syndrome, skeletal dysplasias (such as Morquio's dysplasia and spondyloepiphyseal dysplasia), and rheumatoid arthritis. In affected individuals, the interval between the posterior aspect of the anterior arch of the atlas and the adjacent anterior surface of the odontoid measures 4.5 mm or greater on the flexion lateral cervical spine radiograph.

Children at risk should be screened at about 5 years of age with lateral cervical spine radiographs in neutral and full active flexion and extension. As neurologic changes may not improve despite reduction and stabilization, patients with identified neurologic findings, even if they are transient, should be treated with reduction and posterior fusion from C1 to C2. Those with other associated anomalies may require a more individualized approach.

The treatment of the asymptomatic patient with instability is controversial. Our present position is to follow these children periodically with neurologic evaluation. Sports that involve trauma to the head and neck should be avoided. Fusion is carried out if any neurologic symptoms develop. The opposing argument, based upon reports of sudden death in asymptomatic patients following trauma, calls for fusion in all patients with documented instability.

Torticollis. Torticollis may have a number of etiologies, both congenital and acquired, and the treatment must be individualized. Congenital torticollis is due to muscular contracture of the sternocleidomastoid muscle, pterygium colli, or occipitocervical bony anomalies. Muscular torticollis is by far the most common form. It will respond, in 90% of cases, to conservative treatment consisting of gentle range-of-motion exercises, massage of the tightened muscle, and positioning the child near interesting stimuli in such a way as to favor motion in the direction opposite the deformity. Patients unresponsive to conservative treatment should undergo partial resection of both distal heads of the muscle and should then be placed on an exercise program. Surgery should be performed by 12–18 months of age to allow for maximum remodeling of the facial and cranial molding.

One fairly common, though poorly appreciated, acquired condition is atlantoaxial rotary displacement. This often occurs following trivial trauma or after an upper respiratory tract infection. Apparently there is ligamentous destruction that permits the rotatory subluxation between C1 and C2. Conservative treatment is usually successful; this involves immobilization and analgesia in mild cases and the addition of muscle relaxants and head halter traction in more severe ones. In all cases, immobilization in a cervical collar should be maintained for 6 weeks to allow adequate soft tissue healing. A C1-C2 reduction and fusion is indicated if symptomatic subluxation persists or recurs after adequate immobilization, or if a fixed deformity is associated with a neurologic deficit.

Klippel-Feil Syndrome. The Klippel-Feil syndrome involves a highly variable pattern of congenital fusion of the cervical vertebrae. Treatment must be individualized because of the wide range of anomalies. Patients who have fusion patterns risking neurologic compromise should avoid stressful activities. Mechanical symptoms can usually be treated by conservative means, such as a soft collar, traction, and analgesia. Neurologic symptoms must be carefully evaluated. Often they may occur secondary to associated abnormalities in the brain stem and spinal cord and not from neurologic impingement through the hypermobile segments. When the latter does occur, localized spinal fusions are indicated.

Scoliosis. Scoliosis, the most common spinal deformity, is a lateral curvature of variable etiology. A truly structural curvature demonstrates rotational deformity not seen in the functional curvatures. The modalities of treatment—exercise, bracing, electrical stimulaton, and surgery—must be individualized depending on the nature of the scoliosis and its propensity to progress. Idiopathic scoliosis is the most common form of structural curvature. School screening programs have shown a 2–3% incidence. Some curvatures regress, some remain stable, and others show progression. Curvatures that reach 50–60 degrees by skeletal maturity progress relentlessly throughout life. Therefore, the aim of treatment is to identify the progressive curvatures and prevent them from getting to the lifelong progression range. Children are followed at approximately 3-month intervals. Progressive curves in the 20–40 degree range are treated with either bracing or electrical stimulation in conjunction with an exercise program. These treatment modes do not cure the curvatures but, when successful, prevent further progression. Braces may be either the Milwaukee or low-profile variety, with the former being used for curvatures in the upper thoracic area. They are used 23 hours per day, and a program of exercises in and out of the brace is instituted. Gradual weaning over 1–2 years proceeds at skeletal maturity. Electrical stimulation is used during the sleep hours only and is applied via cutaneous electrodes placed over the convexity of the curvatures. Intermittent pulsation causes contraction of the paraspinal musculature. To date, early results seem comparable to those obtained with braces.

Progressive curvatures greater than 40 degrees in the skeletally immature child or in the 50–60 degree range in the mature individual require surgical stabilization. The goals of surgery are to straighten the spine within safe limits of neurologic toleration, to balance the spine over the pelvis, and to stabilize the spine in this position via bony fusion. Correction is achieved and maintained until bony fusion occurs via internal fixation. The most common variety is the Harrington distraction rod; various modifications in intersegmental wiring allow postoperative care in a removable brace. Severe rigid curvatures may require staged procedures. Anterior releases and fusion with or without internal fixation are followed by posterior fusion and instrumentation.

Neuromuscular curvatures reveal a different pattern and tendency to progression. Bracing is usually not curative but may slow the progression until the spine has reached the more adult size. Children with neuromuscular curvatures do not tolerate braces of the active form, e.g., the Boston or Milwaukee brace, and are best treated with total contact orthosis. The ideal surgical treatment of these children involves fusion and Luque segmental instrumentation. The greater stability permitted by the contoured rods and sublaminal wires at each level permits early mobilization and frees these children from casts, respiratory compromise, and pressure sores. Severe curvatures require staged anterior and posterior procedures. Dwyer or Zielke anterior instrumentation is well suited to the treatment of spina bifida.

Congenital curvatures occur through either embryonic failure of formation or segmentation of the spinal elements. Associated anomalies involve the genitourinary tract, the cardiac system, spinal dysraphism, and diastematomyelia. The tendency to progress varies with the individual anomalies. Some, such as the unilateral unsegmented bar, lead to relentless progression unresponsive to bracing. Early limited in situ spinal fusion is the treatment of choice.

Kyphosis. Kyphosis may occur without associated scoliosis. Etiologies are postural, functional, Scheuermann's disease, and congenital. The treatment varies accordingly. Postural kyphosis does not result in a structural deformity and can be treated with an exercise program. Bracing is not indicated.

Scheuermann's disease kyphosis involves a definite anatomic wedging of one or more vertebral bodies in the thoracic spine area. It is associated with pain, deformity, or both, and treatment depends on the relative severity of each. The onset is usually in the midst of the adolescent growth spurt. Mild pain can be treated symptomatically by reducing activities. If pain reduction is not achieved with rest, bracing is indicated. Mild deformities are initially treated with an exercise program emphasizing thoracic extension exercises and stretching of the compensatory lumbar lordosis. Angular deformities greater than 50 degrees should be treated with bracing. This treatment may effect a permanent cure in this condition, in contrast to the situation in scoliosis.

A Milwaukee brace modified for kyphosis is utilized for thoracic curvatures, while deformities in the thoracolumbar area may be treated with a modified low-profile brace. The brace is worn 23 hours per day, and the exercise program is continued. Full-time use continues until the vertebral body wedging is corrected, which usually takes 1 year. Weaning from the brace over an additional year is then begun.

Surgical correction is reserved for patients who have reached skeletal maturity and demonstrate a significant deformity or have chronic pain. Posterior fusion with compression rods over the entire thoracic spine is the procedure of choice. Some of the more angular and rigid deformities are better treated by staged anterior releases followed by a posterior fusion and instrumentation.

Congenital kyphosis may be of variable severity and is due to failure in either formation or segmentation. The former is the most common noninfectious spinal deformity leading to paraplegia. Accordingly, early recognition of this type of kyphosis and treatment with early spinal fusion are mandatory. Bracing is useless. When the deformity is more severe and angular, anterior interbody fusion is indicated. This is followed by a posterior fusion in the more severe and lengthier curvatures.

Spondylolisthesis. Spondylolysis involves a defect in the pars interarticularis. It almost always occurs at the L5 level and may result in an anterior slipping, or spondylolisthesis, of the spine. Spondylolysis is present in approximately 5% of the population. It is usually asymptomatic and requires no treatment. Nevertheless, about 20% of children with back discomfort have either spondylolysis or spondylolisthesis. Spondylolysis may present as either an acute stress fracture or a well-established nonunion. Symptomatic spondylolysis proved to be due to an acute injury may often be cured— e.g., the stress fracture will heal—with a 6-month antilordotic bracing program. Chronic symptomatic spondylolysis may be treated symptomatically with a combination of rest, exercise, and bracing. A long-term exercise program is continued. Cases refractory to conservative measures should respond to in situ spinal fusion from L5 to the sacrum.

Spondylolisthesis may be asymptomatic or may cause either back pain of variable degree or neurologic impingement with radicular pain. Because symptoms often develop in high-grade slips when surgical fusion is most difficult to accomplish, progressive slips in childhood must be identified. Children should be followed at 6-month intervals with standing lateral radiographs of the spine. Patients in whom progressive slips approach 50% should undergo spinal fusion. The surgical procedure of choice is an in situ fusion extending from the sacrum to either L4 or L5, depending upon the available bone. Severe established slips may require a two-stage procedure. Neurologic evaluation must be performed to determine the need for decompression.

Herniated Lumbar Intervertebral Disc. Lumbar intervertebral disc herniation is uncommon in children. It may present in the second decade of life as low back pain with or without radicular leg pain. Neurologic findings are less common in children than in adults. The initial treatment is conservative and consists of strict bed rest for 2– 3 weeks with symptomatic care of back pain using heat, analgesia, and muscle relaxants. If there is no improvement, myelography and computed tomography scans are performed to document the lesion and its level. The unresponsive herinated disc can be treated with surgical excision. Fusion is not indicated. Chemonucleolysis is not approved for use in children.

Intervertebral Disc Calcification. Cervical intervertebral disc calcification is a definite clinical entity of unknown etiology. The condition seems to be self-limiting, and treatment, accordingly, is symptomatic: neck support, traction, heat, muscle relaxants, and analgesia. Most patients are symptom free within 3–4 weeks.

Intervertebral Disc Space Infection. This represents a pathologic continuum of disc and vertebral body involvement that may occur throughout childhood. Treatment consists of identification of the infecting organism, appropriate antibiotic therapy, rest, and immobilization. Blood cultures and disc space aspiration are performed, though the results may be negative in 50% of cases. As the organism is most often *Staphylococcus aureus*, initial treatment can be aimed at this bacterium. A broader spectrum is necessary when the possibility of another bacterial source exists, e.g., an antecedent urinary tract infection or a history of drug abuse. Four to 6 weeks of antibiotic treatment is appropriate.

Bed rest is continued until the patient is asymptomatic. Bracing is used when discomfort is prolonged, which happens more often in the older age groups. Another relative indication for bracing is a greater bony involvement that might, in the opinion of the treating physician, proceed to clinical deformity.

Spinal Trauma. Spinal fractures are much less common in the pediatric age group than the adult age group. Several peculiarities of the growing child make care of the spinal injury unique. The increased amount of cartilage and the plasticity of the bone may allow a significant ligamentous injury to occur without a noticeable bony lesion, and this will lead to an incorrect evaluation of the stability. In addition, progressive deformity may occur when the vertebral growth plates are asymmetrically loaded. Accordingly, traumatic quadriplegia and paraplegia usually lead to spinal deformity. Careful long-term observation is indicated. Spinal instability should be diagnosed and treated with bracing in the growing child. Spinal fusion is indicated early in the growing unstable spine, and late when the deformity progresses despite bracing.

DISORDERS OF THE SHOULDER GIRDLE

Sprengel's Deformity. This deformity involves a congenitally elevated scapula. Associated anomalies are absent or fused ribs, Klippel-Feil syndrome, congenital scoliosis, and spina bifida in the cervical region. Early treatment involves active and passive range-of-motion exercises. Surgery is indicated when the deformity is cosmetically unacceptable or produces functional disability. The procedure is best done between the ages of 4 and 7 years. In the child over 10 years, treatment may be associated with brachial plexus injuries and with insufficient correction. Muscles are released from their origin over the spine; fibrous, cartilaginous, or bony bridges between the scapula and the spine are excised; and the scapula is brought down to a more normal anatomic position, where the muscles are then reattached.

Congenital Pseudarthrosis of the Clavicle. In this condition there is a failure of normal ossification involving the central portion of the clavicle. It almost always involves the right side. A localized prominence may produce a cosmetic deformity, but there is little or no functional disability. Surgery to trim excessive tissue and provide bone union is rarely, if ever, indicated.

Congenital Deformities of the Anterior Chest Wall

FRANCIS ROBICSEK, M.D.

Sternal Clefts

In the extreme form of a sternal cleft, ectopia cordis, the heart lies exposed with or without its pericardial envelope outside the chest. The initial management of this condition requires coverage with skin with additional surgical procedures later. Because of commonly associated complex intracardiac anomalies, only a few such patients survive into adulthood.

A special form of ectopia cordis is the pentalogy of Cantrell, in which the patient presents a consistent association of anomalies of the abdominal wall, lower sternum, ventral diaphragm, pericardium, and the heart. The syndrome is often associated with omphaloceles of various sizes. Among the intracardiac anomalies, Fallot's tetralogy and ventricular diverticulums are the most common. Operative management includes the repair of intracardiac anomalies if feasible, pericardial closure, retroposition of the heart into the mediastinum, closure of the defect, and reinforcement of the thoracic and abdominal walls. The latter may be accomplished by direct approximation by plastic repair, by the application of prosthetic mesh, or by a combination of these.

Sternal clefts uncomplicated by ectopia cordis may be complete and involve the entire length of the sternum except the xyphoid, or partial, limited usually to the upper third. The prognosis in patients with uncomplicated sternal clefts is uniformly good. However, because the condition is unsightly, and by leaving the heart unprotected, also potentially dangerous, surgical repair is recommended. The technique of the operation is aimed at filling the bone defect created by the non-union of the sternal halves. This can be accomplished either by bilateral costochondral resection, by mobilization and unification of the sternal halves, or by simply bridging the bony gap with autogenous (i.e., fascia, rib grafts) or synthetic (Marlex mesh, Teflon graft) material.

Positional Anomalies of the Sternum

The origin of most if not all positional anomalies of the sternum can be traced to the same factor, overgrowth of the costal cartilages. If the elongated cartilages push the sternum forward, pectus carinatum develops; if the sternum is forced backward, pectus excavatum results. In either case, a psychologically damaging and a physiologically often harmful situation develops. If the deformity is significant enough, it should be surgically corrected, preferably between the ages of 1 and 6 years, but certainly before adulthood.

The treatment of positional anomalies of the sternum is surgical, and while the extent of the procedure has to be individualized case by case, it should follow some definite general principles. (a) The elongated and distorted costal cartilages should be bilaterally resected. (b) The sternum should be brought into proper position by performing a proximal transverse osteotomy, fracturing the posterior lamina and, depending on the nature of the anomaly, either depressing or lifting the breast bone. The sternum should be maintained in its corrected position. The latter may be achieved in excavatum deformities by posterior Marlex mesh support; in carinatum anomalies by resection of the distal sternal body, reattaching the xyphoid process and using the pulley action of the rectus muscles. In all cases the pectoralis muscles should be united in the front of the sternum to further secure its corrected position and to provide a smooth, soft contour to the anterior chest wall.

Jeune's Disease

Jeune's disease, also appropriately named asphyxiating thoracic dystrophy of the newborn, is characterized by broad ribs and narrow and rigid thorax. In milder cases the patient may survive with energetic symptomatic treatment and may later undergo different procedures designed to expand the rib cage. Patients with severe cases usually die shortly after birth.

Bizarre Rib Anomalies

The variety of rib anomalies that occur with or without the presence of positional abnormalities of the sternum or the vertebral column is virtually infinite, and they may vary from absence or prominence of a single rib to a complete "cave-in" of a hemithorax or herniation of the lung. Most of the time their significance is only cosmetic, but in more extensive cases they could lead to respiratory distress syndrome. Surgical repair is tailored to the anatomical features of the patient.

Orthopedic Disorders of the Extremities

H. LEON BROOKS, M.D.

UPPER EXTREMITIES
Congenital Disorders

Congenital Elevation of the Scapulae (Sprengel's deformity). In the presence of a mild deformity and disability, no treatment is indicated. In more severe instances, surgery may be indicated. However, the results of surgical treatment are often disappointing because of the associated malformations and contractures of the soft tissue structures of the region. The presence of a Klippel-Feil syndrome as well as thoracic scoliosis, and renal and cardiac abnormalities should always be remembered in the presence of congenital elevation of the scapula.

Congenital Pseudarthrosis of the Clavicle. This condition is of cosmetic significance only. Function is quite good, and surgery is rarely necessary. Whenever surgery is contemplated, the parents should be warned that they are replacing a bump with a scar. Bilateral congenital pseudarthrosis of the clavicle is usually diagnostic of cleidocranial dysostosis.

Congenital Radioulnar Synostosis. Congenital radioulnar synostosis is usually bilateral. Fortunately, disability is minimal and no surgical procedure is justified. If the pronation deformity is disabling, a corrective osteotomy would be indicated, though rarely.

Congenital Dislocation of the Radial Head. It is not possible to reduce the congenital dislocation of the radial head either manually or surgically. If resection of the radial head is ever contemplated, it should be postponed until after growth is complete.

Congenital Absence of the Thumb. This condition varies from total absence to the presence of a rudimentary thumb. With absence of the thumb, it may be necessary to consider pollicization of one of the remaining digits to allow for the function of opposition. Other procedures performed for the rudimentary thumb do offer some improvement in function.

Syndactyly. This condition occurs most often between the middle and ring fingers. If the deformity is severe, surgery is indicated as early as possible. However, if the development of the fingers is not being retarded by the condition, surgery may be postponed until after the second year.

Gigantism of Fingers (Macrodactyly). This condition may be managed surgically by reduction of the soft tissues and arrest of the phalangeal growth.

Camptodactyly. This contracture of the proximal interphalangeal joint is thought to be related to shortening of the flexor digitorum sublimus. Repetitive stretching exercises of the tendon in the newborn are thought to be the best form of treatment. Other measures, such as casting and tendon lengthening, have not proved to be very successful.

Constriction Bands (Streeter's Dysplasia). This deformity is seen in the neonatal period. It follows a circumferential soft tissue constriction. The venous return is compromised, and in the presence of edema, surgical treatment becomes more urgent. The treatment is usually carried out in two stages. In the absence of vascular compromise, function of the digit or extremity is satisfactory.

Trigger Thumb. This condition presents with the thumb being kept in acute flexion at the interphalangeal joint level. Prior to considering surgical treatment, one should exclude the presence of a congenital clasped thumb, which is associated with the absence of a thumb extensor. Surgical correction by releasing the flexor tendon is very successful.

Lobster Claw Hand. This condition is of two general types. In the first, a deep palmar cleft separates the two central metacarpals. The existing digits tend to be confluent and of equal length. If the appearance and grasp need to be improved, the palmar cleft should be closed. The child usually resists any attempt at prosthetic fitting, because of the excellent sensation and functional length of the hand. In the second type, the central rays are absent. Short radial and ulnar digits remain. If large objects are handled with difficulty, it may be necessary to deepen the web space, to improve grasp and pinch.

Congenital Absence of the Radius. This causes progressive deviation of the hand to the radial side. The early use of a light dynamic splint or serial plaster casts is of benefit. After the hand has been aligned, surgical treatment provides a more permanent correction. Centralization, or placing of the hand on the end of the ulna, is a recommended procedure. The parents, however, should be forewarned that revision surgery may become indicated. Despite surgery, it is recommended that the extremity be splinted at night until skeletal maturity. In the presence of a bilateral deformity, splinting would be the preferable treatment.

Congenital Below-Elbow Amputation. This is the most frequent congenital amputation of the upper extremity. The fitting of a prosthesis early is indicated. This allows for better function as the child grows.

Phocomelia, or Seal Flipper. In this extremely rare condition, a small remnant of the upper extremity, usually the hand, is attached to the shoulder. Prosthetic fittings should be attempted in unilateral cases.

Acquired and Developmental Disorders of the Extremities

Unicameral Bone Cyst. The current recommended treatment is multiple aspirations and injections of methylprednisolone acetate. Because the older form of surgical excision, curettage, and bone grafting was associated with a high recurrence rate, the more conservative aspiration and injection treatment is now favored.

Osteochondritis Dissecans of the Elbow. This usually occurs in athletes who throw frequently, such as pitchers, catchers, and first basemen. Surgical excision of a loose fragment, followed by drilling of the cystic lateral humeral condyle, is recommended.

Madelung's Deformity. When mild, the deformity may be asymptomatic. When moderate or severe, weakness and instability of the wrist joint occur. The deformity may be severe enough to justify the surgery before the distal radial epiphysis has fused. Bowing of the radius is corrected by osteotomy, with shortening of the ulna at the same time.

LOWER EXTREMITIES
Congenital Deformities

The magnitude and duration of treatment as well as the end result often depend on early and accurate diagnosis and the immediate institution of treatment in congenital deformities of the extremities.

Hip. In no other orthopedic disorder are early diagnosis and treatment more rewarding and late diagnosis and treatment more disappointing. Once the diagnosis is made, treatment should be instituted immediately. The principles of treatment involve bringing the femoral head to a position opposite the acetabulum, and maintenance of the reduction until there is adequate capsular and acetabular development. The older the child is at the time of diagnosis, the more difficult the treatment. We will discuss the treatment of the condition in the different age groups.

BIRTH TO TWO MONTHS. In this age group, the use of the Von Rosen splint or the Pavlick stirrup is recommended. The splint should be kept in place for a period of from 8 to 12 weeks. The infant should be checked at weekly intervals. After radiologic confirmation of the reduction and stability of the hip joint, the use of a Freyka pillow at night and during the napping periods is indicated, for 3 more months. In the dysplastic or subluxable type of hip, which does not frankly dislocate, the Freyka pillow may be used for the initial 8 to 12 weeks continuously, and for the following 3 months at night and for the napping periods.

THREE MONTHS TO TWELVE MONTHS. In infants of this age group, shortening of the adductor and iliopsoas muscles prevents appropriate placement of the proximal femur opposite the acetabulum. Because of this, preliminary traction for several weeks, associated most often with adductor tenotomies, allows for adequate reduction of the femoral head into the acetabulum. Once reduction is obtained, the position is maintained using a hip spica. The spica is changed every 6 to 8 weeks. It is usual to keep the patient in the cast for the number of months equal to the time that the hip has been dislocated. Avascular necrosis of the femoral capital epiphysis is a dreaded complication and is associated with forced manipulative reduction, with inadequate stretching of the hip musculature and the presence of the reduced extremity in the frog position.

AFTER TWELVE MONTHS. If the diagnosis is initially made after the age of one year, treatment is more complicated and the results of treatment are more disappointing. Following adductor tenottomy and traction, it usually becomes necessary to perform an open reduction of the dislocated hip, with removal of the limbus. If warranted, it becomes necessary to improve the roof of the acetabulum by performing an innominate osteotomy.

AFTER FOUR TO FIVE. At this stage of life, untreated congenital dislocation of the hip is a major problem. Subluxation is more easily treated with surgical measures such as innominate osteotomy and an open reduction. The frank dislocation requires much more extensive surgery and is associated with less gratifying results.

Metatarsus Adductus. This condition is associated with a C shape of the plantar aspect of the foot, either uni- or bilaterally. It is my opinion that early aggressive management of this condition avoids later heartache for the patient as well as the parents. Soon after birth, if the condition is diagnosed, recommendations are made for the mother to manipulate the foot by stabilizing the heel with one hand and stretching the contracted soft tissues on the medial aspect of the foot. It is my practice to recommend that this be performed each time the diaper is changed. The infant is seen for follow-up assessment. If after a period of three weeks sustained correction is not present, it is recommended that the deformity be corrected with serial casts, which are initially changed at 10- to 14-day intervals and later at 3-week intervals. It may require up to 6 cast changes to achieve the desired correction. Once the correction is obtained, serious consideration should be given to the use of a straight last or reverse last shoe, which should be worn until one feels comfortable that the deformity will not relapse. It is not unusual for the child to need straight or last shoes for several years.

Club Foot (Congenital Talipes Equinovarus). This condition is easily recognizable at birth. It is advisable for the parents to be informed that even with optimal treatment, the foot will usually be smaller than the opposite normal side and that some abnormality of the foot may persist. In the newborn, when the diagnosis is made, aggressive measures should be instituted to correct the deformity as soon as possible after birth, with the application of corrective casts.

The technique of cast application is important. Without appropriate casts, proper correction will not be obtained. The adduction and supination deformities should be corrected initially and the equinus deformity last. The correction of the equinus deformity too soon leads to the characteristic deformity of the boat-shaped foot. Cast changes are performed initially at 10- to 14-day intervals, and subsequently at 3- to 4-week intervals. If complete correction is not obtained by the age of three months, surgical correction of the foot is recommended.

The surgical procedure should be radical and should involve division of all tight ligaments and capsules as well as lengthening of tendons where indicated. After surgical treatment, case immobilization is essential, followed by the use of braces, initially to be worn on a full-time basis, and subsequently as night splints. Failure to continue with appropriate bracing leads to a recurrence of the deformity. In the older child with untreated congenital talipes equinovarus, partially treated or recurrent club feet, extensive surgery in the form of tendon transfers, soft tissue releases, and even bony procedures become indicated. No other orthopedic condition has been more neglected in the past than congenital talipes equinovarus. However, in more recent years, with more aggressive early treatment, the results have become more favorable.

Calcaneovalgus Feet. This deformity presents at birth. In most instances, spontaneous resolution tends to occur. However, the resolution can be accelerated with manipulation of the foot by the parent, stretching the tight peroneal muscles as well as the extensor muscles. If this deformity persists longer than 6 to 8 weeks, manipulation and application of serial corrective casts are indicated. If a significant flat foot occurs, the use of corrective shoes, including a firm medial counter $\frac{3}{16}$-inch arch pad and $\frac{1}{8}$-inch inner heel wedge, helps to correct the deformity in the growing foot. With the presentation of a calcaneovalgus foot, one should rule out the presence of associated neuromuscular disease and hypotonia.

Cavus Feet. This situation, although less common than a flat foot, is often symptomatic of a neurologic disorder, such as myelodysplasia, Charcot-Marie-Tooth disease, Friedreich's ataxia, and other neuromuscular disorders. It is important to exclude these diagnoses when one is presented with a patient with cavus feet. The condition results in difficulty with fitting into shoes, the development of metatarsalgia, plantar callosities, and later, clawing of the toes. Attempts to stretch the plantar fascia by the addition of metatarsal bar pads to the shoes are made but are not very beneficial. In most instances, it becomes necessary to provide shoes with laces to allow more room for the high arch. When cases become very symptomatic, surgical procedures include plantar fasciectomy, as described by Steindler, and calcaneal osteotomies; other bone procedures may be indicated.

Congenital Overlapping Toes. Congenital contracture angulation and subluxation of the fifth toe is a very common familial deformity. It causes disability in only about half the patients concerned, however. When the deformity becomes very bothersome, surgical measures are of benefit. These include reconstructive procedures to reposition the toes, or syndactyly, which involves joining the fifth to the fourth toes.

Tarsal Coalition. With this condition, a bony or cartilaginous fibrous bridge connects two or more of the tarsal bones in the hindfoot or midfoot. Symptomatic measures, using an arch pad or heel cup, are occasionally of benefit. However, in most cases, surgical excision of the congenital bar, or even in certain instances stabilization of the joints of the hindfoot, is required.

Dislocation of the Knee. This deformity is usually seen in a constrained breech delivery with full knee extension. Treatment should begin as early as possible, using daily manipulation with splinting and application of serial casts. Once 90 degrees of flexion has been achieved, the knee is immobilized in this position, with cast changes weekly, until the knee becomes stable. With early treatment, surgery rarely becomes necessary. It is extensive and should be preceded by preoperative arthrography and, in addition, requires lengthening of the quadriceps mechanism. Surgical treatment, however, is usually carried out in those cases with an associated congenital dislocation of the hip.

Polydactyly. This is the most common anomaly of the toes. It consists of the presence of supernumerary digits. It is rare, and it becomes necessary to recommend a surgical procedure when the contour of the foot needs to be improved. However, when surgery is contemplated for supernumerary toes, its effect on the existing function of the extremity must be carefully considered. Interfering with the blood supply or disturbing the anomalous insertions of tendons may increase the disability over and above the existing disability. If a patient has six toes, although the sixth toe may be more nearly normal than the fifth, the sixth would usually have to be amputated. Removal of this toe is usually the most logical and satisfactory approach. If there is an extra metatarsal, amputation must be performed at the tarsometatarsal joint level.

Amputations in the Lower Extremities. When a congenital amputation of the lower extremity exists, early prosthetic fitting is indicated so that the child may reach his developmental milestones at the usual time. The management of the prosthesis often requires a team approach, involving pediatrics, orthopedics, and rehabilitation medicine as well as physical therapy and occupational therapy. Because of growth, changes in the prostheses become frequent in the childhood period. Lower extremity prostheses are best fitted at approximately the age of 10 months, at which time the child is beginning to pull up. This allows for ambulation to be commenced at the normal time.

Congenital Vertical Talus (Rocker Bottom Foot, Persian Slipper Foot, Congenital Convex Pes Valgus). This condition is usually obvious in the newborn nursery. Attempts have been made to apply serial casts, but surgery is almost always required in order to obtain complete correction.

Acquired Deformities

Leg Length Discrepancy. Most frequently leg length discrepancy in children is a result of acquired problems. It is necessary to carefully monitor the discrepancy in leg length. This is most accurately performed by obtaining special x-ray views taken in a longitudinal projection, which are referred to as scanograms. If the discrepancy is no more than $\frac{3}{4}$ inch, leg lengths can be equalized with a shoe lift. If it is greater, surgical measures to equalize the leg lengths need to be considered. These include epiphysiodesis or arrest of growth, or lengthening of the tibia or the femur. The procedure recommended depends on the age of the patient and the amount of inequality as well as other factors. In hemihypertrophy, there is a difference in size not only of the bones but also of the circumferences, which involves muscle size. In this situation, the increased circumference of the limb can, obviously, not be changed. In the presence of hemihypertrophy, intravenous pyelography as well as the evaluation for the presence of vascular malformation is indicated.

Transient Synovitis of the Hip. This condition is usually unilateral. It most commonly occurs in children between the ages of 3 and 5 years. Aspiration of the hip reveals synovial fluid, which does not have the characteristics of a septic arthritis. In the more severe cases with increased pain, bed rest is indicated, with traction on the extremity until the spasm has subsided. With clinical improvement, normal activities are resumed slowly, over a period of several weeks. Follow-up radiologic assessment is indicated in 6 to 12 months to rule out the subsequent development of Legg-Calvé-Perthes disease.

Legg-Calvé-Perthes Disease. This condition is associated with avascular necrosis of the femoral capital epiphysis. The condition is initially treated in the hospital in traction, with bed rest, in order to allow the synovitis to resolve. Subsequent treatment involves maintaining the head of the femur in the acetabulum, in order to allow for reconstitution of the capital femoral epiphysis. The goal of treatment is to maintain a round femoral head. The principle of treatment involves containment of the femoral head within the bony confines of the acetabulum.

Provided containment can be achieved by braces, which position the hip into abduction and internal rotation, full weight bearing is allowed because the femoral head does remain protected and well contained in the acetabulum. The weight-bearing brace used is commonly one such as the Toronto brace or the Scottish Rite brace. It takes up to 2 to 4 years for femoral head reconstitution to be completed. An alternate method of containing the femoral head within the confines of the acetabulum is the use of surgical procedures. These consist of either an innominate osteotomy of the pelvic bone, redirecting the acetabulum over the femoral head, or a varus osteotomy of the proximal femur, redirecting the femoral head into the acetabulum. In late untreated cases of Legg-Calvé-Perthes disease, reconstructive salvage operations are availabe if the hip is symptomatic.

Slipped Femoral Capital Epiphysis. Diagnosis of this condition in the acute stage requires hospitalization, with the use of traction initially until surgery can be undertaken. If the slip is 1 cm or less, stabilization of the femoral head in situ, using threaded pins across the epiphyseal plate, is the treatment of choice. If the slip is greater than 1 cm, with restricted flexion and internal rotation of the hip, in the presence of an acute slip, gentle reduction using either traction or internal fixation under anesthesia is recommended. If the slip is chronic, an extra-articular osteotomy through the subtrochanteric region of the femur is carried out to compensate for the limitation of flexion and internal rotation. Intra-articular procedures are associated with a high incidence of avascular necrosis and are generally not favored. Occasionally a slipped capital femoral epiphysis is associated with a dreaded complication known as acute chondrolysis or acute cartilage necrosis. This is associated with a decreased range of motion and loss of joint space. The use of prolonged skeletal traction and non–weight bearing, crutches, occasionally allow for reconstitution of the joint space, although further reconstructive arthroplasties are required frequently.

Snapping Hip. This condition is occasionally seen in teenagers, particularly when the hip is placed in abduction and external rotation. It is not painful but does worry the patient and parents. Provided other abnormalities are excluded, reassurance is enough to allay any fears on the part of the patient and parents. Very rarely, if the snap becomes particularly bothersome, surgical release of the iliotibial band or fascia lata as it slides over the greater trochanter is beneficial.

Blount's Disease (Tibia Vara). Up to the age of 5, the use of bracing is effective. Beyond that age, in the presence of persistent deformity, repeated osteotomies may become necessary, particularly during the teenage growth spurt.

Osgood-Schlatter Disease. This traction apophysitis occurs classically during preadolescence and adolescent growth spurts. It is associated with the presence of a painful swelling in the area of the tuberosity of the tibia. It does tend to be self-limiting but continues for a period of 6 to 12 months, leaving a painless prominence in the area of the tuberosity of the tibia. Recommended treatment is avoidance of athletic activities as well as jumping and squatting. If the pain becomes less tolerable, immobilization in a cylinder cast or knee immobilizer is beneficial. The use of aspirin for pain relief does reduce the discomfort. Surgery to excise a symptomatic ununited ossicle should only be reserved for those patients beyond the teen years who continue to complain of pain with loss of function in the area of the tibial tuberosity.

Chondromalacia Patellae and Subluxing Patella. This is a problematical condition causing a deep aching pain in the knee and it is often mistaken for an internal derangement of the knee, such as a torn medial meniscus. Tears of the menisci, however, are extremely rare in children. Chondromalacia and a subluxing patella are more common in females than in males. Treatment should be conservative. The use of quadriceps-strengthening exercises of an isometric nature are of great benefit. Isotonic exercises or flexion and extension exercises are contraindicated because they tend to increase pain. In the skeletally mature teenager in whom chondromalacia is associated with a subluxing patella surgery should be considered if there has been a failure of conservative treatment and there is a danger of further deterioration of the undersurface of the patella. Realignment of the quadriceps mechanism, which is affected by various surgical techniques, should be considered. However, the patient should be aware of the need for a prolonged physical therapy rehabilitation program postoperatively.

Baker's Cyst (Popliteal Cyst). This condition presents with a swelling behind the knee, on the medial side. It is common in children under the age of 8 years. It usually disappears spontaneously. If it is large enough to cause symptoms, surgery should be considered.

Osteochondritis Dissecans. Interference with the blood supply to a portion of the femoral condyle leads to an area of avascular necrosis, with the associated separation of the bone and a limp on the affected side. If the condition is diagnosed at an early stage, cast immobilization for 6 to 8 weeks may suffice. Further loosening of the fragments or disruption of the articular surface warrants arthroscopy with possible surgery to replace or drill the affected fragment.

Calcaneal Apophysitis (Sever's Disease). This is a traction type of apophysitis akin to Osgood-Schlatter disease. It affects the os calcis rather than the proximal tibia. It is most common in boys. It is self-limiting and usually improves over the course of 6 to 12 months. Activities that involve stressing the Achilles tendon, such as prolonged running and jumping, tend to produce pain. The use of a heel lift in the shoes tends to decrease the symptoms. No other specific measures are indicated.

Growing Pains. Children between the ages of 3 and 5 years frequently complain of discomfort in the lower extremities, particularly occurring at night. The diagnosis of this condition is by process of elimination. One should be extremely careful not to overlook any serious underlying condition that may progress to irreversible bone or joint damage. The pain usually affects the calves or the front of the thighs and tends to disappear in the mornings. Use of gentle massage or local heat relieves these symptoms. No other specific measures are indicated.

Developmental, Angular, and Torsional Deformities of the Lower Extremities

From birth to adolescence, changes occur in the angulation and torsional alignment of the lower extremities. These give rise to much discussion and lead to much anxiety on the part of parents and grandparents and also lead to difficulty in management as they relate to pediatricians and orthopedists. Whether torsional and angular developmental deformities require treatment depends on personal judgement, slower resolution of the deformity, and asymmetry of one limb. Whenever possible, treatment by reassurance is preferable to the application of devices that not infrequently, when contraindicated, lead to the development of the opposite type of deformity. Proper analysis depends on examination of the

hip, the knee, and tibial torsion as well as the ankles, subtalar joints, and midtarsal joints. It is most important to rule out the presence of metabolic bone disease as well as abnormalities of epiphyseal growth.

Internal Tibial Torsion. This deformity results in a toe-in gait, typically noted when the child first begins to walk. Except in extreme cases, observation until the age of 18 months is appropriate. Should the deformity persist beyond that age, fitting with the Denis Browne type of splint is indicated. The night splint is tolerated very well in the older child. However, parents should understand that it does require several days to a week for the child to adjust to the wearing of the splint. In order to avoid stressing the knees, the bar in the Denis Browne night splint should be the same width as the pelvis, which usually is a maximum of 6 to 8 inches. One should not mistake internal torsion for metatarsus adductus. If metatarsus adductus exists, the attention should be focused on the foot.

Physiologic Bowlegs. It is important to understand that Denis Browne bars are contraindicated for bowing of the tibia alone, because they stretch the medial knee ligaments and accentuate the normal physiologic knock knee that develops later. If the bowleg is unilateral or posteromedial, or is associated with a skin dimple or other musculoskeletal anomalies, other causes for bowlegs such as neurofibromatosis, bone dysplasias, or metabolic bone disease should be excluded. If the physiologic bowleg is not resolved by 24 months of age and a tibiofemoral angle of 20 degrees persists, Blount's disease, or tibia vara, especially in black children, should be suspected.

Knock-knees, or Genu Valgum. Most children have some degree of genu valgum by the age of 30 months, which might become worse until the age of 5. It usually, however, corrects by the age of 6 or 7. Many children with genu valgum tend to have flat feet; therefore, a shoe correction does enable them to track better and to walk with less of a clumsy gait. If the knock-knee deformity is still not corrected by the age of 5, the use of night splints is of benefit. Surgery is almost never indicated in this type of deformity. One should always exclude bone dysplasias and metabolic bone disease in persistent genu valgum.

Femoral Anteversion. As a rule, femoral anteversion resolves spontaneously. It is thought, however, on an empirical basis, that sitting in a W posture causes increased torque on the femoral neck and might prevent spontaneous correction. There is no evidence that persistent femoral anteversion leads to degenerative arthritis of the hip. In extremely rare instances, in a patient who is over 8 years of age and is clumsy and tends to trip, with significant anteversion documented by

CAT scans of the hip, associated with limited ability to rotate the hip externally, surgery in the form of a derotation osteotomy of the proximal femur might be a consideration.

The Hip

LYNN T. STAHELI, M.D.

Hip problems in childhood are unusually serious for several reasons. First, the hip is normally only marginally competent; degenerative arthritis frequently occurs without known cause. Second, hip problems are often more difficult to diagnose than other joint disorders because of the hip's deep location under layers of muscle. Third, the blood supply to the proximal femoral epiphysis is tenuous. Trauma, inflammation, or compression can obstruct flow, cause necrosis, and permanently damage the hip in as short a time as 6–8 hours. Thus, early diagnosis of hip problems is critical. With early diagnosis and skillful management, deformity and disability can usually be prevented.

CONGENITAL DYSPLASIA OF THE HIP (CDH)

CDH includes a variety of deformities, from shallow acetabulum to frank dislocation. Effective management requires early diagnosis, which is not easy. The hip is primarily cartilaginous in the newborn, making radiography unreliable. Physical findings are subtle, and CDH can be missed by even the most skillful examiner. Thus, it is essential that the search for the problem continue throughout infancy.

Newborn Screening. The infant should be quiet and relaxed for the screening examination. The examiner employs Ortolani's or Barlow's maneuvers to detect instability. "Clicks" are insignificant. "Clunks" or "jerks" are signs of instability felt by the examiner as the femoral head slides in and out of the socket. If screening is negative, the hip should be re-examined when the infant is next seen. If a "click" is heard, the infant should be examined at the next two or three visits to be certain that it is insignificant. If a "clunk" is felt, treatment is indicated. If the hip is stable in abduction, a simple, soft abduction splint is applied. If the hip is unstable, a "Pavlik harness" should be used. This harness is the most effective splint available.

If one is uncertain whether it is a "click" or a "clunk," the infant is either treated or referred. It is prudent to overtreat when in doubt. Triple diapers are not helpful and are often harmful. They become compressed between the thighs and provide little or no abduction. More importantly, they create the illusion that treatment is in progress when in fact valuable time is being wasted.

Early Infancy (1–3 Months). The physical findings change during the first weeks after birth. Hip instability signs, which are most reliable in the neonatal period, tend to disappear and are replaced by signs of limited abduction and limb shortening, which become more pronounced with increasing age.

HIGH-RISK INFANTS. The incidence of classic CDH is about 0.1%. The chances increase 30 times when a positive family history is present. It is about 10 times more likely to occur in infants with metatarsus adductus. CDH is found in about 20% of infants with torticollis. Infants at risk should have a single AP radiograph of the pelvis taken at 3 months of age. Some infants with a negative examination will have definite radiographic findings of CDH. Without treatment these children face early degenerative arthritis, perhaps as early as their teen years.

Radiography. Radiography in the newborn period is reliable in only about half of the cases. Reliability rapidly improves over the next 3 months, when it becomes the most definitive diagnostic method. A single AP radiograph of the pelvis is adequate for routine screening and follow-up evaluations. The slope of the acetabulum (acetabular index) is measured as an indicator of acetabular dysplasia. The relationship of the upper femur and acetabulum is assessed for evidence of dislocation. Ossification of the proximal femoral epiphysis, which normally occurs during the first 6 months, is often delayed in CDH. In its absence, the position of the upper femoral metaphysis is compared with the acetabulum. If the hip is reduced, the metaphysis will fall medial to a line (Perkin's) drawn vertically from the lateral margin of the acetabulum and at right angles to a line that passes through both triradiate cartilage clear spaces (Hilgenreiner's). If the epiphyseal ossification center is seen, it should fall in the inner lower quadrant created by the intersection of Perkin's and Hilgenreiner's lines.

The end point of treatment is a normal radiograph. After the hip is reduced, the physical examination becomes normal. Acetabular dysplasia may persist and must be corrected to ensure a lasting satisfactory result. This can only be assessed radiographically.

Older Infants and Children. Limited abduction, shortening of the limb, and limp are classic findings. Whenever the diagnosis is seriously considered, a radiograph should be taken.

Referral

The role of the primary care physician is diagnostic. Treatment should be provided by an orthopedic specialist. Objectives include achieving a concentric reduction, correcting acetabular dysplasia, and avoiding avascular necrosis. At present, Pavlik harness treatment is appropriate in infants under 6 months of age. Traditional traction, closed reduction under anesthesia, and cast immobilization are indicated if dislocation pesists after a trial with the Pavlik harness, and for children first seen after 6 months of age. Open reduction is indicated if closed reduction fails or if the child is seen after about 2 years of age.

SEPTIC ARTHRITIS

Bacterial infection of the hip joint is one of the most urgent problems in orthopedics. It not only can damage the articular cartilage but also can obstruct the circulation to the epiphysis, causing avascular necrosis. The sequelae of necrosis include a severely shortened leg and a fused hip.

Early Infancy. Most sequelae of septic arthritis result from hip infections that occur during the neonatal period or early infancy. At that age diagnosis is difficult; systemic and localizing signs are few. The only reliable sign is "pseudoparalysis" of the involved limb. Spontaneous hip movement is absent. The cause should be determined. Trauma and true paralysis must also be considered.

Joint fluid examination is the only reliable method of establishing the diagnosis. Other studies are unreliable. When in doubt, the joint is aspirated under image intensifier guidance. A negative study should be confirmed by arthrography. After aspiration, dye is instilled into the joint and a permanent radiograph is made. This confirms that the joint was entered.

In later infancy and childhood, diagnosing septic arthritis is less difficult. The patient is often ill, has guarding of the hip, resists rotational movement, and shows an elevated sedimentation rate. Again, these findings mandate the need for a diagnostic arthrocentesis. Studies such as bone scanning delay diagnosis and usually are of little help.

Radiography is of limited value. Fat pad signs are not reliable. It is a common mistake to rely on negative radiographs. Only a negative arthrocentesis documented with an arthrogram can rule out the presence of septic arthritis.

If purulent fluid is obtained from the arthrocentesis, the joint should be surgically drained. An open procedure makes certain the joint is completely evacuated and will remain free of fluid. Incomplete drainage by needle aspiration is too risky to be justified. The potential for disability is too great. About 20% of purulent drainage will be culture and Gram stain negative. This is to be expected. Open drainage and antibiotic treatment should be provided. The antibiotic is selected empirically, using the age of the patient as a guide.

TOXIC SYNOVITIS

Toxic synovitis or "observation hip syndrome" is a benign inflammatory problem of the hip of unknown etiology. It commonly occurs in late infancy and childhood, and in 1 to 3% of cases leads to Perthes disease.

The major diagnostic problem is clearly separating this benign condition from septic arthritis. Differentiation is made by considering several factors: (1) The patient with synovitis is usually not as ill as the child with arthritis. The child's fever, malaise, and activity level are helpful guides. (2) In septic arthritis joint guarding is more pronounced and the patient will usually refuse to walk. (3) The ESR is usually slightly elevated in synovitis and moderately or severely elevated in septic arthritis. Leukocytosis is variable in both. (4) If the diagnosis remains uncertain, an arthrocentesis is indicated. It should be re-emphasized that radiographs and bone scans are seldom helpful in making this differentiation.

Synovitis is managed by rest. Traction on the limb is unnecessary and theoretically harmful. The hip joint capsule is most relaxed and, thus, the joint capacity the greatest, when the hip is flexed, slightly abducted, and laterally rotated. The patient will assume this position while resting. Traction is likely to alter this position, increasing the intra-articular pressure and possibly impairing circulation to the epiphysis.

Bed rest is continued until hip rotation is free and unguarded. A follow-up check should be made in a month or so to ensure that motion has completely returned. Persisting stiffness is an indication for a radiograph to rule out Perthes disease.

PERTHES DISEASE

Perthes disease is commonly referred to as LCP disease, a name derived from the initials of those first describing the disease (Legg-Calvé-Perthes). LCP is an idiopathic avascular necrosis of the femoral capital epiphysis that occurs spontaneously during midchildhood. Healing occurs consistently but slowly over 2 to 3 years. Residual deformity may lead to degenerative arthritis in adult life. LCP tends to occur in some families, in children of delayed skeletal age, and occasionally following toxic synovitis. It affects males most frequently, and in most cases the cause is unknown. During midchildhood, circulation to the femoral epiphysis is even more tenuous than at other ages, being almost totally provided by the lateral retinacular vessels. These may be obstructed by trauma, inflammation, coagulation defects, or other causes.

LCP disease results from one or more ischemic episodes occurring at different sites in the vascular network. In mild cases only the anterior portion of the head is involved; in severe cases the whole head is involved. The disease is also more serious in the older child.

Clinical Features. Onset is usually insidious. It commonly occurs in one hip of a boy between 4 and 8 years of age but may occur in either sex between ages 3 and 14 years. The child presents with a limp and mild discomfort. Often the symptoms are present for months before the family seeks medical attention. The physical findings include limitation of abduction and medial rotation of the affected hip. Radiographic features vary according to the stage of the disease. *Synovitic stage:* This stage has usually passed by the time the child is first seen. If the child is seen very early in the disease process, the radiographs may show slight joint space widening. *Necrotic or collapse stage:* The earliest definitive sign is a crescentic radiolucency just under the subchondral bone of the epiphysis on the lateral projection. More commonly there is a flattening, irregularity, and increased density of the epiphysis. *Fragmentation stage:* Replacement of necrotic bone with preossified fibrous tissue produces a "moth-eaten" appearance characteristic of this stage. *Consolidation stage:* Reossification progresses with increasing homogenicity of the epiphysis. Widening of the neck and head (coxa magna), and flattening of the epiphysis (coxa plana) are frequently seen.

These stages take several years to run their course. Treatment is usually started during the necrotic stage and continues through the fragmentation stage. This requires about 12 to 18 months.

Management. Treatment is controversial, but current management trends are conservative. Individualized management, fewer operative procedures, and shorter treatment periods with less cumbersome braces are currently favored. The first step is restoration of motion by rest. Activity causes microfractures of the soft, ischemic epiphysis. These fractures induce synovitis, which causes stiffness and adductor contracture. Rest reduces this inflammation and allows return of motion. Active motion is encouraged. Traction to immobilize the child and gently stretch the tight adductor muscles is appropriate in some cases. This can be done at home or in the hospital. The objective is to maintain the sphericity of the femoral head during the healing process by providing "containment." The uninvolved firm acetabulum is utilized as a mold to maintain the shape of the head. This requires that the hip be maintained in abduction, usually with an abduction brace. Currently, the smaller, lighter braces are most favored because they allow the child to maintain a nearly normal activity level.

No treatment is required for mild LCP disease. For severe cases, treatment is much less effective. In some cases, maintaining containment by operation is appropriate. The procedures alter the shape of the upper femur or acetabulum so that containment is provided with the child standing in the normal weight-bearing attitude.

SLIPPED CAPITAL FEMORAL EPIPHYSIS (SCFE)

SCFE is a fracture of the capital femoral epiphysis that usually occurs in the pubescent male and gradually produces progressive displacement (chronic slip). Occasionally, acute injury produces varying degrees of slip. Often these are superimposed on the chronic form.

SCFE is a serious condition. The slipping not only produces deformity but also stretches the vessels to the epiphysis. Prognosis depends upon the severity of displacement, which in turn is dependent upon the duration of the problem. Early diagnosis is critical.

SCFE is suspected when the pubertal patient complains of hip or knee pain. As the obturator nerve innervates both the hip and knee, referred pain to the knee is common. The physical examination demonstrates limited medial rotation of the hip. This is best evaluated with the patient prone and the knees flexed to a right angle. Both thighs are then rotated in (feet going out), while the pelvis is held in a level position. Asymmetry of rotation is consistent with the diagnosis. Diagnosis is established by a lateral radiograph. A so-called "frog lateral" of the pelvis is ordered. This view will demonstrate the characteristic posterior displacement of the femoral epiphysis relative to the neck. In addition, diffuse rarefaction of the metaphysis and widening of the physis are seen.

After the diagnosis is established, the patient should be hospitalized without delay, since further slipping can occur at any time and fixation of the epiphysis by operation is essential. Fixation is achieved by passing two or three threaded pins across the physis. This promotes fusion, preventing further displacement.

Idiopathic Cortical Hyperostosis

ROBERT A. SAUL, M.D.

Infantile cortical hyperostosis (Caffey's disease) is usually a self-limited disease of infancy with bone changes, soft tissue swelling, fever, irritability, decreased appetite, and decreased movement of the affected bones. Pseudoparalysis is not an uncommon presenting sign. Radiographically the hyperostotic lesions have affected all bones except vertebrae.

The differential diagnosis, important because minimal therapy is indicated for this condition, includes trauma, battered child syndrome, congenital syphilis, tuberculosis, osteomyelitis, hypervitaminosis A, prolonged prostaglandin therapy, osteoid osteoma, eosinophilic granuloma, leukemia, lymphoma, Hodgkin disease, and Ewing sarcoma. Overly aggressive diagnostic studies have led to inappropriate therapeutic intervention, for example, amputation for a suspected neoplasm that was only cortical hyperostosis. If biopsy is indicated because of the suspicious nature of a lesion, the bone and overlying muscle and skin should all be examined in the biopsy.

The vast majority of affected patients will present before 6 months of age, with approximately 25% having evidence of hyperostosis at birth. The average age of onset is 6 weeks. A thorough radiologic survey should be done to search for involvement in other sites.

The familial nature of infantile cortical hyperostosis—autosomal dominant inheritance with variable expression and incomplete penetrance—emphasizes the importance of adequate delineation of this disorder and appropriate radiographs of family members. In familial cases, sites of involvement include the lower extremity (92%), the upper extremity (61%), the mandible (54%), and the clavicle (41%).

Once the condition is diagnosed, therapy is purely supportive. The disorder is self-limited, and this can be stressed to the family. Most infants do not need any analgesic therapy. Significant irritability affecting feeding or sleeping can be treated with acetylsalicylic acid (10 to 15 mg/kg every 6 to 8 hours). Affected extremities should be handled minimally. Mandibular involvement might mandate feeding assistance. Steroids (prednisone 1 to 2 mg/kg per day) have been used briefly in severe cases, but the efficacy of steroids for this condition is not known and their significant side effects would mandate close observation during the short course of therapy. Long-term sequelae (bowing of the extremities, osseous bridging, osteoporosis, and mandibular asymmetry) can occur. Braces are rarely needed for protection in active children with bowed osteoporotic long bones. Even if the bowing is present, these problems cause little functional disturbance for the child.

Osteomyelitis and Suppurative Arthritis

JOHN D. NELSON, M.D.

When possible, medical and surgical management of bone and joint infections should be a joint effort of the pediatrician and orthopedic surgeon. Because the day-to-day aspects of management are primarily medical, it is generally preferable that the pediatrician be the primary physician and the orthopedic surgeon the consultant.

ACUTE BACTERIAL INFECTIONS

Surgical Management of Arthritis. Surgical evacuation of pus is necessary in all cases of suppurative arthritis. This can often be effected by needle aspiration with or without saline irrigation. (It is inadvisable to irrigate with antibiotic solutions since they are usually irritating to synovium.) In most cases, two or three daily aspirations suffice. If substantial amounts of pus persist after a few days, open surgical drainage is performed.

There are at least three situations in which needle aspiration of joint fluid is not satisfactory. (1) With rare exceptions, open surgical drainage of hip joint pus should be performed immediately. The joint is especially vulnerable to permanent damage from pus itself and from vascular compromise due to pressure. (2) If the history suggests the possibility of a foreign body in the joint, open surgical drainage and exploration are advisable. (3) In my experience, the elbow joint seldom is thoroughly evacuated of pus by needle aspiration. The use of drains and the types of drains employed are a matter of personal preference of the surgeon and have not been subjected to the scrutiny of controlled trials.

Joints should be immobilized in a functional position of extension by sand bags, splints or casts until pain is alleviated and range of motion exercises can be carried out.

Surgical Management of Osteomyelitis. The optimal surgical management of acute osteomyelitis is controversial. The information that follows has been our practice for many years; it is possible that a less aggressive surgical approach would be as beneficial.

If frank pus is encountered in a diagnostic aspiration, the patient undergoes surgical decompression through an oval cortical window. There are exceptions to this. In very young infants, metaphyseal pus often decompresses spontaneously into the contiguous joint, whence it can usually be removed by repeated needle aspirations. If the infected area abuts the growth plate, surgical intervention could conceivably cause damage.

If the diagnostic aspiration yields only bloody material rather than pus, generally antibiotic therapy alone suffices.

The need for casts and immobilization must be determined in individual cases. If there is extensive involvement of a bone in the legs, weight bearing is prohibited to avoid the possibility of pathologic fracture.

Medical Management. Fluid and electrolyte therapy and medication for relief of pain are given as necessary.

Initial antibiotic therapy in about half the cases can be guided by the results of Gram stained specimens of joint fluid or pus interpreted by an experienced microbiologist. Otherwise, initial therapy is empirical and based on likely pathogens at various ages (Table 1).

In the newborn infant, group B streptococci and

Table 1.   ETIOLOGIC BACTERIA IN ACUTE SUPPURATIVE
BONE AND JOINT DISEASES

Ages	Arthritis	Osteomyelitis
Neonates	**Group B streptococci***	*Staphylococcus aureus*
	Staphylococcus aureus	**Group B streptococci**
	Coliform bacilli	Coliform bacilli
	Gonococcus	Pseudomonas
Infants	*Haemophilus influenzae b*	*Staphylococcus aureus*
	Pneumococcus	Streptococci
	Other streptococci	*Haemophilus influenzae b*
	Salmonella	
	Staphylococcus aureus	
Children	*Staphylococcus aureus*	*Staphylococcus aureus*
	Pneumococcus	Streptococci
	Gonococcus	

* The most common causes are shown in bold face type.

staphylococci are the major pathogens, but coliform bacilli must be considered. Initial therapy with methicillin and an aminoglycoside antibiotic is advisable. If cultures confirm group B streptococcal or gonococcal infection, treatment is changed to penicillin G or ampicillin. Pseudomonas infection is rare and part of a picture of sepsis and cutaneous lesions. It is treated with ticarcillin or mezlocillin along with an aminoglycoside.

Arthritis in infancy is most often due to *Haemophilus influenzae* b, but a variety of organisms are encountered. Initial therapy with nafcillin and chloramphenicol or with cefuroxime alone would be appropriate. Osteomyelitis in infancy is usually due to *Staphylococcus aureus* or streptococci. Unless gram-negative bacilli are seen in the Gram stained specimen, an antistaphylococcal penicillin is given initially.

Beyond infancy most cases of arthritis and os-

Table 2.   SUGGESTED DOSAGES OF ANTIBIOTICS TO TREAT
BONE AND JOINT INFECTIONS

Antibiotic	Parenteral Dosage	Oral Dosage*
Beta-lactam Antibiotics		
Amoxicillin	—	125–150 mg/kg/day q6h
Ampicillin	150 mg/kg/day q6h	—
Bacampicillin	—	100 mg/kg/day q6h
Cefaclor	—	125–150 mg/kg/day q6h
Cefazolin or cefuroxime	75–100 mg/kg/day q8h	—
Cefotaxime or moxalactam	100 mg/kg/day q6h	—
Ceftriaxone	50–75 mg/kg/day q12–24h	
Cephalexin or cephradine	—	100 mg/kg/day q6h
Cloxacillin	—	100 mg/kg/day q6h
Dicloxacillin	—	75 mg/kg/day q6h
Methicillin	200 mg/kg/day q6h	—
Oxacillin or nafcillin	150 mg/kg/day q6h	—
Penicillin	150,000 u/kg/day q4–6h	100 mg/kg/day q6h
Ticarcillin or mezlocillin	200–300 mg/kg/day q4–6h	—
Aminoglycosides		
Amikacin or kanamycin†	15–22.5 mg/kg/day q8h	—
Gentamicin	6 (children)–7.5 (infants) mg/kg/day q8h	—
Miscellaneous		
Chloramphenicol	75 mg/kg/day q6h	50–75 mg/kg/day q6h
Clindamycin	30 mg/kg/day q8h	30 mg/kg/day q6h
Vancomycin	40 mg/kg/day q6h	—

* These dosages are greater than those recommended by the manufacturers for less serious infections.
† Manufacturer's note: For kanamycin, IM, 15 mg/kg/day in two divided doses; IM, do not exceed 15 mg/kg/day. For amikacin, IM or IV, 15 mg/kg/day divided into two or three doses. The dose of 22.5 mg/kg/day is higher than that recommended by the manufacturer.

teomyelitis are due to gram-positive cocci, but gonococcal arthritis must be suspected in sexually active youngsters.

Antibiotic therapy is tailored to the culture and susceptibility test results. Suggested dosages are given in Table 2. Customarily, antibiotics are given parenterally for the entire course of treatment. However, several studies have shown that large-dosage oral antibiotic regimens can be successfully employed under rigidly monitored conditions. After several days, when the clinical condition has stabilized, an appropriate oral antibiotic is selected and given in dosages two to three times greater than those recommended for less serious infections (Table 2). Approximately 1 hour after a dose, the serum bactericidal titer against the pathogen isolated from the patient is tested. It should be at least 1:8 against *S. aureus* and *H. influenzae* and 1:32 or greater against streptococci. Approximately 10% of patients have poor gastrointestinal absorption of antibiotics and cannot be treated successfully by the oral route. The large dosages of drugs are well tolerated and do not cause gastrointestinal side effects.

Response to therapy is judged by resolution of fever and local signs and by normalization of the erythrocyte sedimentation rate (ESR). Persistent elevation of the ESR, even though clinical signs have improved, should prompt investigation for undrained pus or sequestrum.

Duration of antibiotic therapy varies with the type of bacteria. For *S. aureus* and coliform bacilli, a minimum of 21 days is suggested, while 10 to 14 days generally suffice for disease due to streptococci or *Haemophilus*. A 3 day regimen has been reported successful for gonococcal arthritis, but most authorities recommend at least 7 days of therapy. Ten to 14 days is adequate for *Pseudomonas* osteomyelitis, provided that thorough surgical debridement has been performed.

SPECIAL SITUATIONS

In children with *sickle cell disease*, aseptic bone infarction can mimic osteomyelitis, and vice versa. Bone infarctions tend to be multiple, there is little fever, no bandemia, and the ESR is normal. Osteomyelitis usually affects one bone, fever is higher, bandemia may be present, and the ESR becomes elevated. When in doubt, a diagnostic aspiration can be done. Infection is usually due to streptococci, *Salmonella*, or other coliform bacilli.

Sacroiliitis is indolent on presentation and occurs in older children. It is almost always staphylococcal.

Discitis, a syndrome of unknown etiology, affects infants and young children and resolves spontaneously within a few weeks. It must be differentiated from vertebral osteomyelitis, which occurs in older children and is associated with more severe symptomatology. It is most often due to staphy-

lococci, but *Pseudomonas* infection occurs in intravenous drug abusers.

Brodie abscess, a subacute or chronic staphylococcal infection, can occur in the metaphysis or diaphysis. It can be difficult to differentiate from bone tumor without surgical curettage. If surgical removal is not done, I treat Brodie abscess with antistaphylococcal antibiotics for several weeks or months until there is roentgenographic resolution of the lesion.

Granulomatous diseases due to mycobacteria, fungi, or *Brucella* tend to be indolent processes that cross the epiphyseal plate and cause disabling sequelae. Cases are treated with long-term antimicrobial drugs.

Chronic staphylococcal osteomyelitis is treated by surgical removal of sequestrum, when necessary, and with prolonged courses of oral antistaphylococcal drugs in dosages adjusted to produce serum bactericidal titers of 1:8 to 1:16. If a thorough sequestrectomy has been done, I treat with antibiotics for at least 3 months; otherwise, I treat for 6 to 12 months, depending on the clinical and roentgenographic responses.

The Treatment of Malignant Bone Tumors

GERALD ROSEN, M.D.

Malignant bone tumors (osteogenic sarcoma and Ewing's sarcoma) are rare in the pediatric population, but their incidence reaches its peak in the second decade of life.

During the past fifteen years dramatic changes in the prognosis for children with malignant bone tumors have taken place. In addition, in recent years the multidisciplinary approach to children with malignant bone tumors has not only given rise to much higher cure rates but also to much more functional end results through the use of limb-sparing surgery in osteogenic sarcoma, and the use of resection surgery and more sophisticated radiation therapy techniques in the treatment of Ewing's sarcoma.

Malignant bone tumors can be divided into two basic groups. The spindle cell sarcomas or classically radio-resistant sarcomas include osteogenic sarcoma, chondrosarcoma, fibrosarcoma, and malignant fibrous histiocytoma of bone. All of these "spindle cell" tumors are managed in a similar way. The treatment for osteogenic sarcoma can be duplicated for the treatment of some of these other spindle cell sarcomas that occur rarely in the childhood and adolescent age group.

The second category of malignant bone tumors in children includes what has been referred to as small round cell tumors, the most common of which is Ewing's sarcoma of bone. Other examples of small round cell tumors include malignant angiosarcoma of bone, primitive neuroectodermal tumors of bone, mesenchymal chondrosarcoma, and primary non-Hodgkin's lymphoma of bone. With the exception of primary non-Hodgkin's lymphomas of bone, all of the small cell sarcomas are managed in a way similar to that of Ewing's sarcoma.

All of the small cell sarcomas of bone are highly malignant and need to be treated in a multidisciplinary fashion with systemic chemotherapy, radiation therapy, and/or surgery. Although the majority of spindle cell sarcomas, including osteogenic sarcoma, are usually highly malignant in children, they occasionally occur in low-grade malignant forms, and it is important to recognize this rare variety, since surgery alone may be curative. However, in the majority of patients with high-grade spindle cell sarcomas (osteogenic sarcoma) multidisciplinary management with surgery and systemic chemotherapy is the treatment of choice.

LOW-GRADE OSTEOGENIC SARCOMAS

Low-grade osteogenic sarcomas are rare in the younger pediatric age group. Occasionally one may be encountered in the child, and it is important to recognize the low-grade histology and good prognosis of this type of tumor with surgery alone. Frequently the tumor arises on the surface of the bone and is referred to as a juxtacortical or parosteal osteogenic sarcoma. The latter term describes the location of the tumor on the surface of the bone, and in itself does not mean the tumor is low-grade. The diagnosis of a low-grade osteogenic sarcoma rests upon histologic interpretation of the biopsy by an experienced pathologist. Even more rare is the low-grade osteogenic sarcoma that occurs in the medullary canal. This type of tumor represents less than 2% of osteogenic sarcomas that occur in the population.

When one encounters a low-grade osteogenic sarcoma, the treatment is merely wide surgical resection of the bone and soft tissues of the involved limb. Occasionally amputations might be required because of the size or location of the lesion.

FULLY MALIGNANT SPINDLE CELL SARCOMAS—OSTEOGENIC SARCOMA

Osteogenic sarcoma is the most common malignant bone tumor seen in childhood and adolescence. Following biopsy and establishment of the diagnosis, a diagnostic work-up including adequate studies of the primary tumor such as arteriography, CT scanning, and nuclear magnetic resonance imaging should be performed to determine the initial extent of the primary tumor in the bone and soft tissues. This will aid in the decision as to whether limb-salvage surgery or amputation is the

treatment of choice. The rest of the diagnostic work-up should include CT scanning of the chest along with standard posterior-anterior and lateral chest x-rays to exclude pulmonary metastases and a bone scan to evaluate the primary tumor and rule out the presence of bony mestastases.

Surgical Management. As will be discussed below, state of the art treatment for patients with osteogenic sarcoma involves the use of preoperative chemotherapy. However, surgical management should be considered prior to the institution of preoperative chemotherapy. Its use should be based upon the age of the patient, site of the tumor, the patient's stature, and the extent of the tumor in the bone or soft tissues at the time of diagnosis prior to the use of systemic chemotherapy.

Surgical management for patients with tumors about the knee can include resection surgery of the knee joint and tumor containing a portion of the bone if the extent of tumor in the soft tissues is not too extensive, the neurovascular bundle is not involved with tumor, and the child has obtained close to his full linear growth.

Resection surgery for tumors in the proximal humerus can be considered even in the smallest child, since limb-salvage surgery for proximal humerus lesions leads to far more functional results than a forequarter amputation. Amputations are usually reserved for patients with very extensive involvement of the soft tissues or involvement of the neurovascular bundle. Treatment planning for the patient with osteogenic sarcoma should be done by the surgeon, pathologist, and pediatric oncologist, and perhaps the patient should be involved in the decision-making.

Preoperative Chemotherapy. Chemotherapy for osteogenic sarcoma is highly specialized and should be performed by oncologists who are fully experienced in this area. The primary preoperative treatment utilized in most treatment protocols includes the use of high-dose methotrexate with leucovorin rescue. Methotrexate is usually given by intravenous infusion in a dose of 12 gm/m^2 over 4 hours, followed by calcium leucovorin rescue (10 mg orally given 24 hours following the methotrexate infusion and every 6 hours for a total of 11 doses, or longer depending upon whether or not the patient has excreted all of the methotrexate by 72 hours. Therefore it is essential that this treatment be given where the serum methotrexate level can be monitored daily. Preoperative chemotherapy has also included alternating the combination of bleomycin (15 mg/m^2/day for 2 days, cyclophosphamide (600 mg/m^2/day for 2 days, and dactinomycin (0.6 mg/m^2/day for 2 days with weekly high-dose methotrexate. Other drugs utilized in preoperative chemotherapy can include doxorubicin at the dose of 30 mg/m^2/day for 3 days. For young children (less than 1 m^2

BSA) the dose of drugs is calculated in mg/kg, converting the dose by dividing the m^2 dose by 30 to arrive at the dose/kilogram. High-dose cis-platinum (120 mg/m^2 or 3 mg/kg in younger children) given with a 6-hour intravenous mannitol diuresis is also of value in the treatment of osteogenic sarcoma, but usually this modality of treatment is reserved for postoperative chemotherapy in patients who do not have a complete response of the primary tumor to preoperative chemotherapy as described above.

Following approximately two months of preoperative chemotherapy the patient can undergo surgery. It is important to note that during preoperative chemotherapy it is extremely important to monitor tumor activity to insure that the tumor is responding and not getting larger. This can be accomplished by following the elevated serum alkaline phosphatase, which will be present in approximately 60% of patients with osteogenic sarcoma, or following the patient with meticulous physical examinations to evaluate pain and tumor size. If the tumor does not respond to preoperative chemotherapy, it may be necessary to expedite surgery.

Postoperative Chemotherapy. Following surgery for the primary tumor the resected specimen has to be carefully analyzed by the orthopedic pathologist. If there is evidence of complete or near-complete tumor destruction by preoperative chemotherapy, that same preoperative chemotherapy, including high-dose methotrexate with leucovorin rescue, bleomycin, cyclophosphamide, dactinomycin, and doxorubicin can be continued postoperatively for a period of 6 to 9 months. If, however, there are still substantial residual cancer cells seen on histologic analysis of the resected primary tumor, postoperative chemotherapy should consist of substitution of cis-platinum at the dose indicated above in combination with doxorubicin at the dose of 30 mg/m^2 (or 1 mg/kg)/ day for 2 days. This combination chemotherapy can be repeated every 3 to 4 weeks for a total of six doses.

The Treatment of Pulmonary Metastasis. Patients presenting with pulmonary metastases on either plain x-ray or CT scan at the initial diagnostic work-up are managed in the same way as are patients with primary tumor only. However, following resection of the primary tumor, bilateral thoracotomies can be performed to remove any residual tumor deposits that remain following preoperative chemotherapy. Again, if the pulmonary metastases show a complete histologic response to preoperative chemotherapy, that same preoperative chemotherapy is continued postoperatively for 6 to 9 months. If, however, there is residual tumor in the pulmonary metastases or the primary tumor following surgeries the patient should be continued on the doxorubicin and cis-platinum combi-

nation chemotherapy for six treatments postoperatively.

With the above approach to treatment approximately 80% of patients with primary tumor only can be expected to be disease-free survivors. Approximately 50% of patients (depending on the extent of disease) presenting with concomitant pulmonary metastasis at the time of diagnosis of their primary tumor can be expected to be disease-free survivors.

A large majority of patients will be able to undergo limb-salvage surgery. Patients should be warned that resection surgery as opposed to amputation (depending upon the experience and skill of the surgical oncologist) may carry with it a 5 to 10% risk of local recurrence, which is a highly ominous event in the prognosis for patients treated for osteogenic sarcoma.

MALIGNANT SMALL CELL SARCOMAS— EWING'S SARCOMA

The management of Ewing's sarcoma should include, in addition to imaging studies performed on the primary lesion, a CT scan of the chest to rule out pulmonary metastases, a bone scan to rule out the presence of distant bone metastases, and a bone marrow aspiration to rule out early bone marrow involvement, which rarely occurs in Ewing's sarcoma but can occur quite early in non-Hodgkin's lymphoma of bone. Electron microscopic studies of the biopsy material can also aid in the subclassification of small cell sarcomas of bone, which may exist under the broad morphologic heading of Ewing's sarcoma. These latter studies may be useful in predicting responsiveness to therapy, since approximately 10–20% of Ewing's sarcomas develop early resistance to chemotherapy and are not permanently locally controlled with radiation therapy to the primary tumor.

Chemotherapy. Chemotherapy for Ewing's sarcoma consists of multi-drug chemotherapy, including cyclophosphamide at the dose of 1200 mg/m^2 on day one, with doxorubicin at the dose of 30 mg/m^2 per day for two consecutive days, methotrexate at the dose of 18 mg/m^2 for two consecutive days, and weekly vincristine for the first 4 weeks of treatment. Three weeks after the first combination of chemotherapy, cyclophosphamide at a dose of 1200 mg/m^2 per day for two consecutive days is utilized. Three weeks after the cyclophosphamide therapy, the first combination chemotherapy—cyclophosphamide for one day, doxorubicin for two days, and methotrexate for two days—is repeated, but without the vincristine. These three treatments make up one cycle of chemotherapy. Each treatment is separated by a rest period of 3 weeks, during which time the blood counts are carefully monitored and the patient transfused as needed to keep the hemoglobin above 10 gm/dl. Platelet transfusions are utilized should the platelet count fall below 20,000 and/or the patient experience bleeding. About one third of patients being treated with this aggressive combination of chemotherapy require hospitalization during periods of neutropenia and fever. If this occurs, drug doses are appropriately reduced.

Because of the immunosuppressive quality of this aggressive combination chemotherapy, irradiated blood products are used for transfusions, since graft vs. host disease has been seen following engraftment from a transfusion in very young patients. Therefore, this type of dangerous combination chemotherapy should be performed only in centers with experience in its use. Following one cycle of combination chemotherapy (the three treatments described above) local therapy can be commenced.

Local Therapy. In the past the prognosis for patients with Ewing's sarcoma has been correlated with the site of the primary tumor and the size of the primary tumor. Tumors of axial origin, such as those of the spine and the pelvis, carried a poor prognosis. This was probably due to the fact that earlier irradiation of the pelvis or spine led to a rapid intolerance for high-dose aggressive combination chemotherapy. Therefore, when radiation therapy is used for primary treatment for tumor at these sites, it may sometimes be preferable to go through two cycles, or six chemotherapy treatments, prior to commencing local therapy.

An additional poor prognostic factor associated with very large, bulky tumors (even though they are readily shrunken with chemotherapy), is that the larger the bulk of tumor, the more likely it is that the primary tumor site harbors resistant clones of cells that may grow back following combination chemotherapy and radiation therapy. Therefore, it has been our preference to try to resect the pelvic tumors that arise in the iliac crest, obviating the problem of local recurrence following radiation therapy. With this approach, the same high cure rate for pelvic Ewing's sarcomas can be achieved as is achieved in those of the distal extremities, i.e., in excess of 80%.

Young children with tumors about the knee, who have complete cessation of growth following full-dose radiation therapy; young children with lesions in expendable bones, such as ribs or fibula; or patients with lesions in the foot might do better with surgical treatment rather than radiation treatment for their primary tumor, since the functional end results with surgery might be better or at least comparable in this group of patients, and there would be no risk of local recurrence of primary tumor following the use of radiation therapy as the only modality of local treatment. However, it is still preferable to use mega-voltage radiation therapy for the majority of tumors in the extremities and in the nonoperable sites such as the spine in children and adolescents who have achieved most of their linear growth. Currently, radiation therapy consists of the use of 4,500 cGy to the entire involved bone, with a boost of 1,500 cGy to the lesional area.

Adjuvant Chemotherapy. Following the commencement of radiation therapy, or two weeks following surgical resection of the primary tumor, chemotherapy should continue until a total of four cycles (twelve treatments) of combination chemotheapy have been given. Whether or not further maintenance chemotherapy is necessary is not known at this point, but its use, particularly to enhance local control in patients who have had radiation therapy for treatment of their primary tumor, may be adopted as a clinical trial in the Children's Cancer Study Group.

With optimal therapy, including the use of surgical resection for pelvic primaries and aggressive combination chemotherapy, between 75 and 85% of patients (depending upon the pimary site) can be expected to be disease-free survivors of Ewing's sarcoma.

Metastatic Ewing's Sarcoma. The patients presenting with evidence of pulmonary metastasis at diagnosis are treated in a way similar to that for patients with primary tumor only. However, at the end of chemotherapy the addition of bilateral pulmonary irradiation (1400–1800 cGy) has produced a disease-free survival rate in this subset of patients equal to that of patients who present with primary tumor only.

NON-HODGKIN'S LYMPHOMA OF BONE (RETICULUM CELL SARCOMA)

Non-Hodgkin's lymphoma of bone in children should be treated as a systemic disease in a fashion similar to that used for non-Hodgkin's lymphoma of other primary sites. This implies the use of radiation therapy to achieve local control and the use of systemic chemotherapy similar to that used in the treatment of high-risk acute lymphoblastic leukemia. This latter type of treatment should include "CNS prophylaxis," usually in the form of intrathecal methotrexate, since non-Hodgkin's lymphoma arising in bone in children is usually highly malignant and may progress to a leukemic picture in the bone marrow or to meningeal disease, such as is seen in acute lymphoblastic leukemia.

With this approach to the patient with non-Hodgkin's lymphoma of bone, prolonged disease-free survival in the majority of children with this disease can be achieved.

14

Muscles

Congenital Muscular Defects

BRUCE O. BERG, M.D.

These abnormalities of muscle include the congenital myopathies and those circumstances in which part or all of the entire muscle is absent. A myopathy is any abnormality of muscle whether it is structural, biochemical, or electrophysiologic and in which there is no related neurologic abnormality. A muscular dystrophy, on the other hand, is a genetically determined primary disease of muscle characterized by muscle fiber degeneration.

Congenital myopathies (see Table 1, pp. 430–431) are apparent at birth or shortly thereafter, and are characterized by weakness and usually hypotonia. Weakness is primarily found in proximal muscles. There is usually decreased muscle bulk, and the stretch reflexes are normal to decreased. Serum creatine phosphokinase is normal to mildly elevated; electromyographic studies may be normal but commonly demonstrate short-duration, low-amplitude polyphasic motor unit potentials. The congenital myopathies are named in accordance with the structural changes demonstrated on muscle biopsy.

Associated skeletal abnormalities, including elongation of facial features, narrow high-arched palate, hip dislocation, lordosis, kyphoscoliosis, and pes cavus, are often present. A variety of orthotic and surgical procedures may be required for improvement or correction of skeletal deformities, particularly those affecting the hips, ankles, and feet.

The congenital absence of muscle may be partial or complete and, though primarily unilateral and involving one muscle, may be bilateral and symmetrical, affecting related muscle groups. The resulting disability is relatively stable. Muscles of the shoulder girdle, upper limbs, and neck are most commonly affected, particularly the sternocostal heads of the pectorals, the trapezius, and the sternocleidomastoids. Occasionally, the congenital absence of pectoral muscles may be accompanied by scoliosis and webbed fingers. No specific treatment is of usefulness, and only a frank discussion of the matter with parents and child is required.

The absence or marked hypoplasia of abdominal muscles may affect respiration, coughing, and defecation. Impairment of normal thoracic excursion may be severe, resulting in pulmonary infection and further pulmonary insufficiency. Anomalies of the genitourinary and gastrointestinal systems are frequently associated with congenital absence of the abdominal muscles. Treatment consists of providing a functional abdominal support, a complete evaluation, and treatment of any concomitant anomaly.

Other skeletal muscles, including the levator palpebri and external ocular muscles, have been reported as congenitally absent. A variety of ophthalmologic surgical procedures are available to effect not only visual but cosmetic improvement.

Torticollis

THOMAS S. RENSHAW, M.D.

Although torticollis, or "wry neck," is usually a benign cosmetic problem secondary to muscle tightness and responds successfully to stretching exercises during infancy, one must realize that there are causes of torticollis for which an exercise program could bring about catastrophic results. These include traumatic or congenital spinal lesions producing instability between the occiput and C-1, or C-1 and C-2, such as congenital hypoplasia or aplasia of the odontoid, nonunion of an odontoid fracture, rupture of the transverse alar ligament of C-1, and subluxation of C-1 and

Table 1.   CONGENITAL MYOPATHIES*

Disease	Clinical Features	Muscle Biopsy
Central core disease	Hypotonia noted at birth or shortly thereafter; motor development delayed. Diffuse weakness, primarily proximal; stretch reflexes normal to reduced. Skeletal abnormalities may occur (hip dislocation, kyphoscoliosis, lordosis, pes cavus). Inherited as autosomal dominant trait, but sporadic cases occur. Serum CPK usually normal; EMG findings nonspecific. Malignant hyperthermia known to occur.	Variability of fiber diameter; often with predominance of type I fibers. Within the fiber, centrally or peripherally, are cores devoid of oxidative enzyme activity. Myofibrillary ATPase activity of cores normal to decreased.
Myotubular myopathy (centronuclear)	Hypotonic at birth with ptosis, external ophthalmoplegia and occasionally facial weakness. Decreased muscle power throughout, greater distally than proximally. Neonatal type described with profound weakness at birth (may die in infancy). Inheritance reported as usually X-linked recessive, but autosomal dominant and recessive traits reported. Serum CPK normal to moderately increased. EMG nonspecific.	Predominance of type I fibers with central nuclei surrounded by clear area. Type I atrophy has been recorded. Increased central staining with oxidative enzymes and pale central area with ATPase reactions.
Congenital fiber type disproportion	Hypotonia and generalized weakness present at birth. Muscle contractures are often present with skeletal abnormalities (high arched palate, congenital hip dislocation, kyphoscoliosis, varus or valgus foot deformities). Rarely, external ophthalmoplegia occurs. Commonly, clinical status remains static or improves.	Type I fibers are more numerous and smaller than type II fibers.
Mitochondrial myopathies	Heterogeneous group of diseases with normal as well as abnormally shaped and enlarged mitochondria within muscle fibers. Symptoms usually begin in childhood but may appear at any time. External ocular muscle weakness a frequent finding. Excessive muscular fatigue following exercise is common. Inheritance is variable. Structural changes of muscle are nonspecific and have been reported in a variety of disorders (hypothyroidism, polymyositis, thyrotoxic myopathy, and spinal muscular atrophy).	Mitochondrial abnormalities suspected on light microscopy by accumulation of subsarcolemmal or intramyofibrillary granules, which are irregular and stain red with modified trichrome stain—"ragged red fibers."
Multicore disease	Several patients described with nonprogressive generalized hypotonia and weakness of trunk and limb muscles, proximal greater than distal. Stretch reflexes are decreased. Serum CPK is normal; EMG demonstrates short duration motor unit potentials or normal findings.	Predominance of type I fibers and numerous small randomly distributed areas of types I and II, with focal decreased oxidative enzyme activity and focal myofibrillary degeneration.
Nemaline myopathy	Hypotonia at birth; some mothers indicate decreased fetal movement. Poor suck, swallow, and respiratory embarrassment; delay in achieving milestones. Elongated face with narrow high arched palate, prognathism, dental malocclusion and pigeon chest. Stretch reflexes reduced to absent. Inherited as autosomal recessive or dominant traits; sporadic cases known to occur. Serum CPK normal to mildly increased. EMG demonstrates brief, low amplitude, abundant, polyphasic motor potentials.	Usually a predominance of type I fibers; about half of type I fibers are small. Subsarcolemmal collection of ("nemaline") rods seen with vesicular nuclei and prominent nucleoli.
Trilaminar neuromuscular disease	Very rare congenital neuromuscular disease with muscular rigidity at birth. Muscles are hard on palpation. Stretch reflexes are normal. CPK in early infancy reported as markedly increased, but decreases near end of first year. EMG has been normal.	About 15% of fibers demonstrate 3 concentric zones of differential (trilaminar fibers). At EM, a sharp delineation is demonstrated between the outer and middle zones, but junction is not defined by membrane.

Table 1.   CONGENITAL MYOPATHIES (*continued*)

Disease	Clinical Features	Muscle Biopsy
Reducing body myopathy	Profound hypotonia with decreased muscle bulk, generalized weakness, and stretch reflexes depressed to absent. Milestones delayed. Serum CPK normal to mildly elevated. EMG demonstrated myopathic potentials.	Variability of fiber size with predominance of type I fibers. Large numbers of fibers contain "reducing bodies" rich in sulfhydryl groups and RNA.
Fingerprint body myopathy	Hypotonia and generalized weakness, usually with sparing of external and bulbar muscles. Stretch reflexes reduced to absent. Muscle bulk reduced. Serum CPK normal to mildly elevated and EMG studies have varied from normal to "consistent with myopathy."	Small type I fibers and hypertrophied type II fibers. EM demonstrates inclusions composed of concentric lamellae resembling fingerprints. Similar structures also found in dermatomyositis, myotonic dystrophy, and oculopharyngeal muscular dystrophy.
Sarcotubular myopathy	One case report of two brothers whose parents were 3rd cousins. Patients were clumsy and had mild weakness of proximal limb muscles and neck flexors. Stretch reflexes were normal to mildly decreased. Serum CPK normal to mildly decreased.	Vacuolar changes seen selectively affecting type II fibers. A "myriad" of small spaces were seen on cross-section in affected muscles and in longitudinal section; vacuolization was segmental.

* From Berg, B.O.: Child Neurology. Jones Medical Publications, 1984, pp. 116–117

C-2. Torticollis can also result from a tumor in the bony vertebral column or spinal cord. Infections in the neck, involving the retropharyngeal space, a disc space, or upper respiratory tract have also caused torticollis. It is, therefore, essential in the evaluation to have good radiographs of the entire cervical spine in both frontal and sagittal planes, as well as dynamic flexion and extension lateral views to assess the stability from the occiput to C-2.

Idiopathic muscular torticollis is a condition that usually presents in early infancy but can develop at any time during childhood. It may be caused by injury to the nerve or vascular supply to the sternocleidomastoid muscle. In children under age 1 year, who have little or no facial asymmetry, an exercise program is almost always successful. The specific exercise is designed to place maximum distance between the ipsilateral sternoclavicular joint and mastoid process and is done by bending the neck laterally *away* from the torticollis and then slowly providing maximal rotation of the head and face to the side of the torticollis. This position should be held for about five seconds and then released and repeated 10 times, at least 4 times a day, or better yet, with each diaper change. Another conservative therapeutic method involves positioning the infant prone in the crib with the normal side toward the wall, which may cause some rotation toward the affected side and help with the stretching exercise program. The exercises are worth trying in children beyond age 1 year, but often by that time surgical treatment will be necessary. There is a high failure rate with the exercise program at any age when the torticollis is accompanied by significant facial asymmetry and/or the restriction of neck rotation exceeds 30° when compared with the normal side.

When surgical treatment is indicated, the treatment of choice is a distal release of both the sternal and clavicular attachments of the sternocleidomastoid muscle. As long as the incision is placed 1.5 to 2 cm above the clavicle, the cosmetic result is quite acceptable. It is rarely necessary to do bipolar tenotomy or a single release at the mastoid area. Surgical results are not age-dependent and a good result may be expected up to and beyond age 10 years. Postoperative management usually consists of a cast or a brace for a period of approximately 4 weeks.

There is a 10 to 20% incidence of congenital hip dysplasia associated with infantile idiopathic torticollis. In addition, approximately 15% of all torticollis is on an ophthalmologic basis, the most common cause being amblyopia.

Congenital Hypotonia

HERBERT E. GILMORE, M.D.

Normal body tone is maintained by the activity of the gamma-motor system. Central control is mediated through the basal ganglia, cerebellum, and brainstem (mainly vestibular) nuclei. Rubrospinal, reticulospinal, and other motor pathways carry impulses from these centers to the cells of the intermediate and anterior horns of the spinal cord. From there they are relayed through the nerve roots, peripheral nerves, and myoneural junction to the muscle spindle and somatic muscle cells. When the activity of any of these areas is disrupted, hypotonia can develop. Infantile hypotonia is caused by many disorders, which affect various levels of the nervous system. Table 1 lists the major diseases affecting each site. Appropriate evaluation of the hypotonic infant is dependent on a clinical and laboratory analysis based on these anatomic considerations. A careful history and thorough physical, neurologic, and developmental examinations are crucial to determine the direction of further laboratory investigations. After a specific diagnosis is established, the appropriate therapy can be instituted.

History

The family history can determine if other family members were hypotonic as infants; the age of onset, duration, and degree of impairment and the areas of involvement in those individuals are useful in determining the underlying disease and the patient's clinical course. The birth history should include a review of any infectious, toxic, or traumatic exposures during pregnancy. The absence of vigorous fetal movements is a symptom of some chromosomal disorders, congenital metabolic diseases, congenital infections, early fetal distress, fetal-onset Werdnig-Hoffmann disease, and arthrogryposis multiplex congenita. Particular note should be made of any difficulties at delivery or evidence for perinatal hypoxia-ischemia. The developmental history is critical in establishing a central nervous system disorder as the cause of infantile hypotonia. The age of onset of smiling; sitting without assistance; reaching for objects; crawling; standing; walking; speaking repetitive syllables, words, phrases, and short sentences; and the age of bowel and bladder control are the major milestones to be noted. Delay in the appropriate onset of these activities suggests central nervous system disease. The history of present illness should include the age at which the symptoms were first noted, the areas of the body most involved, the severity of hypotonia, the presence of deterioration, and progressive involvement of other body parts. Does the infant choke frequently during feeding? Is the hypotonia noted at any particular time of day? Does the older infant have frequent falling that is out of proportion to the level of gait development? Is tremor or dysmetria of the hands noted? Are the parents concerned about the infant's overall development?

Examination

Congenital hypotonia is occasionally noted at birth but is most often recognized by the parents or pediatrician sometime later in infancy. In its dramatic form it is seldom missed: the infant is "floppy," makes few spontaneous movements, and often has sucking and swallowing difficulties; when the infant is lifted up, the head, arms, and legs hang loosely from the trunk; the infant is described as feeling like a "dead weight" or "limp rag." Most often the hypotonia is subtle and first detected when the infant begins to sit, stand, or walk: the infant flops forward when sitting or has "rubbery legs" when standing or walking. Rarely, the hypotonia is so subtle as to be only noted during the physical examination: there is less resistance to passive movements of the limbs; it is easier for the examiner to passively "wave" the infant's hands and feet; often the infant will slip through the examiner's hands when held suspended under the axillae.

During the general physical examination particular note should be taken of the following: the ash-leaf or café-au-lait spots of phakomatosis; malformations associated with particular birth defect syndromes; the ligamentous laxity and double jointedness often seen in connective tissue disorders; the fixed contractures and joint deformity seen in arthrogryposis; the hepatosplenomegaly that is often seen in progressive metabolic disorders; the choreoretinitis or retinal scarring seen in fetal infections (TORCH infections); and the cherry red spot of some lysosomal storage diseases. Male infants with small hands and feet, failure to thrive, and undescended testicles are suspect for Prader-Willi syndrome.

The neurologic examination is critical for determining the anatomic locations of disease and directing further diagnostic investigations. The presence of cranial nerve abnormalities can be particularly helpful in this regard. Fasciculations and atrophy of the tongue are difficult to identify and are best seen in the resting infant with lighting over the surface of the tongue. They can be seen in Werdnig-Hoffmann disease, severe perinatal hypoxia-ischemia, and rarely syringobulbia and brainstem tumors. Strabismus, nystagmus, accentuated or depressed gag and jaw jerk reflexes, and sucking and swallowing difficulties are seen in many central diseases. Facial weakness (facial diplegia), triangle-shaped mouth, or fish mouth suggest a congenital myopathy, myotonic dystrophy, or Prader-Willi syndrome. Extraocular muscle weakness is seen in myasthenia gravis, infantile myotonic dystrophy, and several congenital myopathies.

Muscle bulk, form, and strength should be examined carefully. Infants with hypotonia of central origin do not exhibit early weakness and atrophy; those with anterior horn cell, peripheral nerve, or muscle disease exhibit early, marked weakness and atrophy. These can progress rapidly, resulting in chest wall and extremity deformities (pectus carinatum, pes valgus, claw hand, and so on). The weakness of peripheral nerve disease is proportional to the atrophy and hypotonia; that of muscle disease is in excess. The deep tendon reflexes are normal or only slightly depressed early on in patients with muscle disease; in those with anterior horn cell or peripheral nerve disease they are markedly hypoactive or absent; and in those with central disease they are normal early and accentuated later in infancy. The presence of persistent ankle clonus and Babinski sign suggests central or spinal cord disease. The sensory examination of infants is very difficult and often requires repetitive testing for positive results. It is best performed with the infant resting after feeding, using a pin. It should proceed from the extremities toward the trunk and from the lower extremities upward. An appropriate or startle response should be noted. If performed carefully, the sensory examination can suggest spinal cord, nerve root, or peripheral nerve disease. If spinal cord disease is suspect, a digital rectal examination using the small finger will often demonstrate depressed anal sphincter tone.

The developmental examination should include techniques for determining fine motor adaptive and gross motor delay, as well as the stage of infantile reflex development (automatisms). The presence of the appropriate automatisms at a given age can greatly assist in ruling out central causes of hypotonia. Infants with peripheral nerve or muscle disease do not demonstrate a lag in infantile automatisms.

Some diseases can affect several levels of the nervous system at the same time, resulting in hypotonia with a mixture of central and peripheral symptoms and neurologic findings. Krabbe's disease, infantile metachromatic leukodystrophy, neuraxonal dystrophy, and Leigh's disease can produce progressive encephalopathy affecting the central and peripheral nervous system. Patients with these diseases often have hypotonia and hyperreflexia initially, and several months to years later the reflexes become markedly diminished or are totally absent. Perinatal hypoxia-ischemia can affect the basal ganglia, brainstem nuclei, and spinal cord concurrently, producing a variable clinical picture in addition to hypotonia.

Laboratory Investigations

Despite a careful history and a thorough physical, neurologic, and developmental examination, the clinician often cannot determine the anatomic localization or a specific diagnosis. Laboratory investigations are therefore a necessary and important part of the work-up of patients with congenital hypotonia. The investigator should, however, have at least differentiated peripheral from central disease before laboratory tests are ordered, to avoid inappropriate, costly, and oftentimes painful laboratory procedures. If central disease is suspect, ultrasound and CT scan of the head are invaluable in identifying intraventricular hemorrhage, periventricular leukomalacia, brain tumors, leukoencephalopathies, and other central diseases. If spinal cord disease is suspect, cervical or lumbosacral spine films are appropriate, and a myelogram should be considered. Nerve conduction velocity testing and electromyography (EMG) will identify and differentiate peripheral nerve from muscle disease. Muscle enzyme tests (CPK, SGOT, SGPT) should be performed before the EMG, since needle damage can cause a spurious elevation of these enzymes. Muscle (and often nerve) biopsies are required to differentiate peripheral nerve and muscle disease, since the infant EMG can be difficult to perform and correctly interpret.

Electromyography, nerve conduction velocity, and muscle biopsies are essential for diagnosing Werdnig-Hoffmann disease, congenital myopathies, and hereditary peripheral neuropathies. If progressive metabolic disease is suspect, serum amino acid and lysosomal enzyme and urinary organic acid tests should be performed. Chromosome analysis should be performed in patients with other congenital anomalies. Spinal fluid analysis is required if meningitis, encephalitis, or post-infectious polyradiculoneuropathy is suspected. In the latter disease, the spinal fluid should contain fewer than 10 WBC/ml and more than 60 mg protein/dl. The ability to diagnose this disease accurately in patients younger than 6 months on the basis of spinal fluid protein elevation alone is difficult, since the spinal fluid can normally contain 60 mg/dl or more of protein up to that age. Nerve conduction velocity studies, particularly F-wave determinations, can assist in making this diagnosis. Spinal fluid protein is also markedly elevated in Krabbe's disease, Leigh's disease, and metachromatic leukodystrophy.

If botulism is suspected, serum and stool should be sent for botulin determination; characteristic EMG and nerve conduction abnormalities are often present to assist in making this diagnosis.

Infants suspected of having myasthenia gravis should be given pyridostigmine (Mestinon) 0.05–0.15 mg/kg IM or IV. The onset of action is within 10 minutes and its duration of action is up to several hours. It is therefore more useful than the short-acting edrophonium (Tensilon) test, whose onset of action is within 30 seconds and duration of action only 5 minutes. This does not allow enough time for examination of the uncooperative infant. Tensilon (0.5 mg IV in an infant; 2 mg IV in children under 30 kg) can be used, however, in older children who are cooperative; then particular note should be made of improvement of eye closure, smile, and distal strength. Either test should be performed with equipment for endotracheal intubation and controlled ventilation available.

Clinical Course and Prognosis

The vigor with which one undertakes a diagnostic work-up of the hypotonic infant will depend on the clinical setting, severity, and course of the disease. Infants who present in the newborn period with severe hypotonia often require the full array of diagnostic tests available to arrive at a diagnosis. Infants in whom the hypotonia is mild and who present after one month of age with normal physical and developmental examinations can be followed periodically to determine the course of the hypotonia without any initial laboratory investigation. If other family members have had similar clinical presentations, the diagnosis of benign congenital hypotonia is likely. Infants with mild to moderate hypotonia and additional neurologic findings suggesting a specific anatomic localization or diagnosis should be investigated promptly with the appropriate laboratory tests. Male infants with small hands and feet, failure to thrive, and undescended testicles who later become obese most

likely have Prader-Willi syndrome; the hypotonia in these infants resolves in early childhood and there is no need for further laboratory investigation. Hypotonic infants with fixed joint contractures (arthrogryposis) either had fixed posturing in utero (usually with breech presentation), fetal-onset Werdnig-Hoffmann disease, or a static fetal viral anterior horn cell infection. It is important to differentiate between these, since it is only patients with Werdnig-Hoffmann disease who will progress and often die within one year. Electromyography and muscle biopsy can often differentiate these diseases. Patients with Group II Werdnig-Hoffmann disease (age of onset 2–12 months) may develop the ability to sit and stand but usually never walk and will often die in the first decade; those with Group III (age of onset 1–2 years) can sometimes walk but are often confined to a wheelchair. Neonatal myasthenia gravis is either transient or persistent. The former is due to passive transfer of antiacetylcholine receptor antibody from the myasthenic mother to the child. The time of onset is usually within hours or several days after birth, the patients develop a weak suck and few spontaneous movements, and they have dysphagia and ptosis. The symptoms last for several weeks. The persistent type usually has its onset after many days, and patients require prolonged treatment. Most of the congenital myopathies are benign and transient, but myotubular, mitochondrial, reducing-body, and carnitine-deficiency myopathy and congenital muscular dystrophy are progressive. Most patients with postinfectious polyradiculoneuropathy (Guillain-Barré syndrome) do well, with full recovery of function; a minority will require prolonged ventilatory assistance. Most patients with amino and organic acidopathies and Leigh's disease will improve or stabilize with appropriate dietary changes or restrictions. Patients with progressive metabolic encephalopathy due to lysosomal enzyme disease are usually severely involved and will often progress to a spastic quadriparetic, bedridden state, with all of its attendant complications. Infants with hypotonia due to hypoxia-ischemia, neonatal meningitis, and birth trauma will have a variable course dependent on other associated difficulties such as hydrocephalus and seizures.

Therapy

Therapy for congenital hypotonia is directed at eliminating its cause and alleviating or preventing its effects. Metabolic insults such as hypoxia, hypoglycemia, and acidosis should be corrected promptly. Meningitis and sepsis should be treated with the appropriate antibiotics. Infants with myasthenia gravis should receive 4–10 mg pyridostigmine (Mestinon) syrup orally every 4 hours. Its onset of action is 15–30 minutes and its duration of action is 3–4 hours. If administered parenterally, 1/30 of the oral dose should be given. Patients with transient myasthenia gravis usually do not require treatment longer than 4–6 weeks. Patients with the persistent type require treatment indefinitely. Prednisone (2 mg/kg/day) and/or a thymectomy may be required in cases resistant to pyridostigmine treatment. Patients with polymyositis and postinfectious polyradiculoneuropathy (Guillain-Barré syndrome) can be treated with prednisone starting at 3 mg/kg/day, given daily and tapered over 10 days to 2 mg/kg/day; this dose is then given every other day until improvement is noted, at which time slow tapering can begin. Patients receiving prolonged steroid therapy should have long bone x-rays performed for osteoporosis and femoral head x-rays to determine necrosis; consideration should be given to supplemental calcium and vitamin D treatment in these patients. Other forms of congenital hypotonia have no specific cure, and treatment is directed at appropriate physical and occupational therapy programs, orthopedic procedures (bracing, tendon lengthening, and so on), and fitting of appropriate adaptive equipment (wheelchairs, Bliss Word Board). The parents of infants with progressive Werdnig-Hoffmann disease and muscular dystrophy should be informed that these infants will invariably develop life-threatening swallowing and respiratory difficulties often necessitating nasogastric or gastrostomy tube feedings and ventilatory support. A decision should be made early regarding the appropriateness of such heroic measures. The decision to withhold therapy from these patients often requires the involvement of other family members, hospital ethics committees, lawyers, and occasionally the courts. Intensive psychological and social support should be offered early. The approach to these difficult cases will vary according to physician and parental attitudes and medical and social standards.

Muscular Dystrophy and Related Myopathies

IRWIN M. SIEGEL, M.D.

Muscular dystrophy is the general term for a group of chronic diseases that have in common abiotrophy with progressive degeneration of skeletal musculature, leading to atrophy and weakness, often contracture and deformity, and motor disability.

GENERAL THERAPY

Management of the patient with a muscle disease should be aggressive and multidisciplined. Treatment is best administered by a team including pediatric, neurologic, genetic, physiatric, and orthopedic consultants. Additionally, occupational therapists, physical therapists, and medical social workers or psychologists can assist the patient and the family. Speech and dietary therapy, as well as subspecialty consultation (for instance, gastrointestinal and cardiopulmonary care), provide a thorough approach to the problems of comprehensive management.

Medications. Except in those myopathies due to the absence of a specific metabolite, for which replacement therapy will sometimes help (e.g., muscle carnitine deficiency), or in muscle disease secondary to endocrinopathy (e.g., hypothyroidism) in which appropriate therapy of the primary condition can alleviate the secondary myopathy, there is no effective drug treatment for muscular dystrophy. Although the myotonia of dystrophia myotonica can be relieved by a variety of agents, the dystrophia (weakness) remains. Agents used are phenytoin (Dilantin), 100 mg two to three times a day, or quinine,* 200 mg three times daily. Both procainamide and prednisolone, though mentioned in the literature, have undesirable side effects and are not suggested.

Cardiac. Cardiomyopathy is said to be present in over 80% of patients with Duchenne muscular dystrophy (DMD), but the child may not show clinical evidence of heart disease because his restricted activity maintains a precarious status quo. Treatment is along conventional lines, with the administration of cardiac glycosides and diuretics when indicated.

Respiratory. Pneumonitis, secondary to decreased pulmonary function and poor respiratory toilet with aspiration, is frequently encountered in those in advanced stages of the muscular dystrophies, and periodic evaluation to monitor restrictive pulmonary disease is an integral part of any treatment regimen. Reduction in chest compliance, secondary to progressive weakness of respiratory musculature, requires an ongoing program of pulmonary rehabilitation. This may include diaphragmatic breathing exercises, postural drainage, chest percussion, proper humidification, and training in the use of various respiratory aids. Vigorous treatment of upper respiratory infections requires pharyngeal suction and intermittent positive pressure breathing as well as appropriate antibiotic therapy. Mechanical ventilation of patients in the terminal stages of DMD often can be managed at home without a tracheostomy, utilizing apparatus such as the rocking bed, plastic wrap ventilator, chest-abdomen cuirass respirator, and pneumobelt.

Dietary. Because obesity accelerates functional disability, nutrition should be carefully monitored

---

*This use of quinine is not listed by the manufacturer.

throughout the course of muscular dystrophy but particularly after wheelchair confinement. A well-balanced vitamin-supplemented diet of no less than 1200 calories is suggested. Patients are encouraged to choose fruits and vegetables as alternatives to high-caloric snacks, and high fiber foods and fruit juices to aid in maintaining normal elimination. Only small amounts of dairy products are included because of their mucus-producing tendency.

When deglutition is difficult because of posterior pharyngeal and upper esophageal weakness, swallowing can be assisted by instruction in proper positioning, eating slowly, sitting upright for a time after meals, and introducing soft foods into the diet. Myotonic patients should avoid cold foods or fluids, which may cause pharyngeal myotonia.

Psychosocial. In addition to coping with the psychologic problems imposed by a progressively disabling disease, children with muscular dystrophy face the same problems of peer interaction, body image, family adjustment, and sexuality that all normal youngsters must resolve in the process of maturing. Supportive psychiatric intervention made available at times of psychosocial crises can avert critical emotional damage, and empathic counseling of both the patient and family throughout the course of the illness is an important part of total management.

A higher incidence of mental retardation and decreased intellectual function has been noted in patients with DMD than in normal or other control groups. However, whenever possible, it is desirable to keep the child in the mainstream in the regular neighborhood school. Finally, in the treatment of muscular dystrophy the family is the patient. Group therapy has proved valuable in assisting parents and normal siblings by helping them develop insight and increasing communication through experience-sharing.

MOTOR DISABILITY

Physical Therapy/Occupational Therapy. Because muscular activity enhances protein synthesis (the danger of rapid loss of strength because of inactivity in DMD is well documented), it is imperative that the patient with muscular dystrophy be kept as mobile as possible for as long as feasible. The physical therapist systematically assesses weakness, imbalance, and contracture, and provides submaximal exercise, gait training, and contracture stretching. As the child grows, surface area increases by the square of each linear increment and volume by its cube. This "scale effect" explains why a child with a condition limiting the ultimate muscle mass may eventually lose the ability to ambulate, even though the disease is arrested or only slowly progressive. Gradient measurement of strength and functional ability by the physical

therapist aids in indicating appropriate times for contracture release and bracing.

The occupational therapist determines the patient's ability to attend to the tasks of daily living, assisting him or her through a variety of techniques and devices, such as lift and transfer equipment, clothing adaptations, special mattresses, and so on.

Wheelchair Care. Wheelchair confinement is a critical incident, both physiologically and psychologically, in the life of a patient with muscular dystrophy. Special wheelchair adaptations—for example, balanced forearm orthoses facilitating the use of the hands for feeding, writing, as well as other utilitarian tasks—can be prescribed to increase both comfort and function. Electric wheelchairs are available for those patients with insufficient strength to manage the standard model.

ORTHOPEDIC MANAGEMENT

Orthopedic complications are found in most of the muscular dystrophies. Central core disease (one of the congenital myopathies) can present at birth with congenital dislocation of the hips. Neonatal dystrophia myotonica is frequently complicated by severe clubfeet. In addition to weakness and contracture, particularly of the heel cords, children with dermatomyositis often develop subcutaneous or intramuscular calcification or both. In DMD, lower extremity contracture progresses until equinovarus and weakened pelvic balance, produced by hip flexion contracture, prohibit ambulation. Patients develop a stance and gait typified by hip flexion and abduction, increasing lumbar lordosis, and equinocavovarus. Eventually, they no longer can maintain a line projected from their center of gravity behind the center of rotation of their hips, in front of that of their knees and within their base of support. Ambulation stops at this point.

Properly timed surgery and bracing have helped selected patients to continue standing and walking anywhere from 2 to 5 years, thus significantly delaying confinement to a wheelchair with its inevitable downhill course.

Surgical management should permit early postoperative mobilization, as even brief restraint can lead to rapid loss of strength. Anesthesia must be closely monitored with particular attention to preventing gastric dilatation or potassium overload, to assuring adequate ventilation, and to the singular danger of malignant hyperthermia in this class of disease.

For the patient experiencing increased difficulty with walking because of lower extremity contracture, percutaneous hip flexor, bipolar tensor fascia lata, and heel cord tenotomies, followed by extremity bracing, have proved effective in maintaining ambulation. Percutaneous tarsal medullostomy or osteoclasis with soft tissue release has been successful in treating late equinocavovarus with rigid bony deformity. Isolated forefoot adduction is corrected by percutaneous metatarsal osteotomy. Postsurgical orthotic management employs molded plastic appliances that are considerably lighter than steel or aluminum braces, yet equally sturdy. In those cases of facioscapulohumeral dystrophy in which shoulder weakness significantly interferes with upper extremity function, scapular stabilization has been performed.

Scoliosis. Because paraspinal weakness is symmetric, spinal curvature is unusual in the walking Duchenne dystrophic or the child with limb girdle dystrophy. Asymmetric muscle weakness, leading to scoliosis in the ambulatory patient, can occur in the Becker form of muscular dystrophy, sometimes in childhood dystrophia myotonica, and often with childhood facioscapulohumeral dystrophy. These spinal curves, when severe and progressive, can be surgically stabilized.

Most patients with DMD develop paralytic scoliosis as a complication of wheelchair confinement. A variety of external spinal containment systems, such as thoracic jackets or special wheelchair seating, designed to keep the pelvis level and to shape and hold the spine in the upright extended position, can retard such deformity.

Spinal fusion has been successfully used to correct and stabilize scoliosis in heritable neurologic conditions such as spinal muscular atrophy, familial dysautonomia, Charcot-Marie-Tooth disease, and Friedreich's ataxia. Such surgery is being increasingly performed in properly selected wheelchair-confined Duchenne dystrophics with rapidly decompensating scoliosis.

Fractures. Fractures in muscular dystrophy are most frequently seen in the long bones and are more common in patients falling from wheelchairs than in braced patients still ambulating. Such fractures are usually only slightly displaced, and there is not much pain as there is little muscle spasm. They heal without complication in the expected time and should be treated with minimal splintage (mold and sling for humeral fractures, light walking casts for fractures of the femur), encouraging continued independent function as long as possible.

Myasthenia Gravis

O. CARTER SNEAD III, M.D.

Myasthenia gravis (MG) is a disease of the neuromuscular junction characterized by weakness and fatigability of the skeletal muscles. Strong evidence accumulated over the past 10 years supports an autoimmune character of MG and the pathogenic role of circulating IgG antibodies to the nicotinic acetylcholine receptor (AChR), which mediates neuromuscular transmission.

There are six principles of treatment of MG. First, anticholinesterase drugs are useful to one degree or another in all clinical forms of MG and are the mainstay of treatment in those patients with ocular disease only. Second, patients should be clinically evaluated for strength prior to and 1 hour following administration of an anticholinesterase drug in order to titrate the dose. Third, it is preferable to under- rather than overmedicate a patient with anticholinesterase drug to avoid the risk of "cholinergic crisis"—i.e., acute respiratory failure—secondary to overtreatment. Fourth, any patient with MG, as manifested by bulbar or respiratory muscle weakness, with impending respiratory failure (defined by a vital capacity of less than 10–15 cc/kg) should be intubated and artificially ventilated prior to any attempt to determine whether the crisis is cholinergic or myasthenic. Fifth, plasmapheresis can be life saving in severe generalized MG but does not confer long-term protection. Finally, the presence of thymoma is an absolute indication for thymectomy in patients with MG, but this is the only universally accepted criterion for surgical treatment. There is also some controversy regarding when steroid and other immunosuppressant drug therapy is indicated.

Anticholinesterase Drugs. Edrophonium chloride (Tensilon) is a short-acting (30–60 sec) acetylcholinesterase inhibitor used solely for diagnostic purposes. Any patient receiving this drug intravenously should undergo electrocardiographic monitoring, and an experienced neurologist should be in attendance during the drug administration. The initial dose is 0.15 mg/kg IV, not to exceed 2 mg, administered slowly. If there is no adverse reaction to this test dose within 60 seconds, another 0.2 mg/kg IV should be given slowly, to a maximum dose of 8 mg. Should cholinergic side effects occur at any time during administration of the test dose or diagnostic dose, the edrophonium should be discontinued and atropine sulfate administered in a dose of 0.03 mg/kg IV. Such side effects include abdominal cramps, diarrhea, bradycardia, muscle fasciculations and increased weakness.

Edrophonium is somewhat limited diagnostically because its duration of action is so short that any improvement in weakness it produces may be so fleeting as to be missed.

If edrophonium is to be used as a diagnostic aid in myasthenic crisis, adequate respiratory exchange should be assured prior to drug administration. If the patient is apneic, this means that his ventilation must be controlled. The dosage of drug used in crisis in critical. Theoretically, if the crisis is cholinergic, edrophonium will produce increased oropharyngeal secretions and more res-

438   MYASTHENIA GRAVIS

piratory weakness. If the crisis is myasthenic, improvement in strength and respirations should occur. However, the results may be misleading. One muscle group might improve while another deteriorates, and the severity of the myasthenia may fluctuate. Many clinicians feel that it is preferable to support a patient in crisis with controlled ventilation and careful respiratory care, withdraw all medications, treat the patient acutely with plasmapheresis, and start over with lower doses of anticholinesterase medication.

Edrophonium chloride is available in 1- and 10-ml vials containing 10 mg drug/ml.

Pyridostigmine bromide (Mestinon) is longer acting (6–8 hr), less toxic, and has fewer side effects than the other anticholinesterase drug used to treat patients with MG, neostigmine. The usual starting dose of pyridostigmine is 1 mg/kg PO every 4 hours; however, it should be remembered that continuing anticholinesterase therapy has to be tailored for each myasthenic patient. The peak effect of pyridostigmine is seen at 1 hour. The dose should be titrated upward slowly in 30-mg increments in older children and in increments of 1–2 mg in infants. Any acute muscarinic effects should be treated with atropine, but this drug should not be used routinely. A dosage of pyridostigmine that produces muscarinic side effects, such as salivation, lacrimation, vomiting, or diarrhea, should be reduced. The maximum dose of pyridostigmine generally should not exceed 240 mg every 4 hours. The drug is useful in all variants of MG and is available in 60-mg tablets, 180-mg sustained-release tablets, a syrup with 60 mg/5 ml, and an injectable form, 5 mg/ml in 2-ml ampules.

Neostigmine bromide (Prostigmin) is shorter acting (4–6 hr) and has a higher incidence of side effects than pyridostigmine. The dosage equivalency of these two drugs is 15 mg of neostigmine to 60 mg of pyridostigmine. The usual starting dose of neostigmine is 0.3 mg/kg PO every 3 hours. This drug is also of diagnostic value in patients with MG in whom edrophonium produces transient improvement that is missed. The diagnostic dose is 0.125 mg IM in infants and 0.04 mg/kg in older children. Improvement of symptoms may be seen within 10–15 min of administration of this dose and lasts around 30 min.

Neostigmine bromide is available in 15-mg tablets. Neostigmine methylsulfate is available in injectable form at 1:1000, 1:2000, and 1:4000 concentrations in 1- and 10-ml vials.

Steroids. These drugs are not indicated in neonatal myasthenia, and their usefulness in congenital MG is questionable because the autoimmune basis of this disorder has not been clearly demonstrated. However, if used judiciously, steroids are helpful in the management of juvenile MG. If there is no improvement or if there is worsening of debilitating myasthenic symptoms after 6–12 months of the maximal doses of anticholinesterase medication the patient can tolerate, prednisone therapy should be initiated. This should be done in the hospital, since there may be an initial increase of weakness when steroids are first given. The dose of prednisone is 2 mg/kg/day, up to 100 mg/day. Daily therapy is continued for 7–10 days, and then the drug is given on alternate days for several months. Prednisone is given in conjunction with whatever anticholinesterase therapy the patient has been receiving.

Other Immunosuppressive Drugs. Although cyclophosphamide, methotrexate, and azathioprine have been reported to be of some benefit in selected adult patients, there are few or no data to support their use in children with MG.

Plasmapheresis. Patients with MG who are critically ill and in respiratory failure may benefit from plasmapheresis. Usually a two-volume exchange is used in conjunction with immunosuppressive agents. The procedure is associated with a fall in circulating AChR antibody, with concomitant clinical improvement. The benefit, however, is short lived, and the procedure is fraught with risks in young patients with small blood volumes. This therapeutic modality should be reserved for seriously ill patients with life-threatening MG and should be performed by therapists with extensive experience in plasmapheresis of children. Plasmapheresis is not indicated in neonatal or congenital MG.

Thymectomy. The overall prognosis of survival and remission or improvement in patients with juvenile MG is good. Eighty percent of juvenile myasthenics reach 40 years of age, and there is a 50–60% spontaneous remission rate. Therefore, thymectomy should be reserved for patients with generalized myasthenia that is unresponsive after at least 1 year of aggressive medical management with anticholinesterase drugs and prednisone. Remission after thymectomy is associated with early surgery, presence of bulb signs, absence of ocular signs, onset of symptoms between 12 and 16 years of age, and the presence of other immune disease. Ideally, the surgery should be done in a center where there is a medical/surgical team experienced with plasmapheresis as well as with the drug, respiratory, and surgical management of the myasthenic patient.

Drugs to Avoid in Patient with MG. A number of pharmacologic agents act at the neuromuscular junction and thus could cause an exacerbation of myasthenic symptoms. Such drugs include quinidine, quinine, procainamide, neomycin, kanamycin, streptomycin, polymyxin, lidocaine, curare, succinylcholine, decamethonium, gallamine, propranolol, and other beta-adrenergic blockers. In addition, some authors suggest that phenytoin and chlorpromazine should be avoided. Opiates such as morphine should be used with great caution in patients with MG, since the respiratory depressant action of these compounds may be potentiated by anticholinesterase drugs.

Periodic Paralysis

ROBERT C. GRIGGS, M.D.

Recognition and accurate diagnosis are often the major challenges in the treatment of periodic paralysis. Most patients present in childhood—usually in the first weeks of life for paramyotonia and hyperkalemic periodic paralysis and by adolescence in hypokalemic periodic paralysis. When diagnosis is first considered, careful exclusion of other disorders associated with weakness and abnormality of potassium (K) is necessary. Initial attacks require careful documentation before treatment is initiated. Provocative testing is necessary in most patients to establish diagnosis.

HYPOKALEMIC PERIODIC PARALYSIS

Acute Attacks. During paralytic episodes, potassium is invariably low, and, unless the patient is unable to swallow or is vomiting, potassium should be administered orally. A preparation of KCl that is free of sucrose and other carbohydrate should be chosen. A dosage of 0.5 meq/kg as 25 per cent KCl is usually indicated and may have to be repeated. During severe attacks, serum electrolytes and electrocardiogram (ECG) should be monitored at half-hourly intervals until the attack resolves. The exact dosage of potassium depends on the severity and duration of the attack and on the response to the initial dosage of potassium.

If patients are unable to take oral potassium, intravenous KCl may be necessary. The diluent for such treatment is of concern since both 5% glucose and physiologic saline will cause a transient lowering of serum potassium. A concentration of at least 60 meq/l of KCl must be used if either of these diluents is employed. Intravenous treatment is reserved for severely affected patients and requires careful monitoring of electrolytes, ECG, respiratory function, strength, and urinary output. Intravenous KCl-containing solutions should be administered slowly.

Prevention of Attacks. The prophylactic administration of potassium salts is seldom successful in preventing attacks, even when given in large doses on a daily basis. Patients subject to frequent attacks merit a trial of agents to prevent attacks. I have found that most patients respond to the carbonic anhydrase inhibitor acetazolamide with complete cessation of attacks. Treatment is usually effective within 24 to 48 hours, and attacks recur promptly after treatment is discontinued. The dosage is quite variable (2–20 mg/kg in divided dosages) but is usually that required to produce metabolic acidosis, as indicated by serum chloride elevation and bicarbonate depression. In severe cases, an every-6-hours schedule is necessary.

In occasional patients acetazolamide may produce sufficient hypokalemia to worsen the disorder. In these patients, potassium-sparing agents such as triamterene may be effective. Dietary management, including the avoidance of carbohydrate and sodium loads, may be effective—occasionally as the sole, and often as adjunctive, treatment.

Chronic acetazolamide treatment presents certain hazards, most notably the occurrence of renal calculi. Patients on acetazolamide should have periodic abdominal radiographs and should maintain a high urine output. Sulfonamides should not be prescribed concurrently since a sulfonamide nephropathy may be produced. Frequent but less troublesome side effects include dysgeusia for carbonated beverages, paresthesias, mild anorexia, and osteomalacia.

Treatment and Prevention of Progressive Weakness. Patients with frequent attacks of all types of periodic paralysis may develop persistent interattack weakness after repeated attacks. Acetazolamide prevents and improves such weakness in many patients. Patients unresponsive to acetazolamide may respond to the chloruretic carbonic anhydrase inhibitor dichlorphenamide.

Thyrotoxic hypokalemic periodic paralysis rarely occurs in childhood, and its treatment is markedly different from that of other hypokalemic periodic paralysis. Potassium administration is indicated for acute attacks, but acetazolamide markedly worsens patients. Treatment consists of management of underlying thyrotoxicosis. Propranolol is strikingly effective in preventing attacks, even while patients remain thyrotoxic.

HYPERKALEMIC PERIODIC PARALYSIS

Acute Attacks. Hyperkalemic periodic paralysis is often a misnomer since the serum potassium may remain within the normal range during attacks. The disorder is, therefore, defined by the development of weakness with potassium-loading. Acute attacks are often so mild that treatment is unnecessary. Oral carbohydrate administration in the form of sugar solutions is preferable to potassium-containing fruit juices and soft drinks. Attacks are seldom severe enough to require intravenous therapy. If a severe attack does occur, it will respond to standard measures used to treat hyperkalemia—intravenous glucose, insulin, or sodium bicarbonate.

Prevention of Attacks. Many patients do not require chronic treatment, particularly those with slight, infrequent attacks. Acetazolamide in dosage sufficient to produce a mild kaliopenia (usually 3 mg/kg, 2 or 3 times a day) will prevent attacks and has the added benefit of ameliorating myotonia. Side effects (particularly paresthesias) often limit patient acceptability, and for this reason I have found thiazide diuretics the agent of choice. Chlorothiazide in a dosage of 10 mg/kg in two divided doses prevents attacks; *hypo*kalemia and weakness can develop in these patients as in normal people. Dosage should be kept low enough to prevent this occurrence. Recently, the use of inhaled β-adrenergic agents such as albuterol (1–2 puffs) has been found useful in alleviating attacks.

Normokalemic Periodic Paralysis. There are few, if any, well-documented cases of patients with so-called normokalemic periodic paralysis who have not been found to have features identical to those of hyperkalemic periodic paralysis, and treatment is similar.

PARAMYOTONIA CONGENITA

Myotonia is the more disabling feature of paramyotonia, and episodic weakness is usually mild and infrequent. If the disorder requires treatment, it is important to distinguish the two types: (1) true paramyotonia, and (2) paralysis periodica paramyotonica. Patients with the latter disorder are worsened by potassium administration and respond to agents such as acetazolamide and thiazides, which are kaliopenic. True paramyotonia is worsened by such treatment, and patients may develop quadriplegia with acetazolamide. Tocainide, a drug recently used for treatment of cardiac arrhythmias, is useful for the myotonia and weakness of paramyotonia congenita. Simple maneuvers to avoid cold exposure are usually adequate treatment for mild cases of paramyotonia.

Myositis Ossificans

MARVIN L. WEIL, M.D.

Current therapeutic measures for the three types of myositis ossificans common to children involve symptomatic relief and treatment of complications. Disodium (1-hydroxyethylidene) diphosphonic acid (etidronate disodium), used in adults to inhibit the formation, growth, and dissolution of hydroxyapatite crystals to regulate bone metabolism, is not approved for use in children, since it may modulate bone growth.

The progressive fibrodysplastic form of myositis ossificans has characteristic skeletal formations, with malformation of the big toes, reduction defects of the digits, and baldness. Deafness associated with this condition should be treated in order to minimize the symptoms of mental retardation, which may also occur. Exacerbating factors to be avoided as much as possible include trauma to muscle, intramuscular injections, careless venipunctures, biopsy of lungs, and operations to excise ectopic bone. Dental therapy may result in ossification of the masseter muscles. Surgical removal of the calcified tumor becomes necessary in cases with continued pain or significant functional limitation.

Postparalytic myositis ossificans, which can also occur after long-term coma, may be confused with deep venous thrombosis. Tc-99m diphosphonate imaging can be used to recognize early heterotopic bone formation.

Post-traumatic myositis ossificans is usually treated by nonoperative management. This circumscribed form must be distinguished from osteomyelitis and soft tissue abscesses.

Physical therapy to minimize limitation of movement and appropriate psychotherapy may be indicated in all forms of the disease.

_15_

Skin

Topical Therapy: A Dermatologic Formulary for Pediatric Practice

JO DAVID FINE, M.D.,
and KENNETH A. ARNDT, M.D.

Most common childhood dermatoses can be effectively managed by the pediatrician. Unusual diagnostic or therapeutic problems can be referred to a consultant dermatologist for further evaluation as deemed necessary.

GENERAL PRINCIPLES

Acute Versus Chronic Inflammation. The ability to distinguish between acute and chronic inflammatory states will simplify diagnosis and initial skin care. Acute processes are often exudative, vesicular, and crusted and respond best to wet dressings, powders, lotions, and creams. Chronic eruptions often are dry, scaling, and lichenified and require more occlusive preparations, such as ointments, to lubricate the skin and to enhance the percutaneous absorption of the active ingredients.

Role of Infection. The possibility of primary or secondary infection should be considered when initially evaluating a skin eruption. Information obtained from gross examination of the lesions may be sufficient to make a clinical diagnosis of an infectious process. For example, the presence of honey-colored or yellow crusting or exudate, frequently accompanied by a history of recent exacerbation of an underlying or concomitant dermatosis, suggests secondary bacterial impetiginization. The use of appropriate systemic antibiotics to treat streptococcal and staphylococcal infections will result in marked improvement of the patient. At other times cultures of the lesion (exudate; contents of pustules, vesicles, bullae) or mass (skin biopsy with half the specimen for cultures and half for histology) may be required. Bacterial, fungal,

viral, and occasionally mycobacterial cultures may be indicated.

Surface Area to Volume Ratio. Children have an increased surface area to volume ratio compared with adults. Percutaneous absorption following application of topical agents over large body areas may result in systemic drug levels and subsequent acute toxicity or unwanted systemic effects. The former is seen with boric acid soaks (gastrointestinal symptoms, renal or hepatic failure, cardiovascular collapse, central nervous system stimulation or depression), while the latter is illustrated by adrenal suppression secondary to topical corticosteroid applications. In addition, marked temperature lability may occur when large surface areas are treated with wet compresses. To avoid significant chilling and hypothermia due to surface evaporation of water, only small areas should be treated simultaneously (i.e., a limb or part of the trunk).

Barrier Function and Penetration. In normal skin, intact stratum corneum serves as a barrier to absorption of external agents as well as loss of internal fluids. Barrier function is altered, however, when inflammation is present or when fissures or denuded areas develop. Skin hydration also affects barrier function—substances are absorbed more readily through hydrated than through dry epidermis.

Ointments are more effective vehicles than creams for promoting percutaneous absorption, presumably by increasing surface hydration via occlusion. Similarly, the use of plastic gloves, vinyl exercise suits, or plastic wraps as occlusive dressings with topical corticosteroids will be advantageous in selected nonexudative dermatoses such as psoriasis, chronic eczema, and lichen planus. However, occlusion may also increase skin maceration, particularly in acute vesiculobullous and secondarily impetiginized disorders, and therefore is contraindicated in these situations.

441

When excessive scale is present (i.e., psoriasis), efficacy of corticosteroids may be enhanced by prior or concomitant use of keratolytic agents under occlusion (see "Corticosteroids" later in this article).

Frequency of Application. Little is known about the optimal number of applications needed per day of most types of topical medications for effective treatment of a given skin disease. Some studies suggest that single daily applications of topical corticosteroids, with or without occlusion, may be as effective as multiple daily applications. Despite this, most authorities still recommend the latter approach.

Tachyphylaxis. The continued and uninterrupted use of topical corticosteroids may result in temporary diminution in their effectiveness. This may occur as early as 2 weeks into the course of treatment, but responsiveness returns after corticosteroids have been discontinued for 1 or more weeks. Intermittent use is best both to insure optimal results and to decrease the risk of any adverse effects.

Adverse Systemic Effects. The prolonged use of even low-concentration topical corticosteroids over large surface areas may result in pituitary-adrenal axis suppression. Growth retardation in children has also been reported. Application of potent fluorinated corticosteroids can result in atrophy, telangiectasia, and striae formation within 1 month of use. Areas such as the face and genitals and intertriginous areas are particularly at risk; therefore, corticosteroids must be used judiciously in these sites.

Boric acid compresses may result in significant systemic toxicity and should no longer be used.

Elevated phenol levels in blood and urine may result from application of carbol-fuchsin solution (Castellani's paint) in children. Although an excellent astringent agent for macerated or fissured intertriginous skin folds or web spaces or intertriginous candidiasis, it should be used only in very select situations.

Absorption of silver sulfadiazine (Silvadene) from extensively burned skin may result in hyperosmolality from the propylene glycol in its vehicle and may thereby add to the metabolic instability of such patients.

Appropriate Selection of Quantities by Prescription. Careful thought must be given to the amount of topical medication needed by each patient to ensure that enough is dispensed to last for days or weeks and also to decrease the cost of the prescription. In an adult, 30–60 gm of an ointment or cream are required to cover the entire body in a single application. Most preparations are less expensive when purchased in larger prepackaged containers than in multiple small tubes or jars. If appropriate amounts are dispensed, the overall cost of care is reduced and patient compliance will be improved.

Fixed-Combination Preparations. One can usually provide more versatile and at least as effective therapy by using single-component preparations in concert rather than fixed-combination medications. Furthermore, use of many of the latter may result in unwanted side effects. As an example, an impetiginized inflammatory lesion may be better treated with oral antibiotics and topical corticosteroids than with a fixed combination of neomycin with steroid. Use of neomycin may actually exacerbate some skin disorders as a result of development of allergic contact dermatitis. Positive patch test reactions have been reported in up to 20% of patients subsequent to use of neomycin on inflamed skin.

TYPES OF TOPICAL PREPARATIONS

"Wetness" provides benefit by cooling and drying through surface evaporation of water. *Wet dressings* also clean the skin of surface exudates and crusts and help drain infected sites. They are the principal form of therapy for acute exudative inflammation. *Powders* increase skin surface area, thereby enhancing drying and reducing maceration and friction. They are especially useful in body fold areas. *Lotions* are suspensions of powder in water. After the aqueous phase evaporates, a layer of protective or therapeutic powder is left on the skin.

Creams are emulsions of oil in water; they are less occlusive and more drying than corresponding ointments. *Ointments* either are suspensions of water droplets in oil or are inert bases such as petrolatum. They may not be miscible with water.

Gels are transparent colorless emulsions that liquefy when applied to skin.

Pastes are combinations of powder and ointment and are of stiffer consistency than ointments. Cornstarch is frequently the powder used, as in zinc oxide paste. Since application of cornstarch to intertriginous sites may enhance the overgrowth of yeast, pediatricians should be careful to use zinc oxide ointment rather than paste as a perianal barrier; otherwise secondary *Candida albicans* infection might result.

FORMULARY

This formulary contains a representative list of commonly available topical agents that are beneficial in dermatologic therapy. Although more inclusive lists are available, we believe that this formulary is adequate for general pediatric use.

Acne Preparations

Benzoyl Peroxides. These preparations contain 2.5–10% benzoyl peroxide. They are bacteriostatic for *Propionibacterium acnes* as well as mildly comedolytic. They are usually applied thinly once or twice daily to all acne areas, but should be used less frequently or discontinued if excessive redness or dryness develops. The lower concentrations should be used initially to avoid unnecessary irritation. Higher concentrations of benzoyl peroxide should be used with caution in darker-complexioned individuals, because excessive irritation may lead to postinflammatory hyperpigmentation.

An oil base lotion is Benoxyl (Stiefel), which is available in 5 and 10% concentrations. Benzagel (Dermik, 5 and 10%) and PanOxyl (Stiefel, 5 and 10%) have an alcohol gel base. A lotion with acetone gel base is Persa-Gel (Ortho, 5 and 10%), while an aqueous gel base can be found in Desquam-X (Westwood, 5 and 10% gel, 10% wash) and PanOxyl AQ (Stiefel, 2.5%).

Retinoic Acid (Vitamin A Acid; Tretinoin). This agent is useful in comedonal acne because of its loosening effect on cellular debris impacted within sebaceous gland and follicular ostia. Used nightly or every other night on acne sites (except eye and lip areas), retinoic acid induces comedones to be expelled. A transient flare in activity may be seen approximately 3–6 weeks into treatment. Because of the risk of exaggerated sunburn and possible photocarcinogenicity, retinoic acid preparations should be used with caution, if at all, during summer months. Lower concentrations and creams are initially used; in oilier skin, the gel may be more efficacious. Commonly used forms are Retin-A (Ortho Pharmaceutical) cream (0.05 and 0.1%) and gel (0.01 and 0.025%).

Topical Antibiotics. These agents may be quite effective in mild-to-moderate acne and are used often in conjunction with benzoyl peroxides or retinoic acid. Clindamycin, erythromycin, and tetracycline are all effective against *P. acnes* and may be obtained either commercially prepared and prepackaged or extemporaneously compounded by the physician and pharmacist. Their effectiveness is generally in the order just cited. Topical tetracycline may cause a temporary yellow hue to the skin and also fluoresces when viewed under ultraviolet light; this may make it less desirable for adolescent patients. Although pseudomembranous colitis has been seen in only a very few patients treated with topical clindamycin, its use is contraindicated in patients with ulcerative colitis, Crohn's disease, or pseudomembranous colitis, and its use should be discontinued in otherwise healthy patients who develop persistent diarrhea.

Preparations commercially available include clindamycin (Cleocin-T, Upjohn, 30-ml package, and other preparations), erythromycin (Staticin, Westwood, 60-ml package), and tetracycline (Topicycline, Proctor and Gamble, 70-ml package). Alternatively, one can extemporaneously formulate an approximately 1% clindamycin solution in the following ways: one 600 mg Cleocin hydrochloride capsule in 50 ml of Neutrogena Vehicle/N, or one 600 mg capsule of Cleocin hydrochloride in 54 ml of 70% isopropyl alcohol and 6 ml of propylene glycol.

Acne Cleaners. Many products contain combinations of sulfur, salicylic acid, resorcinol, alcohol, and insoluble or slowly dissolving particles. These have at best only a minor role in acne therapy, providing mild drying and peeling of the skin. It must be emphasized that dryness and superficial peeling are not the desired end-point of topical acne therapy. They are side effects of most of the effective topical agents and are not necessary for successful treatment. We do not suggest these agents routinely, but they may be used at the patient's discretion, with care to avoid excessive dryness and irritation.

Anesthetics (Topical)

Although usually ineffective in alleviating pain or itching of inflamed skin, topical anesthetics may be beneficial in some inflammatory mucocutaneous conditions (aphthous stomatitis, herpes simplex infection of the oral cavity or anogenital area, oral erosive lichen planus). However, benzocaine-containing preparations should be avoided because of their tendency for allergic contact sensitization.

Topical anesthetics include dyclonine hydrochloride (Dyclone) (Dow Pharmaceuticals), 0.5 or 1.0% solution, 30 ml; diphenhydramine hydrochloride (Benadryl elixir) (Parke-Davis), 4 oz; and lidocaine (Xylocaine) (Astra), as a 2% viscous solution (100 ml and 2.5 and 5.0% ointment (35 gm). These agents may be applied locally to the lesion(s) or, in the case of elixirs, may be used as mouth rinses, four to six times daily as needed for symptomatic relief.

Anthralin

Anthralin, a chemical derivative of anthracene, is an effective topical agent used either alone or in conjunction with UVB irradiation for the treatment of psoriasis. Like other tar by-products, anthralin probably is beneficial in psoriasis because of its antimitotic activity. Although used extensively in England and Europe, until recently anthralin was infrequently used in the United States because of its tendency to produce skin irritation and temporary staining. Anthralin is used in concentrations ranging from 0.1 to 2.0%, with usually the lowest concentration initially employed. Although the drug is usually left on the lesions for 4–12 hours prior to bathing, recently it has been shown that anthralin may be just as effective but less irritating if one of the higher concentrations is applied for only 15–30 minutes ("short-contact therapy").

Antibacterial and Antiseptic Agents

Several preparations are available in both liquid and ointment form that contain bacteriostatic or bactericidal agents. Although most pyodermas are better treated with systemic antibiotics (i.e., penicillin for ecthyma and streptococcal impetigo, erythromycin or dicloxacillin for staphylococcal impetigo), localized superficial wounds often may be adequately treated with topical preparations. Such conditions include surgical sites, burns, areas of localized folliculitis, and abrasions.

Combination formulations often broaden the effective antibacterial spectrum. Although a very effective antistaphylococcal agent, neomycin often causes an allergic contact sensitization, with subsequent worsening of the dermatosis. Systemic absorption and toxicity are very improbable for these agents, owing to their poor percutaneous permeability.

Liquids/Surgical Cleansers. Chlorhexidine is antibacterial for both gram-positive and gram-negative organisms; it has immediate as well as continuing antibacterial effects and is not inhibited by the presence of blood. It is available as Hibiclens (Stuart), in a 4-oz package. Povidone-iodine has antibacterial coverage similar to that of Hibiclens. However, bacterial killing with povidone-iodine requires several minutes of direct contact with the skin and may be inhibited by blood. Furthermore, it may leave a slight yellow tint to the skin if it is not thoroughly removed by rinsing. It is available as Betadine (Purdue Frederick), as well as other brands, in the following liquid forms: solution, surgical scrub, shampoo, and douche.

Ointments. Bacitracin is bactericidal, especially for gram-positive organisms like streptococci and staphylococci. It may be dispensed simply in 15-gm tubes or in combination, as in Neosporin ointment (Burroughs Wellcome) (containing 5000 units of polymyxin B sulfate, 400 units of zinc bacitracin, and 3.5 mg of neomycin sulfate per gm), 15 gm; Neo-Polycin ointment (Dow Pharmaceuticals) (containing 8000 units of polymyxin B sulfate, 400 units of zinc bacitracin, and 3 mg of neomycin sulfate per gm), 15 gm; and Polysporin ointment (Burroughs Wellcome) (containing 500 units of zinc bacitracin and 10,000 units of polymyxin B per gm), 30 gm.

Neomycin sulfate is effective against most gram-negative and some gram-positive organisms, but it has a significant potential as a contact allergen. It is available either alone in generic forms (15 gm) or in combination, as noted.

Polymyxin B is effective against most gram-negative organisms, but not *Proteus* and *Serratia*. It is available in combinations, as noted.

Povidone-iodine is also available in ointment form (30 gm) as Betadine or a generic brand.

Gramicidin is bactericidal against gram-positive organisms. It is available in combination with neomycin (Spectrocin ointment, Squibb) and polymyxin B (Neosporin-G cream, Burroughs Wellcome).

Any of these agents can be applied (or used as cleansers if liquid) four to six times daily to the affected sites, as needed.

Antifungal Medications

Dermatophyte Infections. Any agent listed below may be used twice daily for localized dermatophyte infections. Treatment is continued until approximately 2 weeks after all clinical signs of infection are gone—the average duration is about 1 month. However, systemic griseofulvin is necessary for adequate treatment of dermatophyte involvement of hair and nails, when large surface areas of skin are involved, or for recalcitrant, persistently recurrent infection.

Clotrimazole is available as either Lotrimin (Schering) or Mycelex (Miles Pharmaceuticals); cream (30 gm) is usually used, but solution (30 ml) may be preferred for moist, macerated sites, such as interdigital web spaces of toes. Miconazole is similar in structure and mode of action. It is available as Monistat-Derm (Ortho Pharmaceutical), 30 gm of cream or 30 ml of solution. Haloprogin is available as Halotex (Westwood), 30 gm of cream or 30 ml of solution. Newer topical antifungal agents in cream form include econazole (Spectazole, Ortho Pharmaceutical, 15, 30, and 85 gm) and ciclopirox olamine (Loprox, Hoechst-Roussel, 15 and 30 gm). Tolnaftate (Tinactin, Schering) is available as 1% cream in a 15-gm package; as solution, 10 ml; as powder, 45 gm; and as aerosol, 100 gm. Generic brands are also available.

***Candida* Infections.** Clotrimazole, miconazole, econazole, ciclopirox olamine, or haloprogin can be used, as just described.

Nystatin is found in many brands of medications, including Mycostatin (Squibb). The most commonly used forms are ointment, cream, and powder. All are available in 15-gm sizes. The use of topical nystatin in our experience seems to result in a slower clinical resolution of active lesions, and we therefore prefer initially the use of the broader-spectrum antifungal agents previously described.

For *Candida* paronychial infections, any of the above preparations may be tried; occlusion under a fingercot may increase their effectiveness. If this treatment is unsuccessful, 2–4% thymol in absolute alcohol (prescribed 30 ml) may be compounded; this is applied two to three times daily to the nail fold areas until healing is complete. The area must be kept dry at all times during the latter nonaqueous therapy.

For oral *Candida* infection (thrush), nystatin oral suspension (100,000 units/ml; 2 ml for infants, 4–6 ml for older children and adults) may be swished in the mouth four times daily and swallowed. An alternate therapy is 1–2% gentian violet solution painted in the oral cavity one to two times a day.

Iodochlorhydroxyquin (Vioform, CIBA), 3% cream or ointment (30 gm), may be used alone or combined with 1% hydrocortisone (Vioform-Hydrocortisone, CIBA, 20 gm); generic preparations are also available. This agent has mild antifungal and antibacterial properties and is frequently used in diaper dermatitis, especially when the skin is mildly eczematous, impetiginized, or secondarily infected with yeast. Clothing and skin may be stained yellow by its use.

Topical amphotericin B (available as Fungizone cream, ointment, and lotion; Squibb) is effective against *Candida* but not dermatophytes. Its use has no advantage over other anti-*Candida* therapies, and its yellow-orange color may stain.

Tinea Versicolor. This superficial infection, caused by *Malassezia furfur*, may be treated in many ways. Some effective approaches are (1) 2.5% selenium sulfide suspension (available as Selsun, Abbott, and as Exsel, Herbert Laboratories). This lotion is applied daily to all skin areas from the neck to the knees and showered off after 15–30 minutes. This routine is repeated daily for 10–14 days. The scalp also should be shampooed with this solution on the first night of treatment; (2) shampoos containing zinc pyrithione (e.g., Head & Shoulders) applied 5–10 minutes nightly for 10–14 days; (3) 25% sodium hyposulfite (available as Tinver lotion, Barnes-Hind). This is applied twice daily for about 2 weeks to the affected areas; and (4) clotrimazole, miconazole, haloprogin, or tolnaftate preparations.

Antipruritic Agents

If significant itching is present, the use of oral antihistamines as well as topical agents is helpful. For localized pruritic processes, however, drying and cooling preparations can be beneficial when applied four to six times a day. Examples of the latter include (1) Schamberg lotion (somewhat oily), which contains menthol, 0.5 gm; phenol, 1 gm; zinc oxide, 20 gm; calcium hydroxide solution, 40 ml; and peanut oil to make 100 ml. (2) Menthol, 0.25 gm, and phenol, 1 gm in Eucerin cream (Beiersdorf) to make 100 gm (lubricating). (3) Calamine, or phenolated calamine lotion (drying). Caladryl (Parke-Davis) cream or lotion, frequently self-prescribed, should be avoided since diphenhydramine when applied topically is both ineffective and a contact allergen. (4) Sarna lotion (Stiefel), 0.5% each of camphor, phenol, and menthol in an emollient lotion vehicle.

Antiviral Agents

Acyclovir (ACV). ACV is a recently released antiviral compound shown to be effective against herpes simplex. The drug is an acyclic nucleoside of guanine. Following phosphorylation by thymidine kinase it becomes antiviral, exerting inhibition of herpes simplex DNA polymerase. ACV is also somewhat effective against varicella-zoster virus.

This drug may be beneficial topically in the first episode of genital herpes but is ineffective in recurrent disease. It is also effective intravenously in primary genital herpes and may be useful in bone marrow recipients to prevent or attenuate the course of cutaneous herpes infections.

ACV is available as 5% ointment (Zovirax, Burroughs Wellcome, 15 gm).

Burn Preparations

One of the most frequently used agents for first, second, and third degree burns is silver sulfadiazine (available as Silvadene, Marion, in 50- and 400-gm packages). It is bactericidal against a wide spectrum of organisms, allowing wound healing to occur under rather sterile conditions. However, it should be avoided in sulfa-allergic patients because of its potential for systemic absorption and subsequent allergic response.

Corticosteroids

Topical corticosteroids are often the most effective single therapy for a variety of inflammatory and hyperplastic cutaneous disorders. The pediatrician will have most frequent need of them in eczematous dermatitis (including allergic contact dermatitis and atopic dermatitis) and psoriasis. Sensible and effective use of these agents necessitates not only a correct diagnosis but also an understanding of tachyphylaxis, the use of occlusion, and the potential for systemic and cutaneous side effects, all of which have been discussed. Although many preparations exist, it is necessary to become familiar with only a few of these in order to effectively treat steroid-responsive dermatoses.

Table 1 lists the corticosteroids. All of these creams and ointments may be applied thinly two to four times daily to affected skin areas. They are most effective if applied to well-hydrated skin. Corticosteroid solutions are applied one to two times daily after shampooing and drying of the scalp; they are used for 7–14 days as needed and for psoriasis should be occluded overnight by use of a plastic showercap. After a few days of treatment with potent topical corticosteroids, facial, genital, and intertriginous areas are more safely treated with 1% hydrocortisone in order to avoid steroid side effects.

Table 1.   REPRESENTATIVE TOPICAL CORTICOSTEROIDS FOR DERMATOLOGIC DISORDERS

High potency	Fluocinonide 0.05%. Lidex cream, ointment, and gel, and Lidex E cream (Syntex), available in 15-, 30-, and 60-gm sizes.
	Halcinonide 0.1%. Halog cream and ointment (Squibb), Halciderm cream (Squibb), available in 15-, 30-, and 60-gm sizes. Halog also comes as 0.1% solution (2 oz) as well as 240 gm in both cream and ointment.
Middle potency	Betamethasone valerate 0.1%. Valisone (Schering), 15- and 45-gm cream and ointment, 60-ml solution.
	Betamethasone dipropionate 0.05%. Diprosone cream and ointment (Schering), both available in 15- and 45-gm sizes; lotion (0.05%) and topical aerosol (0.1%), available in 20- and 60-ml and 85-gm sizes, respectively. Diprolene ointment (Schering) is available in 15- and 45-gm sizes.
	Fluocinolone acetonide 0.025%. Synalar (Syntex), available in 30-, 60-, and 425-gm in both 0.025% cream and ointment; 2 oz as 0.01% solution.
	Hydrocortisone valerate 0.2%. Westcort cream and ointment (Westwood), in 15-, 45-, and 60-gm cream and ointment.
Low potency	Hydrocortisone 1%. Nutracort (Owen), 120-gm cream and ointment; Hytone (Dermik), (Synacort), (Syntex), 30- and 120-gm cream and ointment; others.

Moist or vesicular lesions (acute inflammatory lesions) are better treated with creams, while corticosteroid ointments are better suited for dry lichenified areas (chronic inflammatory or hyperplastic lesions). If excessive scale is present (i.e., psoriasis, hypertrophic lichen planus), pretreatment or concomitant treatment with Keralyt gel (Westwood, 30 gm) under occlusion (i.e., plastic gloves, bags, or wraps) for 2–4 hours will enhance the effect of subsequent corticosteroid applications.

Emollients

Many emollients are readily available and inexpensive. If hydrophobic (greasy) substances are applied to skin surfaces after adequate hydration (immersion in water for at least 10 minutes), they will add to the surface barrier and impede water loss. In pediatric practice they are most frequently used for children with atopic dermatitis. By decreasing dryness, they help prevent further fissuring, itching, and subsequent inflammation and possibly impetiginization. Some emollients are greasier in texture than others; choice of emollient will depend on expense and cosmetic acceptance. Commonly used emollients include lotions—for example: Alpha Keri (Westwood), U-Lactin (T/I Pharmaceutical), Lubriderm (Ortho), Cetaphil (Parke-Davis), Lubrex (T/I Pharmaceutical), and

Wibi (Owen); creams, such as Nivea (Beiersdorf), Eucerin (Beiersdorf), Carmol (Syntex), and Keri (Westwood); and ointments—Aquaphor (Beiersdorf) and hydrated petrolatum USP.

Keratolytics

Propylene glycol solutions with or without added salicylic acid are excellent agents for loosening and removing scales; they are especially effective when applied to affected skin for 2–4 hours under plastic wrap occlusion after adequate prior hydration by soaks or bathing. Patients with conditions such as ichthyosis (vulgaris and X-linked), psoriasis, hypertrophic lichen planus, and tinea manuum and pedis will benefit from this treatment. Available preparations include Keralyt gel (Westwood, 30 gm) and 40% propylene glycol solution, the latter prepared by a pharmacist. Whitfield's ointment (as half-strength concentration, 3% salicylic acid and 6% benzoic acid, in 30-gm tube) is mainly used either alone or in conjunction with other antifungal creams for the treatment of hyperkeratotic dermatophyte infection of the palms and soles. In isolated cases of dense scalp psoriasis, nightly treatment under a plastic showercap with either Keralyt gel or P & S liquid (Baker) helps in scalp debridement.

Scabicides and Pediculocides

Gamma benzene hexachloride (Kwell lotion or shampoo, Reed and Carnrick, 60 ml, and other generic brands) is effective for both mites (scabies) and lice (pediculosis). When treating scabies, all skin below the angle of the jaw is covered; medication should be applied to dry skin (i.e., the patient should not shower first) and washed off 8 hours later. The treatment may be repeated in 7 days to protect against possible reinfection by hatched larvae. Because of its potential for percutaneous absorption, lindane is contraindicated in pregnant women, in neonates and very young children, and in those with widespread cutaneous disease and an abnormally permeable skin barrier; isolated cases of central nervous system side effects in children have been reported.

Pediculosis pubis is treated by application of lindane to the groin and other affected areas, with rinsing after 8 hours. Pediculosis capitis may be treated with single lindane shampooing, although some advocate repeat treatment in 4–7 days.

Crotamiton (Eurax cream and lotion, Westwood, 60-gm and 2-oz packages) is an alternative to lindane for the treatment of scabies. This is applied twice daily for 2 days.

Six to 10% precipitated sulfur in petrolatum (30 or 60 gm), the initial antiscabetic therapy in pregnancy and infancy, is applied daily for 3 days. It is messy and malodorous but has no risk of systemic side effects.

Another effective agent for the treatment of head lice is malathion (Prioderm lotion, Purdue Frederick, 59 ml). The lotion is applied to dry scalp, left uncovered for 8–12 hours, and then shampooed out. If necessary, the treatment may be repeated in 7 days. Until further data are available, this agent is best avoided in pregnant individuals.

Effective over-the-counter alternate treatments for pediculosis are pyrethrin-containing agents such as A-200 Pyrinate liquid (Norcliff Thayer) and Rid (Pfipharmecs).

Involved eyelashes may be treated by careful application of petrolatum twice daily for 8 days, 0.025% phosphostigmine ophthalmic ointment (5 gm) or yellow oxide of mercury.

Shampoos

Although nonmedicated shampoos are certainly useful in local scalp hygiene, shampoos containing selenium sulfide, zinc pyrithione, tar, or salicylic acid-sulfur are more beneficial for seborrheic dermatitis and psoriasis. These are initially used daily with a second application after the first rinsing; after the scalp improves in appearance, shampooing may be performed every other or every third night as necessary. Useful agents include selenium sulfide, available as Selsun (Abbott) and Exsel (Herbert Laboratories); zinc pyrithione—Zincon (Lederle) and Head & Shoulders (Procter and Gamble); tar (particularly useful in psoriasis)—Sebutone (Westwood), Pentrax (Coopercare), T-GEl (Neutrogena), and others; and salicylic acid-sulfur—Sebulex (Westwood), Vanseb (Herbert Laboratories), TiSeb (T/I Pharmaceutical), and others.

Soaps

Children with eczema or atopic dermatitis may develop skin irritation from harsh soaps. The least irritating soap has been found to be Dove, followed by a group including Aveenobar, Purpose, Dial, Alpha Keri, Neutrogena, Ivory, and Oilatum.

Sunscreens

Sunscreens are agents containing chemicals that absorb ultraviolet light from the sunburn spectrum. Use of sunscreens permits increased exposure time to sunlight without development of sunburn. Their use is especially important in sunlight-aggravated diseases such as lupus erythematosus and polymorphous light eruption. The individual usefulness of a sunscreen to prevent sunburn depends on its relative efficacy in blocking or absorbing UVB radiation (280–320 nm), as well as its SPF (sunlight protection factor) rating. Two of the more effective sunscreens are PreSun 15 (Westwood) and Total Eclipse (Herbert Laboratories). A very effective sunscreen that does not contain para-aminobenzoic acid is TiScreen (T/I Pharmaceutical). Most sunscreens should be reapplied after sweating or swimming. For total sunlight exclusion, sunshades containing opaque substances can be used; these include zinc oxide paste, A-Fil (Texas Pharmacals), and Reflecta. Lipstick sunscreens are also available.

Tar Compounds

Coal tar preparations have long been known to be effective in psoriasis and eczematous dermatitis, although their exact modes of action are still not understood. Tars are anti-inflammatory, inhibit DNA synthesis, and photosensitize to long-wave ultraviolet light (UVA). Among commonly used preparations are the following:

Liquids. For chronic hand or foot eczema, soaks or compresses for 30 minutes twice daily with Balnetar (Westwood, 8 oz) or Zetar emulsion (Dermik, 6 oz) are useful, especially if areas are fissured. When more widespread areas are involved, as in generalized atopic dermatitis or psoriasis, tar baths twice daily, followed by application of other medication or emollients, are beneficial.

Another useful liquid tar preparation for the treatment of scalp psoriasis is T/Gel scalp solution (Neutrogena). This solution contains 2% coal tar extract as well as a keratolytic agent (2% salicylic acid); it is applied to the scalp following shampooing in the evening, occluded overnight with a plastic shower-cap, and rinsed off the following morning.

Gels. Gels are beneficial in psoriasis in conjunction with topical corticosteroids and/or ultraviolet light therapy or both. T/Derm (Neutrogena) or Estar gel (Westwood, 90 gm) is applied daily to the individual lesions. Similarly, tar-containing gels can be applied simultaneously with corticosteroids or Vioform to refractory hand eczema, one to two times a day; the hands are then loosely covered with porous white cotton gloves to decrease the messiness of this combination. These gels contain alcohol and can sting on application.

Oils. Tar body oils (such as T/Derm, Neutrogena) may be useful in the treatment of psoriasis and other inflammatory skin conditions associated with dry skin. They may be applied to the skin following routine bathing.

Ointments and Pastes. In some patients, better response occurs when tar ointments or pastes are used. Two frequently prescribed forms are 5% crude coal tar or Zetar ointment (Dermik). These preparations are quite messy and malodorous and will stain clothing and sheets if not adequately removed; mineral oil may be useful in cleansing them from the skin.

Tar Shampoos. These have been previously discussed. Descriptions of other multicompound formulations containing tar can be found in any of the current dermatology textbooks or monographs.

Wart Remedies

Many modes of therapy are available for warts, depending on type, location, number of lesions, and previous responses to treatment. These include chemicals, liquid nitrogen application, and electrodesiccation and curettage (see also p. 466).

Condylomata acuminata usually respond to application of podophyllin, but there is high potential for cutaneous burns and possible systemic toxicity secondary to overaggressive treatment.

Isolated common warts can be self-treated with daily applications of combined salicylic and lactic acids in collodion (Duofilm, Stiefel, 15 ml; Viranol, American Dermal Corp., 10 ml; Ti-Flex, T/I Pharmaceuticals). Two to four drops daily are applied to the wart after prior hydration (5–10 minutes of soaking in warm water). The lesion is then covered with adhesive or plastic tape for 12–24 hours. If the area becomes red and tender, treatment is withheld for a few days. The resultant whitened surface of the wart is gently filed down daily with a callus file or pumice stone and the medication reapplied. Using this approach, the majority of warts can be cured, but at least 6–12 weeks of daily applications may be required. Plantar warts can be treated similarly or by the daily application of 40% salicylic acid plaster carefully cut to just cover the area of the wart. This is then covered with tape. The wart should be frequently debrided.

Wet Dressings, Compresses

Weeping, exudative, crusted, and vesicular eruptions require the use of wet dressings to aid in drying and surface debridement. As mentioned, boric acid solutions are no longer used because of the risk of absorption and toxicity. We do not use potassium permanganate solutions because of the difficulty in mixing, the potential for chemical burn from undissolved crystals, and the rather dramatic and persistent staining of skin and nails.

Wet dressings of comfortable temperature are applied using several layers of sterile gauze, Kerlix, or clean old linens. The dressings are removed, remoistened, and reapplied every 5–10 minutes for a total of 15–30 minutes three to four times a day as needed. As mentioned, in children only small surface areas are treated simultaneously to avoid chilling due to evaporative heat loss. Solutions include (1) aluminum acetate (Burow's solution)—available as Domeboro powder or tablets (Dome Laboratories, box of 12). Use one tablet or packet to a pint of water (makes a 1 : 40 solution). A fresh solution should be made daily, but it can be refrigerated for storage; however, it should be allowed to warm to room temperature prior to application. (2) Acetic acid solution—0.25–1%. The

higher concentration has been suggested to have the added benefit of killing *Pseudomonas aeruginosa*. (3) Normal saline. (4) Betadine—this is less advantageous than the others because of its color, which may make subsequent wound observation somewhat more difficult unless the wound is first irrigated.

Cosmetic Masking Agents

Some vascular or pigmentary congenital lesions are cosmetically unsightly and deforming. An excellent approach to therapy is the use of Covermark makeup (Lydia O'Leary, 22.5 and 85.5-gm cream). Many of these lesions can be completely masked in this manner.

Skin Diseases of the Neonate

JOAN E. HODGMAN, M.D.

CARE OF THE NORMAL SKIN

The normal skin of the neonate needs no special care. It should be emphasized that the skin's protective function is limited primarily to the outermost layer. Maceration or injury to the stratum corneum destroys this barrier and provides a portal of entry for pathogenic organisms and toxic chemicals. Cleansing of the skin should be gentle, using warm water alone or with mild nonmedicated soap followed by thorough rinsing. It is not advisable to remove vernix vigorously, as this probably provides a protective covering. The initial bath must be postponed until the infant's temperature is stable, and care must be taken to avoid cooling the infant during bathing. Three per cent hexachlorophene is used for the initial bath in many centers to decrease colonization by staphylococcal bacteria. More frequent bathing with hexachlorophene has been associated with neurotoxicity in the premature infant. Daily hexachlorophene baths may be temporarily instituted during outbreaks of staphyloccocal infection for term infants only.

The primary source for colonization by pathogenic bacteria is the hands of nursery personnel. Meticulous handwashing using soaps or detergents containing antibacterial preparations needs to be rigorously enforced for all individuals contacting the infants. The umbilical cord should be carefully cleaned, as it becomes colonized early. The application of triple dye has been effective in our nursery, but alcohol and antibacterial ointments have also been recommended. All normal infants have a thick keratin layer at birth that peels during the first few days. Creams and other emollients should not be used, as they encourage maceration and enhance bacterial growth. Many common practices in the nursery encourage maceration, such as exposure to warm, humid environments, occlusive dressings, and prolonged contact with plastic mattresses. Adhesive tape effectively peels the stratum corneum and should be used sparingly. The common practice of covering puncture wounds with Band-Aids has no justification. We have a rule in our nursery that says, "No blood, no bandage."

The care of the premature infant's skin does not differ essentially from that of the term infant's. The premature skin is more fragile and more permeable than that of the mature infant; consequently, greater care is necessary to prevent injury.

BIRTH TRAUMA

Ecchymoses. Ecchymoses and petechiae are regularly found over the presenting part. After difficult deliveries, hemorrhage and erosions may be present as well. These require no special therapy but should be kept clean and dry.

Caput Succedaneum. Caput succedaneum is an edematous swelling resulting from pressure changes over the presenting part. It usually occurs on the vertex but may involve the genitalia in breech deliveries. Even when alarming, the edema decreases markedly in the first 24 hours following birth, and treatment is unnecessary.

Cephalohematoma. Cephalohematoma is a swelling beneath the scalp resulting from subperiosteal hemorrhage over the skull. The swelling is limited by the suture lines and increases in size during the first few days owing to absorption of fluid. Regression is slow and the edges calcify during healing, leading to a spurious feeling of a central defect in the skull. The condition is benign, and aspiration is contraindicated because of the risk of introducing infection. Subgaleal hemorrhage has been erroneously referred to as giant cephalohematoma. Without the constraint of the periosteum, hemorrhage in this area may be serious enough to induce cardiac failure from hypovolemia and requires urgent transfusion or exchange transfusion.

Pressure Necrosis. Pressure necrosis is seen following prolonged labor and delivery, especially in large infants. The most common sites are the parietal bosses of the skull and the zygoma. With internal fetal monitoring, pressure necrosis of the scalp at the site of monitor placement is a common finding. These sterile abscesses must be differentiated from infections. The presence of normal flora is not an indication for antibiotic treatment. The lesions are indolent and heal slowly. Saline compresses may be useful early to aid in débridement, but then the lesions should be kept clean and dry. Infants may be safely discharged from the nursery during the healing process. Scarring is minimal even with facial lesions.

TRANSIENT LESIONS OF THE NEWBORN SKIN

Milia. Milia are superficial white epidermal inclusions of 1–2 mm, usually limited to the face in term infants. They exfoliate with the normal peeling and require no treatment.

Sebaceous Hypertrophy. Sebaceous hypertrophy occurs primarily in the glands over the nose, which enlarge in response to hormonal changes at birth. They are usually white but become yellow-stained if the infant becomes jaundiced. They are benign and regress spontaneously. An exaggeration of this process has been called acne of the newborn. Although I have heard about this condition, I have never seen a well-developed case. Considering the size of our nursery and the length of my tenure, I have concluded that it is a rarity.

Miliaria. Miliaria crystallina (sudamina) is the sweat rash seen in mature newborn infants. The lesions are small superficial vesicles containing a clear sweat. They are the result of increased sweat production under humid conditions where hygroscopic swelling of the stratum corneum obstructs the follicular outlets. Miliaria crystallina is best treated by decreasing the temperature and humidity of the infant's environment.

Sucking Blisters. Sucking blisters may be noted at birth over the dorsum of the hand and on the fingers. The lesions occur in large, active infants and occasionally are hemorrhagic. They are harmless but must be differentiated from congenital blistering disorders such as epidermolysis bullosa.

Toxic Erythema. Toxic erythema of the newborn is a benign self-limited condition of healthy infants during the first week. It is related to maturity, being uncommon in the preterm infant but seen in 50% of those at term. The lesions usually appear during the first 48 hours but rarely may be present at birth. Sites of predilection are the chest, the buttocks, the shoulders, and the proximal extremities. The central area of the face, the scalp, and the palms and soles are spared. The initial lesion is a blotchy erythematous macule with a central small papulovesicle. Well-developed lesions may appear pustular. The vesicles contain eosinophils, which can be demonstrated by smear. The etiology is unknown, there is no indication of allergy, and treatment is unnecessary.

Pustular Melanosis. Transient neonatal pustular melanosis is another self-limited condition of unknown etiology. It is present at birth and is limited to healthy dark-skinned infants. We see the condition in infants of Mexican extraction as well as in black newborns. Three characteristic types of lesion are present simultaneously: small pustules on a narrow erythematous or nonerythematous base, dried pustules identifiable by their collar of scale, and pigmented macules. Smears show polymorphonuclear leukocytes and debris, and cultures are negative. No treatment is necessary, and isolation of the infant is not required. The pigmented macules may persist for several months but eventually fade.

NEVI

Vascular Nevi. Vascular nevi are among the more common lesions seen in the newborn. The nevus simplex or salmon patch occurs on the nape in at least 40% of infants and has been called the stork bite because of its ubiquity. The same flat capillary nevi may be seen on the face above the eyebrows, on the upper eyelids, around the alae nasi, and on the upper lip. These lesions always regress spontaneously. The nevus flammeus is also a flat capillary nevus, but with a more ominous prognosis. These lesions do not regress and are frequently associated with hemangiomas in the underlying structures. Appropriate ultrasonography should be performed before discharge from the nursery. Ablative treatment has been unsatisfactory and cosmetic cover-up is recommended. The raised capillary nevus or strawberry mark is never seen at birth but may appear in the premature infant during the nursery stay. These lesions ultimately regress, and benign neglect is the most satisfactory therapeutic plan. Eighty per cent of cavernous hemangiomas also regress spontaneously. Steroids have accelerated the regression of these tumors and should be tried early when the tumor is large or in a hazardous location. A small percentage of cavernous hemangiomas are associated with significant complications that may be life-threatening. These vary from sepsis in the infant with large venous lakes to heart failure in the infant with arteriovenous anastomoses. Hypertrophy of the underlying structures may occur, especially when the tumor involves an extremity. Hemorrhage from trapping of platelets within the hemangioma may appear early in infancy. Treatment, which may not be very satisfactory, involves ablating the hemangioma by surgery or radiation.

Sebaceous Nevi. Sebaceous nevi are skin-colored hairless plaques with an orange peel–like surface texture. They occur most commonly on the head, particularly at the hairline. They can safely be ignored during childhood but may develop basal cell carcinomas after adolescence.

Pigmented Nevi. Pigmented nevi in the newborn are considered to pose an increased risk of malignant change, but the actual risk for small lesions is not well defined. Careful notation of size and location during the newborn physical so that changes in the lesions can be detected during follow-up visits should improve our prognostic ability.

DISAPPEARING CONDITIONS

Sclerema Neonatorum. Sclerema neonatorum, a hardening of the subcutaneous tissues, has almost disappeared from the nursery, suggesting that temperature control is important in its genesis. At present, it occurs most frequently in septic infants. Treatment should be directed to the underlying disorder. Administration of steroids, which has been recommended, is not effective.

Subcutaneous Fat Necrosis. Subcutaneous fat necrosis, which has been reported in term infants—particularly the infant of the diabetic—has not been seen in our nursery for at least a decade. The most likely reasons for its disappearance appear to be better temperature control in the delivery room and greater control of the diabetic mother during pregnancy and labor.

Eruptions in the Diaper Region

GARY M. GORLICK, M.D., M.P.H.

GENERAL MEASURES

These measures are aimed at the prevention of the most common diaper rashes as well as their early treatment by simple, effective, and safe measures.

Most importantly, parents must be educated in correct cleaning, bathing, and diaper care of the infant; they in turn must transmit this to the infant's baby-sitters and/or day-care and nursery school personnel, especially when a rash is present. After birth, the umbilicus should be cleaned with isopropyl alcohol tid–qid and continued for approximately 1 week after it has detached and become dry at the stump, to prevent a focus from which bacterial dermatitis might develop. Signs of infection at the umbilicus or circumcision must be brought to the physician's attention and treated. Tub-bathing is not begun until the umbilicus is dry and fully healed. Either type of diaper, permanent (cloth) or disposable, is currently acceptable inasmuch as there is inadequate evidence at this time that one type predisposes to increased incidence of rash. If a disposable type is used, the plasticized outer covering should be folded away from the baby's skin at the back, front, and thigh regions if not pleated. Cloth diapers are best washed in Ivory Snow and rinsed thoroughly. Fabric softeners should not be used if a rash develops. The diaper is to be removed and changed as soon as stooling is noted; with the onset of a rash, quickly changing the diaper after urination also becomes important, as does a change late in the evening hours. The infant's room should not be overheated and should be kept at normal humidity. Skin cleansing is best done with cool or tepid water on a soft and non-traumatic (not heavy and rough-surfaced) washcloth or cotton pledgets. Particular care is necessary to clean and dry all creases well. If soap is used, a mild one is recommended, such as Dove or Neutrogena Baby Soap. Oils should not be used, particularly in the diaper region. Avoid overdressing the infant; consequent heat and sweat retention may lead to miliaria and/or intertrigo. When early chafing or eruption is noted, allow open air exposure as often as feasible, decrease the use of outer plastic pants, and apply a protective ointment such as Desitin, A and D, or zinc oxide to the involved areas.

There appears to be a role for diet management in some diaper eruptions. The infant should have adequate fluid intake. Some rashes respond to water supplements alone. At times, empiric stopping of juices will clear the eruption. The prevention and treatment of diarrheal stools by diet manipulation (e.g., adding banana or rice foods for a binding effect, decreasing or stopping juices or other known diarrhea-producing agents) will often help. Although there is strong evidence against "ammoniacal dermatitis," at least as a primary entity, oral cranberry juice bid–tid may be tried. Any new food introduced and soon followed by a rash should be discontinued and reintroduced carefully when the rash has abated. Cow's milk should not be introduced until an infant is at least 6 to 12 months of age (the American Academy of Pediatrics recommends 12 months) and dermatitis should be carefully watched for on any area of the body including the diaper region. Obesity should be prevented; the friction of opposing skin creates a greater than normal propensity for intertrigo to develop.

Many contactants must be avoided. Oils applied directly to the skin or placed in the bath water should be avoided, as should "bubble-baths" for the young child. The infant's skin should be kept free of cosmetics and other skin and hair preparations. Creams, ointments, oils, talcs, and emollients being used at the time of an eruption may be etiologic and should be empirically stopped. Careful review of all aspects of bathing, cleansing, and diaper care may be necessary to identify contactants that are causing a dermatitis.

SPECIFIC MEASURES

These measures are aimed at the treatment of the conditions listed below. Reference to *Topical Therapy: A Dermatologic Formulary for Pediatric Practice* is herein made for dosage schedules not repeated in this section.

Chafing, Irritant Dermatitis, Intertrigo, and Perianal Dermatitis. Ointments such as Desitin, A and D, Diaparene, and zinc oxide may be applied as often as each diaper change. Talcum powder is useful, especially in the creases, but must not be used if the skin is denuded, and care must be taken that it is not inhaled by the infant, as it is easily airborne. Corn starch is less likely to be inhaled but may enhance the growth of *Candida albicans* (monilial dermatitis).

Monilial Dermatitis. Therapy consists of applying Mycostatin cream or ointment bid–qid to the rash. Another technique is to alternate the application of hydrocortisone cream 1% with either Mycostatin cream or Mycostatin dusting powder at each diaper change. The dusting powder can also be applied bid–tid when the skin is clear in the infant who is prone to repetitions of this condition. Oral Mycostatin is added to the local treatment in the following situations: when thrush is present; when the baby is breast-fed and the mother has monilial mastitis; when the diaper eruption is extensive; when there is nonresponse to local therapy alone; or when the eruption recurs soon after local treatment. One to 2 ml of oral Mycostatin is given tid–qid until finished (60-ml bottle), with particular attention to its contact with all areas of thrush before being swallowed. A mother with active monilial vaginitis may be a source of reinfection and should be treated. The treatment of oral lesions with topical gentian violet is messy and is rarely used today. Oral ketoconazole is *not* to be used for simple monilial dermatitis. In addition to Mycostatin, there are many topical antifungals that are applied bid and are active against *C. albicans*, e.g., clotrimazole (Lotrimin, Mycelex), miconazole (Monistat-Derm), haloprogin (Halotex, Tinactin). As of this writing a topical form of ketoconazole is not available.

Seborrheic, Atopic, and "Psoriasiform" Dermatitis. Apply hydrocortisone cream 1% on a "least-often" as necessary basis, that is, once to qid prn. Stronger topical corticosteroids are rarely necesary, but if they are, use one from the next higher potency group and stop it as soon as response is noted and return to the very safe hydrocortisone 1% cream. Never use fluorinated corticosteroids or oral/parenteral steroids, or occlusive technique, in the diaper region. The therapeutic role of biotin for generalized seborrhea (not Leiner's) is uncertain at the present time.

Bacterial Dermatitis. Controversy exists over the therapeutic effectiveness of topical antibiotics for skin infections. In addition, the potential for allergic contact sensitization is of concern. However, if the diaper dermatitis area is small, topical Neosporin-G *cream* (not ointment) qid alone may suffice. Since *Staphylococcus aureus* is by far the most common cause of diaper area bacterial infection, cloxacillin sodium (Tegopen) is given orally at 25 to 50 mg/kg/day in four divided doses for 7 to 10 days when more than local treatment is necessary.

"Ammoniac Dermatitis." As mentioned before, controversy exists as to whether ammonia causes dermatitis, or if it exacerbates an existing dermatitis. Some clinicians, however, believe the following measures may be efficacious: oral cranberry juice or oral methionine (Pedameth), and/or Caldesene Medicated Powder or Ointment. Pedameth liquid contains 75 mg of racemethionine per 5 ml, and the recommended dosage for infants 2 to 6 months old is 5 ml tid (in formula, milk, or juice) for 3 to 5 days. For infants 6 to 14 months of age the same dosage is given but at a qid frequency and also for 3 to 5 days.

Psoriasis. The ideal therapy for the infant and very young child with psoriasis in the diaper region has not yet been established. Corticosteroids probably should be avoided as much as possible. Treatment with tars such as 2% crude coal tar in a zinc oxide ointment (removed with warm mineral oil) once or twice a day has been effective. Estar, a 5% coal tar, may also be used once or twice a day. Should corticosteroids be used because of nonresponse to the above, it is best to attempt control with mild 1% hydrocortisone ointment. Since this dermatitis is often chronic, it might be best to treat only flare-ups with these specific agents. Preventing Koebner reaction by the most atraumatic hygienic methods is important.

Granuloma Gluteale Infantum. In this uncommon condition symmetrical nodular lesions occur in the diaper region following diaper dermatitis with or without candidiasis, previously often treated with fluorinated steroids. It resolves without therapy, and therefore all agents should be stopped. In some cases it is best to taper corticosteroid agents gradually from those of strongest to those of mildest potency to avoid a "flare-up" when they are abruptly stopped.

Recalcitrant Diaper Eruptions. Rule out pinworms and/or urinary tract infection when appropriate. Rule out *Tinea corporis* infection on rare occasion. Consider dermatitis medicamentosa—especially when Mycolog *cream* has been used, for this contains a potent corticosteroid as well as potential allergic sensitizers. Look for signs of telangiectasis or bleeding within the rash, and for anemia, fever, hepatosplenomegaly, and intractable diarrhea in the child who shows signs of failure to thrive, for these may herald serious systemic conditions such as congenital syphilis, acrodermatitis enteropathica, Wiskott-Aldrich syndrome, or Letterer-Siwe disease.

Agents Not to Be Used. Boric acid, baking soda, mercurials, hexachlorophene, fluorinated corticosteroids, and oral ketoconazole should not be used to treat diaper eruptions. The *cream* form of Mycolog should be avoided; if the physician wishes to use Mycolog, the *ointment* form is strongly advised, as is the precaution to stop as soon as the rash improves and to continue therapy with hydrocortisone cream 1% with or without anticandidal therapy as necessary.

Contact Dermatitis

STEPHANIE H. PINCUS, M.D.

The term contact dermatitis refers to an acute or chronic inflammatory process of the skin that is due to interaction between the skin and an exogenous substance. It is further divided into two types of contact dermatitis: irritant and allergic. The irritant type, sometimes known as primary irritant dermatitis, is the result of damage to the skin by toxic chemicals such as alkalis and detergents. Allergic contact dermatitis refers to the specific lymphocyte-mediated reaction that occurs in sensitized individuals. The most common cause of allergic contact dermatitis is poison ivy exposure. Whenever possible, irritant dermatitis should be distinguished from allergic dermatitis since prevention of these conditions may depend on differing environmental factors.

IRRITANT CONTACT DERMATITIS

Severe irritant dermatitis can develop in all persons exposed to strong acids, potent alkalis, or other toxic chemicals. The treatment of all irritant dermatitis is similar, regardless of the cause. The most important treatment is avoidance of the irritating substance itself. Diaper dermatitis was discussed in the preceding article. The irritant dermatitis seen in older children, again, should be treated by avoidance of the irritating substance and use of emollients such as Nivea cream, Keri cream, and so on. If severe erythema, cracking, or fissuring is present, it may be necessary to add a topical steroid. In such a case, one of the moderate-strength steroid creams, such as triamcinolone cream (0.025 or 0.1%) or betamethasone cream, should be selected. This medication should be applied only as long as necessary. Usually therapy is initiated four times a day and decreased to twice a day as tolerated. In a typical case, treatment for 10 to 14 days is adequate. When the eruption has persisted for a considerable time and resulted in a thickened, lichenified skin, an ointment is preferred. An intermediate-potency ointment such as Valisone is usually adequate. The high-potency fluorinated medications should be reserved for refractory cases since cutaneous atrophy and telangiectasias may result from excess usage.

ALLERGIC CONTACT DERMATITIS

Allergic contact dermatitis is a specific lymphocyte-mediated eruption. It requires that the child be exposed to a sensitizing dose; upon reexposure, the dermatitis typically develops 48 to 72 hours later. The area of dermatitis is confined to the area of contact, and this explains the peculiar distribution sometimes seen. For instance, linear streaks may indicate contact with leaves of poison ivy (e.g., by brushing up against them).

Treatment of acute allergic contact dermatitis depends upon the severity of the eruption. For most cases, topical treatment is adequate. During the acute phase, which is manifested by erythema, weeping, oozing, or vesicle formation, drying may be promoted by the use of cool, wet dressings. Burow solution diluted 1:20 for young children and 1:10 for teenagers should be used. Wet dressings should be applied for 15- to 20-minute periods three or four times a day. Wet dressings will promote evaporative cooling and remove serous exudate and crust. During the acute phase, steroid creams may be applied. In children under the age of 2 years, 1% hydrocortisone is frequently adequate. In older children, it is usually necessary to use a stronger fluorinated steroid, such as 0.1% triamcinolone cream (Kenalog or Aristocort) or betamethasone (Valisone or Benisone). Newer non-fluorinated steroid compounds have been developed to lessen possible atrophy and stria formation. When the weeping and oozing have subsided, steroid cream should be applied three or four times a day. The frequency of application of steroid cream may be gradually tapered after 7 to 10 days. For control of itching, it may be useful to use antihistamines such as Benadryl, Atarax, or Vistaril.

Severe contact dermatitis involving large areas of the body, the face, or the male genitalia requires treatment with systemic steroids. These agents are most effective when given at the onset. Hospitalization may be necessary when there is extensive acute contact dermatitis. The usual initial dose is 1 or 2 mg/kg of prednisone. After 1 day the dose should be reduced to 0.5–1 mg/24 hr. This dose should be maintained for 3 to 5 days and the medication gradually tapered over a 2-week period. Thus, 3 weeks of therapy are usually necessary. A common problem is the exacerbation of contact dermatitis after inadequate courses of systemic steroids (5 to 7 days). When systemic steroids are employed, topical steroids are an adjunctive measure.

A common complication of acute contact dermatitis is development of secondary bacterial infection with *Staphylococcus aureus* or streptococcus. The development of purulent lesions or an exacerbation after initial clearing should suggest secondary infection, as does fever or erythema. In such instances, a culture should be obtained and appropriate systemic antimicrobial therapy given. Topical antibiotics are not adequate to treat such infections. In the treatment of contact dermatitis, it is important to avoid sensitizing agents such as topical antihistamines, topical benzocaine, or topical neomycin, which may lead to the development of a second contact dermatitis. Frequent offenders are topical antipruritic sprays, ointments, and lotions.

Atopic Dermatitis
ALVIN H. JACOBS, M.D.

Atopic dermatitis is a genetically determined abnormality of the skin that often occurs in association with allergic diseases, probably as linked inheritance. It is manifest as dry, itchy skin, which is subjected to many internal and external factors that tend to increase the pruritus, thereby stimulating the "itch-scratch" cycle. These factors include environmental temperature changes, stimulation of sweating, external irritants such as rough clothing, bacterial infection, emotional stress, antigen-antibody reactions, bathing with soap and water, and many others.

In managing patients with atopic dermatitis the physician must recognize that the only primary skin manifestations are pruritus, dryness, and a generalized "goose-pimple" appearance. All other skin findings, such as oozing, weeping, crusting, or cracking, are secondary to scratching, rubbing, and secondary infection.

GENERAL MANAGEMENT

Psychological. Successful management is time consuming for both parents and physician. At the outset the parents must understand that this is a chronic disorder for which there is no complete and quick cure; rather, the therapy is aimed at controlling factors that contribute to the eruption and its attendant discomforts.

During the introductory discussions, the physician must be alert to the mother's emotional reactions to her child's disorder, since in many mothers guilt feelings arise from the fear that they are in some way responsible for the skin problem, as well as from their frequent feelings of rejection of the child and his ugly skin. The mother's emotional involvement is further complicated by the consumption of time in taking care of this crying, fussing, irritable, scratching infant or child. The physician must try to relieve the mother of her guilt feelings and express understanding of the rejection phenomenon. The treatment program must take into account the time the mother will have to devote to the care of her child's skin problem and must allow her periods of relief when she may be away from the child and without anxiety. I feel quite strongly that maternal anxiety transmitted to the infant or child may make the itching worse and aggravate the disease.

Infection. When first seen, most patients with atopic dermatitis have secondary infection, usually due to *Staphylococcus aureus*. This presents as oozing, crusting, and fissuring of the skin. This infection must be adequately treated before other steps will be effective. Locally applied antibiotics are of little use in this situation. Systemic antibiotic therapy should be given for a period of at least 2 weeks to adequately eliminate the secondary infection. Recurrent infection is a common occurrence, requiring prolonged antibiotic therapy with eventual reduction to a maintenance dose. The most useful antibiotic is erythromycin in a dose of 50 mg/kg/day. Occasionally it is necessary to use cloxacillin or cephalexin in the same dosage.

Clothing. The individual with eczema has a tremendous tendency to itch, and anything that irritates the skin will cause him to scratch. He should, therefore, avoid irritating materials, especially woolens. Cotton and some of the softer synthetics are preferable for the atopic patient. Wool-upholstered chairs and wool carpets are also sources of irritation.

Sweating. Another important factor in the stimulation of pruritus is perspiration. Atopic dermatitis is always associated with a degree of sweat retention that will produce itching. Therefore, excessive clothing, high environmental temperatures, and overactivity will increase perspiration and promote itchiness.

Antipruritic Sedation. Since the worst scratching is done at night, it is wise to give these patients nighttime sedation until their skin condition is under control. Diphenhydramine, given in doses of 25–50 mg about 1 hour before bedtime, is an effective antipruritic sedative. In severe cases it is also advisable to give a daytime medication such as hydroxyzine, 10–25 mg three times daily. *Systemic corticosteroids should rarely be given.*

Diet. Dietary management is occasionally helpful, especially in the first 2 years of life. Since cow's milk is the most common allergen in infancy, eliminating it from the baby's diet will often make the dermatitis more easily controllable. At any age skin tests and radioallergosorbent tests are unreliable indicators of foods that might be related to exacerbations of the disease. It is best to rely upon diet history, diet diary, and food challenges.

Hyposensitization. Skin test and hyposensitization therapy are of very little use in the management of the patient with atopic dermatitis, since there seems to be little relationship between the positive tests and causation of flares of the dermatitis.

TOPICAL THERAPY

When eczema is first seen in the acute phase, with inflammation, oozing, and crusting, it is important to recognize that secondary infection is present and that systemic antibiotic therapy must be promptly instituted, as described. Reduction of inflammation and removal of crusts and exudate are best done with intermittent cool wet dressings applied by the open method. Two or three layers of gauze, Kerlix, or linen are thoroughly moistened with Burow's solution and loosely applied to the involved areas without occlusion. One-half to 1 hour of application four times daily is usually sufficient, with remoistening by complete removal of the dressing every 10 minutes to prevent drying and sticking. Burow's solution, 1:40, is prepared by dissolving one tablet or packet (Domeboro tablets and powder packets) in one quart of cool tap water. *Wet compresses should not be used for longer than 3 days.*

At this point, or if the patient is first seen in the dry itchy phase, one may proceed with the modified Scholtz regimen, the prime feature of which is the *complete avoidance of bathing with water.* The dry skin of atopic dermatitis is due to a lack of sufficient water in the stratum corneum. The drier the skin, the greater is the pruritus. Washing with water removes the water-soluble substances that retain the water in the horny layer, thus resulting in increased dryness and itchiness after bathing.

The modified Scholtz regimen is instituted as follows:

1. No bathing with either soap or water is allowed. The only exception to this rule is the use of a moist washcloth to cleanse the groin and axillary areas if necessary.

2. The entire skin surface is cleansed at least twice daily with a nonlipid cleansing lotion consisting primarily of cetyl alcohol, sodium lauryl sulfate, propylene glycol, and water (Cetaphil lotion, Owens Laboratories). The lotion is applied liberally and rubbed in until it foams. It is then gently wiped off, leaving a film of the lotion on the skin. This film aids the retention of water in the horny layer of the skin.

3. No oily or greasy lubricants are allowed, since these will further occlude sweat pore openings and contribute to sweat retention.

4. Inflamed or pruritic areas of the dermatitis are treated by topical corticosteroids in a solution or cream formulation, not an ointment base. In relatively mild or moderate cases, 1% hydrocortisone cream is effective. However, some generic preparations of hydrocortisone do not have a satisfactory base and may even be irritating. Several hydrocortisone preparations have been found to have smooth, nonirritating vehicles (1% Nutracort, 1% Hytone, and 1% Synacort). In more severe cases a medium-strength steroid, such as 0.1% triamcinolone cream, may be used. However, as soon as improvement is evident, one should shift down to hydrocortisone. In any case, only 1%

hydrocortisone should be used on the face, groin, and genitalia.

All acutely inflamed areas can be cleared with the topical steroid preparation. If the entire program is followed, clearing usually occurs in 2–3 weeks. After the acutely inflamed areas have responded, it is possible to maintain the improvement by adhering to the no-bath and Cetaphil cleansing. The topical steroid is then needed only occasionally when there is a brief flare of the dermatitis.

5. When the skin has remained clear of eruption for several months, a brief cool bath is allowed once or twice monthly, always followed immediately by liberal application of Cetaphil lotion. Most patients are eventually able to tolerate a brief, not hot, bath as often as once weekly after they have remained clear for several months. It is essential that they learn never to bathe more often than once weekly and that they continue indefinitely to use the Cetaphil lotion for daily cleansing and lubrication.

Urticaria

VICTOR D. NEWCOMER, M.D.

Urticaria or hives is a vascular reaction pattern of the skin characterized by evanescent wheals, which represent localized leakage of plasma from small blood vessels into the connective tissue of the dermis.

The *single most important step* in the management of acute urticaria is the identification and removal of the causative agent. With a complete history and review of systems, the causative agent can be identified in about 20 to 30% of all patients with urticaria.

Aggravating factors should be avoided whenever possible. The patient should remain quiescent and avoid strenuous activities as much as possible. Excessive heat, sunbathing, and cold showers should be avoided. Vasostimulatory foods and beverages such as tea, coffee, and alcohol should be avoided. Emotional stress should be minimized. Aspirin, which is present in many proprietary preparations, should be avoided, particularly in chronic urticaria, as over 50% of this latter group can be made worse by its administration.

Antihistamines of the H_1 group are the mainstay in the management of urticaria of all types and provide symptomatic relief in about 80% of patients. They are particularly indicated if the sympathomimetics are contraindicated because of cardiovascular problems. They may be divided into six pharmacologic groups. In general, their properties are similar, and there are few comparative studies to give guidance as to which is the most

effective. The choice is largely empirical. Antihistamines block the action of histamine at the receptor site and thereby interfere with the action of histamine on the capillaries. The blocking effect is clinically gradual, and, once obtained, the continued suppression of skin reactivity is of great importance if exacerbations are to be prevented. It is often necessary to maintain the dosage to the point of drowsiness to achieve the greatest benefit. When an antihistamine is ineffective or its side effects are troublesome, one should choose the next agent from another subgroup. Hydroxyzine hydrochloride (Atarax) (0.5 mg/kg q 4–6 h for children) has been used increasingly for urticaria.

Cyproheptadine hydrochloride (Periactin) (0.1 mg/kg q 4–6 h for children) has been especially effective in cold urticaria. The clinical studies reported to date, combining H_1 and H_2 antihistamines, have had mixed results; however, they are worth a trial in those patients with chronic refractory urticaria. β-Adrenergic drugs are the agents of choice in severe and acute attacks on urticaria or where angioedema is developing.

Aqueous epinephrine (Adrenalin) 1:1000, 0.01 ml/kg q 3 to 4 hours subcutaneously, offers prompt relief. Epinephrine suspension (Sus-Phrine) 1:200, 0.005 ml/kg, may be used where prolonged suppression is desired. Ephedrine sulfate, 25 mg qid, may be used but is slower in action. Anxiety and tachycardia are common side effects with the use of all these agents.

Systemic corticosteroids are the drugs of choice in the treatment of severe forms of serum sickness and severe acute attacks of urticaria. Since they require hours for a therapeutic effect, anaphylactic urticaria and angioedema affecting the upper respiratory tract are most effectively treated with the β-adrenergic drugs. Systemic corticosteroids are not advised for chronic recalcitrant urticaria; any possible benefits are more than outweighed by the potential hazards of prolonged treatment. They are of value, however, when used for a short period, in the control of acute, incapacitating exacerbation of chronic urticaria. Topical treatment with steroids is of no value.

The value of *tranquilizers and sedatives* is still debatable, but they may be helpful in patients with an emotional or stress component. Usually, the sedative effect of the antihistamine is all that may be required or tolerated. Doxepin (Sinequan), a tricyclic antidepressant, has been recently recommended as the treatment of choice for chronic urticaria, as it has been found to be safer than systemic steroids and has less of a sedative effect than conventional antihistamines. It is, however, not recommended in patients under 12 years of age. Dosages of 10 mg three times daily are adequate for adults. Hyposensitization has no role in the treatment of urticaria except for insect stings and urticaria due to inhalants such as pollens, dust, and molds. In general, topical agents are of little value in the management of urticaria. Calamine lotion, containing the antipruritic phenol 0.5% and menthol 0.25%, is still used.

Patients who develop hoarseness and do not respond promptly to measures to provide relief from severe pruritus should be admitted to the hospital for close observation and possible endotracheal intubation. *Hereditary angioedema* caused by a low or functional deficiency of an inhibitor of the first component of complement should be ruled out. Diagnosis is made by history and laboratory evidence of a deficiency of C esterase inhibitor and/or low serum complement. In patients with hereditary angioedema, both C4 and C2 levels are low during attacks, and only levels of C4 are low between attacks. During acute attacks, testosterone ethanate* (Danazol) 200 mg three times a day, or stanozolol* (Winstrol) 2 mg three times a day, may be initiated until the attacks subside. After a favorable response is obtained, the dosage may be decreased at intervals of 1–3 months to the smallest possible dose that will continue to suppress recurrence of symptoms. Attacks can be prevented by the use of testosterone ethanate 200 mg a day, or stanozolol, 2 mg a day, in dosages as low as twice a week. Antihistamines, corticosteroids, and epinephrine have no effect. The long-term effects of testosterone ethanate and stanozolol in humans are unknown and as a rule children and pregnant women have not been treated with these agents.

If the larynx is affected repeatedly, a permanent tracheostomy may be required to sustain breathing.

Erythema Nodosum

LAWRENCE SCHACHNER, M.D.

Erythema nodosum is not a simple clinical diagnosis, nor is it an entity whose pathogenesis is well understood. It is believed to be a Type 3 hypersensitivity reaction to a myriad of agents, including infectious diseases, inflammatory diseases, drug reactions, and disorders that may frequently be of undiagnosed or unknown origin. The clinical appearance of erythema nodosum may be mimicked by various focal infections and inflammations of the subcutaneous fat and soft tissues with a predilection for the lower extremities.

On clinical examination in the acute stage, one will note multiple tender red nodular lesions. Although the lesions are most frequent and obtain their greatest size on the lower extremities, more generalized lesions, including facial erythema nodosum, have been seen. A characteristic color change from red to blue to yellow-green before resolution is probably commensurate with the degree of focal subcutaneous hemorrhage. Fever and malaise may precede the cutaneous lesions and/or accompany the acute stage of these lesions. Patients often complain of arthralgias, usually in the lower extremities, during the acute course of this disorder. While all ages and races, and both sexes, may be involved, there is an increased incidence in females versus males and in young people versus old people.

The etiology of erythema nodosum cases seen by a pediatrician may be determined by the ages and even the socioeconomic class of the patients he or she sees. For example, a practitioner who sees many school-age children may see many cases of streptococcus-evoked erythema nodosum. A practitioner who services indigent populations or an area with a recent influx of immigrants from South America or Asia may see a fair amount of tuberculosis-associated erythema nodosum. Similarly, a pediatrician with a large adolescent practice may find many cases of oral contraceptive–associated erythema nodosum.

THERAPY

The initial therapeutic approach should be conservative but strict. At least 2 to 3 weeks of bed rest is usually optimal when patients are seen at the onset of disease. Every 3 hours throughout the day, cool water soaks should be placed wet over the lesions and allowed to dry for 20 minutes. If fever, malaise, or joint pain is significant, salicylates in dosages appropriate for age should be administered. It should be stated here that the most effective therapy for the specific case of erythema nodosum requires discovery of the etiology of the underlying infection.

Of the many etiologies of erythema nodosum, perhaps those most appropriately diagnosed are the infectious diseases. The most common causes, such as group A beta hemolytic streptococcal infection, may be diagnosed by throat culture or streptozyme titer. A purified protein derivative (PPD) test is worth applying to any previously PPD-negative erythema nodosum patient. *Yersinia* species have been associated with gastrointestinal complaints and erythema nodosum.

Lymphogranuloma venereum, cat scratch fever, and deeper fungal infection including coccidioidomycosis, blastomycosis, histoplasmosis, and deep trichophyton infections may also be associated with erythema nodosum. Frequently associated inflammatory disorders include sarcoidosis, regional enteritis, ulcerative colitis, and Behçet's syndrome. Various medications have been associated with eruptions of erythema nodosum, and many contemporary cases have accompanied the use of oral contraceptives, phenytoin, and halogens.

---

* This use of testosterone ethanate and stanozolol is not listed in the manufacturers' directives.

A minimal diagnostic work-up would include a streptozyme test, a PPD, a chest x-ray, skin tests for fungi, and a skin biopsy to rule out the various infections and inflammatory conditions that mimic erythema nodosum clinically but can be distinguished histologically.

Bed rest, wet soaks, and salicylates will usually alleviate pain and tenderness. Rarely, one finds persistent erythema nodosum in a patient whose clinical diagnosis has been confirmed by biopsy and in whom both infectious and noninfectious etiologies have been ruled out. In these rare instances, the use of intralesional corticosteroids may hasten involution of the lesions and relieve discomfort. Although the use of oral corticosteroids has been advocated in the literature, I have not found them to be necessary.

Drug Reactions and the Skin

LAWRENCE SCHACHNER, M.D.

Cutaneous drug reactions include both immunologic reactions of all classes of hypersensitivity and nonimmunologic reactions. The class of hypersensitivity reaction in the immunologic type often determines the appropriate therapy. In Type 1 hypersensitivity reactions, IgE antibodies are produced and reactions ranging from urticaria to angioedema and anaphylaxis may occur. In Type 2 reactions, drugs may form an antigenic complex with the surface of red blood cells or platelets. Thrombocytopenic purpura may be observed. Type 3 hypersensitivity reactions with drugs inducing an antigen-antibody and complement immune complex may result in cutaneous signs such as urticarial vasculitis. Indeed, a Type 3 reaction may be manifested by the persistence of urticarial-wheal type lesions that may progress to purpura. Severe cutaneous reactions of erythema multiforme, Stevens-Johnson syndrome, and toxic epidermal necrolysis might also be examples of Type 3 reactions. Further immune complex–mediated cutaneous reactions to medications include specific reactions, such as fixed drug reaction and erythema nodosum. Type 4 cell-mediated hypersensitivity may occur as an eczematous dermatitis with eruptive distribution in areas where topically applied medications have been used. Photoallergic reactions may be induced by either internal or external use of various medications.

In the pediatric population, the drugs most often associated with immediate or Type 1 hypersensitivity drug reaction are the penicillins, which may also be associated with Type 3 hypersensitivity drug reaction. In addition, numerous other drugs can produce a serum sickness syndrome with urticarial vasculitis and/or angioedematous compo-

nents. These drugs include the commonly used childhood medications phenytoin and the sulfonamides. In Type 2 hypersensitivity reactions, again penicillin and the more rarely used quinidine class drugs may be associated with characteristic reactions. Topical medications, including antibiotics such as neomycin as well as numerous ointments with parabens and ethylenediamine as components, may induce a Type 4 or cell-mediated drug reaction.

Nonimmunologic drug reactions may take several forms. Long-term use of gold- or mercury-based drugs may lead to cutaneous or mucous membrane changes. Drugs may also be capable of a nonimmunologic activation of mast cell– and complement–mediated pathways inducing cutaneous reactions such as acute and chronic urticaria and angioedematous changes.

One may see among the common drug eruptions not only urticarial and vasculitic lesions but also acne type lesions, erythema multiforme, erythema nodosum, exanthem type lesions, eczematous dermatitis, fixed-drug eruptions, lichen planus–like eruptions, lupus-like eruptions, photosensitive eruptions, pigmentary changes, and blistering reactions.

THERAPY

Whenever the diagnosis of a drug eruption is made, if possible, the offending agent should be replaced by a non–cross-reacting medication. Many drug reactions are mild and require little more than discontinuation of the offending medication, followed by simple supportive measures. When pruritus is intense, oral antihistamines as well as mentholated topical preparations can offer considerable relief. The combination of hydroxyzine (Atarax) and pseudoephedrine (Sudafed) has been particularly successful in our more pruritic patients with drug reactions. Mentholated petrolatum or calamine with 0.25% menthol is also quite soothing.

In drug reactions of more emergent nature such as the various severe hypersensitivity reactions, therapy must be individualized. A patient with a Type 1 hypersensitivity reaction of the anaphylaxis class will require emergency preservation of airway supplemental oxygen and intravenous use of epinephrine, Benadryl, and systemic steroids as the clinical manifestations mandate. Patients in whom the drug reaction may provoke considerable loss of cutaneous surfaces, such as drug-induced toxic epidermal necrolysis or Stevens-Johnson type erythema multiforme, may require fluid and electrolyte monitoring identical to patients with extensive burns. Indeed, the epidermal barrier function may be as equally disturbed as in a severe burn. In such patients we have used wet to dry soaks and Silvadene as topical therapy. In severe drug reactions, antibiotic treatment for secondary infection is often necessary. Although controversial, toxic epidermal necrolysis associated with several medications, including Dilantin, and Stevens-Johnson syndrome invoked by a number of medications, may necessitate the use of systemic steroids as a life-saving step.

Lastly, cutaneous reactions to topical medication may be approached as any eczematous dermatitis. In the acute stage, it is important to apply wet to dry soaks to induce drying of the lesions. This may be followed with topical steroid cream preparations to induce added drying and decrease inflammation. Concomitant utilization of oral antihistamines may hasten the patient's relief.

Erythema Multiforme

JAMES E. RASMUSSEN, M.D.

The treatment of erythema multiforme depends upon the severity of the disease. Varieties with only a few papular or bullous lesions, primarily on the extremities, are usually referred to as erythema multiforme minor. Erythema multiforme major encompasses a spectrum of disease ranging from widespread blisters to severe involvement of the ocular and oral mucous membranes (Stevens-Johnson syndrome) to widespread sheet-like necrosis of the epidermis (toxic epidermal necrolysis). Minor varieties usually require no specific therapy since the disease is short term and self-limited and has no common complications. Patients with erythema multiforme major usually require admission to hospital because of the severity of the disease as well as to maintain adequate fluid intake. The care of patients with erythema multiforme major can be divided into general (supportive) care, specific therapy, and management of complications.

General Care. Patients with erythema multiforme major usually have substantial involvement of ocular, oral, and urethral mucosa. These patients usually have decreased fluid intake coupled with widespread loss of the protective epidermal barrier. Therefore, it is necessary to maintain adequate oral or intravenous intake of fluids, electrolytes, calories, and proteins. An occasional patient may also have moderate-to-severe kidney disease such as glomerulonephritis or acute tubular necrosis. Consequently, urine output, specific gravity, hemoglobin, hematocrit, serum electrolyte levels, and total body weight should be monitored diligently. Although most patients do not require intravenous therapy for more than 5–6 days, an occasional patient will have an extended recovery that necessitates parenteral feedings for several weeks.

Local wound care depends upon the extent of the cutaneous erosions. A few small lesions on the extremities can be treated with topical antiseptics such as silver sulfadiazine cream and dressings. In my experience, petrolatum gauze dressings are frequently all that is necessary. More widespread loss of the epidermis will probably require therapy similar to that for an extensive burn. Admission to a burn unit may be useful, but the problem of cross-infection should always be considered in an endemically colonized unit.

Specific Therapy. There is a substantial controversy whether patients with severe erythema multiforme should be treated with systemic doses of corticosteroids. While the majority of clinicians feel that these preparations are definitely helpful, three retrospective analyses have not shown any benefit. In fact, one showed that patients treated with corticosteroids had a greater incidence of bleeding and infection. If corticosteroids are to be used, the dose should be high enough to produce a response (1 mg/kg/day) and the duration short enough not to impede healing—no more than 4–7 days. Topical application of steroids has little or no place in the treatment of erythema multiforme.

Every patient with involvement of the ocular mucosa should be seen by an ophthalmologist. Topical application of corticosteroids and antibiotics is frequently recommended, but whether their use prevents complications and speeds healing is not known.

Complications. Patients with erythema multiforme may suffer a variety of complications, including infection, gastrointestinal bleeding, renal failure, and eye disease. Blood and wound cultures should be done at the first sign of a deterioration in the patient's condition and may be useful on admission as well, since some patients initially have erythema multiforme–associated infection. Prophylactic doses of antibiotics are not generally recommended since they may be associated with overgrowth of antibiotic-resistant organisms. Gastrointestinal bleeding is surprisingly common in this group of patients and can be often massive and life threatening. Whether cimetidine and antacids should be given is not known at this time, but it seems a reasonable precaution. Renal failure can be due to hypovolemia, acute tubular necrosis, or glomerulonephritis. Eye complications, including synechia and xerosis, are common.

Gianotti Disease

SILVIA IOSUB, M.D.

Gianotti disease, or papular acrodermatitis of childhood (PAC), is a distinctive erythematopapular rash with a peculiar distribution on the limbs and face. It is preceded by an upper respiratory tract infection and accompanied by generalized lymphadenopathy, mild constitutional symptoms, and anicteric hepatitis. In the cases described by Gianotti, hepatitis B surface antigen was invariably present and the virus was of the subtype ayw. The skin lesions are monomorphic, flat papules, 2–3 mm in diameter, that are nonpruritic and last 15–20 days.

In the past 10 years cases of PAC-like eruptions have been reported in association with other viruses: Epstein-Barr virus, cytomegalovirus, Coxsackie virus A-16, and parainfluenza virus. These eruptions are called "PAC with [the respective viral condition]." The term "Gianotti-Crosti syndrome" is used when the etiology is unknown.

Since Gianotti disease is self-limited, only symptomatic treatment is indicated.

Papulosquamous Disorders

DEBRA A. HORNEY, M.D.

SEBORRHEIC DERMATITIS

Seborrheic dermatitis of the scalp is best managed by frequent shampooing, preferably with antidandruff or antiseborrheic shampoos. Active agents and shampoos containing these include selenium sulfide (Exsel [prescription], Selsun [prescription], Selsun Blue), zinc pyrithione (Danex, DHS-Zn, Head & Shoulders), and tar derivatives (DHS Tar, Polytar, Zetar).* Combination products including sulfur, salicylic acid, and coal tar are also very effective (Ionil T, Sebulex, Sebutone, Vanseb T, and X Seb T).

Several factors influence the effectiveness of therapy. One is frequency of shampooing. Most patients require daily shampooing. However, this is determined on an individual basis, and some children do well with every-other-day or twice-weekly shampooing. Particularly with black patients, daily shampooing is not well tolerated. The hair of blacks is generally drier and more brittle than the hair of nonblacks. Conditioners, oil sprays, and glycerin-containing preparations are useful to keep the hair better hydrated and less susceptible to breakage.

For best results, the shampoo should be lathered and in contact with the scalp for 5–10 minutes before rinsing. In addition, to prevent the development of tolerance to a given shampoo, three different effective shampoos should be rotated on a weekly basis. Heavy scales and thick crusting of the scalp, as seen in "cradle cap," often require softening with mineral oil or petrolatum for 15–20 minutes prior to shampooing. For persistent

cases, topical application of a steroid lotion or spray may be added to the regimen.

Eyelid dermatitis (blepharitis) may be managed with gentle warm water compresses and cleansing with an amphoteric "no sting" baby shampoo.

Seborrheic dermatitis of the face and intertriginous areas may be treated with 1.0–2.5% hydrocortisone, e.g., Westcort or Tridesilon cream. Because of their cutaneous side effects (atrophy and telangiectasias), fluorinated topical steroid preparations should not be used on the face. Seborrheic dermatitis of the diaper area is often complicated by a candidal infection, which requires appropriate therapy.

PSORIASIS

Psoriasis is a common inherited disorder affecting 1–3% of the population. The nails are affected in 25–50% of patients. Psoriatic involvement of the nail matrix causes small pits in the nail plate, the most characteristic nail change in psoriasis. Other psoriatic nail changes include discoloration, subungual hyperkeratosis, crumbling of the nail plate, and onycholysis (separation of the nail plate from the nail bed). Psoriatic nails are difficult to treat. They should be kept closely trimmed, and subungual debris should be gently removed. Though the response is not dramatic, some patients note improvement with application of Synalar solution, which is massaged into the cuticle and occluded with a Band-Aid or adhesive tape overnight.

Psoriasis of the Scalp. The scalp is often the initial site of psoriatic involvement. The well-demarcated erythematous plaques with thick, adherent silvery scales may be diffuse or localized. Frequent shampooing is the key to effective management. Tar shampoos (Zetar, Polytar, Neutrogena T/gel) are generally best but may be rotated with other keratolytic shampoos (see Seborrheic Dermatitis). When shampooing alone is ineffective, Baker's P & S (phenol, paraffin oil, and saline) solution, mineral oil, or baby oil should be massaged into the scalp at bedtime and the head covered with a shower cap. This will soften the scales, allowing their easy removal in the morning with a tar shampoo. Immediately after shampooing, while the scalp is still wet, apply a steroid lotion (Synalar or Valisone) or aerosol spray (Valisone).

Guttate Psoriasis. The sudden appearance of small guttate (droplike) psoriatic lesions over the trunk and extremities is a common and, sometimes, first presentation of psoriasis in a young child. The eruption is often preceded 1–3 weeks by an upper respiratory infection, such as a streptococcal pharyngitis. A 2–3 week course of erythromycin is warranted even in the absence of etiologic doc-

---

*All shampoos listed are available over the counter unless otherwise indicated.

umentation. Additional topical therapy is discussed later.

Generalized Pustular Psoriasis. This rare, sometimes fatal, form of psoriasis is characterized by an explosive generalized eruption of superficial pustules associated with high fever and toxicity. The cause is unknown, but precipitating factors include acute infection and abrupt discontinuation of systemic or topical steroids. When possible, it is best to admit these very sick patients to a burn unit for total-body whirlpool therapy. Bland emollients and hydrocortisone cream are applied after whirlpool treatments. Short-term use of 13-cis-retinoic acid (Accutane)† (1.0–1.5 mg/kg) early in the course of the disease has shown great promise.

Death, when it occurs, is often associated with electrolyte imbalance or secondary infections.

Psoriatic Arthritis. Psoriatic arthritis occurs in about 5–10% of patients with psoriasis and is seen only rarely in the pediatric patient. This painful arthropathy most commonly affects the distal interphalangeal joints of the hands and feet. There appears to be no relationship between the severity of the cutaneous disease and the development of joint disease. Therapy of psoriatic arthritis consists primarily of aspirin and other nonsteroidal anti-inflamatory drugs, as well as physical therapy to minimize or prevent the flexural deformities that are known to occur.

Topical Therapy

The key to successful therapy of psoriasis is for patients to understand that although there is no cure for the disease, its satisfactory control is largely in their hands. That is, with daily attention to topical therapy, the average psoriatic patient will do well. Various topical agents are used. These include topical steroids, tar derivatives, anthralin, and keratolytic agents, such as salicylic acid.

For infants and young children, and for the face and genital areas in adolescents, 1–2.5% hydrocortisone cream, applied twice daily, is recommended. Otherwise, mid-potency topical steroids (triamcinolone, Cyclocort, Synalar) in an ointment base are good for long-term use. High-potency topical steroids (Lidex, Diprosone, Topicort) should be reserved for recalcitrant disease and short-term use. A steroid ointment under occlusion (e.g., Saran Wrap) at bedtime is helpful for thickened, scaly plaques. Topical steroids should not be used more than twice daily. Other topical preparations, or even bland emollients, may be applied other times during the day.

To enhance penetration of the steroid, a keratolytic agent may be added. Salicylic acid (3–5%) with 25% Lidex cream in Aquaphor or Eucerin base is very effective.

Tar preparations, which decrease epidermal proliferation, remain a highly effective therapeutic modality. LCD (liquor carbonis detergens), 3–10%, in Nivea oil or Eucerin cream, may be applied once or twice daily. Over-the-counter, cosmetically acceptable tar preparations are now available for baths and direct application. Three or four capfuls of Balnetar bath oil (2.5% coal tar) or Zetar emulsion (30% coal tar) is added to the bath water, in which the patient sits for 20 minutes. PsoriGel and Estar gel are applied directly to the lesions but are most effective when mixed with Aquaphor or Eucerin cream to prevent the drying effect of gel preparations. T/Derm body oil (5% coal tar) may be applied directly to psoriatic plaques.

Tar preparations should not be used for inflammatory lesions or acute erythroderma. To avoid a tar folliculitis, the product should be applied down the extremity rather than up. Some tar products may stain hair and fabric.

Phototherapy

Most psoriatic patients are benefited by exposure to sunlight and, accordingly, have less cutaneous disease during the summer months. There is an occasional patient, however, who does worse with sun exposure. In all patients, appropriate sunburn precautions must be taken, since severe sunburn is likely to cause an exacerbation of the disease due to the Koebner phenomenon. Although natural sunlight is superior to artificial ultraviolet therapy, it is frequently helpful for the patient to have access to ultraviolet therapy (UVB) either at home or in the office. To optimize ultraviolet therapy, a tar preparation should be applied at least 2 hours prior to exposure and removed with mineral oil just before the treatment.

Recently, psoralen and long-wavelength ultraviolet light (UVA) have been used successfully in psoriatic patients.‡ However, the long-term toxicity of such therapy has yet to be fully ascertained, and its use in children is not endorsed by the American Academy of Pediatrics.

Systemic Therapy

Only under rare circumstances should systemic therapy for psoriasis be required in children. Systemic steroids result in a dramatic clearing of psoriasis, but once discontinued, or even tapered significantly, there is often a serious rebound in disease activity. Prednisone does, however, have a role in the management of severe exfoliative erythroderma that is unresponsive to intensive topical therapy.

---

† This use is not listed by the manufacturer.

‡ This therapy is still considered investigational.

Methotrexate, a folic-acid antagonist, is highly effective in the management of recalcitrant, widespread psoriasis and psoriatic arthritis. Side effects include gastrointestinal disturbances and bone marrow, renal, and hepatic toxicity. It is used by dermatologists only under extreme conditions in children in a dose of 10–25 mg PO or IM once weekly.

The use of 13-cis-retinoic acid (Accutane) in pustular psoriasis has been described.

LICHEN PLANUS

The etiology of lichen planus is unknown. Thus there is no specific therapy, but the eruption generally resolves within 6 months to 3 years. Treatment is mainly symptomatic, aimed at reducing the pruritus that is the primary complaint in this disease. Orally administered antihistamines and mid- to high-potency topical steroids (Valisone, Lidex cream) are helpful. Hypertrophic plaques, which are recalcitrant to standard therapy, must be treated with Cordran tape or 0.1% triamcinolone ointment covered with Saran Wrap overnight. The rare patient will require a short course of systemic steroids.

A variety of medications have been reported to cause a lichen planus–like drug rash. Thus, suspicious medications should be discontinued or substituted for whenever possible.

Since even minor surface injury is known to aggravate lichen planus, care must be taken to avoid unnecessary trauma. This is especially important in the mouth, where ill-fitting or rough-edged dental appliances and foods such as popcorn or peanuts may cause minor tears in the buccal mucosa along the bite line, where many lichen planus lesions are found. Intraoral lesions may be treated with topical anesthetics (Benadryl elixir mixed in equal parts with Maalox), topical steroids (Kenalog in Orabase), or topical 0.025% Retin-A gel, applied three or four times daily.

PITYRIASIS RUBRA PILARIS

The treatment of pityriasis rubra pilaris (PRP) depends upon suppression of hyperkeratinization. For severe cases, this involves oral vitamin A therapy, 25,000–100,000 units twice daily. An adequate trial requires treatment for at least 3–6 weeks. If the therapy is effective and vitamin A is continued, it is important to watch for signs of vitamin A toxicity (anorexia, pruritus, hair loss, dry skin). To help prevent this, a 1-week drug-free holiday every 4–6 weeks should be considered. 13-cis-Retinoic acid (Accutane)§ may also be effective, but side effects, including hypertriglyceridemia and skeletal hyperostoses, limit its usefulness in PRP. Methotrexate‖ is used in adults, but because of its potential toxicity this drug should be used with great caution in children.

Topical therapy includes mid- to high-potency topical steroid (Synalar, 0.1% triamcinolone, Lidex) in an ointment or emollient base twice daily. Less potent topical steroids should be substituted once a response is seen. For the hyperkeratosis of the palms and soles, keratolytic agents—such as 3–5% salicylic acid or 10–20% urea in Aquaphor or petrolatum—applied two to four times a day are helpful.

Patients and parents should be counseled that PRP tends to be persistent and is characterized by spontaneous remissions and exacerbations.

PITYRIASIS ROSEA

If the rash of pityriasis rosea does not itch, no treatment is required. It is important, however, to advise patients and their parents that the rash may last for 6–12 weeks. Simple lubrication with bland emollients (Lubriderm, Keri lotion, Nivea) or an antipruritic lotion containing menthol and phenol (Sarna lotion) provides relief when pruritus is minimal. For more severe itching, a medium-strength steroid (Synalar, Aristocort, Cordran), applied alone or mixed in equal parts with a bland emollient, may be used twice daily. Antihistamines (hydroxyzine or diphenhydramine) and acetaminophen or aspirin also help relieve pruritus. Early in the course of the disease, exposure to ultraviolet light or sunshine may reduce the pruritus as well as hasten resolution of the eruption.

MUCHA-HABERMANN DISEASE

Mucha-Habermann disease, also known as pityriasis lichenoides et varioliformis acuta or PLEVA, is characterized by crops of scaly papules or papulovesicles that tend to develop central hemorrhagic necrosis and crusts soon after they arise. Lesions may involve the entire body but are most pronounced on the trunk and the flexor aspects of the extremities. The etiology is unknown. Most acute cases resolve spontaneously within a few months and require no therapy other than antihistamines and emollients. Topical corticosteroids and natural or artificial ultraviolet light exposure are sometimes helpful. Likewise, oral administration of erythromycin, 40 mg/kg, or tetracycline, 1 or 2 gm/day, seems to shorten the course or minimize flares in some patients. Tetracycline, however, should not be used in children under 8 years of age because of the possibility of damage to teeth. These antibiotics are used on an empirical basis. The pathogenesis of this disease is not clear.

---

§ This use of Accutane is not listed by the manufacturer.

‖ This use of methotrexate is not listed by the manufacturer.

Chronic Nonhereditary Vesiculobullous Disorders of Childhood

MARY K. SPRAKER, M.D.

The child with a blistering disease, especially when the problem is extensive, is a diagnostic and management challenge for his physician. Therefore, it is important to have a logical approach to assessing this problem. The first step is to make sure that the child does not have an acute blistering disease such as bullous impetigo, the staphylococcal scalded skin syndrome, or toxic epidermal necrolysis; these diseases are discussed at length elsewhere in this text. Genetic blistering diseases are also seen in childhood; they are discussed later in this section under the heading Genodermatoses.

DERMATITIS HERPETIFORMIS

Dermatitis herpetiformis (DH) is an intensely pruritic, chronic recurrent eruption characterized classically by the presence of grouped erythematous papules and vesicles distributed symmetrically over the body, usually on extensor surfaces such as the elbows, knees, sacrum, buttocks, and shoulders. Patients with DH seem to have a gluten sensitivity, since therapy with a gluten-free diet is highly effective. Also, many patients are positive for the HLAB-8 antigen. Therefore it is hypothesized that in genetically susceptible individuals gluten causes the formation of IgA antibodies, which initiate the alternate complement cascade, the end result of which is the inflammatory response we see in the skin. Unlike patients with celiac disease, another gluten-sensitive condition, patients with DH do not have diarrhea or malabsorption.

Treatment consists of medication or dietary restriction. It is said that 75% of patients can be controlled with a strict gluten-free diet that removes the antigen. I encourage all my patients to become familiar with this diet, which requires referral to an experienced dietician, since a strict gluten-free diet is complicated. Because the diet usually takes 4–12 months to control DH, and because it is extremely difficult for adults—let alone children—to follow, I find that therapy with medication is more practical. DH can be treated with either sulfapyridine or dapsone, a sulfone derivative. Either drug can cause a severe hemolytic anemia, which can be idiopathic or related to a glucose-6-phosphate dehydrogenase (G-6-PD) deficiency. Therefore, a G-6-PD level should be established prior to therapy with either drug.

The initial dose of sulfapyridine in children is usually 100–200 mg/kg/day in four divided doses, to a maximum of 2–4 gm daily. When existing lesions have been suppressed, the dosage may be tapered at weekly intervals. Frequently a maintenance dose of 0.5 gm or less may control the disease. Pretreatment and follow-up blood counts must be done at monthly intervals.

The sulfone derivative dapsone is better tolerated, more economical, and probably more effective than sulfapyridine, although some feel that its side effects may be more severe. A G-6-PD level, complete blood count (CBC), renal and liver function studies, and urinalysis must be obtained prior to therapy. The usual starting dose is 2 mg/kg/day, to a maximum of 400 mg daily. Patients respond rapidly within 4–48 hours. Then the dose can be decreased gradually to a minimum maintenance level, often as little as 25–50 mg daily. A CBC should be obtained two times per month for the first 3 months and then every 6–8 weeks. Liver function tests should also be given periodically.

BULLOUS PEMPHIGOID

Bullous pemphigoid is usually a disease of older adults, but occasionally it is seen in young children. The etiology of this rare disease is unknown. The response to therapy is variable, but systemic and often high-dose corticosteroids on a chronic basis are usually required to suppress the eruption. In severe or resistant cases, a combination of sulfones or sulfapyridine in conjuction with systemic corticosteroids may be helpful.

CHRONIC BULLOUS DERMATOSIS OF CHILDHOOD

There is a great deal of controversy regarding this blistering disease. Some argue that it is the most common of the chronic bullous diseases of childhood, and others insist that there is no such disease, that the lesions are merely a form of either dermatitis herpetiformis or bullous pemphigoid. Most pediatric dermatologists believe that chronic bullous dermatosis of childhood is a separate entity because the direct immunofluorescent findings are distinctive: linear deposits of IgA are seen along the basement membrane.

The cause of the disorder is unknown. Like DH, chronic bullous dermatosis of childhood responds to either sulfapyridine or dapsone.

PEMPHIGUS VULGARIS

Fortunately, pemphigus is extremely uncommon in childhood, for it can be severe and sometimes fatal. The disease tends to be chronic, although spontaneous remissions occur rarely. It is usually fatal if not treated aggressively. The treatment of choice is systemic steroids. Because their use will be long term, side effects should be minimized as much as possible. Once the disease is controlled, the dose should be slowly reduced and, preferably, the drug should be given on alternate days. Immunosuppressive drugs such as methotrexate, aza-thioprine, or cyclophosphamide may be used in addition for patients with severe disease that is not controlled with steroids alone or to help reduce the need for high-dose steroids.

HERPES GESTATIONIS

Herpes gestationis is a rare blistering disease that occurs during pregnancy. The mother is primarily affected, but there seems to be an increased risk of fetal morbidity and mortality, and occasionally the infant has a similar dermatitis during the newborn period. The dermatitis clears spontaneously in most mothers within a few days after delivery, but in some it can persist for many months. There may be recurrences during subsequent pregnancies, after oral contraceptive treatment, and sometimes at the time of menstruation.

The mainstay of treatment for the mother is the systemic administration of steroids. These should be withheld during the first trimester of pregnancy, if possible, to avoid potential abnormalities in fetal development. When the disease is controlled, it is preferable to begin alternate-day dosage if possible. Also, the dose should be reduced to a minimum during the final weeks of pregnancy to avoid adrenal suppression in the fetus. There have also been some reports of therapy with pyridoxine, estrogen and progesterone, and plasma exchange. In the infant the disease is self-limited and requires no treatment.

Discoid Lupus Erythematosus

RONALD C. HANSEN, M.D.

The skin lesions of discoid lupus erythematosus characteristically appear in the chronic cutaneous form of the disease but may also be found in systemic and neonatal lupus erythematosus. The lesions should be approached as a separate problem when associated with the systemic disease.

Although the degree of induction or aggravation of the cutaneous lesions by sunlight varies from patient to patient, it is prudent to assume that photosensitivity is a feature in each case. Hence, a sunscreen lotion with a sun protection factor (SPF) of 15 should be applied to all lesional and exposed skin on a daily basis. Caution in sun exposure must be advised as well.

Topical corticosteroid creams are the mainstay of therapy. Here one is forced to use potent fluorinated steroid creams, even on the face, since the disease is difficult to control. It is advisable to review the possibly poor outcome of the lesions, noting that atrophy and telangiectasia are usually the results of the disease rather than of the therapy. Cordran tape is a convenient method by which to occlude a topical steroid.

In refractory cases, intralesional corticosteroid injections can by very beneficial. Intralesional steroids produce temporary atrophy, and this must be discussed in the context of an atrophy and scarring-prone disease such as discoid lupus erythematosus. Antimalarial agents such as hydroxychloroquine (Plaquenil) can be very helpful when the above measures have failed. However, there are finite risks, chiefly retinal toxicity requiring close ophthalmologic follow-up. Hence, antimalarials should be prescribed only by physcians who are knowledgeable about these agents and experienced in the management of childhood lupus erythematosus.

A brief course of systemic steroids is of occasional value in bringing an acute flare of discoid lesions under control, but systemic steroids have no place in chronic therapy of discoid lupus erythematosus in childhood. When systemic steroids are used for other organ system involvement, there is likely to be concurrent improvement in the discoid lesions.

Kawasaki Syndrome

(Mucocutaneous Lymph Node Syndrome)

MARIAN E. MELISH, M.D.

Truly effective therapy for Kawasaki syndrome awaits discovery of its etiology and pathogenesis. For the present, a carefully conducted management program designed to detect complications is indicated. Supportive therapy can be offered based upon a consideration of pathology. Although serious, for most patients the disease is self-limited and can be divided into three stages. Stage I, the acute febrile period, lasts approximately 12 days. Stage II encompasses the period characterized by resolution of fever, desquamation, and thrombocytosis. Arthritis and carditis, when present, usually appear during this period. This period has the highest risk for sudden death due to coronary thrombosis and lasts until approximately day 30 of the illness. Stage III, or the convalescent period, lasts from clinical recovery to the time when the sedimentation rate returns to normal, usually 8–10 weeks from onset. Patients must be carefully monitored throughout their illness with visits to the physician at least two times per week during Stages I and II and weekly through Stage III. An electrocardiogram and a chest radiograph should be obtained at the onset and repeated if there are any clinical signs of cardiac decompensation. Repeated physical examinations are superior to repeat electrocardigrams in detecting cardiac abnormalities, the most important complication of Kawasaki syndrome.

During the acute febrile phase, aspirin in standard antiinflammatory doses of 80–100 mg/kg/24 hr may reduce the duration of fever. We monitor the salicylate level at 48 hours after starting aspirin, aiming for a level between 18 and 28 mg/dl, and we adjust the dose upward or downward as indicated. Once fever, rash, and acute symptoms have been controlled, we decrease the aspirin to a dose of 10 mg/kg/24 hr or less. Low-dose aspirin is more effective in preventing thrombosis during Stages II and III, as it decreases platelet aggregation without stimulating vascular thrombogenic factors. It is important to reduce the aspirin during the period when platelet count is elevated, as most fatalities are due to thrombosis during a period when vasculitis is declining.

If two-dimensional echocardiography is available, patients should be studied during Stage II; approximately 20% of patients have coronary artery dilatation detected by this technique. This will identify a high-risk group that should be followed longer and more carefully. In selected children, especially those with pericarditis, myocarditis, congestive heart failure, or myocardial infarction, cardiac catheterization with selective coronary artery angiography may be indicated. This invasive technique should not be employed routinely, as echocardiography will reveal 80–90% of the abnormalities detected by angiography and carries essentially no risk.

We have been adding dipyridamole (Persantine*), another inhibitor of platelet aggregation, to low-dose aspirin for patients known to have coronary aneurysms. As no dosage recommendations for this drug are available, we calculate the dose using the formula: patient surface area (m^2)/ 1.7 × 150 mg (adult daily dose) = patient's daily dose. The drug is given in three divided doses. In patients with coronary aneurysms, we continue aspirin and dipyridamole for 1 year or until aneurysms resolve on repeat study. For patients with no evidence of heart disease and normal echocardiograms, we continue low-dose aspirin alone for 8–10 weeks until the sedimentation rate is normal.

Cardiac arrhythmias, congestive heart failure due to myocarditis, transient mitral insufficiency, or myocardial infarction must be treated in the hospital with monitoring, digitalis, and antiarrhythmia drugs. Arthritis is self-limited, usually lasting less than 2 weeks, but may require continuing high-dose aspirin. Gallbladder hydrops, presenting clinically as a right upper quadrant mass, can be confirmed by diagnositic ultrasound and monitored until natural resolution occurs. Surgical removal is not necessary as this complication is also self-limited.

Although Kawasaki syndrome is a disease characterized by vasculitis, corticosteroids are specifically contraindicated because of a carefully conducted controlled study indicating that they increase the frequency of aneurysms compared with aspirin or no antiiflammatory therapy. Less carefully conducted studies in Japan have shown a higher mortality rate in steroid-treated children compared with those treated with aspirin.

As the cause of death is nearly always coronary thrombosis, the patient's primary need is for careful monitoring and antiplatelet aggregation therapy throughout the period of greatest risk.

Fungal Infections

LAWRENCE SCHACHNER, M.D.

The use of creams and lotions with combined antifungal and anti-yeast action, such as miconazole (MicaTin) clotrimazole (Lotrimin) and haloprogin (Halotex) have made the treatment of superficial mycosis somewhat simpler. However, their appropriate use, as well as that of griseofulvin in tinea capitis and tinea unguium, can maximize their effectiveness and enhance the rate at which the patient is helped. Adjuncts that enhance the therapeutic action of these medications in specific mycosis, and the substitution of often less expensive preparations such as selenium sulfide (Selsun) or sodium thiosulfate (Tinver) in tinea versicolor have also been very effective.

Specific diagnostic tests for cutaneous fungal infections should not be allowed to become a lost art. Correct performance of potassium hydroxide (KOH) preparations and Wood's lamp examination can lead to immediate and inexpensive confirmation of the diagnosis of cutaneous fungal infections. Fungal cultures, particularly in tinea capitis, can lead to confirmation that a clinical finding such as alopecia is appropriately attributed to a dermatophyte and is not a clinical sign of severe underlying disease.

It is worth reiterating briefly the technique of KOH preparation. Hair specimens, scale from the border of the cutaneous eruption, nail scrapings, or blister roofs are placed on a microscope slide and cover slip. Ten to 20% KOH may be added to the side of the cover slip and will disperse itself equally over the covered material by flowing under the edge of the cover slip. KOH solutions free of dimethylsulfoxide (DMSO) should be heated until they begin to boil. If the KOH solution contains DMSO, the preparation should not be heated. Scanning the field under low power, with the condenser lowered to a position that allows for reduced amounts of illumination, will often aid in finding characteristic hyphae in dermatophytes, or pseudohyphae and budding spores in candidiasis.

---

* This is an investigational use of Persantine.

The Wood's lamp is a valuable diagnostic tool in a number of cutaneous and systemic diseases, not the least of which are tinea capitis and tinea versicolor. In a totally darkened room, the patient's scalp or skin is illuminated with the Wood's lamp. The microsporum species causing tinea capitis reveals a characteristic green fluorescence that is most notable in the areas of inflammation and loss of the acral hair shafts. The Wood's lamp produces an orange or yellow fluorescence over areas of involvement of the skin with tinea versicolor.

There are several media to choose among when preparing fungal cultures. Dermatophyte test medium (DTM) is a reliable diagnostic adjunct. The presence of a dermatophyte is confirmed not only by colony growth but also by the change in color of the media from gold to red in the presence of a dermatophyte. Mycosel agar is another good diagnostic culture medium for identifying dermatophytes and *Candida albicans*.

THERAPY

Two dermatophytoses that always require griseofulvin therapy are tinea capitis and tinea unguium. Tinea capitis, caused by species of *Trichophyton* and *Microsporum*, presents as an inflammatory or noninflammatory scalp disorder featuring scaling and alopecia. Inflammation, when present, can vary from mild to a suppurative boggy mass, replete with pustules and swelling, called a kerion. Griseofulvin should be started in doses of 10 to 20 mg/kg in the microcrystalline forms and half that dose in the ultra-microcrystalline griseofulvins, such as Gris-PEG. Since griseofulvin absorption seems to be enhanced by fatty food, I recommend that it be given after meals including milk or ice cream products. Griseofulvin should be given for a minimum of 4 weeks and preferably for at least 2 weeks after all clinical signs of disease have abated. Additional benefit may be gained by the use of keratolytic shampoos, such as Sebulex, which have been reported to decrease dissemination of spores and infected particles to the patient, and to others who may physically contact the patient. Topical antifungal solutions including clotrimazole, haloprogins, and miconazole preparations may enhance the rate of clinical improvement.

When tinea capitis has evolved to the point of kerion formation, the choice of therapies to clear the infection and minimize permanent hair loss and scalp scarring takes on added importance. In addition to griseofulvin, a course of prednisone at 1 mg/kg/day for 1 to 2 weeks will greatly decrease the inflammation and help attenuate the course of the kerion. Although the subject is certainly controversial, I among others feel that a 10-day course of oral antibiotics such as cloxacillin or erythromycin also may be helpful when kerions are present.

Tinea unguium is a chronic infection of finger- and toenails that is fortunately rare in childhood. Culture and KOH can help distinguish onychomycosis caused by *Trichophyton* or *Epidermophyton* from that caused by *Candida albicans*. The latter often is limited to the nails of the upper extremities, and concurrent paronychial inflammation is characteristic. Topical medications are effective in candidal nail infections, and any of the medications mentioned above, such as clotrimazole or nystatin preparations, would be useful. The onychomycoses due to *Trichophyton* and *Epidermophyton* species require long-term griseofulvin therapy. Similar dosages as for tinea capitis are appropriate; however, therapies must extend for at least 4 to 6 months for potential cure.

Tinea corporis, tinea cruris, tinea faciei, and tinea pedis, when acute, merit wet to dry soaks to decrease the inflammation and the oozing associated with the eczematous state. Tap water soaks are both effective and most inexpensive; if soaks are applied for 20 minutes every 4 hours for 2 days, most patients with these forms of tinea are ready for topical therapy. Most will respond nicely and completely to 2 to 3 weeks of twice-daily therapy with clotrimazole, haloprogin, miconazole, or tolnaftate (Tinactin), though the latter is effective only against dermatophytes and is not active against *Candida albicans*. Recurrences of tinea may be decreased by the prophylactic administration of topical antifungal creams or powders. Only the most chronic severe and unresponsive forms of the above-mentioned tineas will require the addition of griseofulvin.

Tinea versicolor is a common chronic cutaneous infection that may be entirely asymptomatic. Although any of the above-mentioned topical antifungal preparations can be effective, the widespread distribution of the lesions makes selenium sulfide (Selsun) or sodium thiosulfate (Tinver) an effective and less expensive therapeutic approach. Overnight applications of either of these preparations to the entire affected area for a period of 2 weeks often leads to resolution. Pigment changes will take longer to resolve. Prophylactic therapy with these two preparations or with the above-mentioned antifungals can prevent recurrence, especially in more temperate months and climates.

Candidiasis, whether of the oral mucous membrane, the perineum, the flexural surfaces of the body, or the nails or interdigital spaces of the upper extremities, is responsive to nystatin preparations. Oral administration of nystatin suspension is useful not only in thrush but also in decreasing the bowel contamination that can seed candidal diaper dermatitis. The candidal dermatitis of the newborn infant is also nystatin responsive as is candidal vulvovaginitis, which can be treated with vaginal preparations. Much previous enthusiasm for Mycolog cream and similar polyformulary preparations has waned because of the presence of topical corticosteroids and sensitizing compounds in their formulation.

Warts and Molluscum Contagiosum

LAYNE HERSH, M.D.

WARTS

Warts are benign growths caused by the human papilloma virus. Originally warts were thought to be caused by a single DNA virus type; however, there has recently been evidence to suggest at least seven antigenically distinct viruses. Warts often last 1–2 years but may regress spontaneously. The choice of treatment depends on the age of the child and the location of the warts (see also p. 448).

Lesions of the hands and extremities respond best to liquid nitrogen applied with a cotton-tipped applicator. Freezing time varies with the size of the wart but is usually around 15–30 seconds. Parents should be told that a blister may occur and will fall off by itself. In very young children cantharone can be applied sparingly. This works best if the area is then covered with tape for 4–6 hours. Treatments are given once or twice a month, and the wart may take weeks or months to resolve.

Flat warts on the face, arms, and knees, are usually treated with retinoic acid (Retin-A cream or gel) daily until erythema and scaling are produced. If this treatment is too irritating, a light freeze with liquid nitrogen, 5–10 seconds, can be tried instead. Shaving can spread warts and should be avoided.

Plantar warts are notoriously difficult to treat. The least painful way to begin therapy is with 40% salacid plaster, applied daily and secured with tape. As the wart softens it is pared, with a No. 15 blade, once a month. An alternative to the plaster is topical salicylic acid and lactic acid liquid (Duofilm) applied daily. This also works better if occluded with tape.

Condylomata acuminata and penile warts in uncircumcised boys can be treated with 25% podophyllin in tincture of benzoin. Care should be taken to apply the chemical only to the wart. It should be washed off in 2–4 hours to avoid a severe reaction. As the treatment is repeated weekly, the time it is left on can be increased gradually to 6–8 hours. These lesions are rarely encountered in very young children and raise the possibility of sexual abuse.

Treatments still considered experimental include wart vaccine, intralesional bleomycin, topical acyclovir (Zovirax), and topical 5% 5-fluorouracil cream.

Susceptibility to warts and the rate of their resolution depend on the child's immune system. The incidence of warts is higher in immunosuppressed transplant patients and in children with Hodgkin's disease, lymphomas, and leukemias. It has been hypothesized that both cell-mediated immunity (T cells) and complement-fixing antibodies (B cells) may play an important role in the immune response.

MOLLUSCUM CONTAGIOSUM

Molluscum contagiosum is a viral infection of the skin characterized by a pearly-white papule with central umbilication. The treatment usually includes cantharone, with or without occlusive tape, for 4–6 hours or a light liquid nitrogen freeze of 5–10 seconds. Occasionally it may be preferable to use a local anesthetic and open each papule with a No. 11 blade, then curette out the contents of the sac. Treatment can be repeated once or twice a month, depending on the number of lesions and the rate of appearance of new papules.

Scabies and Pediculosis

SIDNEY HURWITZ, M.D.

SCABIES

The treatment of scabies consists of topical application of 1.0% gamma benzene hexachloride (lindane; available as Kwell, Scabene), 10% crotamiton (Eurax), 6–10% precipitate of sulfur in petrolatum, or a suspension of benzyl benzoate in a 12.5–25% concentration. Application of lindane from the neck down in older children and adults and to the entire body, including the head and neck, in infants and young children is curative in 96% of patients. The medication is applied to dry skin for a period of 6–12 hours and is then removed by a thorough washing (shower or bath). One application is usually curative, but, when necessary, lindane may be reapplied in 1 week for another 6–12 hours. The vulnerability of small infants to percutaneous absorption of this potentially neurotoxic substance warrants caution in prescribing lindane for infants and small children. Although most cases of adverse reaction have been caused by misuse of the preparation, the problem of possible toxic effects is more acute in infants and small children, owing to a relatively greater skin surface and possibly higher blood level accumulations in this age group.

For infants and small children (those 1 year of age or younger), alternative therapy includes 10% crotamiton cream or lotion (Eurax) applied twice a day for 5 days or 6% sulfur in petrolatum applied nightly for 3 nights. Again, the therapy may be repeated in 1 week if necessary.

Pruritus, due to hypersensitivity to the mite antigens, may persist for days or weeks despite adequate therapy. It may be treated by oral doses of antihistamines or hydroxyzine, by topical application of antipruritic lotions containing menthol or phenol (Cetaphil or Keri lotion with 0.25% menthol), or by topical application of pramoxine, available as Prax or Pramosone (1% hydrocortisone in combination with pramoxine), in cream or lotion. Postscabietic nodules, which represent a hypersensitivity to the mite, frequently persist for many weeks to months. Although therapy is not necessary, they can be treated with variable degrees of success by application of topical corticosteroids alone or in combination with tar formulations (Estar gel, PsoriGel, or Fototar cream), intralesional steroids, or corticosteroids under occlusion.

When treating an individual patient, the entire family and close personal contacts should be examined and, if affected, treated appropriately. Since the hypersensitivity state and associated pruritus and nodular lesions frequently do not cease immediately after eradication of the infestation, the patient and his family should be alerted to this possibility so that they will not be tempted to continue excessive, unnecessary, and potentially hazardous therapy.

PEDICULOSIS

Head Lice. Pediculosis capitis, except under crowded and unsanitary conditions, is the most common form of louse infestation. Lindane (Kwell, Scabene) is a highly effective treatment. One tablespoon, approximately 15 ml, of 1% shampoo is massaged into the scalp for 4 minutes and followed by a thorough rinsing. If the lotion is used, it may be applied to the scalp, left on overnight, and then washed out carefully. A second treatment may be repeated after 1 week if viable eggs persist. Other members of the family should be examined, and those with evidence of infestation should be treated. Pyrethrins (RID, A-200) are also effective and are available as over-the-counter formulations. It should be noted, however, that corneal damage, namely ulceration and scarring, has been reported with the use of A-200, which contains 5% denatured kerosene.

An alternative treatment for pediculosis capitis is malathion (Prioderm) in a 0.5% lotion. Prioderm lotion has the advantage of being ovicidal. It is best applied to dry hair and rubbed in gently until the hair and scalp are thoroughly moistened; the hair is allowed to dry naturally, and the lotion should be shampooed out after a period of at least 8 hours. Since nits are firmly attached to the hair shaft, their removal may be facilitated by the use of a fine-toothed comb or tweezers or by soaking the hair with a 1:1 white vinegar–water rinse or a 3–5% acetic acid solution followed by wrapping with a damp towel soaked in the same solution. Many pyrethrin products are sold with a plastic nit comb. Although none of these combs will remove all the nits, closely spaced teeth are helpful.

Pediculosis Pubis. Pediculosis pubis normally involves the hairs of the pubic region but may also involve the eyelashes, beard, mustache, and axillary and other body hairs. Infestation of the pubic region is most frequently seen in adolescents and young adults as a result of transmission by sexual intercourse, but the lice may also be transmitted by clothing, bedding, or towels. The treatment of pediculosis pubis is similar to that of pediculosis capitis. Sexual contacts should be treated simultaneously, but other household members need not be treated. At the conclusion of therapy, treated individuals should change their underclothing, pajamas, sheets, and pillowcases. These articles should be washed and dried by machine, ironed, or boiled to destroy remaining ova and parasites.

Pediculosis Palpebrarum. Pediculosis of the eyelashes may be treated by petrolatum applied thickly to the eyelashes twice daily for 8 days, followed by mechanical removal of remaining nits. Although this appears to be the treatment of choice, physostigmine ophthalmic preparations (Eserine) are also effective when applied topically to the eyelid margin twice daily for 24–48 hours). Because of the parasympathetic effect of physostigmine, miosis is a possible side effect. Fluorescein eyedrops may also be utilized to treat pediculosis of the eyelids.

Pediculosis Corporis. The body louse generally lives in clothing or bedding, lays eggs along the seams of the clothing, and visits the human host only long enough to feed. This disorder is rarely seen in children, except under conditions of poor hygiene. The treatment of pediculosis corporis mainly consists of proper hygiene, with frequent showers or baths and frequent changes of underclothes and bedding. Underclothing and bedding should be laundered with hot water or boiled; drycleaning destroys lice in articles that cannot be laundered. Pressing woolens with a hot iron with special attention given to the seams of the clothing, is also satisfactory. All likely contacts (members of the household and close contacts in an institution) should be examined and treated if there is evidence of infestation.

Disorders of Pigmentation

SIDNEY HURWITZ, M.D.

Alterations in skin color may be generalized or localized and may result from a variety of defects ranging from absence of melanocytes and effective melanization of melanosomes to overproduction of melanin and increased numbers of melanocytic cells. Although chiefly of cosmetic significance, these disorders can be persistent and extremely annoying, both cosmetically and psychologically, to affected individuals.

HYPERPIGMENTED LESIONS

Disorders of hyperpigmentation may be external or internal in origin. Those of particular interest in the pediatric age group include freckles (or ephelides), lentigines, café-au-lait spots, postinflammatory melanosis (postinflammatory hyperpigmentation), melasma (chloasma), and inherited pigmentary disorders such as incontinentia pigmenti.

Freckles. Freckles (ephelides) are red or light brown well-circumscribed macules, usually less than 5 mm in diameter, which appear in childhood, especially on sun-exposed areas of the skin. Freckles are best managed by avoidance of sun exposure and appropriate covering make-up (when desired). Although sunscreens do not prevent freckle formation, they permit a more uniform tan in which freckling is less prominent. Gentle peeling with 50% trichloroacetic acid, cryotherapy with carbon dioxide slush or liquid nitrogen, and judicious use of monobenzyl ether of hydroquinone (Benoquin, Eldoquin, Eldopaque, or Solaquin) may make many of these lesions less conspicuous. The possibility of contact dermatitis and occasional persistent hypopigmentation, however, warrants caution in the use of these physical or chemical methods.

Lentigines. Lentigines are small, smooth, freckle-like pigmented macules that usually appear in childhood but may increase in number up to adulthood. Treatment of lentigines is ordinarily not indicated. When desired, however, excision by a small punch biopsy or by shaving, cryosurgery, or electrodesiccation may be performed. The *Peutz-Jeghers* and *multiple lentigines (leopard) syndromes* have lentigines as a major component.

Café-au-lait Spots. These spots are large, round or oval, flat lesions of light brown pigmentation found in 10–20% of normal individuals. The presence of six or more café-au-lait spots greater than 1.5 cm in diameter is presumptive evidence of neurofibromatosis. Large, often unilateral café-au-lait spots with irregular borders are characteristic of patients with the *McCune-Albright syndrome*, a disorder that consists of polyostotic fibrous dysplasia, endocrine dysfunction, sexual precocity in girls, and abnormal cutaneous pigmentation. The cutaneous lesions are present early in life and frequently are the first sign of this disorder.

Postinflammatory Melanosis. Postinflammatory melanosis (postinflammatory hyperpigmentation), one of the most common causes of hyperpigmen-

tation, is characterized by an increase in melanin formation following cutaneous inflammation. If areas of postinflammatory hyperpigmentation can be protected from further ultraviolet exposure, fading occurs gradually over a period of months. In cases in which hyperpigmentation is prolonged and therapy is desired, topical applications of a low-potency steroid (hydrocortisone in a 1.0% concentration) may be helpful. In patients who desire more active therapy, hydroquinone preparations may hasten improvement.

Melasma. Melasma (formerly referred to as chloasma) is a patchy dark-brown to black hyperpigmentation located primarily on the cheeks, the forehead, and occasionally the temples, upper lip, and neck. Seen in up to 20% of women who take anovulatory drugs or who are pregnant, this disorder has been termed "the mask of pregnancy." Since sun exposure tends to trigger and intensify this hyperpigmentation, the disorder characteristically becomes more prominent in the summer months. Once melasma has developed, it generally tends to persist for long periods, and treatment is generally not very satisfactory. Treatment consists of discontinuation of potentially responsible medications, protection from sun or ultraviolet exposure by the use of appropriate clothing and sunscreen preparations, and the topical application of hydroquinones.

Incontinentia Pigmenti. Incontinentia pigmenti (Bloch-Sulzberger disease) is a rare hereditary disorder thought to be transmitted as an X-linked dominant trait, lethal in males, that affects the skin, central nervous system, eyes, and skeletal system. Although cutaneous lesions may constitute the only manifestation, approximately 80% of children with incontinentia pigmenti have other defects (cataracts, microcephaly, spastic paralysis, strabismus, alopecia, delayed or impaired dentition, epilepsy, and mental retardation).

DISORDERS OF HYPOPIGMENTATION

Vitiligo. Vitiligo is a common, genetically determined, patterned loss of pigmentation that follows the destruction of melanocytes and is characterized by oval or irregular ivory-white patches of skin surrounded by a well-demarcated or hyperpigmented, often convex, border. Although there is no completely satisfactory treatment of vitiligo, partial and even complete repigmentation can occasionally be accomplished by the administration of psoralen compounds (Trisoralen, Elder) followed by gradually increasing exposure to sunlight or long-wave ultraviolet light. Since treatment is long and difficult, psoralen therapy should be carefully monitored by physicians experienced in the use of photosensitizing drugs. When treatment of vitiligo is unsatisfactory, the depigmented lesions can be hidden by the use of cosmetic makeups or aniline dye stains such as Neodyoderm or Vitadye.

Albinism. Albinism is an uncommon inherited disorder manifested by congenital hypopigmentation of the skin, hair, and eyes. It occurs in two forms, oculocutaneous and ocular. Except for contact lenses and tinted glasses to ameliorate photophobia, there is no effective treatment for patients with ocular forms of albinism. Since early actinic changes, keratoses, basal cell tumors, and squamous cell carcinomas are common, even in children and adolescents, those with cutaneous albinism must learn to avoid sunlight exposure and to use protective clothing and sunscreen preparations on exposed surfaces.

Partial albinism (piebaldism) is an uncommon but widely distributed dominantly inherited disorder. Commonly associated with a white lock of hair above the forehead (the "white forelock") in 85–90% of affected individuals, partial albinism is characterized by congenital patterned areas of depigmentation and varying shades of normal skin color that are usually present at birth. Treatment consists of the cosmetic masking of areas of leukoderma with aniline dyes (as in the treatment of vitiligo), the protection of hypopigmented and depigmented areas from sun damage by proper clothing, and the use of appropriate sunscreen preparations on exposed surfaces.

Chédiak-Higashi Syndrome. The Chédiak-Higashi syndrome is a rare autosomal recessive, lethal disorder characterized by diffuse oculocutaneous hypopigmentation, photophobia, hepatosplenomegaly, abnormal granulation of leukocytes, and recurrent pyogenic infections. Most patients die in early childhood of overwhelming infection, hemorrhage, or a lymphoma-like process; over 50% succumb before the end of the first decade of life. Management consists of supportive measures to prevent recurrent infection and combined prednisone and vincristine therapy for the lymphoma-like phase of the disorder.

Waardenburg Syndrome. The Waardenburg (Klein-Waardenburg) syndrome is a rare autosomal dominant disorder characterized by congenital deafness, lateral displacement of the medial canthi and lacrimal puncta of the lower eyelids (dystopia cantharum), broad nasal root, white forelock, heterochromia iridis, and, in some patients, skin lesions resembling those of piebaldism. Here again, protection with sunscreens is obligatory and cosmetic cover-ups (as in patients with vitiligo) may be utilized.

Tuberous Sclerosis. Tuberous sclerosis is an autosomal dominant disorder of variable penetrance characterized by hypopigmented macules; central nervous system involvement, sclerotic calcification in the brain visible as "tubers" by x-ray, retinal phakomas, rhabdomyomas of the heart, renal cysts and tumors, cysts of the bones and lungs, adenoma sebaceum, fibromas of the fingers, toes, and gums, and shagreen patches (flesh-colored to yellowish or yellowish orange, slightly elevated plaques of dermal connective tissue). Although lance-ovate lesions resembling in shape the leaf of the mountain ash tree ("ash leaf spots") are highly characteristic of this disorder, only 18% of the hypopigmented lesions of tuberous sclerosis have this configuration.

Hypomelanosis of Ito. Hypomelanosis of Ito (incontinentia pigmenti achromians) is a neurocutaneous syndrome characterized by distinctive macular, linear, or irregular whirls or swirls of hypopigmentation. There is no known therapy for the hypopigmentation other than cosmetic coverups (as described in the section on vitiligo).

Pityriasis Alba. Pityriasis alba is a common cutaneous disorder characterized by discrete asymptomatic hypopigmented patches on the face, neck, upper trunk, and proximal extremities of children and young adults. Most cases appear following sun exposure and result from a disturbance in pigmentation of the affected areas. Low-potency topical corticosteroids (hydrocortisone) and lubrication followed by sun exposure appear to diminish the dry skin and fine scaling and enhance repigmentation of involved areas.

Postinflammatory Hypopigmentation. Postinflammatory hypopigmentation may be associated with a wide variety of inflammatory dermatoses or infections. This relatively common pigmentary deficiency may be noted following involution of certain inflammatory skin disorders, particularly burns, bullous disorders, infections, eczematous or psoriatic lesions, and pityriasis rosea. Since the defect is primarily epidermal, postinflammatory hypopigmentation generally improves in time without active therapy.

Photodermatoses

SUSAN E. KOCH, M.D.

Photosensitivity disorders are uncommon in pediatric practice. The causes of these disorders vary from inherited metabolic defects, such as the porphyrias, to environmental agents. These conditions are distinguished by their typical distribution involving primarily sun-exposed areas: face, anterior chest, dorsal forearms, and hands. Exclusion of an airborne source of contact dermatitis is critical.

Environmental Agents. Abnormal sensitivity to sunlight may be caused by a variety of environmental agents. Topical preparations such as coal tar, hexachlorophene, halogenated salicylanilides, and sunscreens can cause photosensitivity reactions. Skin contact with certain plants may cause phototoxic reactions that resolve with avoidance of further exposure. These are known as phyto-photodermatoses. The plants responsible include lime, celery, carrots, figs, and wild parsnips, all of which contain furocoumarins. Careful interview of the patient and his parents will elucidate these precipitants in most cases.

Oral medications responsible for phototoxic and photoallergic reactions include tetracyclines, phenothiazines, sulfonamides, griseofulvin, quinine, nalidixic acid, isoniazid, diphenhydramine, and psoralens. The use of these agents is limited in children and adolescents. Discontinuation of the offending agent when possible usually results in a reversal of the photosensitivity state.

Sunburn. The sunburn reaction is caused primarily by short-wave or UVB radiation, which causes redness and in severe cases blistering of exposed skin. The intensity of this reaction is maximal 24 hours after exposure. Treatment measures include cool compresses or baths and appropriate doses of aspirin. The systemic use of corticosteroids should be reserved for severe cases. Preventative measures for susceptible individuals, i.e., the use of topical sunscreens, are beneficial. Light clothing may not be effective in screening harmful rays.

Polymorphous Light Eruption. Altered tolerance to sunlight in this condition commonly begins in childhood and may have a familial basis among American Indians. Delayed onset of symptoms up to 72 hours after exposure and patchy involvement of sun-exposed areas may make diagnosis difficult. Typically, eczematous patches, papules, or blistering occurs several hours after sun exposure, associated with itching or burning of the skin. Symptoms are most prominent in the spring and early summer. Because UVB radiation is often responsible, regular topical use of sunscreens may be beneficial. Severe cases may require avoidance of midday sun and systemic therapy with antimalarial drugs such as chloroquine* and hydroxychloroquine* during the spring and summer months. The major problem with antimalarial therapy is the potential for retinal toxicity. For this reason patients should be carefully selected, and pretreatment and interval ophthalmologic examinations are mandatory. The response to therapy may require several weeks.

Topical corticosteroid treatment may be beneficial in acute reactions but is not useful as a preventative for long-term therapy. Paradoxically, the use of an oral photosensitizing agent, psoralen, followed by UVA light, may induce inherent photoprotective mechanisms, such as thickening and increased pigmentation of the skin, that result in an increased tolerance to sunlight. However, recent reports of the development of skin tumors in patients given such therapy cause concern about its use in the pediatric age group.

Porphyrias. These disorders of heme synthesis encompass a unique subset of photodermatoses in which a metabolic derangement results in the production of endogenous photosensitizers. Patients with these disorders are sensitive to the upper UVA spectrum and the visible spectrum (390–600 nm). Porphyria cutanea tarda is an autosomal dominant disorder characterized by increased skin fragility, blistering, and altered skin color. The disorder usually occurs in adults but has rarely been reported in children. Precipitating drugs such as anticonvulsants, oral contraceptives, and griseofulvin should be discontinued. Phlebotomy leads to remission, but it may take months. Oral antimalarial therapy with chloroquine* may also be used. Chloroquine acts as a chelating agent and thereby enhances renal excretion of porphyrin. Low biweekly doses may induce a chemical and clinical remission. The risk of retinal toxicity should be considered prior to its use.

Erythropoietic protoporphyria is the most common variety of porphyria occurring in children. Subjective symptoms of burning and itching occur during or soon after sun exposure and are followed by the development of redness, hive-like lesions, blisters, and purpura. Chronic skin changes such as depressed scars, cobblestone-like thickening, and pigment changes ultimately result. High protoporphyrin levels in red blood cells and plasma are diagnostic. Oral administration of the naturally occurring compound beta-carotene is safe and effective in these patients. The recommended dosage for children 1–8 years of age is 30–60 mg/day; for children 9–16 it is 90–120 mg/day. Capsules may be opened and mixed with orange or tomato juice to facilitate administration in the younger age group. The goal of therapy is maintenance of blood carotene levels between 600 and 800 µg/100 ml during the spring and summer months. A beneficial response occurs after 6 weeks of therapy. Sunscreens are of limited value in these patients since the UVB spectrum does not trigger the adverse reaction.

Congenital erythropoietic porphyria, or Günther's disease, is a rare automsomal recessive condition associated with a mutilating form of blistering photodermatitis, hemolytic anemia, keratoconjunctivitis, and mahogany-stained teeth that fluoresce under Wood's light. Therapy for this condition consists primarily of strict sun avoidance, protective clothing, and physical sunscreens. Beta-carotene may be helpful in some cases. Splenectomy for hemolytic anemia may decrease the photosensitivity.

Lupus Erythematosus. The role of light in the exacerabtion of lupus erythematosus is variable. Topically applied corticosteroids are often helpful in controlling local disease. The lesions respond

---

* This use is not listed by the manufacturer.

* This use is not listed by the manufacturer.

best to potent therapy with fluorinated cortico-steroids, but careful monitoring is necessary to prevent overuse, which may result in skin atrophy. Systemic antimalarial therapy may be indicated for extensive scarring disease. It cannot be overemphasized that the use of these oral agents must be limited to selected patients.

SUNSCREENS

In recent years a variety of sunscreens have become available. Knowledge of the uses and limitations of the sunscreens is necessary in the treatment of photodermatoses. Topical agents include the physical sunscreens (titanium oxide, zinc oxide), which block both visible and ultraviolet light, as well as the chemical sunscreens, which absorb ultraviolet light.

The electromagnetic spectrum involved in photosensitivity disorders includes the ultraviolet spectrum (200–400 nm) and the visible spectrum (400–760 nm). Short-wave ultraviolet light, or UVC (200–290 nm), is screened by Earth's atmosphere and generally is not considered important in the photodermatoses. The UVB band (290–320 nm) is responsible for the sunburn reaction, induction of skin cancers, and certain photosensitivity disorders. Long-wave ultraviolet light, or UVA (320–400 nm), is implicated in a variety of disorders, including many of the drug-induced photodermatoses. Para-aminobenzoic acid (PABA) and its esters provide excellent protection against UVB radiation with few side effects. They are not effective in the treatment of those disorders related to UVA. Non-PABA sunscreens containing benzophenones, cinnamates, and sulfonic acid derivatives are protective in the UVB and, to a certain extent, the UVA spectrum. Complete protection against UVA light is currently not afforded by any of the chemical sunscreens. Adverse effects from these products include local irritation of the skin and the development of photocontact and allergic contact dermatitis. The latter reactions are more common with sunscreens containing PABA and its derivatives. The discoloration of clothing that occurs with PABA can be avoided by the use of PABA esters.

Physical sunscreens (titanium oxide and zinc oxide) are opaque, and their photoprotective properties result from the scattering of both ultraviolet and visible light. Their use is limited to small areas of skin, such as the nose, because of their cosmetic unacceptability and their occlusive properties.

Nevi and Nevoid Tumors

ARTHUR J. SOBER, M.D.

A nevus is a proliferation of one or more cutaneous elements within the skin. These lesions may be either congenital or acquired. For therapeutic considerations, nevi are subdivided into those of melanocytic (nevocytic) origin, those of vascular origin, and those originating from other cutaneous elements. A 10× hand lens and bright room illumination are most helpful in facilitating diagnosis. Consultation with a dermatologist may be useful if the diagnosis is unclear.

MELANOCYTIC NEVI

Junctional, compound, and *dermal nevi* usually require no therapy as long as they can be reliably distinguished from cutaneous melanoma (relatively rare in prepubertal children). When treatment of these nevi is indicated for cosmetic considerations alone, or for chronic irritation, then total excision or shave excision can be performed at the discretion of the physician. Histopathologic examination of all melanocytic nevi removed for whatever reason is essential since an unsuspected melanoma may occasionally be removed as a "benign" nevus.

Halo nevi occur frequently in pediatric populations and are usually of no pathologic significance. The pigmented center should be carefully examined to eliminate the rare possibility of halo melanoma.

Congenital melanocytic nevi fall into two categories: (1) giant—about which there is general agreement that a malignant potential exists that may express early in life, and (2) congenital nevi of the smaller variety—about which there is debate about the malignant potential. The presence of hair is of no help in the management of pigmented nevi. For giant congenital nevi, early full-thickness removal of the entire lesion is recommended. This usually can be accomplished by a combination of staged excisions and grafting. Dermabrasion is not recommended since this procedure will not remove the nevus cells located in the lower reticular dermis or subcutaneous fat. Melanomas have been observed arising in the dermis of giant congenital nevi.

For the smaller congenital nevi, I have in general been recommending prophylactic removal at an age convenient for surgery, since I have seen melanomas arising in association with them. The overall frequency of such occurrences is not clear. The risk of melanoma development in a small congenital nevus which is not removed is at present unknown but is probably relatively low. Other experts on melanomas feel strongly that the prophylactic removal of congenital nevi of the smaller type is unwarranted. I have been recommending full-thickness excision with close margins. Therapeutic recommendations for congenital nevi of the smaller type are evolving, so the reader should check the current literature for subsequent opinions.

Spitz nevi (benign juvenile melanoma, compound spindle cell nevus, epithelioid cell nevus, and so on) need no therapy if recognizable as such. Since this lesion may be difficult for the pathologist to distinguish from malignant melanoma, the slides of any lesion diagnosed as malignant melanoma in a prepubertal child should be sent to an expert melanoma pathologist for confirmation. The physician and patient may be rewarded with the good news that the previously diagnosed "melanoma" was actually a benign lesion (Spitz nevus). No treatment is needed for Spitz nevi, but simple excision with close margins is adequate should removal be desired. Any confusion on clinical grounds with malignant melanoma (since some Spitz nevi may be darkly pigmented) warrants a biopsy.

Therapy is unnecessary for a *blue nevus*, a benign lesion, unless the physician suspects malignant melanoma in which case excisional biopsy with narrow margins is the procedure of choice.

No treatment is needed for a *mongolian spot*, since these lesions usually disappear spontaneously. Of those that fail to disappear, most occur in covered locations and require no therapy. For the rare patient with a mongolian spot of cosmetic concern, the lesion can be effectively covered with an opaque cosmetic (Covermark) matched in color to the patient's skin and applied daily.

VASCULAR NEVI

A plethora of diagnostic terms for these lesions in part contributes to the management confusion.

Capillary nevi (salmon patches, plane nevus, nevus flammeus, telangiectatic nevus, port-wine nevus) usually require no treatment. With the exception of port-wine lesions, capillary nevi on the eyelids fade rapidly and almost all will disappear by the end of the first year of life. Patches on the forehead fade more slowly. Over 50% of lesions on the nape of the neck are still visible at age 1 year, but these present little cosmetic problem. Port-wine lesions increase in size with the growth of the child and have little tendency to fade. Involvement of the trigeminal area may be associated with Sturge-Weber syndrome. Opaque cosmetics matched to the skin tone (Covermark) have been remarkably helpful in hiding the disfigurement. Therapy with the argon laser (especially on the deeper-colored lesions) appears promising.

Cavernous nevi (hemangioma, angiomatous nevi) in the majority of patients require no active therapy. Most important in the management of these lesions is to establish a trusting rapport with the parents. The management of each lesion should be individualized and therapy based on the likelihood of resolution with good cosmetic results without treatment. Regular followup is advised at frequent intervals during periods of rapid growth and at progressively longer intervals when resolution is occurring. Serial photographs of the lesion are helpful in following the course and in the instruction of other parents in what they should expect from their own child's lesion.

The nevi composed of superficial vessels alone can be expected to resolve with good cosmetic results in at least 90% of patients. Those nevi with deeper vessel involvement will involute less frequently, but still the majority (50 to 70%) will undergo complete resolution. Folds of atrophic skin may remain after the deeper lesions have involuted. Resolution is less likely to be complete when mucosal surfaces are involved or when the lesion is large. Fewer than 10% of cavernous nevi ultimately result in any cosmetic handicap, according to Rook. Surgical excision in selected cases may be of use in the late management of noninvoluting lesions.

Therapeutic intervention is triggered by the presence of complications, which include hemorrhage, ulceration, malignant change, encroachment on a vital structure, or thrombocytopenia. Severe hemorrhage following trauma is rare. Ulceration is of no immediate significance but may result in a more conspicuous scar. Local care includes wet to dry dressings with saline or Domeboro solution three to four times daily followed by local application of bacitracin ointment. Malignant change is extremely rare. Thrombocytopenia and encroachment on vital structures have led to the use of systemic prednisone (2 mg/kg/24 hr per one source or $\geq$ 20 mg/24 hr per another source), with improvement usually noted in 2 to 3 weeks. After 3 to 4 weeks of the high doses, the steroid levels can be tapered over an additional 4 weeks. Relapse may require reinstitution of systemic steroids. Therapy also may be necessary for complications resulting from internal organ involvement (rare) by a vascular nevus associated with a cutaneous nevus. X-ray therapy is no longer recommended for management of hemangiomas.

Treatment of *lymphangiomas* by surgery is deceptive, with recurrences frequently resulting even with full-thickness excision and grafting. Lymphangiomas are often best left without treatment.

NEVI OF OTHER CUTANEOUS ELEMENTS

Nevus sebaceus—prophylactic excision with close margins after puberty is recommended to prevent the subsequent development of basal cell carcinoma. Otherwise careful follow-up is necessary. Parents should be informed of the possibility of malignant degeneration.

Connective tissue nevi (shagreen patch, and so on)—other stigmata of tuberous sclerosis should be sought. Examination of the entire skin with long-wave ultraviolet light (Wood light) is recommended. Management is that of the underlying disease. The connective tissue nevus per se needs no treatment.

Epidermal nevi—excision where possible is recommended since these lesions may give rise to basal cell carcinomas. Dermabrasion frequently results in recurrence of the lesion.

Other Skin Tumors

MARY K. SPRAKER, M.D.

Most skin tumors are uncommon in children, but when a lesion does occur it is important that it be diagnosed accurately since some of these tumors indicate underlying systemic disease, some require surgical intervention, and an occasional lesion is malignant.

FACIAL LESIONS

The following lesions are most frequently found on the face and therefore may be confused with acne if they are not carefully examined.

Angiofibromas, inaccurately called *adenoma sebaceum* in the older literature, are the small (1–4 mm) pink or flesh-colored papules seen in association with tuberous sclerosis. They generally begin during early childhood but occasionally are not present until puberty. As the patient ages, the lesions become somewhat larger. They can be effectively treated with cryosurgery, electrodesiccation and curettage, or dermabrasion if removal is necessary for cosmetic reasons. Occasionally a lesion may be solitary; in that case it is not associated with tuberous sclerosis.

Although *trichoepitheliomas* may occur as solitary lesions in early adult life, the other form of the disorder, which is dominantly inherited, begins during childhood or at puberty and is associated with multiple lesions. Small (2–5 mm) flesh-colored papules and nodules are seen on the central area of the face. Solitary lesions should be excised, but with multiple lesions excision is unnecessary. Instead, they are treated with electrodesiccation, cryotherapy, or dermabrasion. While most trichoepitheliomas are benign, there is disagreement in the literature about whether some of these lesions eventually evolve into basal cell carcinomas.

Trichofolliculomas also occur on the face. These flesh-colored papules or dome-shaped nodules classically have a central pore with a protruding tuft of fine hair. The lesion is best treated by surgical excision.

Syringomas frequently first appear during adolescence. Small (1–3 mm) skin-toned or yellowish papules or nodules are seen. They occur on the lower eyelids in more than half the affected patients. Other common locations include the sides of the neck, trunk, extremities, and genital area. It is estimated that one-fifth to one-third of children with Down's syndrome have syringomas. Treatment is necessary only for cosmetic reasons

and consists of destruction by electrodesiccation, cryotherapy, or surgical excision.

Basal cell carcinomas are slow-growing, locally invasive but rarely metastasizing malignant skin tumors that are all too common in older adults but are also seen occasionally in children. They occur most commonly in individuals with fair skin who have been exposed to the sun. Over the past decade we have been seeing more adolescents with basal cell carcinomas of the face; these lesions are frequently mistaken for acne. The lesions begin as small (2 mm) erythematous papules that have a clear or translucent quality and often contain telangiectasias. They enlarge slowly and may undergo some central necrosis and crusting. Occasionally basal cell carcinomas are pigmented and resemble nevi, or they may be sclerosing and resemble scars.

In the *basal cell nevus syndrome,* multiple basal cell carcinomas are associated with other abnormalities including temporal bossing, dental cysts, bifid ribs, intracranial calcifications, ovarian fibromas, and, rarely, medulloblastoma. The disorder is inherited in an autosomal dominant fashion. Skin lesions usually first appear at puberty, although they may occur much earlier.

It is important that basal cell carcinomas be completely removed, since the carcinoma may recur locally if the excision is not complete. The lesions can be surgically excised or removed by curettage and electrodesiccation.

RED-BROWN LESIONS

Pyogenic Granulomas. These solitary, red-to-brown, vascular pedunculated nodules, 5 mm–1 cm in diameter, may develop rapidly on any cutaneous surface. The lesions are round and well circumscribed and clinically may resemble small capillary hemangiomas. The etiology is unclear, but it is thought that trauma to the skin in the presence of pyogenic bacteria causes a reactive proliferative vascular process. These lesions are usually easy to treat. They can be shaved or snipped off parallel to the skin and the base electrodesiccated. The specimen is usually sent for a pathologic examination to confirm the diagnosis and to differentiate this benign lesion from other conditions, including a Spitz nevus or amelanotic melanoma.

Urticaria Pigmentosa. It is not uncommon for the pediatric dermatologist to see children with one or two localized lesions of urticaria pigmentosa known as *mastocytomas.* These red-brown or yellow-brown papules or nodules urticate when rubbed (Darier's sign). They are composed of collections of mast cells in the dermis that release histamine when the skin is traumatized, resulting in the characteristic urtication. Children with just a few of these lesions rarely have systemic symptoms.

Other children, however, have myriads of smaller yellow to red-brown macules or papules that are also composed of mast cells and therefore urticate with stroking. When the disease is this extensive it is known as *urticaria pigmentosa*. Many children have only cutaneous symptoms of the disease, consisting of itching and, sometimes, blister formation. Approximately 10% of patients, however, have systemic involvement, since mast cells can also accumulate in almost any body organ or tisssue, including the bones, liver, spleen, and lymph nodes. Patients with systemic symptoms may have flushing attacks, hypotension, headaches, tachycardia, pruritus, diarrhea, and, rarely, blood clotting abnormalities. These symptoms can be severe and life threatening.

Patients with cutaneous disease alone generally require no therapy unless the lesions are symptomatic; then antihistamines usually help to control pruritus or blistering. The prognosis in most patients is excellent since the lesions resolve spontaneously in time. Children with numerous lesions should avoid aspirin, codeine, morphine, procaine, and polymyxin B because these nonspecific releasers of histamine may cause systemic symptoms. Patients with systemic symptoms may be treated with oral cromolyn, cimetidine combined with an H_1 antihistamine or UVA light therapy with psoralen. Children with many cutaneous lesions should have a complete blood count periodically to check for the presence of mast cell leukemia, which has been reported in a small number of patients.

Juvenile Xanthogranulomas. These yellow to red-brown papules and nodules can be solitary or multiple. They may occur anywhere on the body but are common on the head and neck. They resolve spontaneously after several years. In most patients this is a benign and self-limited problem. However, the disease can also occur in other body organs, including the lung, pericardium, meninges, liver, spleen, and testes. Systemic involvement usually is asymptomatic and requires no treatment or evaluation. However, if lesions are present in the eye, glaucoma or hemorrhage may occur in the absence of treatment. Therefore, any child with this disease should be examined by an ophthalmologist.

Eccrine Poromas. This benign cutaneous tumor, which arises from the sweat duct unit, usually occurs in older adults but has been reported in adolescents. Firm, reddish nodules, 2–12 mm in diameter, are usually seen on the dorsal surface of the foot. The treatment of choice is surgical excision.

FLESH-COLORED LESIONS

Follicular Cysts. This lesion, which is also known as an *epidermal* or *sebaceous cyst*, is a discrete, slowly growing, elevated, firm nodule that may occur anywhere on the body but is commonly seen on the face, scalp, and back. The cyst contains a cheesy white material that has a sour odor. The treatment is surgical excision. The entire cyst, with its epidermal lining, must be removed to prevent recurrence.

Pilomatrixomas. These uncommon solitary deep nodules occur only in children and adolescents. A 0.5–2 cm flesh-colored or reddish-blue nodule is seen on the face, neck, or upper extremities. Treatment is surgical excision.

Neurofibromas. These soft polypoid lesions, which "buttonhole" or invaginate into the underlying dermis when pressure is applied to their surface, may first appear in childhood. Solitary lesions may occur in otherwise normal individuals. However, when multiple lesions are present they are a cutaneous marker for the dominantly inherited disease *neurofibromatosis*.

Connective Tissue Nevi. These single or multiple, slightly raised, skin-colored oval lesions may occur anywhere on the body and may be sign of an inherited condition. Biopsy shows them to be composed of collagen or elastic fibers. The *shagreen patch* seen in tuberous sclerosis is actually a large connective tissue nevus. In the *Buschke-Ollendorff syndrome*, multiple widespread connective tissue nevi are present in association with osteopoikilosis.

Lipomas. These benign nodules, which are soft and rubbery in consistency, may occur on any part of the body. They are composed of mature fat cells. Treatment is not required unless the lesions are large enough to cause a cosmetic problem.

Recurring Digital Fibromas of Childhood. These smooth, shiny, erythematous nodules occur on the distal phalanges of infants and young children. Although there have been some cases of spontaneous resolution, surgical excision is usually recommended. These lesions recur unless excised and dissected down to the periosteum.

Dermatofibromas. Dermatofibromas are small (1 mm–3 cm) dermal nodules that are fixed to the skin but move freely over the subcutaneous fat. They may occur anywhere on the body. They range from flesh colored to brown. Treatment is unnecessary unless there is a cosmetic problem.

SCARS AND KELOIDS

Damaged dermis heals with a *scar* that is initially pink. The color gradually fades to a permanent white, and the scar appears shiny. New scars may be elevated or hypertrophic before they finally flatten and contract, within 6 months to 1 year after the original injury. They must be differentiated from *keloids*, which are an exaggerated connective tissue response to skin injury. Keloids appear long after the original injury and slowly increase in size beyond the area of the original wound. While hypertrophic scars usually require no therapy, as they will flatten in time, keloids do not resolve spontaneously and may continue to enlarge slowly. They can be treated with intralesional injections of corticosteroids; if this fails, surgery can be attempted if it is needed for cosmetic reasons. Surgical excision must be done with care, and intralesional steroids are usually injected both at the time of excision and periodically during the postoperative period to prevent recurrence of the keloid.

The Genodermatoses

SIDNEY HURWITZ, M.D.

The genodermatoses are a group of cutaneous disorders with genetic rather than environmental causes. These include the ichthyoses, ectodermal dysplasias, disorders of collagen and elastic tissue, and diseases of metabolism. Their management requires knowledge of the conditions and their clinical features and of the genetic risks for patients and their families. An important aspect of therapy of the genodermatoses is genetic counseling so that families of affected individuals can evaluate the risk of future pregnancies for themselves and their offspring.

Ichthyosis. Ichthyosis refers to a group of hereditary cutaneous conditions characterized by dryness and scaling. The management of all forms of ichthyosis consists of retardation of water loss, rehydration and softening of the stratum corneum, and alleviation of scaliness and associated pruritus. Ichthyosis vulgaris and sex-linked ichthyosis can be managed quite well by topical application of emollients and the use of keratolytic agents to facilitate the removal of scales from the skin surface. Limited baths with a mild soap or prolonged baths followed by the application of petrolatum and hydration of skin by frequent use of lubricating creams or lotions are helpful. Urea, in concentrations of 10–25%, has a softening and moisturizing effect on the stratum corneum and is helpful in the control of dry skin and pruritus. Propylene glycol (40–60% in water), applied overnight under plastic occlusion, helps hydrate the skin and assists in the desquamation of scales.

Salicylic acid is an effective keratolytic agent, and concentrations between 3 and 6% promote shedding of scales and softening of the stratum corneum. When these agents are used to cover large surface areas for prolonged periods, however, care should be taken to ensure that salicylate toxicity does not occur. Keralyt gel (Westwood Pharmaceuticals), a proprietary preparation containing 6% salicylic acid in propylene glycol, is frequently helpful following hydration of the involved area. Alpha-hydroxy preparations, such as lactic, glycolic, or pyruvic acid, are also beneficial for the treatment of ichthyosiform dermatoses (lactic acid is available as LactiCare lotion). Oral doses of vitamin A have been used in the treatment of lamellar ichthyosis but appear to be ineffective except in larger doses. The hazards of toxicity, therefore, preclude its use in infants and small children with this disorder.

Topically applied vitamin A acid (tretinoin, Retin-A), although potentially irritating, is beneficial in the treatment of lamellar ichthyosis and epidermolytic hyperkeratosis. Drugs that, it is hoped, will revolutionize the therapy of ichthyosis are the synthetic retinoids. Although not recommended for the management of ichthyosis, 13-*cis*-retinoic acid (Accutane, Roche) has been used experimentally. Unfortunately, long-term management is necessary for individuals with ichthyosis, and complications seen in association with this disorder preclude long-term use for the ichthyosiform dermatoses.

Palmoplantar Keratodermas. Palmoplantar keratodermas are a large, heterogeneous group of disorders with punctate or diffuse thickening of the stratum corneum of the palms, soles, or both. Management is similar to that of the ichthyoses, but the palmoplantar keratoses are more difficult to treat. The mechanical removal of thickened stratum corneum can be accomplished by soaking the hands or feet in water for 15–20 minutes, followed by the application of an effective keratolytic agent such as Keralyt gel (with occlusion) and gentle rubbing with a pumice stone while the skin is wet. Salicylic acid (10%) in Aquaphor under occlusion is also helpful in the therapy of this disorder.

Hidrotic Ectodermal Dysplasia. This dysplasia is an autosomal dominant disorder of keratinization characterized by dystrophy of the nails, hyperkeratosis of the palms and soles, and defects of the hair. *Anhidrotic ectodermal dysplasia* is a sex-linked recessive disorder in which more than 90% of affected patients have been male. It is characterized by partial to complete absence of eccrine sweat glands, hair and dental abnormalities, and associated congenital defects. Therapy of anhidrotic ectodermal dysplasia is directed toward temperature regulation, restriction of excessive physical exertion, choice of a suitable occupation, and avoidance of warm climates. Cool baths, air conditioning, light clothing, and reduction of the causes of normal perspiration are beneficial. Dental supervision may help to preserve teeth and reduce cosmetic disfigurement.

Aplasia Cutis Congenita. Aplasia cutis congenita is a localized congenital absence of the epidermis, dermis, and, at times, the subcutaneous tissue. Whether this disorder is inherited is uncertain, but a number of familial cases suggest an autosomal mode of inheritance. The disorder is present at birth, and, although it generally occurs on the scalp, it may also involve the skin of the face, trunk, and extremities. Treatment during the newborn period consists of control of secondary infection. As the child matures, most scars become inconspicuous and require no correction. Obvious scars may be treated by multiple punch-graft hair transplants or surgical excision with plastic repair when the child becomes older.

Pachyonychia Congenita. Pachyonychia congenita is an unusual congenital and sometimes familial disorder inherited in an autosomal dominant fashion and characterized by dyskeratosis of the fingernails and toenails, hyperkeratosis of the palms and soles, follicular keratosis (especially about the knees and elbows), hyperhidrosis of the palms and soles, oral leukokeratosis, and, in some instances, epidermal inclusion cysts and steatocystoma multiplex. The lesions persist for life, and treatment is directed toward relief of the hyperkeratosis by the use of oral vitamin A in large doses, 20% urea in an emollient cream, 60% propylene glycol in water under occlusion, or 6% salicylic acid in a gel containing propylene glycol (Keralyt gel), which aids in the debridement of the excessive keratin. The nails may be treated by surgical avulsion, with scraping of the matrix, to prevent regrowth.

Acrodermatitis Enteropathica. Acrodermatitis enteropathica is a hereditary disorder that appears in early infancy and is characterized by acral and periorificial vesicobullous, pustular, and eczematoid skin lesions, alopecia, nail dystrophy, diarrhea, glossitis, stomatitis, and frequent secondary infection due to bacterial or candidal organisms. Diiodohydroxyquin is no longer considered the treatment of choice for this disorder. Zinc gluconate or zinc sulfate is highly effective in dosages of 5 mg/kg/day given two or three times a day. With adequate therapy (100–200 mg/day) most patients improve in temperament, showing a decrease in irritability (usually within 1 or 2 days). The appetite improves in a few days, and diarrhea and skin lesions begin to respond within 2–3 days after the initiation of therapy. Hair growth begins after 2 or 3 weeks of therapy, and an increase in the growth rate of the infant generally occurs in approximately 2 months.

Familial Benign Pemphigus. Familial benign pemphigus (Hailey and Hailey disease) is an autosomal dominant genodermatosis characterized by recurrent vesicles and bullae that most often appear on the sides and back of the neck, the axillae, the groin, and the perianal region. Exacerbations commonly occur during the hot summer months, in the form of small vesicles or, more usually, superficially crusted erosions in intertriginous areas. Therapy should be directed at relief of the precipitating factors: heat, humidity, and friction. Although topical antibiotics may be helpful in some cases, systemic antibiotics chosen on the basis of bacterial culture and sensitivity studies seem to be most effective in the treatment of this disorder. Topical and systemic corticosteroids may also be useful in some cases. Systemic corticosteroids, however, are not generally recommended, since the disorder frequently recurs when the dosage levels are reduced. In persistent cases, when patients have been disabled by painfully eroded plaques unresponsive to other therapeutic measures, excision of the involved regions, followed by split-thickness skin grafts, has been helpful.

Epidermolysis Bullosa. Epidermolysis bullosa (EB) is a term applied to a group of inherited disorders characterized by bullous lesions that develop spontaneously or as a result of varying degrees of trauma.

Mild cases of the dystrophic and nondystrophic types of EB may be compatible with a nearly normal existence. Severe disease, however, remains a challenge and requires cooperation by the patient, parents, and physician. Nursing care and adequate dental attention for patients with severe EB are time consuming and difficult. Since lesions result from mechanical injury, measures should be taken to relieve pressure and to prevent unnecessary trauma. A cool environment, avoidance of overheating, and lubrication of the skin to decrease friction help control blister formation. Extension of blisters may be prevented and pain may be reduced by aseptic aspiration of blister fluid.

A water mattress with a soft fleece covering limits friction. Daily baths, nonadherent dressings such as petrolatum-impregnated gauze, and topical antibiotics control infection and promote spontaneous healing. Large denuded areas may be treated by the open method (as in the treatment of burns) with intravenous fluids and systemic antibiotics. Prophylactic antibiotics also help reduce the risk of glomerulonephritis secondary to cutaneous streptococcal infection.

Dysphagia is a major symptom of esophageal involvement in recessive dystrophic EB. Softening of the diet may improve symptoms, but if conservative management fails bougienage or surgery, or both, may be considered. Restoration of function in severe fusion and flexion deformities of the hands and feet will be helped by physiotherapy and plastic surgery. A recent development in the management of severe recessive dystrophic EB has been the use of oral phenytoin (Dilantin)* in dosages of 2.5–5.0 mg/kg/day, to a maximum of 300 mg/day (a dosage high enough to obtain serum

---

* This use is not listed in the manufacturer's directive.

levels of 5–12 μg/ml). Early trials suggest that up to two-thirds of patients with recessive dystrophic EB are likely to benefit from this form of therapy, but the results of double-blind studies are still awaited.

It is the responsibility of the physician to inform parents of the risks associated with transmitting genetic abnormalities. Support and information groups are beneficial to many families who have children with epidermolysis bullosa. The Dystrophic Epidermolysis Bullosa Research Association is an international group dedicated to research and support for patients with all forms of EB and their families. For information regarding this organization one should contact Arlene Pessar, R.N.; D.E.B.R.A. of America, Inc.; 2936 Avenue W; Brooklyn, N.Y. 11229, USA.

Disorders of the Hair and Scalp

ANNE W. LUCKY, M.D.

INFECTIOUS DISEASES

Bacterial Folliculitis and Impetigo of the Scalp. Scalp folliculitis is most commonly caused by *Staphylococcus aureus* and less commonly by Group A *beta hemolytic streptococci*. It is often found in association with seborrheic or atopic dermatitis of the scalp. Clinically the primary lesions are pustules surrounding hair follicles, but secondary erythema, oozing, crusting, edema, tenderness, and ultimately, abscess formation with cervical lymphadenopathy are common. Predisposing factors include occlusion by greasy hair preparations, impetigo elsewhere, and trauma. Bacterial folliculitis must be distinguished from a kerion, a hypersensitivity reaction to fungal infection. A diagnosis of folliculitis is confirmed by culturing the pustules. Fungal and bacterial disease may coexist. Treatment should be tailored to the particular bacterial organism found on culture using systemic antibiotics such as erythromycin in doses of 30 to 50 mg/kg/day or dicloxacillin in doses of 25 to 75 mg/kg/day orally. A 10 to 14 day course is usually sufficient but may be prolonged if infection lingers. Adjunctive local care should consist of a keratolytic shampoo (see seborrheic dermatitis) when scale is present and warm soaks with an antiseptic such as Burow's solution to remove accumulated crusts. The family should be instructed in careful hygiene, separating the infected patient's personal items (i.e., towels, combs, and hats) from those of other family members until infection has cleared. Resistant or recurrent cases may result if pathogenic organisms are harbored in the nasopharynx or on the skin of the patient or close contacts. Nasopharyngeal colonization re-

quires topical therapy with an antibiotic ointment such as bacitracin or polymyxin (Polysporin).

Seborrheic Dermatitis, Eczema, and Psoriasis. Seborrheic dermatitis (cradle cap) and atopic dermatitis (eczema) involving the scalp are similar clinically and pathogenetically and will be considered together. "Cradle cap" of infancy is responsive to therapy. If scaling and pruritus persist or appear in later childhood we often consider that the entire picture had been a manifestation of atopic dermatitis. The typical lesions are adherent, greasy, white to yellow scales, which appear first in patches on the scalp and eventually may cover the entire scalp surface. The scalp is pruritic, and secondary excoriations with infection are frequent. There is erythema, scale, fissuring and weeping behind the ears. Greasy yellow scales and erythema can be found in the eyebrows, along the nasolabial folds, in the neck folds, axillae, and groin. Severe infantile seborrheic dermatitis occurs between the ages of three weeks and three months. Treatment of seborrhea and eczema consists of antiseborrheic shampoos that may contain any of a number of products to reduce itching, scaling, and erythema. Such products include sulfur and salicylic acid, pyrithione zinc, coal tar, and selenium sulfide. The shampoo should be applied daily to the scalp and left on for at least 5 minutes before washing off. This should be continued until all scale is removed. Shampooing can be reduced in frequency as clinical improvement occurs. Excessive use of antiseborrheic shampoos may dry out the scalp and produce scaling that can be confused with the original pathologic process. In persistent cases, overnight applications of a phenol and saline solution (Bakers P&S) are helpful in removing excessive scale. If antiseborrheic shampoos irritate the scalp, a mild, bland shampoo plus topical steroid lotions such as 1% hydrocortisone lotion or, in severe cases, 0.1% triamcinolone lotion will hasten resolution and rapidly bring relief of pruritus.

Psoriasis may appear in childhood as single or multiple stubborn plaques of erythema and scale in the scalp or as generalized scaling. Erythematous plaques with silvery scale may be present on elbows, knees, genitalia, and intergluteal clefts and diaper area in infants. Nails are often studded with 1 mm pits. Psoriasis is usually not as pruritic as atopic dermatitis. Scalp lesions may be the only sign of psoriasis in childhood. Treatment of scalp psoriasis is similar to that outlined for seborrheic dermatitis with tar shampoos and topical steroids being especially useful.

Tinea Capitis (Scalp Ringworm). Tinea capitis is fungal infection of the scalp and hair shaft. Tinea capitis due to *Trichophyton tonsurans* must always be considered in the differential diagnosis of seborrheic dermatitis. *Trichophyton tonsurans* is now the infective agent in over 90% of cases in most areas of the U.S.A., whereas *Microsporum audouini* once was the primary dermatophyte. A few cases acquired from kittens and puppies are caused by *Microsporum canis*. The most common presentation is diffuse scaling mimicking seborrheic dermatitis with patchy and diffuse hair loss. Since *T. tonsurans* invades the hair shafts (endothrix infection), hairs become fragile and break at the level of the scalp, leaving characteristic "black dots." *T. tonsurans* differs from *Microsporum* infections because it does *not* fluoresce with a Wood's light and is *not* limited to prepubertal children. *T. tonsurans* is a chronic disorder, carried asymptomatically by many children. It can produce lesions on the skin (tinea corporis) which serve as reservoirs of infection. In some cases, an inflammatory reaction, a kerion, may occur. A kerion is a boggy, erythematous, tender mass studded with perifollicular pustules. These pustules may be sterile or contain *S. aureus*. A kerion is the host's cellular immune response to the fungal infection. Systemic symptoms such as fever, diffuse maculopapular rash (or "id"), leukocytosis, and lymphadenopathy may accompany a kerion.

The only effective treatment is systemic griseofulvin. Topical antifungal agents are ineffective. Griseofulvin (microsize) is given in a single daily dose of 15 to 20 mg/kg/day. It is available as a suspension (Grifulvin V, 125 mg/tsp) or as capsules which may be opened and fed to young children who cannot swallow the tablets. Absorption is enhanced by a fatty meal (i.e., milk, ice cream, yogurt). Adjunctive therapy includes 2.5% selenium sulfide lotion (Selsun Brown, Excel) used as a shampoo twice weekly. This acts as a sporicidal agent and reduces shedding of spores significantly. With systemic griseofulvin treatment it usually takes 6 to 8 weeks for fungal cultures to become negative. In refractory cases, the dose of griseofulvin should be raised and the length of treatment increased. Complete blood counts and liver function tests may or may not be measured when treatment is initiated, but should certainly be followed with prolonged therapy or therapy at increased dosage. Treatment of a kerion requires griseofulvin and systemic antibiotics if secondary infection with *S. aureus* is documented. Systemic or intralesional glucocorticoids have been advocated by some physicians to hasten resolution of kerions, but there are no data to support the contention that kerions resolve faster or that scarring is reduced. Ketoconazole is a relatively new systemic antifungal agent that may be useful for tinea capitis but is not yet approved for this purpose.

SCARRING ALOPECIAS

Cutis Aplasia Congenita. Congenital absence of the skin in single or multiple patches on the scalp leaves a thin, shiny, parchment-like hairless scar that is prone to breakdown and secondary infection and crust formation. Such lesions are often mistaken for trauma secondary to a fetal monitor. Underlying bony defects may be present and skull x-rays should be taken. In later life, excision of small lesions that do not have underlying skeletal defects may be warranted for cosmetic purposes. Nonhealing lesions may require excision and primary closure or grafting in infancy.

Nevus Sebaceus of Jadassohn. Nevus sebaceus is a hamartoma of the epidermis. There is overgrowth of sebaceous and apocrine elements and underdevelopment of hair follicles. Such lesions are present at birth and are usually found on the scalp and face. Nevus sebaceous is one of the main causes of localized congenital alopecia. The lesions are yellow to orange pebbly plaques that become more prominent at puberty. In the third and fourth decades of life tumors such as basal cell epitheliomas or squamous cell carcinomas may develop. Because of the cosmetic appearance and the malignant potential, excision (under local anesthesia when possible) is recommended either in infancy or in the preteen years.

Other Scarring Alopecias. Scarring alopecias may occur as a result of a number of infections and inflammatory disorders affecting the scalp such as bacterial folliculitis and tinea capitis. Systemic disorders such as lupus erythematosus, morphea, and lichen planus can result in permanent hair loss. Scarring alopecia of unknown etiology leaving a "footprint in the snow" pattern has been termed pseudopelade of Brocq. Traction from tight braids or pony tails may at first cause transient hair loss, but eventually will permanently destroy hair follicles. No therapy short of localized hair transplantation is effective.

NON-SCARRING ALOPECIAS

Alopecia Areata. Alopecia areata is one of the most common causes of alopecia in childhood. There is a spectrum from single to multiple coin-sized areas of spontaneous complete hair loss (alopecia areata), to total loss of all scalp hair (alopecia totalis), to universal loss of scalp and body hair (alopecia universalis). Occasionally diffuse hair loss precedes the patchy lesions. Histopathologically, alopecia areata is characterized by swarms of lymphocytes surrounding the hair bulb. Other autoimmune disorders such as vitiligo, Hashimoto's thyroiditis, diabetes, and hypoparathyroidism may be associated with alopecia areata. Many patients will have characteristic linear pitting of the nails. Alopecia areata has spontaneous remissions and exacerbations. Theories that alopecia areata is a psychosomatic disorder related to stress have not been well substantiated. As a rule, the younger the child and the more extensive the hair loss, the less likely it is that regrowth will occur.

Loss in the ophiasis pattern, around the margins of the scalp, also indicates a poor prognosis.

Treatment must be individualized and is often not successful. Therapy with intralesional steroids (triamcinolone acetonide, 1 ml of 5 to 10 mg/ml suspension) can be successful in limited cases, but may require multiple and repeated courses of therapy. No more than 10 mg of triamcinolone should be given every 4 to 6 weeks to avoid systemic effects from the intralesional steroids. High-potency topical steroids may be useful in a child too young or too afraid to cooperate with intralesional injections. Systemic steroids are *not* recommended in growing children. There are serious side effects, not the least of which is growth retardation. Even if systemic steroid therapy is successful in allowing regrowth of hair, when the steroids are tapered hair loss usually recurs. Newer forms of therapy promoted in the recent literature include topical 1% or 3% minoxidil which will soon be available, and sensitization to dinitrochlorobenzene (DNCB) or squaric acid ester. This form of therapy has raised questions about potentially stimulating the immune system and causing malignancy. Simple irritation of the scalp with such substances as topical retinoic acid (Retin-A) or anthralin have met with fair success. Although some groups have advocated the use of systemic psoralens and ultraviolet A light (PUVA), the efficacy and safety of this procedure in childhood has not yet been established. Psychological adjustment of the child to alopecia areata is best reflected by the attitude of the parents and the physician. Support and encouragement without specific therapy is often the best treatment.

Traumatic Hair Loss. Traumatic hair loss is usually either self-induced by compulsive hair pulling (trichotillomania) or inappropriate use of hair cosmetics or hair styling. Hair loss secondary to trauma is usually nonscarring and is a combination of traction from the bulb and breakage of the shaft. Repeated trauma to the hair bulb may eventually cause permanent scarring alopecia. Trichotillomania appears as isolated or multiple areas of alopecia. It is identified by the presence of fractured, unevenly broken off, short hairs. There are some pathognomonic histologic features, and thus scalp biopsy may be useful. It may be a sign of underlying emotional or psychologic conflict and if persistent and severe, the child and family should be referred for appropriate counseling. It is often impossible to obtain a positive history of compulsive hair pulling from parent or child. Traction alopecia occurs primarily in small children whose hair is kept in tight braids or pony tails. Rubber bands can sever the hair shafts, but the traction itself will cause disruption of the hair bulb and a permanent hair loss pattern, especially around the scalp margins. The only treatment is advice on hair styling. Overzealous cosmetic treatments can produce broken hairs, secondary to increased fragility. Home permanent waves, chemical hair straighteners, blow dryers, and hot combs are major causes of traumatic hair loss. In this condition the number and density of hairs in the scalp are normal but the hairs are broken. Discontinuation of all treatment to the hair except a mild shampoo and conditioner is warranted. Conditioners render the hair easier to comb with fewer tangles. Hair is more fragile when wet and thus combing should be done after drying.

Diffuse Hair Loss. Diffuse hair loss may result from a wide variety of causes. Normal hair loss occurs at the rate of 100 hairs per day. Thinning of the scalp hair may not be noticeable until a large percentage of scalp hair is gone, and thus increased shedding of hair may be the initial complaint. Telogen effluvium is the term used for the phenomenon of a large number of hairs going into the resting (telogen) stage of growth at the same time and then falling out. Telogen effluvium may follow 2 to 3 months after a severe illness with high fever (e.g., typhoid fever, scarlet fever, or Kawasaki disease). It is physiologic in infants and their mothers approximately 3 months postpartum. Occasionally alopecia areata may begin with diffuse hair loss. Endocrine causes such as hypo- or hyperthyroidism and excessive levels of androgens from ovarian or adrenal origin may present with diffuse hair loss. Female pattern baldness or so-called "androgenetic" alopecia consists of thinning of the hair predominantly over the crown of the scalp. It may be a familial trait or result from elevated circulating plasma androgens in teenage girls. Deficiencies of trace elements such as zinc or iron, essential fatty acids, proteins, or multiple nutritional losses such as seen in marasmus or anorexia nervosa can produce diffuse hair loss. Finally, a careful history of drug exposure including thallium, mercury, propranolol, and chemotherapy or radiation therapy must be considered in differential diagnosis. Treatment depends on discovering the underlying cause.

Disorders of Sebaceous Glands and Sweat Glands

ALAN R. SHALITA, M.D.

DISORDERS OF SEBACEOUS GLANDS

Acne Vulgaris. The primary lesion of acne is a microcomedo not visible to the naked eye. This is the precursor of the more mature, visible lesions—open comedones (blackheads), closed comedones (whiteheads), papules, pustules, and nodulocystic lesions. Therapy, therefore, should be directed against the pathogenic factors and the primary lesions.

Since the microcomedo, the primary lesion, results from abnormal follicular keratinization, initial therapy should include the topical application of tretinoin, the only drug that effectively interrupts this process. Treatment is begun with either the 0.05% cream or the 0.01% gel (the cream being less drying). Despite the different concentrations of active ingredient, these two preparations are of approximately equal effectiveness because of better penetration of the drug from the gel vehicle. Patients should be warned that there may be initial redness and peeling from this drug and, in some cases, an actual worsening of the condition for the first 2–4 weeks of treatment. Excessive irritation can be countered by alternate-day application.

For comedonal acne, tretinoin alone is usually sufficient. In mild forms, such as that seen in prepubertal children, a less potent agent, such as 0.5–3% salicylic acid in alcohol, used as a cleanser, may be sufficient. In more advanced forms of comedonal acne, particularly those that have not responded to low concentrations of tretinoin, the dosage may be increased to 0.1% cream or 0.025% gel. Those patients whose acne remains refractory should be tried on the 0.05% liquid, the most potent and irritating form of tretinoin.

Most patients with acne also have one or more inflammatory lesions (papules, pustules, cysts) accompanying the comedones. For these patients the addition of a topical antibacterial agent is useful. Topical benzoyl peroxide (2.5–10%) or a topical antibiotic (erythromycin, clindamycin) is useful for this purpose. In general, one recommends the use of tretinoin once a day and a topical antibacterial at another time of day. For patients whose skin is too sensitive for this sequential regimen, tretinoin and the antibacterial agent may be alternated on different days. Cream forms of meclocycline and erythromycin are available for those patients who do not tolerate the hydroalcoholic vehicles.

Most recently, 5% benzoyl peroxide and 3% erythromycin have been combined in one formulation, a hydroalcoholic gel that requires mixing at the time of dispensing and must be refrigerated to maintain its freshness. This preparation may also be used in a sequential regimen with tretinoin.

For more severe inflammatory acne, the addition of systemic broad-spectrum antibiotics is indicated. Tetracycline* or erythromycin is the initial drug of choice at a dosage of 1 gm/day. The dosage may be reduced after 1 month according to the patient's response. Patients must be cautioned to take these drugs on an empty stomach in order to maximize absorption, i.e., 1 hour before or 2 hours after meals. Patients should also be warned not to take these medications with vitamin preparations

containing minerals or with iron supplements. Vaginal candidiasis is a not-infrequent complication in women but can usually be treated with local antimonilial therapy without decreasing the antibiotic dosage. Photosensitivity may also occur but is not common.

Minocycline is better absorbed than tetracycline or erythromycin, giving high skin tissue levels and superior clinical response. Less attention is required to when the drug is taken, and it is not photosensitizing. It may cause a dose-related vertigo, but this is usually alleviated by reducing the dose from 50 mg qid to 50 mg tid or bid. The therapeutic advantages of minocycline must be weighed against its cost.

Patients who do not respond to these treatment programs should be considered candidates for treatment with isotretinoin. Isotretinoin (13-cis-retinoic acid) has proved to be dramatically effective in treating patients with severe nodulocystic acne who have not responded to conventional therapy, including systemic antibiotics. The drug is administered in a dose of 1 mg/kg for 4–5 months. Although more than 90% of patients will show a good to excellent response, the time frame is variable, and some patients may not exhibit maximum therapeutic response until after the drug has been discontinued. Some patients may even have flares of their disease during treatment.

Isotretinoin causes numerous side effects, and the prescribing physician should be thoroughly familiar with the latest package insert at the time of prescription. The drug is teratogenic and therefore is contraindicated in pregnant women. All female patients of childbearing age should be adequately advised of this fact, and a pregnancy test should be obtained before therapy is initiated. Ideally, one would not begin treatment in women until the first menses after a negative pregnancy test.

The most common side effect of isotretinoin is dryness, manifested as cheilitis, xerosis, and conjunctivitis. This may be managed with simple emollients. Muscle aches and bone pain are not uncommon but usually respond to simple analgesia. Bony exostoses have been reported but do not appear to be clinically significant at this time.

A variety of laboratory abnormalities have also been reported in patients receiving isotretinoin. The most important and consistent of these is triglyceride elevation. Therefore, triglycerides should be monitored biweekly until stabilized.

Further, it should be noted that patients receiving both tetracyclines and isotretinoin may have an increased risk of developing pseudotumor cerebri. It is therefore recommended that these drugs not be given concomitantly. Rather, flares of acne during isotretinoin treatment may be managed with intralesional injection of triamcinolone ace-

---

* Use of tetracycline during tooth development (through eighth year) may cause permanent tooth discoloration.

tonide (5 mg/cc) or short courses of prednisone (20–30 mg/day tapered to 0 over 10–14 days).

Older teenaged females with refractory acne may have an underlying endocrine problem. Elevations of ovarian or adrenal androgen may be treated with oral contraceptives or low-dose dexamethasone (0.25–0.5 mg/day).

Local treatment in the physician's office is frequently of significant adjunctive benefit. Large inflammatory lesions may be treated by the intralesional injection of triamcinolone acetonide (2.5–5.0 mg/cc), and comedones may be removed by acne surgery. Although these procedures do not affect the overall course of the disease, they enhance patient compliance by providing more rapid improvement in clinical appearance.

Finally, patients should be instructed in the proper use of cleansers. In general, they should avoid harsh, abrasive cleansers and use nonirritating preparations, particularly if under treatment with agents that are already causing peeling. Greasy hair pomades, oily make-up, and heavy "moisturizing" lotions and creams should also be avoided. Astringent cleansers may be used to remove excess oil.

Neonatal Acne. Mild acne may occur in infants during the first 6 months of life as a result of stimulation of the sebaceous follicles by maternal androgen. Usually this requires no treatment, but the judicious use of a mild salicylic acid cleanser may be efficacious. Rarely, benzoyl peroxide or the topical application of erythromycin may be necessary for a brief period.

DISORDERS OF SWEAT GLANDS

Hyperhidrosis. Hyperhidrosis occurs in both generalized and localized varieties. Generalized hyperhidrosis usually occurs in association with an internal disorder, such as hypothalamic lesions, thyrotoxicosis, fever, lymphomas, or pheochromocytoma. Localized hyperhidrosis is generally restricted to the palms and soles or the axillae. It most frequently occurs in relation to stress or anxiety and causes considerable embarrassment and discomfort, but it is not an indicator of pathology.

Localized hyperhidrosis may be treated with oral anticholinergic drugs, but their benefit is limited by their side effects. Solutions of 15–25% aluminum chloride in absolute ethanol are usually effective. Commercially available aluminum salt preparations are beneficial in the early stages, but there is frequent escape from their sweat-inhibitory effects. Iontophoresis has been reported to be beneficial in patients refractory to aluminum salts. Recently, it has been suggested that some patients may be helped by counseling to reduce stress and by biofeedback training.

Miliaria. There are two common types of miliaria, miliaria crystallina and miliaria rubra. Miliaria crystallina occurs after damage to the epidermis from sunburn or mild thermal burn. This produces occlusion of the sweat pores, and sweating then results in small retention vesicles. The lesions are generally asymptomatic and will resolve either spontaneously or following treatment with a mild exfoliating agent, such as 3% salicylic acid in 70% alcohol.

Miliaria rubra (prickly heat) is an erythematous rash, consisting of papules or vesicles, that is associated with increased heat, humidity, and sweating. The lesions are frequently pruritic or produce a stinging sensation. A variety of factors that produce sweat duct occlusion in the mid or lower epidermis appear to be pathogenic.

Treatment involves placing the patient in a cool, dry environment whenever possible. Soothing, drying lotions such as white shake lotion may be beneficial, as is the liberal application of zinc stearate powder or talcum powder.

Hypohidrotic Ectodermal Dysplasia. Hypohidrotic ectodermal dysplasia is a congenital disease that is usually inherited as an X-linked recessive trait, thus affecting only males. These individuals have markedly decreased or absent sweating associated with a variety of defects in the teeth, hair, and nails. Infants with this condition may present with high fever and require immediate attention to prevent damage to the central nervous system. Proper counseling is most important. Patients must avoid strenuous exercise and heat. Fever should be treated with antipyretics and with cooling baths and alcohol sponging.

Miscellaneous Dermatoses

STEPHEN E. GELLIS, M.D.

Juvenile plantar dermatosis is a condition seen in children aged 3–10 that appears symmetrically in the weight-bearing areas of the feet as shiny and fissured skin. It is thought to result from the chronic exposure of the feet to a humid environment produced by occlusive footwear. The condition may also have an association with atopic dermatitis. Treatment consists of the avoidance of occlusive footwear such as running shoes and rubber boots. The purchase of well-aired shoes and the placement of insoles may be helpful. In acute flare-ups, topical steroids and soaks in an oil and tar preparation (Polytar, Balnetar) are somewhat useful.

Perioral dermatitis is an eruption of unknown etiology that appears as small asymptomatic papules and scaling surrounding the skin of the nose and mouth. It is usually seen in young females and younger children and may be a variant of acne. A brief course of tetracycline, 250 mg twice a day for 3 weeks, will clear most cases. For children under age 12, tetracycline should not be prescribed because of its potential for producing dental staining. In this age group, topical keratolytics such as benzoyl peroxide and topical antibiotics may be tried. Topical steroids may aggravate the condition and should be avoided.

Keratosis pilaris is a common condition in children who have either a personal or a family history of atopy. It consists of keratotic papules 1–2 mm in size over the extensor aspect of the arms, the thighs, and occasionally the cheeks. At times, entrapped hairs may be seen within the papules. The eruption is more prominent in dry environments. Treatment consists of the use of emollients, particularly those containing urea or lactic acid (U-Lactin, Nutraplus, Lacticare, Aquacare). Increasing the humidity in the bedroom at night with a vaporizer or humidifier is also effective. In extensive cases, a keratolytic gel (Keralyte), applied with plastic occlusion overnight, will remove the keratotic papules temporarily. Manual removal by rubbing with a pumice stone while the skin is wet may also be tried.

16

The Eye

The Eye

ROBERT W. LINGUA, M.D.

EVALUATION OF THE NEWBORN

The Term Infant

Neonatal Ophthalmia. The first ocular therapeutic intervention occurs at birth, with the instillation of an antimicrobial drug to prevent ophthalmia neonatorum. Silver nitrate, 1% (bacteriocidal), although still widely accepted as adequate for the prevention of gonococcal conjunctivitis, has been replaced by 0.5% erythromycin ointment (bacteriostatic) or 1% tetracycline, particularly when infants are considered to be at risk for chlamydial infection. Therapy can be more specific when a particular agent is identified on smears or cultures or when a characteristic lesion was noted in the birth canal.

INFECTION IN THE BIRTH CANAL. Mothers discovered to have a gonococcal process at the time of birth are treated with systemic doses of penicillin (aqueous crystalline), as are the infants (20,000–50,000 U IV, given once, for low- to normal birthweight infants, respectively). An active herpetic lesion in the birth canal is best avoided by cesarean section; if the lesion is discovered after birth, antiviral trifluridine (Viroptic) is added to the usual antibacterial prophylactic (the eye may serve as a point of entry for systemic disease), ophthalmologic consultation is requested for evaluation of the cornea and retina, and careful monitoring for systemic involvement is begun.

CONJUNCTIVITIS IN THE NEWBORN. Initial therapy of ongoing conjunctivitis detected in the newborn of an asymptomatic parent is chosen on the basis of a presumptive diagnosis appropriate to the clinical and historical features. The time of onset of the discharge is useful as a general guide to which organism may be the offending agent, but it is not to be considered diagnostic or used as the sole basis for selecting initial therapy. Ocular hyperemia without a copious discharge or lid erythema or edema in the first 24–48 hours of life is most likely a sign of the chemical conjunctivitis caused by the silver nitrate prophylaxis, if that was the chosen method. No treatment is recommended. Chemical conjunctivitis has not been recognized after erythromycin or tetracycline prophylaxis. Follow-up evaluation in 48 hours is recommended to be sure that these findings were not the prodrome of a more significant infection. Conjunctivitis in the immediate postnatal period that is characterized by intense ocular hyperemia, thick and copious yellow discharge, and lid edema is considered hyperacute and gonococcal in origin until cultures prove otherwise. When gonococcal conjunctivitis is strongly suspected, smears and cultures are taken, and irrigation, one of the most important therapeutic maneuvers, is begun and repeated every 2 hours until clinical improvement is observed. The child should be isolated, with secretion precautions taken, until the diagnosis is proved incorrect by laboratory testing or until systemic therapy has been given for 24 hours. Several doses of erythromycin ophthalmic ointment may be used as initial broad-spectrum therapy if there is a delay in obtaining laboratory results. The ultimate choice of the antibiotic is based on the smears. For gram-negative intracellular diplococci, erythromycin ointment may be continued, but the mainstay of therapy is systemic penicillin (aqueous crystalline C, 50,000 U/kg/day in two doses for 7 days). The parents should also be evaluated for infection. Methods of instilling the prophylactic agent at birth vary; therefore, a hyperacute conjunctivitis occurring up to a week after birth may still represent gonococcal disease if subtherapeutic doses were given in the nursery. For all other bacterial infections (staphylococcal, streptococcal), topical therapy with erythromycin ointment tid for 2 weeks will suffice. Any infant

483

not responding in 48 hours or in whom corneal involvement is suspected may be referred for ophthalmologic consultation. In stubborn cases, scrapings of the conjunctival epithelial should be taken since a finding of chlamydial infection at this time can be of diagnostic assistance should the infant later develop a pneumonitis.

CHLAMYDIAL INFECTION. Chlamydial pneumonitis can occur in infants after chlamydial conjunctivitis. Oral doses of erythromycin, 30–50 mg/kg/day for 14 days (3 weeks if a pneumonitis coexists), are suggested. When the conjunctiva is markedly inflamed and the discharge is copious, concurrent topical 0.5% erythromycin ointment is added bid for several days, until the lids open and close freely and the clinical signs improve. Both parents of infants in whom a definitive diagnosis has been established should be treated. A more persistent chlamydial infection, lymphogranuloma venereum, which is increasing in incidence, requires 3 weeks of oral erythromycin therapy.

HERPETIC DISEASE. Any evidence of vesicular lesions on the infant should prompt a reevaluation of both the parents and the infant for other signs of herpetic disease. When the mother is discovered to have an asymptomatic lesion in the birth canal, or if a lesion is discovered on the infant, even at a site remote from the eye, antiviral prophylaxis is suggested (Viroptic) and the infant should be monitored for systemic involvement. Antiviral agents may cause ocular hyperemia, corneal epithelial defects, and tearing when used for long periods, and consultation with an ophthalmologist is advisable when they are given either prophylactically or therapeutically.

The Premature Infant

The premature infant who requires intensive care presents additional ophthalmologic concerns. When intubation and pancuronium bromide (Pavulon) administration are required, or in other situations of depressed neurologic function, lid function and therefore ocular lubrication may be compromised, leading to corneal scarring. Ocular ointments are preferable (e.g., Lacri-Lube q 4 h) to liquid preparations since the latter are of only brief benefit and evaporate quickly in the warmth of an isolette. Antibiotic preparations are not required unless secondary infection has ensued.

In the infant considered at risk for retinopathy of prematurity, ophthalmologic consultation is required to monitor the process. Vitamin E is given to replenish the low levels commonly seen in premature infants, although the administration of pharmacologic doses to protect against an increased incidence or severity of the retinopathy has yet to be uniformly accepted. An increase in the incidence of sepsis and necrotizing enterocolitis has been reported in association with large oral doses of vitamin E. Vitamin E sufficiency is considered to exist at the 0.6–0.8 mg % plasma level. Many premature infants have levels at the 1.0–1.2 mg % level. Regardless, when supplemental vitamin E is administered, plasma levels should be monitored twice a week to insure that the concentration does not exceed 3.5 mg %, above which the side effects of this agent are much increased.

Agents given to dilate the pupil for an examination of the retina should be used with discretion. Phenylephrine (Neo-Synephrine) may raise the systolic pressure 20 mm Hg, according to some reports, and has also been associated with ventricular hemorrhage. Blanching of the eyelids after its use is common and is not pathologic. The cycloplegic preparations have also been associated with significant elevations in blood pressure. To reduce the potential for side effect in low-birth-weight infants, one drop of 2.5% Neo-Synephrine and 1% cyclopentolate (1% Cyclogyl), once in each eye, is sufficient. A combination preparation can be made up by the pharmacy in an aseptic way to contain a net concentration of 2.5% phenylephrine, 0.5% Mydriacil, and 0.5% Cyclogyl by combining 7 cc of 1% Mydriacil, 3.5 cc of 10% Neo-Synephrine, and 3.5 cc of 2% Cyclogyl. One drop of the combination is adequate for indirect ophthalmoscopy, and the potential for side effects is minimal.

CONGENITAL OPACIFICATIONS OF THE VISUAL AXIS

Two ophthalmic surgical emergencies of infancy are congenital glaucoma and the total and dense congenital cataract.

The uncontrolled intraocular pressure of glaucoma exerts pressure on the vasculature of the optic nerve. If it is not relieved, permanent visual compromise can occur. Since this form of glaucoma is unresponsive to topical medication, the treatment is surgical; a goniotomy or trabeculotomy may be performed to establish an outflow path for the aqueous humor. When early diagnosis allows prompt intervention, the prognosis is very good.

For complete neuroanatomic development to occur along the visual pathways, a formed image must be carried to the visual cortex from the eye. Therefore, clearing an obstructive cataract from the visual axis and prompt optical rehabilitation are essential in the first 10 weeks of life, or a permanent reduction in the child's visual acuity will result.

Infants who have had surgery for cataract or glaucoma may require topical hypotensive agents that can affect other medical conditions. Timoptic (beta blocker), one such preparation, can aggravate asthmatic symptoms. Echothiophate iodide, a pseudocholinesterase inhibitor, can cause prolonged apnea if a child taking this preparation is given succinylcholine (Anectine) anesthesia for surgery.

ASSESSMENT OF THE EYE IN THE AMBULATORY SETTING

Vision and Ocular Alignment. A constant misalignment of the eyes requires evaluation regardless of age, whereas an intermittent deviation with a normal retina can be observed if it does not persist beyond 6 months of life. In the child older than 6 months, any misalignment, intermittent or not, requires evaluation and treatment. When medical means (drops, patching, glasses) fail to achieve alignment, surgical intervention is frequently indicated.

A nonsurgical alternative now under investigation by a national study group has been demonstrated to accomplish alignment with reduced anesthetic risk and at lower cost to both patient and provider. Injecting botulinum toxin to the extraocular muscles allows a temporary paralysis of the "overacting" muscle to result in a planned contraction of its opposing "weak" muscle, leading to a long-term change in eye position. In older children the procedure is performed in the office under eyedrop anesthesia; younger children are brought to an outpatient facility where the injection can be given under ketamine sedation. The injection is performed under electromyographic guidance. Therefore, the patient must be awake, or under the influence of ketamine, so that activity at the myoneural junction allows proper localization of the muscle with an electrode needle. Once this method is approved by the Food and Drug Administration, it is this author's opinion that it will replace surgery for the treatment of routine primary strabismus. In more complex forms of abnormal motility, involving vertical and oblique misalignments and restrictions or paralyses of muscle function, surgery will continue to be the preferred therapy.

The timing of surgical intervention is based on the stage of binocular development and the risk that amblyopia will develop. When a misalignment of the visual axes threatens or has led to amblyopia, and the visual loss has been restored with patching, an alignment procedure may be performed. In children with early-onset strabismus, alignment is necessary before 2 years of age, since clinical studies have demonstrated that normal binocularity and depth perception fail to develop if it is delayed beyond this time. Children reach visual maturity at 8–10 years of age. Before this time, misdirection of the visual axes does not cause double vision as it does in the visually mature patient. Rather, active cortical suppression of the visual input along one of the visual pathways occurs and, if continued, leads to amblyopia. If the amblyopia is not treated by the time the child reaches visual maturity, the loss of vision from central suppression becomes permanent. Conversely, any visual loss that occurs owing to strabismus or any other situation that causes one eye to be "favored" by the brain (unequal refractive errors, cataract, hazy cornea, severe ptosis) will result in amblyopia. These losses can be reversed with therapy as long as the child is visually immature.

Learning disabilities in children with normal vision and ocular motility are apparently not helped by eye exercises or glasses, according to a joint statement by the American Academy of Pediatrics and the American Association for Pediatric Ophthalmology and Strabismus.

EYE PREPARATIONS IN STRABISMUS MANAGEMENT

A history of topical drug use may have important clinical implications. Children who are under the care of an ophthalmologist for strabismus may be using several topical preparations, either diagnostically or therapeutically. Atropine preparations are used, briefly or for extended periods, in one eye or both, in the quantification of a refractive error to assist in amblyopia management. When such preparations are used unilaterally, the clinical picture is of a fixed and dilated pupil. Because this may erroneously indicate intracranial damage after trauma, an identification band (plastic hospital variety) may be worn when the pupil is under the drug's influence. In an emergency setting, a pupil that has not received atropine, yet is unilaterally dilated, will constrict to topical pilocarpine if the etiology is third nerve compromise. If the eye is under the influence of atropine, the pupil will not constrict to pilocarpine regardless of the intracranial status. Echothiophate iodide, which induces an accommodative spasm, is used in certain types of accommodative esotropia. It also causes an intensely miotic and poorly reactive pupil, may cause ocular hyperemia, and, because of the plasma pseudocholinesterase inhibition, must be stopped at least 2 weeks prior to the use of succinylcholine in anesthesia for elective surgery. In situations requiring emergent anesthesia when the patient is known or suspected to have used echothiophate iodide, Anectine is avoided to prevent prolonged apnea. The effectiveness of prolonged use of cycloplegic preparations (atropine, Cyclogyl) to retard the progress of myopia is without clinical or scientific confirmation.

OCULAR AND PERIOCULAR INFLAMMATION

Steroid compounds came into use in ophthalmology because they reduce ocular inflammation in certain disorders when opacity and limitation of acuity could be the result of an untreated inflammatory process. For example, in intraocular inflammation, where the inflammatory cells and debris can clog the drainage pathways for the aqueous humor and cause a secondary glaucoma, steroids prevent the vision-threatening complications by reducing the inflammatory response. However, they can also enhance viral replication and cause a rise in intraocular pressure when administered for prolonged periods. When they are used for over a year, as in certain cases of juvenile rheumatoid arthritis, steroid-induced cataracts may result. Because of these potential complications, extreme care should be exercised and concurrent ophthalmologic evaluation is suggested when steroids are used to treat conjunctivitis unresponsive to antibacterial therapy. The ability of these drugs to reduce the discomfort of any ocular inflammation makes them popular choices when we want our patients to feel better, but they should not be used until fluorescein staining of the cornea rules out a herpetic process. Close observation is necessary during the initial days of use, since a herpetic lesion may present in the mildest of ways and become characteristic only after 24–48 hours. Each episode of herpetic keratitis additively induces corneal opacity; it is one of the major causes of blindness, often requiring corneal transplantation in later years.

Disorders of the Eyelids

Focal Lesions

HORDEOLUM AND CHALAZION. The suggested treatment regimen is warm compresses, to promote drainage, followed by a topical antibiotic tid for 2 weeks. The common lid flora are all sensitive to sulfa compounds. A firm swelling in the lid left after the process resolves may slowly absorb over several months. Antibiotic-steroid preparations in an otherwise quiet eye may help reduce the amount of swelling and avoid surgical removal. Persistence of these masses, though not functionally significant, may be of cosmetic concern, and incision and curettage may be performed electively. When inflammation spreads from the site of the mass across the lid, with early signs of cellulitis, oral amoxicillin is added to the regimen, but its use in quiet masses does not improve their rate of absorption.

Vesicular Lesions. Vesicular lesions of the eyelid may be seen in children with herpes simplex, herpes zoster, and varicella syndromes. Fluorescein staining of the cornea is performed when any vesicular lesion is near the eye or if the eye is red in a patient with distant lesions. Any corneal staining seen in association with vesicles of the skin is to be considered herpes simplex, and ophthalmologic confirmation should be sought. Topical antiviral preparations (in preferential order) are Viroptic (trifluridine), Vira-A (vidarabine), and Stoxil (idoxuridine); these should be given promptly. The slit-lamp examination will assist in diagnosis and evaluation for intraocular inflammation.

Lesions distributed along one or more divisions of the trigeminal nerve signal herpes zoster infection. The pain may be severe and require extensive analgesia. Topical antibiotic preparations applied to the skin may prevent secondary infection, scab irritation, and scratching, which can aggravate scarring. Ophthalmic preparations are suggested for use on the skin about the eye, since the skin preparations contain vehicles that are irritating to the eye and this irritation may erroneously indicate ocular involvement. Unlike in herpes simplex eye disease, steroids play an important role in the initial therapy, and concurrent ophthalmologic care is advised.

Molluscum contagiosum in the vicinity of the eyelids appears as pseudovesicular and umbilicated. Although a self-limited process, it may cause an ocular hyperemia, which does not per se require treatment. When persistent, expression of the lesions hastens their resolution.

Blepharitis. Flaking at the base of the lids with secondary inflammation, seborrheic blepharitis, can cause significant ocular irritation (frequent blinking) and secondary bacterial conjunctivitis. Treatment involves debridement of the flakes and administration of topical antibacterial compounds. Even after the acute episode is controlled, the condition will usually recur if periodic lid hygiene is not performed. A suggested regimen consists of lid scrubs with a dilute solution of baby shampoo, followed by a sulfa eyedrop, in the morning, and repeat scrubs in the evening, followed by polymixin-bacitracin ophthalmic ointment. Since the ointments may blur the vision for an hour or two, we restrict their use to bedtime unless the condition is severe. After 1 or 2 weeks, lid scrubs alone three times a week will keep the seborrhea under control. If scalp seborrhea is also present, treatment of the head will not control the eye condition.

Pediculosis. Lice and their larvae may look like flakes to the naked eye and, therefore, must be considered in the differential diagnosis of blepharitis. Again, treating the scalp and other affected areas with Kwell will not help the eyelashes. Physostigmine ointment (Eserine) is applied three times daily, paralyzing the lice to allow their easy removal (or they may spontaneously fall off). Some suggest that any sterile ophthalmic ointment (Lacri-Lube) will smother the lice and accomplish the same end. Since only the adult forms are affected by this treatment, repeated use (for at least 10 days) is required until all the nits hatch; otherwise, reinfection of the lids and other areas will occur. Temporary side effects of Eserine are miosis, photophobia, and ocular hyperemia.

Allergic Blepharitis. After an encounter with a substance to which the child is allergic, or after an insect bite, edema of the upper and lower eyelids may completely shut the eye and alarm the parents. Usually the eye is quiet and noninflamed beneath the lids and the lids themselves are edematous but not hyperemic. This allergic state can be treated with oral Benadryl, and ocular medications are not required unless superinfection ensues. Cold compresses may alleviate the swelling, which subsides in 24–48 hours.

Orbital and Periorbital Cellulitis. Children who present with preseptal cellulitis are treated for impending orbital cellulitis. They should be hospitalized and given intravenous ampicillin and chloramphenicol for 10 days, although the latter may be discontinued if clinical improvement is seen in 3–5 days. When one is sure that the preseptal inflammation originated from a previously diagnosed stye or nasolacrimal obstruction, oral antibiosis may be instituted, and signs of clinical improvement after 24 hours will avoid hospitalization. Amoxicillin is adequate in these circumstances.

Treatment of frank orbital cellulitis requires hospitalization. Broad-spectrum intravenous antibiotics are given to cover *Haemophilus influenzae* (ampicillin and chloramphenicol) or *Staphylococcus* and *H. influenzae* (methicillin and chloramphenicol) until blood culture results are received. Definitive therapy should continue for a full 10-day course. When intravenous antibiotics fail to control the process, orbital and sinus drainage may be required; computed tomography will assist in localization of the abscess.

Topical antibiotics are unnecessary, unless (1) the process began after trauma, in which case topical sulfa preparations to combat the normal flora are sufficient; or (2) the process began with a membranous, acute conjunctivitis, in which case Neosporin is prescribed. Supportive measures include elevation of the head of the bed, warm compresses, and analgesics. It is not uncommon for an otitis to coexist.

LACRIMAL SYSTEM

The flow of tears is normally directed across the eye into the puncta at the nasal aspect of the upper and lower eyelids and thence into the lacrimal sac, where they turn inferiorly, pass through the nasolacrimal duct, and enter the nose beneath the inferior turbinate. When the valve of Hasner at the distalmost aspect of the nasolacrimal duct fails to open completely, a partial or complete obstruction will result, and signs of tearing, and mucus accumulation, with or without secondary infection, will ensue owing to the reflux. A child with a partial obstruction will intermittently show signs of the syndrome when reflex tearing occurs in emotional upset, during an upper respiratory infection, or in situations that encourage evaporation of the ocular surface, such as wind or dry heat.

When tearing alone exists and when mucus accumulation is slight and infrequent, no topical medication is necessary. When mucus accumulation is heavy enough to glue the lids closed in the morning and separating them is traumatic to both parent and child, Polysporin ointment may be instilled at bedtime. When secondary conjunctivitis, often characterized by a greenish hue to the discharge, exists, more frequent administration is required and a 10% sulfacetamide solution is also used twice daily. Bleph-10 does not sting upon administration and is easier for the parents to instill regularly. As ointment blurs the vision and leads to frequent hand-eye contact, it is used three times daily only in stubborn cases. We prefer not to use compounds containing a steroid because of the chronicity of the treatment. Parents should understand that the antibiotic is employed for the secondary infection and is not therapeutic for the obstruction. Massage of the sac is thought to produce hydrostatic pressure against the distal occlusion and aid in its opening, but because one cannot measure pressure in the duct, this claim is not proven. Evacuation of static mucus in the sac with digital pressure, to reduce the likelihood of inspissation and either dacryolith formation or dacryocystitis, is indicated. Extending the duration of lacrimal sac evacuation into a massage is optional.

When topical therapy is unsuccessful in controlling bacterial growth in the lacrimal sac, signs of dacryocystitis will develop. Oral amoxicillin may be instituted, along with frequent warm compresses, topical Polysporin, and sac expression, in the older infant. An improvement in clinical signs in 24 hours will militate against hospitalization and intravenous antibiotics. In the newborn, hospitalization for preseptal cellulitis is recommended because of the risk of sepsis.

Spontaneous opening of the occlusion can be awaited in the first year of life, although elective probing of the duct may be undertaken any time after the fifth month and is recommended in children with complete obstructions who have had repeated episodes of conjunctivitis. When dacryocystitis requiring parenteral medication occurs in the first 6 months, probing of the duct is usually accomplished prior to discharge from the hospital. Partial occlusions can be successfully probed at any age. Relief of complete obstruction should be encouraged prior to 18–24 months of life, since accelerated growth of the nasal structures may reduce the success of probing and make more invasive surgery necessary. When probing fails, silicone intubation is indicated.

CONJUNCTIVITIS

Allergic Conjunctivitis. Cold compresses have been recommended in the past but are usually of only brief benefit. Over-the-counter preparations of decongestant-only formulas sting upon administration, and the child may complain more about the drops than about the ocular hyperemia that prompted the parents to seek consultation. Antihistamine-decongestant preparations are little better. In general, for mild allergic states, reassurance, avoidance of known allergens, and awaiting the seasonal passage of the syndrome is suggested. When the condition is severe, mild topical steroid preparations may be used. A formulation that penetrates the eye inefficiently, such as Pred Mild, should be chosen, and the cornea should be observed carefully. A not-infrequent severe atopic condition of the upper tarsal conjunctiva, giant papillary conjunctivitis, causes a marked foreign body sensation, limiting the child's ability to open the lids, and interferes with schooling because of the protracted course. Eversion of the eyelids reveals the characteristic cobblestoning of the conjunctiva. Topical chromolyn sodium 4% has been of benefit in reducing the symptoms, if not the signs, of this condition. It is no longer an investigative drug and is available as Opticrom* 4%. Ulcerations of the cornea (so-called shield ulcers) may accompany the disorder, so when strong topical steroids are instituted, close supervision of the cornea is mandatory. Fortunately, the condition is self-limiting, and if the cornea remains uninvolved, is not visually disabling. For most allergic states, the child will be most comfortable in cool, air-conditioned environments.

Bacterial and Viral Conjunctivitis. In any acute conjunctivitis, less irritating 10% sulfacetamide solution (Bleph-10) is a good first-choice medication. After 48 hours, the condition may appear to have worsened clinically, and a distinction between an allergic reaction to the medication, an unsuspected, untreated condition, and the natural course of the illness will have to be made. Repeat staining of the cornea is suggested; and, rather than risking conjunctivitis medicamentosa from multiple prescriptions, it is often wise to stay with the original preparation and add a nighttime or morning ointment (Polysporin). Unless frequent broad-spectrum coverage with a solution is required, it is worthwhile to avoid the possibility of a neomycin reaction or sensitization. Combination antibiotic-steroid preparations give the greatest relief and the quickest clinical reversal of signs but

are employed only when close supervision of the cornea, to avoid aggravation of an occult herpetic process, is feasible.

Focal Inflammations on the Bulbar Conjunctiva. Following an upper respiratory infection, a child may present with a small localized swelling and hyperemia of the conjunctiva just adjacent to the cornea (phlectenule). The cornea shows no epithelial defect on staining, and the process is unresponsive to topical sulfa preparations. Today, this most frequently represents a focal allergic response to by-products of *Staphylococcus*; the tubercle bacillus was the most common cause in years past. Topical antibiotic and steroid preparations (Blephamide, Vasocidin) hasten resolution and can safely be used with close supervision of the cornea.

TRAUMA

When penetration is known to have occurred, the eye is shielded, Valsalva maneuvers are discouraged, and intravenous antibiotics are begun (methicillin, gentamicin). X-ray or computed tomography scanning of the orbit for retained foreign bodies is part of the initial management.

Minor superficial lacerations about the eyelid are adequately treated with Polysporin. The parents should be informed that the ophthalmic ointment is preferable to the less expensive, over-the-counter preparation for the skin, since the former will not irritate the eye should it enter between the lids.

Corneal Abrasion. Traumatic abrasions of the cornea may be treated with frequent applications (every 2 hours) of an ointment (Polysporin, erythromycin) when the child rejects a patch. When an accompanying iritis is diagnosed, placing the ciliary body at rest with a topical cycloplegic (Cyclogyl 1%, homatropine HBr 2%) may reduce the photophobia and pain. If the child will accept a patch, a drop of 10% sulfacetamide and patch-closure of the lids will suffice. Reexamination with fluorescein in 24 hours usually allows discontinuance of the patch and transition to topical ointments.

Removal of corneal foreign bodies is first attempted by irrigation with a sterile eye rinse. If this is unsuccessful, light brushing with a cotton-tipped applicator may remove the foreign body after topical anesthesia (Ophthane, Ophthetic) is achieved. Slit-lamp examination will disclose a rust ring if iron is present; in such cases, an ointment is preferable. Management of more advanced ocular injuries requires ophthalmologic consultation, and further discussion is beyond our present purpose.

Chemical Injuries. Chemical injuries to the ocular surface may be severely vision threatening, so the offending agent should be presented to the evaluating physician to establish its pH. Acid injuries are rarely deeply penetrating and heal in

---

* Safety and efficacy in children below 4 years of age have not been established.

response to traditional abrasion therapy. When the conjunctival fornices are involved, and after fluorescein reveals closure of any corneal epithelial defects, topical steroids may help prevent scarring. Alkaline burns (lye, ammonia) may be severely disabling. If there is any history of chemical invasion of the lids, irrigation is the key first maneuver. Sweeping the conjunctival fornices after topical anesthesia will remove any residual solids that, with slow dissolution, may be sources of continued injury. When the substance is known to have contained lye, at least a liter of irrigation fluid should be administered after placement of a lid speculum and topical anesthetics. Evaluation of the extent of injury with fluorescein staining will guide treatment. When the damage is minor and restricted to the conjunctiva, antibiotic or antibiotic-steroid solutions are used. When the cornea is involved, ophthalmologic management after immediate irrigation is wisest because of the probable resulting visual loss.

Thermal Injuries. Thermal injuries, such as cigarette burns, are treated as corneal abrasions. The speed of lid closure usually restricts most thermal injuries to the eyelids. First-degree burns heal well with exposure or, at most, a mild sulfa ointment. Second-degree burns, because of the thinness of the skin, may rapidly convert to third-degree burns, leading to lid cicatrization and requiring more advanced therapy; therefore, close observation is recommended.

17

The Ear

Foreign Bodies in the Ear

VICTOR E. CALCATERRA, M.D.

Removal of foreign bodies from the external ear canal is made difficult by the extreme sensitivity of the medial portion of the canal. In addition, it is often children too young to cooperate who accidentally insert a foreign body into the ear. The situation may be complicated by the development of a secondary external otitis.

Different methods of removal are dictated by the location of the foreign body and the ability of the patient to cooperate. As in cerumen removal, irrigation with water by a syringe is often a useful method but should be avoided if the foreign body consists of a material that swells with water. If purulent material from an accompanying external otitis or other debris is present, it may obscure visualization of the foreign body and cleaning of the canal with an angled tube-suction device will be necessary. Extraction can be done using either an otoscope with an operating head or a hand-held aural speculum with appropriate lighting, such as a headlight or head mirror. Various instruments for extraction can be used. A small alligator-jaw ear forceps is most useful for removing foreign bodies. Larger or friable foreign bodies are best removed with a currette. Often a large angled tube-suction device may be sufficient to pull out the foreign body. Complete cooperation of the patient is essential, and it may therefore be necessary to use general anesthesia in children.

Secondary lacerations of the ear canal usually heal without difficulty. Secondary infections respond well to otic drops.

Otitis Media

JEROME O. KLEIN, M.D.

Antimicrobial treatment of otitis media is based on the bacteriology of the specific disease. *Streptococcus pneumoniae* is the most important cause of otitis media in all age groups. Until recently, *Haemophilus influenzae* was considered a pathogen only in preschool children; new information indicates that this organism is also a significant cause of otitis media in older children, adolescents, and adults. *Branhamella catarrhalis* was found to be an important cause of otitis media in recent studies from Pittsburgh and Cleveland, but these data require corroboration from other centers. Of lesser importance as causes of otitis media are group A beta-hemolytic streptococci, *Staphylococcus aureus*, and anaerobic bacteria.

Choice of Initial Therapy

Some children with acute otitis media improve without the use of antimicrobial agents. Studies employing a placebo control suggest that the number of cases of bacterial otitis media that resolve spontaneously may be as large as one third of enrolled children. Without treatment, however, many children will have persistent acute signs and some may develop suppurative complications. The limited incidence of suppurative complications of otitis media in areas in which antimicrobial agents are used extensively in comparison with the period of time when these drugs were unavailable, or with areas of the world in which drugs are not available today, speaks for their beneficial effects.

The preferred antimicrobial agent for the patient with otitis media must be active against *S. pneumoniae* or *H. influenzae*. Amoxicillin or ampicillin is the drug of choice for initial treatment of otitis media, since each is active in vitro and in vivo against these organisms and each is less expensive than alternative drugs. The current incidence of ampicillin-resistant *H. influenzae* is low and does not require a change in initial therapy. Other drugs that are satisfactory include trimethoprim-sulfamethoxazole (TMP-SMZ), the fixed combination preparation of erythromycin and sulfisoxazole (Pediazole), cefaclor and combinations of a sulfonamide and penicillin G (administered by mouth or as single intramuscular dose of the

Table 1. DAILY DOSAGE SCHEDULE FOR ORAL ANTIMICROBIAL AGENTS USEFUL IN OTITIS MEDIA

Drug	Dosage/kg/24 hr
Penicillin G	50,000 units in 4 doses
Penicillin V	50 mg in 4 doses
Ampicillin	50–100 mg in 4 doses
Amoxicillin	40 mg in 3 doses
Amoxicillin and clavulanic acid	40 mg in 3 doses
Cefaclor	40 mg in 3 doses
Erythromycin	40 mg in 4 doses
Sulfisoxazole*	120 mg in 4 doses
TMP-SMZ*	8 mg TMP 40 mg SMZ in 2 doses

* Manufacturer's warning: Not recommended for infants less than 2 months of age.

benzathine salt), sulfonamide and penicillin V, or sulfonamide and erythromycin. TMP-SMZ, cefaclor, and the combination of erythromycin or clindamycin and a sulfonamide are acceptable combinations for the child with allergy to penicillin. If the child has had a major reaction to a penicillin (an immediate or accelerated reaction), crossreactivity of penicillins and cephalosporins should be considered and use of the cephalosporin avoided.

With appropriate antimicrobial therapy, most children with acute otitis media are significantly improved within 48 to 72 hours. If there is no improvement the patient should be reexamined. Tympanocentesis to identify the microbiology of the middle ear infection should be performed for children who are toxic; the appropriate antimicrobial agent may be chosen on the basis of review of Gram's stain and subsequent results of culture of the fluid. A change in initial antimicrobial regimen should be considered if signs persist but the child is not toxic and tympanocentesis is not performed. The new regimen should include drugs that are effective for all strains of *H. influenzae*, including those that produce beta-lactamase, and the pneumococcus. If ampicillin or amoxicillin was given initially, then the new combination of amoxicillin plus clavulanic acid (Augmentin), TMP-SMZ, erythromycin-sulfisoxazole, or cefaclor should be administered.

Management of the Child with Recurrent Episodes of Acute Otitis Media

The bacteriology of middle ear infection in children who have recurrent episodes of acute otitis media is qualitatively similar to that for the first episode; the predominant pathogens are *S. pneumoniae* (though of different serotypes) and *H. influenzae*. Two methods of prevention should be considered: immunoprophylaxis (use of pneumococcal vaccine) and chemoprophylaxis (use of a modified course of an antimicrobial agent).

Chemoprophylaxis. Although available studies do not provide conclusive evidence of the validity of chemoprophylaxis, the data are persuasive that children who are prone to recurrent episodes of acute infection of the middle ear are benefited. While we await definitive studies of chemoprophylaxis for recurrent otitis media, I believe it is reasonable to consider the following program:

1. Criteria for usage: children who have had three documented episodes of acute otitis media in 6 months or four episodes in 12 months.

2. Antimicrobial agents: sulfisoxazole and ampicillin (amoxicillin has advantages of ease of administration) were the drugs used in published studies and provide advantages of demonstrated efficacy, safety, and low cost.

3. Dosage: half the therapeutic dose—amoxicillin 20 mg/kg or sulfisoxazole* 50 mg/kg—administered once a day at bedtime offers maximal compliance. Administration at any single time during the day would probably be satisfactory.

4. Duration: during the winter and spring when respiratory tract infections are most frequent, for a period up to 6 months.

5. Observations during prophylaxis: children should be examined at one-month intervals to determine if middle ear effusion is present. Management of the middle ear effusion should be considered separately from prevention of recurrences of the acute infection.

6. Management of acute infections during prophylaxis: acute infections should be treated with an alternative regimen. Amoxicillin plus clavulanic acid would be an appropriate drug to use as an alternative without regard to initial therapy. If a sulfonamide is used for prophylaxis, ampicillin or cefaclor would also be appropriate. If ampicillin is used for prophylaxis, erythromycin-sulfisoxazole, TMP-SMZ, or cefaclor would be adequate to treat the acute infection.

Immunoprophylaxis. The currently licensed pneumococcal vaccines contain purified polysaccharide antigens of the types of pneumococci most frequently associated with otitis media. Each antigen produces a satisfactory, independent antibody response in children over 2 years of age. Children less than 2 years of age do not respond adequately to many of the serotypes of the vaccine. Children over 2 years of age respond to the vaccine with higher serum titers. The vaccine is of little value in infants. Available data suggest that the older children who still have problems with recurrent acute otitis media have received some benefit from the use of the vaccine. I recommend its usage in children over 2 years of age, although I recognize that it will only prevent a fraction of cases of acute otitis media.

* Manufacturer's warning: Not recommended for infants less than 2 months of age.

Management of the Child with Persistent Middle Ear Effusion

Many children have fluid that persists in the middle ear for weeks to months. Most children with middle ear effusion have some impairment of hearing; the audiogram reveals a conductive loss in the range of 15 to 40 dB. With such deficits, the softer speech sounds and voiceless consonants may be missed. The results of more than a dozen studies suggest that children with histories of recurrent episodes of acute otitis media score lower on tests of speech and language than do disease-free peers. These data are controversial, but the physician must consider the consequences of prolonged periods of impairment of hearing due to middle ear fluid in the young child.

Medical Therapy. No medical therapy has been found to be uniformly effective in ridding the middle ear of fluid. Nasal and oral decongestants, administered either alone or in combination with an antihistamine, are very popular for this purpose. The results of clinical trials, however, indicate no significant evidence of efficacy for any of these preparations used alone or in combination for relief of signs of disease or decrease in time spent with middle ear effusion. Use of steroids and prostaglandin inhibitors is under investigation.

Surgical Management. The value of myringotomy for persistent middle ear effusion alone is of benefit in some children, but in many the fluid reaccumulates once the incision heals.

Adenoidectomy alone or in combination with tonsillectomy may benefit some children with recurrent and persistent otitis media, but we await data from the ongoing prospective, randomized trial at Children's Hospital in Pittsburgh for definitive information on the efficacy of the procedure.

Tympanostomy or ventilating tubes allow for egress of secretions produced by the middle ear mucosa and maintain ambient pressure in the middle ear and mastoid. The procedure has not been tested adequately in controlled and randomized trials. Nevertheless, insertion of tubes in children who have had persistent middle ear effusion appears to be beneficial in most children; hearing is restored and permanent structural changes that might occur due to persistent fluid are prevented.

Labyrinthitis

STEVEN D. HANDLER, M.D.

Purulent Labyrinthitis. Purulent labyrinthitis occurs when bacterial agents invade the inner ear from adjacent sources, such as the middle ear or meninges, or through hematogenous spread. Proper management requires treatment of the bacterial source of the inner ear infection. If a purulent acute otitis media is the cause of the infection, wide-field myringotomy for drainage and intravenous antibiotics are required. Chronic otitis media requires intravenous doses of antibiotics and surgical drainage in the form of a middle ear exploration and mastoidectomy. Meningitis as a cause of purulent labyrinthitis is treated aggressively with intravenous antibiotics. If the purulent labyrinthitis persists, with symptoms of incapacitating vertigo and permanent sensorineural hearing loss, a labyrinthectomy may be indicated.

After the acute process has been treated, full audiometric testing is mandatory to determine the presence and nature of any hearing loss. Children who are too young or not cooperative enough to undergo conventional audiometric testing should be evaluated with brainstem evoked audiometry. Persistent serous otitis media is managed with myringotomy and ventilation tube placement. Persistent tympanic membrane perforation requires surgical closure with tympanoplasty and possible ossicular reconstruction. Sensorineural hearing loss must be detected and followed closely. Hearing aid amplification is required in some cases of unilateral and in almost all cases of bilateral sensorineural hearing loss in children. If any vestibular imbalance is present, the child must be monitored carefully when he engages in activities in which any vestibular dysfunction might be dangerous, e.g., swimming.

Viral Labyrinthitis. Viral labyrinthitis occurs when viral agents invade the inner ear. In cases of prenatal viral labyrinthitis there is no active treatment for the infection, which has usually subsided by the time the diagnosis is made.

Complete audiometric and, if indicated, vestibular evaluation should be performed. Appropriate habilitative measures (e.g., special education, amplification with hearing aids) must be started as soon as possible to maximize speech and language development.

Postnatal viral labyrinthitis is usually associated with viral upper respiratory infections. The treatment of this condition is supportive. Vertiginous symptoms are treated with bed rest, fluids, and antivertigo or sedative drugs, if necessary. Once again, hearing and vestibular evaluations are required after the resolution of the acute infection. Appropriate intervention can then be planned, with special schooling, close observation in swimming activities, amplification with hearing aids, and so forth.

Serous Labyrinthitis. Serous labyrinthitis is a sterile inflammatory process that is usually secondary to an adjacent infection such as otitis media or meningitis. The treatment requires proper diagnosis and treatment of the adjacent infection, i.e., otitis media or meningitis. Recovery is usually complete, with normal hearing and absence of vertigo.

Syphilitic Labyrinthitis. Treponemal infection of the labyrinth occurs in syphilitic labyrinthitis. Treatment requires high doses of penicillin and a long course of corticosteroids. While the vertigo and hearing loss often stabilize on this regimen, the latter may progress once the steroid doses are tapered or stopped.

Perilymph Fistulas. Perilymph fistulas are an infrequent cause of labyrinthitis. In addition to treatment for bacterial or viral labyrinthitis, middle ear exploration and closure of the fistula are required for control of the vertigo and stabilization of the hearing loss.

Injuries of the Middle Ear

VICTOR E. CALCATERRA, M.D.

Perforations of the Tympanic Membrane

A sudden increase of pressure in the ear canal can produce a blowout or rupture of the tympanic membrane. This typically occurs either from a sharp blow over the pinna, such as from a slap, or from a nearby explosion, such as a land mine. Direct tympanic membrane injuries occur from sharp, penetrating objects. No treatment is necessary because the perforation usually heals. Unless there is an infection with otorrhea, otic drops are unnecessary and should be avoided, since they will cause severe pain when instilled in an uninfected middle ear. If, however, there is purulent discharge indicating an infection, a culture is advised, and antibiotics are prescribed based on the sensitivities. If the perforation is extremely large and especially if fragments of the tympanic membrane are displaced deeply into the middle ear, an attempt should be made to realign the torn fragments into normal position and to maintain their position with a patch of gelfoam. If the tympanic membrane has not healed after several months, a tympanoplasty will usually be successful and will restore hearing to normal.

Fractures

Fractures involving the middle ear are commonly part of a larger fracture of the temporal bone and base of skull. Injuries to the facial nerve, tympanic membrane, and ossicles must be considered. A hemotympanum is very common and will usually disappear in a few weeks, presumably by clearance through the eustachian tube. Tears and perforations of the tympanic membrane usually require no treatment, and otic drops should be avoided. Infections should be treated with systemic antibiotics. Facial nerve function should be as-sessed as early as possible in a fracture involving the temporal bone and middle ear. Immediate and complete paralysis suggests transection of the nerve, which usually requires surgical exploration and repair of the nerve.

Ossicular Discontinuity

Discontinuity of the ossicles from trauma is recognized by a persistent conductive hearing loss after the tympanic membrane has healed. The stapes and incus are usually affected and may be either displaced or fractured. Treatment is surgical realignment of the ossicles.

Occasionally the stapes, including the footplate, is dislocated from the oval window, allowing leakage of perilymph from the inner ear into the middle ear, resulting in a sensorineural hearing loss and dizziness. Treatment involves surgically plugging the oval window with fat and replacing the stapes by interposing a prosthesis from the incus. If there is only a crack or minor defect in the stapedial footplate, the leak may be corrected by a soft tissue patch without a stapedectomy.

Hearing Loss

ARNOLD E. KATZ, M.D.,
and HUBERT L. GERSTMAN, D. Ed.

MEDICAL AND SURGICAL MANAGEMENT OF CONDUCTIVE HEARING LOSS

The external and middle ears compose a system that gathers and transmits sound to the inner ear. This system is connected and suspended in an optimal manner so that its mass and tension characteristics efficiently transmit sound. Addition of mass (e.g., wax, fluid, tumors) or alterations in tension (e.g., otosclerosis, adhesions) impair the efficiency of the system and result in hearing loss. Conductive hearing impairments are usually treatable, medically, surgically, or both. They are also frequently effectively treated with amplification (hearing aids).

Congenital Conductive Hearing Loss

Congenital conductive hearing losses may be unilateral or bilateral. Although the maximum conductive loss can be no greater than 60 decibels or so, bilateral losses in this range can impair greatly the child's ability to develop speech. The severity of congenital impairment must be considered in outlining therapy. Surgical correction of total aplasia of the external auditory canal or middle ear is fraught with the real possibility of facial nerve injury. Surgical correction of anomalies of the ossicles is accompanied by a much smaller risk of facial paralysis. These risks must be fully discussed with the patient's family. In unilateral conductive losses, surgery should probably be delayed until the child is able to participate in the selection of therapy. Amplification is frequently a good choice.

Inflammatory Conductive Hearing Loss

External Otitis. This infection may cause a conductive hearing loss, depending on how much inflammation and debris are in the canal. When the canal is filled with debris, pain is usually a major symptom and must be controlled with salicylates or codeine. Removal of debris is accomplished with a gentle suction and small wisps of cotton wound on metal cotton carriers. A wick must also be inserted so that the otic drops used will reach the site of infection. The otic drops usually employed and quite effective contain hydrocortisone, polymyxin B, and neomycin; 4 drops four times a day. After the swelling of the canal has decreased, the wick may be eliminated; however, the drops should be continued at least 3 days after the relief of pain. Recurrences may be prevented by routine use of acid-alcohol drops (mix white vinegar and rubbing alcohol 50/50) after swimming or bathing. Any signs of systemic involvement necessitate the culturing of the exudate and the immediate institution of systemic antibiotics. *Staphylococcus aureus* group A, beta-hemolytic streptococcus, micrococci, diphtheroids, and *Pseudomonas aeruginosa* are the organisms most usually encountered.

Secretory Otitis Media. The therapy of this most common cause of hearing loss must be based on the knowledge of the natural history of this disease. By far most of these patients will experience spontaneous remission without any treatment. Medical or surgical therapy should not be instituted until the patient has been followed for at least 1 month without improvement in symptoms.

If the fluid persists for over a month, one must then ask how this fluid is affecting the patient. If speech has developed normally and the child is doing very well in school, one can feel comfortable about following the child. It would be wise to advise the school that the child may suffer from an intermittent increase in the severity of the hearing problem. He or she should be seated in the front row with the better ear toward the teacher, and any deterioration of the child's work should be brought to the attention of parents and physician.

If speech or school work is suffering (even if the hearing loss is 25 decibels or less) aggressive therapy should be instituted in the following order:

1. The child should be instructed to perform the Valsalva maneuver several times a day.

2. The chewing of sugarless gum should be recommended.

3. If the child is atopic, antihistamines or decongestants or both may be of value. If there is no response to these for 1 month, they should be discontinued. If the fluid clears while the child is taking this type of medication, parents should be instructed to reinstitute this therapy at the first sign of a running nose or other clinical symptoms of increased antigenic exposure. No group of drugs has enjoyed such widespread advocacy without demonstration of efficiency in these cases as have antihistamines and decongestants. It is highly likely that if these drugs are effective, they are only of value in a minority of patients with this disease. It has been estimated that less than 30% of patients with chronic secretory otitis media have an underlying allergic etiology.

4. Although advocated by some, the efficiency of prophylactic antibiotics in this disease has not been established. If the fluid is associated with recurrent attacks of acute suppurative otitis media, trimethoprim/sulfamethoxazole or sulfisoxazole,* 100 mg/kg/24 hr, may be of value.

5. Myringotomy with aspiration of fluid and placement of a ventilating tube is remarkably effective in immediately relieving the hearing loss caused by this disease. Unfortunately, the ventilating tubes remain effective for only about 6 months to a year. Occasionally, after the tubes are obstructed or expelled, the fluid re-collects. In these patients, replacement of the tubes is sometimes necessary. It must be remembered, however, that amplification (hearing aids) remains a viable option in the treatment of these very difficult management problems. Adenoidectomy, with or without tonsillectomy, probably does not affect the natural history of this disease.

Acute Suppurative Otitis Media. Treatment of this entity is discussed on page 49.

Chronic Suppurative Otitis Media. Intermittent foul-smelling drainage from one or both ears usually heralds a perforation of the tympanic membrane or a cholesteatoma. Both of these conditions are usually accompanied by a conductive hearing loss and the patient should be referred to an otolaryngologist. Surgery is indicated to remove the infected bone of the middle ear and mastoid, which frequently accompanies this disease.

Trauma Causes of Conductive Hearing Loss

Foreign Bodies. These may cause a conductive hearing loss in various ways. Their presence may prevent sound from reaching the tympanic membrane. They may also cause a conductive hearing loss by perforating the tympanic membrane or fracturing or dislocating the ossicles. If there is no damage to the tympanic membrane or ossicles, removal of the foreign body will restore hearing.

---

* Sulfisoxazole is contraindicated in infants less than 2 months of age.

If there is middle ear damage, further surgery may be necessary to restore hearing. Foreign bodies in the ear of an uncooperative child should be removed by an otolaryngologist, frequently with general anesthesia.

Trauma to the Tympanic Membrane or Ossicles. Blast injuries or penetrating wounds to the external ear can result in conductive hearing loss. Immediate treatment should include examination under an otoscope, if possible, and assessment of the amount of hearing loss. Most traumatic perforations heal spontaneously. Parents should be advised to keep water out of the ear during bathing or washing the child's hair. This is best accomplished by placing a cotton ball to which has been applied a small amount of petroleum jelly in the external canal to seal it. Do not fill the canal with petroleum jelly. Dry cotton will act as a wick and allow water to contaminate the middle ear. Antibiotic drops are also helpful in preventing or treating an ear infection while the tympanic membrane is healing.

If a conductive hearing loss persists after the eardrum is healed, one must suspect ossicle damage. Exploratory tympanotomy with an ossiculoplasty may be necessary to restore the hearing.

Fractures of the External Auditory Canal. Fractures of the external auditory canal may accompany other types of facial and temporal bone trauma. Trauma to the mandible may result in a posterior displacement of the anterior wall of the canal with obstruction. Sound is prevented from vibrating the tympanic membrane, and a conductive hearing loss will result.

If this fracture is diagnosed early (within 7 to 10 days) it can be reduced easily with a nasal speculum. The speculum is inserted into the canal and opened. If weeks elapse between the time of the fracture and the time of the diagnosis, much more extensive surgery is necessary to enlarge the canal.

Neoplastic Causes of Conductive Hearing Loss

Benign and malignant tumors of the external and middle ears may reach sufficient size to cause a conductive hearing loss. If the tumor is benign (e.g., osteoma), local surgical excision is indicated. If it is malignant, treatment of the malignancy must assume prime importance. Treatment of the malignancy will probably necessitate sacrifice of hearing in the affected ear. Malignancy must be suspected in a chronic external otitis with pain and blood-tinged purulence, and a biopsy must be performed on the canal. Even in the absence of the hallmarks of malignancy, a firm, granular-appearing external canal should have a biopsy to rule out an early squamous cell carcinoma or rhabdomyosarcoma.

Conductive Hearing Loss—General Considerations

In general, pure conductive hearing loss is defined by the fact that the patient has normal "cochlear reserve." When the sound is loud enough, the hearing loss is compensated for by amplification. Thus, when medical or surgical treatment fails to fully restore hearing, a mild amount of gain in a hearing aid may be safely used. In chronic otitis, as in other conditions characterized by intermittent reductions in hearing acuity, a hearing aid is sometimes utilized on an "as needed" basis.

Except in rare cases, "pure" conductive pathologies seldom require significant other supportive treatment. However, if the illness is a concomitant, subsequent or consequent condition to etiologies affecting motor speech, language, or cognitive development, the matter requires prompt treatment and frequent follow-up visits and supportive training. For instance, a cleft palate problem invariably is accompanied by some otitis media. Such a child already is impaired to a degree by a communication deficit. The added illness hinders perceptual skill to the extent that loss of acuity affects perception. Therefore, particular attention must be paid to the status of the middle ear.

When conductive pathology is overlaid on a significant sensorineural hearing loss, the conductive components must be remedied so as to allow other habilitation training and amplification to be optimal. The fitting of hearing aids requires attention to the amount of gain, the intensity of sound to be allowed into the auditory system, the frequency range or spectrum to be admitted, and the varied patterns in the different portions of the frequency bands amplified. These specific differences in amplification properties are fitted to the patients' perceptions of clarity, intelligibility, pitch, quality, and sound comfort in search of a perfect union of person to machine. The compensation for conductive loss may be markedly different than that for sensorineural loss; thus additional or intermittent conductive impairment may be doubly disturbing to the basic sensorineural patient.

SENSORINEURAL HEARING LOSS

Medicine's best contribution to the area of sensorineural hearing loss is probably in its prevention. Immediate treatment of toxic conditions, conservative use of ototoxic medications, genetic counseling for parents who have already produced hearing-impaired offspring, and efficient treatment of upper respiratory infections or other diseases apt to produce damage to the cochlea or the auditory nervous system are the most productive for management of those at high risk.

Except for that caused by certain specific disease

states (e.g., viral labyrinthitis) and certain medications (aspirin may produce ototoxic reactions that are reversible when use is discontinued), sensorineural hearing loss is permanent, irreversible, and frustrating.

Audiologic and Other Management

Audiologic evaluation, coupled with variously required other evaluations, such as those performed by psychologists and speech/language pathologists, contributes to the diagnosis regarding site-of-lesion and, more importantly, regarding degree of impairment. An understanding of specific effects of patterns of hearing loss contributes more to habilitation and rehabilitation than any other single factor.

Once the basic diagnostic activity is under way, management plans may begin for infant stimulation, specifically of language. Later, stimulation for speech and consideration of cognitive development may be included in the management plan. Before the child is at the preschool level, treatment proceeds on several fronts, including any medical and surgical intervention that is necessary, fitting of hearing aids when appropriate, counseling of parents, plans for preschool educational programs, and general long-term plans.

In addition to hearing aids, specific activities may also take place in the area of auditory training, which teaches the child to differentiate specific warning sounds in the environment and later other alerting sounds and the various meanings of sounds that the child may be capable of heeding on both an uncompensated and a compensated basis. Other training forms take advantage of the visual modality for the benefit of communication and the other sensory modalities in training for speech production.

Training in sign language contributes to children's ability to develop symbolic behaviors, to increase their use of language, and to maintain other such linguistic shortcuts in categorizing their experience to the benefit of cognitive skills.

18

Infectious Diseases

Neonatal Septicemia, Meningitis, and Pneumonia

BISHARA J. FREIJ, M.D.,
and JOHN D. NELSON, M.D.

Systemic bacterial infections are major causes of morbidity and mortality during the first four weeks of life. Optimal outcome depends on early diagnosis, prompt institution of effective therapy, and careful monitoring for the development of complications of the underlying illness or toxicity from drug therapy. A high index of suspicion is essential to make an early diagnosis because the signs and symptoms are usually nonspecific and the clinical condition of untreated newborns with systemic bacterial infections can deteriorate rapidly. Consequently, many neonates treated for presumed bacterial infections are eventually found to have nonbacterial problems.

The choice of specific antimicrobial agents should be based on knowledge of the common etiologic agents of neonatal sepsis and their patterns of in vitro susceptibilities. Because these vary among institutions, it is essential to know the recent historical experience of the nursery at which the infant is being treated. The dosage and frequency of administration of antibiotics vary with the infants' weights, postnatal ages, and the presence of associated problems such as renal failure. To ensure adequate therapeutic concentrations of antibiotics in body fluids and to avoid toxic concentrations, monitoring of serum concentrations is desirable for antibiotics such as vancomycin, aminoglycosides, and chloramphenicol that have a narrow therapeutic range or erratic serum concentrations. Careful attention to fluid and electro-

lyte balance, correction of acidosis and hypoxia, provision of adequate caloric intake, and other supportive measures are as critical as the choice of correct antimicrobial agents in optimizing outcome.

SEPTICEMIA

Antimicrobial Therapy. Sepsis in the first few days of life ("early-onset") is usually caused by organisms acquired in utero or during passage through the birth canal. These include group B *Streptococcus, Escherichia coli,* and, less frequently, enterococci, *Listeria monocytogenes,* and gram-negative enteric bacilli such as *Klebsiella-Enterobacter* species and *Proteus mirabilis.* If sepsis develops after the fourth day of life ("late-onset"), nosocomial infection with *Staphylococcus aureus,* coagulase-negative staphylococci, *Pseudomonas aeruginosa,* or enteric bacilli should be considered in addition to bacteria responsible for early-onset sepsis.

Initial, empiric antimicrobial therapy includes a beta-lactam antibiotic in combination with an aminoglycoside. Ampicillin is preferred to penicillin G because of its broader spectrum of activity. It is active in vitro against streptococci, *Listeria, Proteus,* and approximately half of *E. coli* strains. The recommended dosage schedule and frequency of administration to neonates of different body weights and postnatal ages for commonly used antibiotics is summarized in Table 1. Therapeutic drug monitoring for ampicillin or penicillin G is not necessary because of their high therapeutic index (the margin between therapeutic and toxic doses).

The aminoglycosides are active against most gram-negative enteric bacilli and *Pseudomonas.* The choice of a specific aminoglycoside varies in different nurseries. Gentamicin is the most commonly

Table 1. RECOMMENDED DOSAGE SCHEDULE OF SELECTED ANTIBIOTICS

	Daily Dosage (mg/kg)			
	Age 0–7 Days		Age >7 Days	
Antibiotic	*Weight <2 kg*	*Weight >2 kg*	*Weight <2 kg*	*Weight >2 kg*
Amikacin	15 (2)*	20 (2)†	30 (3)†	30 (3)†
Ampicillin‡	50 (2)	75 (3)	75 (3)	100 (4)
Carbenicillin	200 (2)	300 (3)	300 (3)	400 (4)
Cefotaxime	100 (2)	100 (2)	150 (3)	150 (3)
Chloramphenicol	25 (1)	25 (1)	25 (1)	50 (2)
Erythromycin	20 (2)	20 (2)	30 (3)	30–40 (3)
Gentamicin	5 (2)	5 (2)	7.5 (3)	7.5 (3)
Kanamycin	15 (2)	20 (2)	30 (3)	30 (3)
Methicillin†	50 (2)	75 (3)	75 (3)	100 (4)
Moxalactam	100 (2)	100 (2)	150 (3)	150 (3)
Nafcillin†	50 (2)	50 (3)	75 (3)	75 (4)
Penicillin G†	50,000 U (2)	50,000 U (3)	75,000 U (3)	100,000 U (4)
Ticarcillin	150 (2)	225 (3)	225 (3)	300 (4)
Tobramycin	4 (2)	4 (2)	6 (3)	6 (3)
Vancomycin	30 (2)	30 (2)	45 (3)	45 (3)

* Numbers in parentheses indicate the number of divided doses per 24 hours.
† This dose of amikacin exceeds the manufacturer's maximum recommended dose of 15 mg/kg/day.
‡ Dosage is doubled for treating meningitis.

used aminoglycoside. Amikacin can be used for infections caused by gentamicin-resistant strains of coliform bacilli. Moxalactam or cefotaxime therapy can be used for gram-negative enteric infections in place of aminoglycosides, and they are the drugs of choice for infections caused by aminoglycoside-resistant coliforms. Monitoring the prothrombin time and giving weekly injections of vitamin K are advisable when moxalactam is used.

Because of their low therapeutic index, serum concentrations of the aminoglycosides should be carefully monitored. Dosage adjustment is essential in neonates with impaired renal function. In these infants, two or three specimens of serum at different times following an intravenous or intramuscular dose allows estimation of drug half-life and determination of appropriate intervals of administration. Recommended peak serum levels (measured about 30 to 60 minutes after an IM or IV dose) are 5–8 μg/ml for gentamicin or tobramycin and 15–25 μg/ml for amikacin or kanamycin. Trough (predose) levels should be less than 2 μg/ml for gentamicin or tobramycin and less than 10 μg/ml for amikacin or kanamycin.

If *S. aureus* is suspected to be the causative agent, as in infants with soft tissue or bone and joint infections, methicillin or nafcillin should be used. In infants with impaired renal function, nafcillin is preferred because it is cleared mainly by the liver. In nurseries with significant problems with methicillin-resistant strains of *S. aureus*, vancomycin is recommended for antistaphylococcal coverage. Vancomycin should be infused slowly over 60 minutes or longer. Shorter periods of administration are sometimes associated with the development of a histamine-like reaction characterized by flushing, pruritus, and a rash involving the upper arms, upper body, neck, and face, which persists for a few hours. Careful monitoring of serum concentrations of vancomycin is recommended, especially in infants with impaired renal function. A peak serum concentration of 15–30 μg/ml is desirable. If vancomycin is administered in conjunction with an aminoglycoside, there is an increased risk of nephrotoxicity.

Coagulase-negative staphylococci are being increasingly recognized as primary neonatal pathogens, especially in low birth weight infants, and should not be dismissed as contaminants when isolated from blood cultures. Risk factors for developing infections with these bacteria include invasive procedures, central vascular catheters, and total parenteral nutrition. Vancomycin is the antibiotic of choice for these infections. Nafcillin or methicillin can be used if the isolate demonstrates in vitro susceptibility to these agents. Removal of vascular catheters is often required to eliminate the source of these organisms.

If *Pseudomonas* sepsis is suspected, treatment should consist of carbenicillin or ticarcillin and an aminoglycoside. Ticarcillin has somewhat greater in vitro activity against *Pseudomonas*.

When the etiologic agent is identified, the initial antibiotic regimen can be modified according to the results of in vitro susceptibility tests. While studies in laboratory animals with group B streptococcal sepsis indicate that the addition of an aminoglycoside to ampicillin enhances killing of bacteria and prolongs survival compared with ampicillin alone, there are no clinical trials documenting a similar effect in humans. Neonates with group B streptococcal sepsis can be treated with ampicillin or penicillin alone. Determination of the minimal inhibitory concentration (MIC) and minimal bactericidal concentration (MBC) detects tolerant strains of group B *Streptococcus* that are inhibited but not killed by normally achievable concentrations of ampicillin or penicillin. Treatment with ampicillin and an aminoglycoside overcomes the tolerance. Tolerant strains of *S. aureus* have also been described, and these can be treated with methicillin and an aminoglycoside. The precise clinical significance of bacterial tolerance is not known. If a gram-negative enteric isolate is susceptible to both ampicillin and aminoglycosides, treatment with ampicillin alone is preferred because of its wider margin of safety.

Blood cultures should be repeated 24 to 48 hours after the initiation of antimicrobial therapy. Persistently positive blood cultures may be due to errors in antibiotic dosage, infection with resistant organisms, or an occult focus of infection such as an abscess requiring further intervention. The optimal duration of antimicrobial therapy is generally 7 to 10 days in infants with uncomplicated sepsis who respond rapidly to therapy.

Bacterial cultures are frequently sterile in infants being treated for presumed sepsis. If a nonbacterial cause is found or the infant looks well, antibiotic therapy can be discontinued after 72 hours. If bacterial sepsis is still suspected but no pathogen is isolated, the infant is customarily treated for a minimum of 7 days.

Supportive Therapy. Maintaining adequate tissue perfusion and correcting metabolic abnormalities such as acidosis and hypoglycemia are critical for a good outcome. Septic infants are frequently hypoxic and may require oxygen administration and occasionally mechanical ventilation. Caloric needs are increased during infection, and nutritional support is important.

The role of fresh frozen plasma and exchange transfusions in neonates with severe sepsis is not well defined yet, although anecdotal reports suggest that they may be useful. The use of irradiated granulocyte transfusions may be life saving in infants with severe sepsis and neutropenia (absolute neutrophil count less than 1500 per mm^3) and depleted bone marrow reserves.

MENINGITIS

Antimicrobial Therapy. Meningitis is caused by the same organisms responsible for neonatal sepsis. Initial empirical therapy is therefore the same as for sepsis and consists of ampicillin and an aminoglycoside. Ampicillin dosage is doubled (Table 1) in order to achieve cerebrospinal fluid (CSF)

concentrations that exceed the MBC of group B *Streptococcus* or other susceptible bacteria. By contrast, aminoglycoside dosages should not be increased because of their low therapeutic index. This results in small aminoglycoside CSF concentrations relative to the MBC of coliform bacteria.

A lumbar puncture should be repeated 24 to 36 hours after initiation of therapy. Typically, infants with group B streptococcal or *Listeria* meningitis have sterile CSF cultures within 24 to 48 hours, while infants with coliform meningitis require 3 to 4 days and occasionally longer before the CSF becomes sterile. Persistently positive cultures may be due to an error in antibiotic dosage or infection with resistant organisms. If both these possibilities are ruled out, computed tomography of the head should be performed to look for evidence of ventriculitis, subdural empyema, or brain abscess.

The high frequency of neurologic complications, especially in infants with longer durations of positive CSF cultures, have prompted evaluation of alternative methods aimed at increasing the CSF concentration of aminoglycosides without reaching toxic serum concentrations. Daily lumbar intrathecal administration of gentamicin in infants with coliform meningitis does not sterilize the CSF more rapidly or improve outcome compared with systemic therapy alone. Intraventricular instillation of gentamicin did not hasten bacteriologic cure and was associated with increased mortality in one study.

A controlled treatment trial evaluating the efficacy of moxalactam for treatment of neonatal coliform meningitis revealed that while the antibiotic achieved concentrations in the CSF much larger than the MBC of the infecting organisms, this was not associated with more rapid sterilization of the CSF, reduced mortality, or decreased neurologic complications in survivors. Moxalactam or cefotaxime can be used as alternatives when aminoglycosides are contraindicated or when the organisms are resistant.

The duration of antimicrobial therapy is customarily two weeks for uncomplicated group B streptococcal or *Listeria* meningitis and three weeks for coliform meningitis. The overall case fatality rate is about 20%, with most deaths occurring in premature infants. Neurologic sequelae are found in about 40% of survivors.

Brain abscess complicating meningitis is infrequent, except in the case of *Citrobacter diversus* infection, in which it occurs in about 70% of patients. The duration of antimicrobial therapy for brain abscess is variable and depends on the rate of response to medical therapy. If the abscess is amenable to surgical drainage, antibiotics are continued for 5 to 7 days after excision. If surgery is not performed, antimicrobial therapy is required until resolution is demonstrated by computed tomographic scanning.

Coagulase-negative staphylococci are the most frequent cause of central nervous system infection in neonates with ventriculoperitoneal shunts. Vancomycin is the drug of choice for these infections. If these organisms demonstrate in vitro susceptibility to the antistaphylococcal penicillins, methicillin or nafcillin may be used at double the dose used for sepsis.

Supportive Therapy. Intravenous fluids should be restricted to about 60 to 70% of the usual daily maintenance requirement to avoid fluid retention and hyponatremia secondary to inappropriate secretion of antidiuretic hormone. Convulsions can usually be controlled with intravenous diazepam followed by the administration of phenobarbital with or without dilantin. Hydrocephalus is a common complication that may require surgical intervention. Hearing loss is an important complication, and all infants should be evaluated with auditory brainstem evoked potentials following recovery from meningitis.

PNEUMONIA

Antimicrobial Therapy. The initial therapy of pneumonia developing during the first week of life consists of ampicillin and an aminoglycoside. If group B *Streptococcus* or ampicillin-susceptible gram-negative organisms are the etiologic agents, ampicillin alone is adequate. If *S. aureus* pneumonia is suspected, methicillin or nafcillin should be used instead of ampicillin. For pneumonias caused by ampicillin-resistant coliforms, gentamicin alone is effective. *Pseudomonas* pneumonia is best treated with carbenicillin or ticarcillin and an aminoglycoside.

If *Haemophilus influenzae* is isolated, ampicillin is used if the strains are beta-lactamase negative. Beta-lactamase positive strains of *H. influenzae* can be treated with cefotaxime or moxalactam. Chloramphenicol is best avoided in neonates because of its very erratic serum concentrations and the potential for CNS and myocardial toxicity (the "gray baby syndrome").

Chlamydial pneumonia is treated with erythromycin given orally. Ampicillin or amoxicillin therapy is probably effective, but there is limited experience.

The duration of antimicrobial therapy depends on the etiologic agent. In general, pneumonias caused by *S. aureus, Pseudomonas,* or coliforms are treated for three weeks, those due to group B *Streptococcus, Listeria,* or chlamydia are treated for 10 to 14 days, and those due to *H. influenzae* or *S. pneumoniae* require 7 to 10 days of therapy. If an infant does not improve in response to antimicrobial therapy, a lung biopsy may be necessary to establish an etiologic diagnosis especially in infants whose original cultures failed to identify the causative agent.

Supportive Therapy. Oxygen and assisted ventilation are often required in neonates with pneumonia. Frequent monitoring of arterial blood gas levels, chest physiotherapy, and attention to fluid and electrolyte balance are essential for a good outcome.

Pleural empyema can complicate pneumonia due to any bacteria but is most frequently seen in association with *S. aureus* pneumonia. Closed chest tube drainage should be instituted with large caliber tubes. This drainage procedure relieves dyspnea, allows the lung to re-expand, and prevents the eventual formation of a restrictive pleural peel. These tubes should be maintained until drainage becomes minimal, which is usually 5 to 7 days after insertion. Direct instillation of antimicrobial agents into the pleural space is unnecessary and potentially harmful because of the irritative effect.

Bacterial Meningitis and Septicemia Beyond the Neonatal Period

RALPH D. FEIGIN, M.D., *and* JOSEPH P. NEGLIA, M.D.

Bacterial meningitis continues to be a significant problem. *Haemophilus influenzae, Streptococcus pneumoniae,* and *Neisseria meningitidis* are the most frequent pathogens in the normal child over one month of age and *H. influenzae* is responsible for more than 60% of cases.

Diagnosis is dependent upon careful examination of the cerebrospinal fluid (CSF), using Gram stain, culture, cell count, protein, and glucose (with simultaneous serum glucose for comparison). Countercurrent immunoelectrophoresis and latex particle agglutination tests of CSF, blood, and urine have been useful in rapid diagnosis of infection caused by these pathogens; results are not dependent upon the presence of viable organisms. These tests can be particularly valuable in patients who have received prior antibiotic therapy.

Initial Therapy

Ampicillin and chloramphenicol are recommended. Ampicillin is administered intravenously at 300 mg/kg/24 hr in six divided doses and chloramphenicol at 100 mg/kg/24 hr in four divided doses. Chloramphenicol may be discontinued once susceptibility to ampicillin has been established. Tube dilution sensitivity tests should be performed upon all isolates obtained from blood and CSF. Sensitivity of *H. influenzae*, type b, to ampicillin should not be inferred on the basis of beta-lactamase testing alone, as ampicillin resistance may be conferred by plasmids other than those that control beta-lactamase activity. Moxalactam (150 mg/kg/24 hr) in four divided doses has also been effective in treatment of meningitis due to *H. influenzae* (both ampicillin resistant and sensitive strains) Cefotaxime (200 mg/kg/day in 4 divided doses) and ceftriaxone (150 mg/kg/day in divided doses q 12 hr) have also been employed successfully in a relatively small number of cases. They have not been proved to be superior to chloramphenicol for ampicillin-resistant strains of *H. influenzae* but can be used in cases of *H. influenzae* resistant to both ampicillin and chloramphenicol. Penicillin G (300,000 u/kg/24 hr) in six divided doses is the drug of choice for meningitis due to *S. pneumoniae* or *N. meningitidis*. In documented penicillin allergy, chloramphenicol may be used as a single drug for suspected or proven meningitis.

Intravenous antibiotics should be continued until the patient is afebrile for 5 days, but for at least 7 to 10 days in all cases. If clinical improvement is not noted within 24 hours or if the rate of improvement is slower than anticipated, repeat CSF examination is indicated. We favor re-examination of CSF at conclusion of therapy in all cases, since it permits the physician to document bacteriologic sterility at the time of discharge. This is not mandatory, however. At the end of treatment, CSF white blood cell counts and protein concentrations generally have not returned to normal and the CSF/serum glucose ratio may remain depressed. In all cases, CSF culture, Gram stain, and CIE should be negative. Retreatment is mandatory if they are not, and also may be suggested if more than 10% of CSG cells are polymorphonuclear or if the CSF glucose or CSF/blood glucose ratio is less than 20 mg/dl or 20% respectively.

Supportive Care

The blood pressure, pulse rate, and respiratory rates of all children with suspected or proven bacterial meningiitis should be monitored closely. Vital signs should be taken every 15 minutes until stable and then every 4 hours for the first several days. Temperature should be taken rectally every 4 hours.

A complete neurologic examination should be performed at admission and daily thereafter. A rapid neurologic examination to assess level of consciousness, pupillary response to light, extraocular motility, symmetry of movement, and activity of the deep tendon reflexes should be performed 6 to 12 times a day for the first several days.

The patient should be NPO for at least the first 24 hours, since vomiting may ensue and aspiration is best avoided. Also, careful measurement of intake and output can be achieved more readily if the child is receiving fluid intravenously.

Prospective studies have documented that almost 60% of children with bacterial meningitis develop the syndrome of inappropriate antidiuretic hormone secretion (SIADHS). In an attempt to determine the presence and severity of SIADHS, body weight, serum electrolytes, and serum and urine osmolarities should be measured at the time of admission. The studies may be repeated several times during the first 24 to 36 hours in the hospital and daily for several days thereafter. Urine should be obtained sequentially and careful measurement made of volume and specific gravity. The syndrome, when present, is best treated by fluid restriction. A multiple electrolyte solution containing 40 meq/l of Na^+ and Cl, 35 meq/l of K^+ and 20 meq/l of lactate or acetate should be administered initially at a rate of 800 to 1000 ml/m²/24 hr. Fluid restriction is continued until the measurements detailed above prove that inappropriate secretion of ADH is not a factor or that its effect has dissipated. The best indication of fluid retention in excess of solute is an increase in body weight or decrease in serum sodium concentration. As the serum sodium increases toward normal, fluid administration may be liberalized progressively to normal maintenance levels of 1500 to 1700 ml/m²/24 hr.

Head circumference should be measured and the head transilluminated at the time of admission and every day thereafter. This permits assessment of the development of subdural effusions or may suggest other causes of an enlarging head. Recent experience has shown transillumination to be a more reliable indicator of the presence of a small subdural effusion than is computed tomography (CT).

Computed tomography of the head may be recommended for children with bacterial meningitis in whom one or more of the following is documented: (1) focal or lateralizing neurologic signs; (2) focal seizures; (3) persistent increase in intracranial pressure with increasing head circumference that is unrelated to cerebral edema or to inappropriate secretion of antidiuretic hormone and does not respond to fluid restriction; or (4) suspicion of the presence of an intracranial process that antedated the meningitis or that appears to be concurrent with the meningitis.

Ultrasonography may be used to detect ventricular enlargement in children with open fontanels. This is less cumbersome and far less costly than CT scan and may be used to sequentially follow the course of ventricular enlargement.

The treatment of subdural effusions has been the subject of much debate. Recent studies suggest that treatment should consist of subdural paracentesis only, to curtail specific symptoms of increased intracranial pressure or when one suspects the effusion to be responsible for seizure activity or focal neurologic signs. In most cases of meningitis, subdural taps are not required. When vigorously sought, the frequency of subdural effusions found in young children with bacterial meningitis is such that they can be considered part of the general disease process rather than a persistent or troublesome complication of meningeal infection.

Seizures occur before hospitalization or during the first several days of treatment in approximately 30% of afflicted children. When seizures are noted, a patent airway must be maintained and appropriate anticonvulsants administered. Initially, sodium phenobarbital, 7 to 10 mg/kg/dose, may be administered intravenously. Phenytoin, 5 mg/kg/24 hr, in two divided doses, may be used for seizure control. Phenytoin generally does not depress the respiratory center to the same extent as phenobarbital and may inhibit antidiuretic hormone release. If necessary, diazepam, 1 mg per year of age to a maximum of 10 mg, may be given intravenously as a bolus. Shock and/or disseminated intravascular coagulation may complicate meningitis and may necessitate vasopressor therapy.

Fifteen to 20% of children with bacterial meningitis will develop some auditory nerve function deficiency. Detailed neurologic, psychometric, and auditory evaluation is necessary to permit early corrective measures.

Children with invasive *H. influenzae* infection, including *H. influenzae* meningitis, frequently carry the organism in their nasopharynx after a course of systemic antibiotic therapy. Prior to discharge, those children who are returning to a home in which another child 4 years of age or less resides should be given rifampin, 20 mg/kg/dose, once daily (maximum 600 mg) for 4 days to avoid reintroduction of the organisms in the household.

Prophylaxis is indicated for household contacts of children with *H. influenzae* or *N. meningitidis* disease and for day care center contacts when two or more cases of invasive *H. influenzae* disease have occurred in a day care center within a period of 30 days. Rifampin is the current drug of choice given as 20 mg/kg/24 hr in one daily dose for 4 days for contacts of the child with *H. influenzae* infection and as 20 mg/kg/24 hr in two divided doses for 2 days for contacts of the child with *N. meningitidis* infection. The dose for children under 1 month of age who are contacts of a patient with *N. meningitidis* infection is decreased to 10 mg/kg/24 hr (same schedule).

Four meningococcal vaccines are currently licensed in the United States: monovalent A, monovalent C, bivalent A and C and quadrivalent A, C, Y, and W135. Vaccine may be given to child contacts of patients with Type A, C, or W135

meningococcal disease in the doses recommended by the manufacturer. Group A vaccine is effective in children 3 months old and older; the other vaccines are effective in those 2 years of age and older. Safety of these vaccines in pregnant women has not been established. No highly immunogenic serogroup B vaccine has been prepared to date.

Septicemia

Septicemia beyond the neonatal period may be caused by any microorganism. In general, a careful history and physical examination will provide clues to a bacteriologic diagnosis. In the infant, the neonatal history may suggest specific infection with *S. agalactiae* (group B beta-hemolytic streptococci), *S. aureus*, *Pseudomonas*, or other enteric pathogens. Sepsis in patients with impetiginous lesions or a history of recent surgery may be due to *S. aureus* or *S. pyogenes*. Infection with *S. pneumoniae*, *H. influenzae*, or other encapsulated pathogens is more likely in patients who have been splenectomized. Infection with *S. pneumoniae* or *Salmonella* is more frequent in children with sickle-cell disease or other hemoglobinopathies than in the normal population.

Whenever septicemia is suspected, two or three sets of blood cultures should be obtained over a period of several hours and antibiotic therapy should be initiated. A careful search should be made for the focus of infection. When, following careful physical examination, no source is discernible, a chest radiograph should be obtained and cultures of urine and CSF (if indicated) should be performed. Countercurrent immunoelectrophoresis on blood, CSF, and urine also may be helpful in establishing a specific bacteriologic diagnosis.

Until a bacteriologic diagnosis is established, ampicillin, 200 mg/kg/24 hours in six divided doses, and gentamicin, 5 to 7.5 mg/kg/24 hr in three divided doses, or kanamycin, 20–30 mg/kg/24 hr* in two or three divided doses, should be provided intramuscularly or intravenously to cover enteric microorganisms. Alternatively, penicillin G, 100,000 to 200,000 u/kg/24 hr intravenously in six divided doses, and chloramphenicol, 100 mg/kg/24 hr in four divided doses, may be utilized.

Shock and bleeding are common in septicemia, particularly when gram-negative organisms are recovered. In these patients, gentamicin or kanamycin should be given intravenously over a period of 30 minutes to 1 hour. If renal failure ensues, the usual first dose of aminoglycoside may be given but subsequent dosage must be altered. Subsequent adjustments are best made by measuring the concentration of the specific aminoglycoside in the blood. When this cannot be done, an

---

*This dose of kanamycin exceeds that recommended by the manufacturer.

appropriate dosage interval can be estimated by using the patient's serum creatinine concentration or calculated creatinine clearance.

Cefotaxime (200 mg/kg/24 hr) or cefuroxime (200 mg/kg/24 hr) each in 4 divided doses, may be used but should not be employed alone if septicemia due to *Pseudomonas aeruginosa* is suspected.

When the cause of septicemia is due to *S. pneumoniae, S. pyogenes, S. agalactiae, N. gonorrhoeae, N. miningitidis,* or a penicillin sensitive *S. aureus,* generally penicillin may be utilized alone. Selected strains of *S. pneumoniae* have increased resistance to penicillin, and rare strains will not respond to clinical dosages. *Haemophilus influenzae* septicemia may be treated with ampicillin if the organism proves susceptible (see section on meningitis) or with chloramphenicol. Moxalactam has been shown to be effective in the treatment of both ampicillin-sensitive and ampicillin-resistant *H. influenzae* infections (150 mg/kg/24 hr in four divided doses intravenously). Cefotaxime, cefuroxime, and ceftriaxone may also be useful under these circumstances. The treatment of *Salmonella* septicemia must be guided by the sensitivity of the microorganism. In general, ampicillin or chloramphenicol may be utilized; chloramphenicol is preferred if *S. typhosa* is identified.

Penicillin-resistant staphylococcal infection should be treated with methicillin administered intravenously in a dosage of 200 mg/kg/24 hr in six divided doses. Oxacillin and nafcillin, 200 mg/kg/24 hr in six divided doses, are suitable alternatives. A cephalosporin or clindamycin will provide effective coverage for patients allergic to penicillin. Cephalosporins should not be given to patients who have had anaphylaxis or exfoliative dermatitis following exposure to penicillin. Peak serum concentrations of cefazolin generally are higher than concentrations of other cephalosporins when equivalent doses are employed. The drug can be provided in a dose of 50 mg/kg/24 hr in four divided doses intravenously. Cefotaxime, a new semisynthetic cephalosporin, also may prove useful in the treatment of septicemia. Cefotaxime (100 mg/kg/24 hr in four divided doses) provides better coverage against *Enterobacteriaceae* than other cephalosporins and reaches higher CSF concentrations. Clindamycin can be administered in a dose of 30 mg/kg/24 hr in three divided doses intravenously.

When *Pseudomonas* is identified, carbenicillin, 400 to 600 mg/kg/24 hr, in four divided doses intravenously, can be used alone *but preferably should be provided in combination with gentamicin.* Ticarcillin may be used instead of carbenicillin in a dose of 200 mg/kg/24 hr in four divided doses intravenously. Piperacillin† and mezlocillin, two new semisynthetic penicillins, also are effective in the treatment of *Pseudomonas* and *Klebsiella* infections and may be given intravenously in dosages of 300 mg/kg/24 hr in six divided doses.

A *syndrome* of pneumococcal bacteremia has been described in children between 6 and 24 months of age who do not appear to be seriously ill. These children frequently have temperatures in excess of 39.7°C (103.5°F) and white blood cell counts of 15,000 per mm^3 or greater with no focus of infection discernible by history or physical examination. We recommend a blood culture in these children, as it is important to identify children who are truly bacteremic. Recent studies have shown that a skilled clinician can differentiate children who may have bacteremia from those who do not as effectively as any single laboratory test. The decision to initiate outpatient treatment for suspected bacteremia should be made by the clinician on a case by case basis. When recall of patients is less than optimal or when a question of the necessity for antibiotics is entertained, we advocate initiation of penicillin or amoxicillin therapy.

Endocarditis

THOMAS G. CLEARY, M.D.,
and STEVE KOHL, M.D.

Although endocarditis is an infrequent pediatric problem, corrective surgery for congenital heart disease, use of intravascular catheters, rheumatic fever, drug abuse, and sepsis continue to put children at risk of this life-threatening disease.

Principles of Antibiotic Therapy

Bactericidal rather than *bacteriostatic* agents should be used. Drugs such as chloramphenicol, tetracycline, clindamycin, and erythromycin, which slow growth of bacteria but do not consistently kill, are generally inadequate as single agents because of the risk of relapse. Therapy is generally continued for 4 to 6 weeks, although 8 to 12 weeks may be required in selected cases. No compromise in treatment plan should be made once the diagnosis is certain. Rapid improvement of the sort often seen with viridans streptococci should not tempt the physician to utilize less than optimal therapy. Traditionally, dosage has been monitored by the serum bactericidal titer (SBT). The SBT is determined by testing the ability of serial dilutions of the patient's serum to kill a standard inoculum of the bacteria isolated from the patient's blood. Although this is a crude, poorly standardized test, it is appropriate to use when serum antibiotic concentration data cannot be accurately deter-

---

†Manufacturer's note: Dosages in infants and children under 12 years of age have not been established.

mined. Recent data suggest that maintaining peak titers of $\geq$ 1:64 and trough titers of $\geq$ 1:32 predicts bacteriologic cure. Lower serum bactericidal titers are sometimes associated with failure to kill the pathogen. We do not recommend using the SBT to guide lowering antibiotic dosage, since the failure to adequately treat these infections represents a greater risk than drug toxicity. Lowering antibiotic dosages is most safely done with the aid of directly measured serum antibiotic concentrations. The concentration of antibiotic obtained shortly after the end of drug infusion (peak) is used to adjust the mg/kg/dose; the concentration found just before the dose (trough) is used to adjust the interval between doses. Both peak and trough drug concentrations should be followed regularly during the course of therapy for endocarditis because changes in hemodynamic status and renal function (sometimes associated with endocarditis-induced glomerulonephritis) alter drug distribution and excretion. In the occasional child who has fungal endocarditis there currently is no satisfactory way of predicting adequacy of therapy.

Optimal drug selection is based on the sensitivity data obtained by inoculating the bacteria isolated from the patient's blood in serial dilutions of a potentially useful antibiotic to define the lowest antibiotic concentration that inhibits bacterial growth (minimal inhibitory concentration, MIC) and the lowest concentration that kills the bacteria (minimal bactericidal concentration, MBC). Combinations of antibiotics are often used in endocarditis therapy. This is particularly appropriate when the organism isolated from the patient's blood is resistant to usual first-line antibiotic choices, when a very unusual organism with unpredictable antibiotic sensitivity is isolated, and when the organism has a marked disparity between the MIC and the MBC (tolerance). Tolerance (MBC/MIC > 16) is a clinically significant problem, particularly with enterococcal and *S. aureus* endocarditis. The antibiotic choice in these settings is guided by determining the killing of the organism in the face of serial dilutions of each of the prospective drugs in a checkerboard fashion. Synergistic combinations are preferred over those which show antagonism or simple additive killing.

Microbiology

Empiric antibiotic therapy is based on predicted bacteriology. The alpha hemolytic streptococci, particularly *S. sanguis* I, *S. sanguis* II, *S. mutans*, and *S. milleri* (*M.G.-intermedius*), are the most common organisms causing endocarditis. *S. mitior* (*mitis*) and pyridoxal-dependent *S. mitior* are of special concern because unlike most viridans streptococci they are relatively resistant to penicillin.

For viridans streptococci which have low MIC's to penicillin ($\leq$ 0.1 μg/ml), regimens of proven efficacy (95% cure) include intravenous aqueous crystalline penicillin G given at a dose of about 25,000–35,000 units per kg/dose (maximum 20 million units/day) every 4 hours for 4 weeks or intravenous aqueous crystalline penicillin G for 4 weeks combined with intramuscular streptomycin at a dose of 15 mg/kg/dose (maximum of 500 mg/dose) given every 12 hours during the first two weeks of penicillin therapy. Shorter courses of therapy and regimens including procaine penicillin have been inadequately studied in children to be recommended. In the penicillin-allergic patient, cephalothin 100–150 mg/kg/day in 6 divided doses intravenously (maximum 12 gm/day), or vancomycin, 40 mg/kg/day in 4 divided doses intravenously (maximum 2 gm/day), are appropriate alternative agents. For viridans streptococci having relatively high MIC's (> 0.1 μg/ml) to penicillin the regimen that includes both penicillin for four weeks and streptomycin for two weeks is favored.

Enterococci (*S. faecium*, *S. faecalis*, *S. durans*) are usually treated with combinations of antibiotics because of "tolerance" to penicillin. All enterococci are resistant to $\geq$ 0.2 μg/ml of penicillin G. *S. faecium* has a higher MIC to penicillin and is more resistant to kanamycin, tobramycin, and gentamicin than *S. faecalis*. Although many enterococci show high-level in vitro resistance to streptomycin (MIC > 2000 μg/ml) and do not respond in vitro to penicillin and streptomycin in a synergistic fashion, failures on penicillin-streptomycin regimens are uncommon. We prefer to treat enterococcal endocarditis with combinations of ampicillin or penicillin and gentamicin because gentamicin is synergistic with penicillin and serum concentrations of gentamicin can be easily measured. Generally, a dose of 1 to 2 mg/kg/dose (maximum 100 mg/dose) is given intravenously every 6 to 8 hours. Vancomycin combined with an aminoglycoside is appropriate for the penicillin-allergic patient. Cephalosporins are *not* adequate because they appear to be ineffective in enterococcal endocarditis. Desensitization to penicillin is another option in the penicillin-allergic patient. Those who have been symptomatic for over 3 months prior to diagnosis are at a high risk of relapse. Thus, although many patients with enterococcal endocarditis can be treated with 4 weeks of therapy, those with very subacute courses should be given 6 weeks of therapy.

Staphylococcus aureus endocarditis is generally treated with nafcillin at a dose of 25–35 mg/kg/dose (maximum 2 gm/dose) given intravenously every four hours for a total of 4 to 6 weeks. We do not use methicillin in this setting because of the nephrotoxicity associated with prolonged courses of methicillin therapy. Although the data in humans suggest no advantage with combined therapy, many infectious disease specialists recommend adding an aminoglycoside to the regimen during the first one to two weeks of therapy. *S. aureus* organisms that exhibit "tolerance" to penicillins should be treated more aggressively than those that do not. We use nafcillin for 6 weeks along with gentamicin in the first 2 weeks in this setting. Methicillin-resistant *Staph. aureus* (MRSA) represents a relatively new problem currently occurring in hospital-acquired staphylococcal endocarditis related to intravenous devices and in some drug addicts. MRSA is resistant to nafcillin and oxacillin as well as methicillin. Vancomycin is the drug of choice for MRSA. Cephalosporins are not recommended despite occasional in vitro sensitivity because treatment failures appear to be common. For the rare *S. aureus* that is sensitive to penicillin G, doses of penicillin similar to those used with viridans streptococci may be used. *Staphylococcus epidermidis*, particularly when acquired in a hospital, is often multiply resistant to antibiotics. Because these infections may be very difficult to cure, two or three drug regimens should be routinely used. When the organism is sensitive to semisynthetic penicillin, nafcillin, rifampin and gentamicin can be used. Vancomycin is generally substituted for nafcillin when the organism is resistant to semisynthetic penicillins or when the patient is allergic to penicillins.

Gram-negative enteric rod endocarditis is usually treated with an aminoglycoside (gentamicin, tobramycin, or amikacin) plus a penicillin (carbenicillin, ticarcillin, pipercillin, or mezlocillin) or a cephalosporin (cephalothin, moxalactam, cefotaxime, or cefoperazone). Prognosis in these patients is generally worse than for patients with the more common gram-positive cocci.

Fungal endocarditis (typically due to *Candida* sp.) has a very poor prognosis. Amphotericin B, at a maintenance dose of 0.5–0.6 mg/kg/day given intravenously over six hours (maximum dose 30 mg/day)* and 5-fluorocytosine at a dose of 150 mg/kg/day orally in four divided doses are given for candida species. Although optimal duration is uncertain, we generally continue therapy for a very prolonged period (6–12 weeks). We discontinue 5-fluorocytosine if the organism is resistant or if the patient develops toxicity (particularly, bone marrow depression). Dosage needs to be lowered when renal function is impaired. Levels of 5-fluorocytosine should always be kept below 100 μg/ml. Valve replacement is usually indicated

---

* Total daily dosage of amphotericin B should not exceed 1.5 mg/kg.

in candida endocarditis and should be done within a few days of starting antifungal therapy.

When the diagnosis of endocarditis seems clear-cut but no cultures are positive, we give combined ampicillin-gentamicin therapy for a 4- to 6-week period, since many of the culture-negative cases are due to routine pathogens that the laboratory has failed to isolate.

Supportive Measures

Nonantibiotic medical measures such as digitalization, maintenance of fluid and electrolyte status, diuretics, and anticoagulants may be required. Daily physical exam, close monitoring of hemodynamic data, and frequent laboratory evaluation are essential. A team approach involving cardiologists, cardiac surgeon, infectious disease specialist, medical microbiologist, and general pediatrician is needed to give the patient the best chance for cure.

Aggressive surgical management is indicated in cases of uncontrolled infection, heart failure unresponsive to medical management, multiple large emboli, and fungal endocarditis, and in most cases of early prosthetic valve endocarditis. Some experts also recommend an aggressive surgical approach in the settings of gram-negative endocarditis, *S. aureus* infection of aortic or mitral valve, left-sided vegetations large enough to be seen on M-mode echocardiography, aortic insufficiency with mild heart failure, or with new conduction abnormalities that are persistent and unrelated to drugs or ischemia in a patient with aortic valve involvement. Late prosthetic valve endocarditis can sometimes be treated without removal of the prosthetic device. The major infectious indication for cardiac surgery is continued bacteremia despite optimal antibiotic therapy. Repeat blood cultures during the course of therapy and after therapy is completed are essential, as most relapses occur within two months after the end of therapy. Fortunately, prosthetic devices inserted shortly after institution of adequate antibiotic therapy generally do not become infected.

Antibiotic Prophylaxis. Antibiotic prophylaxis continues to be controversial both because no regimen has ever been shown in controlled studies to affect the incidence of endocarditis in humans and because failures are well documented with recommended prophylactic regimens. Prophylaxis has been recommended for those who have valvular heart disease, prosthetic heart valves, idiopathic hypertrophic subaortic stenosis, mitral valve prolapse, and congenital heart disease (excluding isolated secundum atrial septal defect). Although oral prophylaxis is adequate for most patients, recent recommendations have favored parenteral rather than oral therapy in those patients who are at highest risk of endocarditis (Table 1).

Table 1. PROPHYLAXIS FOR PATIENTS AT RISK OF BACTERIAL ENDOCARDITIS*

Area of Operation or Instrumentation	Regimen		
	Parenteral	*Oral*	*Penicillin Allergic*
Teeth or Upper Respiratory Tract	Ampicillin: 50 mg/kg (max. 1 gm) IM or IV 30–60 min before and 8 hr after procedure OR Penicillin G: 50,000 U/kg (max. 2 × 10^6 U) IM or IV 30–60 min before and 8 hr after procedure PLUS Gentamicin: 2 mg/kg IM or IV 30–60 min before and 8 hr after procedure	Penicillin V: 1 gm PO 60 min before and 0.5 gm PO 6 hr after procedure for those <60 lb; twice these doses for those >60 lb	Vancomycin: 20 mg/kg (max. 1 gm) IV infused during the hour before and 8 hr after procedure OR Erythromycin: 20 mg/kg (max. 1 gm) 60 min before and 10 mg/kg PO (max. 500 mg) 6 hr after procedure
Gastrointestinal or Genitourinary Tract	Ampicillin: 50 mg/kg (max. 1 gm) IM or IV 30–60 min before and 8 hr after procedure PLUS Gentamicin: 2 mg/kg IM or IV 30–60 min before and 8 hr after procedure	Amoxicillin: 1.5 gm PO 60 min before and 0.75 gm PO 6 hr after procedure for those <60 lb; twice these doses for those >60 lb	Vancomycin: 20 mg/kg (max. 1 gm) IV infused during the 1 hr before and 8 hr after procedure PLUS Gentamicin: 2 mg/kg IM or IV 30–60 min before and 8 hr after procedure

Staphylococcal Infections

PAUL G. QUIE, M.D.

Staphylococci cause a wide variety of serious infectious diseases. *Staphylococcus aureus* is an opportunistic pathogen associated with both abscess-type lesions such as boils and osteomyelitis and toxin-related diseases such as toxic shock syndrome. *S. epidermidis* is primarily a nosocomial pathogen colonizing vascular catheters and other foreign bodies and producing systemic disease.

Superficial staphylococcal skin infections may not require antibiotic therapy and *S. epidermidis* bacteremia may clear with removal of foreign bodies, but most staphylococcal infections require treatment with penicillinase-resistant antibiotic agents. Staphylococcal abscesses frequently require incision and drainage in addition to antimicrobial agents. Staphylococci may develop tolerance for antibiotics and persist in tissues so that long-term therapy is frequently necessary.

Selection of the antimicrobial agent and the route of administration for treating staphylococcal disease will be conditioned by the severity of infection, the patient's age, and the antibiotic sensitivity of the strain causing infection (Table 1).

SERIOUS INFECTIONS

In general, systemic administration of bactericidal antibiotics is necessary for treatment of serious staphylococcal disease. Since most staphylococci are penicillin resistant, a semisynthetic beta-lactamase–resistant penicillin is the drug of choice. Nafcillin and oxacillin are highly effective beta-lactamase–resistant penicillins.

Hypersensitivity reactions such as skin rash, leukopenia, and nephropathy occur in 0.1% of treated children. Renal reactions consisting of hematuria and dysuria usually do not appear until high-dose intravenous therapy is continued for 10 days or more. These toxic or irritative reactions disappear when dosage of the drug is reduced or therapy is changed to a non-penicillin drug.

First-generation cephalosporins such as cephalothin and cephapirin, as well as clindamycin and vancomycin, are effective antistreptococcal agents useful for treating patients allergic to penicillin. Cephalosporins should not be used for central nervous system staphylococcal infections since they diffuse poorly into cerebrospinal fluid.

The newer cephalosporins such as cefamandol, cefotaxime, and cefuroxime are not first-choice antibiotics for treating staphylococcal infections. In vitro sensitivity data show them to be less effective than less expensive first-generation cephalosporins.

The aminoglycosides, gentamicin and amikacin, are effective antistaphylococcal agents used in combination with beta-lactamase–resistant penicillins for initial therapy of serious staphylococcal infections. Aminoglycosides have bactericidal activity and synergism can be demonstrated between other antistaphylococcal agents and aminoglycosides against most strains of *S. aureus* in vitro. It is reasonable, although controversial, to initiate therapy with a combination of aminoglycoside and nafcillin, clindamycin, or vancomycin when life-threatening *S. aureus* infection is suspected. The serious side effects of ototoxicity and nephrotoxicity restrict use of aminoglycosides to special circumstances once the in vitro antibiotic sensitivities of the infecting *Staphylococcus* are known. Aminoglycoside therapy can be stopped and the primary antistaphylococcal agent continued when patients improve clinically.

Vancomycin is an important antistaphylococcal agent. It is frequently used for treating systemic infections with *S. epidermidis* because of the frequent resistance of these organisms to penicillins, cephalosporins, and aminoglycosides. Vancomycin must be administered intravenously for treating staphylococcal infection since it is not absorbed from the gastrointestinal tract. This property makes it useful for oral treatment of *Clostridium difficile* toxin–related pseudomembranous enterocolitis.

Vancomycin has been considered a highly toxic agent with serious side effects of ototoxicity and nephrotoxicity; however, these reactions were related to impurities in older preparations of the drug. Vancomycin is now highly purified and therapy is relatively free from serious side effects in patients with normal renal function.

Antibiotics may be administered by the intravenous route either continuously or intermittently. However, practical considerations usually make intermittent administration over a 10- to 20-minute period at 4- to 6-hour intervals the preferred schedule.

Rifampin is a valuable antibiotic for treating severe staphylococcal infections. *S. aureus* resistant to beta-lactamase antibiotics are usually exquisitely sensitive to rifampin and synergistic or additive effects of rifampin can be demonstrated in vitro. Rifampin should always be used with another antibiotic, since staphylococci rapidly develop resistance to rifampin. Rifampin is able to penetrate phagocytic cells, and since *S. aureus* may survive intracellularly, this property provides a clinical advantage.

Trimethoprim-sulfamethoxazole is another effective oral antistaphylococcal combination with an excellent spectrum of activity against beta-lactamase–producing *S. aureus*. The drug has only been available in oral form for several years but recently it has been licensed for intravenous administration to very sick patients.

Combination therapy with rifampin and trimethoprim-sulfamethoxazole has recently been shown to be effective therapy for serious staphylococcal infections.

MILD TO MODERATE STAPHYLOCOCCAL INFECTIONS

Oral administration of antibiotics is acceptable when treating soft tissue infections that are considered mild or moderate. Cloxacillin and dicloxacillin are the beta-lactamase–resistant penicillins of choice, since absorption from the gastrointestinal tract is reliable and adequate serum levels are attained. Cephalexin or erythromycin may be used for patients allergic to penicillin.

Clindamycin is highly effective for treating staphylococcal infections in pediatric patients. The frequent occurrence of colitis limits its usefulness in adults, but this complication is much less frequent in pediatric age patients. Clindamycin is concentrated in phagocytes, which is a therapeutic advantage in certain clinical situations.

Duration of therapy is arbitrary, but the notorious difficulty in eradicating staphylococci from necrotic lesions and the frequency of recurrences dictates at least two weeks for most lesions. Nonspecific agents still being used for staphylococcal lesions include vaccines, toxoids, gamma globulins, and bacteriophages. None has survived the rigor of controlled trials and their use is not recommended.

SPECIFIC STAPHYLOCOCCAL INFECTIONS

Bullous Impetigo and Staphylococcal Scalded Skin Syndrome. *S. aureus* bullous impetigo can usually be treated with hygenic measures and topical antibiotic therapy. However, when extensive lesions are present, systemic antibiotics are necessary. Oral therapy with a beta-lactamase–resistant antibiotic such as dicloxacillin should be used. When large areas of the body are denuded, the disease is described as "scalded skin syndrome" and intravenous therapy with nafcillin should be used. Cephalothin or clindamycin may be used in patients allergic to penicillin. Once patients are stabilized, oral therapy is effective.

Abscesses. Furuncles and other skin lesions are the most common clinical infections caused by *S. aureus*. These lesions are often self-limited and heal spontaneously, but if there are systemic symptoms or cellulitis is present, antibiotic therapy and incision and drainage are indicated. Antibiotic choice is similar to that described for patients with *S. aureus* impetigo and scalded skin syndrome. Recurrent furunculosis is a difficult clinical problem and often requires prolonged antibiotic therapy; fortunately the oral route is satisfactory. Several family members may be involved and exquisite hygiene for all family members is necessary. Artificial colonization of the nasal mucosa with a strain of *S. aureus* of low virulence (502A, available from Henry Shinefield, M.D.) may interfere with autoinoculation by a patient's or family's more virulent resident strain. Care must be taken to assure that patients are immunologically normal before this form of therapy is employed.

Metastasis of *S. aureus* from skin lesions to bone or soft tissues such as liver, kidney, lung, and brain may occur. Deep abscesses require intravenous

Table 1. DOSAGE SCHEDULE OF DRUGS USEFUL IN TREATMENT OF STAPHYLOCOCCAL INFECTIONS

Antibiotic	Oral (for mild to moderate infection)	
	1 Month to 50 kg	*>50 kg or Maximum*
PENICILLINS		
Benzyl (Penicillin G)	50,000–150,000 units/kg/24 hr (4)	1.6–4.8 million units/24 hr (4)
Phenoxymethyl (Penicillin V, V-Cillin, Pen-Vee K, others)	50–100 mg/kg/24 hr (4)	1–4 gm/24 hr (4)
Methicillin (Staphcillin)	—	—
Oxacillin (Prostaphlin)	50–100 mg/kg/24 hr (4)	1–2 gm/24 hr (4)
Nafcillin (Unipen)	50–100 mg/kg/24 hr (4)	1–2 gm/24 hr (4)
Cloxacillin (Tegopen)	25–50 mg/kg/24 hr (4)	1–4 gm/24 (4)
Dicloxacillin (Dynapen, Pathocil, Veracillin)	12.5–25 mg/kg/24 hr (4)	0.5–2 gm/24 hr (4)
CEPHALOSPORINS		
Cephalothin (Keflin)	—	—
Cephapirin (Cefadyl)	—	—
Cefazolin (Ancef, Kefzol)	—	—
Cephalexin (Keflex)	25–50 mg/kg/24 hr (4)	1–4 gm/24 hr (4)
Cephradine (Anspor, Velosef)	25–50 mg/kg/24 hr (4)	1–4 gm/24 hr (4)
OTHERS		
Erythromycin lactobionate (Erythrocin-Lactobionate-IV) *AND* Erythromycin gluceptate (Ilotycin Gluceptate)	—	—
Erythromycin stearate and estolate (Erythrocin, E-mycin, Ilosone, others)	25–50 mg/kg/24 hr (4)	1–2 gm/24 hr (4)
Clindamycin (Cleocin)	10–20 mg/kg/24 hr (4)	600–1200 mg/24 hr (4)
Vancomycin (Vancocin)	—	—
Gentamicin (Garamycin)	—	—
Rifampin		10–20 mg/kg/day

Note: Numbers in parentheses: Number of doses into which the daily dose should be equally divided.

antibiotic therapy and drainage of accessible lesions after localization. If abscesses are present in the vicinity of foreign bodies, removal is necessary to prevent chronic suppuration. *S. epidermidis* may be the basis for suppurative lesions or bacteremia associated with vascular catheters and other foreign bodies and intensive prolonged antibiotic therapy is necessary for *S. epidermidis* as well as *S. aureus*. Appropriate antibiotics need to be administered for 6 to 12 weeks in order to eradicate staphylococci from deep-seated abscesses. Since many strains of *S. epidermidis* are insensitive to beta-lactamase–resistant penicillins, vancomycin therapy is necessary.

Septicemia, Osteomyelitis and Endocarditis. Staphylococcal bacteremia is a relatively frequent occurrence and septicemia (symptomatic bacteremia) and endocarditis are constant threats. Secondary bacteremia, i.e., when a focus of infection is defined, can be treated by drainage, removal of vascular catheters or foreign bodies, and conventional antibiotic therapy for one to two weeks. Oral therapy with cloxacillin, clindamycin, or cephalexin is satisfactory. It must be remembered that patients with congenital or postoperative heart lesions and drug abusers are highly susceptible to endocarditis. *S. aureus* septicemia or endocarditis must be treated promptly and aggressively with intravenous antibiotics. The necrotizing properties of *S. aureus* lesions are especially dangerous when they involve the heart valves or brain and combination therapy with nafcillin (vancomycin in penicillin sensitive individuals) and gentamicin should be given intravenously for maximum bactericidal action. Vancomycin should be the antibiotic of first choice when treating *S. epidermidis* endocarditis. Since many patients with staphylococcal endocarditis have artificial valves or other heart prostheses, removal of these foreign bodies may be necessary for cure.

Poor response to antibiotic agents that should be satisfactory by in vitro sensitivity testing may result from occult staphylococcal lesions or from "tolerance" of *S. aureus* to the agent. Tolerance, defined as dissociation between minimal inhibitory and minimal bactericidal concentrations of an antibiotic is usually associated with beta-lactam antibiotics that primarily act on staphylococcal cell

Table 1. DOSAGE SCHEDULE OF DRUGS USEFUL IN TREATRMENT
OF STAPHYLOCOCCAL INFECTIONS (*Continued*)

Parenteral (for severe infection)			
<1 Week	*1 to 4 Weeks*	*1 Month to 50 kg*	*>50 kg or Maximum*
100,000 units/kg/24 hr IV every 12 hr	100,000–250,000 units/kg/24 hr IV every 6 hr	200,000–400,000 units/kg/24 hr IV every 4 hr	8–24 million units/24 hr IV every 4 hr
	—	—	—
50–100 mg/kg/24 hr IV every 12 hr	100–200 mg/kg/24 hr IV every 6 hr	200–300 mg/kg/24 hr IV every 4 hr	6–12 gm/24 hr IV every 4 hr
50–100 mg/kg/24 hr IV every 12 hr	100 to 200 mg/kg/24 hr IM or IV every 6 hr	100–200 mg/kg/24 hr IV every 4 hr	4–8 gm/24 hr IV every 4 hr
40–60 mg/kg/24 hr IV every 12 hr	60 to 100 mg/kg/24 hr IM or IV every 6 hr	100–200 mg/kg/24 hr IV every 4 hr	4–8 gm/24 hr IV every 4 hr
—	—	—	—
40 mg/kg/24 hr IV every 12 hr	60 mg/kg/24 hr IV every 6 hr	100 mg/kg/24 hr IV every 4 hr	6–12 gm/24 hr IV every 4 hr
40 mg/kg/24 hr IV every 12 hr	60 mg/kg/24 hr IV every 6 hr	100 mg/kg/24 hr IV every 4 hr	6–12 gm/24 hr IV every 4 hr
40 mg/kg/24 hr IV every 12 hr	50 mg/kg/24 hr IV every 8 hr	50 mg/kg/24 hr IV every 6 hr	3–6 gm/24 hr IV every 6 hr
—	—	—	—
Not recommended	10–20 mg/kg/24 hr IV every 8 hr, infuse over 0.5–1 hr	10–20 mg/kg/24 hr IV every 6 hr, infuse over 0.5–1 hr	1.5–4 gm/24 hr IV every 6 hr, 1 gm diluted in 100 ml
—			
Not recommended	20–40 mg/kg/24 hr IV every 6 hr, infuse over 30 min	20–40 mg/kg/24 hr IV every 6 hr, infuse over 30 min	1.2–2.4 gm/24 hr IV every 6 hr, 1 gm diluted in 100 ml
30 mg/kg/24 hr IV every 12 hr, infuse over 30 to 60 min	45 mg/kg/24 hr* IV every 8 hr, infuse over 1 hr	40–60 mg/kg/24 hr* IV every 6 hr, infuse over 1 hr	2 gm/24 hr IV every 6 hr, infuse over 1 hr
5 mg/kg/24 hr† IV every 12 hr	7.5 mg/kg/24 hr† IM every 8 hr	5 mg/kg/24 hr† IM every 8 hr	5 mg/kg/24 hr† IM every 8 hr

Note: Numbers in parentheses: Number of doses into which the daily dose should be equally divided.
* These doses may exceed the manufacturer's recommended dosage.
† May be given IV slowly over 20 to 30 minutes.

walls. If tolerance is suspected, rifampin or an aminoglycoside should be added to the therapeutic regimen.

Infections of the Central Nervous System. Neurologic procedures using plastic tubes to relieve congenital or acquired obstructions to the flow of cerebrospinal fluid have resulted in susceptibility of the CNS to staphylococcal infections. Infections secondary to neurologic procedures are usually caused by *S. epidermidis*, and vancomycin is used for initial therapy. *S. aureus* infections of the CNS may be related to primary lesions at a distant site. High-dose intravenous nafcillin or vancomycin is necessary to treat *S. aureus* meningitis or brain abscess. Intrathecal medication should not be used. It is necessary to remove CNS shunts that have become infected with staphylococci. Antistaphylococcal therapy should be continued for at least two weeks after an infected shunt is removed, and if signs and symptoms of increased intracranial pressure dictate that a new shunt is needed, antibiotics should be continued for several days after the surgery.

Toxic Shock Syndrome. The toxic shock syndrome is secondary to infection with a toxin-producing strain of *S. aureus*. It occurs most frequently in young menstruating women presumably because tampon use favors *S. aureus* replication and production of toxin that is absorbed through mucous membranes and results in shock, rash, and severe diarrhea. Supportive therapy and replacement of fluid and electrolytes are critical in toxic shock syndrome. Antistaphylococcal therapy is aimed at preventing recurrences in toxic shock syndrome associated with menstruation. When the syndrome occurs in young children or males, identification of the site of infection, drainage, and therapy with beta-lactamase–resistant antibiotics are necessary. Shock may be associated with other serious staphylococcal infections as a consequence of massive fluid accumulation in local infections, a direct effect on cardiac function, or activation of complement and coagulation systems; therefore aggressive intravenous therapy with nafcillin or other beta-lactamase–resistant antibiotics is mandatory.

Pyomyositis. Pyomyositis is a staphylococcal disease associated with the tropics and primarily affects malnourished individuals. However, pyomyositis does occur in the United States. Staphylococci are present in the muscle or fasciae in this disease, and although there may be few objective signs of infection aside from muscle pain and swelling, a fatal outcome is frequent. When *S. aureus* organisms are identified, the infected site *must* be drained surgically and the patient treated aggressively with intravenous nafcillin or other beta-lactamase antibiotics.

Streptococcal Infections

MICHAEL A. GERBER, M.D.

The most common group A streptococcal infections in children are pharyngitis and impetigo. These infections are significant not only because of the acute morbidity associated with them but also because they may be followed by nonsuppurative sequelae. Streptococcal pharyngitis may be followed by acute rheumatic fever or acute glomerulonephritis, and impetigo may be followed by acute glomerulonephritis.

There are several reasons for attempting to diagnose and treat streptococcal pharyngitis. (1) It is important for the prevention of nonsuppurative sequelae. It has been established that eradication of the streptococci from the upper respiratory tract of a patient with acute pharyngitis will prevent that patient from developing acute rheumatic fever. Although acute rheumatic fever has become a rare disease in this country, there are data that suggest that the dramatic decline in the incidence of this disease is due, at least in part, to efforts to diagnose and treat streptococcal pharyngitis. Antibiotic therapy has not, however, been shown to be effective in preventing the other nonsupportive sequelae of streptococcal pharyngitis—poststreptococcal glomerulonephritis. (2) Antibiotic therapy helps to prevent the suppurative sequelae of streptococcal pharyngitis such as peritonsillar abscess, retropharyngeal abscess, and cervical lymphadenitis. These complications were relatively common in the preantibiotic era, but their incidence has declined markedly with the use of antibiotic therapy. (3) Eradication of the infecting streptococci from the patient's upper respiratory tract with antibiotic therapy prevents spread of that organism to other individuals. (4) Antibiotic therapy, particularly if begun early in the disease, can shorten the clinical course of the illness.

It is extremely difficult to distinguish streptococcal pharyngitis from other forms of acute pharyngitis on the basis of clinical findings alone. Therefore, an accurate diagnosis depends on a throat culture. Since group A streptococci are the only important bacterial cause of acute pharyngitis in children in this country, routine throat cultures should be processed for the detection of only this organism. One of the problems with the throat culture is that it cannot distinguish between patients with bona fide streptococcal infections and those who are streptococcal carriers with acute upper respiratory symptoms caused by other agents such as viruses. Patients who are streptococcal carriers are not dangerous to themselves or to others. They do not develop acute rheumatic fever, and they rarely spread the organism to contacts. They do not need to be identified or treated. In order to minimize the number of streptococcal carriers who are tested and subsequently treated with antibiotics, throat cultures should be performed selectively. The patient's age, the season, the presence of specific clinical findings that suggest a streptococcal etiology, the presence of specific clinical findings that suggest a viral etiology, and an awareness of what pathogens are present in the community should all be taken into consideration when deciding whether or not to perform a throat culture on a patient with a sore throat. In addition, unless there is a history of rheumatic fever in the immediate family, only symptomatic household contacts of a patient with acute streptococcal pharyngitis should be cultured and, if positive, treated.

Another problem with the throat culture is the fact that it takes 24 to 48 hours before the results are known. This delay has led many physicians to initiate antibiotic therapy prior to knowing the results of the throat culture. Since the majority of children with acute pharyngitis do not have streptococcal infections, this approach results in a large number of children receiving an unnecessary course of antibiotic therapy. In addition, once antibiotic therapy has been initiated, many physicians are reluctant to discontinue it, even when the throat culture is reported to be negative. On the other hand, those physicians who wait the 24 to 48 hours for the results of the throat culture before initiating antibiotic therapy may be faced with the problem of poor compliance in a patient who may already be improving. Although the antibiotic therapy of streptococcal pharyngitis can be delayed for several days and still prevent acute rheumatic fever from developing, waiting 24 to 48 hours before initiating antibiotic therapy may deprive the patient with streptococcal pharyngitis of the symptomatic benefit afforded by early antibiotic therapy. Early antibiotic therapy may not only allow the patient to return to school or day care 24 to 48 hours sooner but, in addition, may also allow a parent to return to work 24 to 48 hours sooner.

The most effective treatment for streptococcal

pharyngitis is a single intramuscular injection of benzathine penicillin G, 600,000 units for patients less than 60 pounds and 1.2 million units for patients more than 60 pounds. Preparations containing procaine penicillin in addition to benzathine penicillin G are associated with decreased pain at the injection site. If such mixtures are used, care must be taken to provide the required amount of benzathine penicillin G. Alternatively, oral penicillin V may be given. The dosage for both children and adults is 125–250 mg, 3 or 4 times daily for a full 10 days. Studies have also suggested that a dosage of 250 mg of penicillin V, 2 times daily, is effective in the treatment of children. Shorter courses of therapy have been associated with a significantly higher treatment failure rate, and, therefore, patients should be encouraged to take the penicillin V for the entire 10 days, even though they will likely be asymptomatic after the first few days. Twenty-four hours after initiation of appropriate antibiotic therapy, the patient can be considered no longer contagious and may return to school or day care.

Antibiotics other than penicillin offer no advantage in the treatment of streptococcal pharyngitis, and their use should be limited to patients who are allergic to penicillin. Erythromycin is the drug of choice for patients who are allergic to penicillin. Erythromycin estolate (20 to 40 mg/kg/day) in 2 to 4 divided doses or erythromycin ethyl succinate (40 mg/kg/day) in 2 to 4 divided doses may be given. Studies have suggested that erythromycin estolate is both more effective and better tolerated than erythromycin ethyl succinate. The maximal dose of erythromycin is 1.0 gm/day, and the erythromycin should be given for a full 10-day course. Although erythromycin-resistant strains of group A streptococci are prevalent in some areas of the world, they are still rare in this country. A 10-day course of oral cephalosporins is an acceptable alternative for the patient allergic to penicillin. However, cephalosporins are more expensive and should not be used in patients with immediate hypersensitivity reactions to penicillin (e.g., anaphylaxis).

Certain antibiotics are not recommended for the treatment of streptococcal pharyngitis. Tetracyclines and trimethoprim-sulfamethoxazole have been shown to be ineffective in the treatment of this disease. The sulfonamides, although effective as continuous prophylaxis for prevention of recurrent attacks of rheumatic fever (see below), should not be used for the treatment of streptococcal pharyngitis, for they will not eradicate the streptococci from the upper respiratory tract. Penicillinase-resistant penicillins are considerably more expensive and offer no advantage over penicillin V, even in patients who harbor penicillinase-producing staphylococci in their upper respiratory tract, and, therefore, they should not be used.

Scarlet fever is simply streptococcal pharyngitis with a rash, and the antibiotic therapy should be identical to that for routine streptococcal pharyngitis.

Recent reports have noted a higher incidence of failures to eradicate group A streptococci from the upper respiratory tract following recommended doses of appropriate antibiotics, despite demonstrated sensitivity of group A streptococci to these antibiotics. Evidence suggests that most of the patients with treatment failures are streptococcal carriers and not truly infected. Routine reculturing of asymptomatic individuals who have completed a full course of appropriate antibiotic therapy is, therefore, not indicated. Reculturing of asymptomatic individuals, and retreating if positive, should be considered if compliance is questioned, if there is a history of rheumatic fever in the immediate family, if there is a lot of poststreptococcal glomerulonephritis in the community, if there is an outbreak of streptococcal pharyngitis in a closed or semiclosed community, or if there has been intrafamily "ping-ponging" of streptococcal pharyngitis.

Patients who have had rheumatic fever are at high risk of developing a recurrent attack of acute rheumatic fever with any symptomatic or asymptomatic streptococcal upper respiratory tract infection. For this reason, prevention of recurrent rheumatic fever depends upon continuous antibiotic prophylaxis. The most effective protection from rheumatic recurrences is afforded by long-term continuous antibiotic prophylaxis, perhaps for life if heart disease is present. The most effective form of prophylaxis is 1.2 million units of benzathine penicillin G, given intramuscularly every 4 weeks. Successful oral prophylaxis depends primarily upon the compliance of the patient. Oral penicillin V (125 or 250 mg twice daily) and oral sulfadiazine (1.0 gm/day for patients more than 60 pounds; 0.5 gm/day for patients less than 60 pounds) are equally effective. Prophylaxis with sulfonamides is contraindicated in late pregnancy. For the exceptional patient who is allergic to both penicillin and sulfonamides, erythromycin (250 mg twice daily) should be used.

Impetigo is a common superficial infection of the skin caused by group A streptococci. Although streptococcal impetigo is usually a mild and occasionally self-limited disease, antibiotic treatment is indicated in order to prevent local extension of the lesions and to prevent transmission of the infection to others. However, there is no evidence that antibiotics can prevent the only nonsuppurative sequelae of impetigo, acute glomerulonephritis. Intramuscular benzathine penicillin G is the most effective form of therapy in a dose of 600,000 units for patients less than 60 pounds and 1.2 million units for patients more than 60 pounds. If compliance is assured, a 7-day course of oral penicillin V (or erythromycin in the patient allergic to penicillin) is an effective alternative. Penicillinase-producing staphylococci that may be present in the streptococcal impetigo are usually commensals and do not interfere with the efficacy of penicillin therapy. Therefore, penicillinase-resistant penicillins offer no advantage over penicillin V. Topical antibiotic therapy of impetigo is not as effective as systemic antibiotic therapy, and the use of topical antibiotics in a patient who is receiving systemic antibiotics is unnecessary. However, in a patient with a solitary lesion or a few small lesions, topical antibiotics alone may be sufficient therapy. Bacitracin is the topical antibiotic of choice. Although cleanliness and good hygiene are important in preventing streptococcal impetigo, scrubbing with hexachlorophene and removing crusts does not appear to be beneficial and may actually delay healing of lesions. During epidemics of streptococcal impetigo, especially in association with poststreptococcal glomerulonephritis, prophylactic benzathine G should be considered as a means of reducing the number of new cases.

Group B Streptococcal Infections

BASCOM F. ANTHONY, M.D., *and* KWANG SIK KIM, M.D.

The group B streptococcus is a leading cause of life-threatening, invasive infection in the immediate newborn period ("early-onset" disease) and for several weeks after birth ("late-onset" disease). Otherwise, it is a rare cause of serious disease except in parturient and postabortal women and diabetics and other chronically ill adults.

Antibiotic Therapy. Significant resistance to penicillin has not been documented in human isolates of group B streptococci. Approximately 5% are penicillin-tolerant, i.e., they resist normal killing by penicillin in vitro, but the clinical importance of this phenomenon is unknown. Penicillin G, ampicillin, and many other beta-lactam agents are active against group B streptococci. These include several newer cephalosporins, with the exception of moxalactam, which is notably inactive. Most strains are sensitive to vancomycin, erythromycin, and chloramphenicol and resistant to tetracycline. Although only marginally susceptible or resistant to gentamicin, group B streptococci are killed in vitro and in experimental animals by the synergistic combination of this aminoglycoside with penicillin G or ampicillin.

Therefore, the regimen of intravenous ampicillin and gentamicin that is commonly used to treat suspected neonatal sepsis provides effective initial therapy of group B streptococcal disease. For this purpose, we prefer gentamicin to kanamycin because of greater streptococcal resistance to the latter drug. Once group B streptococci have been isolated from blood or other normally sterile body fluids, penicillin G is considered the drug of choice and is seldom contraindicated in newborn infants. The continuation of gentamicin beyond this point is recommended only if continuing bacteriologic assessment or clinical observations indicate that the infection has not responded to initial treatment. Such findings should also trigger a search for occult infection requiring surgical drainage and a reappraisal of antibiotic therapy (e.g., measuring bactericidal levels in CSF, testing for tolerance, and so on).

Newborns should receive penicillin G intravenously in a dose of 150,000 to 200,000 units/kg/day given in two or three doses. The dosage should be doubled for meningitis and divided into three or four doses. A minimum of 10 to 14 days of intravenous therapy is recommended for group B streptococcal bacteremia and pulmonary disease. When meningitis is present, at least two to three weeks' treatment is advisable, with repeated lumbar puncture to document a bacteriologic response. A similar duration of therapy is recommended for group B streptococcal arthritis, and three to four weeks is recommended for documented osteomyelitis.

Similar regimens of treatment are recommended for serious group B streptococcal infections outside the newborn period. When penicillin allergy exists, chloramphenicol (for meningitis), vancomycin, or a carefully selected cephalosporin is a reasonable alternative.

Adjunct Therapy. Despite appropriate antibiotics and vigorous supportive care, these infections are often lethal, especially in small, high-risk newborns. Further improvement in outcome may require augmenting the natural defenses of the infant. The deficiencies that are best documented in group B streptococcal sepsis are exhaustion of neutrophile stores and a lack of type-specific antibody. Granulocyte transfusion, if available, should be considered for the severely ill infant with neutropenia. Preparations of human immune serum globulin, containing significant levels of type-specific antibody and modified for intravenous use, are now available. Theoretically, both phagocytes and plasma factors may be provided by exchange transfusion with fresh, antibody-containing blood. There is compelling experimental evidence for such measures, but their value has not been established in controlled studies of infants with group B streptococcal infection.

Prevention. The efficacy and feasibility of specific preventive measures is not proven. The most promising chemoprophylactic regimen is ampicillin or penicillin treatment of the mother during labor, which appears to interrupt vertical transmission of group B streptococci. It has been recommended that this be limited to women who are known to be streptococcal carriers and who develop premature labor (<37 weeks), prolonged rupture of membranes (>12 hours), or evidence of amnionitis. The effect of prophylactic penicillin administered to infants shortly after birth is more controversial and has little effect on neonatal infection acquired before birth. Immunization of pregnant patients with purified group B streptococcal vaccines is under active study.

Listeria monocytogenes Infection

ITZHAK BROOK, M.D.

Listeria monocytogenes represents a bacterial species consisting of gram-positive to gram-variable motile, asporogenous, acapsular aerobic to microaerophilic rods. The organism is widely spread in water and soil and causes diseases in various mammals, fish, and birds.

Although colonization with the organism is common, it causes disease in humans in a sporadic way, attacking primarily, although not exclusively, neonates, pregnant women, immunocompromised hosts, and older individuals.

Inapparent infections during pregnancy are transmitted transplacentally or during delivery. Listeriosis of the newborn can manifest itself in a serious generalized infection, in which respiratory distress and heart failure are the main symptoms, with appearance of miliary granulomatosis of almost all internal organs and skin.

Central nervous system infection, which can be purulent meningitis, encephalitis, and brain abscess, is another serious neonatal problem. Bacteremia usually accompanies central nervous infection; however, listerial endocarditis with embolization is rare.

Because of the severity of listerial disease, the pediatrician must suspect and diagnose the infection rapidly in susceptible hosts. Therapy of suspected sepsis in a neonate, as in the compromised host, is often initiated without knowledge of the etiology.

Listeria monocytogenes is susceptible in vitro to clinically attainable serum concentrations of a number of antimicrobial agents including penicillin, ampicillin, tetracycline, erythromycin, sulfonamides, cephalosporins, chloramphenicol, and aminoglycosides. Ampicillin and penicillin are the drugs of choice for the treatment of listeriosis, although resistant strains may occur. In vitro susceptibility to these drugs is usually below 1 μg/ml,

and resistance to them is rare. Clinical failures in the treatment of listeriosis with penicillin can be partially ascribed to inadequate drug dosage or to its administration too late or for too short a time. The cephalosporins diffuse poorly into CSF and are not suitable for treatment of meningitis. The third-generation cephalosporins that have good penetration into CSF do not suppress the growth of *Listeria*.

We must remember that an unusual gap exists between the minimal bactericidal concentration and minimal inhibitory concentration of both penicillin and ampicillin. Bactericidal concentrations are not attainable in the cerebrospinal fluid. Additional evidence of the inefficacy of ampicillin alone is the high relapse rate in renal transplant patients with *Listeria* meningitis treated for 2 weeks with ampicillin.

Synergistic bactericidal activity between penicillin or ampicillin and streptomycin or gentamicin has been demonstrated in vitro, in vivo, and in clinical conditions. Combination therapy is thus recommended for patients with septicemic listeriosis, especially newborns, and patients with endocarditis or with immunosuppression for whom antimicrobial therapy must be bactericidal to be effective.

Initial therapy of listeriosis in the first week of life should be ampicillin 100–200 mg/kg/day IV or IM in two to three divided doses, and 200 mg/kg/day in three divided doses in the second through fourth week of life. The dose for older children and immunocompromised children should be 200 to 300 mg/kg/day in four to six divided doses. In severe cases of endocarditis or encephalitis a dose of 300–400 mg/kg/day in four to six divided doses may be needed. The treatment of all age groups should be maintained for a period of up to 4 weeks, depending on the patient's age and the form of disease.

Addition of gentamicin 5–7.5 mg/kg/day in three divided doses is desirable early in the disease. Despite the low concentration of aminoglycosides in the cerebrospinal fluid, their use is indicated because of their synergism with penicillin or ampicillin. The patient's postnatal age and renal status may influence the route and the dose of administration of the drugs, especially the aminoglycosides. Careful monitoring of serum levels may be required in certain cases. Two weeks of parenteral therapy are generally recommended for patients without meningitis. In meningitis, a longer course may be needed. The length of therapy should be decided after several lumbar punctures to ensure bacterial cure.

Combined therapy is warranted until all previously positive cultures become negative. Following that, ampicillin therapy can be continued alone for 2 weeks. In endocarditis or osteomyelitis, the ampicillin-gentamicin combination should be given for about 2 weeks; thereafter, ampicillin alone should be continued for 4 weeks. Therapy should be continued for at least 1 week after defervescence. Listeriosis of immunocompromised patients typically relapses; therefore, prolonged therapy for as long as 6 to 8 weeks may be indicated.

Other antimicrobial agents can be used in patients with penicillin allergy or penicillin resistant strains. Erythromycin, chloramphenicol, tetracycline, and sulfonamines have all been used successfully. However, these are bacteriostatic drugs and are less effective than penicillin or ampicillin. Recent in vitro work showed excellent activity of trimethoprim sulfa and rifampin against listeria. Chloramphenicol, because of its excellent penetration into the cerebrospinal fluid, is preferred for the therapy of intracranial infections. Tetracyclines can be used for children older than 8 years.

Supportive measures are important, particularly in listeriosis of the newborn. Patients with meningitis may also require respiratory assistance.

The ability to prevent fetal disease by antimicrobial therapy in the pregnant mother with positive endocervical cultures of listeria is unclear. Symptomatic maternal listeriosis may be treated with ampicillin or erythromycin.

Diphtheria

HORACE L. HODES, M.D.

By far the most important agent for the treatment of diphtheria is diphtheria antitoxin. It must be administered on the basis of a clinical diagnosis alone, since it is not safe to wait for the result of bacteriologic studies. Since diphtheria antitoxin is a horse serum, it can be given only after a negative skin or conjunctival test for sensitivity. The antitoxin is diluted 1:100 for the skin test and 1:10 for the conjunctival test. Antitoxin can neutralize only toxin that is free in the circulation. It has no effect on toxin that has become attached to cells—a process that takes place rapidly. Antitoxin should be given intravenously in one injection. It is diluted 1:20 in 5% glucose in water and administered at a rate that does not exceed 1 ml per minute. All of the antitoxin is given in one administration; it is not divided and it is not repeated. The amount of antitoxin given varies with the severity of the clinical disease and with the duration of illness before treatment is begun. If the disease is of 48 hours' duration or less, we recommend that 40,000 units be given intravenously in the average case of diphtheria of the pharynx or larynx. In more severe cases, or when the duration of the disease is three days or longer, we recommend that 80,000 units be given. In extremely severe diphtheria,

such as "bull neck" diphtheria, we recommend the use of 100,000 to 120,000 units of antitoxin.

The value of prompt antitoxin treatment cannot be overemphasized. It is borne out by the high case fatality rate among patients whose treatment is begun more than three or four days after the onset of disease. One excellent study showed that 1473 patients who received antitoxin on the first or second day of illness had a case fatality rate of 1.3%, while the 1189 who were treated on the fourth day or later had a case fatality rate of 16.9%.

Penicillin and erythromycin have a definite antibacterial action against Corynebacterium diphtheriae, and one of these drugs should be given in addition to antitoxin. Penicillin is useful also because it is effective against the streptococci that frequently are found in the throats of patients with diphtheria, and it decreases the number of persons who remain carriers of C. diphtheriae after they recover from diphtheria. A dose of 50,000 units/kg/day of crystalline penicillin G is given intravenously in four divided doses for 4 days. For the next 10 days 300,000 to 600,000 units of procaine penicillin G daily is given by intramuscular injection. For patients who are penicillin sensitive, 40 mg/kg/day of erythromycin may be given orally or parenterally for a total of 14 days. After completion of the course of antibiotic therapy, eradication of C. diphtheriae should be documented by three consecutive negative throat cultures. If this has not been achieved, a second 5-day course of oral penicillin or erythromycin should be given and the cultures repeated.

It should be noted that antibiotics cannot be used as a substitute for antitoxin, since diphtheria toxin is the cause of the life-threatening nature of diphtheria.

Complications. Diphtheritic myocarditis is the most serious complication of diphtheria. Some evidence of myocarditis can be found in the first week of illness in 50% of diphtheria patients if frequent electrocardiograms are made. Minor electrocardiographic changes are not necessarily indicative of significant myocarditis unless clinical signs are also evident. However, they should always be regarded as a danger signal, and all patients showing them should be cared for in a cardiac unit. The severity of the illness and the degree of toxemia are in general related to the incidence of severe myocarditis and circulatory failure. Patients with myocarditis should have continuous cardiac monitoring. Atrioventricular block and left bundle branch block have been associated with a mortality of over 50%. Arrhythmias are treated with procainamide, lidocaine, and isoproterenol. For congestive heart failure, short-acting digitalis preparations are given, and fluid and salt are restricted.

Treatment of respiratory obstruction requires

expert clinical judgment. The clinical appearance of the patient, his ability to rest quietly and to sleep, and the state of his blood gases must be closely watched to determine whether intervention is needed. Laryngeal, tracheal, and bronchial obstruction by pseudomembranes may require treatment by intubation, aspiration, bronchoscopy, or tracheostomy.

All patients with diphtheria should be kept in bed until it is certain that all danger of cardiac damage has passed. During the first two weeks of illness all exertion should be avoided. Patients with very severe diphtheria are often unable to swallow, and they should receive intravenous infusions of approprite solution during the first few days of illness.

Weakness or paralysis of pharyngeal muscles may occur early in diphtheria. Usually this complication is mild and requires no special treatment. However, sometimes swallowing difficulties are severe. In such cases measures to prevent aspiration, such as pharyngeal suction, are required.

Peripheral neuritis involving the extremities is a late complication and is usually mild and self-limited and requires no specific treatment. In rare instances respiratory muscles are affected, and the patient may require respiratory assistance. Complete recovery from peripheral neuritis nearly always occurs, however.

Diphtheria of the skin is very rarely accompanied by toxic symptoms and needs no specific treatment. For the rare patient who exhibits toxicity, antitoxin should be used.

Some patients who recover from diphtheria with the aid of antitoxin are found to have a positive Schick test. It is therefore recommended that all patients be given diphtheria toxoid after the first week of illness. A second dose should be given one month later and a third dose a month after that. Because they may have a severe reaction to toxoid preparations intended for infants and small children, patients 12 years of age or more should receive "adult type" toxoid, which contains only 1 to 2 Lf of diphtheria toxoid (less than 1/10 of the quantity of toxoid in the "pediatric type").

Contacts. Household contacts and other close contacts of a diphtheria patient who show clinical evidence of diphtheria should be cultured and treated with antitoxin and penicillin or erythromycin at once. Close contacts who are asymptomatic and have been immunized previously should be cultured and they should receive a booster dose of either pediatric or adult type diphtheria toxoid, depending on their age. They should also be observed carefully for 7 days. If toxogenic *C. diphtheriae* is isolated, the contact should be treated with penicillin or erythromycin.

Asymptomatic close contacts with a negative or doubtful history of previous immunization should be cultured and given 40 mg/kg/day of erythromycin by mouth for 7 days or one dose of 600,000 to 1,200,000 units of benzathine penicillin intramuscularly. Immunization with DTP should be started if they are under 12 years old, and pediatric type diphtheria toxoid and tetanus toxoid (Td) if they are over 12 years of age. They also should be observed daily for 7 days. We do not believe that the prophylactic use of antitoxin is warranted because of the risk of allergic reactions to horse serum.

Medical and nursing attendants of a diphtheria patient should be considered to be close contacts, and they should be treated accordingly.

Pertussis

MELVIN I. MARKS, M.D.

Pertussis continues to be a major problem in developing countries and in other poorly immunized populations. The term "pertussis" is reserved for respiratory infection due to the bacterium *Bordetella pertussis*; however pertussis-like syndromes are occasionally noted in association with infection due to *B. parapertussis*, *B. bronchiseptica*, *Chlamydia trachomatis*, adenovirus, and combinations of these microorganisms. The age of the patient, immunization status, virulence of the bacteria, and stage of the disease are major determinants of the clinical expression.

Supportive Care. The younger the patient, the more important the supportive care in cases of pertussis due to *Bordetella pertussis*. In fact, respiratory compromise due to obstructive secretions, aspiration of secretions and/or vomitus, and central nervous system complications (apnea, seizures) are the major causes of severe morbidity and death in this infectious disease. These are most prevalent in infants in the first year of life, particularly those under 6 months of age. Hence, these patients with pertussis need to be assessed very carefully for two features. One is the severity of the clinical disease, and the other is the ability of the family to provide appropriate supportive care. There should be no hesitation about admitting such patients to the hospital. This should probably be done with all infants under 6 months of age and with many under one year of age. For example, a brief period of in-hospital training may be necessary to help parents learn how to observe the child and how to manage the secretions, vomiting, and paroxysmal episodes.

These patients most commonly come to medical attention during the early paroxysmal stage. During this stage, a variety of stimuli will precipitate a paroxysm in infants, which is often followed by vomiting and occasionally by apnea, cyanosis, and severe distress. It is important, therefore, to provide the most comforting, quiet environment. This is often achieved by the parent or nursing staff, provided these caretakers have appropriate expectations about the clinical expression of disease and its complications. Pollutant-free air and a solicitous, caring observer are most important. Infants are often most calm in the arms of their mother or other caretakers in such a situation. Invasive procedures, such as blood taking, suctioning, and measurement of vital signs, should be kept to a minimum and are probably best done immediately after a paroxysm, when there is some refractoriness to further coughing. Suctioning should be gentle and should be used in addition to the head down position for handling excessive secretions and vomitus. Adequate hydration and nutrition are important, since excessive secretions and vomiting can disturb fluid and electrolyte balance and the nutritional status of the host in a dramatic fashion. Humidified oxygen should be administered to patients with cyanosis and apnea and when blood gas levels indicate true hypoxemia. The risks and benefits of masks, tents, and other methods for administering oxygen need to be weighed carefully in such cases. Humidified air in a mist tent is contraindicated.

Respiratory isolation is important, since pertussis is so highly contagious. Nonetheless, immune individuals (e.g., the child's mother) who are providing constant care for the patient should avoid wearing masks if possible. Similarly, isolation should be carefully done but should not be a deterrent to observation. Infants with paroxysmal pertussis under six months of age and those with apnea should never be left alone, because apnea, convulsions, and aspiration are frequent and life-threatening complications.

Antibiotic Therapy. Erythromycin is the most active drug against *B. pertussis* in vitro and in vivo and should be administered in all cases. This is done primarily to reduce contagiousness, although administration of the drug may reduce the severity of the disease if given during the catarrhal phase. The appropriate dosage of erythromycin is 50 mg/kg/day given orally in divided doses every 6 hours, for 14 days. Respiratory isolation can be relaxed after approximately 5 days of erythromycin therapy, since the bacteria will be eliminated from the nasopharynx during this period of time in almost all patients. Fourteen days of therapy are recommended, since bacteriologic relapses have been reported with shorter durations. Although tetracycline, chloramphenicol, trimethoprim-sulfamethoxazole, ampicillin, and newly developed cephalosporins (cefoperazone, moxalactam and cefotaxime) are active in vitro against *B. pertussis*, there is limited clinical experience with these agents and additional side effects are expected with their use, particularly in infants.

Occasionally Useful Therapy. Adrenal corticosteroids have been used in infants with particularly severe paroxysmal disease in an effort to reduce the host's inflammatory response, which is thought to be mediated by toxins elaborated by these bacteria. Although preliminary studies indicate this, and some bronchodilators, such as albuterol* and salbutamol*, reduce the severity of paroxysms and other complications of the disease, there are insufficient controlled studies to justify their use on a routine basis. Currently, prescription of these pharmacologic agents should be limited to hospitalized infants with severe paroxysmal disease and with careful observation for the known toxicities of these agents. Corticosteroids (betamethasone in oral doses of 0.075 mg/kg/day or hydrocortisone in intramuscular doses of 30 mg/kg/day) can be given for two days and then in gradually tapered dosages for one week. Albuterol* can be given at a dosage level of 0.5 mg/kg/day during the severe paroxysmal stage.

Knowledge of the complications of pertussis is important in order to diagnose and manage bronchopneumonia, otitis media, and convulsions. Other manifestations of the disease, such as rectal prolapse and petechiae, may be referable to the extreme pressures developed during the paroxysmal stage and may occasionally be attributed to therapies as well.

Prevention. Avoidance of exposure and appropriate immunization with pertussis vaccine are most effective. Exposed susceptible individuals under 6 years of age should receive a booster dose of vaccine if their primary series of immunizations (three doses, each separated by at least 4 weeks, plus a booster dose at 1 year and 18 months) is incomplete, or if more than two years has elapsed since immunization. Immunization can be initiated shortly after birth in epidemic situations and in highly endemic regions. Erythromycin can also be administered at the time of exposure or at the earliest onset of catarrhal symptoms in exposed susceptible individuals at any age. To avoid outbreaks in closed populations erythromycin and strict respiratory isolation may be necessary for all subjects over 6 years of age. Immune globulin has no proven value in the prevention or treatment of pertussis.

Pneumonia

MARGARET H. D. SMITH, M.D.

Respiratory pathogens causing pneumonia vary with the age of the child; the child's exposures, activities, and hobbies; and the child's immune

---

* The safety and efficacy of these agents in children less than 12 years of age have not been established.

status. On the other hand, the great variety of available chemotherapeutic agents make etiologic diagnosis highly desirable, hence history, awareness of community infectious problems, and relevant, reliable diagnostic procedures are more important than ever before. Rapid, practical, specific diagnosis of viral infections will be most welcome when available, since many of the bronchopneumonias of early childhood are undoubtedly due to respiratory viruses, which we cannot, at present, diagnose specifically outside of research institutions.

Newborns

Pneumonia in the neonate is usually due to organisms from the mother's vaginal flora, i.e., gram-negative rods or Group B streptococcus. Treatment is presented in Table 1. Ampicillin and gentamicin give wide coverage for these organisms. Because of rapidly maturing renal function in the first days of life, the recommended dosage regimen differs slightly for infants less than one week of age as compared with those one week and older; furthermore some clinicians differentiate between

very small premature infants and infants born at term.

Pneumonia arising in infants older than one week may be due to chlamydial infection acquired from the mother but may also be nosocomial in origin, due to staphylococci or to gram-negative rods that may be highly resistant to the usual drugs. In this situation history and accurate bacteriologic diagnosis are essential.

Pneumonia due to Group B streptococcus can often be treated with penicillin G or ampicillin alone; however, some strains display a wide divergence between the minimal inhibitory concentration (MIC) of the penicillin and its minimal bactericidal concentration (MBC). If these determinations are *not* available, or *until* the results are available, or *if* there is a wide discrepancy between MIC and MBC, many clinicians prefer to use both a penicillin and an aminoglycoside together.

Pneumonia due to gram-negative organisms displaying a high degree of resistance to penicillins and aminoglycosides may warrant the use of chloramphenicol, despite the "gray baby syndrome," which the latter can cause. Newborns receiving

Table 1. DRUGS AND DOSAGE SCHEDULES FOR ANTIMICROBIALS USEFUL FOR BACTERIAL PNEUMONIA IN NEWBORNS

Pathogen, Proven or Provable	Antimicrobial Drug	Dosage		Duration of Treatment	Comments
		1 Week of Age	1–4 Weeks		
Group B streptococcus	Penicillin G	25,000 to 50,000 units/kg IV q 12 h	35,000–70,000 units/kg IV q 8 h	10–14 days	
	or Ampicillin*	25–50 mg/kg IV or IM q 12 h	50–100 mg/kg IV or IM q 8 h	10–14 days	
Escherichia coli, Enterobacter sp.	Gentamicin	2.5 mg/kg IV or IM q 12 h	2.5 mg/kg IV or IM q 8 h	10–14 days	Do peak and trough drug levels.
	Tobramycin	2 mg/kg IV or IM q 12 h	1.2 mg/kg IV or IM q 8 h	10–14 days	Do peak and trough drug levels.
	Amikacin } Kanamycin	7.5 mg/kg IV or IM q 12 h	7.5 mg/kg IV or IM q 8 h	10–14 days	Do peak and trough drug levels.
Staphylococcus aureus	Oxacillin	25–50 mg/kg IV or IM q 12 h	25–70 mg/kg IV or IM q 8 h	21 days minimum	
	or Vancomycin	15 mg/kg IV q 12 h	15 mg/kg IV q 8 h		
Pseudomonas aeruginosa	Gentamicin or amikacin *and*	as above	—	10 days minimum	Use ceftazidime when available.
	Mezlocillin	75 mg/kg IV or IM q 12 h	75–100 mg/kg q 8 h		
	or ticarcillin	75 mg/kg IV or IM q 12 h	75–100 mg/kg IV or IM q 8 h		
Chlamydia trachomatis	Erythromycin	10 mg/kg PO q 12 h	10 mg/kg PO q 8 h		
Gram-negative bacilli resistant to usual drugs	Chloramphenicol	12.5 mg/kg IV or PO q 12 h	12.5–25 mg/kg IV or PO q 12 h		Do peak and trough drug levels.

* Many clinicians recommend adding an aminoglycoside because of possible tolerance. See text.

this drug should be watched with particular care, and drug levels should be measured.

Children Between 1 Month and 5 Years of Age

While viruses frequently cause pneumonia in this age group, bacteria are common too, particularly *Streptococcus pneumoniae* and *Haemophilus influenzae*. Treatment is presented in Table 2. Since ampicillin is effective against both, it is the drug of choice until or unless *S. pneumoniae* has been identified as the etiologic agent. Since some 20% of *H. influenzae* strains are resistant to ampicillin in the United States, chloramphenicol may have to be used in certain patients. In known pneumococcal pneumonia, intravenous penicillin G is the drug of choice at the start, followed by oral penicillin V for a week or two as the patient improves. (Benzathine penicillin gives low levels and should not be used.)

If *Staphylococcus aureus* is suspected, because of the presence of lobar pneumonia in a child less than 6 months old or because of pneumatoceles or purulent empyema, oxacillin should be used parenterally as initial therapy followed by oral oxacillin or cloxacillin for a period of weeks during convalescence. Should clinical response be poor or should the patient have had exposure, direct or indirect (e.g., mother, a nurse in an intensive care unit), to methicillin-resistant staphylococci, then vancomycin, or vancomycin plus rifampin, should be substituted.

Chlamydia trachomatis and, rarely, *Bordetella pertussis* can cause diffuse, severe pneumonia with intractable cough in infants during the early months of life. Both are best treated with erythromycin. The drug is usually given orally, since it is extremely irritating when given intramuscularly.

Children of 5 Years and Above, Including Adolescents

In this age group viral pneumonias are much less common than in the younger child, unless an epidemic of influenzae A is in progress, in which case amantadine may need to be considered for treatment as well as prophylaxis. Otherwise, the two major pathogens are *Streptococcus pneumoniae*, best treated with penicillin G, and *Mycoplasma pneumoniae*, for which erythromycin is appropriate. Tetracyclines may also be used for patients above 8 to 10 years, in whom tooth staining is no longer a problem.

It is in this age group that thought must be given to rarer pathogens associated with hobbies and travel, such as psittacosis (best treated with tetracyclines or chloramphenicol), *Francisella tularensis* (treated with streptomycin or gentamicin), *legionella* (treated with erythromycin for milder cases; add rifampin or tetracyclines for severe cases).

Immunosuppressed Children

Pneumonia in the immunodeficient or immunosuppressed child poses a challenge, first from the viewpoint of etiology (is it due to cytomegalovirus, unusual bacteria, fungi, or a protozoan, namely *Pneumocystis carinii*, or to toxicity from antineoplastic drugs?) and second, from the viewpoint of finding an appropriate, well-tolerated treatment regimen. Among the bacteria most often

Table 2.   DRUGS AND DOSAGE SCHEDULES FOR ANTIMICROBIALS USEFUL FOR PNEUMONIA
IN *CHILDREN AND ADOLESCENTS*

Pathogen, Proven or Provable	Antimicrobial Drug	Dosage	Duration	Comments
Streptococcus pneumoniae	Penicillin G	37,500 units IV q 6 h (after improvement use Pen V PO same dose)	10 days total	
Haemophilus influenzae (or any pneumonia in a child <4 years of age)	Ampicillin *and* Chloramphenicol *or* Cefuroxime alone	25 mg/kg IV or IM q 6 h 25 mg/kg IV or PO q 6 h 25–50 mg/kg IV or IM q 8 h	7–10 days 7–10 days	Select single appropriate drug based on susceptibility.
Chlamydia trachomatis	Erythromycin	10 mg/kg PO q 6 h	10 days	Many formulations available; check tablet size, concentration of syrup, etc.
Mycoplasma pneumoniae	Erythromycin	10 mg/kg PO q 6 h	14 days	"
Legionella sp.	Erythromycin	10 mg/kg PO q 6 h	14 days	"
Staphylococcus aureus	Oxacillin	25–50 mg/kg IV or IM q 6 h (after improvement use 12.5–50 mg/kg PO q 6 h *or* cloxacillin 12.5–50 mg/kg PO q6 h)	15–30 days	If organism reported to be methicillin-resistant use vancomycin and rifampin.
Klebsiella pneumoniae	Gentamicin*	2.5 mg/kg IM or IV q 6 h	14 days	

* Manufacturer's note: Maximum recommended daily dose is 7.5 mg/kg.

Table 3.   DRUGS AND DOSAGE SCHEDULES FOR SOME OF THE ANTIMICROBIALS USEFUL FOR BACTERIAL PNEUMONIA IN THE CHILD WITH *IMMUNOSUPPRESSION* OR *CYSTIC FIBROSIS*

Pathogen, Proven or Probable	Antimicrobial Drug	Dosage	Duration	Comments
Entirely unknown	Mezlocillin or ticarcillin	50–75 mg/kg IV q 6 h	2–3 weeks minimum	
	and			
	Amikacin	5–10 mg/kg IV or IM q 8 h	2–3 weeks minimum	
	or			
	Gentamicin	1–2.5 mg/kg IV or IM q 8 h	2–3 weeks minimum	
	and			
	Vancomycin	10 mg/kg IV q 6 h	2–3 weeks minimum	
*Pneumocystis carinii**	Trimethoprim/ sulfamethoxazole	2.5 mg TMP, 12.5 mg/kg SMX PO q 12 h	2–3 weeks minimum	
Pseudomonas aeruginosa	Ticarcillin	75–100 mg/kg IV q 4 h	3–4 weeks minimum	Use ceftazidime when available. Cystics metabolize rapidly and need larger than usual doses. Check peak and trough levels.
	and			
	Tobramycin†	2–3 mg/kg IM or IV q 8 h		
	or			
	Gentamicin†	1–2.5 mg/kg IM or IV q 8 h		
Bacteroides fragilis	Chloramphenicol	25 mg/kg IV or PO q 6 h		Do peak and trough levels.
	Clindamycin	6–10 mg/kg IV or IM q 6–8 h 2.5–7.5 mg/kg PO q 6 h		
Bacteroides, other sp.	Penicillin G	37,500 units IV q 6 h		
Enterobacter sp., *Escherichia coli*	Gentamicin	1–2.5 IV or IM q 8 h		
Mycobacteria ("atypical," environmental)	INH	5 mg/kg IV or PO q 12 h		
	and			
	Rifampin	20 mg/kg PO q 24 h		Substitute ansamycin for rifampin if available.
	and			
	Streptomycin	10–15 mg/kg IM q 12 h		

* *Pneumocystis carinii* is a protozoan but is included here for convenience.
† Manufacturer's note: Maximum recommended daily dose is 7.5 mg/kg.

implicated are the gram-negative bacilli, followed by *Staph. aureus* and, less often, mycobacteria. Since *Pneumocystis carinii* (a protozoan) is more frequent than mycobacteria, a rational, empiric regimen to start with includes an aminoglycoside, oxacillin, and trimethoprim-sulfamethoxazole, but this must often be adjusted to cover *Pseudomonas*, methicillin-resistant staphylococci, and other organisms, depending on the results of culture. See Table 3 for details of treatment.

Children with Cystic Fibrosis

The realization that recurrent pulmonary infections are, in large measure, responsible for the downhill course in these patients has led in recent years to aggressive efforts at prophylaxis and therapy. As yet, the best approach is not defined. *S. pneumoniae, H. influenzae* and staphylococci are frequently recovered from respiratory cultures of

these patients, but it is often difficult to differentiate invasive organisms from commensals. Later in the course, mucoid strains of *Pseudomonas* predominate. Not only is it difficult to deliver adequate doses of antimicrobial drugs to the damaged bronchial lumen and alveoli where the organisms are multiplying, but these patients metabolize the drugs themselves, particularly aminoglycosides, differently; thus it is essential to start with a larger drug dosage than usual and to monitor peak and trough drug levels. See Table 3 for details of treatment.

Adjuncts to Antimicrobial Therapy

The *cephalosporins* and *cephamycins* are in general more expensive than the penicillins and other, more established microbial agents. Also, many of them cross the blood-brain barrier poorly, so that in a child with any kind of infection, in whom prevention of meningitis is one of the goals of treatment, this group of drugs falls short. However, as prices fall, and as we become more familiar with the newer compounds, drugs such as cefuroxime, cefotaxime, and others may become drugs of choice. They should even now be used for patients with known *sensitivity to penicillin*, for patients with *H. influenzae* infection in which the organisms are *multiply resistant* to ampicillin and chloramphenicol, and in situations where chloramphenicol levels cannot be measured.

Oxacillin is recommended over methicillin, because of the latter's greater nephrotoxicity, and over nafcillin, because of this compound's tendency to produce local necrosis at the site of injection.

Management of the pediatric patient with pneumonia includes attention to fluid and electrolyte balance; oxygen when needed for cyanosis or dyspnea; drainage of pleural fluid or empyema if respiration is impeded by the large accumulation of fluid. A semi-sitting position in an infant seat can be of great help to a dyspneic infant, as can a rectal tube when abdominal distention is severe.

Follow-up of the child after a bout of pneumonia is controversial. Some clinicians recommend a chest roentgenogram a month or so later; others prefer to avoid the extra radiation, since the yield of significant findings is very low. At least it should be considered.

Meningococcal Disease

NELL J. RYAN, M.D.

The general principles of treatment of meningococcal disease should include measures to control the process already underway and measures to prevent the development of complications that further compromise the patient. Serious and potentially fatal complications of meningococcal disease include endotoxic shock, disseminated intravascular coagulation, hemorrhage into the adrenals, and cerebral edema. Unless the disease is rapidly fulminant, these complications can be prevented or reversed by prompt and adequate treatment of the infectious process. The following management is effective in achieving this goal.

The single most important therapeutic consideration is the prompt institution of adequate and specific antibiotics. Aqueous penicillin G is the drug of choice. The initial dose is 6 million units/m^2 intravenously followed by 16 million units/m^2/24 hours in 6 divided doses. Intravenous administration is continued for 10 days and until the patient has been free of fever for at least 72 hours. The patient who is allergic to penicillin can be effectively treated with chloramphenicol. The in-

itial dose is 50 mg/kg IV, and treatment consists of 100 mg/kg/24 hours given in four divided doses. Close observation of the patient is essential. The child should, if at all possible, be admitted to a pediatric intensive care unit and the following parameters monitored hourly: temperature, pulse, respiration, blood pressure, and neurologic vital signs. Baseline complete blood cell count, platelet count, blood chemistries, and coagulation studies should be obtained and monitored as clinically indicated. Fluids should be restricted to 1000 cc/m^2/24 hours for the first 72 hours. This will prevent cerebral edema, which is emerging as the major cause of death in meningococcemia and meningococcal meningitis; the endotoxin affects the endothelial cells, which results in altered brain capillary function, leading to cerebral edema. Fluids must, therefore, be given cautiously even in those patients with hypotension as a result of endotoxic shock. The plasma volume is not diminished in endotoxic shock, and transfusions do not always increase the peripheral circulation. The aggressive use of fluids to treat the endotoxic shock and vascular failure will potentiate the cerebral edema and can be fatal.

If the patient presents with or develops endotoxic shock, steroids are of benefit. Hydrocortisone is given in an initial dose of 10 mg/kg IV and maintained at a dose of 10 mg/kg/24 hours given every 4–6 hours and continued as clinically indicated. If the plasma volume is decreased, fresh frozen plasma in increments of 5 cc/kg is indicated. Electrolytes should be corrected and maintained. Increased intracranial pressure (manifested by a tight, bulging fontanel or spread sutures in the infant and young child and papilledema in the older child) is treated with dexamethasone. The initial dose consists of 1 mg/kg up to a maximum of 20 mg IV. The maintenance dose is 1 mg/kg/24 hours (maximum 20 mg) given in 4 divided doses and maintained for 72 hours. Disseminated intravascular coagulation, a consumption coagulopathy, can usually be controlled or reversed by the prompt treatment of the infection. Platelet transfusions and infusions of fresh frozen plasma may be necessary to support the patient until the disease process can be controlled. Heparin 100 units/kg IV every 4 to 6 hours is recommended if widespread thrombosis (purpura fulminans) is present.

Prophylaxis. There is an increased risk of severe meningococcal disease in close family, day care, and school contacts of the index case. Prophylactic antibiotics are recommended for household and immediate (same classroom on a regular basis) day care contacts of the index case. Prophylaxis is not recommended for hospital personnel unless extremely close contact such as mouth to mouth resuscitation occurred. Rifampin is the drug of choice. The dose for adults is 600 mg orally twice a day for two days. For children, the dose is 10 mg/kg orally twice a day for 2 days.* The dose should not exceed 1200 mg/day.† This dose is cut in half for neonates. If the organism is known to be sensitive to sulfonamides, a sulfonamide such as sulfadiazine‡ is recommended. The dose is 100 mg/kg/24 hours given in four divided doses.

Prevention. The efficacy of group-specific meningococcal vaccines has been documented. Vaccines against groups A, C, and Y have been shown to be effective in clinical trials. Group A vaccine is effective in children above 6 years of age, and group C vaccine is effective in children over 2 years of age. A single dose of serogroup C vaccine is about 70% effective in preventing meningococcal infections for a period of 6 to 9 months in children over 2 years of age.

Infections Due to *Escherichia coli, Proteus, Klebsiella-Enterobacter-Serratia, Pseudomonas,* and Other Gram-Negative Bacilli

HARRIS D. RILEY, JR., M.D.,
and MICHAEL J. MUSZYNSKI, M.D.

Although the management of infections due to these organisms must be individualized, certain generalizations can be made. Few infections that the physician is called upon to treat pose as difficult a problem as do those due to gram-negative coliform bacilli. Infections with these organisms are increasing in frequency, particularly as a hospital-associated phenomenon. Although new antibiotics have become available to which certain of these organisms are susceptible, the susceptibility of a given strain is unpredictable, and susceptible strains may develop resistance relatively rapidly. Furthermore, most of the antimicrobials that have activity against these organisms are accompanied by a significant risk of toxicity.

The fact that infections due to these organisms are particularly common in postoperative patients and in those debilitated by other disorders or therapies compounds the difficulties by limiting the choice of available therapeutic agents and makes evaluation of antibacterial treatment more perplexing. Because of the variability in response to therapy, careful bacteriologic study and in vitro susceptibility tests should precede initiation of therapy.

In general, comparatively large doses of the selected antimicrobial agent(s) should be utilized and should be continued for relatively long periods. Infection, especially bacteremia, due to these and other gram-negative bacteria, may be accompanied by clinical shock secondary to the elaboration of endotoxins. Appropriate supportive therapy for this complication is an important phase of the total management.

Antimicrobial agents of choice against the relatively common gram-negative bacilli are shown in Table 1. The most reliable guide to the choice of an antimicrobial agent is the results of in vitro antibiotic susceptibility tests. However, in many instances, particularly in infants and children, treatment must be initiated after appropriate cultures are obtained but before the results of these studies are known. Table 1 can be used as a general guide in such situations. The choice of a particular drug depends upon many different circumstances: epidemiologic information, particularly whether the infection is community- or hospital-acquired; the clinical picture, including the site of infection and presence of underlying disease; the frequency of resistance to various antimicrobials among various organisms in the local area; and others.

The dose, route of administration, and other details of therapeutic use of the various antimicrobial agents useful in the treatment of infections due to these organisms are listed in Table 2. Since these infections occur frequently in the neonatal and infancy periods, the difference in the pharmacology and metabolism of drugs in patients in these age groups, as well in patients with impaired renal function, should be recalled. The dosage schedule for newborn and low birth weight infants is also included.

INFECTIONS

Escherichia coli Infections

Escherichia coli are gram-negative motile rods normally found as part of the bacterial flora of the gastrointestinal tract. They have the capacity to produce a powerful endotoxin, which enters the circulation and induces shock and the clinical pathologic picture of the Shwartzman phenomenon.

Infection in the Neonate. Gram-negative bacilli, particularly *E. coli*, are among the most common causes of septicemia and meningitis of the neonate. In most areas of the United States, *E. coli* and *Klebsiella-Enterobacter-Serratia* account for a large segment of the cases. *E. coli* bacilli also are a significant cause of pneumonia in this age group and have been shown along with other gram-negative enteric organisms to be a cause of otitis media in infants less than 6 weeks of age. *E. coli* also produces urinary infection often associated with jaundice in infants less than 2 months of age.

---

* Manufacturer's precaution: Data not available to determine dosage for children under 5 years of age.

† Exceeds manufacturer's maximum daily dose of 600 mg/day.

‡ This use is not listed in the manufacturer's directive.

Text continued on page 528

Table 1.   ANTIMICROBIAL AGENTS FOR INFECTIONS DUE TO GRAM-NEGATIVE BACILLI OF RELATIVELY COMMON CLINICAL OCCURRENCE*

Organism	Drug	
Escherichia coli[†]		
Community-acquired	Ampicillin Kanamycin Tobramycin Gentamicin	Cephalosporin[1] Chloramphenicol Tetracycline
Hospital-acquired	Ampicillin Gentamicin Kanamycin Amikacin[3] Quinolones[2]	Tobramycin[3] Cephalosporin[1] Ticarcillin Chloramphenicol
Enterotoxigenic and enteroinvasive[‡]	Polymyxin (oral) Neomycin (oral) Kanamycin (oral)	Ampicillin Gentamicin (oral)
Enterobacter species	Gentamicin Tobramycin[3] Cephalosporins Carbenicillin or ticarcillin Nalidixic acid Kanamycin	Polymyxin or colistin Chloramphenicol Ticarcillin Amikacin[3] Tetracycline
Klebsiella pneumoniae	Gentamicin with or without a cephalosporin Tobramycin[3] Kanamycin	Tetracycline Cephalosporin[1] Chloramphenicol Amikacin[3]
Proteus mirabilis	Ampicillin Penicillin G Cephalosporin[1] Gentamicin	Kanamycin Tobramycin[3] Nalidixic acid Chloramphenicol
Indole-positive *Proteus* (*P. vulgaris, P. morganii,* *P. rettgeri*)	Gentamicin Kanamycin Tobramycin Chloramphenicol Carbenicillin or ticarcillin	Nalidixic acid Tetracycline Amikacin[3] Sisomicin[2,3] Cephalosporin[4]
Pseudomonas aeruginosa[†]	Tobramycin[3,5,6] Polymyxin or colistin Ticarcillin Gentamicin[6]	Pipercillin Azlocillin Mezlocillin Aztronam[2] Tobramycin[3,5] Imipeneum-cilastin Amikacin[3,5,6] Carbenicillin
Serratia marcescens	Tobramycin Amikacin[3] Gentamicin Kanamycin Trimethoprim-sulfamethoxazole	Chloramphenicol Nalidixic acid Carbenicillin Ticarcillin Cephalosporin[1]

* In most instances, drug of first choice is listed first. Susceptibility tests are important in determining therapy for infections due to any of these organisms. However, in many instances, drug of choice depends on susceptibility results.

† For treatment of urinary tract infections, see text.

‡ Indications tentative.

[1] Refers to one of the cephalosporins, administered parenterally or orally depending upon drug and nature of infection. See text and Table 2 for further details and information on new cephalosporins.

[2] Investigational drug.

[3] See text for discussion of indications and use.

[4] Cefoxitin appears to be the most effective cephalosporin.

[5] Combination of gentamicin or other aminoglycoside and carbenicillin or ticarcillin is usually synergistic. Both can be used in serious life-threatening infections. Use of carbenicillin or ticarcillin alone is associated with emergence of resistant *Pseudomonas* and super-infection with resistant *Klebsiella*.

[6] Synergistic with carbenicillin and ticarcillin against many strains.

Table 2.   DAILY DOSAGE SCHEDULE FOR ANTIMICROBIAL AGENTS*

Drug	Oral	Intramuscular	Intravenous	Intrathecal	Adult or Maximum Dose
Penicillin G[1]	500,000–2,000,000 U in 5 doses ½ hr a.c.	20,000–50,000 U/kg in 4–6 doses	20,000–100,000 U/kg in 4–6 doses		20–100 million U/24 hr
Neonate & Prem.[2]	50,000 U/kg in 4 doses	20,000–50,000 U/kg in 2–4 doses	20,000–50,000 U/kg in 4 doses		
Chloramphenicol[3]	50–100 mg/kg in 4 doses[4]		50–100 mg/kg in 3–4 doses (10% solution)		3–4 gm/24 hr; maximum in child 2.0 gm/24 hr
Neonate & Prem.[2,4]	25[a]–50[b] mg/kg in 4 doses		15[a]–25[b] mg/kg in 2–4 doses (0.5 mg/ml)		
Tetracycline[5,c]	20–40 mg/kg in 4 doses	12 mg/kg in 2 doses	12 mg/kg in 2 doses (1 mg/ml)		2.0 gm/24 hr
Neonate & Prem.[2]	10–20 mg/kg in 4 doses	6 mg/kg in 2 doses	6 mg/kg in 2 doses (1 mg/ml)		
Kanamycin[6]	100 mg/kg in 4 doses	30 mg/kg in 3 doses	30 mg/kg in 3 doses (2.5 mg/ml)		Oral, 3–4 gm/24 hr IM, 1.0–1.5 gm/24 hr
Neonate & Prem.[2,17]	50 mg/kg in 4 doses	15–20 mg/kg in 2–3 doses (see text)	(see text)		
Neomycin[d]	100–150 mg/kg in 4 doses[f]				Oral, 6.0 gm/24 hr IM, 1.0 gm/24 hr
Neonate & Prem.[2]	50 mg/kg in 4 doses				
Streptomycin sulfate[7,d]		20–40 mg/kg in 2–3 doses		1.0 mg/kg or 20 mg/24 hr (5 mg/ml)	2.0 gm/24 hr
Neonate & Prem.[2]		10–20 mg/kg in 2 doses			
Sulfonamides[8]	120–150 mg/kg in 4 doses		120 mg/kg (24 mg/ml) in 2–4 doses		3–4 gm/24 hr
Neonate & Prem.[2,4]	50 mg/kg/day[e] in 2–3 doses				
Polymyxin B[9]	15–20 mg/kg in 4–6 doses	2.5–5.0 mg/kg in 4–6 doses	2.5–5.0 mg/kg in 3 doses (0.4 mg/ml 5% dextrose in endocarditis)	<2 yrs, 2 mg/24 hr or every other day	Oral, 500 mg/24 hr Parenteral, 200 mg/24 hr
Neonate & Prem.[2]	10–15 mg/kg in 4 doses	3[a]–4[b] mg/kg in 4 doses		>2 yrs, 5 mg/24 hr (0.5–1.0 mg/ml)	Intrathecal, 10 mg/24 hr
Colistin[9]	15–30 mg/kg in 4 doses	5.0–8.0 mg/kg in 3 doses	1.5–5.0 mg/kg in 2–4 doses	<1 yr, 2 mg/24 hr[14] >1 yr, 5 mg/24 hr	5.0 mg/kg/24 hr IM
Neonate & Prem.[2]	10–20 mg/kg in 4 doses	1.0–2.0 mg/kg in 2–4 doses			
Novobiocin[10]	20–45 mg/kg in 4 doses				Oral, 2.0 gm/24 hr
Neonate & Prem.[2,4]	10–15 mg/kg in 2–3 doses				
Gentamicin[11]	5–10 mg/kg in 1 dose[26]	3–7.5 mg/kg in 3 doses		1–2 mg/24 hr	IM, 5 mg/kg/24 hr[11]
Neonate & Prem.[2,12]		5(3–7.5) mg/kg in 2–3 doses[18]			
Cephalothin[13]		80–160 mg/kg in 4–6 doses	80–160 mg/kg in 4–6 doses or in continuous infusion		Parenteral, 2–6 gm/24 hr
Neonate & Prem.[2]		50–100 mg/kg in 2–3 doses	50–100 mg/kg in 4 doses or in continuous infusion		

Table continued on following page

Table 2.   DAILY DOSAGE SCHEDULE FOR ANTIMICROBIAL AGENTS* (continued)

Drug	Oral	Intramuscular	Intravenous	Intrathecal	Adult or Maximum Dose
Ampicillin[15]	100–200 mg/kg in 4 doses	150–400 mg/kg in 4 doses	150–400 mg/kg in 4 doses		Oral, 2–6 gm/24 hr Parenteral, 2–4 gm/24 hr
Neonate & Prem.[2]	25–200 mg/kg in 4 doses	50–200 mg/kg in 2–3 doses[19]			
Paromomycin[9]	50–100 mg/kg in 4 doses[f]				2.0 gm/24 hr
Neonate & Prem.[2]					
Cephaloridine		50–100 mg/kg in 3 doses	30–100 mg/kg in 2–3 doses		4.0 gm/24 hr
Neonate & Prem.[2]					
Nystatin	1,000,000–2,000,000 U in 3–4 doses				
Neonate & Prem.[2]	400,000 U in 4 doses				
Amphotericin B[16]			1 mg/kg given over 6–8 hr period		1 mg/kg
Neonate & Prem.[2]					
Methenamine mandelate	100 mg/kg first dose; then 50 mg/kg/24 hr in 3 doses				4 gm/24 hr
Nitrofurantoin	5–7 mg/kg/24 hr; reduce dosage after 10–14 days to 2.5–5.0 mg/kg/24 hr				400 mg/24 hr
Neonate & Prem.[2]	Contraindicated				
Carbenicillin	100 mg/kg/day in 4 doses		400–600 mg/kg in 4–6 doses		40 gm/24 hr
Neonate & Prem.[2]			300 mg/kg/24 hr		
Carbenicillin indanyl sodium	30–50 mg/kg in 4 doses				2–3 gm (max)
Cephalexin	50–100 mg/kg/24 hr in 4 doses				12 gm/24 hr
Nalidixic acid[g]	12 mg/kg/24 hr				4.0 gm/24 hr
Cefazolin		50–100 mg/kg in 3 doses	50–100 mg/kg in 3 doses		6.0 gm/24 hr
Neonate & Prem.[2]		Not recommended	Not recommended		
Tobramycin		8–10 mg/kg in 3 doses	8–10 mg/kg in 3 doses		5 mg/kg/24 hr
Neonate & Prem.[2]		5 mg/kg in 2–3 doses	5 mg/kg in 2–3 doses		
Clindamycin	10–25 mg/kg in 4 doses	10–40 mg/kg in 4 doses	10–40 mg/kg in 4 doses		4.8 gm/24 hr
Neonate & Prem.[2]	Unknown	Unknown	Unknown		
Cloxacillin	50–100 mg/kg in 4 doses				4.0 gm/24 hr
Neonate & Prem.[2]	Not recommended				
Dicloxacillin	25–100 mg/kg in 4 doses				4.0 gm/24 hr
Neonate & Prem.[2]	Not recommended				
Methicillin		100–300 mg/kg in 4–6 doses	100–300 mg/kg in 4–6 doses		12.0 gm/24 hr
Neonate & Prem.[2]		50–200 mg/kg[20] in 2–3 doses	50–100 mg/kg[20] in 2–3 doses		

Table 2.   DAILY DOSAGE SCHEDULE FOR ANTIMICROBIAL AGENTS* (*continued*)

Drug	Oral	Intramuscular	Intravenous	Intrathecal	Adult or Maximum Dose
Nafcillin	50–100 mg/kg in 4 doses	100–200 mg/kg in 4–6 doses	100–200 mg/kg in 4–6 doses		12.0 gm/24 hr
Neonate & Prem.[2]		75–100 mg/kg in 2–4 doses[20]	75–100 mg/kg in 2–4 doses[20]		
Oxacillin	50–100 mg/kg in 4 doses	100–200 mg/kg in 4–6 doses	100–200 mg/kg in 4–6 doses		12.0 gm/24 hr
Neonate & Prem.[2]		50–200 mg/kg in 2–4 doses[20]	50–200 mg/kg in 2–4 doses[20]		
Penicillin V	25,000–400,000 U/kg in 4 doses				6.4 million U/24 hr
Neonate & Prem.[2]	25,000–200,000 U/kg in 3 doses				
Amoxicillin	40–100 mg/kg in 3 doses				3.0 gm/24 hr
Neonate & Prem.[2]	40–100 mg/kg in 3–4 doses				
Amikacin		20 mg/kg in 2–3 doses	20 mg/kg in 2–3 doses		
Neonate & Prem.[2]		Initial dose, 10 mg/kg[21]	Initial dose, 10 mg/kg[21]		
Ticarcillin			300 mg/kg in 4–6 doses		
Neonate & Prem.[2]			Initial dose, 100 mg/kg[22]		
Lincomycin	30–60 mg/kg in 4 doses	20 mg/kg in 2 doses	20 mg/kg in 2 doses		Oral, 2 gm/24 hr IM, 8.0 gm/24 hr IV, 8.0 gm/24 hr
Cefaclor	40 mg/kg in 3 doses				2–3 gm/24 hr
Cefadroxil[h]	40 mg/kg in 2 doses				2 gm
Neonate & Prem.	Not recommended				
Cephradrine	40–60 mg/kg in 4 doses	50–100 mg/kg in 4 doses	50–100 mg/kg in 4 doses		2–3 gm
Neonate & Prem.	Not recommended	Not recommended			
Cephapirin		40–80 mg/kg in 4 doses	40–80 mg/kg in 4 doses		
Cefamandole[23,24]		50–150 mg/kg in 4–6 doses	50–150 mg/kg in 4–6 doses		4–6 gm
Cefoxitin		50–150 mg/kg in 3–4 doses	50–150 mg/kg in 3–4 doses		12 gm
Neonate & Prem.		Not recommended	Not recommended		
Hetacillin	50–100 mg/kg in 4 doses				
Cyclacillin	0.5–1.0 gm in 4 doses				2 gm
Neonate & Prem.	Not recommended				
Bacampicillin	25–50 mg/kg in 2 doses				3.2 gm
Cefotaxime		150–200 mg/kg in 4 doses	150–200 mg/kg in 4 doses		
Ceftriaxone		75 mg/kg in 2 doses	75 mg/kg in 2 doses		
Cefuroxime		75 mg/kg in 3 doses	75 mg/kg in 3 doses		
Cinoxacin for UTI only > 12 y.o.	1000 mg in 2–4 doses				
Doxycycline	4–5 mg/kg in 2 doses				
Erythromycin	30–50 mg/kg in 4 doses		40–70 mg/kg in 4 doses		
Neonate & Prem.[2] and <4 mos	20–40 mg/kg in 3 doses				

Table continued on following page

Table 2.   DAILY DOSAGE SCHEDULE FOR ANTIMICROBIAL AGENTS* (*continued*)

Drug	Oral	Intramuscular	Intravenous	Intrathecal	Adult or Maximum Dose
Flucytosine	150 mg/kg in 4 doses				
Ketoconazole	5–15 mg/kg in 1 dose				
Metronidazole	20–30 mg/kg in 3 doses		20–30 mg/kg in 3 doses		
Neonate & Prem.[2]	Not recommended		15 mg/kg loading dose then 15 mg/kg in 2 doses		
Mezlocillin		300 mg/kg in 6 doses	300 mg/kg in 6 doses		24 gm
Neonate & Prem.[2]		≤2000 gm: <1 wk, 150 mg/kg in 2 doses; >1 wk, 225 mg/kg in 3 doses >2000 gm: <1 wk, 150 mg/kg in 2 doses; >1 wk, 300 mg/kg in 4 doses	<2000 gm: <1 wk, 150 mg/kg in 2 doses; >1 wk, 225 mg/kg in 3 doses >2000 gm: <1 wk, 150 mg/kg in 2 doses; >1 wk, 300 mg/kg in 4 doses		
Miconazole			30 mg/kg in 3 doses		
Minocycline	4–5 mg/kg in 2 doses				
Neonate & Prem.[2]	Not recommended				
Moxalactam[2,24,25]		100–200 mg/kg in 4 doses	100–200 mg/kg in 4 doses		
Neonate & Prem.[2,10]		100 mg/kg in 2 doses, >1 wk, 150 mg/kg in 3 doses	100 mg/kg in 2 doses, >1 wk, 150 mg/kg in 3 doses		
Piperacillin *Not recommended <12 y.o.		100–300 mg/kg in 4 doses			20 gm
Rifampin	15 mg/kg in 1 dose				
Meningococcal prophylaxis × 2 da	1200 mg in 2 doses; 1–12 y.o., 20 mg/kg in 2 doses; <1 y.o., 10 mg/kg in 2 doses				120 mg/kg
Haemophilus prophylaxis × 4 da	20 mg/kg/da in 1 dose				1200 mg/kg
Trimethoprim *Not recommended <12 y.o.	200 mg/kg in 2 doses				
Trimethoprim (TMP)-sulfamethoxasole (SMX)	5–10 mg/kg TMP 25–50 mg/kg SMX } in 2 doses		5–10mg/kg TMP 25–50 mg/kg SMX } in 3 doses		
Neonate & Prem.[2] and <2 mos			2 mg/kg TMP, 10 mg SMX loading dose, then 2 mg/kg TMP, ł0 mg/kg SMX in 2 doses		
Pneumocystis prophylaxis	5 mg TMP/25 mg SMX/kg in 1 dose		5 mg TMP/25 mg SMX/kg in 1 dose		
Pneumocystis treatment	20 mg TMP/100 mg SMX/kg in 3 doses		20 mg TMP/100 mg SMX/kg in 3 doses		
Vancomycin	50 mg/kg in 4 doses		40 mg/kg in 2–3 doses		
Neonate & Prem.[2]			30 mg/kg in 2 doses		

Table 2.   DAILY DOSAGE SCHEDULE FOR ANTIMICROBIAL AGENTS* (continued)

Drug	Oral	Intramuscular	Intravenous	Intrathecal	Adult or Maximum Dose
Azlocillin			300–600 mg/kg divided q 4 hr		
Neonate & Prem.			<1 wk, 100–150 mg/ kg in 2 doses >1 wk, 200 mg/kg in 2 doses		
Cefoperazone[24,25] Not yet approved for pediatric use					2–4 gm/day divided q 6–12 hr

* Some of these agents may be administered by other routes. For intrapleural, intra-articular, intraperitoneal, ocular, aerosol, and topical use, see Report of the Committee on the Control of Infectious Diseases, American Academy of Pediatrics, Evanston, Ill., 1964. Some, such as neomycin, are specifically contraindicated by the intrapleural and intraperitoneal routes.

[1] Phenoxymethyl penicillin or phenethicillin is preferred for oral therapy. Procaine penicillin should not be used in neonates. Sodium penicillin contains 1.5 meq. of sodium, and potassium penicillin G, 1.69 meq. of potassium per 1.0 million units. The latter should be avoided intravenously in neonates and in patients with impaired renal function.

[2] If renal output is reduced, decrease the dose still further.

[3] Should not be used for minor infections or when less hazardous agents are effective. Observe for bone marrow depression.

[4] Avoid during first week of life unless essential. Desirable to follow treatment with serial blood levels to avoid "gray" syndrome.

[5] Any of the tetracycline group of antibodies may be used.

[6] With parenteral administration, auditory nerve and renal injury may occur; frequent audiometric and renal tests are essential. Manufacturer's note: The intravenous dose of kanamycin should not exceed 15 mg/kg/24 hr.

[7] Auditory nerve damage can occur.

[8] A soluble sulfonamide should be used. Manufacturer's precaution: Systemic sulfonamides are contraindicated in infants under 2 months of age.

[9] Observe for renal and neural toxic effects.

[10] Severe skin and liver toxicity occasionally occurs. Manufacturer's warning: Use should be avoided in premature and newborn infants because it affects bilirubin adversely.

[11] In general, dose by the intramuscular route should not exceed 5 mg/kg/24 hr for no longer than 7 to 10 days except in serious or life-threatening situations. Observation for vestibular and renal toxicity should be carried out. Desirable to follow therapy with serial blood levels if renal function impaired. The intrathecal use of gentamicin is not mentioned in the manufacturer's instructions.

[12] For neonates, see No. 18.

[13] Doses up to 200 mg/kg/24 hr in infants and children have been utilized without untoward effect.

[14] For intrathecal use, colistin without dibucaine should be used.

[15] In severe infections, may be necessary to increase oral and intramuscular dose as much as 3 times that listed.

[16] Fever, thrombophlebitis and renal, hepatic, and bone marrow damage may occur.

[17] Infants <7 days, <2000 gm, 15 mg/kg in 2 doses; >2000 gm, 20 mg/kg in 2 doses. Infants >7 days, <2000 gm, 20 mg/kg in 2 doses; >2000 gm, 20 mg/kg in 3 doses.

[18] Dose should be given in 2 divided doses in infants <7 days and in 3 divided doses in infants >7 days.

[19] In infants <7 days, 50–100 mg/kg in 2 doses; >7 days, 100–200 mg/kg in 3 doses.

[20] In infants <7 days, 50–100 mg/kg in 2 doses; >7 days, 100–200 mg/kg in 3–4 doses. Pediatric IV doses not known due to rarity.

[21] After initial loading dose of 10 mg/kg, follow with 7.5 mg/kg dose every 12 hr. (Can be given IM or IV.)

[22] After initial loading dose of 100 mg/kg, dose is as follows: <2000 gm = 225 mg/kg in 3 doses during first week of life; 600 mg/kg in 6 doses after 7 days of age; >2000 gm, 300–400 mg/kg in 4–6 doses; 600 mg/kg in 6 doses after 2 weeks of age. Can be given IM or 15–20 minute IV infusion.

[23] CSF penetration not adequate. "Break-through" meningitis may occur during during therapy.

[24] Bleeding due to hypoprothrombinemia is a possible complication. Administer prophylactic vitamin K.

[25] Displaces bilirubin from albumin. Use with caution with patients under 2 weeks of age.

[26] Oral preparation is an investigational drug.

[a] Premature.

[b] Full-term.

[c] First dose should be doubled. Do not use sulfonamides in premature infants or infants under 2 months of age.

[d] In general, limit parenteral therapy to 10 days.

[e] Manufacturer's warning: The use of drugs of the tetracycline class during tooth development (last half of pregnancy, infancy, and childhood to the age of 8 years) may cause permanent discoloration of the teeth. This adverse reaction is more common during long-term usage of the drugs but has been observed following repeated short-term courses.

[f] May exceed manufacturer's recommended dosage.

[g] Manufacturer's warning: Do not administer to children less than 3 months of age.

[h] Safety and dosage in children have not been established.

Supportive measures are critically important in the neonate with a systemic infection, irrespective of type or cause. In general, antimicrobials should be administered by the intravenous route because the depressed infant has decreased gastrointestinal absorption and microcirculatory changes in sepsis can lead to poor absorption of intramuscular drugs. Re-establishment and maintenance of body temperature in a heated environment are important, and urinary output should be monitored. Intravenous fluid and electrolyte therapy should be meticulously provided by standard methods. The complications of hyponatremia, hypoglycemia, or hypocalcemia may mimic or complicate septicemia. Thus, appropriate diagnostic biochemical determinations must be repetitively carried out and appropriate replacement therapy instituted. Lumbar punctures should be performed at frequent intervals in meningitis due to *E. coli* or other gram-negative enteric bacilli until sterilization of the cerebrospinal fluid has occurred, which is usually by the fourth or fifth day of therapy. Treatment should be continued for 3 total weeks or 2 weeks post–cerebrospinal fluid sterilization.

Antibiotic therapy is of cardinal importance in the management of infections due to *E. coli*. Because of changing patterns of resistance, in vitro susceptibility studies are essential. Kanamycin had been the drug of choice for *E. coli* infections in the neonate; however, in recent years kanamycin-resistant strains of *E. coli* have become more widespread. In many geographic areas, more than 40% of strains are resistant. In hospitals in which the majority of *E. coli* strains remain susceptible to kanamycin, this drug may be used. The intramuscular or intravenous dosage is as follows: infants 1 to 7 days of age weighing less than 2000 gm, 7.5 mg/kg every 12 hours; infants 1 to 7 days of age weighing more than 2000 gm, 10.0 mg/kg every 12 hours*; infants 8 to 30 days of age weighing less than 2000 gm, 10 mg/kg every 12 hours*; infants 8 to 30 days of age weighing more than 2000 gm, 10 mg/kg every 8 hours.*

In most areas, gentamicin plus ampicillin is currently the preferred combination of drugs for *E. coli* septicemia or meningitis of the neonate. For infants under 1 week of age, the dosage is 5 mg/kg/24 hr in equally divided doses every 12 hours. Beyond 1 week of age, the dosage is 5 to 7.5 mg/kg/24 hr in divided doses every 8 hours for both full-term and low birth weight infants. For intravenous administration, the dose is diluted in sterile normal saline and infused over a 1- to 2-hour period. If necessary, the drugs can be given intramuscularly except to infants with poor circulation. If renal function is impaired, the dosage of kan-

amycin or gentamicin must be reduced and serum levels monitored to avoid potential toxicity.

Ampicillin administered parenterally may be effective in infections caused by susceptible strains, especially those that are community-acquired. The daily dose administered intravenously for infants 1 to 7 days of age is 50 to 200 mg/kg in two doses, and for infants 8 to 30 days of age, 75 to 250 mg/kg divided into three doses. A combination of ampicillin and kanamycin or gentamicin is preferred initially because of possible synergism in action. Other drugs listed in Table 1 may be used if susceptibility studies show the organism to be sensitive. Amikacin and tobramycin are effective, but their use should be reserved for strains resistant to other antibiotics. Two of the newer cephalosporins, cefuroxime and cefamandole, show increased activity against *E. coli*. However, CSF penetration is poor with cefamandole, and "breakthrough" meningitis during therapy is a possibility. Cefuroxime achieves excellent CSF concentrations, but is not adequate as a single agent for the treatment of neonatal infection due to its limited activity against many *Enterobacteriaceae*. In addition, cefuroxime is not currently approved by the Federal Food and Drug Administration for use in patients less than three months of age.

Third generation cephalosporins such as moxalactam, cefotaxime, and ceftriaxone may be useful. Moxalactam should be used with caution in infants under two weeks of age as it significantly displaces bilirubin from albumin (even more so than sulfonamides). Experience with cefotaxime and ceftriaxone in the therapy of neonatal sepsis is limited. Neither agent should be used singly in the empirical therapy of neonatal sepsis and meningitis, since neither is active against *Listeria*. General supportive care depends on the underlying problem. Serious *E. coli* infections in older infants and children should be treated with parenteral gentamicin. Ampicillin given intravenously in a dose of 200 mg/kg/24 hr at 4- to 6-hour intervals plus gentamicin, 3 to 7.5 mg/kg/24 hr in three divided doses is the initial treatment of choice. Other drugs may be used depending upon the results of susceptibility tests.

Urinary Tract Infection. *E. coli* remains the most common cause of primary uncomplicated urinary tract infection. The strains are usually quite susceptible to the sulfonamides or to ampicillin. Sulfisoxazole*, 150 mg/kg/24 hr in four divided doses for a period of 2 weeks, affords effective therapy in most patients. Ampicillin, 50 to 100 mg/kg/24 hr orally in four divided doses, is equally effective but not superior. Amoxacillin (20–40 mg/kg/24hr in three divided doses) is often used instead of ampicillin, since gastrointestinal side effects (es-

---

* These doses exceed the manufacturer's maximum recommended daily dosage of 15 mg/kg/day.

* Contraindicated in infants younger than 2 months of age.

pecially diarrhea) are less frequent. The sulfonamides are still preferred for urinary tract infection of this nature since they are usually effective, and the cost and incidence of associated untoward reactions are low.

Because these drugs are effectively concentrated in the renal parenchyma and urine, favorable treatment response may be observed even when in vitro susceptibility testing shows the organism to be resistant. For this reason, if a favorable clinical response has been achieved after 48 to 72 hours and pyuria has been diminished and the urine sterilized, treatment may be continued with the drug initiated. If this has not been accomplished by this time, it is likely that the organism is resistant.

In recurrent disease the infecting E. coli is likely to be sulfonamide-resistant, and antibiotic susceptibility data must be used as guidelines for selecting alternative drugs. However, the trimethoprim-sulfamethoxazole combination or cephalosporins administered orally are often useful in such situations.

It is most important to ensure that the patient demonstrates both a clinical and bacteriologic cure and that an asymptomatic bacteriologic relapse does not occur. If the repeat urine cultures at 48 to 72 hours are sterile, treatment should be presumed effective. After the 2-week course of therapy, repeat urinalysis and quantitative urine cultures should be performed within several days and repeated at monthly intervals thereafter for 3 months and again at 6 months and a year. Shorter courses of antimicrobial administration may be effective in uncomplicated lower urinary tract infections. However, differentiation between upper and lower urinary tract infection in children and infants is often difficult. Short courses of antimicrobial therapy in these patients with UTI may be associated with unacceptable rates of relapse of infection. Drugs for oral therapy of UTI in children over 12 years include trimethoprim alone or cinoxacin,* a nalidixic acid derivative. If urinary tract infections recur, especially if polymicrobial in type, the presence of abnormalities of the urinary tract, especially those producing obstruction, should be suspected.

Diarrheal Disease. The association of E. coli with diarrheal disease has been known for years. Numerous outbreaks of diarrhea occurring in nurseries have been investigated, and certain antigenetically distinct strains of E. coli have been connected to these epidemics.

In recent years, the possible pathogenic mechanisms for the diarrhea associated with E. coli have been elucidated by the demonstration of the toxigenic and invasive properties of some of the strains. Stool isolates of E. coli can be characterized

as being (1) enteropathogenic; (2) enterotoxigenic (ETEC), by their ability to produce toxins; or (3) enteroinvasive (EIEC), by their capacity to penetrate mucosal cells. It is now known that strains may have none, one, two, or all three of these characteristics. Recent evidence also suggests that the intestinal mucosal adherence of some E. coli strains may be related to their pathogenicity.

E. coli. has been shown to cause diarrhea by two separate mechanisms: enterotoxin production and mucosal invasion. Strains with invasive capacity produce the characteristic findings of bacterial dysentery, namely local inflammation with hyperemia, ulceration, and intraluminal exudate composed of polymorphonuclear leukocytes. Enterotoxigenic E. coli causes diarrhea by two means: (1) production of an antigenic heat-labile toxin that resembles cholera toxin, in that is activates cellular adenyl cyclase, thereby increasing intracellular cyclic adenosine monophosphate and promoting secretion of sodium and water; (2) production of a nonantigenic heat-stable toxin, the exact action of which is undefined. Heat-labile enterotoxin has been shown to cause diarrhea in humans; heat-stable enterotoxin, although known to be a major cause of diarrhea in animals, has also recently been shown to be associated with diarrheal disease in humans.

Supportive therapy for E. coli–mediated diarrhea, irrespective of pathogenesis, consists mainly of maintaining adequate fluid and electrolyte intake. Patients with evidence of dehydration should be hospitalized and managed with intravenous fluids and electrolyte therapy, details of which are described elsewhere. In these patients, it is important to determine serum electrolyte concentrations since hypo- and hypernatremia occur fairly commonly.

Infants who are not dehydrated can be managed as outpatients. The details of management are described in other sections but two points must be mentioned. Homemade salt solutions should *not* be prescribed because of the risk of inducing hypertonic dehydration. Evidence is accumulating that certain commercially available oral rehydration fluids can be used successfully in the outpatient treatment of mildly dehydrated children. Adsorptive agents that firm the stool or narcotic-containing agents that decrease bowel motility have *no* place in treatment of diarrheal disease in infants and young children. None of these agents is specifically directed toward the primary cause of the diarrhea. None has been shown to decrease the fluid and electrolyte loss across the bowel mucosa in E. coli diarrhea, but by decreasing bowel motility they may mask the amount of fluid accumulated in the bowel lumen. They may also allow heavier colonization of the offending organism with greater enterotoxin production in the jejunum.

---

* Contraindicated in infants younger than 3 months of age. Use in prepubertal children is not recommended.

Deaths or severe central nervous system depression have occurred when atropine- or diphenyoxylate-containing antidiarrheals have been used in infants and children.

The effectiveness of antimicrobial therapy in *E. coli* diarrhea is open to some question. Specific antimicrobial therapy appears to shorten the severity and duration of diarrhea. Neomycin sulfate oral solution is the drug of choice in areas where neomycin resistance is not encountered frequently. It is administered in a dose of 100 mg/kg/24 hr divided into doses every 6 to 8 hours for 5 days. This dose is higher than that recommended by the manufacturer but has been found safe and effective. Continuation of therapy for more than 5 days is not advised because the bacteriologic cure rate is not improved and because neomycin may cause a malabsorptive state. Colistin sulfate oral suspension is the alternative drug of choice and is given in doses of 10 to 15 mg/kg/24 hr every 6 to 8 hours for 5 days. Antibiotic susceptibility testing should be performed because when resistant organisms are involved, treatment has resulted not only in failure but also spread of the infection, presumably by suppression of competing normal bacterial intestinal flora.

Controlled studies have not been performed to date evaluating the effectiveness of antibiotic therapy in the treatment of diarrhea due to enterotoxigenic and enteroinvasive strains. Because the bacteria remain within the intestinal lumen in enterotoxigenic *E. coli* disease, it seems logical to speculate that nonabsorbable antibiotics might be useful in treatment. However, in an outbreak of diarrheal disease due to a strain of *E. coli* elaborating a heat-stable enterotoxin but which did not belong to an enteropathogenic serotype, oral colistin therapy was ineffective in eradicating the organisms from the stools of culture-positive infants and in preventing illness or shortening the carrier state. It is reasonable to presume that drugs effective against these strains in vitro might be beneficial in decreasing the severity and duration of diarrhea in those patients, as it has been shown to be with *Shigella* dysentery. If strains susceptible to ampicillin are involved, this drug should be administered at a dose of 100 mg/kg/24 hr in 4 to 8 divided doses, preferably intravenously. In a double-blind, placebo-controlled study of 110 older patients with "traveler's diarrhea," a 5-day course of oral trimethoprim/sulfamethoxazole or trimethoprim alone significantly reduced the gastrointestinal distress and number of diarrheal stools in a majority of the patients.

It is not clear at this time whether older children with *E. coli* diarrhea should receive antimicrobial therapy.

Outbreaks of *E. coli* diarrhea in newborn nurseries can be catastrophic. Such outbreaks can be controlled by use of rapid fluorescent antibody techniques to detect the presence of organisms in the stool, and to follow such infants by segregation of colonized infants and treatment with oral neomycin or colistin in the dosages mentioned.

Other Infections. A variety of other infections, including pneumonia, peritonitis, and abscesses, may be caused by *E. coli*. The information in Tables 1 and 2 can be used for selection of antimicrobial therapy pending susceptibility test results. Surgical intervention and supportive measures depend upon the disease. *E. coli*, including nonenteropathogenic strains, has been causally linked to necrotizing enterocolitis in neonates. Therapy for *E. coli* infections, other than uncomplicated urinary tract infections, should be provided by the parenteral route.

Proteus-Providencia-Morganella Infections

The variable, unpredictable response to antibacterial therapy of *Proteus* and *Morganella* infections is striking, and prolonged therapy is often necessary. In addition to in vitro susceptibility studies, *Proteus* isolates should also be classified as to species because of the variability in the susceptibility of various species and strains to different antibacterial agents. For example, *P. mirabilis* is usually susceptible to ampicillin (or occasionally to large doses of penicillin G), and it is the drug of choice in most infections due to this species. Many strains of *P. mirabilis* are also susceptible to gentamicin, cephalosporins, including many third-generation cephalosporins, ticarcillin, and kanamycin. Indole-positive species such as *P. vulgaris* and *Morganella morganii*, for practical purposes, are always resistant to ampicillin and penicillin G. The drug of choice must be governed by the results of in vitro susceptibility tests as well as the clinical condition of the patient. Many strains are susceptible to gentamicin, kanamycin, tobramycin, and nearly all to amikacin; these are usually the drugs of choice in infections due to these species. Some strains are susceptible to the carbenicillin and ticarcillin and others to one of the cephalosporins, particularly the second and third generation agents.

Most strains of *P. vulgaris* are two- to four-fold more sensitive in vitro to tobramycin than to gentamicin. In vivo, however, strains resistant to gentamicin are likely to be resistant to tobramycin. Amikacin and sisomicin show increased activity against most strains of indole-positive *Proteus*. The use of these two agents should be reserved for infections due to organisms resistant to other available agents. Cefoxitin and cefotaxime also show activity against certain strains of indole-positive *Proteus*. Cefuroxime, cefoperazone, and ceftazidime are much less active. Alternate drugs for infections due to susceptible strains are listed in Table 1. Some strains of *Proteus* are moderately susceptible to novobiocin, but this drug has a significant toxicity risk, and the response to therapy is often variable. Although in vitro the infecting organism is rarely susceptible, clinical results in certain refractory infections, especially of the urinary tract, with cycloserine* have been encouraging. This drug is potentially toxic and should be used with caution. The usual dose is 10 mg/kg/24 hr.

Organisms of the genus *Providencia* were formerly known as *P. inconstans* and included with "paracolon bacilli." They are easily differentiated from *Proteus* and *Morganella* by their lack of urease. Members of the group have been isolated from human feces during outbreaks of diarrhea but also in normal individuals. They are primarily associated with urinary tract infections but may also cause sepsis and localized infections. *Providencia* organisms are highly resistant to antibiotics except for carbenicillin and ticarcillin and the aminoglycosides; some strains are inhibited by cefamandole or cefoxitin and some by trimethoprim-sulfamethoxazole.

Providencia stuartii has recently emerged as a hospital pathogen in burned patients, appearing first in burn wounds but subsequently as a cause of pulmonary and urinary infections.

Klebsiella-Enterobacter-Serratia Infections

Klebsiella-Enterobacter-Serratia organisms have variable susceptibility to antimicrobial agents and must be tested in vitro. Frequently, however, antimicrobial therapy must be instituted before results of antibiotic susceptibility tests are available. An aminoglycoside antibiotic, such as gentamicin, amikacin, or tobramycin (the choice depending upon the susceptibility patterns of organisms in the local area), is usually the drug of choice with certain exceptions. For example, many strains of *K. pneumoniae* are susceptible to cephalothin and some strains of *Enterobacter* are inhibited by carbenicillin and ticarcillin and by cefamandole, moxalactam and cefotaxime and other third-generation cephalosporins. Trimethoprim-sulfamethoxazole and second and third generation cephalosporins inhibit some strains of *Serratia*. In contrast to *Klebsiella* and *Enterobacter*, almost all strains of *Serratia* are resistant to the polymyxins. For serious *Klebsiella* infections, it is usually desirable to add a cephalosporin. Other drugs for treatment of infections due to members of the *Klebsiella-Enterobacter-Serratia* group, depending upon susceptibility results, are shown in Table 1.

Pseudomonas Infections

The *Pseudomonas* group is composed of gram-negative, motile rods, which are nonfermenters and occur widely in soil, water, sewage, and air.

P. aeruginosa is the member of the genus most commonly pathogenic for human beings. *Pseudomonas* occurs in several antigenic types and several phage types that are equally pathogenic. Because of its ability to form a pigment that colors inflammatory exudate blue or green, the epidemic spread of *P. aeruginosa* in hospital wards has long been recognized. It is found in small numbers in the intestinal tract and on normal skin, particularly when other coliforms are suppressed.

P. aeruginosa is resistant to the more commonly used antimicrobial agents and therefore assumes prevalence and importance when more susceptible bacteria of the normal flora are suppressed. Although most strains of *P. aeruginosa* are susceptible to the polymyxins, these agents have been relatively ineffective in eradicating bacteremia and deepseated tissue infections. Gentamicin and other aminoglycosides and carbenicillin or ticarcillin are usually more effective but the polymyxins still have a place in selected infections, particularly in urinary tract infections or in bacteremias arising from the urinary tract. In other instances, the organism may be eradicated but the ultimate results are often unsatisfactory because of the poor host defenses in debilitated patients.

Carbenicillin is effective against susceptible strains but some 30% of strains are resistant to it. It must be given in relatively large doses intravenously. During prolonged therapy with carbenicillin alone, organisms initially susceptible may become resistant. Most strains of *Pseudomonas* are inhibited by gentamicin but recently an increasing number of strains have been found to be resistant. Ticarcillin, a semisynthetic penicillin similar to carbenicillin, has excellent activity against *Pseudomonas* with 90% or more of isolates being susceptible. Presumptive therapy for systemic *Pseudomonas* infection is a combination of tobramycin and ticarcillin. The two drugs appear to act synergistically in vitro, and coadministration may delay emergence of *P. aeruginosa* resistant to ticarcillin.

Tobramycin has been found to be two to four times more active against *Pseudomonas* than is gentamicin. It is particularly valuable in treatment of infections due to gentamicin-resistant strains. When tobramycin is used in combination with ticarcillin, higher antibacterial serum titers are achieved than with either agent alone. See Table 2 for dosage.

The broad-spectrum ureidopenicillins, mezlocillin and azlocillin, have good activity against *P. aeruginosa*. In general mezlocillin is equal to ticarcillin in activity, and azlocillin is approximately twice as active. The minimal inhibitory concentrations (MIC) of the new piperazine penicillin, piperacillin, for *P. aeruginosa* are four-fold lower than those of mezlocillin or ticarcillin. Advantages

---

* Manufacturer's precaution: Safety and dosage of cycloserine have not been established for pediatric use.

of these newer agents over carbenicillin and ticarcillin include greater CSF penetration, lower sodium load, and a broader antimicrobial spectrum. Piperacillin and azlocillin are generally reserved for use against isolates with high MICs to ticarcillin and, like ticarcillin, are used in combination with an aminoglycoside. Adverse reactions with piperacillin (fever, rash, lymphadenitis, eosinophilia) have been reported to occur with greater frequency in patients with cystic fibrosis.

The recently marketed ticarcillin/clavulanate combination may prove useful in the therapy of *Pseudomonas* infections. Clavulanic acid is an effective inhibitor of beta-lactamase. Isolates highly resistant to ticarcillin may be inhibited by ≤ 64 μg/ml of ticarcillin in the presence of clavulanic acid. Most efficacy studies have been performed with adult patients, and there is presently no indication by the FDA for its use in patients under 12 years of age.

Aztreonam is a monobactam antimicrobial currently undergoing extensive safety and efficacy testing in adults, children, and infants. It is a bactericidal agent highly active against most Enterobacteriaceae, *P. aeruginosa*, *Enterobacter spp.*, and *Serratia marcescens*. Similar to some of the newer cephalosporins, aztreonam is not active against facultative aerobic gram-positive or anaerobic bacteria. As with the antipseudomonas beta-lactams, it is frequently synergistic with aminoglycosides against *P. aeruginosa*.

Imipenem (thienamycin) is a novel, broad-spectrum beta-lactam antibiotic with activity against many aerobic and anaerobic gram-positive and gram-negative bacteria, including *P. aeruginosa*. Of the pseudomonads, on *P. maltophilia* and *P. cepacia* are resistant. This experimental agent may prove useful as an alternative to antibiotic combinations currently employed to provide initial broad-spectrum coverage (especially in situations in which infection with *P. aeruginosa* is a possibility).

Antibiotics in the quinolone class (e.g., ciprofloxacin, enoxacin, ofloxacin, amifloxacin) are under investigation as orally effective agents against *P. aeruginosa* and other gram-negative as well as gram-positive bacteria.

Amikacin inhibits many strains of *P. aeruginosa*. It may be used alone or in combination with carbenicillin or ticarcillin. At the moment, its most valuable use is in the treatment of *Pseudomonas* infections due to strains resistant to gentamicin or to other agents.

Pseudomonas is a preeminent opportunist, and the vast majority of infections caused by it occur in hospitals, particularly those housing patients with serious diseases. Since 1961 the incidence of *P. aeruginosa* bacteremia has increased and the respiratory tract has become an increasingly important source of infection. The use of gentamicin, carbenicillin, and colistin has not changed the outlook of *Pseudomonas* bacteremia. A polyvalent vaccine has proved useful in burned patients and further attention needs to be given to immunoprophylaxis. At the present time, control of the underlying disease condition contributes most toward survival of patients with bacteremia and other serious *Pseudomonas* infections.

The pseudomallei group of the genus *Pseudomonas* consists of *P. cepacia*, *P. mallei* and *P. pseudomallei*. The former is the cause of glanders, a severe infectious disease of horses that can be transmitted to man. Human infections can usually be treated with sulfonamides.

Melioidosis due to *P. pseudomallei* is a disease resembling glanders in man and occurs chiefly in Southeast Asia but perhaps also in the Western hemisphere. *P. pseudomallei* is susceptible to many antibiotics in vitro. Tetracycline, chloramphenicol, or gentamicin, alone or in combination, may be the treatment of choice. Tetracycline/streptomycin and chloramphenicol/streptomycin combinations have also been used. Trimethoprim-sulfamethoxazole may be effective.

Outbreaks of nosocomial bacteremia due to *P. cepacia* secondary to contaminated antiseptics and disinfectants used in cleaning equipment or in skin asepsis for intravenous infusions have been described. Environmental isolates are frequently sensitive to chloramphenicol and trimethoprim/sulfamethoxazole and occasionally to kanamycin. *Pseudomonas cepacia* has been isolated with increasing frequency from the sputum of cystic fibrosis patients. Such patients are usually adolescents and young adults with a history of long-term, intensive antipseudomonas therapy. Cystic fibrosis patients who acquire *P. cepacia* tend to have a poorer prognosis than those from whom *P. cepacia* has never been isolated. Cystic fibrosis isolates of *P. cepacia* are often resistant to standard antipseudomonas agents as well as to chloramphenicol and trimethoprim/sulfamethoxazole. The new third-generation cephalosporin ceftazidime demonstrates good in vitro activity against all *P. cepacia*, but early trials in cystic fibrosis patients with this difficult organism have been disappointing. Certain other pseudomonads may cause infections in humans. These include *P. fluorescens*, *P. maltophilia*, and *P. putida*. Less frequent are *P. acidovorans*, *P. alcaligenes*, *P. putrefaciens*, *P. pseudoalcaligenes*, *P. testosteroni*, *P. dimunita*, and *P. mendocina*. These organisms vary widely in their antimicrobial susceptibility, and treatment should be guided by in vitro susceptibility tests.

Aeromonas and *Plesiomonas* Infections

The *Aeromonas* and *Plesiomonas* genera have characteristics in common with both the Enterobacteriaceae and *Pseudomonas* in that they ferment carbohydrates and are oxidase positive. They may be easily mistaken in the laboratory for *E. coli* unless oxidase testing or selective media are used. The most important members are *A. hydrophila*, *A. Sobria*, and *P. shigelloides*. These organisms are found in natural water sources and soil and are frequent pathogens for cold-blooded marine and freshwater animals. In man, *A. hydrophila* has been associated with cellulitis and wound infections (especially those acquired in natural water environments), hepatobiliary infection, and septicemia, mainly in immunocompromised patients. Both *Aeromonas* and *Plesiomonas* have been implicated as etiologic agents in patients with gastroenteritis. Enteropathogenic strains of *Aeromonas* have been described. Diarrhea is usually mild and clinically indistinguishable from certain types of gastroenteritis, although a dysentery-like illness requiring hospitalization can occur.

Resistance to cephalosporins and penicillins is common. The latter has led to the incorporation of ampicillin into isolation media to select for *Aeromonas*. Most stains of *Aeromonas* and *Plesiomonas* are susceptible to chloramphenicol and tetracycline, with variable sensitivity to the aminoglycosides. Of the newer cephalosporins, only moxalactam demonstrates reasonable activity. Most strains are susceptible to the monobactam aztreonam, and trimethoprim/sulfamethoxazole may be effective against selected isolates. Whether or not antimicrobial therapy will alter the clinical course of gastroenteritis related to these agents is not yet known.

Noncholera Vibrio Infections

Noncholera vibrios are commonly found in the coastal waters of the world. *Vibrio parahaemolyticus* is the most important species. Illnesses have been reported after ingestion of incompletely cooked or raw seafoods (especially oysters) contaminated with these organisms. Gastroenteritis is the most common presentation. Wound infection and bacteremic illness have been described with other halophilic vibrio species.

Noncholera vibrios are inhibited by a variety of antibiotics. Gentamicin is the drug of choice against infections due to *V. parahaemolyticus*, but ampicillin, tetracycline, chloramphenicol, cephalothin, and kanamycin are frequently effective. Most strains of *V. fetus* are inhibited by tetracycline, chloramphenicol, ampicillin, streptomycin, and kanamycin.

Campylobacter Infections

Campylobacter organisms are small, curved, gram-negative rods that were previously classified among the vibrios. *Campylobacter fetus* (formerly *C. fetus*, subspecies *fetus*) is best recognized as a cause of puerperal infection. Reports of bacterial endocarditis, thrombophlebitis, and meningitis can also be found in the literature. Most isolates were found to be sensitive to aminoglycosides and tetracycline. Chloramphenicol and clindamycin may be effective as well. Clinical experience and pharmacokinetic data with clindamycin in neonates are limited. *C. fetus* is generally resistant to cephalosporins, colistin, polymyxin B, rifampin, and vancomycin. Sensitivity to erythromycin is variable.

Campylobacter jejuni (formerly *C. fetus*, subspecies *jejuni*) is now known to be a common cause of infectious diarrhea. The illness typically presents in early childhood and is usually self-limited; however, cases of rather severe colitis have been described. The onset is acute with diarrhea, fever, vomiting, and abdominal pain. Septic complications such as bacteremia, arthritis, and osteomyelitis have been reported occasionally. Uncomplicated *Campylobacter* enteritis usually does not require antimicrobial therapy. Whether or not treatment early in the disease may affect the clinical course is still unclear. Erythromycin therapy (40 mg/kg/24 hr divided every 6 hr for 7 days) shortens the duration of excretion of organisms in the stool and is the drug of first choice. Chloramphenicol, gentamicin, and tetracycline may also be effective.

Infections Due to Other Gram-Negative Bacilli

Other Enterobacteriaceae. Certain other members of the Enterobacteriaceae sometimes cause infection in humans. *Arizona* organisms are now considered among the *Salmonellae*. However, nosocomial infections caused by members of this group, notably *Arizona hinshawii*, have been described.

Edwardsiella. *Edwardsiella* includes a group of motile, lactose-negative organisms that resemble salmonellae in some biochemical features and sometimes in pathogenicity for humans. They ferment only glucose and maltose. *E. tarda* has been isolated from a variety of mammals and reptiles. It is occasionally found in the human intestinal tract, especially in acute gastroenteritis, and it can produce serious septic infections. However, people are likely only accidental hosts. Tetracyclines, chloramphenicol, kanamycin,* and ampicillin are the drugs of choice.

Citrobacter. The *Citrobacter* group is composed of Enterobacteriaceae previously designated as *Escherichia freundii* and the Bethesda-Ballerup of "paracolon" organisms. *Citrobacter* strains occur infrequently in normal feces. They have been recovered from urinary tract infections in various septic processes. *Citrobacter* is also an occasional cause of neonatal meningitis. A significant number of these infants will develop brain abscesses often despite early and appropriate antimicrobial ther-

---

* Other aminoglycoside antibiotics may also be effective but clinical experience to date is limited.

apy. Nosocomial outbreaks have been reported. Drugs of choice are aminoglycosides or third generation cephalosporins. Some strains are susceptible to chloramphenicol and tetracycline.

Other Gram-Negative Bacilli. *Acinetobacter.* *Acinetobacter lwoffi* (previously *Mimi polymorpha* and *Achromobacter lwoffi*) neither ferments nor oxidizes carbohydrates, whereas *Acinetobacter calcoaceticus* (previously *Herellea vaginicola* and *Achromobacter anitratus*) utilizes glucose oxidatively and produces acid from 10% (but not from 1%) lactose-containing medium. These organisms are frequently antibiotic-resistant, and antibiotic susceptibility tests are required as a guide to therapy. Drugs likely to be effective are gentamicin, tobramycin, polymyxins, and new experimental agents aztreonam and imipenem. Ceftazidime (a soon-to-be-available third-generation cephalosporin) has shown promise as an effective agent against *Acinetobacter spp.* and other nonfermenters.

Moraxella. Moraxella† are similar to *Acinetobacter* but are oxidase-positive and highly susceptible to penicillin. They are primary animal parasites, most commonly present on the mucous membranes. Most of these organisms do not utilize carbohydrates.

Alcaligenes.* *A. faecalis* fails to ferment or oxidize any of the usual carbohydrates; it is usually motile. It may occasionally be confused on initial isolation with other nonlactose fermenters, chiefly *Salmonella* or *Shigella*. These organisms are not uniformly sensitive to any antibiotic; tetracycline and chloramphenicol are usually the most effective.

Flavobacterium. Flavobacteria† are widely distributed in soil and water and are encountered as opportunistic pathogens in humans. *F. meningosepticum*, which has high virulence for the neonate, has an unusual antibiotic susceptibility pattern for a gram-negative bacillus. It is usually susceptible in vitro to erythromycin, novobiocin, and rifampin, and to a lesser degree to chloramphenicol and streptomycin, but is resistant to gentamicin and polymyxins. Trimethoprim/sulfamethoxazole and cefoxitin may also be effective.

Streptobacillus moniliformis. *Streptobacillus moniliformis*, the cause of one type of rat-bite fever, is carried by many rats presumably as a saprophyte. Penicillin G is the treatment of choice, but streptomycin and tetracycline are also therapeutically effective. The wound should be immediately cleansed with soap and water. Tetanus prophylaxis should be carried out by standard methods.

Calymmatobacterium (Donovania) Granulomatis. Granuloma inguinale is an indolent, ulcerative disease, caused by a gram-negative bacillus that is antigenically similar to, but not identical with, *Klebsiella pneumoniae* and *K. rhinoscleromatis*. It can be treated successfully with tetracyclines, chloramphenicol, or streptomycin. Penicillin G is not effective.

Bartonella bacilliformis. *Bartonella bacilliformis* is a gram-negative, very pleomorphic, motile organism which causes in humans two different clinical manifestations of the same geographically restricted bacterial disease.† The collective designation of the two syndromes is Carrión disease.

Penicillin, streptomycin, and chloramphenicol are dramatically effective in Oroya fever and greatly reduce the fatality rate, particularly if blood transfusions are also given. Control of the disease depends upon the elimination of the sand fly vectors. Insecticides, DDT, insect repellents, and elimination of breeding areas are of value. Prevention with antibiotics may be useful. Chloramphenicol should be used when the patient is also suffering from secondary *Salmonella* infection.

Others. There are a few other gram-negative bacilli which very rarely cause human infection but have been reported to do so. The type of infection they cause is variable but may be bacteremic or localized in various organ systems. Selection of antimicrobial therapy is based on in vitro susceptibility test results. The agents that are usually effective are listed here, but some of the newer agents mentioned, especially the newer aminoglycosides and cephalosporins, may prove useful with further experience.

Actinobacillus actinomycetemcomitans	Tetracycline Streptomycin Chloramphenicol
Actinobacillus lignieresii	Kanamycin
Bordetella bronchiseptica	Tetracycline Polymyxins Chloramphenicol
Chromobacterium violaceum	Kanamycin or gentamicin Tetracycline Chloramphenicol
Comamonas terrigenia	Chloramphenicol Tetracycline
Enterobacter agglomerans	Gentamicin Chloramphenicol Colistin Kanamycin
Haemophilus aphrodilus (HB group)	Penicillin G Gentamicin Cephalothin Chloramphenicol Tetracycline

---

* Also "nonfermenter."

† Recently cases of anemia with *Bartonella*-like bodies have been reported from Southeast Asia.

Infections Due to Anaerobic Cocci and Gram-Negative Bacilli

ITZHAK BROOK, M.D., M.Sc.

The recovery of a child from an anaerobic infection depends on prompt and proper management. The strategy for therapy of anaerobic infections consists of surgical drainage of pus, débridement of any necrotic tissue, and appropriate antibiotics. Certain types of adjunct therapy such as hyperbaric oxygen may also be useful. Antimicrobial therapy is in many patients the only form of therapy required, whereas in others it is an important adjunct to a surgical approach.

Surgical therapy may be the only therapy required in some cases, as for localized abscesses or decubitus ulcers without signs of systemic involvement. In the treatment of such lesions, antibiotics are indicated whenever systemic manifestations of infection are present or when suppuration has either extended or threatened to spread into surrounding tissue. Antibiotics are needed in the majority of cases, however. Selection of antimicrobial agents is simplified when a culture result of a reliable specimen is available. This may be particularly difficult in anaerobic infections because of the problems encountered in obtaining appropriate specimens. Because of this difficulty, many patients are treated empirically on the basis of suspected, rather than established, pathogens. Fortunately, the types of anaerobes involved in many anaerobic infections and their antimicrobial susceptibility patterns tend to be predictable. Some anaerobic bacteria have become resistant to antimicrobial agents, however, and many can become resistant while a patient is receiving therapy.

Aside from susceptibility patterns, other factors influencing the choice of antimicrobial therapy include the pharmacologic characteristics of the various drugs, their toxicity, their effect on the normal flora, and their bactericidal activity.

Since anaerobic bacteria generally are recovered mixed with aerobic organisms, selection of proper therapy becomes more complicated. In the treatment of mixed infection the choice of the appropriate antimicrobial agents should provide for adequate coverage of most of the pathogens. Some broad-spectrum antibacterial agents possess such qualities, while for some organisms, additional agents should be added to the therapeutic regimen.

Antimicrobial Drugs

Penicillins. Penicillin-G is the drug of choice when the infecting strains are susceptible to this drug. These include the majority of anaerobic strains other than those belonging to the *B. fragilis* group. Other strains that may show resistance to penicillins are growing numbers of *Bacteroides,* such as the *B. melaninogenicus* group and *B. oralis,* strains of clostridia, *Fusobacterium* species, and microaerophilic streptococci. Some of these strains show minimal inhibitory concentration (MIC) in dosages of 8 to 32 units/ml of penicillin G. In these instances, administration of very high dosages of penicillin G may eradicate the infection. Ampicillin, amoxicillin, and penicillin generally are equally active, but the semisynthetic penicillins are less active than the parent compound. Methicillin, nafcillin, and the isoxazolyl penicillins have unpredictable activity and frequently are inferior to penicillin G against anaerobes. Carbenicillin and ticarcillin are active against *B. fragilis* because of the high serum level that can be achieved; however, penicillin G is also active against *B. fragilis* in this concentration. Resistance to these agents is present in up to 30% of *B. fragilis* strains.

Chloramphenicol. Although it is a bacteriostatic drug, chloramphenicol is one of the antimicrobial drugs most active against anaerobes, and resistance to this drug is rare. Although several failures to eradicate anaerobic infections, including bacteremia, with chloramphenicol have been reported, this drug has been used for over 25 years for treatment of anaerobic infections. It is regarded as a good choice for treatment of serious anaerobic infections when the nature and susceptibility of the infecting organisms are unknown. Because of its good penetration through the blood-brain barrier it is used in infections of the central nervous system. The toxicity of chloramphenicol must be borne in mind, however. This includes the low risk of aplastic anemia, dose-dependent leukopenia, and "gray baby syndrome" in the newborn.

Cephalosporins. The antimicrobial spectrum of the first-generation cephalosporins against anaerobes is similar to that of penicillin G, although they are less active on a weight basis. Similar to what is seen with penicillin G, most strains of the *B. fragilis* group and many of the *B. melaninogenicus* group are resistant to cephalosporins as a result of cephalosporinase production. Cefoxitin, a second-generation cephalosporin, is relatively resistant to this enzyme and is therefore effective against the *B. fragilis* group. Cefoxitin is active in vitro against at least 95% of strains of *B. fragilis* at a level of 32 µg/ml, but cefoxitin is relatively inactive against most species of *Clostridium* (including *C. difficile*) other than *Clostridium perfringens*. Clinical experiences with cefoxitin in anaerobic infections have shown it to be effective in eradication of these infections. It has often been used for surgical prophylaxis because of its activity against enteric gram-negative rods. Third-generation cephalosporins, with the exception of moxalactam, have similar activity against anaerobes as the first-generation cephalosporins.

Clindamycin. Clindamycin has a broad range of activity against anaerobic organisms and has proved its efficacy in clinical trials. Approximately 95% of the anaerobic bacteria isolated in clinical practice are susceptible to easily achievable levels of clindamycin. *B. fragilis* is generally sensitive to levels below 3 μg/ml. There are, however, reports of resistant strains associated with clinical infections, although these are uncommon.

Several reports have described the successful use of this drug in the treatment of anaerobic infection. Clindamycin does not cross the blood-brain barrier efficiently and should not be administered in cases of central nervous system infections. Because of its effectiveness against anaerobes it is frequently used in combination with aminoglycosides for the treatment of mixed aerobic-anaerobic infections of the abdominal cavity and obstetric infection. The primary manifestation of toxicity with clindamycin is colitis. It should be kept in mind that colitis has been associated with a number of other antimicrobial agents, such as ampicillin and all the cephalosporins, and has been described in seriously ill patients in the absence of previous antimicrobial therapy. The occurrence of colitis in pediatric patients is very rare, however.

Metronidazole. This drug shows excellent bactericidal activity against most obligate anaerobic bacteria, such as *B. fragilis,* other species of *Bacteroides,* fusobacteria, and clostridia. Occasional strains of anaerobic gram-positive cocci and nonsporulating bacilli are highly resistant. Microaerophilic streptococci, *Propionibacterium acnes,* and *Actinomyces* species are almost uniformly resistant. Aerobic and facultative anaerobes, such as coliforms, are usually highly resistant. Over 90% of obligate anaerobes are susceptible to less than 2 μg/ml metronidazole.

Clinical experience in adults and limited experience in children indicate its efficacy in the treatment of infections caused by anaerobes, including intraabdominal sepsis, infections of the female genital tract, and especially infections of the central nervous system. However, it does not seem to be as effective in therapy of anaerobic gram-positive pulmonary infection. Because of its lack of activity against aerobic bacteria, additional antimicrobial agents effective against these organisms should be administered whenever they are also present. The use of metronidazole seems advantageous in central nervous system infections because of its excellent penetration into the central nervous system. Until the Food and Drug Administration approves the use of this drug for children, however, it should be used only in seriously ill patients, following the regulations of the Food and Drug Administration.

Tetracyclines. Tetracycline has presently limited usefulness because of the development of resistance to it by virtually all types of anaerobes. Presently only about 45% of all *B. fragilis* strains are susceptible to this drug. The new tetracycline analogues, doxycycline and minocycline, are more active than the parent compound. The use of tetracycline is not recommended before 8 years of age because of its adverse effect on teeth.

Other Drugs

Vancomycin is effective against all gram-positive anaerobes, but is inactive against gram-negative ones. Little clinical experience has been gained in the treatment of anaerobic bacteria using this agent.

Clavulanic acid is a new beta-lactamase inhibitor that resembles the nucleus of penicillin but differs in several ways. Clavulanic acid irreversibly inhibits beta-lactamase enzymes produced by some Enterobacteriaceae, staphylococci, and beta-lactamase–producing *Bacteroides species* (*B. fragilis* group and strains of *B. melaninogenicus* and *B. oralis*). When used in conjunction with a beta-lactam antibiotic, it may prove to be effective in treating infections caused by beta-lactamase–producing bacteria. Its usefulness in the therapy of human infections is currently being evaluated. Clavulanic acid and other beta-lactamase inhibitors may prove to be effective adjuncts to penicillins in the treatment of resistant organisms.

Haemophilus influenzae Infections
JANET R. GILSDORF, M.D.

Haemophilus influenzae type b is the most common cause of serious systemic bacterial infections in children. Invasive diseases caused by this organism are limited almost exclusively to children between 2 months and 6 years of age; approximately 75% of illnesses occur before the age of 18 months. Although the encapsulated type b *H. influenzae* is responsible for the majority of invasive bacteremic diseases caused by this organism, the nonencapsulated, nontypable *H. influenzae* is an important cause of local, mucosa-associated infections, such as otitis media and sinusitis.

GENERAL ANTIBIOTIC THERAPY

The antibiotic therapy of invasive *Haemophilus influenzae* type b disease is in a period of transition. New drugs are available that offer the same therapeutic efficacy as ampicillin and chloramphenicol but with decreased toxicity and at lower cost. In addition, carefully monitored home antibiotic therapy, using either oral or parenteral drugs, may be considered in selected patients.

In many invasive *H. influenzae* infections, empiric

antibiotic therapy is initiated before the etiologic agent is identified. This empiric therapy is broad spectrum—designed to treat the most likely infecting organisms until more definitive therapy, based on culture and sensitivity test results, can be chosen.

Bacteremic Infections Without Meningitis. Empiric therapy for patients with possible bacteremic *H. influenzae* infections without meningitis (Table 1) should include a parenteral antimicrobial agent that will be effective against ampicillin-resistant strains and that will achieve bactericidal levels in the cerebrospinal fluid (CSF), as central nervous system (CNS) seeding may accompany any bacteremic *H. influenzae* type b infection. Such empiric therapy should include parenteral chloramphenicol, 75–100 mg/kg/day divided into four doses, or one of the third-generation cephalosporins, such as ceftriaxone, 50–75 mg/kg/day divided into one or two doses; cefotaxime, 100–150 mg/kg/day divided into four doses; or cefuroxime, 100–150 mg/kg/day divided into three doses. If the organism is known to be ampicillin sensitive (β-lactamase negative), parenteral ampicillin, 100–200 mg/kg/day in four to six divided doses, may be used. Adequate treatment of meningitis requires higher doses of these antibiotics, as a variable percentage of the serum antibiotic concentration is found in the CSF.

Antibiotic Resistance. The prevalence of ampicillin-resistant strains may be as high as 30% in some areas of the United States. The majority of ampicillin-resistant strains may be rapidly identified by their production of β-lactamase. However, rarely, ampicillin resistance is mediated by another mechanism, possibly alteration of penicillin-binding proteins. These organisms produce no β-lactamase and can be identified only by standard sensitivity testing. Chloramphenicol-resistant strains remain rare and are often ampicillin resistant as well. However, because of the possible increased spread of chloramphenicol-resistant strains, sensitivity testing to chloramphenicol should be done on all invasive *H. influenzae* type b strains.

Chloramphenicol. Serum chloramphenicol levels following oral administration of this drug may be identical with or higher than those following the same dose of intravenous chloramphenicol. Thus, oral chloramphenicol is adequate therapy in patients tolerating oral feedings. The use of chloramphenicol requires the ready availability of reliable and timely tests for monitoring serum levels of this drug after two or three doses. Peak serum levels (drawn 30 minutes following completion of an intravenous infusion or 90 minutes following an oral dose) should be maintained between 15 and 25 µg/ml to assure an adequate therapeutic level and to avoid toxicity. Limited data are available on the clinical use of trough

Table 1. THERAPY OF *HAEMOPHILUS INFLUENZAE* TYPE B SYSTEMIC INFECTIONS

Infection	Empiric Drugs (Prior to Confirmation of *H. influenzae* Type B Infection)	Comments	Subsequent Drugs (After Confirmation of *H. Influenzae* Type B Infection)	Duration of Therapy
Meningitis	Chloramphenicol, 75–100 mg/kg/day IV in 4 doses or Ceftriaxone, 100 mg/kg/day IV in 2 doses or	Monitor serum levels to maintain peak at 15–25 µg/ml	Ampicillin, 200–300 mg/kg/day IV in 4–6 doses for ampicillin-sensitive strains or Chloramphenicol, 75 mg/kg/day PO in 4 doses or	10–14 days (including 5 afebrile days) As above
	Cefotaxime, 200 mg/kg/day IV in 4 doses or Cefuroxime, 200 mg/kg/day IV in 4 doses		Ceftriaxone } Doses or } same Cefotaxime } as for or } empiric Cefuroxime } therapy	As above As above As above
Bacteremic nonmeningeal infections	Chloramphenicol, 75–100 mg/kg/day IV in 4 doses or Ceftriaxone, 50–75 mg/kg/day IV in 1 or 2 doses or Cefotaxime, 100–150 mg/kg/day IV in 4 doses or Cefuroxime, 100–150 mg/kg/day IV in 3 doses	Monitor serum chloramphenicol levels to maintain peak at 15–25 µg/ml	Ampicillin, 100–200 mg/kg/day IV in 4–6 doses for ampicillin-sensitive strains or Chloramphenicol, 75 mg/kg/day PO in 4 doses or Ceftriaxone } Doses or } same Cefotaxime } as for or } empiric Cefuroxime } therapy	Varies with clinical entities *Note:* oral antibiotics may be used to complete therapy in some clinical entities (see text)

serum levels (drawn immediately prior to administration of a dose), but a trough level between 5 and 10 µg/ml assures continuous levels of chloramphenicol above the minimal inhibitory concentration of the drug for most strains of *H. influenzae* b. Serum chloramphenicol levels may vary widely and may be affected by the concurrent administration of anticonvulsive drugs or rifampin.

MENINGITIS

Empiric therapy for bacterial meningitis in children should include an antibiotic effective against ampicillin-resistant *Haemophilus influenzae*. Such drugs include chloramphenicol, 75–100 mg/kg/day divided into four doses, or one of the new cephalosporins—such as ceftriaxone, 100 mg/kg/day divided into two doses; cefotaxime, 200 mg/kg/day divided into four doses; or cefuroxime, 200 mg/kg/day divided into four doses. If the infecting organism is known to be ampicillin sensitive, therapy with ampicillin, 200–300 mg/kg/day in four to six divided doses, may be used.

With appropriate antibiotic treatment, a clinical response (decreased temperature, normalized peripheral blood leukocyte count, and improved neurologic status) should be noted in 24–36 hours. Failure of a patient to respond clinically to initial antibiotic therapy within 48 hours is an indication for repeat lumbar puncture. If the CSF is not sterile, a resistant organism should be suspected and alternate antibiotic therapy instituted. If a multiply-resistant organism is suspected, trimethoprim-sulfamethoxazole—20 mg trimethoprim and 100 mg sulfamethoxazole/kg/day in four divided doses—could be considered, although sufficient data are not available documenting its efficacy.

Initial fluid management should not exceed maintenance requirements, and the osmolality of serum and urine should be monitored for evidence of inappropriate antidiuretic hormone secretion. This entity is managed by decreasing fluid intake to about 75% of maintenance levels. Rarely, endotoxemia and septic shock may occur; they are treated with plasma expanders, oxygen administration, and other supportive measures.

Antibiotic therapy for uncomplicated *H. influenzae* meningitis should continue for 10–14 days, and the patient should be afebrile for 5 days before the discontinuation of therapy. If the patient's disease course is uncomplicated, repeat lumbar puncture is not necessary, either during therapy or when treatment is terminated. Relapse is rare, usually occurring 48–96 hours after antibiotic therapy is stopped. If recurrent infection occurs more than 5–7 days following the end of therapy, reinfection rather than relapse is likely. Typical CSF findings from a lumbar puncture done at 10–12 days after the initiation of therapy include an elevated protein and lymphocytosis, although about 30% of patients may have persistent neutrophils. Decreased CSF glucose or polysaccharide antigen in the CSF may persist for weeks.

Acute Complications. In all children, the possibility of increased intracranial pressure should be considered and its signs sought for by repeated physical examination, careful neurologic examination, frequent monitoring of vital signs, and daily measurement of head circumference. Once increased intracranial pressure is recognized, therapy should be instituted immediately. Severe intracranial hypertension may require insertion of an intracranial pressure monitoring device to check on the adequacy of therapy with mannitol or other osmotic agents. Airway maintenance and oxygen administration are important. Anti-inflammatory agents such as steroids have been used, but there are no data to support their efficacy. Seizures may occur early as a result of small areas of infarction secondary to cerebral vasculitis. Phenobarbital or phenytoin (Dilantin) is used to control seizures. An inappropriate antidiuretic hormone effect is managed with fluid restriction and careful monitoring of serum and urine osmolality. Ventriculitis, especially in infants younger than 6 months of age, may cause prolonged fever and hydrocephalus. Disseminated intravascular coagulation occurs uncommonly and is managed with fresh frozen plasma, platelet transfusions, and supportive measures as necessary.

Secondary and Persistent Fevers. Fever persists beyond 10 days after the initiation of therapy in about 10% of patients. These prolonged (persistent) fevers may be due to drug fever, subdural effusions, nosocomial infections, unrecognized and undrained secondary foci (septic arthritis, pleural or pericardial empyema), or recurrent meningitis. Secondary fever occurs in 20–50% of patients and may be associated with intercurrent viral illness, drug fever, phlebitis, or subdural effusion.

Occurrence of subdural effusions during the resolution of meningitis is common. If the effusions as seen on computerized tomographic (CT) scans are large or are associated with increased irritability, neurologic deficit, persistent seizures, or persistent fever, the fluid should be evacuated and cultured. Rarely, subdural effusions contain infected loculated fluid. Such subdural empyemas should be surgically drained to shorten the duration of hospitalization and decrease morbidity. Increasing head size may indicate subdural effusion, communicating hydrocephalus, or inadequately treated ventriculitis. Brain abscess secondary to *H. influenzae* meningitis is rare but is more common than with other meningotrophic organisms and is usually apparent on CT scan (demonstrating enhancement of the vascular rim). Surgical drainage or prolonged antibiotic therapy, or both, may be required.

Outcome. The mortality rate of *H. influenzae* type b meningitis is 3–7%, and the morbidity rate is up to 50%. About 10% of patients may suffer unilateral or bilateral deafness, and a comprehensive hearing evaluation should be done during recovery from the infection. Other neurologic sequelae include seizure disorders, learning disabilities, mental retardation, blindness, and spastic di- or quadriplegia. Cranial nerve palsies are generally transient.

EPIGLOTTITIS

Acute epiglottitis, which is nearly always caused by *H. influenzae* type b, is a true medical emergency requiring immediate measures to maintain an adequate airway. Nasotracheal intubation, orotracheal intubation, and tracheostomy have been used successfully and have comparable rates of morbidity. The use of a technique for which there is readily available expertise and back-up is more important than the specific procedure. Most patients with epiglottitis have an associated *H. influenzae* bacteremia, so initial antibiotic therapy should follow the guidelines for bacteremia without meningitis and should be continued for at least 7 days. In most instances, with adequate therapy the signs and symptoms of the acute infection abate within 48 hours and the tracheal cannula may be removed 2–3 days after the initiation of antibiotic therapy. Secondary foci of infection are uncommon but may include pneumonia and rarely meningitis.

SEPTIC ARTHRITIS

The mainstay of treatment of septic arthritis is adequate joint drainage, which may be accomplished using various methods depending on the joint involved and the age of the patient. Septic arthritis of the hip is a surgical emergency and should be externally drained at the time of diagnosis. Infections of the shoulders, knee, and elbows may also require surgical drainage, particularly in young infants; however, repeated needle aspirations along with appropriate antibiotic therapy have been used successfully.

Initial empiric antibiotic therapy of patients with septic arthritis should include antimicrobial agents that are effective against the most likely pathogens and that achieve adequate bactericidal levels within the joint spaces. Coverage for *H. influenzae* type b is accomplished by following the guidelines for therapy of bacteremic *H. influenzae* type b infections without meningitis. If β-lactam antibiotics (ampicillin or the new cephalosporins) are used, they should be given intravenously until the child is afebrile, the erythrocyte sedimentation rate is significantly decreased, and local inflammation has decreased (usually 5–7 days). Then oral antibiotics (ampicillin, 100–150 mg/kg/day in four divided doses; or cefaclor, 80–100 mg/kg/day in four divided doses*) may be used to complete a minimum antibiotic course of 2–3 weeks. Antibiotic therapy needs to be continued until the sedimentation rate returns to normal. Peak serum bactericidal levels $\geq 1:8$ assure continued adequate therapy. Undrained septic arthritis may require a longer period of treatment with parenteral β-lactam antibiotics. If chloramphenicol is given, the oral drug may be used to complete the entire 2–3 week course, with careful monitoring of serum drug levels and hematopoietic status. A decreased reticulocyte count is the first indication of marrow suppression; however, the drug may be safely continued until the peripheral leukocyte count is below 3000 cells/mm^3.

OSTEOMYELITIS

Haemophilus influenzae type b osteomyelitis tends to be a less destructive process than that caused by staphylococci, and thus surgical drainage may not be necessary. In most instances the extremity is immobilized, often with casting. The initial antibiotic therapy is identical to that recommended for septic arthritis. Parenteral administration of ampicillin or the new cephalosporins should be continued until the child is afebrile, all local signs of inflammation have abated, and the erythrocyte sedimentation rate has significantly decreased (1–3 weeks). Oral therapy with amoxicillin (100–150 mg/kg/day in four divided doses) for infections caused by ampicillin-sensitive strains may then be continued for an additional 2–4 weeks, until the erythrocyte sedimentation rate is normal. As a guide to adequate therapy, the peak serum concentration of oral amoxicillin (drawn 2 hours after an oral dose) should be 8–20 µg/ml with a bactericidal titer $\geq 1:8$. For infections caused by ampicillin-resistant organisms, the entire course of therapy may be accomplished with parenteral new cephalosporins or oral chloramphenicol.

PNEUMONIA

Haemophilus influenzae pneumonia is commonly segmental or lobar and may be associated with pleural effusion. Initial antibiotic therapy should include antimicrobial agents that assure adequate bactericidal levels in lung tissue; it is accomplished using the guidelines for bacteremic *H. influenzae* type b infections without meningitis.

After the child has clinically stabilized, is no longer tachypneic, and tolerates oral feedings (3–5 days), oral amoxicillin may be used for infections caused by ampicillin-sensitive strains. For ampicillin-resistant strains, oral chloramphenicol or cefaclor* (40 mg/kg/day in four divided doses) may be

---

* Manufacturer's recommended daily dose for serious infections is 40 mg/kg/day, to a maximum of 1 gram/day.

used. Effective treatment of uncomplicated pneumonia is achieved with 10–14 days of total antibiotic therapy. However, in the presence of large pleural effusions, prolonged antibiotic therapy may be necessary. Needle aspiration of large pleural effusions should be performed early to assess sterility, and empyema should be treated with a closed chest tube until drainage decreases substantially (usually 2–3 days).

CELLULITIS

The most serious aspect of this illness is the associated bacteremia, seen in 70–80% of patients, and the possibility of a secondary focus of infection, such as meningitis, septic arthritis, or pericarditis. Most infants defervesce within 18–24 hours of appropriate antibiotic therapy; persistence of fever more than 48 hours after starting treatment suggests the possibility of a resistant organism or the occurrence of a secondary focus of infection. The empiric antibiotic therapy of *Haemophilus influenzae* type b cellulitis is outlined in the guidelines for treatment of bacteremic infections without meningitis. After the child is afebrile and inflammation has decreased (2–4 days), a 7–10 day total antibiotic course may be completed with an oral antibiotic, such as amoxicillin (100–150 mg/kg/day in four divided doses) for ampicillin-sensitive organisms, or chloramphenicol (75–100 mg/kg/day in four divided doses) for ampicillin-resistant organisms.

Periorbital cellulitis may be associated with underlying sinusitis or orbital cellulitis; CT scans may be useful in defining the extent of the infection.

BACTEREMIA WITHOUT APPARENT FOCUS

Occult *Haemophilus influenzae* type b bacteremia occurs among infants under 2 years of age presenting with high fever, leukocytosis with a marked shift to the left, and no apparent focus of infection on initial evaluation. Many of these children ultimately develop clinically apparent pneumonia or otitis media. The child with *H. influenzae* bacteremia but without an identifiable source of infection is at increased risk of invasive disease, particularly meningitis, and should be treated as if he had a systemic infection, with admission to the hospital and initiation of appropriate therapy. If the CSF cultures are sterile, no secondary foci of infection are found, and the child is afebrile and clinically improved, the antibiotics are discontinued after 7 days.

UNCOMMON SYSTEMIC INFECTIONS

The following may be complications of acute *H. influenzae* type b bacteremia.

Pericarditis. *H. influenzae* type b pericarditis is generally associated with another focus of infection, such as meningitis, septic arthritis, facial cellulitis, or pneumonia. In these patients the duration of antibiotic therapy is dictated by the primary site of infection. Pericarditis may be a life-threatening infection, and the patient should be carefully monitored for evidence of cardiac tamponade. Early surgical drainage of the pericardial empyema will decrease morbidity.

Endocarditis. *H. influenzae* type b endocarditis may occur in children with cyanotic congenital heart disease; these children have persistent *Haemophilus* bacteremia and low-grade fever. Most case reports document successful therapy with 6 weeks of intravenous ampicillin or with intravenous or oral chloramphenicol if the organism is ampicillin resistant.

CNS Shunt Infections. Patients with indwelling ventricular drainage systems may be at increased risk for meningitis following *H. influenzae* bacteremia. These patients have been successfully treated with 2–3 weeks of chloramphenicol without replacement of the shunt apparatus. However, sterilization of the ventricular fluid obtained from the shunt reservoir during antibiotic therapy must be documented.

Neonatal Sepsis. *H. influenzae* both type b and nontypable species, may produce a clinical picture similar to that of group B streptococcal sepsis in neonates. These premature or term infants present with apparent respiratory distress syndrome and may develop shock within the first 24 hours. Optimal antibiotic therapy for preterm infants includes the newer cephalosporins such as cefotaxime, 50 mg/kg/day in two daily doses for infants younger than 7 days of age and 75 mg/kg/day in three daily doses for babies 1–4 weeks of age. For term infants, the dose of cefotaxime is 75 mg/kg/day in three daily doses for neonates younger than 7 days of age and 100 mg/kg/day in four daily doses for babies 1–4 weeks of age. Ceftriaxone, 50 mg/kg once a day, may also be used in neonatal infections. If the organism is shown to be ampicillin sensitive, ampicillin—100 mg/kg/day in two divided doses for babies from birth to 7 days of age and 150–200 mg/kg/day in three to four divided doses for neonates beyond 7 days of age—may be used. Therapy should continue for 14 days in infants showing a rapid clinical response; prolonged clinical illness requires longer therapy and a search for another focus of infection. Chloramphenicol is not used in the neonatal period.

MUCOSAL SURFACE INFECTIONS

The following respiratory mucosal infections are generally caused by nonencapsulated, nontypable *H. influenzae* but may occasionally be caused by encapsulated type b organisms.

Otitis Media. Approximately one-third of all otitis media infections are due to *H. influenzae*, and approximately 30% of these may be due to ampicillin-resistant organisms. In general, oral amoxicillin (40 mg/kg/day in three divided doses) remains the drug of choice for otitis media of unknown etiology. In patients who fail to respond to this therapy (i.e., show continued fever, irritability, and poor feeding), several alternative antimicrobial agents may be used, all of which appear to have equal efficacy against *H. influenzae*. These include cefaclor (40 mg/kg/day orally in three divided doses), erythromycin-sulfisoxazole* (40 mg/kg/day of erythromycin in three or four divided doses), trimethoprim-sulfamethoxazole (6–8 mg/kg/day of trimethoprim in two divided doses), or amoxicillin-clavulanic acid (40 mg/kg/day of amoxicillin in three divided doses). Antihistamines, decongestants, and nasal drops have not been shown to be effective in preventing acute otitis media or in facilitating drainage of the middle ear effusion following acute infection. However, these agents may provide symptomatic relief for children with viral upper respiratory infections often associated with acute otitis media. In most instances, the antibiotic therapy is continued for 10 days, with a follow-up evaluation 2–3 weeks after discontinuation of therapy. Asymptomatic sterile middle ear effusions may persist for at least 4 weeks following acute infection in half of adequately treated patients.

Sinusitis. The antimicrobial therapy for *H. influenzae* sinusitis is identical to that for acute otitis media. However, adequate resolution may require continued antibiotic therapy for 2–3 weeks, along with the use of systemic or topical decongestants. If clinical improvement does not occur within 48–72 hours, surgical drainage may be indicated.

Bronchiectasis. Long-term (6 weeks) administration of amoxicillin or another of the drugs used to treat acute otitis media usually results in symptomatic improvement of children with chronic pulmonary disease and bronchiectasis. In controlled studies, long-term sulfonamide administration has decreased the frequency of recurrences in individuals with *Haemophilus* bronchiectasis.

Conjunctivitis. Systemic antibody therapy is generally not required for *H. influenzae* conjunctivitis unless it is associated with periorbital cellulitis. Topical antibiotic ophthalmic drops (such as gentamicin or sulfacetamide) every 2 hours or ointment every 4–6 hours for 5–7 days generally controls this infection.

PROPHYLAXIS OF CONTACTS

Clusters of systemic *H. influenzae* type b infections have recently been recognized among household and day care contacts of children with invasive *H. influenzae* b disease, and the asymptomatic nasopharyngeal carriage rates of *H. influenzae* b may be much higher in contacts than in the general population. Rifampin has been shown to eliminate

the nasopharyngeal carrier state, at least in the short term, from household and day care contacts.

Household Contacts. Among household contacts of a child with systemic *H. influenzae* b infection, the risk of the occurrence of secondary disease in children under 4 years has been well documented and is significantly higher than for age-matched children in the general population. The risk is particularly great for children under 1 year (6%). Thus, the American Academy of Pediatrics Committee on Infectious Diseases has recommended that rifampin prophylaxis be used in all household contacts of children with invasive *H. influenzae* type b disease if any of the household members are under 4 years of age.

Day Care Contacts. The risk of occurrence of secondary invasive disease among day care contacts is less well understood, and the efficacy of rifampin in preventing secondary disease in the day care setting has not been established. Thus, prophylaxis of day care contacts needs to be considered on an individual basis for each day care situation. Notification of the day care facility and parents of the other children must be accomplished to assure prompt evaluation of febrile illnesses in the contacts. An outbreak of multiple cases of invasive *H. influenzae* b infections in a day care setting may indicate the presence of as yet unrecognized risk factors among these children. Thus, rifampin prophylaxis should be instituted when an outbreak is suspected (more than one case within 60–90 days), and all day care children and adult caregivers should be treated simultaneously.

Administration of Rifampin. Rifampin is given at a dose of 20 mg/kg once a day for 4 days to children and 600 mg once a day for 4 days to adults. No pediatric suspension of rifampin is commercially available, so liquid preparations must be freshly made up by a pharmacist or the correct daily dose of the powder must be prepared to be administered in a suitable vehicle such as applesauce or ice cream. Rifampin is available in 300-mg and 150-mg capsules. Contraindications to rifampin use include pregnancy and known allergy to rifampin. All household contacts are treated simultaneously and as soon as possible following diagnosis of the index case. If the patient's household has children younger than 4 years, the patient should receive 4 days of rifampin upon hospital discharge. No data are available to suggest that rifampin may protect the patient from reinfecting himself. The risk of spread to contacts from patients with systemic nonmeningeal *H. influenzae* b infections (such as pneumonia, cellulitis, etc.) is identical with that from children with meningitis, and the prophylaxis recommendations apply to situations involving all forms of invasive *H. influenzae* b infections.

---

* Manufacturer's warning: Not recommended for use in infants under 2 months of age.

PREVENTION OF *HAEMOPHILUS INFLUENZAE* TYPE b INFECTIONS

A vaccine consisting of the capsular polysaccharide of *H. influenzae* b (PRP) is available for use in older children. This vaccine is ineffective in inducing protective immunity in children under age 18 months and appears to be about 90% effective for children over age 24 months. The duration of immunity following immunization between 18 months and 24 months of age remains uncertain, and reimmunization may be required to assure protection. Current recommendations include immunization of all children at age 24 months. Higher priority should be given to children among certain high-risk groups, such as those in day care, and possibly to children with asplenia syndromes, including sickle-cell disease, and with lymphoid malignancies prior to the initiation of chemotherapy. However, the efficacy of the vaccine in these immunocompromised children has not been established. In addition, clinical trials are underway to investigate the efficacy of the capsular polysaccharide covalently linked to various carrier proteins in inducing protective immune responses in younger children.

Tetanus Neonatorum

JAMES M. ADAMS, M.D.

Although neonatal tetanus is now rare in the United States, it is most prevalent among infants delivered at home and in segments of the population with inadequate maternal immunization. It must be differentiated primarily from neonatal seizures, but birth trauma, hypoxic injury, septicemia, and other diseases of the perinatal period are common in this group of patients and may coexist with neonatal tetanus.

General Supportive Care. Programs for outpatient management of tetanus have been implemented in developing nations, but the disease should be considered an indication for hospitalization of the newborn infant even if initial spasms are mild. The baby should be admitted to a neonatal intensive care unit or a unit able to provide electronic cardiac monitoring, a controlled thermal environment, skilled nursing care, and mechanical ventilatory support, if necessary.

The infant should be placed initially in a servo-controlled or manually controlled incubator, protected from light and noise. This environment reduces the spasm-provoking external stimuli that reach the baby. Swaddling and minimal handling and disturbance of the infant further reduce the tendency of environmental stimuli to provoke self-perpetuating spasms. Such minimal intrusion into the environment of the infant requires close observation by trained personnel as well as careful electronic monitoring. Swaddling may result in overheating if the temperature of both the infant and its environment is not properly monitored and controlled.

Serum electrolytes, blood urea nitrogen, albumin, and urine specific gravity determinations aid in guiding metabolic and nutritional management. All infants should receive 1 mg of vitamin K_1 initially, and a VDRL specimen should be obtained. Prophylactic eye care should be administered with erythromycin ointment.

Fluids should be administered intravenously initially as 10% glucose in water with appropriate electrolytes at an infusion rate of 100 to 125 ml/kg/24 hr. Once spasms are controlled, or if mechanical ventilation has been instituted and the condition stabilized, enteral feedings can be initiated by nasogastric tube if bowel sounds are present. A formula of 24 calories per ounce should be given initially at 25 ml/kg/24 hr by continuous nasogastric infusion and advanced progressively until intravenous fluids can be discontinued. For long-term growth and nutrition, formula intakes of 140 to 150 ml/kg/24 hr will be necessary. When the infant's course is stabilized on full milk drip feedings, intermittent gavage may be attempted. This feeding program is designed to avoid gastric distention, impairment of mobility of the diaphragm, and regurgitation. In term infants, if the formula utilized meets the recommendations of the American Academy of Pediatrics Committee on Nutrition, vitamin and mineral supplementation will not be required unless specific deficiencies are identified.

Bacteriologic Management. Because septicemia or meningoencephalitis cannot be ruled out during the initial hours of hospitalization, ampicillin (150 mg/kg/24 hr) and kanamycin (15 mg/kg/24 hr) should be administered parenterally following blood and cerebrospinal fluid cultures. When a diagnosis of tetanus has been confirmed, these antibiotics may be discontinued and 100,000 units/kg/24 hr of aqueous penicillin G given alone to finish a 10-day course of therapy.

Human tetanus immune globulin, 500 units, should be given in divided doses intramuscularly. All babies should receive an initial dose of diphtheria-tetanus vaccine prior to discharge, as no permanent immunity results from *Clostridium tetani* infections treated with antitoxin. The initial immunization should be delayed, however, until 4 to 6 weeks after administration of antitoxin.

Positive cultures of *C. tetani* from the umbilicus are rarely obtained, even with anaerobic techniques. Antibody tests may confirm the diagnosis, but results are usually not available in the early days of the disease.

Control of Tetanic Spasms. Various tranquilizers and sedating drugs have been utilized to control the violent spasms of tetanus. At best, these agents can be expected to modify the frequency or severity of the spasms rather than abate them. In general, slightly better results can be expected from combination regimens and very high dosage ranges. The incidence of apnea, retention of pulmonary secretions, and other complications of central nervous system depression, however, is also increased. The potential for addiction with these drugs, particularly chloral hydrate, must be considered.

Phenobarbital 10–15 mg/kg/day may be given by nasogastric tube in two or three divided doses. Chloral hydrate, 40 to 60 mg/kg/day, may be added. Good results have been achieved abroad using a continuous infusion of diazepam, 20–40 mg/kg/day. This is combined with phenobarbital, 10 mg/kg/day. The safety of parenteral diazepam in the neonate has not been established, however, and respiratory depression requiring mechanical ventilation should be anticipated in some patients receiving this high-dose regimen.

During the recovery phase of the disease, intermittent spasms, usually less severe, may require continuation of phenobarbital or diazepam, 2–4 mg/kg/day per nasogastric tube, for muscle relaxation.

Pulmonary Care. Virtually all deaths in tetanus neonatorum are respiratory. Specific pulmonary complications include apnea, hypoventilation, hypoxemia, pneumothorax, infection, and airway obstruction from retained secretions. Constant observation of color, respiratory rate, heart rate, and work of breathing is necessary. Arterial blood gases should be obtained as a guide to respiratory management and warm, humidified oxygen given as necessary to maintain PaO_2 at 60 to 80 torr. Transcutaneous oxygen monitoring is helpful in determining trends in oxygenation during spasms and at rest. Indications for mechanical ventilation are (1) apnea, (2) $PaCO_2$ persistently greater than 50 to 60 torr, (3) recurrent hypoxemia during spasms, and (4) continuous or rapidly recurring spasms.

Infants should initially be ventilated in conjunction with neuromuscular blockade. Pancuronium bromide is given intravenously in an initial dose of 0.05 mg/kg. This may be increased to 0.1 mg/kg, given as frequently as needed to keep the infant quiet and immobile. Complete muscular paralysis is not necessary. As lung function in these babies is essentially normal but chest compliance and airway resistance subject to change throughout the course, we prefer a volume-controlled ventilator. As the infant receiving neuromuscular blockade is at the mercy of the environment, strict attention must be paid to suctioning, changes of position, chest percussion, and maintenance of sterile technique.

Infants should be maintained on mechanical ventilation until respiratory compromise is no longer produced by residual spasms. This may require 3 to 4 weeks. Tracheostomy should be the exception rather than the rule in neonatal tetanus. Modern neonatal intensive care has produced a low incidence of complications of prolonged endotracheal intubation, and tracheostomy itself is not without serious consequences in this age group.

Pulmonary infection is a constant threat, and the clinician should be alert to changes in temperature control, glucose metabolism, or pulmonary function as early warning signs. If changes in pulmonary function suggest pneumonia, complete blood count, blood culture, chest radiograph, and Gram's stain, and culture of tracheal secretions should be performed. Gram's stain may aid in the initial choice of antibiotics, but in most instances appropriate therapy would include methicillin (200 mg/kg/24 hr) and gentamicin (5.0–7.5 mg/kg/24 hr).

Infant Botulism

STEPHEN S. ARNON, M.D.

Infant botulism, the recently recognized infectious form, occurs when ingested spores of *Clostridium botulinum* germinate, colonize the intestine, and produce in vivo the most potent poison known, botulinal toxin. The generalized flaccid paralysis produced by the toxin's blockade of peripheral cholinergic synapses, most notably the neuromuscular junction, constitutes the central challenge of management. Meticulous supportive care (nutritional, respiratory, nursing) is the basis of therapy. In the absence of complications, all hospitalized infants have recovered without residua.

In severely paralyzed patients the need for immediate hospitalization with intensive care will be obvious, even if the diagnosis is not. ("Suspected sepsis" remains the most common admission diagnosis.) However, even the mildly weak and hypotonic infant should be observed where a respirator is immediately at hand, as the severity of paralysis may increase within hours, and aspiration, upper airway occlusion, or diaphragmatic paralysis may suddenly occur. Cardiac and respiratory monitoring should begin at admission, and prophylactic intubation is prudent.

The intensity of supportive care a patient requires will vary during the several weeks of hospitalization while the motoneurons regenerate new myoneural junctions and thereby restore movement. Some patients need total ventilatory and nutritional sustenance. Transcutaneous monitoring of blood oxygen tension is desirable because an affected infant will be unable to squirm or otherwise signal distress should the position of the endotracheal tube change. Similarly, cough and postural reflexes are generally absent, and if the patient is not carefully positioned after each handling, breathing difficulties may ensue. Few patients have needed tracheostomy despite prolonged intubation, and tracheostomy should not be considered a necessary part of management.

Gavage feeding permits easy supplying of fluid, electrolyte, and caloric needs and may stimulate peristalsis, thereby hastening the elimination of *C. botulinum* toxin and organisms from the gut. The presence of gastric atony and of possible gastroesophageal reflux mandates close watch for residual volumes. However, with an infusion pump and crib blocks even quite paralyzed patients have been successfully fed by gavage. The patient should receive mother's milk if available; if not, a formula milk without added iron is the next choice. Intravenous feeding ("hyperalimentation") has been used as a last resort but brings with it the need for repeated phlebotomy (thus, nosocomial anemia) as well as the hazard of infection.

The currently available botulinal antitoxin is a horse serum product that is not used in infant botulism for several reasons. Most importantly, experience has shown that patients recover completely without it. Also, evidence of its therapeutic efficacy is lacking. In addition, its use may induce lifelong hypersensitivity. Finally, serum sickness and anaphylaxis often occur when equine antitoxin is given to older children and adults. A human-derived botulism immune globulin, when developed, may have therapeutic benefit.

Antibiotics are used in infant botulism only to treat secondary infections, which occur most frequently in the lungs or urinary tract. Antibiotic therapy directed against *C. botulinum* organisms in the gut lumen has been tried but has failed to eradicate the bacteria or to stop excretion of toxin. Furthermore, it is possible that antibiotics effective against *C. botulinum* might be more effective against other gut anaerobes and may thereby create a larger ecologic space for *C. botulinum*. Also, clostridiocidal antibiotics may actually increase the pool of toxin in the gut available for absorption, as botulinal toxin is liberated with bacterial cell death and lysis. For this reason, when antibiotics are needed to treat the common secondary infections of infant botulism, it may be desirable to use the combination drug trimethoprim-sulfamethoxazole (Bactrim, Septra), to which *C. botulinum* is resistant. This drug is approved for use in infants over 2 months of age. Aminoglycoside antibiotics, often begun at admission when infant botulism is mistaken for "sepsis," may exacerbate the paralysis by further blocking neuromuscular transmission.

During recovery, patients fatigue easily when muscular action is sustained, a consideration particularly important in deciding when to resume oral feeding, because of the hazard of aspiration. Patients should not be fed by mouth until they are fully able to gag and swallow. Tube feeding has been continued uneventfully at home by some parents. Patients are usually ready for discharge when gag reflex, swallowing, and coughing ability are adequate to protect the airway.

Some practical measures deserve mention. Bladder atony is often present, and frequent emptying by Credé's method will reduce risk of urinary tract infection. Since *C. botulinum* toxin and organisms remain in patients' feces for weeks (and might be fecally-orally transmitted to other infants), scrupulous hand washing by all who handle the infant is mandatory. For the same reason, the patient's linen should be bagged separately and autoclaved. (Spores of *C. botulinum* are very heat-resistant.) Staff personnel with open lesions on their hands should not change the patient's diapers.

Normal bowel action may take weeks to return and may be impeded by an inspissated bolus of feces, a possibility detectable by digital examination. During convalescence, a stool softener may be beneficial. Cathartics and enemas intended to reduce the quantity of intraluminal *C. botulinum* are ineffective, and repeated purgation is potentially dangerous. Once discharged, close contact with other infants (e.g., same crib) should be avoided for about 3 months or until excretion of organisms has ceased. The possibility of nosocomial infant botulism will exist as long as some hospital dietetic departments use honey as the carbohydrate source in lactose-free ("CHO-Free") infant feeds.

Physicians who suspect infant botulism should contact their state health department to arrange for diagnostic testing of feces and serum.

Shigellosis

LARRY K. PICKERING, M.D.

Shigellosis is defined as infection of the gastrointestinal tract by shigella organisms. Bacillary dysentery is a form of shigellosis characterized by passage of stools of small volume that contain blood, mucus, and inflammatory cells. Shigella are divided into four serogroups and at least 40 serotypes: (a) group A, *S. dysenteriae*, (b) group B, *S. flexneri*, (c) group C, *S. boydii*, and (d) group D, *S. sonnei*. Currently, *S. sonnei* accounts for between 60 and 80% of cases of shigellosis reported in the United States, and *S. flexneri* serotypes account for most of the remaining cases. *S. boydii* and *S. dysenteriae* are rare causes of diarrhea in the United States. Shigella is a highly infectious organism; the infectious dose for healthy adults is 10 to 100 organisms.

Table 1. ANTIMICROBIAL THERAPY OF SHIGELLOSIS

Antimicrobial Agent	Dose	
	Children	*Adults*
First choice: Trimethoprim (TMP)-sulfamethoxazole (SMX) (Bactrim, Septra)	TMP (10 mg/kg/ 24 hr plus SMX (50 mg/ kg/24 hr) orally for 5 days; give in 2 divided doses	TMP (160 mg) plus SMX (800 mg) orally for 5 days every 12 hr
Alternates: Ampicillin or	50–75 mg/kg/24 hr orally for 5 days; give in 4 divided doses	500 mg orally for 5 days; give in 4 divided doses
Tetracycline	Not recommended	2.5 gm orally in a single dose one time

Antimicrobial therapy is administered to patients with shigellosis to abbreviate the clinical course and/or decrease excretion of the causative organisms. A stool culture should be obtained and antibiotic susceptibility testing of the suspected pathogen performed to ensure optimal therapy. The organisms do not survive well in fecal specimens, so that freshly passed stool specimens should be plated directly onto culture media such as xylose-lysine-deoxycholate, salmonella-shigella, and MacConkey agars. Changing susceptibility patterns often make the initial selection of an antimicrobial agent difficult. Antimicrobial agents should not be used routinely or liberally for gastroenteritis of unknown etiology. In addition, antidiarrheal agents with antiperistaltic activity should not be used in patients with shigellosis, since they may prolong the fever, diarrhea, and excretion of the organism.

Several antibiotics have been used successfully in eradicating clinical symptoms and fecal shedding of *Shigella*. Approximately half of the *S. sonnei* strains are resistant to ampicillin, whereas *S. flexneri* strains have remained relatively susceptible to ampicillin. Table 1 outlines suggested antimicrobial therapy for children and adults who are presumed to have shigellosis or from whom *Shigella* organisms are isolated from stool. Trimethoprim plus sulfamethoxazole is the treatment of choice for shigellosis because of the increasing frequency of ampicillin resistance among *Shigella* isolates. In children with known ampicillin-susceptible strains, ampicillin is the treatment of choice and can be given either orally or intravenously. Single-dose tetracycline therapy is effective in the treatment of *Shigella* infection in adults, but it must be limited to adults because of the side effects, including discoloration of teeth, that occur in children under 8 years of age who receive tetracycline. Patients who are transient asymptomatic carriers may be managed without antimicrobial therapy if they understand and employ excellent standards of personal and public hygiene. Treatment of these patients, however, may reduce fecal shedding of the organism and prevent spread of infection.

Sulfonamides are as effective as ampicillin if the organism is susceptible, but most *Shigella* strains are resistant to sulfonamides. Nonabsorbable antibiotics such as neomycin, kanamycin, and gentamicin will not alter the course of the disease or the fecal excretion of *Shigella*. Amoxicillin is not as effective as ampicillin in the treatment of shigellosis and should not be used. In shigellosis caused by antibiotic-resistant strains, nalidixic acid (55 mg/kg/24 hours given four times daily for 5 days to children) may be effective, but has not been approved for this use.

The prognosis for an uneventful recovery from shigellosis is excellent in the majority of infected patients. Mortality in the United States is less than 1%. Complications may include dehydration and electrolyte imbalance or the rare problems of perforation of the colon, generally following a procedure such as sigmoidoscopy; rectal prolapse due to unrelenting diarrhea; and bacteremia. The extraintestinal complications of Reiter's syndrome and hemolytic-uremic syndrome can be initiated by *Shigella* infections.

Typhoid Fever

SANDOR FELDMAN, M.D.

Modern sanitation has dramatically reduced the incidence of typhoid fever in this country. In 1984, approximately 370 cases were reported in the United States. However, worldwide, in underdeveloped countries *Salmonella typhi* remains a significant health problem. Typhoid fever is still to be suspected in children with prolonged high fevers (39–41° C), headache, nausea, anorexia, malaise, irritability, cough, abdominal pain, leukopenia, splenomegaly, or rose spots. Constipation is common, but diarrhea is relatively uncommon. *S. typhi* can be isolated from blood and bone marrow. Later in the course of infection the organism can be isolated from urine and stool. Elevated O-antigen agglutinating antibody ($\geq 1:320$) or rising O- and H-antigen agglutinating antibodies to *S. typhi* are suggestive of typhoid fever.

Therapy. Initial therapy should be intravenous chloramphenicol, 50–100 mg/kg/day (maximum of 2 gm/day) in four divided doses, or ampicillin, 100–200 mg/kg/day in four divided doses. Within 3–5 days there will usually be defervescence of fever, and the symptoms will have begun to ameliorate. At that time, if the oral fluid intake is adequate, antibiotic therapy may be changed to the oral route. Amoxicillin, 100 mg/kg/day in three divided doses, may be substituted for ampicillin. Antibiotic therapy should continue for 14 days. Alternatively, trimethoprim-sulfamethoxazole* (TMP-SMZ)—trimethoprim, 10–12 mg/kg/day and sulfamethoxazole, 50–60 mg/kg/day in two divided doses—has been found to be effective therapy for salmonellosis, including *S. typhi*. Intravenous TMP-SMZ requires 125 ml of diluting fluid for each 80 mg TMP. Children receiving this antibiotic intravenously should have careful monitoring of fluid intake.

Many of the cephalosporins have demonstrated in vitro activity against *S. typhi* and the other *Salmonella* serotypes. Clinical studies are lacking to support their use. In some instances these antibiotics have been ineffective, despite in vitro activity. However, preliminary observations suggest that cefoperazone and some of the newer third-generation cephalosporins may be useful in the treatment of *S. typhi* and the nontyphoidal *Salmonella* species.

Salmonellae, including *S. typhi*, have shown some resistance to ampicillin, chloramphenicol, and TMP-SMZ. Simultaneous resistance to the three antibiotics is increasing. Antibiotic-resistant *Salmonella* species are imported from third world countries. Antibiotic sensitivity to *Salmonella* isolates are required to ensure appropriate therapy.

Treatment for less than 14 days increases the risk of relapse, while treatment for more than 14 days does not decrease this risk. Relapse rates are reported to be from 10 to 20%. Relapse appears to occur less often following treatment with ampicillin (amoxicillin) or TMP-SMZ than with chloramphenicol.

In the United States, children with typhoid fever should be hospitalized for enteric isolation and nursing care. Careful handwashing measures are necessary to decrease the likelihood of intrafamily spread and spread to hospital personnel. During the initial stage of therapy, intravenous fluids may be required, with careful monitoring of fluid and electrolyte balance. The diet should be bland and well balanced and include a generous amount of fluids.

Avoid antipyretic therapy with acetaminophen or salicylates as they can produce hypothermia. Tepid sponge baths can be used to control fever. Physical activity should be markedly limited during the acute phase of the illness and curtailed during convalescence.

Recently a placebo-controlled trial, jointly undertaken by the United States and Indonesia, revealed that dexamethasone 3 mg/kg initially, followed by 8 doses at 1 mg/kg every 6 hours for 48 hours significantly reduced the mortality in severely toxic, stuporous, and delirious patients. The routine use of steroids for fever and symptomatic control is not indicated.

Complications. Complications tend to occur during the 3rd and 4th weeks of illness and are more frequent in the untreated or in those whose therapy was started late. Recurrence of fever usually heralds the onset of relapse or other complications. Gastrointestinal hemorrhage and intestinal perforation are the most severe life-threatening complications. Intensive supportive therapy, antibiotics, and blood products are administered as indicated. Failure of medical management to stabilize the patient may require surgical intervention. However, mortality rates after surgical intervention are high. Sound clinical judgment will be necessary to guide the medical and surgical management of this complication.

Acute cholecystitis with gallstones may require surgery. *S. typhi* involving the lungs, liver, bones, joints, and so on will require prolonged antibiotic therapy.

Chronic Carriers. Chronic carriage is defined as fecal excretion of Salmonella for at least one year. Overall, the carriage rate of *S. typhi* is 2%; however, the rate is much lower in children. The most common source of the organism is the gallbladder with the presence of gallstones. Cholecystectomy should be considered.

Ampicillin, 100–200 mg/kg/day or trimethoprim-sulfamethoxazole* (trimethoprim, 8 mg/kg/day, and sulfamethoxazole, 40 mg/kg/day) for 3 to 4 weeks has been used successfully to treat *S. typhi* carriers. Failures are common.

Vaccination. Typhoid vaccine in the United States is indicated for those persons exposed to documented typhoid carriers, i.e., household contacts, travelers to endemic areas, and laboratory workers with frequent contact with the organism. A heat-phenol–inactivated vaccine is available commercially in the United States. The acetone-inactivated vaccine is used by the United States military. An oral live attenuated typhoid vaccine is presently under investigation and appears to confer immunity for at least 3 years.

The heat-phenol–inactivated vaccine is given subcutaneously in two doses: (1) 0.5 ml/dose 3 weeks apart for children 10 years or older, and (b) two doses 0.25 ml/dose 3 weeks apart for those children 6 months to 10 years. A booster dose of either 0.5 ml or 0.25 ml, depending on the child's age, should be given every 3 years for the child at high risk for typhoid fever. Adverse effects are

---

* This use of trimethoprim-sulfamethoxazole is not listed in the manufacturer's directive.

* This use of trimethoprim-sulfamethoxazole is not listed in the manufacturer's directive.

pain at the site of injection, fever, malaise, and headaches and may require dose reduction.

Salmonellosis

SANDOR FELDMAN, M.D.

For the past several years there has been an increase in the occurrence of nontyphoidal salmonellosis in the United States. Man usually acquires the infection through contact with infected domestic animals and pets or food such as poultry, meat, eggs, and milk products. Multiple-drug–resistant *Salmonella* from antimicrobial drug–fed animals resulted in a four-state outbreak of gastroenteritis. Water-borne salmonellosis is uncommon in this country. There are three primary species: *S. typhi* (one serotype), *S. choleraesuis* (one serotype) and *S. enteritides* (over 1700 serotypes). In the latter group, serotypes *S. typhimurium*, *S. enteritides*, and *S. heidelberg* are the most common isolates. Children less than 5 years of age, particularly those under 1 year of age, have the highest incidence of salmonellosis.

Gastroenteritis (Enterocolitis). This acute-onset syndrome is the most common presentation of *Salmonella* infection. Within 4–48 hours of ingestion of the contaminated food there is nausea, vomiting, headache, malaise, and fever. These symptoms usually resolve and are followed by abdominal cramps and diarrhea. The latter may vary from a few loose stools to a fulminant diarrhea. The mainstay of therapy is fluid and electrolyte replacement with either oral (clear liquids) or intravenous fluids, depending on the child's clinical condition. Abdominal cramps may be treated with infrequent doses of paregoric. In general, antispasmodics and analgesics should be avoided, since overdose for this self-limiting symptom has been reported. Over-the-counter antidiarrheals play no role in the management of gastroenteritis. Usually within a week the diarrhea resolves. Once the child's appetite is regained and the stool frequency has decreased, a soft, bland diet can be instituted.

Antimicrobial therapy is not indicated in this self-limiting form of salmonellosis. However, ampicillin, trimethoprim-sulfamethoxazole* (TMP-SMZ), or chloramphenicol therapy should be considered in that order of preference and depending upon in vitro susceptibility tests for patients at increased risk for disseminated infections. Examples are newborns, infants during the first year of life, children with hemoglobinopathies, such as sickle cell disease or congenital immunodeficien-

cies, and children receiving prednisone, antimetabolites, and/or radiation therapy. Bacteremia in conjunction with gastroenteritis may occur in 9% or more of infants under 1 year of age. Antibiotic therapy should be administered only during acute phase of the infection.

Enteric Fever. Nontyphoidal enteric fever presents clinical features indistinguishable from typhoid fever. Antibiotic therapy is the same as that discussed in the section entitled typhoid fever. Resistance of nontyphoidal *Salmonella* to ampicillin, chloramphenicol, and TMP-SMZ is increasing, particularly when the strain is imported from outside the United States. Antibiotic sensitivities are required to ensure proper therapy for *Salmonella* infections. As with *S. typhi*, first- and second-generation cephalosporins are not indicated in the treatment of *Salmonella* infections. Some of the newer third-generation cephalosporins may prove to be useful in the near future. Gastrointestinal hemorrhage and intestinal perforation are uncommon complications following nontyphoidal salmonellosis.

Bacteremia. This is characterized by a hectic fever pattern for days to weeks and chronic bacteremia without the constitutional symptoms of enteric fever or gastroenteritis. *S. choleraesuis* is frequently the causative serotype. Therapy is similar to that for typhoid fever and requires monitoring with blood cultures. Dissemination to other organ systems can be expected in about 10% of patients.

Local Infections. Localized infections of almost any organ system can occur following salmonellosis. Osteomyelitis in children with sickle cell anemia is well known. Surgical drainage of abscesses is indicated. Intravenous antibiotic therapy with either ampicillin or chloramphenicol may be prolonged, depending on the infected organ. Antibiotic therapy should be continued for at least one week after the signs of infection have disappeared.

As with the treatment of all *Salmonella* infections, antibiotic sensitivities are required because of the increasing resistance. TMP-SMZ* is an alternative to ampicillin and chloramphenicol.

Salmonella meningitis, occurring chiefly in neonates and infants under 1 year of age, has a mortality rate of 85% and relapses occur frequently. The duration of antibiotic therapy in children with meningitis should be at least 14 to 21 days with parenteral ampicillin, 200–300 mg/kg/day, or chloramphenicol, 100 mg/kg/day. Several cases have been successfully treated with TMP-SMZ* (trimethoprim, 10–20 mg/kg/day, and sulfamethoxazole, 50–100 mg/kg/day). Chloram-

---

* This use of trimethoprim-sulfamethoxazole is not listed in the manufacturer's directive.

* This use of trimethoprim-sulfamethoxazole is not listed in the manufacturer's directive.

phenicol should be avoided in the newborn because of the high risk of the gray baby syndrome.

Chronic Carriers. Chronic carrying of nontyphoidal *Salmonella* occurs in less than 1% of infected children. Intrafamily spread can usually be prevented by hand washing measures. Antibiotic therapy is not usually indicated.

Campylobacter Infections

DANIEL E. TORPHY, M.D.

Campylobacter are curved or spiral gram-negative rods that were classified as *Vibrio fetus* and "related vibrios" for many years. They were discovered in 1909 and became well known in veterinary medicine as a common cause of abortion and infertility in sheep and cattle.

Human infection with *Campylobacter* was reported in 1947 and sporadically thereafter until 1972, when a method of isolating *Campylobacter* from stool samples was described. Subsequent studies from many countries and in patients of all ages have established *Campylobacter* as an important human pathogen.

The taxonomy of *Campylobacter* is unsettled and can be confusing. Only three species seem to cause human disease. *C. jejuni* is a frequent cause of gastroenteritis and is isolated almost exclusively from stool samples using selective media. Some isolates reported as *C. jejuni* turn out to be *C. coli* on closer study. *C. fetus* subsp. *fetus* (also called *C. fetus* subsp. *intestinalis*) infections are much less common than those due to *C. jejuni* and usually involve adults. They are usually isolated from blood or other, normally sterile, body fluids and not from stool.

Campylobacter are found in the feces of cattle, sheep, dogs, cats, and domestic and wild fowl. Outbreaks have been traced to water and raw milk. Spread from person to person and mother to infant occurs.

Gastroenteritis

C. jejuni accounts for 5% or more of acute gastroenteritis and is most frequent in the summer-autumn in temperate climates. Children and young adults are most commonly affected, but infants as young as 2 days with *C. jejuni* gastroenteritis have been reported. Typical patients have diarrhea, fever, and abdominal cramps. Stools may contain blood or mucus, and vomiting, malaise, headache, and myalgias are common. Abdominal pain may be severe and has resulted in surgery for suspected appendicitis or intestinal obstruction. Fever will usually last 2–4 days and diarrhea for a week. Fatalities are rare, but dehydration is not uncommon. A few patients develop chronic or recurrent diarrhea, and antibiotic treatment for these patients is clearly indicated. Pancreatitis, mesenteric adenitis, seizures, pneumonia, and arthritis may complicate *C. jejuni* gastroenteritis.

Maintenance of fluid balance, as with any enteritis in children, is of primary importance. Treatment with erythromycin 40 mg/kg/day in divided doses for 5 days eliminates *C. jejuni* from the stool, but controlled studies have not proved that the clinical course is improved. Certainly patients with persistent or recurrent *C. jejuni* enteritis should be treated. Treatment of all children with *Campylobacter* enteritis has been advocated to prevent secondary spread. Treatment seems reasonable if significant diarrhea is still present and hygiene is inadequate.

More than 95% of isolates are susceptible in vitro to erythromycin. Tetracycline is a reasonable alternative in older children, although more isolates are resistant. In vitro studies would be useful in unresponsive cases, as would culture for *Salmonella*, *Shigella*, *Yersinia*, and other pathogens, which also might be present and causing enteritis.

Drugs that decrease intestinal motility such as diphenoxylate and opiates should not be used. They have been associated with an increase in the duration and severity of symptoms in some patients and with at least two deaths.

Extraenteric Infections

C. jejuni can, rarely, cause extraenteric infections, including meningitis. *C. fetus* subsp. *fetus* infections, while rare, include endocarditis, meningitis, pericarditis, thrombophlebitis, arthritis, pneumonia, hepatitis, and other focal infections. Recurrent or chronic bacteremia with intermittent fever for a month or more with eventual localization may occur. Most *C. fetus* subsp. *fetus* infections occur in adults, usually older men who are debilitated or immunocompromised or who have a serious, underlying chronic disease. The first reported human infections with *Campylobacter* involved pregnant women and their newborn infants. Perinatal infections are rare and often result in spontaneous abortion or neonatal death with meningitis.

Extraenteric infections will usually require hospitalization and parenteral treatment with erythromycin or an aminoglycoside. Gentamicin, 5–7.5 mg/kg/day in divided doses every 8 hr for several weeks, should be considered along with adequate drainage if the infection is localized. Controlled studies of antibiotic treatment in these infections are not available. Chloramphenicol or another antibiotic with good CNS/CSF penetration and to which the isolate has demonstrated susceptibility should be considered in treating *Campylobacter* meningitis.

Yersinia enterocolitica Infections

GARY P. WORMSER, M.D.

Yersinia enterocolitica is a small gram-negative coccobacillus in the family Enterobacteriaceae. Although the first clinical isolation occurred in the United States, it is a much more common pathogen in other temperate countries around the world. In parts of the Federal Republic of Germany and Canada, for example, it rivals *Salmonella* and surpasses *Shigella* as a cause of acute diarrheal illness. Evidence also indicates that the organism is growing in importance and in frequency as a human pathogen.

Y. enterocolitica strains are susceptible in vitro to numerous antimicrobials, the most active of which are trimethoprim-sulfamethoxazole, tetracycline, the aminoglycosides, and second or third generation cephalosporins (Table 1). Most strains show considerable resistance to penicillin and cephalothin. Two distinct β-lactamases are found in *Y. enterocolitica*, which may account for the observed sensitivity patterns to the β-lactam antibiotics. Rare strains may also carry R plasmids coding for resistance to chloramphenicol, sulfonamides, streptomycin, kanamycin, and tetracycline.

Few data exist, however, on the clinical efficacy of antimicrobials on any of the manifestations of yersiniosis. A recent placebo-controlled double-blind evaluation of oral trimethoprim-sulfamethoxazole in the treatment of *Y. enterocolitica* gastroenteritis in children failed to demonstrate any clinical or microbiologic benefit from therapy. However, this investigation left open the question of whether therapy given early in the course of disease is beneficial, since the patients were not entered until day 11 or 12 of illness. Future controlled clinical trials with be required to resolve

Table 1.   SUSCEPTIBILITY OF *YERSINIA ENTEROCOLITICA* TO ANTIMICROBIALS IN VITRO

Active Against Most Strains
Trimethoprim-sulfamethoxazole
Tetracycline
Aminoglycosides
Chloramphenicol
Second generation cephalosporins or cephamycins
   (cefamandole, cefoxitin)
Third generation cephalosporins (cefotaxime,
   cefoperazone, moxalactam)
Variably Active
Ampicillin
Carbenicillin
Inactive Against Most Strains
Penicillin
Oxacillin
First generation cephalosporins
Erythromycin
Clindamycin

Table 2.   RECOMMENDATIONS FOR THE TREATMENT OF *YERSINIA ENTEROCOLITICA* INFECTIONS

Manifestation	Treatment
Gastroenteritis	Give antibiotics if any of the following is observed: if patient is moderately to seriously ill and not better when diagnosis is made* if patient is chronically symptomatic if patient is bacteremic if patient is immunodeficient if patient has thalassemia or an iron overload state
Mesenteric adenitis and/or terminal ileitis	give antibiotics if patient is not better when diagnosis is made*
Bacteremia	Give antibiotics
Suppurative focus	Give antibiotics
Nonsuppurative complication	Do not give antibiotics; use anti-inflammatory agent

* Most patients are already improving when the diagnosis is made and will not benefit from antimicrobial therapy.

this issue. Meanwhile, it is reasonable to consider empiric use of antibiotics for moderately to seriously ill patients who can be diagnosed early. Even when the diagnosis is made promptly, however, little justification can be given for treating the patient who is already improving.

Patients with bacteremia or with sites of infection other than the gastrointestinal tract should always be treated, but data to suggest the agent of choice or the optimum duration of therapy are limited. Gentamicin, streptomycin, tetracycline, trimethoprim-sulfamethoxazole, and chloramphenicol have all been used successfully. Based on in vitro susceptibilities, second or third generation cephalosporins should work; however, since resistance to some of these agents is easily induced in vitro, watching for this potential problem will be necessary in patients receiving these drugs.

There is no convincing evidence that antibiotics prevent or ameliorate the nonsuppurative complications of *Y. enterocolitica* infection. Also, few data are available on the use of nonantibiotic treatment modalities in yersinial enteritis, but experience with other invasive intestinal pathogens suggests that antimotility drugs should probably be avoided.

Recommendations, largely empiric, for the treatment of yersiniosis are given in Table 2. Trimethoprim-sulfamethoxazole (for children over 2 months of age) given over 7–14 days may be considered the preferred agent for outpatient management. Either intravenous trimethoprim-sulfamethoxazole or parenteral aminoglycoside therapy may be considered the preferred treatment for inpatients, and probably should be given for at least 2 weeks in bacteremic cases. In all cases close attention must be paid to careful hygienic practices to limit secondary spread of this communicable disease, remembering that fecal carriage may persist for several weeks after resolution of symptoms.

Brucellosis

MOSES GROSSMAN, M.D.

Brucellosis is a contagious disease of animals, principally ungulates, that is occasionally transmitted to man. The infective organism (a gram-negative bacillus) is transmitted through handling of infected meat (in slaughter houses) and infected placentae (farms, veterinarians) and by ingestion of nonpasteurized milk or milk products from infected animals. Human infection is rare in the United States (less than 200 cases a year) and is particularly rare in children. Brucellosis is often featured in the differential diagnosis of prolonged fever despite its rare occurrence. Diagnosis depends on culturing the organism from blood, bone marrow, or a focal infection site, or on a fourfold increase in agglutination titer measured in paired specimens of sera.

Specific antimicrobial treatment serves to shorten the course of the disease and to prevent complications. The drug of choice by virtue of greatest clinical experience is tetracycline, 30–40 mg/kg/24 hr given orally in four divided doses (maximal adult dose 2 gm/24 hr) for a period of some three weeks. Seriously ill patients or those with localizing infections (osteomyelitis or endocarditis) do better if they receive streptomycin 20–30 mg/kg/day intramuscularly in two divided doses (maximum 1 gm/day) in addition to tetracycline. Children under the age of nine years should not receive tetracycline. The best alternate drug is probably trimethoprim-sulfamethoxazole* (10 mg/kg/day trimethoprim and 50 mg/kg/day sulfamethoxazole in two divided doses given orally). Ampicillin may also be effective. Response to treatment is apt to be slow. Relapses with a recurrent positive blood culture may occur and require retreatment. Besides specific antimicrobial therapy, children require supportive therapy, attention to nutrition, and an individualized approach to bed rest and school attendance depending on the severity of the disease.

---

* This specific use is not listed by the manufacturer. Also, this drug is not recommended for infants less than 2 months of age.

Tularemia

WALTER T. HUGHES, M.D.

Francisella tularensis is one of the most virulent bacteria causing human disease, but it is remarkably susceptible to antibiotics introduced during the acute stage of the infection. Type A strains are found only in North America, are associated with rabbits and tick vectors, account for 70 to 90% of all cases of tularemia, and without treatment 5 to 7% of infected patients will die. Type B strains are less virulent, rarely cause fatal disease, and are associated primarily with rodents and aquatic animals.

Streptomycin, gentamicin, tetracycline, and chloramphenicol have been used successfully for the treatment of tularemia. In most cases streptomycin is the drug of choice, given in the dosage of 20–30 mg/kg/day in two equally divided doses intramuscularly for 7 to 10 days. The total daily dose should not exceed 2.0 grams. Ototoxicity, which is primarily vestibular, is the most serious adverse effect; nephrotoxicity is rarely a problem with the usual doses.

Gentamicin is an alternative to streptomycin and may be equally effective, although comparative studies in children have not been done. The dose of gentamicin is 5.0 mg/kg/day in two or three equally divided doses intramuscularly or intravenously. Vestibular and auditory ototoxicity and nephrotoxicity are adverse side effects encountered in a few patients. Both streptomycin and gentamicin are bactericidal for *F. tularensis* and relapses rarely occur after a course of treatment. Other aminoglycosides have not been adequately tested to judge their effectiveness in tularemia.

Tetracycline and chloramphenicol are also effective in the treatment of this infection; however, they are bacteriostatic and relapses occasionally occur with courses of treatment of less than two weeks. Tetracycline may be given orally in the dose of 30 mg/kg/day in four equally divided doses (not to exceed a total dose of 2.0 gm). The intravenous tetracycline preparation is given in the dose of 20 mg/kg/day in four equal doses (not to exceed a total dose of 2.0 gm). Tetracycline should be avoided in infants and children less than 9 years of age because of the staining effect on developing teeth. Chloramphenicol is given in the dosage of 50 to 100 mg/kg/day in four equally divided doses (not to exceed a total daily dose of 2.0 gm), orally or intravenously. Aplastic anemia is a rare complication of chloramphenicol therapy. The course of treatment with either tetracycline or chloramphenicol is usually about 2 weeks.

Despite the high virulence of *F. tularensis*, man-to-man transmission rarely occurs. The Centers for Disease Control recommends drainage-secretion precautions for open lesions. No isolation is required for pulmonary or other systemic forms of the disease. Laboratory personnel should be forewarned of specimens sent for culture, since once the organism replicates in culture, it is hazardous.

Defervescence occurs in about 48 hours with most cases treated early in the course of the infection. In nonfatal cases in which treatment is started late in the infection, e.g., with chronic draining lesions, little impact of antibiotic therapy may be evident and slow recovery can be expected. Relapses are more likely in patients treated early in the course with bacteriostatic drugs for less than two weeks. Lifelong immunity follows the primary infection. The overall mortality rate in treated cases of tularemia is less than 1.0%.

Prevention. Documented cases should be reported to the local health department so that high-risk areas may be identified for the institution of control measures. A live attenuated tularemia vaccine (investigational) is available from the Immunobiologics Branch, Centers for Disease Control, Atlanta, Georgia, for use under special conditions.

Impervious gloves should be used in handling rabbits and other wild animals killed by hunters or found dead of unknown causes. Meat to be consumed should be thoroughly cooked. *F. tularensis* survives freezing. One should avoid drinking raw water from creeks, rivers, or lakes.

Children in tick-infested areas should be disrobed and inspected at least daily for adherent ticks. Hairy portions of the body are prime sites. The tick should be removed with forceps or a gloved hand. An attempt should be made not to burst the tick, since infected tissues and fluids may be expelled, sometimes reaching the eyes. Domestic pets should be regularly inspected and deticked. Tick repellents such as diethyltoluamide or dimethylphthalate may be used for the prevention of tick adherence.

The use of antibiotics prophylactically for tick bites or contact with suspect animals is not warranted and when used may only serve to prolong the incubation time.

Plague

HEINZ F. EICHENWALD, M.D.

Plague, a potentially very severe disease caused by *Yersinia pestis*, continues to occur in various parts of the world, including the western United States and Canada. In its classic form, the infection is transmitted from rats to humans by the flea, a mechanism that still operates in developing countries. In the United States, however, the epidemiologic situation is now far more complex and involves a number of species of wild rodents, various types of fleas, and presumably some environmental factors.

Plague pneumonia is a dangerous complication of bubonic disease and is of considerable epidemiologic interest because patients thus affected become highly contagious, spreading the organism via the air. The inhalation of *Y. pestis* by exposed individuals results in primary pneumonic plague, a rapidly fatal illness.

TREATMENT

Two groups of antimicrobial agents are highly efficacious: the aminoglycosides, such as streptomycin and gentamicin, and the tetracyclines. In fact, the aminoglycosides are so effective that huge numbers of bacteria are killed within hours after treatment has begun, resulting in the massive release of endotoxin and other bacterial products. This phenomenon has led to an apparent paradox in therapy: to avoid endotoxemia, tetracycline is used for the first 2 or 3 days of treatment because it is *less* effective than an aminoglycoside. In severely ill patients, however, especially those with hemorrhagic or pneumonic disease, streptomycin or gentamicin should be used for the initial 5 days, followed by tetracycline for an additional 5-day period. Some experts recommend tetracycline as the initial drug even in these severely ill patients.

If streptomycin is employed, the usual daily dosage is 30–40 mg/kg in two or three doses administered IM or infused slowly IV. Gentamicin dosage is 5–7.5 mg/kg/day given every 8 or 12 hours IM or IV. Dosage of tetracycline is 30–50 mg/kg/day, with an initial loading dose of 30 mg/kg. Because of the hazards of IV administration of this drug, it is best given orally, but if this is not possible a slow IV infusion should be employed.

Ten days is the usual duration of therapy; some investigators recommend that medication be continued for a week after body temperature has returned to normal.

Various other antimicrobial agents also have been successfully employed, but there is less experience with their use. Chloramphenicol is administered in a dosage of 50 mg/kg/day orally or IV in four equal doses; sulfonamides* in a dosage of 75 mg/kg/day have also been reported to be effective, but their use is not recommended at present.

Nonspecific therapy consists of the administration of appropriate fluids during the active phase of the illness to prevent the patient from becoming excessively dehydrated, and the management of septic shock.

---

* Manufacturer's warning: Sulfonamides are not indicated in infants younger than 2 months of age.

PREVENTION

Persons in contact with a patient with plague, especially in cases of plague pneumonia, should be quarantined and given prophylactic treatment with tetracycline (20–25 mg/kg/day) or sulfonamides* (75 mg/kg/day).

Persons caring for plague patients usually are advised to wear a face mask and goggles, but whether these precautions prevent infection is not known. It seems more prudent to protect these individuals with chemoprophylaxis. Discharges from the patient, including feces, should be handled carefully and decontaminated because they usually contain plague bacilli.

A plague vaccine has been produced but its efficacy remains in question. In those areas of the world where the chain of transmission includes rats and fleas, flea control followed by eradication of all rats in the community offers the best prospect for the elimination of plague.

Tuberculosis

LAURA S. INSELMAN, M.D.

Although the overall case rate of tuberculosis in the United States has declined in recent years, its incidence has actually increased in many large cities throughout the country. This apparent resurgence is due, in part, to the large influx of foreign-born into the United States in the late 1970s, but it is also recognized in the native-born population. It has occurred in both children and adults and appears to continue on its upward trend at present, at least in New York City. In addition, an increasing proportion of extrapulmonary tuberculosis has been identified in all age groups. Many of these cases have manifestations that differ from earlier classical descriptions of the disease—miliary tuberculosis in a completely asymptomatic child, clinically advanced tuberculous meningitis with repeatedly normal cerebrospinal fluid examinations, and growth of tubercle bacilli in a pleural effusion.

Chemotherapy for tuberculosis is directed towards the eradication of the tubercle bacilli in both extracellular and intracellular sites harboring large and small numbers of organisms, the prevention of the emergence of drug-resistant strains of *Mycobacterium tuberculosis*, and the prevention of the complications of tuberculosis. To accomplish this, two drugs, at least one of which is bactericidal, are used to treat most types of pulmonary and localized extrapulmonary tuberculosis. Three drugs are employed for more intensive initial therapy for widespread pulmonary involvement, as, for example, endobronchial tuberculosis, and for systemic disease. These guidelines are based on the number of bacilli anticipated in a lesion, with more drugs required for larger numbers of organisms.

Short-Course Chemotherapy. Until recently, daily treatment for 1 to 2 years was the recommended therapeutic regimen for pulmonary tuberculosis. Short-course chemotherapy using two bactericidal drugs, isoniazid and rifampin, either as a daily or an intermittent regimen for nine months, appears to be as effective as longer treatment for uncomplicated pulmonary tuberculosis, at least in adults. This regimen results in sputum conversion in more than 90% of patients by the third treatment month (compared to 73% by six months in 1981 with the longer regimen), has a reported relapse rate of 1–2% after completion (compared to 7% in 1982 with the longer regimen), improves patient compliance, and is less costly.

Extensive clinical data on the use of short-course chemotherapy in childhood is not yet available. Although further evaluation is needed, even in adults, recent studies suggest that short-course chemotherapy may be effective in children, and guidelines of The American Thoracic Society, Centers for Disease Control, and American College of Chest Physicians indicate that it could be used in children with uncomplicated pulmonary tuberculosis.

Short-course chemotherapy has not been investigated for treatment of extrapulmonary tuberculosis, for which the longer regimen is presently recommended. The shorter regimen should not be used when sterilization of the sputum or clinical response in the early phase of treatment fails to occur; when either isoniazid or rifampin cannot be utilized because of drug toxicity or intolerance; when drug-resistant bacilli are present; or when "complicated" pulmonary disease, such as tuberculous empyema, and other medical conditions, such as diabetes mellitus, silicosis, malignant disease, and immunosuppression, occur.

Dosage guidelines (Table 1) for the short-course daily regimen in adults consist of isoniazid, 5–10 mg/kg/day (maximum 300 mg/day), and rifampin, 10 mg/kg/day (maximum 600 mg/day), both given orally for nine months. The short-course intermittent regimen for adults consists of oral isoniazid and rifampin prescribed in the above doses daily for one month, after which each is given twice weekly for an additional eight months at dosages of 15 mg/kg/dose (maximum 900 mg/dose) for isoniazid and 10 mg/kg/dose (maximum 600 mg/dose) for rifampin. Suggested dosages in children consist of isoniazid,† 10–15 mg/kg/day (maximum

---

* Manufacturer's warning: Sulfonamides are not indicated in infants younger than 2 months of age.

† The hepatic toxicity of isoniazid and/or rifampin may be increased and may cause one or both to be discontinued when administered concomitantly. The Centers for Disease Control recommends that the isoniazid dose not exceed 10 mg/kg/24 hr and that the rifampin dose not exceed 15 mg/kg/24 hr when these drugs are used concurrently.

Table 1. SUGGESTED DOSAGES FOR SHORT-COURSE CHEMOTHERAPY

	Daily Regimen	Intermittent Regimen
Children		
Isoniazid*	10–15 mg/kg/day†	20–40 mg/kg/dose‡
Rifampin*	10–20 mg/kg/day§	10–20 mg/kg/dose‖
Adults		
Isoniazid*	5–10 mg/kg/day†	15 mg/kg/dose‡
Rifampin*	10 mg/kg/day§	10 mg/kg/dose‖

* The hepatic toxicity of isoniazid and/or rifampin may be increased and may cause one or both to be discontinued when administered concomitantly. The Centers for Disease Control recommends that the isoniazid dose not exceed 10 mg/kg/24 hr and that the rifampin dose not exceed 15 mg/kg/24 hr when these drugs are used concurrently.
† Maximum, 300 mg/day.
‡ Maximum, 900 mg/dose.
§ Maximum, 600 mg/day.
‖ Maximum, 600 mg/dose.

300 mg/day), and rifampin,† 10–20 mg/kg/day (maximum 600 mg/day), for the daily regimen, while those for intermittent therapy include isoniazid,† 20–40 mg/kg/dose (maximum 900 mg/dose) and rifampin,† 10–20 mg/kg/dose (maximum 600 mg/dose) (see note on p. 552), each given twice weekly after a one-month course of the daily dosages (see footnote on page 552). Both the daily and intermittent regimens are prescribed for at least nine months in children and adults, with a minimum of six months after the sputum culture no longer grows *Mycobacterium tuberculosis*. Use of isoniazid and rifampin may be supplemented with other antituberculous agents, if indicated.

The following recommendations for chemotherapy of children with tuberculosis are based on the more established longer treatment regimens. These guidelines may be individualized when appropriate. The short-course regimen is mentioned as a possible alternative when applicable, as in treatment of tuberculous mediastinal lymphadenopathy, pneumonia, pleural effusion, and chronic pulmonary tuberculosis.

TYPE OF TUBERCULOSIS

PPD Conversion

The presence of a positive reaction to an intermediate strength Mantoux test and the absence of radiographic changes and physical signs or symptoms suggestive of tuberculosis indicate that exposure to tuberculosis, i.e., infection without disease, has occurred. Pulmonary tuberculous lesions are presumably present but are too small to be radiographically identified and cause clinical manifestations.

A positive tuberculin skin test in a child indicates recent exposure to tuberculosis. Any child with a positive tuberculin skin test reaction who never received previous therapy for tuberculous infection or disease or previous immunization with the bacillus Calmette-Guérin (BCG) antigen is considered a recent PPD converter and should receive appropriate evaluation and treatment.

Therapy consists of isoniazid, 10–15 mg/kg/day (maximum 300 mg), given daily for 12 months. Isoniazid is prescribed prophylactically to prevent the development of widespread extrapulmonary tuberculosis, which could originate from the radiographically unidentifiable pulmonary lesions and spread hematogenously. Such systemic disease, particularly meningitis and miliary tuberculosis, is more likely to occur in children. In addition, prophylactic isoniazid may prevent the further development of pulmonary lesions. Prophylactic treatment extended beyond one year does not provide greater protection and, when given for less than one year, is not considered effective and long-lasting.

Pulmonary Tuberculosis

Mediastinal Lymphadenopathy. Enlarged tuberculous hilar lymph nodes are present radiographically as part of the primary tuberculous complex, which also consists of the primary tuberculous lesion in the lung parenchyma and its associated lymphatic vessels. If calcification occurs in the primary lesion, the Ghon complex is formed. Mediastinal lymphadenopathy without the radiographically identifiable primary parenchymal lesion is the most frequent type of pulmonary tuberculosis in children.

Treatment consists of isoniazid, 10–20 mg/kg/day (maximum 300 mg), either alone or with rifampin, 15–20 mg/kg/day (maximum 600 mg); ethambutol,‡ 15–25 mg/kg/day (maximum 1500 mg); or para-aminosalicylic acid, 200 mg/kg/day (maximum 12 gm). Two drugs are used if the primary parenchymal lesion is present; otherwise, isoniazid alone may be prescribed. Each drug is given for 12 months. Short-course chemotherapy with isoniazid and rifampin may be considered for treatment of tuberculous mediastinal lymphadenopathy in children.

Pneumonia. A radiographic tuberculous pneumonic process indicates local and/or bronchogenic extension of the primary tuberculous complex. The treatment regimen includes isoniazid, 15–20 mg/kg/day (maximum 500 mg), and rifampin, 15–20 mg/kg/day (maximum 600 mg). Each drug is prescribed for 12–18 months but could be tried in a short-course regimen. Streptomycin, 20–40 mg/kg/day (maximum 1 gm), may be added for one month if extensive pneumonia is present.

Pleural Effusion. A tuberculous pleural effusion

---

‡ Manufacturer's warning: Ethambutol is not recommended for children under 13 years of age.

can result from extension of a subpleural site of infection but could also represent a hypersensitivity reaction to tuberculin. The effusion usually has small numbers of tubercle bacilli, and therefore cultures may not always indicate the presence of the organisms.

Treatment consists of isoniazid, 15–20 mg/kg/day (maximum 500 mg), and either rifampin, 15–20 mg/kg/day (maximum 600 mg); ethambutol,* 15–25 mg/kg/day (maximum 1500 mg); or para-aminosalicylic acid, 200 mg/kg/day (maximum 12 gm). Each drug is prescribed for 12–18 months, but isoniazid and rifampin could be used in a short-course regimen. Occasionally, in order to enhance resorption of the fluid, prednisone, 1–2 mg/kg/day (maximum 60 mg), is given for 6–12 weeks or until the effusion has diminished.

Endobronchial. Endobronchial tuberculosis results from erosion of tuberculous caseous lymph nodes into a bronchus, causing partial or complete airway obstruction. A sinus tract may form, allowing passage of caseous material into the bronchus. Isoniazid, 20 mg/kg/day (maximum 500 mg), and rifampin, 15–20 mg/kg/day (maximum 600 mg), are prescribed for 12–18 months, and streptomycin, 20–40 mg/kg/day (maximum 1 gm), is given for one month. In order to reduce the size of the enlarged caseous lymph nodes and thereby decrease the airway inflammation, prednisone, 1–2 mg/kg/day (maximum 60 mg), may be added for 6–12 weeks or until wheezing and dyspnea subside. Short-course chemotherapy has not been evaluated in children with endobronchial tuberculosis and should not be used in its treatment at present.

Miliary. Lymphohematogenous dissemination of *Mycobacterium tuberculosis* from a tuberculous pulmonary site can result in diffuse, nodular, millet-sized lesions throughout both lungs and other organs. Treatment for miliary tuberculosis is the same as that for endobronchial disease, except that isoniazid and rifampin are given for 18–24 months. If acute respiratory distress occurs, prednisone is prescribed until dyspnea or cyanosis resolves. Miliary tuberculosis is a systemic form of tuberculosis, for which short-course chemotherapy is not utilized.

Chronic. Chronic pulmonary tuberculosis usually occurs in adolescents and adults but may be manifested in the younger age group. It occurs in individuals who have been previously infected with *Mycobacterium tuberculosis* and may result from either reactivation of the latent infection, i.e., endogenously acquired, or from acquisition of a new infection, i.e., exogenously acquired. Isoniazid, 10–20 mg/kg/day (maximum 300 mg), and

either rifampin, 15–20 mg/kg/day (maximum 600 mg), or ethambutol,* 15–25 mg/kg/day (maximum 1500 mg), are prescribed for 12–18 months. The use of short-course chemotherapy may be indicated.

Extrapulmonary Tuberculosis

Meningitis. Tuberculous meningitis results from hematogenous spread of tubercle bacilli. Like miliary tuberculosis, it has a 100% mortality rate if untreated and is particularly likely to occur in children under four years of age.

Treatment includes the use of four drugs: isoniazid, 20 mg/kg/day (maximum 500 mg); rifampin, 15–20 mg/kg/day (maximum 600 mg); streptomycin, 20–40 mg/kg/day (maximum 1 gm), and prednisone, 1–2 mg/kg/day (maximum 60 mg). Isoniazid and rifampin are prescribed for 18–24 months, and streptomycin is given until one month following a satisfactory clinical response. Prednisone is utilized for 6–12 weeks in order to decrease the intracranial pressure.

Skeletal, Superficial Lymph Nodes, Gastrointestinal, Renal, Pericardial, Dermatologic, Endocrinologic, Genital, Ophthalmologic and Upper Respiratory Tract. Chemotherapy of each of these forms of extrapulmonary tuberculosis is similar and consists of isoniazid, 15–20 mg/kg/day (maximum 500 mg), and either rifampin, 15–20 mg/kg/day (maximum 600 mg), ethambutol,* 15–25 mg/kg/day (maximum 1500 mg), or para-aminosalicylic acid, 200 mg/kg/day (maximum 12 gm). The drugs are prescribed for 24 months for renal tuberculosis, 18–24 months for skeletal tuberculosis, and 12–18 months for the other forms of extrapulmonary disease.

In addition, therapy is directed at the specific organ system involved. For example, in skeletal tuberculosis, accessible abscesses are surgically drained, and such weight-bearing structures as the hip and vertebrae are immobilized. The presence of a paravertebral abscess, spinal cord compression, or progression of the disease process despite chemotherapy is an additional indication for surgery. In tuberculosis of the superficial lymph nodes, surgical excision of the nodes is combined with antituberculous chemotherapy if the size of the nodes is increasing or, in order to prevent spread of tubercle bacilli, if spontaneous drainage will occur. Pericardial surgery may be necessary in tuberculous pericarditis if tamponade or constriction develops. In renal tuberculosis, intravenous pyelography, ureteral calibration, urinalyses, urine cultures, and renal function tests are performed periodically during and for approximately 10 years following chemotherapy to evaluate the development of complications. Follow-up after completion of chemotherapy for the other organ systems is

---

* Manufacturer's warning: Ethambutol is not recommended for children under 13 years of age.

also indicated to detect complications and permanent changes resulting from tuberculosis.

Special Situations

Congenital Tuberculosis. Chemotherapy for a newborn with congenital pulmonary tuberculosis includes isoniazid, 15–20 mg/kg/day, and rifampin, 15–20 mg/kg/day, for 12–24 months. Streptomycin, 20 mg/kg/day, may also be prescribed for two months. Treatment for congenital systemic and extrapulmonary tuberculosis is directed along the previously mentioned guidelines for these conditions. Short-course chemotherapy has not been evaluated for congenital tuberculosis and is not presently recommended in this age group. As with any serious infectious disease in the newborn, the presence of central nervous system involvement, even if asymptomatic, must be determined.

Newborn Infant of Tuberculous Mother. The neonate and mother are separated after delivery until the neonate is adequately protected, either with isoniazid prophylaxis or with BCG immunization, and until the mother's treatment renders her noninfectious. These measures are employed to prevent the newborn from acquiring tuberculosis.

If the infant's initial tuberculin skin test reaction and chest x-ray are negative, then either isoniazid prophylaxis or BCG immunization is administered. If isoniazid is used, it is prescribed for one year at a dose of 10–15 mg/kg/day. Conversion of the tuberculin skin test reaction is evaluated every three months by Mantoux testing, and, if it occurs, necessitates further investigation for the possible development of tuberculous disease despite isoniazid prophylaxis. If the skin test remains negative, isoniazid is frequently continued for one year even if the mother is theoretically noninfectious without bacilli in her sputum. This protection is employed because the mother may still shed bacilli with subsequent respiratory tract infections.

If the initial tuberculin skin test reaction and chest x-ray are negative and BCG immunization is used, the infant and mother are separated until the infant's tuberculin skin test reaction becomes positive. If either the initial tuberculin skin test reaction or chest x-ray are positive, then the infant is evaluated and treated for congenital tuberculosis.

Antituberculous drugs are secreted in breast milk, although in small amounts. Thus, recommendations regarding breast feeding for a noninfectious mother taking antituberculous chemotherapy should be individualized, with evaluation of the advantages of breast feeding and the possible risks of drug toxicity to the infant.

Pregnancy. Although guidelines for chemotherapy of tuberculosis during pregnancy are not well established, at least two drugs are used for treatment of intrapartum active pulmonary disease. Possible drug combinations include isoniazid, ethambutol, and if extensive disease is present, rifampin; isoniazid and rifampin; and isoniazid, para-aminosalicylic acid, and streptomycin. All these drugs cross the placenta. However, only streptomycin has a definite adverse effect, ototoxicity, on the fetus.

Therapy for other manifestations of tuberculosis during pregnancy varies according to individual circumstances. Isoniazid prophylaxis for a recent tuberculin skin test conversion or antituberculous chemotherapy for untreated, inactive pulmonary disease may be given either during or after pregnancy. The risk of developing tuberculosis is greatest during the first year after infection and may, therefore, necessitate the use of isoniazid prophylaxis in some instances. Isoniazid prophylaxis is often begun after the first trimester. Therapy is not necessary in pregnant women with long-standing tuberculin skin test conversions or with previously treated, inactive pulmonary disease.

The presence of tuberculosis during pregnancy is not an indication for a therapeutic abortion. When the disease is properly treated during pregnancy, the mother and fetus have an excellent prognosis. After delivery, the mother and newborn are separated, and the infant is evaluated and treated as previously described.

Exposure in the Home. Any child who has been in contact with an adult in the home with active tuberculosis should be evaluated for exposure or disease due to tuberculosis. If the Mantoux intermediate tuberculin skin test reaction and chest x-ray are negative, isoniazid prophylaxis, 10–15 mg/kg/day (maximum 300 mg/day), is prescribed for at least three months. Tuberculin skin test conversion may not have occurred yet, and isoniazid is employed to prevent the development of infection. If the skin test reaction remains negative and if exposure to active tuberculosis is no longer present, isoniazid can be discontinued. If the skin test reaction becomes significant, which, in this setting, is interpreted as having at least 5 mm of induration, then additional evaluation and therapy are necessary.

Exposure Outside The Home. Mantoux tuberculin skin testing is sufficient evaluation of a child exposed to active tuberculosis in a school, camp, or day care center. If the tuberculin skin test reaction is negative, no treatment is necessary, provided that the contact with active tuberculosis is broken. If the tuberculin skin test reaction is positive and the chest x-ray is negative, isoniazid prophylaxis is prescribed for one year. Usually an adult, rather than another child, with active tuberculosis is the source of exposure in these settings.

Drug Resistance. Both primary and secondary antituberculous drug resistance have become increasingly important in the United States, particularly with the recently arrived foreign-born from Southeast Asia and the Caribbean. Drug resistance is prevented by the simultaneous use of at least two antituberculous agents, usually isoniazid and rifampin. If resistance to either one occurs, two new bactericidal drugs to which the tubercle bacillus is sensitive are either substituted or added, and treatment is prescribed for at least 18 months. The drug that demonstrates in vitro resistance may still be included because its in vivo activity may differ.

If prophylaxis is prescribed for exposure to an isoniazid-resistant strain of *Mycobacterium tuberculosis*, rifampin, 15–20 mg/kg/day (maximum 600 mg), may be included with isoniazid for 12 months. Administration of rifampin alone for chemoprophylaxis of tuberculous infection is a possible alternative but has not been evaluated at present.

Characteristics of Antituberculous Drugs

Isoniazid. Since its introduction in 1952, isoniazid has become the primary drug in the treatment of tuberculosis in children. It is a hydrazide of isonicotinic acid, is bactericidal, and affects both intracellular and extracellular organisms. It exerts its action in cavities, caseous tissue, and pulmonary alveolar macrophages by possible inhibition of the biosynthesis of mycolic acids in the mycobacterial cell wall and inhibition of enzymes within the bacilli. Peak plasma concentrations of 3–5 μg/ml are attained by 2 hours after ingestion, with therapeutic levels persisting until 6–8 hours. The drug easily penetrates almost all tissues and fluid collections, including cerebrospinal fluid. It is metabolized by the liver and excreted by the kidney.

Isoniazid is administered orally or, for widespread disease, intramuscularly, as one daily dose, usually in the morning. It is prescribed in lower doses for treatment of PPD conversion and mediastinal lymphadenopathy and in higher doses for therapy of pulmonary, extrapulmonary, and systemic disease. Dosages of isoniazid for the daily and intermittent short-course regimens differ, with higher doses in the intermittent regimen following the initial one month daily treatment, whereas the dose remains unchanged in the daily regimen.

Adverse effects of isoniazid include neurotoxicity and hepatotoxicity. Peripheral neuritis associated with isoniazid administration is due to increased pyridoxine excretion and is prevented by the daily ingestion of 10 mg of pyridoxine (maximum 50 mg) for every 100 mg of isoniazid administered. Pyridoxine supplementation is prescribed in adolescents and adults, including pregnant women, but is unnecessary in young children with adequate nutrition and without predisposition to peripheral neuropathy. Isoniazid-induced neurotoxicity may also cause convulsions, optic neuritis, tremors, ataxia, toxic encephalopathy, and memory disturbances.

Hepatotoxicity resulting from isoniazid alone or in combination with rifampin has a much lower incidence in children than adults, even when both drugs are used. The hepatic injury usually occurs within the first three months of therapy and is transient, with the elevated liver enzyme levels frequently returning to normal despite continuation of the drug. In general, isoniazid is administered if the serum aspartate aminotransferase (glutamic oxaloacetic transaminase) level is below three times normal and clinical manifestations of liver disease are absent. The risk of isoniazid-associated hepatitis is increased with alcohol ingestion.

Other side effects of isoniazid include hematologic reactions, with anemia, agranulocytosis, and thrombocytopenia; vasculitis, including a lupus erythematosus-like syndrome; hypersensitivity, with skin rashes, fever, and eosinophilia; gastrointestinal disturbances; and arthritic symptoms of arthralgias and joint pains. Isoniazid potentiates the actions of carbamazepine, phenytoin, and barbiturates, resulting in toxicity of the central nervous system (somnolence, confusion, ataxia) and liver. Dosages of these drugs are often decreased during their administration with isoniazid. Metabolic acidosis, hyperglycemia, seizures, and coma can result from isoniazid overdose.

Rifampin. The combination of isoniazid and rifampin has become the most effective treatment of tuberculosis in children. Rifampin is produced by *Streptomyces mediterranei* and was introduced as an antituberculous agent in the 1960s. It is bactericidal to intracellular and extracellular organisms, causing suppression of mycobacterial RNA chain formation by inhibiting the DNA-dependent RNA polymerase. It penetrates easily into most tissues, macrophages, and fluid collections but only across an inflamed blood-brain barrier. Peak serum levels of 7 μg/ml are attained by 3 hours following ingestion. The drug is metabolized by the liver and excreted by the kidney and gall bladder.

Rifampin is administered orally in one daily dose, usually in the morning. Its absorption may be delayed by para-aminosalicylic acid, and administration of both drugs should be separated by 8 to 12 hours.

The primary adverse effect of rifampin is hepatotoxicity, as discussed with isoniazid. Rifampin causes secretions, including urine, stool, saliva, sweat, tears, and sputum, to become a benign red-orange color and may discolor contact lenses. It can also cause gastrointestinal disturbances; hematologic reactions, with anemia, thrombocytopenia and leukopenia; hypersensitivity, with dermatitis, fever, eosinophilia, stomatitis, hemolysis, and renal insufficiency; neurotoxicity, consisting of drowsiness, ataxia, confusion, and headache; and cell-mediated immunosuppression. Intermittent therapy may result in the hepatorenal syndrome.

Rifampin enhances the hepatic metabolism of coumarin, quinidine, digoxin, oral contraceptives, corticosteroids, oral hypoglycemic agents, and methadone, resulting in a decrease in their serum levels and subsequent effects. Increased serum rifampin concentrations caused by diminished hepatic uptake of rifampin occur with probenecid. Rifampin overdose can result in a red-orange discoloration of skin and secretions but not sclera; gastrointestinal irritation; angioedema; somnolence; diffuse pruritus; and elevated liver enzymes.

Ethambutol. Ethambutol* is frequently used as the third antituberculous agent in multidrug regimens. It is also prescribed with rifampin or isoniazid for an 18-month regimen if one of these two drugs cannot be employed because of intolerance or resistance. Ethambutol is a synthetic alcohol that is bacteriostatic to intracellular and extracellular organisms, causing inhibition of RNA synthesis. It attains peak serum levels of 5 μg/ml within 4 hours after ingestion; concentrates within erythrocytes, which may act as its storage for entry into the plasma; and is excreted by the kidney.

Ethambutol is administered orally in one daily dose, usually in the morning. It is prescribed in high doses (25 mg/kg/day) for the first 6–8 weeks and in low doses (15 mg/kg/day) subsequently.

Adverse effects of ethambutol include ocular toxicity, which may result in unilateral or bilateral optic neuritis, diminished visual acuity, central scotoma, absence of green color perception, and a defect in the peripheral visual field. The incidence and intensity of the ocular toxicity are related to the dose and duration of therapy, usually not occurring with the lower dosage and subsiding upon discontinuation of the drug. Visual acuity and red/green color perception, even in young children, should be tested before, during, and after administration of ethambutol.

Other side effects of ethambutol include hyperuricemia, which usually occurs by the third week of treatment and results from diminished renal clearance of urate; gastrointestinal irritation; hypersensitivity, with fever, dermatitis, and joint pain; and central nervous system alterations, with headache and mental confusion. Ethambutol has no known drug interactions.

Streptomycin. Streptomycin is often used in multidrug regimens for treatment of extensive pulmonary and systemic tuberculosis. As an ami-

noglycoside and a product of *Streptomyces griseus*, it inhibits ribosomal protein synthesis. It is bactericidal to extracellular organisms in cavities and, to a lesser degree, to intracellular organisms, where its action is primarily bacteriostatic. It does not easily penetrate fluid collections and crosses the blood-brain barrier only if the barrier is inflamed. Cell membrane transport of streptomycin is oxygen dependent, and the drug's antitubercular activity is markedly diminished in the anerobic milieu of a tuberculous abscess. Peak serum levels of 25–50 μg/ml are attained within 2 hours after administration, and the drug is excreted by the kidney.

Streptomycin is administered intramuscularly either once daily or, in severe disease, as a 12–hour regimen initially for a few days and then once a day. Adverse effects of streptomycin include ototoxicity and nephrotoxicity, which are more likely to occur with increased dose and duration of therapy. Ototoxicity may be manifested as vestibular, with vomiting, vertigo, tinnitus, headaches, and nystagmus, and as auditory, with hearing loss, which may be irreversible. Audiograms and tests of vestibular function should be performed before, during, and after therapy with streptomycin.

Although nephrotoxicity is less likely with streptomycin than with other aminoglycosides, albuminuria, cylinduria, and oliguria can occur. Additional side effects of the drug include hypersensitivity, with fever, dermatitis, eosinophilia, and stomatitis; hematologic reactions, with agranulocytosis, anemia, and thrombocytopenia; and peripheral neuritis. Streptomycin may potentiate the effects of neuromuscular blocking agents, ethacrynic acid, and cephalosporins. Elevated serum levels of streptomycin occur with probenecid and result in enhancement of its effects.

Para-aminosalicylic Acid. Para-aminosalicylic acid, a derivative of aminosalicylic acid, is bacteriostatic to extracellular organisms and diffuses readily into most tissues, particularly caseous areas and fluid collections, but not into cerebrospinal fluid or macrophages. Its primary effect is to elevate serum isoniazid concentrations by competition with isoniazid for hepatic acetylation, but its competitive inhibition of folate biosynthesis probably also contributes to its effects. The drug is metabolized by the liver and excreted by the kidney.

Para-aminosalicylic acid is administered orally, usually in three divided doses to decrease gastrointestinal irritation, and is better tolerated when given after meals. Peak serum levels of 75 μg/ml are attained by 2 hours after ingestion of 4 grams of the drug.

Adverse effects of para-aminosalicylic acid include gastrointestinal disturbances, for which reason it has been replaced to a great extent by rifampin and ethambutol; hepatotoxicity; hema-

---

* Manufacturer's warning: Ethambutol is not recommended for children under 13 years of age.

tologic reactions, with agranulocytosis, anemia, thrombocytopenia, and eosinophilia; hypokalemia; and thyroid imbalance. Its actions are potentiated with probenecid and diminished with salicylates.

Adrenocorticosteroids. Controversy exists regarding the beneficial effects of the anti-inflammatory actions of corticosteroids in tuberculosis. However, in combination with antituberculous drugs, corticosteroids are used to treat tuberculosis in children in certain situations. They are often employed to diminish intracranial pressure in tuberculous meningitis, decrease the alveolocapillary block causing cyanosis in miliary disease, promote fluid absorption in symptomatic pleural and pericardial tuberculous effusions, and enhance shrinkage of tuberculous lymph nodes in endobronchial disease.

The drugs are administered intravenously or intramuscularly in divided doses initially if the patient is seriously ill or orally as one daily dose for less symptomatic disease. Prednisone is frequently used as the oral preparation.

Adverse effects of corticosteroids include pituitary-adrenal suppression, growth inhibition, osteoporosis, behavioral disturbances, cataracts, myopathy, electrolyte imbalance, and peptic ulcer. Corticosteroids enhance the action of neuromuscular blocking agents and decrease the effect of calcium salts. Rifampin, barbiturates, and phenytoin cause suppression of the effects of corticosteroids.

Other Drugs. Experience with dosage and toxicity of pyrazinamide, cycloserine, ethionamide, capreomycin, and viomycin is limited in children. Pyrazinamide is becoming increasingly important in short-course chemotherapy for adults. It is bactericidal to intracellular organisms, attains peak plasma levels of 45 μg/ml within 2 hours after oral ingestion, crosses the blood-brain barrier, and is excreted by the kidney. Its dose is 20–30 mg/kg/day (maximum 3 gm/day), administered in 3 or 4 divided doses, or 2–2.5 gm three times a week. Side effects include hepatotoxicity, which is rare, even when the drug is given with isoniazid and rifampin; hyperuricemia; gastrointestinal irritation; and arthralgia.

Supportive Therapy

General supportive measures, including adequate nutrition and unnecessary exposure to other infections, which may further compromise the body's defense mechanisms, are important in the care of a child with tuberculosis. Unless the child is acutely ill, bed rest is not required.

The need for hospitalization varies according to the type and extent of disease. Ideally, all children with recent PPD conversions or with tuberculous disease should be hospitalized to obtain appropri-

ate culture material, ascertain tolerance and compliance with medications, investigate household contacts for exposure to tuberculosis, identify and initiate treatment of the index case, and remove all sources of active tuberculosis from the environment before returning the child home. In addition, hospitalization provides an opportunity for family education concerning the importance of the medications and follow-up care. However, this may not be practical, and the decision to hospitalize children with recent PPD conversions or asymptomatic pulmonary tuberculosis may have to be individualized. All children with symptomatic pulmonary, extrapulmonary, or systemic tuberculosis should be hospitalized until the previously mentioned goals have been accomplished and the disease is under control.

If acid-fast bacilli are present on sputum smears, isolation is required until further smears are negative, which usually occurs by two weeks after antituberculous therapy has begun. Isolation is unnecessary for children without sputum or without an open wound growing tubercle bacilli.

Prevention

The best prevention of tuberculosis is the minimization of exposure by identification and treatment of the index case and chemoprophylaxis of infected individuals. All cases of tuberculosis should be reported to the local health department.

BCG Vaccine. The protection afforded by the BCG vaccine, a derivative of *Mycobacterium bovis*, is controversial. The vaccine varies in potency, efficacy, and immunogenicity and has resulted in serious reactions, including BCG osteomyelitis, dissemination of BCG infection, and death. In addition, conversion of the Mantoux tuberculin skin test reaction caused by the immunization results in loss of negativity of the skin test as an index of subsequent exposure to active tuberculosis.

In the United States, the vaccine is employed only when compliance with isoniazid prophylaxis cannot be assured in an individual with a negative Mantoux tuberculin skin test and negative chest x-ray who has repeated exposure to active tuberculosis. It is administered intradermally at doses of 0.05 ml for neonates and 0.10 ml for older children and adolescents. If the Mantoux tuberculin skin test reaction does not become significant 6–8 weeks later, BCG is readministered, and the tuberculin skin test is repeated 6–8 weeks after that time. The size of the induration of the skin test reaction resulting from a BCG immunization usually measures 5–9 mm in diameter. The vaccine is not used for patients with burns, skin infections, or immunosuppression or during pregnancy.

Leprosy

ROBERT H. GELBER, M.D.

Leprosy (Hansen's disease) is a chronic infectious disease caused by *Mycobacterium leprae*. It is only rarely fatal but, owing to the predilection of the causative agent for peripheral nerves, may cause insensitivity, myopathy, and their resultant deformity. The World Health Organization estimates that there are 12–15 million cases worldwide.

The successful treatment of leprosy requires long-term compliance with an appropriate antimicrobial regimen, recognition of and considered intervention for a variety of immunologically determined reactional states, patient cooperation in protecting insensitive parts from further damage, and skilled reconstructive and cosmetic surgery for established disabilities and deformities. Compliance in any disease requiring prolonged therapy is often inadequate. This may be an especial problem in leprosy because of the lack of troublesome symptoms both initially and especially after some months or years of treatment and, also, because of reactional symptoms often perceived by the patient to be the result of therapy itself. Because of social stigma, patients and their parents are often fearful of institutionalization and rejection by other family members and friends and do not seek medical attention for a diagnosis that they suspect or reject the diagnosis and therapy when offered by a professional.

Sociocultural fears and expectations decidedly affect patients' lives. Many patients believe their disease is a result of some wrongdoing. Upon diagnosis patients frequently remove themselves from the life of their families. They may begin to use separate dishes and toilet facilities and to sleep alone. Because of the belief in certain cultures that the disease is in the blood and because in some countries it had been the practice to separate children at birth from affected parents, patients frequently believe that they should not parent children. Children with established deformities become stigmatized and often are ridiculed by their peers. Both functional and cosmetic repairs are integral to the success of medical therapy and in allowing patients to live normally in society. Education and counseling are necessary initially and on a continuing basis to help patients comply with therapy and not allow certain cultural and psychosocial aspects of the diagnosis themselves to contribute to the debilitation of the patient.

Chemotherapy

Dapsone. Because of the enormous numbers of *M. leprae* and the lack of cell-mediated immunity, the lepromatous form of leprosy presents the

Table 1. PEDIATRIC DOSAGE OF THE MOST IMPORTANT ANTIMICROBIALS FOR LEPROSY

	2–5 Years of Age	6–12 Years of Age	13–18 Years of Age
Dapsone	25 mg three times weekly	25 mg/day	50 mg/day
Rifampin*	150 mg/day	300 mg/day	600 mg/day

* Dosage is 10–20 mg/kg, not to exceed 600 mg/day.

greater therapeutic difficulty. Dapsone (4,4'-diaminodiphenylsulfone, or DDS) is still the agent of choice for treating all forms of leprosy (Table 1). It is the only agent approved for general use as treatment of leprosy in the United States and has the virtues of being relatively safe, effective, and inexpensive. Dapsone is available in 25-mg and 100-mg tablets. In lepromatous leprosy administration of dapsone should be initiated and maintained as a single adult daily dose of 100 mg for lifetime. Suggested pediatric doses are the following: for ages 2–5 years, 25 mg three times weekly; for ages 6–12 years, 25 mg daily; and for ages 13–18 years, 50 mg daily. Although previously leprologists had built up to the maintenance dose slowly and discontinued dapsone during reaction, particularly erythema nodosum leprosum, these measures no longer appear reasonable. Dapsone is cross-allergenic with sulfonamides and should not be initiated in patients with a history of sulfa allergy. It may cause a hemolytic anemia, particularly in G6PD-deficient patients, and may result in dose-related methemoglobinemia and sulfhemoglobinemia in certain patients. Early in therapy, a syndrome termed the sulfone syndrome, associated with an initially morbilliform rash followed by an exfoliative dermatitis, and at times a mononucleosis-type blood picture, fever, lymphadenopathy, hemolytic anemia, and hepatic dysfunction, uncommonly occurs and may require corticosteroids in addition to discontinuation of dapsone.

Dapsone monotherapy of lepromatous leprosy may result in the development of dapsone-resistant relapse. This becomes clinically apparent with the development of new lesions despite continued dapsone administration at a minimum of five years after the initiation of dapsone therapy. The risks of developing dapsone-resistant relapse vary between 2.5 and 40 per cent in different series. It appears that lower dosage regimens and intermittent adherence to therapy predispose to such relapse. Furthermore, even after 10 or more years of dapsone therapy, lepromatous leprosy patients harbor viable dapsone-sensitive *M. leprae* "persisters," capable of causing clinical relapse if therapy is discontinued; hence the recommendation for lifetime antimicrobial therapy of lepromatous disease.

In certain remote regions where patients do not have access to medical facilities and cannot be expected to take medication regularly, the repository sulfone DADDS,* 225 mg intramuscularly every 77 days in adults and proportionally less according to weight in children, might be substituted for dapsone in all forms of leprosy. However, resulting plasma levels of DDS are sufficiently low and the potential for developing dapsone resistance is of sufficient magnitude that treatment of the lepromatous form of the disease with this agent alone should be avoided if at all possible.

Because of the dual problems of bacterial resistance and persistence, borderline and lepromatous leprosy ideally should be treated with at least two agents, generally dapsone and rifampin. On the other hand, tuberculoid leprosy patients, in whom neither dapsone resistance nor persisters are generally problems, require in most instances only monotherapy with dapsone. Tuberculoid leprosy patients may be treated for five years with dapsone alone.

Rifampin. Rifampin has proved in both animal and human studies to be significantly more potent than dapsone against *M. leprae.* It is available in 150-mg and 300-mg capsules. A single daily adult dose of 600 mg is recommended, and proportionately less is used for children, generally 150 mg daily for ages 2–5 years; 300 mg daily for ages 6–12 years; and 600 mg daily for ages 13–18 years, depending on body weight (10–20 mg/kg, not to exceed 600 mg/day). Rifampin turns the urine an orange-red color. It may be hepatotoxic and should be avoided in all patients with established liver dysfunction. Discontinuation of rifampin followed by reinstitution has been associated with severe and even fatal episodes of thrombocytopenia and renal failure. There is no available information on what duration of rifampin together with dapsone will prevent drug-resistant relapse, and whether such combination chemotherapy for any duration will allow discontinuation of therapy without subsequent relapse from "persisters." Furthermore, the cost of rifampin, about $300 per adult patient-year, is prohibitively expensive in most developing nations where leprosy is a problem. At present, then, it is recommended that in lepromatous leprosy rifampin be administered for at least two to three years, depending on local financial resources, together with dapsone, which should be continued indefinitely.

Second-Line Drugs. Particularly because of allergy to sulfones and in the therapy of sulfone resistance, other second-line antimicrobial agents may be necessary to treat leprosy.

Clofazimine† (B663, or Lamprene) appears as potent as dapsone aginst *M. leprae.* It is an investigational drug at this time. In adults 100 mg orally twice or three times weekly is an effective alternative to dapsone administration. Its administration is unfortunately associated with a red-black discoloration, which may be unnoticeable in blacks and other dark-skinned persons but it cosmetically unacceptable to many people with lighter complexions. Clofazimine-induced gastrointestinal side effects of a mild to moderate degree affect some patients.

Ethionamide‡ is even more active than dapsone against *M. leprae* and, when utilized, should be given in a once daily adult dosage of 250–375 mg and proportionally less in children. Unfortunately, gastrointestinal intolerance to ethionamide is common, as is liver dysfunction, particularly when it is used together with rifampin. Indeed, if such a combination is utilized, liver function tests should be carefully monitored.

Streptomycin in a daily adult dose of 1 gm (and proportionally less in children) intramuscularly is as potent as dapsone against *M. leprae.* However, because of its potential for nephrotoxicity and eighth-nerve damage, no more than one year's therapy can be recommended. Hence, streptomycin should be used only with another agent that can be administered on a longer-term basis.

On therapy, tuberculoid macules may resolve somewhat, disappear entirely, or remain unchanged. Their anesthesia or hypoesthesia may also variably respond to therapy. Lepromatous infiltration does not begin to show noticeable improvement for a few months. Effective antimicrobial therapy will, however, prevent new lesions from appearing and the progressive neuropathy of untreated disease. It is important that both clinician and patient understand these expectations.

The Chemotherapy Recommendations of the World Health Organization

Because of growing concerns with the emergence of secondary and even primary dapsone resistance, the World Health Organization in 1981 developed some novel treatment recommendations. They suggest triple drug therapy for adults with multibacillary leprosy with rifampin, 600 mg once monthly (supervised); dapsone, 100 mg daily; clofazimine, 300 mg once monthly (supervised) plus 50 mg daily, or, if clofazimine is unacceptable cosmetically, ethionamide, 250–375 mg daily. The WHO recommends this therapy be maintained for at least two years, preferably until skin smears are

---

* DADDS is not available in the United States.

† Clofazimine is available from the National Hansen's Disease Center, Carville, Louisana.

‡ This use of ethionamide is not listed by the manufacturer.

bacteriologically negative, and then discontinued. For adult patients with paucibacillary disease, they recommend dapsone, 100 mg daily, and rifampin, 600 mg monthly (supervised), for a total of six months. Our own experience suggests that primary dapsone resistance is most uncommon and what little is found is only partially resistant but sensitive to levels achieved by generally recommended dapsone doses. Furthermore, patients harboring partially dapsone-resistance strains respond clinically in dapsone. We recommend dapsone sensitivity studies be done on newly diagnosed patients, and, if high-level dapsone-resistance is found, multibacillary patients receive rifampin daily and clofazimine three times weekly and paucibacillary patients receive rifampin daily alone.

Monthly rifampin and the reduced duration of therapy recommended by the WHO for both tuberculoid and lepromatous leprosy are largely a result of important economic considerations in developing countries. Because these are not particularly relevant in the United States and Western Europe and because there is limited clinical experience with these reduced durations and none with the WHO-recommended regimens, most authorities in the United States and Europe have not adopted monthly rifampin or these reduced courses of therapy.

Reactions and Their Treatment

About 50% of patients with lepromatous leprosy may develop the syndrome of erythema nodosum leprosum (ENL) generally within the first few years of antimicrobial therapy. This syndrome may consist of one or a number of the following manifestations: crops of erythematous painful skin papules that remain a few days and may pustulate and ulcerate, and are most commonly found on the extensor surface of the extremities; fever that may be as high as 105°F (40.5°C); painful neuritis that may result in further nerve damage; lymphadenitis; uveitis; orchitis; and occasionally large joint arthritis and glomerulonephritis. Histopathologically, this syndrome is secondary to a vasculitis and is probably the result of immune complexes. The clinical manifestations may be mild and evanescent or severe, recurrent, and occasionally fatal.

Patients with borderline leprosy may develop signs of inflammation, usually within previous skin lesions, and painful neuritis, which may cause further nerve damage and occasionally fever; these are called nonlepromatous lepra reactions. If they occur prior to therapy, they are termed "downgrading reactions"; if they occur during therapy, usually within a few weeks or months of the start of treatment, they are termed "reversal reactions." Therapy is required in the presence of neuritis, with skin inflammation of a sufficient extent that ulceration appears likely, or for cosmetic reasons, especially if lesions involve the face.

Because the majority of cases of childhood leprosy are indeterminant or tuberculoid and because the described reactional states occur in borderline and lepromatous leprosy, reactions are not really as much a problem in affected children as they are in adults.

Corticosteroids are effective in ENL and generally even the most severe cases can be controlled in adult doses of 60 mg prednisone. In this respect we have not found alternate-day steroids useful. Individual ENL papules resolve in a matter of days, and control can be best judged by the assessment of the prevention of new manifestations. When episodes are controlled, steroid doses can be tapered and then discontinued generally in 1 to 4 weeks. If ENL appears to be recurrent, thalidomide is the drug of choice for its control and prevention. The dosage must be individualized, and the minimal amount necessary to control ENL manifestations is advised; generally in adults 100–400 mg in a single evening dose is sufficient. In the United States thalidomide is available only through the National Hansen's Disease Center, Carville, Louisiana, and a number of regional Hansen's disease centers. An occasional patient, despite thalidomide therapy, may require small doses of corticosteroids to prevent recurrent ENL.

Because of thalidomide's potential for causing severe birth defects, including phocomelia, it should not be administered to women in the childbearing years. Side effects include tranquilization, to which tolerance generally develops rapidly, and constipation.

Clofazimine (an investigational drug), although slow in onset and only moderately effective in adult doses of 300 mg per day, may enable one to reduce the steroid requirement for therapy of ENL.

Thalidomide is of no value for lepra reactions. Corticosteroids are usually effective in controlling these reactions in adult doses of 40 to 60 mg prednisone per day but generally must be maintained at a lowered dose for a few months to prevent recurrence. Clofazimine may be of some value in decreasing the steroid requirement in these reactions in the same dose as for treating ENL but is not as effective in nonlepromatous lepra reactions.

Rehabilitation

Follow-up visits should always include examination of the feet, and plantar ulcers must be vigorously treated with specific antibiotics, débridement, and either bed rest or a total-contact walking cast until healed. Judicious use of extradepth shoes with molded inserts or specially molded shoes is crucial to prevent recurrence.

Tendon transfers to permit substitution of inner-vated for denervated muscles may provide patients with more functional use of hands, correct foot drop and enable them to close their eyes so that corneal trauma and its sequelae will not lead to blindness. If maximal results are to be expected, reconstructive surgery should not be initiated until patients have received at least 6 months of therapy directed against *M. leprae* and at least six months have passed since signs of reaction have abated. When possible, mechanical devices may help the severely deformed, and special job training may be necessary to prevent trauma and further disability.

Prophylaxis

The close, prolonged intimate contact of house-hold members of lepromatous patients poses some risk for the development of subsequent disease (about 10% in endemic countries and 1% in non-endemic locales). Although tuberculoid leprosy is not contagious, family members of tuberculoid patients may be incubating disease obtained from the same source. We recommend that household contacts of patients be examined annually for 5 to 7 years, preferably by a physician experienced in leprosy. Health workers and casual contacts appear to be at no significant risk. Therefore, when patients are hospitalized, no isolation requirements are necessary.

Trials of chemoprophylaxis with sulfones have at most been marginally effective. Thus, they are not generally recommended. BCG vaccination has been successful in some locales and not in others. It is not generally recommended. However, in the future vaccines utilizing heat-killed *M. leprae* alone and combined with BCG or *M. leprae* products may prove more efficacious in inducing the necessary protective cellular immunity. Specific and sensitive serodiagnosis of leprosy has recently become possible owing to the presence of circulating antibodies, particularly of the IgM class, directed at an *M. leprae*–specific phenolic glycolipid in nearly all lepromatous patients and about two-thirds of tuberculoid patients. It is hoped that early serodiagnosis during the long incubation period may soon prove feasible and useful in leprosy control.

Nontuberculous (Atypical) Mycobacterial Infections

THEODORE P. VOTTELER, M.D.
F.A.A.P., F.A.C.S.

Submandibular lymphadenitis is the usual presentation of nontuberculous mycobacterial (NTM) infection in children. The next most common sites of lymphadenitis are preauricular or intraparotid nodes. The facial node is the third most common site, but probably all nodal areas within the body have been described to contain NTM infections. Human tuberculous cervical lymphadenitis involves the posterior cervical or supraclavicular lymph nodes often associated with lung disease on chest roentgenogram.

Surgical Management. Nontuberculous mycobacterial infections are usually resistant to drug therapy. Therefore, surgical excision of all involved tissue is the primary method of management, producing excellent results if all involved tissue can be excised.

LYMPHADENITIS. Surgical excision of all involved lymph nodes with associated sinus tract and involved skin is curative. In the usual submandibular site, the mandibular branch of the facial nerve is to be anticipated in the surgical field, adjacent or adherent to the submandibular nodes or tract. Use of the nerve stimulator to protect and preserve the nerve is mandatory. Preoperative instructions to the anesthesiologist to avoid anesthetic muscle relaxant techniques negating the use of the nerve stimulator is wise. Although adjacent, the submandibular gland is not involved and need not be removed. Wide excision of the entire nodal area is not required, merely removal of all enlarged nodes, preferably by blunt dissection. Primary skin closure is utilized without drainage despite the presence of pus. Incision and drainage of the initial presenting abscess should be avoided to prevent a chronic draining sinus. Intraparotid or preauricular lymph nodes should be removed by similar techniques, utilizing nerve stimulation as required. Removal of adjacent parotid gland tissue by parotidectomy is unnecessary. Removal of involved lymph nodes in other sites of the body should not present unusual technical problems for the experienced surgeon. Persistent drainage after surgery should alert the physician to inadequate node removal rather than being taken as an indication for antibiotic usage.

SKIN. Chronic ulceration caused by NTM infections may be identified by smear or punch biopsy. Excisional therapy with primary closure should be curative.

SOFT TISSUE. Rarely, soft tissue lesions due either to inoculation from puncture wounds or to systemic bacteremia are identified, but these should also respond to excisional therapy. Tenosynovitis requires excision of involved tissue plus prolonged drug therapy, as described below.

PULMONARY DISEASE. The rare pulmonary disease due to NTM infection in childhood usually responds to prolonged drug therapy. Lobectomy or segmentectomy may be utilized to excise localized disease, however. The roentgen features used to differentiate NTM infection from human tuberculosis are not specific, and diagnosis is based on bacteriologic confirmation.

Medical Management. Although surgical excision is the primary mode of therapy for NTM infections, drug therapy with the various antituberculosis drugs may be indicated in certain situations. Disseminated disease in the immunocompromised patient, bone joint, and pulmonary disease, although rare, will require maximum therapeutic dosages of standard antituberculosis drugs—isoniazid, rifampin, and possibly streptomycin, all in dosages appropriate for human tuberculosis. Rifampin and isoniazid in combination are probably the drugs of choice to initiate therapy. Ethambutol is not recommended by the manufacturer for children at this time. Hepatotoxicity occurs with these drugs and should be considered throughout the therapeutic regimen. Skin disease due to *Mycobacterium chelonei* and *M. marinum* have been reported to respond to minocycline, 2.0 mg/kg daily orally, when surgical excision cannot be performed.

Length of therapy will depend on response of the lesion under treatment, but duration should be a minimum of one year after resolution of the adenitis or drainage. Antibiotics should not be utilized to replace inadequate surgical procedures unless specific circumstances so dictate this mode of therapy, i.e., parental refusal, excess anesthetic risk, or lack of surgical expertise.

Human-to-human transmission has not been documented, but draining wounds require proper disposal of infected material. Disseminated disease in the immunocompromised patient suspected to be due to NTM bacteria will require proper isolation techniques until the causative organism is identified and proper therapy instituted.

Day care or school authorities may prevent attendance when tuberculosis is mentioned by parents. They should be contacted directly by the physician when NTM infections have been documented to prevent erroneous isolation precautions.

Adolescent Syphilis

JOAN E. MORGENTHAU, M.D.

Syphilis still ranks third among *reportable* infectious diseases in adolescents. It is exceeded only by gonorrhea and chickenpox. In a recent year, of 3031 cases of primary and secondary syphilis in individuals between birth and age 19 reported to the Centers for Disease Control Center, 2872 (94.7%) were in adolescents between the ages of 15 and 19. In this age group, the male/female ratio is 2.5 to 1, and the incidence is highest in large cities in which male homosexuals make up over 50% of the reported cases. Adolescents at risk in addition to the gay community include prostitutes, those living in group homes or under detention, and victims of rape, sexual abuse, and incest. In excess of 95% of the cases are sexually transmitted, and the presence of other sexually transmitted diseases should alert the health professional to the possibility of syphilis. Because syphilis is highly contagious in its primary and secondary stages, health care workers should take particular care against accidental contamination during treatment.

The health provider should be aware that most states specifically permit the treatment of sexually transmitted diseases in minors without parental consent. Although the age may vary in different jurisdictions, the concept of the emancipated or mature minor is often invoked. In the case of minors with a sexually transmitted disease public health issues have been considered paramount. If the adolescent is assured of confidentiality, at both the individual and agency level, he is more likely to present himself for treatment early in the course of the disease. This permits appropriate case finding with the recommendation that sexual contacts of a case of infectious syphilis, within the preceding three months, be treated with the same regimen as the case of early syphilis.

Treatment schedules and criteria for reexamination and retreatment vary little among authors around the world. While the mechanism of the action of penicillin on the etiologic organism, *Treponema pallidum,* is not completely understood, four decades of clinical experience have confirmed the absolute superiority of penicillin therapy in all stages of the disease. The spirochete has yet to develop penicillin resistance, and therefore penicillin is the drug of choice in all stages of the infectious process, including the prophylaxis of incubating disease. Penicillin acts on dividing cells, and a level of 0.031 IU/ml can be taken as the theoretical and practical therapeutic level in the serum. This concentration should be maintained at a constant rate for at least 7–10 days in early syphilis and up to 3 weeks in cases of late disease. Increasing the concentration of the penicillin does not increase the rate of immobilization of the spirochetes. A single injection of 2.4 million units of benzathine penicillin G will maintain therapeutic levels in the serum for 2–3 weeks. The use of probenecid will enhance these levels by decreasing renal excretion, by blocking active transport of penicillin out of the cerebrospinal fluid, and by competitively decreasing binding of penicillin to serum albumin, thus promoting penetration of the blood-brain barrier.

What difference of opinion exists seems to be in relationship to the efficacy of benzathine penicillin G in the treatment of neurosyphilis. Although controlled clinical trials are completely lacking, most physicians believe that patients with symptomatic neurosyphilis should be managed differently from other patients with syphilis of more than one year's duration because of suboptimal levels of the antibiotic in the CSF. Although it may not be necessary to achieve maximum treponemicidal levels of penicillin in the CSF to cure neurosyphilis, since suboptimal levels may work in concert with a variety of host defenses, many clinicians prefer to hospitalize such patients and treat them with high doses of intravenous or intramuscular penicillin therapy.

When using penicillin therapy in the treatment of syphilis, the clinician should be aware of the possibility of a Jarisch-Herxheimer reaction. While this reaction is not well understood, it occurs within 2 to 12 hours after the initial dose of penicillin, most frequently in cases of early syphilis when there are large numbers of treponemes present. In some series of secondary syphilis, it has been seen in up to 90% of the cases. The symptoms, which are flulike in character, including fever, chills, headache, and myalgias, may last for 24 hours and are usually treated symptomatically. Some physicians report success in preventing the Jarisch-Herxheimer reaction by the use of prednisone, 5 mg, orally four times daily for 24 hours prior to the penicillin injection and continuing for the first day or two after treatment. The Jarisch-Herxheimer reaction is not dose dependent but is rather an all or none reaction to the initial injection of penicillin in the treatment of syphilis.

It should be remembered that from 30–40% of untreated cases will develop late syphilis within 2 to 20 years.

Early Syphilis. Included in this category is primary, secondary, and latent disease of less than 1 year's duration. The treatment of choice is benzathine penicillin G, 2.4 million units IM (1.2×10^6 in each buttock). Penicillin-allergic patients can be treated with tetracycline hydrochloride, 500 mg PO qid × 15 days. Tetracycline appears to be effective but has been evaluated less extensively than penicillin. Patient compliance needs to be carefully monitored. Tetracycline should *not* be used in cases in which the possibility of pregnancy exists. Erythromycin 500 mg PO qid × 15 days may be used. If compliance, including serologic follow-up, cannot be assured, the patient should be referred to an allergist for penicillin desensitization.

Syphilis of More Than One Year's Duration (excluding Neurosyphilis). This category includes latent syphilis of indeterminate duration, cardiovascular syphilis, and late benign disease. The treatment of choice is benzathine penicillin G, 2.4 million units IM once a week for three successive weeks (total of 7.2×10^6). The optimal treatment regimens for late syphilis are less well researched than those for early disease. For penicillin-allergic patients there is no good clinical data on alternative treatment. Cerebrospinal fluid should be examined prior to and following treatment, and one of the following regimens may be used: tetracycline hydrochloride, 500 mg PO qid × 30 days, or erythromycin, 500 mg PO qid × 30 days.

Neurosyphilis. There are no adequate, controlled clinical trials; however, published studies suggest that a total dosage of 6.0–9.0 million units of penicillin G over a 3–4 week period results in satisfactory results in 90% of patients with syphilis of the central nervous system. Close follow-up, both laboratory and clinical, is essential.

Potentially effective treatment may be achieved with aqueous crystalline penicillin G, 12–24 million units IM per day plus probenecid, 500 mg PO qid × 10 days; benzathine penicillin G, 2.4 million units IM weekly × 3; aqueous penicillin G sodium, 24 million units IV per day × 14 days.

Rape. Although the incidence of syphilis in those reporting rape is less than 1%, prophylactic treatment, if desired, can be given. A broad-spectrum antibiotic will also be effective against some of the other sexually transmitted diseases. Treatment options include (1) tetracycline, 0.5 gm PO qid × 7 days; (2) doxycline, 100 mg PO bid × 7 days; (3) amoxicillin, 3.0 gm or ampicillin, 3.5 gm PO each with 1.0 gm probenecid as a single PO dose.

Pregnancy. Patients who have received prior adequate treatment need not be retreated unless there is clinical or serologic evidence of reinfection or the treatment history is uncertain. The treatment of choice is benzathine penicillin G in a dosage appropriate for the stage of the disease. Tetracycline should *not* be used in pregnant patients.

Follow-up and Retreatment. All patients with syphilis should be carefully followed to establish adequacy of treatment and absence of reinfection. Nontreponemal tests such as the VDRL or RPR should be used as the treponemal tests, as the FTA may remain positive for life. In adequately treated primary syphilis the serology reverts to normal within 1 year; in treated secondary syphilis the serology reverts to normal within 2 years; and in treated early latent syphilis the serology reverts to normal within 4 years. Serology should be repeated at 3, 6, and 12 months after early syphilis; serology should be repeated at these intervals and at 24 months after late syphilis. Patients with neurosyphilis should have periodic serologies and CSF exams for 3 years. The serologic response to treatment is usually correlated with the duration of the disease prior to treatment.

Reinfection. Infection with the *T. pallidum* does not confer lasting immunity, and there is no test currently available to measure immune response in this disease. Retreatment should be considered when (1) clinical signs or symptoms persist or recur; (2) there is a 4-fold increase in titer with a nontreponemal test (this does not occur with a false biologic positive); and (3) an elevated nontreponemal titer does not show a 4-fold decrease within 1 year.

Retreatment should follow the schedule recommended for syphilis of more than one year's duration. The CSF should be examined before deciding on the treatment regimen. In general, patients should only be retreated once, since a persistent nontreponemal serology (especially with a low titer) is an indication of serofastness and there will be no response to further treatment.

Congenital Syphilis

HUGH E. EVANS, M.D.

Maternal Disease. The mother with a positive VDRL titer should be treated unless she is known to have received standard antibiotic therapy or the test result is thought to be a biological false positive. Benzathine penicillin G, given as a single intramuscular dose of 2.4 million units in the 1st trimester, should prevent fetal infection. In spite of such treatment, congenital infections have occurred. If the mother has early syphilis, aqueous procaine penicillin G, 600,000 units daily, intramuscularly, for 8 days is recommended. Latent syphilis is treated with either 2.4 million units of benzathine penicillin G weekly for 3 weeks or 600,000 units of parenteral procaine penicillin G daily for 15 days. Neurosyphilis should be treated with procaine penicillin G 600,000 units twice daily for 2–3 weeks.

If penicillin allergy is known, erythromycin stearate, 500 mg orally four times a day for 15 days, is recommended. Placental passage is unpredictable, and clinical and serologic outcomes have been variable. While tetracycline is as effective as penicillin, it is hepatotoxic to the mother and has adverse effects (osseous, dental) on the fetus. Cephalosporins may prove to be an alternative in this setting.

Newborn. In most cases the newborn of a mother known to have been appropriately treated with penicillin should not require therapy. Since congenital syphilis has occurred in spite of such treatment and documentation of maternal therapy may be uncertain, each neonate at risk should be evaluated and most should be treated. The adverse effects of therapy are negligible and outweighed by the potential benefits. If any drug other than penicillin was used in treatment of the mother, there is then no doubt at all about the need to treat the infant.

If the infant is symptomatic (jaundice, hepatosplenomegaly, skin rashes, snuffles, bone changes on x-ray), 10 days of treatment with aqueous crystalline penicillin G or procaine penicillin G in a dose of 50,000 units/kg, in two divided doses or once daily as a single dose, respectively, is required. If neurosyphilis has been excluded, one intramuscular dose of benzathine penicillin G, 50,000 units/ kg would be sufficient. Since criteria for neurosyphilis vary, one should assume the infant to have neurosyphilis even though this is a rare manifestation at present.

In theory, an asymptomatic neonate of a penicillin-treated mother, or one whose mother is serofast, need not be treated but should be clinically and serologically re-evaluated at 1, 2, and 4 months. Sequential testing will show a reduction in antibody titer. In practice, many of these infants are born to mothers of lower socioeconomic groups and their mothers have had little or no antenatal care. Compliance with a program of multiple follow-up visits is unlikely in this context. Treatment with benzathine penicillin G (as above) may be the more prudent and cost-effective approach in such cases. If the mother's treatment status is uncertain, the asymptomatic infant with a positive serology should have skeletal x-rays and a cerebrospinal fluid examination. It is rare for a neonate to require antibiotics other than penicillin, which remains the drug of choice in virtually all types of syphilis since *Treponema pallidum* is as exquisitely sensitive to this agent as it was over 40 years ago. The current reports of fetal and neonatal deaths due to congenital syphilis reflect mainly inadequate antenatal care. The latter may be due in turn to socioeconomic factors, cultural differences, and an "attitudinal barrier." Inadequate control programs and surveillance also contribute to this adverse outcome.

Infancy. The treatment regimen for congenital syphilis diagnosed in infancy but after the neonatal period is the same as that recommended for newborns. For older children, calculation of the dose should be modified so that adult levels are not exceeded.

Leptospirosis

RALPH D. FEIGIN, M.D.

Leptospirosis is a disease caused by a single family of organisms of which there are multiple serogroups and serotypes. In the last decade, the dog has been incriminated as an important vector as well as a reservoir of this disease.

To be of maximum therapeutic benefit an antimicrobial agent must be administered before the invading organisms damage the endothelium of blood vessels and various organs or tissues. One problem in evaluating the efficacy of therapy to date has been that, generally, leptospirosis is a self-limited disease with a favorable prognosis. Even patients with severe icteric leptospirosis may recover without specific treatment.

Most claims of the beneficial value of antimicrobial agents in human leptospirosis are based on the response of individual patients rather than on controlled studies. However, when penicillin therapy was given to 28 patients prior to the fourth day of illness and compared with a control group of 33 patients who were given only supportive care, the duration of fever and the incidence of jaundice, meningismus, renal involvement, and hemorrhagic manifestations were diminished in the treated group. Therefore, when a diagnosis of leptospirosis is considered possible or probable and the patient has been ill for less than 1 week, treatment with penicillin or tetracycline (avoid the latter in children less than 8 years of age) should be initiated. Parenteral aqueous penicillin G (6 to 8 million units/m^2 of body surface/24 hr in six divided doses) provides optimal blood and tissue concentrations of penicillin. For patients who are sensitive to penicillin, tetracycline (20 to 40 mg/kg/24 hr) should be provided intravenously or orally in four divided doses for 1 week. Do not give tetracycline intravenously in excess of 1 gm total dose.

A sudden increase in body temperature, drop in systemic blood pressure, and exacerbation of other symptoms may accompany the initiation of penicillin therapy (a Herxheimer reaction). This reaction generally subsides spontaneously and is not a contraindication to continued treatment.

The management of leptospirosis requires careful attention to supportive care. Profound fluid and electrolyte changes may be noted, particularly significant hyponatremia. Thus, fluid and electrolyte balance must be accorded meticulous attention. Dehydration, cardiovascular collapse, and acute renal failure require prompt, specific treatment. In some cases, acute renal failure may be prevented by ensuring adequate renal perfusion and appropriate fluid administration early in the disease when prerenal azotemia and shock may be seen. If prerenal azotemia is suspected, diuresis may be attempted with the administration of a fluid or colloid load designed to expand extracellular volume and replace extracellular fluid deficits. In patients who do not respond to such therapy, acute tubular necrosis should be suspected, and appropriate fluid restriction should be initiated. Urine output, urine specific gravity, serum and urine osmolalities, and accurate measurement of body weight should be monitored sequentially. Children should receive sufficient fluid to replace insensible water loss plus their urine output. This may require adjustments of fluid intake on an hourly basis. Generally, a multiple electrolyte solution containing 5% or 10% glucose and 40 meq of sodium and chloride per liter, 35 meq of potassium per liter, and 20 meq of lactate or acetate per liter administered at a rate calculated as above is appropriate fluid therapy. If azotemia is severe or prolonged, peritoneal dialysis or hemodialysis should be instituted. Exchange transfusion has been suggested for patients with marked hyperbilirubinemia.

The use of corticosteroids in the treatment of severe cases has not been evaluated critically. Their use has been suggested in patients with impending hepatic coma. Anecdotal reports also suggest that they may be of value in patients with profound hypotension or shock.

Hemorrhagic manifestations of disease may be related to disseminated intravascular coagulation or thrombocytopenia without disseminated intravascular coagulation, or may merely reflect friability of blood vessels due to the severe vasculitis. Platelet transfusions have been used for patients with thrombocytopenia but generally the lifespan of the infused platelets is short. Heparin has been used for the treatment of disseminated intravascular coagulation, but there is little evidence to suggest that such therapy is beneficial.

When uveitis is present, ophthalmologic consultation should be sought. Conjunctival suffusion is common with leptospirosis and clears without specific topical therapy.

Rat Bite Fever

MOSES GROSSMAN, M.D.

The clinical term rat bite fever refers to two separate and similar syndromes, both induced by bites of infected rodents. The microorganisms involved are *Spirillum minor* and *Streptobacillus moniliformis*. The syndrome caused by the former is also known as sodoku; the latter one produces a syndrome also known as Haverill fever or streptobacillary fever. Specific etiologic diagnosis may be attained by darkfield examination, inoculation of laboratory animals, or serologically.

Antimicrobial therapy is important. Untreated the disease lasts longer and may have a distinct mortality. The drug of choice is penicillin for both microorganisms and for all forms of the disease. The traditionally recommended regimen is 20,000 to 50,000 units of procaine penicillin per kg per 24 hours divided into twice daily doses for seven days. While there is no published experience with using oral penicillin there is every reason to believe than an oral regimen of penicillin would be effective if compliance could be assured. Patients allergic to penicillin should be given tetracycline as an alternate drug of choice (30–50 mg/kg/24 hr) in divided doses. In children younger than nine years it is inadvisable to use tetracycline. Erythromycin might be a third choice drug, particularly in the spirillary form of the syndrome.

In addition to antimicrobial therapy, local care of the ulcerated area at the site of the bite and attention to tetanus prophylaxis are important adjuncts to treatment.

Pneumocystis carinii Pneumonitis

WALTER T. HUGHES, M.D.

Pneumonitis caused by *Pneumocystis carinii* is usually fatal if untreated. With specific antimicrobial therapy about 75% of patients can be expected to recover if treatment is begun early. Since the infection usually occurs in immunocompromised patients and a definitive diagnosis requires an invasive procedure, such as open lung biopsy or percutaneous needle aspiration, management requires close attention to complications from the underlying primary disease and the diagnostic procedures. Thus, associated or secondary viral, bacterial, or fungal infections may occur and pneumothorax or pneumomediastinum may complicate the diagnostic procedure. Hypoxia with low arterial oxygen tension (PaO$_2$) is regularly present, while carbon dioxide retention is unusual and the arterial pH is frequently increased. Unlike other infections in the immunosuppressed host, *P. carinii* infection remains localized entirely to the lungs.

When *P. carinii* pneumonitis is recognized as the first illness of an infant or child, careful search should be made for an underlying disease.

Specific Therapy. Trimethoprim-sulfamethoxazole (TMP-SMZ)* and pentamidine isethionate are equally effective in the treatment of *P. carinii* pneumonitis but TMP-SMZ is the drug of first choice because of its low toxicity and easy availability.

TMP-SMZ may be given orally or intravenously. The oral dose is 20 mg trimethoprim and 100 mg sulfamethoxazole per kg/day, divided into four parts at 6-hour intervals. It is advisable to give half of the calculated daily dose initially as a loading dose when the oral route is used. TMP-SMZ is available in tablet form ("regular size" with 80 mg trimethoprim, 400 mg sulfamethoxazole and as a "double-strength" tablet with twice these amounts). An oral suspension contains 40 mg trimethoprim and 200 mg sulfamethoxazole per 5 ml. The intravenous preparation is available in 5.0-ml am-

pules containing 80 mg trimethoprim and 400 mg sulfamethoxazole. Each 5.0-ml ampule must be added to 125 ml of 5% dextrose in water. The dosage for intravenous use is 15.0 mg trimethoprim and 75.0 mg sulfamethoxazole per kg/day divided in three to four equal doses. Each dose is infused over a 60 minute period. From available data, peak serum levels of 3 to 5 µg/ml of trimethoprim and 100 to 150 µg/ml of sulfamethoxazole seem to be the optimal ranges.

The adverse and toxic side effects are essentially those of sulfonamides, and although uncommon they include transient maculopapular rash, nausea, vomiting, diarrhea, neutropenia, agranulocytosis, aplastic anemia, megaloblastic anemia, hemolytic anemia, methemoglobinemia. Stevens-Johnson syndrome, allergic reactions, toxic nephrosis, and drug fever. Folic acid deficiency has occurred rarely. It is reversible by folinic acid, 10 to 25 mg daily. Folinic acid does not interfere with the therapeutic effects of the drug. Patients with acquired immune deficiency syndrome (AIDS) have a higher rate of adverse reactions than other patients.

Pentamidine is the drug of second choice because of its high frequency of adverse effects. The drug was approved by the Federal Drug Administration in 1984 and is marketed in the United States by LyphoMed (Melrose Park, IL).

Pentamidine is administered as a single daily dose of 4 mg/kg IM for 10 to 14 days. If improvement is apparent after 5 days of treatment, this may be reduced to 3 mg/kg/day. The total dosage should not exceed 56 mg/kg. IM injections should be given deeply into the anterolateral aspect of the thigh. Each 100 mg of the drug should be dissolved in 1 ml of sterile distilled water. Filtration of the drug in solution through a Millipore filter (0.22-micron pore size) immediately before injection is advisable to ensure sterility for the immunosuppressed host. Pentamidine can be given IV, but some report that severe adverse reactions are more frequent than with the IM route; more recent studies have found this not to be the case. If the IV route is used, the drug should be infused over a period of one hour.

Adverse effects include induration, abscess formation, and necrosis at injection sites; nephrotoxicity; hypoglycemia or, rarely, hyperglycemia; hypotension; alteration in liver function; tachycardia; hypocalcemia; nausea and vomiting; skin rash; anemia; hyperkalemia; and thrombocytopenia.

Isolation. Recent studies indicate that *P. carinii* is transmitted by the airborne route. It is advisable to use respiratory isolation procedures to separate active cases of *P. carinii* pneumonitis from other compromised individuals at high risk for this infection.

Supportive Measures. Oxygen should be ad-

---

* Manufacturer's precaution: Not recommended for infants less than 2 months of age.

ministered by mask as needed to maintain the PaO_2 above 70 mm Hg. The fraction of inspired oxygen (FIO_2) should be kept below 50 volumes % if possible, to avoid oxygen toxicity, since oxygen therapy usually is required for relatively long periods.

Assisted or controlled ventilation is indicated in patients with arterial oxygen tension less than 60 mm Hg at FIO_2 of 50% or greater. Those with acutely elevated $PaCO_2$, without pH changes and with or without hypoxemia, should be considered candidates for ventilatory therapy.

Patients receiving immunosuppressive drugs should have these discontinued if the status of the primary disease permits. Corticosteroids are of no benefit and may be deleterious to the course of the pneumonitis.

Fluid and electrolyte quantities are calculated by the patient's needs, but the solution should contain 5 or 10% glucose to help prevent hypoglycemia during pentamidine therapy. Metabolic acidosis must be corrected.

Bacterial pneumonia or sepsis may occur in association with *P. carinii* pneumonitis, in the seriously ill patient with marked neutropenia (absolute neutrophil count less than 500/cu mm) or evidence of bacterial infection, antibiotics should be given. Oxacillin, 200 mg/kg/day, and gentamicin, 5 to 7 mg/kg/day, are administered IV until the results of cultures are known.

Efforts should be made to improve the nutritional status of the patient by dietary means even during the acute stage of the disease. Multivitamins should be given empirically. The value of IV alimentation has not been determined.

Give blood transfusion if hemoglobin level is less than normal. The hemoglobin content must be sufficient to result in an arterial oxygen content of 15 to 20 ml/dl of blood at an arterial oxygen tension of 100 mm Hg.

Pneumothorax may be a complication of the diagnostic procedures. If it is less than 15% with no adverse effect on respiration, close observation is adequate. If it is more extensive, insertion of a thoracotomy tube with a water seal drainage system is necessary.

Parameters to Monitor. *Serum immunoglobulins:* At the onset of the illness, administer immune serum globulin (165 mg/ml) 0.66 ml/kg if the immunoglobulin G level is below 300 mg/dl.

Roentgenograms of chest should be done daily until there is clinical evidence of improvement. If needle aspiration of the lung, lung biopsy, or endotracheal brush catheter technique has been used as a diagnostic procedure, chest roentgenograms should be made at 30 minutes, 4 hours, and 12 hours after the procedure to detect pneumothorax.

Hemoglobin, WBC count and differential, and platelet estimate daily.

Measure body weight, intake and output daily.

Arterial blood gases: Measure pH, $PaCO_2$, PaO_2, and base excess or deficit initially and as often as necessary, based on severity of clinical course.

Serum electrolytes: Measure sodium, chloride, potassium, and carbon dioxide content every 3 days, or more frequently if indicated.

Total serum proteins, albumin, and globulin: Monitor every 3 days. Hypoalbuminemia may occur.

Blood pressure, pulse and respiratory rate: Monitor every 4 hours, or more often if the condition is critical.

For patients receiving pentamidine: Check *blood urea nitrogen (BUN), creatinine, and urinalysis* every 3 days. If the BUN exceeds 30 mg/dl or serum creatinine is greater than 1.5 mg/dl, withhold pentamidine for 1 or 2 days; monitor *blood glucose* 4 to 6 hours after each injection of pentamidine. Administer glucose if blood glucose value is less than 40 mg/dl; monitor *serum glutamic oxaloacetic transaminase (SGOT)* every 3 days; withhold pentamidine for 1 to 2 days if evidence of hepatic toxicity exists; and monitor *serum calcium and phosphorus* every 3 days. If the serum inorganic phosphate level becomes increased and the calcium level becomes decreased from normal values on the basis of renal insufficiency, give calcium lactate, 15 to 20 gm/day, or calcium carbonate, 5 to 8 gm/day orally. The diet should be low in phosphate, and 25,000 to 50,000 units of vitamin D is given orally. For patients with renal impairment and receiving trimethoprim-sulfamethoxazole, the dosage should be regulated on the basis of serum drug levels. Measurement of serum levels of the sulfonamide is adequate. The level of free sulfonamide should be maintained with peak values between 100 and 150 μg/ml measured 2 hours after the oral dosage.

Experimental studies suggest that diaminodiphyenylsulfone (dapsone) may be effective in *P. carinii* pneumonitis.

Expected Course. Fever, tachypnea, and pulmonary infiltrates usually persist with little change for 4 to 6 days. If no improvement is apparent after a week of therapy, concomitant or secondary infection most likely exists. These infections have included bacterial pneumonia or sepsis, systemic candidiasis, aspergillosis, cryptococcosis, histoplasmosis, and cytomegalovirus inclusion disease, as well as other viral infections. *P. carinii* pneumonitis may recur several months after apparent recovery in 10 to 15% of cases.

Prevention. *P. carinii* pneumonitis can be prevented by chemoprophylaxis with TMP-SMZ.† Dosage is one fourth the therapeutic dose, 5 mg/kg of trimethoprim and 25 mg/kg of sulfamethoxazole per day in two divided doses. The protection

---

† This use is not listed by the manufacturer.

is afforded only while the patient is receiving the drug.

Measles

EDWARD A. MORTIMER, Jr., M.D.

Measles is an acute, systemic viral infection that in the past affected nearly all children in the United States and therefore was classified as one of the usual childhood diseases. A severe disease, it is characterized by a course of approximately 7 days with high fever; moderately severe respiratory symptoms, including coryza, conjunctivitis, and cough; the classical enanthem (Koplik's spots); and a characteristic rash. Besides the severity of the acute illness the importance of the disease in the United States has been measured by its complications, particularly otitis media, pneumonia, measles encephalitis and, rarely, subacute sclerosing panencephalitis. In the past in the United States mortality was largely a result of pneumonia; perhaps because of better nutrition, antibiotics, and other factors, deaths from the disease declined remarkably even before widespread use of the vaccine.

Even today, however, the situation in the remainder of the world is very different. WHO estimates for 1980 indicate that of the 103 million babies born in the Third World annually, 2,200,000 (2.1%) succumb to measles before their fifth birthdays. Undoubtedly complicating factors such as low birth weight, malnutrition, recurrent diarrhea, and other infections contribute to this high mortality. Thus, measles remains a severe disease.

Control of Measles

The control of measles and its associated morbidity and mortality is dependent on prevention by active immunization, which is achieved with live, attenuated measles vaccine, for the reason that therapy for the established disease provides only symptomatic relief. Passive immunization employing immune serum globulin is of value in individual children in some circumstances but is of no use as a routine measure.

Live, Attenuated Measles Vaccine. Primary prevention of measles is achieved by a single injection of live, attenuated measles vaccine. The United States Public Health Service and the American Academy of Pediatrics recommend that all children, with the rare exceptions of those with specific contraindications, receive measles vaccine. Properly administered measles vaccine results in seroconversion and clinical protection in more than 95% of recipients. Available preparations include monovalent measles vaccine, measles vaccine combined with live, attenuated rubella vaccine (MR), and the familiar MMR, which combines live, attenuated measles, mumps, and rubella vaccines. There is no biologic advantage to administering measles vaccine in monovalent form.

The optimum age for routine administration of measles vaccine in the United States is considered to be 15 months of age. Although it was originally recommended that measles vaccine be given at 9 months of age, this recommendation was subsequently changed to 12 months of age and more recently to 15 months. The reason for this is that small traces of maternal transplacental antibody appear to interfere with acquisition of immunity, and this effect persists in a few children even beyond 12 or 13 months. However, under epidemic conditions or in countries where measles is endemic, the vaccine may be administered to infants as young as 6 months; it should be readministered at 15 months to those who received it prior to 12 months.

Because measles vaccine produces a "mild" measles infection, side effects may be anticipated in some recipients. The most frequent of these is fever, usually appearing about 6 days after inoculation. Although fever is usually slight and lasts only a few days, in approximately 10% of children it may reach 103°F (39.4°C) or more. Less commonly, transient, nondescript rashes occur. An important question is whether the neurologic sequelae of the disease (acute encephalitis and subacute sclerosing panencephalitis [SSPE]) occur following measles vaccine. Although there have been isolated anecdotal reports of acute encephalitis following the vaccine, their rarity suggests that they may well represent coincidence and not causation. Similarly, it is impossible to determine whether the very few cases of SSPE reported in children who received measles vaccine are a consequence of the vaccine or stem from unrecognized measles in infancy. If measles vaccine causes SSPE, the rate is only a small fraction of that from natural measles, for the reason that the incidence of SSPE in the United States has declined remarkably following widespead use of the vaccine.

VACCINE FAILURES. Vaccine failures, as evidenced by clinical measles in a previously immunized child (or failure of serologic conversion in studies of efficacy), have been reported in 5 to 10% of children. Many, if not most, of these can be attributed to any one of three factors: improper handling of the vaccine, administration at too young an age, or simultaneous use of immune serum globulin. The vaccine is susceptible to inactivation by light or by warmth during transport or storage (breaks in the "cold chain"); it should always be transported and stored until use at or below 45°F (8°C). The vaccine also should not be directly exposed to bright light unnecessarily, although the current preparation is less sensitive to light than earlier measles vaccines.

As noted above, administration of properly stored and handled vaccine may nonetheless be associated with failure to immunize because of persistent maternal antibody; the younger the infant, the higher the proportion of failures. Many of the cases of measles occurring during outbreaks in previously immunized persons are so explained. For this reason it has been a recommended (and frequently mandatory) policy to re-immunize all children who received measles vaccine prior to their first birthdays, and it is considered acceptable to re-immunize those who were vaccinated between 12 and 14 months. (Deleterious effects resulting from revaccination of a person successfully immunized in the past have not been observed and would not be expected logically, and therefore serologic testing prior to revaccination is unnecessary.)

Some vaccine failures are attributable to the simultaneous administration of immune globulin to many children who received measles vaccine prepared from the less attenuated Edmonston B strain of virus between 1963, when it was first licensed, and 1975, when it was replaced by the further attenuated vaccine. Immune globulin was given to ameliorate the excessive reactions from the Edmonston B vaccine, and, indeed, some physicians continued to use it in conjunction with the further attenuated vaccine. Unfortunately, although the immune serum globulin reduced reaction rates, it also prevented the acquisition of active immunity in some children, particularly those who received the further attenuated vaccine. For this reason children who received this latter vaccine plus immune serum globulin should be considered candidates for re-immunization.

Recipients of Killed Measles Vaccine. A unique problem is presented by those individuals, now young adults, who received killed measles vaccine during the years it was licensed (1963–1967). Up to 1 million children received the killed vaccine. The vaccine was abandoned when it became apparent that protection was transient and that children exposed to measles 2 or more years later experienced a severe type of measles with high fever, unusual rash, edema, pneumonitis, and other findings (atypical measles). Such persons also exhibit greater reactivity to subsequent live measles vaccine; a few have quite severe reactions resembling atypical measles. However, because atypical measles with the wild virus is far more severe than the vast majority of reactions to the live vaccine in these persons, most authorities advise administering the live vaccine with adequate warning to the patient. Re-immunization is particularly important for those who travel to other countries where measles is common.

Effects on Measles Epidemiology. The widespread use of measles vaccine for more than two decades has changed the usual age distribution of the disease markedly. Although there are many fewer cases of measles (2543 in 1984, and many younger physicians have never seen a case), two shifts in age incidence have resulted from vaccine use. Initially there was a shift of the peak incidence from elementary school age to adolescents and young adults who escaped natural measles and did not receive the vaccine. Although outbreaks of measles continue to be observed at such sites as college campuses, the proportion of cases in children less than 5 years old with measles has increased, presumably because the vaccine is not mandated prior to school entry. Rates in elementary school age children continue to be low. For these reasons many colleges now require proof of measles immunity before entry, and special efforts should be made to immunize young children earlier than school entry, by insisting, for example, upon full immunization prior to entrance into day care programs.

Contraindications to Measles Vaccine

Egg Sensitivity. Live measles vaccine is propagated in chick embryo cell culture. Until recently it was believed that there was insufficient egg protein in the vaccine to cause concern. However, in recent years 3 cases of potentially serious immediate allergic reactions to the vaccine have been unquestionably related to egg sensitivity. Therefore, rare cases of children with a clear-cut history of immediate anaphylactic type response to egg ingestion should not receive measles vaccine.

Immunocompromised States. Children with congenital immune deficiencies and those whose immune systems are compromised by immunosuppressive therapy should not receive measles vaccine because of the risk of enhanced infection with the vaccine virus. However, because recipients of the vaccine do not transmit the virus, immunodeficient persons are not jeopardized by the immunization of others, including siblings.

Neomycin Allergy. Measles vaccine contains small amounts of neomycin but no other antibiotic. The rare individual who has experienced an anaphylactic response to topical or systemic neomycin should not receive the vaccine. Contact dermatitis from topical neomycin is not a contraindication, although such persons may develop a small, transient nodule at the injection site.

Pregnancy. Although there is no evidence that measles vaccine (or any live vaccine, including that for rubella) is deleterious to the fetus, pregnant women should not receive measles vaccine on theoretical grounds and to avoid confusion about causation of any adverse outcome of the pregnancy.

Prior Receipt of Immune Serum Globulin. Human immune serum globulin contains substantial amounts of measles antibody, which may interfere with a measles vaccine "take." Therefore, administration of the vaccine to any child who has received immune serum globulin should be deferred for at least 3 months after receipt of the globulin.

Acute Illness. Because children repetitively display evidence of mild, transient respiratory infections with little or no fever and because there is no evidence of deleterious interaction between such illnesses and the receipt of measles vaccine or of interference with acquisition of immunity, whether to administer measles vaccine in the presence of such symptoms should be determined by individual circumstances.

Passive Immunization

Immune serum globulin (ISG) will prevent or modify measles in exposed susceptible individuals, depending on the dose administered and on its administration as soon as possible after exposure (no later than 6 days). Preventive doses of ISG (0.25 ml/kg intramuscularly, maximum dose 15 ml) should be given to all infants between 6 and 24 months of age and to all nonimmune immunodeficient persons exposed to measles, because of the high incidence of complications in such children. An alternative approach for certain susceptible individuals exposed within the previous 72 hours is to administer measles vaccine, because vaccine-induced immunity appears promptly, often prior to the development of the clinical disease. This approach is of particular utility during outbreaks of measles when the presence and timing of exposure are uncertain.

For unimmunized children older than 2 years who are exposed to measles, a modifying dose of ISG may be given (0.04 ml/kg body weight as a single injection). This dose may be expected to ameliorate the severity of the disease if given within 6 days and nonetheless permit the development of active immunity. Unless such children develop modified (mild) measles, they should receive measles vaccine 3 months after receipt of ISG.

ISG should not be used to control measles outbreaks in schools or communities. Instead, all persons at risk of exposure born since 1957 should receive measles vaccine unless thay have proof of physician-diagnosed measles or immunization with live measles vaccine age 12 months or older. In such situations ISG should only be given to individuals for whom the vaccine is contraindicated and to infants 6 to 24 months of age with documented exposure to the disease.

Management of Measles

The treatment of measles is symptomatic only. ISG will not modify the course or prevent complications once symptoms have begun. Prophylactic antibiotics are of no utility in preventing secondary infection. Acetaminophen, 5 mg/kg, may be given as often as every 4 hours for symptomatic relief. Symptoms of the disease are such that bed rest during the febrile stages is not difficult to enforce. Mild cough suppressants may be given but usually appear to have little effect.

A frequent problem that has arisen since the advent of the vaccine is that of misdiagnosis, because an increasing number of physicians have never seen measles. If there is doubt, a quick way to obtain diagnostic help is to have the patient seen by an older physician who had past experience with outbreaks of the disease.

An important part of the management of measles is recognition and treatment of complications. The most common of these is bacterial otitis media, which requires appropriate antimicrobial therapy. In the past, mastoiditis frequently ensued. Pulmonary complications include bronchiolitis, especially in infants, and pneumonia, which may be lobar or bronchopneumonic in distribution. Suspicion of pneumonia usually arises when the patient worsens late in the course of the disease or fever fails to subside with full appearance of the rash. A chest X-ray may be required for diagnosis. Pneumonia may be bacterial in origin, especially if lobar in type, and should be treated with antimicrobial drugs. Rarely, pneumothorax or pneumomediastinum occurs. Occasionally, inflammation of the upper airway progresses to obstructive laryngotracheitis and may require tracheostomy.

Other rare complications include appendicitis, presumably secondary to lymphoid hyperplasia; abdominal pain and vomiting in the course of measles or early in convalesence suggest this possibility. Acute measles encephalitis, estimated to occur in about 1 per 1000 cases, usually appears near the end of the course of the disease or early in convalesence. Persistent or recurring fever, somnolence, irrational behavior, vomiting, and convulsions are frequent manifestations. Treatment is symptomatic; neurologic consultation is advisable.

Rubella and Congenital Rubella

PHILIP R. ZIRING, M.D.

The decline in the incidence of rubella and congenital rubella since licensure of live attenuated rubella virus vaccines in 1969 has been one of the most notable achievements of modern medicine. The last major epidemic of rubella in the United States in 1964 was accompanied by rubella infection in one in every 100 pregnancies and the birth of approximately 20,000 infants with rubella-associated defects. More than 100,000,000 doses of rubella vaccine have been administered in the

United States since 1969, which brought the predictable seven-year cycles of rubella epidemics to a conclusion. So dramatic has this change been that by 1983 there were only 6 cases of congenital rubella nationwide reported to the Centers for Disease Control.

We will consider rubella and congenital rubella in this section because, despite their low incidence, they are matters for pediatricians to remain concerned about. Sporadic cases of rubella still occur, especially in clusters among older adolescents and young adults who have not had the disease or been immunized and in susceptible persons immigrating to the United States. There is a great need to maintain a high level of awareness about the importance of immunization and the safety and efficacy of rubella vaccine. Furthermore, we have an ongoing concern for the thousands of patients with congenital rubella, many of whom were victims of the 1964 epidemic who are now entering the third decade of life and who are at risk for developing new clinical manifestations of this disorder.

Rubella

In general, rubella (German measles, three-day measles), can be considered among the mildest viral illnesses. In fact, a significant percentage of adults and even larger numbers of children may undergo infection that is completely asymptomatic. Though often pruritic, the rash generally responds to simple antihistamine treatment. There may be an associated sore throat, tender lymphadenopathy, and low-grade fever, which is responsive to analgesics. It is most important to recall that the patient is highly contagious for a period of time beginning a few days prior to the onset of rash until one to two weeks after the rash clears. During this time it is important to avoid exposure of the patient to a woman who may be in early pregnancy and whose rubella susceptibility status is unknown. The most important common complication of rubella is postinfectious arthralgia or arthritis, principally involving the small joints of the hands and feet. Though these joint symptoms sometimes are quite painful and may recur periodically for an extended period of time, they always clear completely without residua. Thrombocytopenia of mild degree is not uncommon and usually resolves without treatment. Thrombocytopenic purpura is a rare complication, which should prompt thorough hematologic investigation to insure that there is no other underlying cause. A course of prednisone may be initiated if significant thrombocytopenia is persistent. Postinfectious encephalitis is seen in rubella far less often than in measles and usually responds to simple supportive measures.

Congenital Rubella

It is most useful to consider the clinical manifestations of congenital rubella in three stages: those that are present and identifiable at birth, those that are developmental and appear only as the infant grows older, and those late manifestations that may not be clinically apparent until the second decade of life or beyond.

Disorders Apparent in the Neonatal Period. The rubella-associated birth defects that are apparent at birth are a result of rubella virus interference with cell growth and cell division in the fetus. They include defects of the eye (cataract, glaucoma, and retinopathy), of the heart (stenosis of the main pulmonary artery and/or its branches, patent ductus arteriosus, and other less common heart defects less commonly seen), central nervous system (sensory neural hearing loss and other evidence of brain injury), bone marrow (anemia, thrombocytopenia and defects of the immune system), and general intrauterine growth retardation. The management of these disorders is little different from that used when such defects result from other diverse etiologies.

A few clinical issues are especially worth remembering. For example, surgery for congenital glaucoma must be performed promptly after diagnosis in the neonatal period to guard against permanent visual loss from high intraocular pressure. Surgery for congenital cataracts, on the other hand, can often be deferred until as late as one year of age when optimum surgical results are often obtained. Surgery for a uniocular rubella cataract has rarely been rewarded by useful vision in the operated eye. Sensory neural hearing loss is the most common clinically significant consequence of rubella infection during the first four months of pregnancy and must be ruled out in every infant suspected of having congenital rubella. The hearing loss may be unilateral or bilateral and range in severity from mild to profound, and may be manifest in hearing at all frequencies. Early diagnosis through testing of infants by skilled audiologists followed by early amplification with hearing aids and enrollment in auditory training programs can often spell the difference between an individual capable of speech and one unable to communicate orally.

Developmental Disorders. As the infant passes beyond the neonatal period, other disorders of a developmental character may appear. Mental retardation is more likely and more severe the earlier in pregnancy the infection takes place and is often complicated by the presence of impairment of vision and/or hearing. The enrollment of these infants in preschool enrichment programs often helps them to make maximum use of their residual abilities and assists the family with needed training and support.

Symptoms of spastic cerebral palsy are usually not apparent until the first year of life. In such cases, close follow-up by neurologists, orthopedists, physiatrists, and physical, occupational, and speech therapists skilled in the management of physically handicapped children can often be helpful in management related to ambulation, sitting, feeding, and other skills of daily living.

Behavioral disorders occur commonly and are often complicated by the presence of sensory defects or mental retardation. Extreme restlessness and hyperactivity or symptoms of autism often prove difficult to manage. The results of the use of stimulant medication, tranquilizers, or barbiturates have generally been disappointing. More success has followed the use of mild sedatives such as diphenhydramine (Benadryl) or psychotropic agents such as thioridazine (Mellaril). Consultation with child psychiatrists and behavioral psychologists may also be helpful.

Late Manifestations of Congenital Rubella. Clinical disturbances of endocrine function in children and young adults with congenital rubella, with onset not until the first or second decade of life, are now well recognized. Patients with hypo- or hyperthyroidism have been described, with identification of rubella virus antigen in the thyroid gland of at least one child with Hashimoto's thyroiditis. The most common endocrine disturbance seems to be insulin-dependent diabetes mellitus, with up to 20% or more of patients having some evidence of this disorder by the second decade of life. Recent interest has been focused on the association of insulin-dependent diabetes mellitus in children with congenital rubella, predominantly with certain HLA phenotypes, especially DR3 and B8. In such cases, the rubella infection of the islet cells in utero seems to have acted as a "trigger" in the expression of insulin-dependent diabetes mellitus in children who are so genetically predisposed. Early diagnosis of these disorders through measurement of antibodies directed against thyroid and islet cells is now becoming more commonplace. The interpretation of such tests and their therapeutic implications may often best be carried out in consultation with a pediatric endocrinologist.

Several patients with congenital rubella were reported a few years ago with progressive rubella panencephalitis, a degenerative disorder of the central nervous system apparently caused by an exacerbation of rubella infection within the brain. Though few patients have been so identified thus far, it is important to be alert to the existence of this entity in patients with congenital rubella who undergo deterioration in behavior, intellectual performance, or motor function or develop seizures.

Prevention of Rubella. As noted, immunization of most children at approximately 15 months of age and selected adults who are shown to be rubella seronegative has resulted in a dramatic decline in the incidence of rubella and congenital rubella. The RA 27/3 strain of virus grown in human diploid cell culture may be given alone or in combination with other live attenuated virus vaccines (measles, mumps). A single inoculation of this vaccine produces durable immunity, although the antibody levels achieved may be lower than that following natural rubella infection. The immunity so induced is protective and may well be lifelong. Ongoing surveillance conducted by the Centers for Disease Control in Atlanta of the risk to the fetus of inadvertent rubella immunization of a susceptible woman in early pregnancy has taken place since the introduction of the vaccine. It has been well established that vaccine virus so inoculated can be recovered from the fetus, but evidence is still lacking that this vaccine virus is teratogenic. Numerous such pregnancies have gone to term with no evidence of congenital rubella birth defects present in the offspring. Pregnant women so exposed should be counseled regarding the *theoretical* risks such vaccination poses; but they may be reassured at this time regarding the lack of known association with congenital rubella birth defects. Side effects of vaccination are similar (though generally milder) than those seen in natural rubella, with transient arthralgias and arthritis being the most common clinical conditions observed.

Varicella and Herpes Zoster

ANNE A. GERSHON, M.D.

Varicella and herpes zoster are both caused by the same agent, varicella-zoster (VZ) virus. Varicella occurs when susceptible individuals are exposed to the virus. Herpes zoster is seen in persons who have had varicella previously. It is due to reactivation of latent VZ virus acquired during varicella. Varicella might thus be thought of as secondary to exogenous exposure to VZ virus and zoster as secondary to endogenous exposure to the agent.

VARICELLA (CHICKENPOX)

Symptomatic Treatment. Since varicella is commonly a mild self-limited disease in children, therapeutic aims usually are to treat symptoms such as fever and itching. Antipyretics (see below), oral antihistamines, baking soda baths, and calamine lotion applied to skin lesions are most often used. To minimize secondary bacterial infection of skin lesions the patient's fingernails should be cut short, and daily bathing is advised.

Complications.   BACTERIAL SUPERINFECTION. The most common sites for bacterial superinfection are the skin and the respiratory tract. Skin infections may progress from superficial to deep, resulting in cellulitis. On occasion deep vein thrombosis or gangrene may develop. Bacterial infection of the skin that appears to be progressive should be treated vigorously with warm soaks and appropriate antibiotics, usually penicillin or a penicillinase-resistant semisynthetic penicillin. If cellulitis is present, blood cultures as well as cultures of the local site should be obtained. If an extremity is involved, it should be elevated. Deep-seated infections or gangrene due to staphylococci or group A beta-hemolytic streptococci may require protracted intravenous antibiotic therapy as well as surgical management. If deep vein thrombosis is present, anticoagulants should be considered. "Bullous varicella" represents a form of the staphylococcal scalded skin syndrome and should be treated as such.

Superinfection of the respiratory tract may be due to *Haemophilus influenzae*, pneumococcus, or staphylococcus. Pneumonia following varicella in an otherwise normal child should be regarded as bacterial until proved otherwise, and it should be treated vigorously with broad-spectrum antibiotics until the infecting organism can be identified.

ENCEPHALITIS. Encephalitis is an unusual complication of varicella in normal children and may be life-threatening. Two types have been described: cerebral, usually associated with seizures and altered mental status; and cerebellar, usually associated with ataxia. Cerebellar involvement carries a good prognosis; complete recovery is the rule. In contrast, the cerebral form is often severe, resulting in either death or brain damage. Varicella encephalitis may occur just before or up to two weeks after onset of the rash. It must, of course, be distinguished from other types of viral or toxic encephalitis, and bacterial meningitis should be ruled out. There is no proven specific therapy.

Reye's syndrome has been reported to follow varicella roughly once in every ten thousand cases. To decrease or avoid this complication it seems reasonable not to administer aspirin to children with fever due to varicella. While a causative role for aspirin in Reye's syndrome has not been established, it seems prudent to control fever due to varicella with acetaminophen or tepid baths until the etiology of Reye's syndrome is better understood.

OCULAR LESIONS. Ocular lesions may occur in varicella. They are usually superficial and heal spontaneously. No specific therapy is recommended, but in severe cases an ophthalmologist should be consulted.

MISCELLANEOUS. Miscellaneous complications such as thrombocytopenia, glomerulonephritis, arthritis, and clinical hepatitis are rare following varicella. Such entities should be treated as in any other patient with these manifestations. Subclinical elevations of liver enzymes are not uncommon during varicella; this benign form of hepatitis resolves spontaneously.

Varicella in the Immunocompromised

Varicella may be severe or fatal in immunocompromised patients. At particular risk are those with no prior history of varicella and any of the following: (1) malignant disease being treated with chemotherapy and/or radiotherapy, (2) organ transplantation, (3) congenital or acquired defects in cell-mediated immunity, and (4) receipt of prednisone at doses greater than 1.5 mg/kg/day. Infants born to women with the onset of varicella 5 days or less prior to delivery may also develop severe varicella.

Those at high risk to develop severe varicella should be passively immunized following close exposure to a person with varicella or herpes zoster (see below). During the potential incubation period of varicella, it is advisable to taper steroid dosage to physiologic levels and to withhold chemotherapy and/or radiotherapy even if passive immunization has been given.

Two types of severe varicella have been observed in high-risk children. One is rapidly fatal, with high fever and disseminated intravascular coagulation. The other is initially indolent, but new crops of vesicles continue to develop for up to two weeks. Dissemination of virus may result in pneumonia, encephalitis, and/or hepatitis. Varicella pneumonia is usually manifested by dyspnea, hypoxia, and bilateral fluffy pulmonary infiltrates. Respiratory failure and death may ensue. Treatment includes oxygen and respiratory assistance if necessary and antiviral chemotherapy (see below). Blood gas levels should be monitored closely. Steroids are of unproven value. Passive immunization is probably not useful once varicella has developed, although this is a controversial issue.

Passive Immunization Against Varicella. This is best accomplished by administration of varicella-zoster immune globulin (VZIG). VZIG is prepared from plasma from normal individuals with high antibody titers to VZ virus. VZIG has now replaced zoster immune globulin (ZIG), which was prepared from plasma of donors convalescing from zoster. This is because (1) the two preparations are equally effective, and (2) donors for VZIG are easier to recruit in greater numbers than donors for ZIG. VZIG is licensed and available through regional offices of the American Red Cross. Supplies are not unlimited, so VZIG should not be used indiscriminately. It costs about $75 for a vial containing 1.25 ml.

VZIG should be given to high-risk susceptibles (i.e. no prior history of clinical varicella) within 72 hours of close exposure to VZ virus (such as occurs in a household or when young children play closely indoors for more than 1 hour). VZIG is given IM, 1.25 ml for every 10 kg of body weight; up to a maximum of 6.25 ml.

VZIG usually modifies but does not prevent varicella in high-risk patients. Modified disease is manifested by mild illness—few lesions, little or no fever, and perhaps a prolonged incubation period. Subclinical infection detected serologically following VZIG has been identified. Rarely a high-risk patient develops severe varicella despite appropriate passive immunization with VZIG. In such an instance, there should be no hesitation to administer antiviral chemotherapy as well.

Passive immunization against varicella may also be accomplished by administering plasma from a person with zoster (ZIP). This method is less safe than VZIG, since it carries the risk of transmission of hepatitis and potentially AIDS. Immune globulin (IG) contains too little antibody to VZ virus to be of practical use for passive immunization. VZIG has not been shown to have any role in the prevention of zoster. Patients developing zoster already have high circulating titers of VZ antibody.

Antiviral Chemotherapy

Two drugs are currently being used, although neither is licensed for this particular indication. While both are efficacious against chickenpox and zoster, neither drug prevents development of latent infection.

Vidarabine (adenine arabinoside or Ara-A) for IV use has been available for approximately the past 10 years. It exerts its antiviral effect by interfering with synthesis of both viral and host DNA. While it is relatively nontoxic, it causes some adverse effects, probably because it inhibits host DNA synthesis. Toxic effects are, in order of their frequency, rash, nausea and vomiting, and neurologic symptoms ranging from tremors to frank but self-limited psychotic signs such as hallucinations.

Despite its toxicity, however, there is good evidence that Ara-A is effective for treatment of severe varicella. It is given IV, 10 mg/kg/day over a 12-hour period for 7 or more days, depending on the response of the patient. It may be expected to hasten the healing of lesions and decrease the incidence of complications such as pneumonia, encephalitis and hepatitis.

The other useful antiviral drug, acyclovir (ACV), has also been licensed for IV use to treat severe herpes simplex infections, but it too has been employed successfully to treat severe VZ virus infections, particularly in immunocompromised patients. It is very well tolerated; the only side effects reported with any frequency have been phlebitis due to the high pH of the IV solution, and reversible elevation of the creatinine clearance.

ACV is probably well tolerated because, unlike Ara-A, it interferes mainly with synthesis of viral DNA. It requires the presence of a virus-induced enzyme, thymidine kinase, to exert its antiviral effects, which probably explains its relative lack of toxicity for the host. Synthesis of DNA is impaired only in virus-infected cells. Unfortunately, however, the enzyme is not required for viral replication, and therefore resistance to ACV may occur. The full clinical implications of this resistance are not yet known. At this time no clinical VZ infections have been caused by virus resistant to ACV, but in the future this may become a problem.

Antiviral therapy is most successful when it is administered as *early* in the course of the illness as possible, usually within 3 days of onset. Some patients cannot respond to antiviral therapy because the illness is too fulminant. For those with the more indolent form of illness, the decision as to when to begin antiviral therapy may be difficult. When it is clear that therapy is needed, it may be too late. For this reason and also since ACV is so well tolerated, our approach is to hospitalize all immunocompromised patients with varicella for IV ACV therapy. This does not apply, however, to those who have received VZIG appropriately or those who have had varicella vaccine (see below) unless they appear very ill. The aim today is to treat the patient with potentially severe varicella before the disease has had an opportunity to progress to complications such as pneumonia.

ACV is administered IV, 1500 mg/m^2/day in 3 divided doses for 5 to 7 days, depending on the condition of the patient. At this dosage, peak serum levels of ACV can be expected to be more than 5 times the in vitro inhibitory concentration of ACV for VZ virus (about 5 μM). Our opinion concerning ACV is that while there are fewer published articles concerning its efficacy than there are for Ara-A, there is a great deal of favorable anecdotal information as well as data on drug levels. ACV is better tolerated and easier to administer than Ara-A. Consequently we feel that it is the drug of choice for potentially severe or severe varicella. There are no data concerning use of both Ara-A and ACV together, and therefore this combination is not recommended.

The role of antiviral therapy in treatment of isolated encephalitis has not been established. It is controversial as to whether patients with isolated varicella encephalitis should be given antiviral therapy or not. Our usual policy is to administer antiviral therapy if the patient with encephalitis is immunocompromised.

Other experimental forms of therapy for varicella in the immunocompromised include interferon, transfer factor, and irradiated (3000 R) lymphocytes from an immune individual. ACV that may be administered by mouth has recently been licensed. Despite the appeal that this drug might theoretically have for treatment of chickenpox, it cannot be recommended at this time except on an experimental basis.*

HERPES ZOSTER (SHINGLES)

This syndrome is not uncommon in children who have already had chickenpox. It is usually mild and self-limited, requiring no specific therapy.

Some persons with herpes zoster, especially those who are immunocompromised, may manifest dissemination of VZ virus, clinically suggestive of coexistence of varicella and zoster. In such instances, treatment with ACV or Ara-A as outlined above should be considered. The mortality (roughly 1–2%) for untreated disseminated zoster in immunocompromised patients does not seem to be as high as for varicella in these patients (roughly 10–15%). Therefore the decision concerning which zoster patient to treat may be exceedingly difficult. Those presumed to be severely immunocompromised are usually treated even at an early stage of illness. As for varicella, the best therapeutic effects are seen when treatment is begun within 3 days after onset of zoster. Antiviral therapy has no effect on the incidence of postherpetic pain, although the duration of pain may be shortened. Postherpetic pain is rare in children; it is a serious problem, however, for older adults.

Ocular lesions due to zoster are often deep seated and difficult to treat. An ophthalmologist should be consulted for this complication. Facial zoster may be associated with some degree of mild encephalitis and abnormal spinal fluid. In otherwise normal patients this is usually self-limited; antiviral chemotherapy should be considered for immunocompromised patients with this complication.

Varicella Vaccine. A live attenuated vaccine was developed in Japan about 10 years ago. This vaccine is not yet licensed in the United States, but it is available on a research basis. The vaccine is well tolerated and immunogenic in normal children and adults, and in children with leukemia in remission. It appears to confer significant protection against disease caused by the wild virus. Breakthrough cases of varicella have occurred following exposure of leukemic vaccines to wild

VZ virus, but these cases have almost always been mild. Licensure of the vaccine for normal and immunocompromised varicella susceptibles is expected in the United States by 1987.

Herpes Simplex Virus Infections

JOSEPH W. ST. GEME, JR., M.D.

Herpes simplex virus (HSV) is one of the most prevalent of the human herpesviruses. The other members of this family of viruses are varicella-zoster virus, cytomegalovirus, and Epstein-Barr virus.

Primary Gingivostomatitis. This condition may last 1 week and be so painful that nutrition is impaired. Therapy is often unsatisfactory. Topical dental analgesic solutions, chilled fluids, soft foods, and systemic analgesic-antipyretic medications constitute the bulwark of symptomatic treatment for this ordinarily self-contained illness. Systemic dissemination may occur in immunodeficient individuals and require chemotherapy with parenteral adenine arabinoside or oral or parenteral acyclovir (acyloguanosine), a highly specific anti-DNA virus purine analog.

Recurrent Herpes Labialis. Topical antiviral solutions, lotions, and ointments containing iododeoxyuridine and adenine arabinoside are of equivocal therapeutic value. Immediate treatment of recurrent lesions with topical or oral acyclovir at the first appearance of symptoms in nonimmunocompromised patients may ultimately prove beneficial. Immunocompromised children with limited infections should be treated swiftly with acyclovir. Topical application of acetone or alcohol may hasten the resolution and desiccation of vesicular lesions. These organic solvents may also diminish the quantity of HSV in these lesions because of the suceptibility of virions with abundant lipid envelopes to degradation by such chemicals.

Keratoconjunctivitis. Serious, destructive primary or secondary (reactivation) ophthalmic infections may occur due to HSV type 1. Occasionally, HSV type 2 may produce the same process in the newborn infant. Treatment of this illness marked the initial success with specific antiviral chemotherapy. Unless deep stromal tissues are affected, HSV keratoconjunctivitis responds nicely to therapy with topical 0.1% iododeoxyuridine ophthalmic solution. Occasional mutant strains of HSV, which do not elaborate the thymidine kinase enzyme necessary to activate this pyrimidine analog, are resistant to iododeoxyuridine and can be treated effectively with topical adenine arabinoside.

Vulvovaginitis, Cervicitis, and Prepucitis. Vul-

---

* Safety and efficacy of oral acyclovir in children have not been established.

var and vaginal lesions are particularly distressing. Unfortunately, topical therapy with iododeoxyuridine, adenine arabinoside, and adenine arabinoside 5'-monophosphate is ineffective. Oral and/or topical acyclovir treatment of primary infections is effective. Immediate acyclovir therapy of recurrent infections is moderately successful. Protracted, continuous oral acyclovir treatment suppresses recurrence but only for the duration of treatment. In general, HSV type 2 is less susceptible to these antiviral agents than is HSV type 1. Photodynamic inactivation of HSV with neutral red and other photoactive dyes, thought initially to be efficacious, has proved to be inadequate and, because of HSV mutagenic potential, may be hazardous. It is frustrating that genital HSV infections, so discomforting to women in particular and potentially threatening to the offspring of pregnant women, cannot be managed with any modality more salutary than sitz baths.

Meningoencephalitis. Following definitive diagnosis, therapy should be instituted for 10 days with parenteral adenine arabinoside at a dosage of 15 mg/kg body weight/24 hr over 12 hours in concentrations not exceeding 0.7 mg/ml of standard intravenous solution. Such treatment may reduce mortality from 70 to 30% and improve the quality of survival for those individuals who escape the lethality of this neurotropic virus. Ultimately, parenteral acyclovir may become the preferred treatment. Preliminary data from Sweden and the United States suggest that parenteral acyclovir, 10 mg/kg body weight every 8 hours for 10 days is more effective than adenine arabinoside.

Perinatal Infection. Recent collaborative study data indicate that the mortality and morbidity of these infections, particularly the moderately serious nondisseminated neonatal meningoencephalitis, can be attenuated by parenteral adenine arabinoside therapy at a dosage of 15 mg/kg body weight/24 hr over 12 hours, as described above. With localized meningoencephalitis, mortality was reduced from 50 to 10% and morbidity from 83 to 50% with adenine arabinoside therapy. Specific diagnosis is simpler in these perinatal infections because the predominant HSV type 2 can be isolated from the cutaneous vesicular lesions, conjunctiva, oropharynx, urine, and spinal fluid of these infants. The risk of transparturient transmission of this perinatal viral pathogen can be modified by cesarean section if the amniotic membranes remain intact. It is also comforting that the majority of the maternal infections seem to occur at some time other than the final few weeks of pregnancy.

Because so many of these genital infections during pregnancy represent reactivation of HSV type 2 in immune women, the duration of lesions is shorter and quantity of virus is less, and specific maternal IgG-neutralizing antibody is transferred to the infant across the placenta. Consequently, the risk of HSV transmission from women with primary lesions to their offspring, which is 50%, falls to 5% in women with secondary reactivated lesions.

Eczema Herpeticum. This unusual infection represents the topical inoculations of the eczematous skin of an infant or child with HSV type 1 as a result of contact with a person who has recurrent herpes labialis or is a silent virus shedder. The vesicular and vesiculoulcerative lesions may persist for a week or more. Infrequently, HSV disseminates to noneczematous skin and other somatic sites. Mortality and morbidity are very low unless the afflicted child is malnourished or immunodeficient. In these more precarious situations, one should consider treatment with large doses of standard gamma globulin, 0.5 ml/kg body weight, and parenteral adenine arabinoside* or acyclovir in addition to wet-to-dry sterile saline dressings of the cutaneous lesions.

Mumps

STEPHEN R. PREBLUD, M.D.

Mumps (epidemic parotitis) is caused by an RNA virus belonging to the myxovirus group, which also includes the influenza and parainfluenza viruses. The virus causes a generalized disease that is usually clinically apparent. However, approximately 30% of affected individuals may have subclinical infection. Immunity is generally long-lasting, even following subclinical infection.

Cases of uncomplicated mumps require only supportive therapy, which includes rest, hydration, and management of fever and the discomfort associated with salivary gland inflammation. While alteration in the diet is frequently not necessary, avoidance of acid foods, such as citrus juices, minimizes secretion of the glands' digestive enzymes and may help decrease the pain. Aspirin or acetaminophen is usually adequate analgesic-antipyretic therapy. The dose of aspirin is 65–100 mg/kg per day, and the dose of acetaminophen is 30–40 mg/kg per day, divided into 4–6 doses. There is no association between the level of the patient's activity and the risk of mumps-related complications. However, normal outside activities should be limited to avoid unnecessary spread of disease.

Complications

Epididymo-orchitis. Epididymo-orchitis is the most frequently observed complication associated with mumps infection. Treatment usually involves

---

* This use of adenine arabinoside is not listed by the manufacturer.

bed rest, analgesia, and elevation of the affected testicle. The efficacy of ice packs is subjective. Surgical intervention is not ordinarily necessary. However, hospitalization may be indicated when parenteral analgesics are required. Because of its lack of efficacy, mumps immune globulin is no longer available. Administration of standard immune globulin is not indicated.

Meningitis and Encephalitis. Central nervous system involvement, manifest most often as aseptic meningitis and less frequently as encephalitis, is a relatively common complication. The literature does not always distinguish between aseptic meningitis and encephalitis, hence the commonly used term meningoencephalitis. Therapy is generally supportive and includes bed rest, oral fluids as tolerated, and analgesic-antipyretic medication. Hospitalization may be indicated because of diagnostic uncertainties or excessive fluid loss due to vomiting. Parenteral hydration should take into account maintenance fluid needs plus losses associated with emesis. However, as is the case with bacterial meningitis, signs of inappropriate antidiuretic hormone release during the first few days of the illness may necessitate some restriction and electrolyte alteration of fluids. While a lumbar puncture may be necessary diagnostically, its use solely to help relieve headache is not warranted.

Deafness. Mumps-associated deafness is a rare but significant residuum of mumps infection. The virus had been isolated from perilymph fluid. It is estimated to occur once in every 15,000 to 20,000 cases of mumps. It may occur with or without meningoencephalitis. Onset is usually one week after parotitis. The hearing loss is usually unilateral and is often permanent.

Pancreatitis. Clinically apparent pancreatitis is estimated to occur in 1% of mumps infections. However, mild elevation of pancreatic enzymes in the absence of symptoms may occur in up to 40% of patients. Parotitis may or not be present. Occasionally, the pancreatitis can result in transient glucose intolerance. Treatment includes bed rest, fluids, and relief of discomfort as necessary. Use of insulin is individualized.

There are some epidemiologic and virologic data suggesting that mumps infection may be involved in the manifestation of diabetes mellitus after a latent period of several years. Other data, however, do not support this possible association.

Congenital Infection. Maternal mumps infection is associated with an increased risk of fetal wastage. However, although mumps virus has been isolated from a fetus, there is no convincing evidence that fetal infection is associated with congenital abnormalities. Aqueductal stenosis and subendocardial fibroelastosis, previously thought to be due to congenital mumps infection, are no longer felt to be related to intrauterine infection with mumps virus.

Other Complications. Some other complications reported to have occurred with mumps infection are arthritis, mastitis, myocarditis, hepatitis, nephritis, oophoritis, thyroiditis, and thrombocytopenia. Death occurs rarely. Some possible complications only temporally associated with mumps infection are Guillain-Barré syndrome, myelitis, and neuritis. There are also some data suggesting that there may be an association between mumps infection and ovarian carcinoma.

Prevention

The administration of over 60 million doses of the Jeryl Lynn strain of live attenuated mumps vaccine in the United States since 1967 has been associated with a 98% decrease in the reported incidence of mumps. This vaccine has been shown to induce antibodies in over 95% of vaccinees in clinical trials. The vaccine is noncommunicable. Side effects of vaccination occur very infrequently. Parotitis, rash, pruritus, purpura, and orchitis have been temporally associated with mumps vaccination but are uncommon and usually mild and of brief duration. Very rarely, febrile seizures, unilateral nerve deafness, and encephalitis within 30 days of vaccination are reported. Obviously, temporal association does not necessarily indicate true cause and effect. No vaccine-associated deaths have been reported. Epidemiologic studies indicate that the risk of infection following vaccination is reduced by at least 85%. Vaccine-induced immunity is expected to be lifelong.

Since young children are at highest risk for mumps infection, mumps vaccine is recommended for all children 12 months of age or older. Mumps vaccine combined with measles (and rubella) vaccine should not be administered until 15 months of age. The vaccine can be particularly beneficial for older children and adolescents and adults, especially males, who have not had mumps. While many individuals with a negative history of mumps infection are in fact immune (in part because of subclinical infection), there is no increased risk of side reactions following vaccination of an immune person. Serologic and skin tests for immunity may be misleading, unreliable, or simply unavailable and should not be obtained prior to immunization.

The only means of possibly preventing mumps infection after exposure may be vaccination. Immune globulin administration is not recommended. While mumps vaccine given shortly after exposure may not provide protection, there is no contraindication to its use. Disease severity is not altered, and protection against future exposures can be provided if the exposure in question does not result in infection.

As is the case with any live vaccine, there are

some contraindications to vaccination. Since vaccine virus can cross the placenta, pregnant women should not be vaccinated. Other contraindications include anaphylactic allergy to vaccine components, especially neomycin; recent administration of immune globulin; severe febrile illnesses; and immune deficiency conditions. Egg allergy is not a contraindication to vaccination unless the patient has a history of a prior anaphylactic reaction following exposure to egg white. However, even in this case, vaccine may be administered following a protocol of skin testing. If such testing is positive, vaccine may be injected in incremental amounts.

Like measles and rubella vaccines, mumps vaccine suppresses cellular immunity for a few weeks following administration. Practically, this means that tuberculin skin testing should be done prior to vaccination, at the time of vaccination, or at least 4 weeks later.

Influenza

JOHN M. ZAHRADNIK, M.D.

Yearly influenza illnesses continue to exert significant medical, social, and economic problems within nearly every community. Symptomatology and physical signs frequently mimic illness caused by other viruses, but in general the result is a spectrum of illness, extending from the asymptomatic child to the more classical complaints of fever, malaise, myalgia, headache, sore throat, arthralgia, and upper respiratory tract symptoms. Epidemiologic and virologic information disseminated by local and state health departments and from the Centers for Disease Control are invaluable aids that can guide therapy. Current recommendations include prophylactic immunization with the current influenza virus vaccines and both the therapeutic and prophylactic use of amantadine.

Treatment. Uncomplicated influenza virus infection in children usually requires no specific therapy. However, therapeutic relief of some symptoms may include the use of acetaminophen for fever, glyceryl guaiacolate for cough, or if needed, an antitussive such as dextromethorphan and plenty of fluids to maintain hydration. The use of aspirin treatment for an influenza-like illness in children, including teenagers, during the influenza season is inappropriate, as a strong association between salicylate usage and the subsequent development of Reye's syndrome has been demonstrated. In addition, parents and children should be discouraged from self-medicating with non-prescription pharmaceuticals containing salicylates.

Amantadine hydrochloride (Symmetrel) has been effective in reducing the duration of fever and other systemic symptoms associated with type A influenza virus infections, when administered within 24 to 48 hours after the onset of symptoms. It has been evaluated and approved for use in children 1 year of age and older at a dose of 4.4–8.8 mg/kg body weight/24 hours in two divided doses, administered for 48 hours after resolution of the systemic symptoms (usually a total of 5 days). The drug is available as a syrup containing 50 mg/5 ml and as 100 mg capsules. The total daily dosage should be limited to 150 mg/24 hours in children under 9 years of age and 200 mg/24 hours for those 10 years of age and older (100 mg twice daily). It is especially recommended for high-risk children who are unvaccinated, as an adjunct to late immunization and as supplemental protection in patients in whom a poor immune response to vaccination may be expected (i.e., those with a severe immunodeficiency). A reduction of the dosage should be considered in those children with impaired renal function. The prophylactic use of amantadine should be continued daily for the duration of influenza A activity in the community (usually lasts 6–12 weeks within a given community). It is not effective against influenza B.

Ribavirin (Virazole), another antiviral agent, has been successfully used in the treatment of acute influenza infection, including influenza B, when administered as an aerosol, and should be available in the near future.

Complications. Respiratory tract complications, including croup or laryngitis, may be helped with cool mist therapy. Secondary bacterial infections, such as otitis media, sinusitis, or pneumonia, may develop; and appropriate antibiotic treatment should be instituted against the most likely respiratory tract pathogens, Streptococcus pneumoniae, Haemophilus influenzae or Staphylococcus aureus.

Convulsions may occur on occasion, and a bacterial central nervous system infection should be ruled out. Reye's syndrome, an acute noninflammatory encephalopathy with an altered state of consciousness, occurs primarily in school-aged children but can be a serious complication at any age following either influenza A or B. Management of this condition is discussed in another section.

Acute myositis is seen primarily in children, usually following an influenza B infection. It is usually a self-limited complication with complete recovery.

Immunization. Influenza virus vaccine is especially recommended for children with chronic or acute conditions that make them susceptible to serious complications of influenza. Such conditions include (1) cardiac disease, including congenital heart disease and rheumatic heart disease; (2) chronic bronchopulmonary disease, such as asthma, bronchiectasis, chronic bronchiolitis, cystic fibrosis, or other instances in which the pulmonary system is compromised (i.e., neonatal intensive care unit graduates with a history of pulmonary disease); (3) chronic metabolic diseases, including diabetes mellitus; (4) renal dysfunction, such as chronic glomerulonephritis or nephroses; (5) anemia, including sickle cell disease; (6) immunosuppression; and (7) chronic neurologic disorders, especially those involving ventilation. In addition, it seems appropriate that children being treated with long-term aspirin therapy (i.e., Kawasaki's disease, rheumatoid disorders) should also receive influenza virus vaccine.

Primary immunization requires two injections of inactivated, split virus vaccine administered 4 weeks apart for children up to age 12 years. The dosage for children under 36 months of age is one-half (0.25 ml) that given to older children (0.5 ml). Children over 12 years can usually be protected with one 0.5 ml dose of either the split virus or whole virus preparation. In previously vaccinated children, only a single booster dose is necessary in subsequent years unless a major shift in the virus occurs that necessitates that the new influenza virus antigen be added to the vaccine preparation. There has been no increased risk of Guillain-Barré syndrome observed in association with influenza virus vaccine since surveillance began in 1978. Vaccine should not be given to children who have allergies to eggs, as the preparation is initially grown in embryonated hen's eggs and may contain some residual host protein.

Rabies

PAUL F. WEHRLE, M.D.

Rabies is present as a viral zoonosis in many species of animals. Among domestic animals, dogs have until recently served as the most important source of infection for man. Improved dog control and rabies immunization requirements prior to dog licensure have substantially reduced this hazard. Only approximately 100 cases of canine rabies have been reported annually in the United States during recent years. In contrast, the disease in wildlife, particularly among bats, skunks, foxes, and raccoons, has been recognized more frequently. The popularity of some of these species as household pets and the increased interest in outdoor recreational activities provide a greater opportunity for contact with man. Wild animals, with more than 85% of reported animal rabies, now represent the greatest rabies exposure hazard for man in the United States. There is no reason to believe that sylvatic rabies among wild animals throughout the United States will change signifi-

cantly in the future, except to increase in some species, such as raccoons. Of the individual states only Hawaii remains consistently rabies-free.

In the United States approximately 25,000 persons receive rabies prophylaxis each year. This may be an important reason that annually only 0 to 5 cases of human rabies have been reported; one to three cases each year follow exposure in foreign countries.

Management After Exposure

Evaluation of Animal. If saliva from an animal is introduced by bite or contact with mucous membranes or recently abraded skin, the animal must be evaluated. Rabies virus is present in saliva up to two weeks before clinical signs appear. For domestic animals consideration should be given to the species of the animal, its potential exposure to rabies infection, its immunization history, and the circumstances of the bite. A provoked bite by a well cared for and previously immunized pet should cause little concern other than for the mechanical injury itself, while a bite by a dog not available for examination and of unknown origin in a rabies endemic area requires prophylaxis. A bite by a wild animal or a bat always requires prophylaxis, as does a bite by an animal found to be rabid by laboratory identification of rabies virus antigen.

Local and state health officials are excellent sources of information concerning the current prevalence of rabies in particular animal species. If assistance in determining the probability of infection is required, consultation is advisable. Some species, for example, rodents, are seldom if ever a source of concern, while bites of skunks and bats always require prompt attention and prophylaxis. Local and regional rabies prevalence data are often helpful in reaching postexposure treatment decisions.

NOTE: A useful guide for management following exposure is presented in Table 1. This guide has been prepared by the Immunization Practices Advisory Committee (ACIP) and is available from the Centers for Disease Control (CDC), Atlanta, Georgia 30333 as MMWR 33:393–402, 1984. Telephone consultation also is available to supplement local or state resources at (404) 329-3095.

Local Treatment. Careful irrigation and thorough washing of the wound is the most important single prophylactic measure. Although many substances have been used, soapy water is effective and should be used as promptly as possible for primary treatment. Such washing has been shown, in the experimental model, to reduce the risk of rabies by 80–90%. Tetanus prophylaxis may also be indicated.

Rabies Immunizing Products. Two different

Table 1. RABIES POSTEXPOSURE PROPHYLAXIS GUIDE—JULY 1984

The following recommendations are only a guide. In applying them, take into account the animal species involved, the circumstances of the bite or other exposure, the vaccination status of the animal, and presence of rabies in the region. Local or state public health officials should be consulted if questions arise about the need for rabies prophylaxis.

Animal Species	Condition of Animal at Time of Attack	Treatment of Exposed Person*
Domestic Dog and cat	Healthy and available for 10 days observation	None, unless animal develops rabies†
	Rabid or suspected rabid	RIG§ and HDCV
	Unknown (escaped)	Consult public health officials. If treatment is indicated, give RIG§ and HDCV
Wild Skunk, bat, fox, coyote, raccoon, bobcat, and other carnivores	Regard as rabid unless proven negative by laboratory tests¶	RIG§ and HDCV
Other Livestock, rodents, and lagomorphs (rabbits and hares)	Consider individually. Local and state public health officials should be consulted on questions about the need for rabies prophylaxis. Bites of squirrels, hamsters, guinea pigs, gerbils, chipmunks, rats, mice, other rodents, rabbits, and hares almost never call for antirabies prophylaxis.	

* *All bites and wounds should immediately be thoroughly cleansed with soap and water.* If antirabies treatment is indicated, both rabies immune globulin (RIG) and human diploid cell rabies vaccine (HDCV) should be given as soon as possible, *regardless* of the interval from exposure. Local reactions to vaccines are common and do not contraindicate continuing treatment. Discontinue vaccine if fluorescent-antibody tests of the animal are negative.

† During the usual holding period of ten days, begin treatment with RIG and HDCV at first sign of rabies in a dog or cat that has bitten someone. The symptomatic animal should be killed immediately and tested.

§ If RIG is not available, use antirabies serum, equine (ARS). Do not use more than the recommended dosage.

¶ The animal should be killed and tested as soon as possible. Holding for observation is not recommended.

types of immunizing products are available for use in humans. These are inactivated rabies vaccines, which induce an active immune response. This response requires 7–10 days to develop and persists for at least a year. Also, globulins that contain pre-formed antibody are available. These provide prompt or immediate passive protection, which persists for several weeks. Both types of product should be used concurrently for rabies postexposure treatment when prophylaxis is indicated.

Passive Immunization. There is a delay of several days in antibody response following active immunization, and the incubation period for rabies may be as brief as 10 days. Therefore, if rabies prophylaxis is indicated, antirabies serum (ARS) or rabies immune globulin (RIG), human, should be administered. The latter product, since it is derived from human plasma, gives more lasting protection and is relatively free from reactions. It is the preferred product, when available.

RIG is administered as a single dose as soon as possible after the bite has occurred. The recommended dose is 20 IU/kg or approximately 9 IU/lb body weight. Whenever possible, half of the dose of RIG should be thoroughly infiltrated in the area around the wound, avoiding tendons and other structures potentially damaged by direct injection. The remainder is to be administered intramuscularly. Since passive antibody has been shown to suppress active antibody following vaccines, excessive doses of RIG should be avoided, and the recommended dosage followed closely.

If ARS must be used because RIG is not available, the package insert should be consulted for detailed instructions and precautions.

Postexposure Immunization. Presently two vaccines are available, both prepared in human diploid cell culture. These are inactivated human diploid cell vaccines (HDCV) prepared from fixed rabies virus grown in WI-38 or in MRC-5 human diploid cell cultures. The vaccine virus is chemically inactivated and supplied in 1-ml single dose vials containing the lyophilized vaccine; only the accompanying diluent should be used for reconstitution.

Since the incubation period for rabies may be as short as 10 days or as long as more than one year following exposure, postexposure antirabies immunization should always include both passively administered antibody (preferably RIG) and vaccine (HDCV), with only one exception: persons who have been previously immunized with rabies vaccine and have a prior laboratory documented rabies antibody titer should receive only vaccine. Although treatment should be instituted as soon as possible after exposure, if delay has occurred, treatment should be given regardless of the interval between exposure and treatment. If several months have elapsed, treatment may be unnecessary but should at least be considered, since the incubation period may be prolonged and treatment may still be of benefit.

HDCV. Single 1-ml doses of vaccine should be given intramuscularly, e.g., deltoid region, beginning as soon as possible after the exposure. After the initial dose, additional doses are given on days 3, 7, 14, and 28. A sixth dose 90 days after the initial dose has been recommended by the World Health Organization. Routine postvaccination serologic testing for rabies antibody is no longer recommended. Although antibody response has been reported following intradermal inoculation of this vaccine, the data available presently do not permit reliance on this route for postexposure prophylaxis.

Should RIG (or ARS) be unavailable at the time the series is instituted, it may be given up to 8 days after the first dose of vaccine. After that time it is considered unnecessary, since antibody response to HDCV should be present. It should be emphasized that only a single dose of RIG is needed.

ADVERSE REACTIONS TO HDCV. Although local and systemic reactions to HDCV have been infrequent, some patients (1 per 625 treated) have reported systemic allergic reactions, including urticaria and anaphylactic shock. A similar frequency of fever and headache has also been reported. Whether these are due to the vaccine or simply associated temporally is unknown. No deaths or cases of postvaccinal encephalopathy have been reported. In no instance was it necessary to discontinue the postexposure prophylaxis regimen. Physicians should be alert to the possibility of reactions with any vaccine, including HDCV.

Pre-exposure Immunization

Persons in high rabies risk groups such as veterinarians, animal handlers, spelunkers, and persons living in or visiting countries where rabies is a serious problem should consider pre-exposure prophylaxis. The use of vaccines prior to exposure may provide protection for those with unexpected or unrecognized exposure and, in addition, eliminates the need for RIG and decreases the number of doses of vaccine required should exposure occur.

Three 1-ml intramuscular injections of HDCV should be given intramuscularly in the deltoid area on days 0, 7, and 28. This can be expected to dependably stimulate antibody in recipients. All who receive pre-exposure immunization should be re-evaluated periodically regarding the degree of continuing risk. Antibody testing and/or additional doses of HDCV may be indicated.

Accidental Inoculation with Live Virus Rabies Vaccines Intended for Animals

Persons vaccinating animals with modified live rabies vaccines for animal use should have received pre-exposure rabies immunization. For those accidentally exposed by direct inoculation with attenuated live rabies vaccines intended for animals, and who have not received prior pre-exposure immunization, the post-exposure routines indicated above may be considered. This may be unnecessary, since the risk, if any, must be extremely small indeed. The possibility of vaccine-induced rabies exists, even though none has been reported in humans.

Treatment of Clinical Rabies

Since at least one and perhaps three patients have recovered from clinical rabies following intensive therapy, life support measures are indicated. Vaccine, RIG, monitoring of intracranial pressure, and other measures may be utilized. Regional health resources and the Centers for Disease Control, Atlanta, Georgia, should be consulted for advice from those experienced in rabies treatment. Protection (vaccine, clothing, gloves) should be provided for those caring for these patients. (No rabies has been reported in staff.)

Tetanus Prophylaxis

Since tetanus has been reported following animal bites and since the injury often fulfills the criteria for "tetanus prone wounds," the tetanus immunization history should be verified. A tetanus toxoid booster dose is indicated, with or without human hyperimmune globulin, depending on prior tetanus toxoid immunization status.

Infectious Mononucleosis

MARIE F. ROBERT, M.D.
and WARREN A. ANDIMAN, M.D.

The Epstein-Barr virus is the etiologic agent of heterophile-positive infectious mononucleosis (IM). The virus is also associated with a spectrum of syndromes including subclinical infection (as occurs in most children throughout the world), chronic mononucleosis, a variety of lymphoproliferative disorders and polyclonal B cell lymphomas that occur in individuals with discrete forms of immunoincompetence, and with two human cancers—Burkitt lymphoma and nasopharyngeal carcinoma.

IM is generally a benign, self-limited disease of adolescents and young adults. It is characterized by fever, lymphadenopathy, pharyngitis, and an absolute lymphocytosis with many atypical forms. Hepatitis and splenomegaly are not uncommon. Disorders of the hematopoietic system sometimes result from the production of antibodies to erythrocytes, granulocytes, and platelets by cells of the B-cell lineage. The nervous system may become involved as a result of invasion by virus-transformed B cells.

Aspirin and saline gargles may reduce the pain associated with the pharyngitis and tonsillitis of IM. Occasionally, codeine is required to relieve these symptoms. Some patients with IM have severe tonsillopharyngitis and dysphagia. In such individuals, it is imperative to pay heed to the adequacy of the airway. Prednisone or an equivalent steroid preparation has been used to treat this complication with favorable results. In older individuals, it is administered in a dose of 10 mg four times daily for one to two days, after which the dose is tapered rapidly over the course of 5 to 7 days. It is rarely necessary to administer steroids for a longer time. Corticosteroids have also been advocated to treat the hemolytic anemias, thrombocytopenias, and some of the neurologic complications of IM, e.g., Bell's palsy, transverse myelitis, meningoencephalitis and Guillain-Barré syndrome. The use of steroids under these circumstances has not been subjected to double-blind placebo-controlled trials. One study reports a more rapid fall in temperature and a greater subjective feeling of well-being in patients receiving a short course of steroids. The hepatitis of IM and the height of the heterophile antibody response are not affected by the use of steroids.

Acyclovir* has been shown to reduce the replication of Epstein-Barr virus in productive cell lines in vitro. It does not prevent the continuous outgrowth of latently infected transformed cell lines. The drug has been used in one small clinical trial involving hospitalized patients with severe disease. Drug recipients shed less virus and regained weight faster than placebo controls, suggesting a more rapid resolution of pharyngitis. The drug had no effect on splenomegaly, lethargy, lymphadenopathy, or fever or on the ability to recover virus-transformed cell lines from peripheral blood.

Activity in the course of IM should be determined by the severity of symptoms. Complete bed rest is usually not necessary. Vigorous activities and contact sports should be avoided in the presence of splenic enlargement, which occurs in approximately 50% of patients. Splenic rupture is a very rare but potentially fatal complication of IM. Penicillin or other antibiotics should be used only when concurrent throat cultures are positive for Group A, beta-hemolytic streptococcus. Ampicillin should be avoided whenever possible because of the frequent occurrence of skin rash in IM patients treated with this antibiotic.

In contrast to the vast majority of IM patients who recover completely, a very small group of patients develop a chronic mononucleosis syndrome characterized by persistent or recurrent fatigue, myalgia, low-grade fever, slight sore throat, adenopathy, weight loss, sleep disturbances, and psychoneurotic symptoms. This constellation of findings may persist for several years. Many of these patients have abnormal serologic responses to the virus. Unconfirmed and unpublished observations suggest that some patients with chronic IM experience brief alleviation of their symptoms when treated with acyclovir and that shedding of virus may be interrupted temporarily. These trials need to be extended before specific recommendations can be made.

Epstein-Barr virus–associated lymphoproliferative diseases, including lymphoma, occur in some persons with defects in cell-mediated immunity. The immunodeficiency may be congenital (e.g., X-linked lymphoproliferative syndrome) or acquired (e.g., post organ transplant; AIDS). These individuals fail to mount normal cytotoxic T cell or natural killer cell responses to the virus. Some patients who develop Epstein-Barr virus–associated lymphoproliferations following receipt of an allograft and administration of immunosuppressive therapy experience remission of their polyclonal B cell proliferations if their immunosuppressive drugs are reduced in dosage or stopped. It has been reported that some of these patients, especially those with polyclonal lymphomas, also respond to acyclovir. The monoclonal lymphomas do not appear to respond to either treatment modality. There is no evidence to date that patients with X-linked lymphoproliferative syndrome who develop multisystem lymphoproliferations with virus-containing lymphocytes will respond to acyclovir. Some of these neoplasms may respond to traditional chemotherapeutic regimens, but these have not been widely tested.

Cat Scratch Disease

ANDREW M. MARGILETH, M.D.

Cat scratch disease is usually a benign self-limited illness. The specific treatment is difficult, as no chemotherapeutic agent has been effective. Patients should be reassured that the disease is self-limited, with spontaneous resolution expected over a 2- to 4-month period. Supportive care for such symptoms as headache, malaise, and fever is indicated. Analgesics are helpful for the lymph node tenderness, which usually decreases and disappears over a period of 1 to 2 weeks.

Patients should be cautioned about trauma to the enlarged lymph node, since abscess formation may follow direct injury to the nodes. Application of warm moist soaks to the primary inoculation

---

* Safety and efficacy of oral acyclovir in children have not been established.

skin site and/or to the adenitis may help make the patient more comfortable and possibly shorten duration of the primary skin lesion as well as the lymphadenitis. Most importantly, the patient should be followed closely and re-examined at 3- to 4-week intervals to ensure that the adenopathy is gradually decreasing.

In a small percentage (12 to 15%) of patients the lymphadenitis may progress to suppuration. When suppuration becomes painful, needle aspiration (using a 19-gauge needle and aseptic technique) is indicated. We recommend using the side or backdoor approach by inserting the needle through 1 to 2 cm of normal subcutaneous tissue before entering the abscess. This should avoid chronic sinus tract drainage in the event that a tuberculous lesion is present. Aspiration will relieve the patient's pain and provide material for culture. Reaspiration of a suppurative node is occasionally necessary and is easily done as an office procedure. Incision and drainage are not recommended, since chronic sinus tract formation may persist for 3 to 7 months. Surgical excision of involved nodes is usually not indicated unless one suspects a noninfectious etiology such as a neoplasm.

In the patient with the oculoglandular disease of Parinaud due to cat scratch disease treatment should be symptomatic. Secondary infection of the eye is rare. Surgical removal of the conjunctival granuloma or polyp appears to shorten the course of the illness.

In the rare (1%) patient who develops encephalopathy and/or encephalitis, supportive care is the primary treatment, since spontaneous recovery over a 5- to 10-day period is expected. Complete recovery from this complication has occurred in 99% of reported patients. Therefore invasive procedures should be avoided. Initially an electroencepalogram is usually abnormal. Recently CAT scans have shown transient nonspecific abnormalities suggestive of cerebritis.

Lyme Disease

FREDERIC P. ANDERSON, M.D., M.P.H.

Lyme disease is caused by the *Ixodes* spirochete carried by the deer tick, *Ixodes dammini*, on the East coast, *Ixodes pacificus* on the West coast, and *Ixodes ricinus* in Europe. It is highly endemic along the coastline of southern New England and the offshore islands, but its habitat appears to be expanding; cases of Lyme disease have been reported in 14 states from coast to coast and as far south as Tennessee.

A case may present at any of three stages, each requiring its own therapeutic decision. The initial insult occurs at the time of the tick bite, which is usually acquired in a sylvan environment. If the rate of spirochetal carriage in the area is known (it may range from 15 to 100% of specimen deer ticks), the decision may be made to treat the patient presumptively.

The second and more usual stage of presentation is following the development of erythema chronicum migrans (ECM). Approximately one-third of patients recall having had a tick bite 3–32 days prior to the development of a papule that expands centrifugally into the typical rash accompanied by systemic signs of infection.

Tetracycline is the drug of choice. It is given orally at a dose of 250 mg four times daily for at least 15 days and longer if the symptoms persist. Concern naturally arises with the use of tetracycline in regard to enamel staining and hypoplasia of immature teeth. Although incorporation of the drug into dental enamel probably continues until age 10, the cosmetic implications are negligible after 8 years of age. Indeed, even in younger children, the therapeutic advantages of tetracycline may outweigh the small risk of enamel damage inherent in a single 15-day course. Fortunately, Lyme disease is uncommon in the very young.

Penicillin V may be used at a dose of 50 mg/kg/day in four oral doses for at least 15 days. Penicillin G should not be used because of its significantly inferior efficacy. For the child deemed too young for tetracycline and allergic to penicillin, erythromycin, 30 mg/kg/day for at least 15 days, can be substituted. Though in vitro studies suggest a high degree of potency, clinical studies show erythromycin to be inferior to the aforementioned antibiotics in its ability to halt the disease process and to prevent subsequent manifestations of Lyme disease. As many as 14% of adult patients treated with penicillin V or tetracycline experience a Jarisch-Herxheimer–like reaction manifested by increased fever, rash, and pain during the first 24 hours of therapy. This has not been observed with erythromycin therapy, presumably because of a slower rate of spirochetal killing.

Experience to date suggests that patients treated with tetracycline at the ECM stage will not develop major late disease manifestations (myocarditis, meningoencephalitis, or recurrent arthritis), while 7.5% of patients receiving penicillin V and 14% of those treated with erythromycin develop subsequent problems. In untreated patients, for comparison, approximately two-thirds develop major late manifestations, most commonly arthritis.

The third and most serious stage of presentation of Lyme disease involves patients seen for neurologic, cardiac, or joint disease. This group includes those with untreated ECM and those who failed to respond to therapy at that stage. An undetermined but possibly major portion of their number is composed of those whose earlier disease was never made manifest and in whom Lyme disease is recognized only in the course of evaluation for neurologic, joint, or cardiac disease.

Neurologic manifestations include meningoencephalitis, cranial neuritis (especially Bell's palsy), and radiculoneuritis commencing several weeks after the ECM phase is completed. If Bell's palsy alone is seen and the patient has not previously received antibiotics, he is treated with oral antibiotics as described for ECM. If his symptoms have been present for less than 24 hours, a short course of oral prednisone (2 mg/kg/day) may be added. If he has already received appropriate oral antibiotics earlier or has more extensive neurologic involvement, he should be treated with intravenous penicillin G, 5–20 million units per day, until the symptoms have ameliorated and the pleocytosis has cleared; treatment should continue for at least 10–20 days. In cases of penicillin allergy, tetracycline, 50 mg/kg/day, or erythromycin, 40 mg/kg/day, for 30 days may be substituted, although there is little available evidence concerning their efficacy at this stage.

Cardiac manifestations, commonly atrioventricular conduction abnormalities, occur within several weeks of ECM and may result in complete heart block and inadequacy of perfusion. Treatment is the same as for the neurologic manifestations, with the addition of aspirin, 100 mg/kg/day, or prednisone, 2 mg/kg/day.

Musculoskeletal pains involving tendons, bursae, muscles, and synovia may begin coincident with ECM, but frank pauciarticular arthritis usually does not develop until 1–24 months have passed. Whereas adults may experience continuous symptoms with progressive joint destruction, children usually have intermittenly painful swollen joints (usually the knees), with spontaneous remissions and exacerbations. Significant symptomatic relief may be afforded by aspirin (80–100 mg/kg/day), tolmetin sodium (10–30 mg/kg/day), or prednisone (1–2 mg/kg/day). If oral antibiotics have not previously been given, the child should be treated as outlined for ECM. If antispirochetal therapy has failed, tetracycline, 50 mg/kg/day for 30 days, may be given or intravenous high-dose penicillin G may be employed as described for neurologic symptoms. Experience suggests that only 50% of patients with arthritis will respond with permanent cessation of symptoms. Although spirochetes have been identified in the synovia of patients with arthritis, it is not clear that the pathologic process relates to infection of the joint in all cases or whether an immunopathic process succeeds the infectious one, rendering further antiinfective therapy ineffective.

Primary prevention is limited to careful perusal of the naked child by parents if he is known to have been exposed to the tick vector of the illness.

Cytomegalovirus Infections

JAMES BARRY HANSHAW, M.D.

Congenital Infection. Approximately 90% of congenital cytomegalovirus infections are asymptomatic; the remaining 10% may have mild to severe, even fatal, cytomegalovirus disease. Although several drugs such as adenosine arabinoside and acyclovir have been used experimentally in patients, there is no evidence of any lasting effect on the progression of the disease. The arabinosides can induce a diminution in virus excretion in some patients. However, in view of their unproved efficacy, they cannot be recommended. There is little evidence that acyclovir will be useful in cytomegalovirus infections. Interferon and transfer factor are still regarded as experimental therapeutic modalities.

Most infants with symptomatic infection do not require therapy. Exchange transfusion is rarely necessary for indirect hyperbilirubinemia. Neonatal sepsis, an unusual complication of cytomegalic inclusion disease, is usually due to enteric organisms or a streptococcal infection. Thus, the therapy would not be different from that used in other neonates with sepsis. Since congenital cytomegalic inclusion disease may be a cause of spastic quadriplegia, mental retardation, and obstructive hydrocephalus, long-range measures dealing with these chronic problems must be planned on an individual basis. It is especially important to identify deafness in early life in order to maximize hearing and speech as the child matures.

Acquired Infection. Clinically apparent disease due to cytomegalovirus infection occurs in patients with primary or iatrogenic immune deficiency as well as in individuals who have been previously well. Infection may result in a variety of abnormalities, including an infectious mononucleosis-like illness (cytomegalovirus mononucleosis), infectious polyneuritis, hepatomegaly with abnormal liver function tests, and pneumonitis. The last manifestation is more often associated with a deficiency of cellular immunity such as that induced by immunosuppressive therapy in allotransplantation. In such instances the pneumonitis may be benefited by a temporary reduction of immunosuppressive therapy. Some young adult patients with cytomegalovirus mononucleosis have persistent fatigue over months but rarely for more than a year. Such patients may require 15 or more hours of sleep per day. Although satisfactory controlled studies have not been done, it would appear that improvement is often correlated with extended periods of bed rest. Conversely, attempts to increase activity level frequently results in clinical relapse.

Prevention. Cytomegalovirus mononucleosis may occur in previously healthy young adults or following the transfusion of fresh blood. The greater the number of transfusion units, the higher the probability of cytomegalovirus transmission. Because of the lability of cytomegalovirus, this complication of transfusion can be diminished significantly by using citrated or deglycerolated blood that has been stored or frozen for more than 72 hours or by using seronegative donors. This is especially important in preterm infants.

Although there is no available vaccine for the prevention of cytomegalovirus infection, live virus vaccine trials are currently under way in this country and abroad. Induction of passive immunity using high-titered antibody is now under study and may prove useful in the prevention of disease in immunocompromised patients.

Mycoplasma Infections

GAIL H. CASSELL, M.S., PH.D.,
KEN B. WAITES, M.D.,
and CATHERINE V. JEWETT, M.D.

Of the twelve species of mycoplasmas isolated from the respiratory or genitourinary tract of humans, three are a significant cause of disease: *Mycoplasma pneumoniae, Mycoplasma hominis,* and *Ureaplasma urealyticum.* Concepts regarding the pathogenic potential of all three have changed dramatically during the last decade.

RESPIRATORY DISEASE

Most medical textbooks and reviews in the literature emphasize the benign, often subclinical course of *M. pneumoniae* infection. Indeed, most clinical infections consist of nothing more serious than upper respiratory tract infection. The most frequent clinical presentation of *M. pneumoniae* infection is the syndrome of tracheobronchitis associated with an influenza-like illness. Clinically apparent pneumonia develops in only 3 to 10% of infected persons. Nevertheless, *M. pneumoniae* probably accounts for up to 20% of all pneumonia cases in the general population and for up to 50% in closed populations. It is estimated that 500,000 cases of pneumonia and 11,500,000 cases of tracheobronchitis due to *M. pneumoniae* occur annually in the United States. A mycoplasmal etiology should be considered in the differential diagnosis of pneumonia in any age group (not just in individuals 6–21 years of age, as is commonly done). Viral and bacterial pneumonia can occur concomitantly with mycoplasmal infection. Although severe mycoplasmal respiratory disease has been uncommon, recent reports suggest that the disease spectrum is wider than previously thought and that severe pulmonary involvement can occur in otherwise healthy children and adults of all ages. The severe disease, often mimicking necrotizing bacterial pneumonia, can initially cause diagnostic confusion. Lung abscesses, pneumatoceles, extensive lobar consolidation, pleural effusion (up to 20% of cases), and relapsing or recurrent pneumonia may occur. Reduced pulmonary clearance has been observed as late as one year after infection. Finally, *M. pneumoniae* has been associated with exacerbations of chronic respiratory disease, in particular, chronic bronchitis and asthma, but the role of this organism in sustaining the chronic state or initiating exacerbation is unknown. A number of nonpulmonary complications occur in association with *M. pneumoniae* infection. These include CNS disease, carditis, mucocutaneous lesions, gastrointestinal symptoms, joint manifestations, nephritis, and hematologic disorders.

Contrary to popular belief, controlled therapy trials indicate treatment with either erythromycin (30–60 mg/kg/day) or tetracycline* (25–50 mg/kg/day) markedly reduces the duration of symptoms of the respiratory disease.

Erythromycin is the drug of choice, especially in children less than 8 years old, owing to the bone and tooth toxicity of tetracycline in young children. It has been noted that patients sometimes relapse following the 5- to 7-day courses of antibiotics that are commonly prescribed. This may be due to the continued presence of the mycoplasma; thus 14 to 21 days of therapy is more appropriate.

The effect of antibiotic therapy on extrapulmonary complications is debatable. Since most cases involving complications are not diagnosed until late in the course of disease, the benefit of early treatment is unknown. Corticosteroids in conjunction with antibiotic therapy appear to be helpful in patients with severe pneumonia and erythema multiforme, but controlled, prospective studies are needed before their true value can be assessed.

GENITAL TRACT INFECTION

The pediatrician may be faced with basically three groups of patients in whom disease due to *U. urealyticum* and *M. hominis* is likely to occur: the sexually active adolescent, the neonate, and the child with hypogammaglobulinemia. Genital mycoplasmal colonization of many (up to 70%) sexually active teenagers in good health suggests that after puberty and sexual contact these organisms may exist as commensals in some members of this

---

* Manufacturer's warning: Tetracycline should not generally be used in children under 8 years of age.

population; however, both organisms have been associated with specific urogenital and systemic diseases in both males and females. *M. hominis* causes pyelonephritis and pelvic inflammatory disease as well as septicemia in susceptible persons. *U. urealyticum* is the etiologic agent in over 20% of cases of nongonococcal urethritis and can also be responsible for acute prostatitis and pyelonephritis. *M. hominis* infection of the neonate can result in subcutaneous abscesses or a pyogenic meningitis. Both organisms have been isolated from the lungs of neonates with congenital pneumonia in the absence of other pathogens. Infant colonization by genital mycoplasmas at birth tends to be transient, but older children with no history of sexual contact may have prolonged lower genital tract carriage of these organisms.

The final group of patients who are at high risk for systemic mycoplasma infections are individuals with immunodeficiencies, particularly hypogammaglobulinemia. Several mycoplasmal species, including *M. pneumoniae*, *M. hominis*, and *U. urealyticum*, have been isolated from septic joints in both children and adults with this disorder. Due to the severity of polyarticular joint destruction, prompt diagnostic joint aspiration and antibiotic therapy should be instituted.

Many infections due to mycoplasmas are discovered accidently, either by observing the presence of *M. hominis* growing on blood agar or because of treatment failure with antibiotics directed at common bacterial pathogens but ineffective against mycoplasmas. Tetracyclines are the preferred drugs to treat urogenital tract infections in children over 8 years of age. Both *M. hominis* and *U. urealyticum* are generally sensitive to all drugs in the tetracycline group, but in recent years increasing reports of resistant strains of ureaplasmas (up to 10%) and *M. hominis* (up to 40%) have been reported. Oral tetracycline (25–50 mg/kg/day) or doxycycline (4 mg/kg/day) is usually adequate for local urogenital infections with either organism. The duration of therapy necessary to resolve symptoms and eradicate the organism may vary, but an initial treatment for 10 days is recommended. Treatment failure with tetracycline may indicate a resistant strain; therefore, repeated cultures with appropriate antibiotic sensitivities should be obtained and alternative drugs employed. *U. urealyticum* is sensitive to erythromycin (although resistant strains have been reported) and resistant to clindamycin, lincomycin, and aminoglycosides. There is variable sensitivity to chloramphenicol. Erythromycin (40 mg/kg/day) is the preferred drug for ureaplasma infections in infants and young children. *M. hominis* is resistant to erythromycin and sensitive to tetracyclines, clindamycin, and lincomycin. It may be moderately sensitive to chloramphenicol and aminoglycosides. Clindamycin (8–16 mg/kg/day) is a useful drug for neonatal *M. hominis* infections not involving the CNS.

In infants and children, severe systemic infections due to *M. hominis*, such as CNS invasion, warrant aggressive antibiotic therapy, preferably guided by antibiotic sensitivity testing of isolates. In view of the life-threatening nature of CNS infections, a 2-week course of parenteral tetracycline is justified.

The child with mycoplasmal arthritis may require prolonged parenteral antibiotic therapy followed by oral medication for several weeks to months to eradicate the organism. Until antibiotic sensitivities are available, treatment with tetracycline as well as an additional drug (erythromycin, clindamycin, or chloramphenicol) is justified, the choice depending on which species of mycoplasma is isolated.

Viral Pneumonia

WALLACE A. CLYDE, JR., M.D.

Viruses are the most common infectious agents causing pneumonia in children less than 4 years old. While a host of different types are capable of producing pneumonia, by far the most common ones are respiratory syncytial virus, parainfluenza virus types 1, 2, and 3, influenza viruses A and B, and adenovirus types 1, 2, and 5 (in decreasing order of importance). Viruses remain a significant cause of pneumonia in school-age children, in whom respiratory syncytial virus and influenza viruses play an important role. Other viruses are prominent causes of pneumonia in selected situations, for example, herpesviruses and cytomegalovirus in newborns and adenovirus types 3, 4, and 7 in military recruits. There is evidence that rotavirus infection of infants is often accompanied by pneumonia.

Since the ability to exclude treatable forms of pneumonia is limited, antimicrobial therapy is often employed empirically. If this course is chosen, judgment should be made as to the most likely etiologic agents and treatment begun while other diagnostic studies are pending. In the neonate, a penicillin and an aminoglycoside are appropriate. For the older infant, a broad-spectrum penicillin can be used. In school-age children, erythromycin would be the first choice. In all cases, if diagnostic studies are negative and/or if no response occurs in 48 hours, re-evaluation is indicated. If positive cultures are obtained, antimicrobial realignment should be done according to sensitivity data.

An additional judgment should be made based on severity of a given episode of pneumonia. In mild disease, no treatment need be given pending diagnostic studies if parents are alerted to watch for the signs of air hunger or increasing fever. In moderate disease, empirical antibiotics should be started. In severe disease, hospitalization is prudent for initial management; supportive therapy with humidified oxygen should be given, along with ventilatory assistance if deterioration occurs in clinical or laboratory status. In each instance, close follow-up of cases is important, since rapid changes in both directions are characteristic of childhood pneumonia. All cases of pneumonia occurring in the first month of life should be hospitalized for intravenous therapy.

While specific diagnosis of and therapy for all types of viral pneumonia are not available, many clinical microbiology laboratories are initiating facilities for this, and several new antiviral drugs are available. Rapid diagnostic tests are commercially available for herpesviruses, influenza viruses, and respiratory syncytial viruses; these viruses can be treated respectively with adenosine arabinoside or acyclovir, rimantidine, and ribavirin (experimental, but effective). More progress in rapid diagnosis and specific therapy of viral infections can be expected in the near future, which will broaden the clinician's effectiveness in managing these diseases.

Viral Hepatitis

MYRON J. TONG, PH.D., M.D.

The agents that are primarily hepatotropic and cause viral hepatitis include the hepatitis A virus (HAV), hepatitis B virus (HBV), and the non-A non-B viruses. The hepatitis A virus causes acute hepatitis and is transmitted by the oral-fecal route. The hepatitis B virus causes acute and chronic hepatitis and is transmitted by blood and body secretions. There are two or more non-A non-B viruses that may cause acute and chronic hepatitis that are transmitted by blood and body secretions. However, there are as yet no serologic tests for these viruses, and the diagnosis is made by exclusion of hepatitis A and hepatitis B. Epidemics of non-A non-B hepatitis spread by the oral-fecal route have been reported ouside of the United States but have not yet been a problem in this country.

Immunoprophylaxis Against Hepatitis A Infection. Since HAV infection is transmitted by the oral-fecal route, prophylaxis should be provided to households as well as sexual contacts of the index case. The efficacy of standard immune globulin (IG) has been well established and is recommended for persons living in the same household. Also, personnel working in day care centers, preschools, or institutions for custodial care where cases of hepatitis A infection are iden-

tified should also receive IG. However, routine use of IG in casual contacts in schools, offices, and factories is not warranted, since spread of the HAV is unlikely under these circumstances. The recommendation for prophylaxis of IG is 0.02 ml/kg body weight by the intramuscular route and should be given within two weeks of exposure.

Perinatal transmission of the hepatitis A virus does not occur when the mother has acute hepatitis A during pregnancy. Therefore, immunoprophylaxis is not needed for infants born to such mothers even if the acute HAV is detected at term.

Immunoprophylaxis Against Hepatitis B Infection. There are two modes of immunoprophylaxis against HBV infection. Passive immunization is by hepatitis B immune globulin (HBIG), which contains high titer anti-HBs. HBIG is recommended for postexposure prophylaxis following (1) parenteral exposure, such as an accidental needle puncture previously used on an HBsAg positive patient, (2) direct mucous membrane contact, and (3) oral ingestion of HBsAg positive blood or blood products. Ideally HBIG should be given within 24 hours of exposure or certainly within 7 days at a dose of 0.06 ml/kg body weight. A second dose of HBIG should be given one month later. An alternative is to begin the HBV vaccine at another site at the time of the first HBIG administration followed by additional doses of HBV vaccine 1 and 6 months later. The latter is recommended if the recipient works in or resides in a high-risk area, since vaccination against hepatitis B will provide prolonged protection by active production of anti-HBs. Spouses of patients with acute hepatitis B should be tested for HBsAg and anti-HBs and if negative, should receive HBIG, since they are at high risk for developing acute hepatitis B infection. Children of a parent who develops acute hepatitis B may need HBIG, especially if the child is young and if there is potential exposure of blood or body fluids (i.e., saliva) from parent to child.

Active immunization against hepatitis B infection is provided by hepatitis B vaccine, which has been available in the United States since July 1982. Experience to date with the hepatitis B vaccine has confirmed its safety, immunogenicity, and efficacy in adults as well as in infants. The hepatitis B vaccine prevents acute and chronic HBV infection and is recommended for individuals at increased risk, such as health care professionals who are exposed to blood or blood products and patients with thalassemia or hemophilia who receive multiple transfusions. Also, the hepatitis B vaccine is recommended for staff and residents in institutions for the mentally disabled, for intimate contact with carriers, for homosexual males, and for seronegative children in familes in which parents or siblings are HBV carriers. The recommended

Table 1. RECOMMENDATIONS FOR INFANTS BORN TO HBsAg POSITIVE MOTHERS*

Hepatitis B immune globulin (HBIG)	0.5 ml by the intramuscular route within 24 hours of birth
Hepatitis B vaccine	0.5 ml (10 μg) by the intramuscular route concurrently with the HBIG at another site, or within 7 days of birth; repeat at 1 and 6 months.

* Includes mothers with acute hepatitis B during the third trimester of pregnancy and chronic HBsAg-positive carrier mothers regardless of HBeAg status.

schedule *for adults* is three 20-μg doses of the hepatitis B vaccine at 0, 1, and 6 months; *for children* (birth to 10 years) the recommended schedule is three 10 μg doses at 0, 1, and 6 months. Anti-HBs may be tested one month after the last dose of the hepatitis B vaccine. Over 90% of infants and heterosexual adults should respond to vaccination with production of anti-HBs. After hepatitis B vaccination, anti-HBc should not be detected and if present, indicates HBV infection via another source during immunization.

Prophylaxis Against Perinatal Transmission of the Hepatitis B Virus.   In order to prevent perinatal transmission of the HBV in infants born to HBsAg-positive mothers, immunoprophylaxis must be given to the newborn infants. When hepatitis B immune globulin (HBIG) was administered to infants born to HBsAg-positive HBeAg-positive mothers within 24 hours of birth and at 3 and 6 months, 71% of infants were protected from HBV infection during the neonatal period. However, 20 to 25% of the treated infants still became HBsAg positive during the first year of life, and another 20% did not have the desired passive-active response and became infected by the HBV after the passively administered anti-HBs had waned in the infant's circulation. More recent studies have shown that use of HBIG in conjunction with the hepatitis B vaccine protected 85 to 93% of such infants from becoming infected by the HBV. More importantly, these infants had high-titer anti-HBs at 1 to 2 years of age, which ensured continual protection against future HBV infection. Simultaneous administration of the

Table 2. HIGH-RISK PREGNANT WOMEN WHO SHOULD BE TESTED FOR HBsAg

1. Immigrants from highly endemic areas, such as Asia, Africa, Haiti, and various Pacific islands
2. Those with acute or chronic liver disease or contacts with persons with acute or chronic hepatitis B
3. Health professionals exposed to blood or to patients in institutions for the mentally retarded
4. Those who have been illicit injectable drug users
5. Those who have been rejected as blood donors

HBIG and the hepatitis B vaccine at different sites did not interfere with production of anti-HBs in the infants.

The current recommendations for infants born to HBV carrier mothers are shown in Table 1. (a) In order to detect asymptomatic HBV carriers during pregnancy, women who are considered high risk should be screened for HBeAg during the pre-natal period (Table 2). Screening of pregnant women who are not high risk is optional. (b) Newborn infants who are born to HBsAg-positive mothers, regardless of the HbsAg status of the mother, should receive 0.5 ml of HBIG by the intramuscular route as soon after birth as possible but certainly within 24 hours of birth. (c) The first dose of the hepatitis B vaccine at a dose of 0.5 ml (10 μg) may be administered concurrently with the HBIG at another site or within 7 days of birth, and again 1 and 6 months later. (d) At 3 months of age, the infant should be tested for HBsAg and if positive, no further therapy should be given. Approximately 5 to 15% of infants will become infected by the HBV in spite of administration of HBIG and HBV vaccine at birth. (e) At 1 year of age, the infant should be tested for presence of anti-HBs. If positive, he is protected from HBV infection. Current studies have shown that 85 to 93% of infants will develop anti-HBs.

In mothers who develop acute hepatitis B during the third trimester of pregnancy or delivery period, the recommendations are that the infants should receive 0.5 ml of HBIG within 24 hours after birth, and that the hepatitis B vaccine should be administered as recommended for infants born to HBV carrier mothers. The protection rate for these treated infants is 90%.

Enteroviruses

GILBERT M. SCHIFF, M.D.

Approximately 70 specific serotypes of enteroviruses have been detected. They are members of the picornavirus group, are 270–300 angstroms in size, contain single-stranded RNA, are stable at acid pH and room temperature, and are resistant to lipid solvents. The enteroviruses are classified according to pathogenicity for experimental animals and other biochemical, physical, and molecular criteria. At present three poliovirus, 23 coxsackie A virus, 6 coxsackie B virus, and 32 echovirus serotypes are recognized. In addition, more recently identified viruses are classified as the "newer, higher numbered enteroviruses," i.e., enteroviruses 68–72. The newest member, Enterovirus 72, is the hepatitis A virus.

Prevention. Passive immunization with human immune globulin (IG) is effective in the prevention of clinical hepatitis A infection (Enterovirus 72). Use of pooled human IG (0.2 ml/kg intramuscularly) for passive protection against other enteroviruses is possible but would appear to be of value only in certain situations, such as severe enteroviral outbreaks in nurseries.

Wide-spread use of inactivated poliomyelitis vaccine and oral live, attentuated poliomyelitis vaccine (OPV) has been highly effective for the control of poliomyelitis. An increased danger of paralytic poliomyelitis following administration of OPV to infants with agammaglobulinemia is recognized. Because OPV is given at such a young age, the congenital immune deficiency may not be recognized. Therefore, OPV should not be administered to an infant with a family history of agammaglobulinemia until the condition can be ruled out.

Attenuated viral vaccines for other enteroviruses are not available. Preliminary evaluation of hepatitis A vaccines have started. Other enteroviral vaccines undoubtedly could be developed but require more aggressive efforts to document specific needs and cost effectiveness. The multiplicity of enteroviral serotypes tends to direct attention towards the development of broad-spectrum antiviral therapy to counter the medical problems caused by these viruses.

Treatment. At the present time no specific antienteroviral therapy is available. Supportive therapy is the keystone for treatment and varies according to the clinical manifestations. Passive antibody therapy in severe neonate enteroviral infections (when specific maternal antibody is absent) and in chronic enteroviral infections in agammaglobulinemic children remains on an experimental basis. If nothing else, this type of therapy may terminate viremia and prevent continued seeding of organs. There are a number of newer antiviral agents that have been shown to be effective against a broad spectrum of enteroviruses in tissue culture systems and some animal models. Some of these drugs are ready for evaluation in well-controlled human studies.

A recurring problem has been the use of corticosteroids as part of the treatment regimen in such illnesses as severe neonatal viral myocarditis and meningoencephalitis, myopericarditis in older children, and acute hemorrhagic conjunctivitis. On the basis of animal experiments, we generally accept the fact that viruses and corticosteriods or other immunosuppressive agents are not good bedfellows. In reality, there have been no well-controlled human studies to suggest that such is the case. However, in general, I recommend avoidance of these agents in the presence of documented active viral diseases whenever possible. In myopericarditis, which we tend to see in active adolescents and young adults, and in cases of myocarditis in infants and older children, the treatment is bed rest, relief of pain, and if congestive failure occurs, the careful use of cardiac glycosides and diuretics. The heart in infants with myocarditis is frequently very sensitive to cardiac glycosides and only low doses are necessary, especially the initial dose. As mentioned, I prefer avoidance of corticosteroids or immunosuppressive agents in acute myocarditis despite some clinical studies that suggest a favorable effect of corticosteroids alone or in combination with azathioprine. These studies lacked proper controls and laboratory diagnosis. Better clinical studies and additional data are needed.

In patients with meningoencephalitis, treatment for cerebral edema is frequently required, and urea, mannitol, or large doses of corticosteroids have been used. Again, I recommend that the latter be avoided because of the potential overall adverse effects of corticosteroids in the presence of acute viral infections.

Acute hemorrhagic conjunctivitis is usually self-limited and is generally an illness that occurs in adolescents and adults. There is the potential for this illness to become a greater problem in children of all ages. The supportive treatment usually includes local application of broad-spectrum antibiotics and sulfonamides to prevent or treat secondary bacterial infection. Corticosteroids have been used to reduce inflammation and relieve pain. However, relapses are four to five times more frequent after their use, and development of chronic conjunctivitis and corneal ulceration has been reported among patients who received corticosteroids. I recommend avoidance of corticosteroids for this condition.

Finally, the role of laboratory diagnosis in relation to treatment should be emphasized. Prompt diagnosis of viral etiology can result in avoiding the unnecessary use of antibiotics in many patients. Aseptic meningitis is a typical example of a situation in which this phenomenon may be operative. Initial examination may not be conclusive, and antibiotics should be intelligently initiated to "cover all fronts." But once an enteroviral etiology has been established, antibiotics should be discontinued.

Aseptic Meningitis

SHELDON L. KAPLAN, M.D.

Aseptic meningitis is not a specific diagnosis but rather a syndrome that is characterized by an abrupt onset of meningeal irritation and a CSF pleocytosis. It generally has a benign clinical course. Although there are numerous infectious and noninfectious causes of aseptic meningitis, a viral infection is the most common etiology. Once the diagnosis of viral meningitis is suspected, the age of the patient will determine how the physician will approach the managment of this condition. Since in young children, particularly under a year in age, viral meningitis may not be easily distinguished from bacterial meningitis on the basis of historical or physical finding or from the results of cerebrospinal fluid (CSF) examination, antibiotics such as ampicillin and chloramphenicol may be administered intravenously for 48 to 72 hours, at which time CSF culture results are available. Antibiotics administered prior to hospitalization may alter the biochemical, morphological, and cultural results of the CSF examination and confuse its interpretation. In children who have not received antibiotics and who have negative CSF cultures by 72 hours, antibiotics can be discontinued. Although antiviral therapy is not currently recommended for viral meningitis, such treatment is available for herpes encephalitis, which in an early phase may present like viral meningitis. The value of vidarabine or acyclovir in treating aseptic meningitis associated with genital herpes infections is unknown.

Older children with viral meningitis generally do not require hospitalization, but antipyretics and analgesics may allow symptomatic relief. Avoidance of light is helpful if the patient has photophobia, and elevation of the head may help relieve headaches. Infants and children with more severe symptoms are usually admitted to the hospital initially for supportive care. Serum electrolytes may reveal hyponatremia, which can result from the inappropriate secretion of antidiuretic hormone. In such patients, mild fluid restriction is warranted. Intravenous fluids may be required for provision of maintainance fluid rates if the child has persistent nausea and vomiting. Meningitis due to enteroviruses can be associated with a disseminated infection, including myocarditis, pericarditis, hepatitis, and so on, which must be recognized for optimal management of the patient. Enteric or excretion isolation is recommended for patients with viral meningitis.

The majority of children with viral meningitis appear to recover uneventfully. Some children continue to complain of headaches, weakness, fatigue, dizziness or other similar problems for variable periods of time after the meningitis. Younger children and especially those under 3 months of age with enteroviral meningitis may suffer neurologic sequelae despite the fact that their general and neurologic examination is completely normal at discharge. Delayed language and speech development, behavior problems, and other developmental abnormalities may become evident years following the episode of meningitis. Therefore such children deserve careful follow-up and periodic psychologic evaluation as they enter the school-age years. Seizures during the acute illness appear to be correlated with an increased risk for these neurologic sequelae.

Encephalitis Infections— Postinfectious and Postvaccinal

MARVIN L. WEIL, M.D.

Postinfectious and postvaccinal encephalitis refers to a group of immune disorders of the brain and spinal cord that can complicate viral and bacterial infections as well as immunization with live and inactivated viral and bacterial vaccines. Treatment involves relief of specific symptoms and modulation of the immune system in some instances. Although a diverse group of agents and antigens can elicit this type of encephalomyelitis, manifestations of these disorders are limited to a number of symptom complexes, each with its own requirements for therapy.

Acute disseminated encephalomyelitis, which is sometimes hemorrhagic, may occur after rubeola, rubella, varicella, variola, Epstein-Barr virus, mumps, and influenza as well as after vaccinia or rabies immunization. Onset is usually abrupt, with seizures requiring anticonvulsant medication such as lorazepam, dilantin, phenobarbital, or paraldehyde. Somnolence and coma may ensue as the result of either diffuse brain involvement or elevated intracranial pressure. The hemorrhagic encephalomyelitis variant should be treated promptly with steroids (e.g., dexamethasone, 1.5 mg/kg/day), since this may result in prompt improvement. Symptoms of increased intracranial pressure should receive appropriate attention. Supportive therapy is important during the first 7 days, since patients surviving the first week generally recover to a variable degree.

In some cases of postvaccinal encephalomyelitis due to vaccinia, virus can be isolated, suggesting a mixed process involving both the acute infection and the immune response. In such cases, immunosuppressants such as dexamethasone may be contraindicated.

Focal neurologic syndromes associated with these conditions such as tranverse myelitis, optic atrophy, or acute cerebellar ataxia should be treated with appropriate supportive measures. Inappropriate antidiuretic hormone secretion should be treated by limitation of free water. Postencephalomyelitic sequelae such as static neurologic deficits, seizures, and cognitive and psychiatric disturbances require long-term treatment.

Symptoms of acute parainfectious encephalopathy (e.g., Reye's syndrome) should be treated appropriately and not confused with this condition.

Cerebral Edema and Increased Intracranial Pressure

Appropriate therapy for increased intracranial pressure requires almost continuous careful, accurate, and perceptive clinical and technological monitoring. Prompt recognition of changes in clinical status is essential, so that appropriate therapeutic responses can avert added morbidity or mortality. A therapeutic regimen based on physiologic priinciples is essential, since each patient may present a different array of problems.

The cranial vault of the older child or adult has a fixed volume occupied by brain parenchyma (approximately 80%), cerebrospinal fluid (approximately 10%), and vascular bed (approximately 10%). Space-occupying lesions or brain swelling causes encroachment on the cerebrospinal fluid space and the vascular bed except for more rigid vessels such as the dural sinuses. Small increases in the volume of this encroachment lead to minimal increases in intracranial pressure until there is no further room for expansion and cerebral compliance is lost. Beyond this point, any small increase in intracranial volume, by either enlargement of a space-occupying mass, increase in the size of the edematous brain, or vasodilatation, results in a marked increase in intracranial pressure. Physiologic changes that result in vasoconstriction decrease the volume of the vascular bed and lower intracranial pressure. This can improve cerebral perfusion pressure and cerebral perfusion, provided vasoconstriction does not become excessive and produce ischemia by impedance of cerebral blood flow. Blood supply to cerebral tissue (average value about 50 ml/100 gm/min) is determined by the size of the vascular bed and its resistance to blood flow, and the cerebral perfusion pressure (mean arterial pressure [diastolic blood pressure plus about 1/3 of the pulse pressure] minus the intracranial pressure). Normal cerebral perfusion pressure, about 38 torr for newborns and 50 torr for older children and adults, is maintained by cerebral blood vessel autoregulation. Loss of autoregulation results in the linear transfer of mean arterial pressure to the cerebral vasculature with increased capillary pressure as well as increased intracranial pressure. Once brain compliance is lost, physiologic changes that result in increased blood flow by means of vasodilatation or increased mean arterial pressure result in an elevation of intracranial pressure and a reduction in perfusion pressure.

Therapy of increased intracranial pressure may require surgical reduction of any intracranial mass lesions. Different types of cerebral edema, vasogenic, cytotoxic, interstitial, or a combination, respond to treatment modalities in different ways. Vasogenic edema results from breaks in the tight junctions of the microvasculature with leakage of plasma and plasma proteins into the interstitial spaces of the brain. Steroids, which can cause tightening of these junctions in the cerebral microvasculature, may be of benefit. Hyperosmolar agents such as mannitol and urea are of benefit in that they shrink the remaining normal brain, while they may fail to produce an osmolar gradient at sites of vascular damage. Hyperosmolar agents may prove harmful in the presence of widespread vasogenic edema. Cytotoxic edema involves the accumulation of intracelluar water; hence, it is more responsive to mannitol and other hyperosmolar agents. Steroids, which are effective in preventing hypoxic damage to mitochondria, have little benefit in treatment if given after the hypoxic event. Drugs such as furosemide, which reduce cerebrospinal fluid production, may also improve intracranial pressure.

Management. With due regard for the concepts outlined above, the following method is recommended for the management of intracranial hypertension:

Keep the head of the bed elevated to about 30 degrees if this is not contraindicated in order to promote venous drainage and minimize venous back-pressure to the head. Avoid neck flexion and compressive tracheostomy ties, which may impede venous drainage from the brain. Maintain the blood pressure below 140 systolic if possible without compromising cerebral perfusion pressure. This assumes importance when autoregulation of cerebral blood flow is lost. Dexamethasone, 1.5 mg/kg/day, is beneficial for tumor or abscess edema. Benefits of steroids in traumatic or posthypoxic cerebral edema have not been clearly established in controlled studies, but many centers continue to use them. It is generally advisable to discontinue their use at the earliest opportunity, especially after about 5 days, in order to minimize complications of steroid therapy. Normovolemic hydration is preferred to partial dehydration in order to avoid iatrogenic hypotension. The initial serum osmolality is maintained at around 300 mOsm.

Controlled hyperventilation to a $Paco_2$ of 23–25 torr may be necessary to keep the intracranial pressure below 20 torr for young children and adults and below about 8–12 torr in infants with open fontanels. $Paco_2$ values below 23 are not recommended, since they are of little additional benefit and may cause added cerebral ischemia. Supplemental oxygen should be used if necessary to keep the Pao_2 above 90 torr. A Pao_2 below 50 torr may result in a severe increase in intracranial hypertension. Even short bouts of hypoventilation may result in severe exacerbations of intracranial hypertension. Positive end-expiratory airway pressure (PEEP) may be increased as needed to keep

Table 1. GLASGOW COMA SCALE

Best Motor Response	
Obeys	6
Localizes	5
Withdraws	4
Abnormal flexion	3
Extensor response	2
Nil	1
Verbal Response	
Oriented	5
Confused conversation	4
Inappropriate words	3
Incomprehensible sounds	2
Nil	1
Eye Opening	
Spontaneous	4
To speech	3
To pain	2
Nil	1

the FiO_2 below 50% in order to avoid oxygen toxicity; however, PEEP above 6 torr should be avoided in order to minimize pulmonary embarrassment of venous return from the brain.

Intracranial pressure monitoring by epidural, subdural, subarachnoid, or intraventricular devices has been an important advance in the management of intracranial hypertension. Patients who achieve a Glasgow Coma Scale of 7 (Table I) or less should be considered as candidates for intracranial pressure monitors.

If, despite the above therapy, the intracranial pressure rises above 20 torr; spontaneous waves (of Lundberg) over 20 torr last for more than 5 minutes; waves over 20 torr triggered by turning or suctioning do not subside in 5 minutes; or any pressure occurs over 30 torr, then give furosemide, 0.5 mg/kg IV, and if necessary, mannitol, 0.5–1.0 gm/kg IV as a 20% solution. If benefits fail to last more than 3 hours, an intravenous drip of mannitol at 0.05 to 0.15 gm/kg/hr may be tried. Serum osmolality should be maintained at 320 milliosmoles or less to avoid rebound phenomenon. The serum glucose may be maintained at about 200 mg/dl to minimize the amount of mannitol required.

Should the above measures prove ineffective at keeping the intracranial pressure below 20 torr and the cerebral perfusion pressure at about 50 torr, pentobarbital is recommended, although its use remains controversial. Some centers have been unable to duplicate the beneficial results claimed by others. Should pentobarbital be used, a loading dose of 5 mg/kg is given IV as 50–100 mg bolus doses, followed by 0.5–3.0 mg/kg/hr IV to achieve a blood level of 25–40 μg/ml. If the intracranial pressure continues to be elevated, the infusion rate is increased until the pressure is controlled, or the EEG demonstrates burst suppression, or the cardiac index falls below normal (2.7 liters/min/m²). Excessive doses of pentobarbital should be

avoided, since they may result in excessive cerebral vascular resistance and augment cerebral ischemia.

If the intracranial pressure continues to be elevated, hypothermia with a core temperature of 32° C is recommended to lower intracranial pressure and decrease cerebral metabolism. Temperatures below this limit may result in cardiac arrhythmias.

The use of pentobarbital or hypothermia may decrease the need for mannitol therapy. Should the intracranial pressure rise during such treatment and the serum osmolality is less than 320 mOsm, mannitol 0.5 gm/kg IV may be given.

The detrimental effects of even transient episodes of elevated intracranial pressure with concomitant reductions in perfusion pressure can not be overemphasized. Pancuronium (Pavulon), 0.06–0.1 mg/kg, may be used in conjunction with pentothal when intubation is required or when suction is necessary in restless, struggling patients or those who develop dystonic posturing during nursing or other procedures.

Psittacosis

(Ornithosis)

CAROL F. PHILLIPS, M.D.

Psittacosis is a zoonotic disease caused by *Chlamydia psittaci*. It was originally thought that this organism was transmitted only by psittacine birds, but it is now known that it can be carried by other species. Therefore, the term "ornithosis" is preferred. The organism is acquired by inhaling infected particles shed in bird secretions or droppings. The incubation period is 8–10 days (range, 5–16 days). A history of employment in the breeding or marketing of pet birds or the poultry industry, or the recent acquisition of a pet bird, is suggestive. The disease may be transmitted by healthy birds. One hundred and sixteen cases were reported from 25 states in 1979, mostly from the western United States. There was no seasonality. Patients ranged in age from 5 to 89 years, but 76% of patients were 20–59 years old. Many cases may be mild and not diagnosed.

The clinical picture consists of fever, which is frequently high, chills, pneumonia, severe headache, weakness, mental confusion, and myalgia. Splenomegaly, photophobia, anorexia, and nausea and vomiting are less frequent. Rarely, endocarditis, hepatitis, arthritis, severe anemia, pulmonary embolism, erythema nodosum, or disseminated intravascular coagulation occur. Without therapy the patient remains quite ill for 2–3 weeks. The mortality rate is now less than 1%.

The white blood cell count is not helpful. Chest X-ray usually shows an atypical pneumonia, but lobar consolidation can be seen. The organism can be isolated from blood or sputum, but the diagnosis is usually made by demonstrating a fourfold or greater increase in the psittacosis complement fixation (CF) titer in paired blood specimens. A presumptive diagnosis can be made with a compatible clinical picture and a single CF titer of 32 or higher. There is no prolonged immunity. Relapses and reinfections occur even in patients with high CF titers.

The treatment of choice is tetracycline, 30–40 mg/kg/day. If the patient is less than 8 years old, therapy with erythromycin, 40 mg/kg/day, could be instituted. There are isolated case reports of the efficacy of erythromycin, but experience is limited. Therapy should be continued for 3 weeks.

Bed rest, oxygen, adequate fluids, and antipyretics are supplemental therapy. The disease is rarely communicable from person to person. Hospitalized patients should be placed on respiratory isolation.

Rickettsial Diseases

PAUL J. HONIG, M.D.

The rickettsial infections are spread by the bites of blood-sucking arthropods. There are four major diseases: (a) typhus, (b) Rocky Mountain spotted fever, (c) scrub typhus, and (d) Q fever. The primary rickettsial disease found in the United States is Rocky Mountain spotted fever (1000 cases/year), with scattered outbreaks of rickettsialpox having been reported recently. The typhus group, which occurs infrequently, and Q fever will not be discussed.

RICKETTSIALPOX

Although the illness is usually mild, the duration of symptoms can be shortened with antibiotic treatment. Patients respond in 1 to 2 days to oral doses of tetracycline (25–50 mg/kg/24 hr) every 6 hours (usually given for a total of 5 days). Children under 8 years of age, who have mild symptoms, should not be treated because of the effects of tetracycline on the teeth. Children with more severe symptoms or high fever who are under 8 years of age may benefit from as little as two days of tetracycline therapy, however.

ROCKY MOUNTAIN SPOTTED FEVER

Since no test is available that will confirm the diagnosis of Rocky Mountain spotted fever early in the course of the disease, treatment must be initiated presumptively. The disease can be aborted if antibiotics are started in time (by the first day or two of the exanthum). Oral doses of chloramphenicol, 50 mg/kg/day in children under 8 years of age, or tetracycline, 50 mg/kg/day in

older youths, are recommended. (It is important to remember that chloramphenicol and tetracycline will only suppress the growth of the rickettsia. Final eradication of the rickettsia depends upon a normal functioning immune system.)

When the disease is diagnosed late in the course (clinically toxic, obtunded, or hyponatremic), hospitalization is necessary. Supportive measures are in order. Hypovolemic shock due to chronic leakage of fluid from damaged vessels must be watched for closely. Although antibiotics, such as intravenous chloramphenicol, 50 mg/kg/day, will arrest the growth of rickettsia, the natural course of the disease will not be altered when severe vascular damage has already occurred. If the diagnosis is in doubt, broader antibiotic coverage for sepsis is advisable.

Prevention of this disease is important. Children and their dogs should be routinely inspected for ticks if they play in wooded areas. Insect repellents are somewhat effective. If a tick is found attached to the skin, attempts should be made to induce the tick to release voluntarily. Various methods have been recommended. These include application of chloroform or liquid nitrogen to the tick; touching the tick with a hot, previously lighted match; or covering the tick with nail polish, mineral oil or petrolatum. Prophylactic antibiotic therapy (tetracycline) should be considered when children who live in endemic areas are bitten by ticks, especially if new cases of Rocky Mountain spotted fever are currently being diagnosed. Treatment can be instituted as soon as the biting tick is discovered or following the first signs of illness.

Chlamydia

MARC O. BEEM, M.D.

Chlamydia trachomatis is uniformly sensitive to erythromycin, the tetracyclines, and the sulfonamides, and the mainstay of treatment for all *C. trachomatis* infections is the systemic administration of one of these antimicrobial agents. To achieve microbial cure and avoid clinical relapse, patients should be treated for the full periods indicated. Additionally, treatment is indicated for the mother and her sexual partner in the case of infant infection and for the sexual contacts of older patients.

TYPICAL DRUG REGIMENS EMPLOYED

Erythromycin
Erythromycin ethylsuccinate:
Infants—40 mg/kg/day divided into four doses.
Adults—500 mg qid.
Tetracyclines (not indicated in patients who are younger than 8 years of age or who are pregnant)

Tetracycline HCl:
Children—50 mg/kg/day divided into four doses.
Adults—500 mg qid.
Doxycycline:
Children—4.4 mg/kg/day divided into two doses.
Adults—100 mg q 12 h.
Sulfonamides (not indicated in infants younger than 2 months of age)
Sulfisoxazole:
Infants—150 mg/kg/day divided into four doses.
Adults—1 gm qid.

TREATMENT PROGRAMS FOR SPECIFIC CONDITIONS

Inclusion Conjunctivitis
Neonatal
Erythromycin or sulfisoxazole, in dosages as outlined above, for 2 weeks.

Older child or adult
One of the above antimicrobial agents is given for 2 weeks. This assures adequate treatment of the genital infection that may also be present.

Topical medications are not needed. Although this route of medication has long been employed in the treatment of chlamydial conjunctival disease, it often fails to bring about complete resolution of the conjunctival disorder and does not treat the respiratory or genital aspects of the infection.

Chlamydial Pneumonia of Infancy
Erythromycin or sulfisoxazole, in dosages as outlined above, for 2 weeks.

These patients may have episodes of accentuated respiratory distress associated with increased lower respiratory tract secretions and paroxysms of staccato coughing. These aspects of the illness are greatly helped by chest physical therapy. Occasional infants may have disease of a severity that requires supplemental oxygen; on rare occasions assisted ventilation may be necessary.

Uncomplicated Urethral, Endocervical, or Rectal Infections
Tetracycline in dosages as outlined above should be given for at least 7 days. If this cannot be used, erythromycin is the drug of choice since it, like tetracycline, is effective against the genital mycoplasma, *Ureaplasma urealyticum* (another possible cause of nongonococcal urethritis). The treatment interval of sexual partners should overlap that of the patient.

Legionella Infections

GARY D. OVERTURF, M.D.

Numerous species of *Legionella* may cause clinical infections, including *L. pneumophilia, L. micadei, L. bozemani, L. damoffi, L. gormanii, L. jordanis, L. longbeachae,* and *L. wadsworthii.* Infections appear to be more frequent among debilitated or immunocompromised infants or children. In normal ambulatory children with abnormal chest radiographs, *Legionella* species are implicated in only 1 to 2% of the pneumonias.

Supportive Therapy. Supportive therapy with fluids and colloids for hypotension, and ventilatory support for respiratory failure are sometimes needed in patients with *Legionella* infection. Antipyretics may be used but have little sustained effect on the temperature. Corticosteroids have no role as primary treatment. Immunosuppressive agents may be continued with effective antimicrobial chemotherapy if necessary for control of the primary disease. Pleural effusions are usually not a management problem, but open drainage for empyema may be necessary.

Isolation. Person-to-person transmission has not been conclusively documented. Only secretion precautions are necessary. Infected water is the usual vehicle implicated in hospital outbreaks. A cluster of hospital cases should prompt a review of drinking (potable) water treatment, showers, respiratory therapy equipment, and air conditioning systems.

Specific Therapy. Although a minority of patients with *Legionella* pneumonia slowly recover after 6 to 8 days of illness, antibiotics are indicated in all patients with pneumonia. It is probable that most children have self-limited illness and will not come to recognition.

In children, erythromycin is the preferred drug, although no prospective comparative studies of antibiotics have been performed. Case fatality rates have been lowest with use of either erythromycin or tetracycline. Use of erythromycin lowers the case fatality rate approximately fourfold over that of patients given no therapy. Results of tetracycline therapy have been variable. Results of in vitro susceptibility testing do not necessarily predict clinical response. Many drugs active in vitro do not work clinically. The ability of antimicrobials to enter alveolar macrophages and monocytes where *Legionella* reside is important. Penicillins, cephalosporins (including cefoxitin and newer cephalosporins) and aminoglycosides have no role in treatment of legionnaires' disease.

Erythromycin should be given for 3 weeks to prevent relapse (Table 1). Administration of the drug intravenously is recommended for moderately or severely ill children for the first several days of therapy or until a clinical response occurs. Thereafter, an oral preparation can be given. Patients frequently cannot tolerate high oral doses because of gastrointestinal side effects. Use of rifampin orally in combination with erythromycin should be considered if the patient is critically ill, is heavily immunosuppressed, or has pulmonary cavities. Rifampin should not be given alone because of the possibility of resistance emerging

Table 1. THERAPY FOR *LEGIONELLA* INFECTIONS

	Drug	Route	Doses per Day	Total Daily Dose
Mild illness with no respiratory compromise	Erythromycin	Oral	4	30–50 mg/kg/day
	Alternative—doxycycline*	Oral	1–2	5 mg/kg/day first day followed by 2.5 mg/kg/day daily
Moderate to severe illness	Erythromycin	IV	4	30–50 mg/kg/day for children under 50 kg; 4 gm/day maximum
	Alternative—erythromycin	IV	4	As above
	with rifampin†		1–2	10–20 mg/kg/day for children over 5 years not to exceed 600 mg/day‡
	Alternative—doxycycline*	IV	1–2	5 mg/kg first day, 2–4 mg/kg/day 12 hours later, and then daily for children under 50kg; 200 mg first day and then 100–200 mg daily in children over 50 kg
	with rifampin†	Oral	1–2	Doses as above

* Tetracyclines may not be effective in all cases; tetracyclines should not be used in children younger than 8 years of age for even short courses unless clearly indicated.

† Rifampin should not be used as a single agent; erythromycin with rifampin is preferred for pulmonary abscess.

‡ Not FDA approved for children under 5 years of age.

during therapy. Cavitary disease or empyema generally requires therapy of more than 3 weeks' duration. If erythromycin cannot be given, doxycycline is given in two doses the first day and then daily thereafter for 3 weeks. In moderately to severely ill patients, rifampin should be given with doxycycline for at least the first week of therapy.

The clinical response to erythromycin therapy is usually prompt clinical improvement within 1 to 2 days and defervescence in 3 to 4 days. Pulmonary infiltrates may continue to progress, and clinical and radiographic evidence of pulmonary consolidation may develop despite clinical response. It is unusual for fever, leukopenia, or confusion to persist for more than 3 or 4 days of erythromycin therapy. A few patients may complain of persistent fatigue and weakness for several months after completion of effective therapy.

In patients who develop respiratory failure and require ventilatory support, restrictive lung disease may develop. Otherwise, chest radiographs usually show resolution of infiltrates in 2 or 3 weeks (or up to 3 months) after initiation of therapy; a few patients are left with residual pulmonary scarring.

Systemic Mycoses

HENRY G. CRAMBLETT, M.D.

After 20 years, amphotericin B remains the treatment of choice for systemic mycoses, although its use causes considerable toxicity. Amphotericin B is still the most effective drug for the treatment of disseminated candidiasis, cryptococcal infections, and aspergillosis.

Because of its proved efficacy in these diseases amphotericin B should be administered to any patient with sufficient indication for this antibiotic. It is emphasized that amphotericin B should be used primarily for treatment of patients with progressive and potentially fatal fungal infections. It is extremely unlikely that serious difficulty will be experienced with this drug if one is aware of its dangers and exercises certain precautions and prudence in its use.

Amphotericin B is either fungistatic or fungicidal depending upon the concentration obtained in body fluids at the site of the infection and the susceptibility of the fungal agent. The drug probably acts by binding to sterols in the fungus cell membrane with a resultant change in membrane permeability which allows leakage of a variety of small molecules.

There is considerable disagreement about how to administer a therapeutic regimen. However, I believe it to be prudent to follow the manufacturer's recommendations in this regard.

Adverse Reactions

Anemia. Anemia that is self-limited and of mild severity may occur during the course of amphotericin B therapy. This effect is not an indication for discontinuance. The anemia is probably the result of mild hemolysis or shortened life-span of erythrocytes due directly to the systemic fungal infection plus suppression of red blood cell production by amphotericin B. The anemia is normocytic, normochromic, and not accompanied by reticulocytosis.

Fever. Fever occurring during the course of

therapy is not unusual and may at times be associated with thrombophlebitis or at other times may be associated with the actual administration of amphotericin B. Therapy of fever includes aspirin and the usual antipyretic measures. If fever does not respond to the foregoing measures, it may be necessary to interrupt the intravenous therapy by infusing drug-free fluid for 1 to 2 hours.

Thrombophlebitis. If the same vein is used continuously for administration of the antibiotic, thrombophlebitis will inevitably result. It may be necessary to resort to the use of intravenous catheters for the administration of the drug because of this problem.

Central Nervous System Effects. Seizures, apnea, and cyanosis may occur during intravenous administration of amphotericin B. The exact mechanism by which this occurs is not known. To date, no serious sequelae of these episodes have been reported.

Nephrotoxicity. Four major anatomic changes in the kidneys in association with or after amphotericin therapy have been described. For the most part these effects seem to be at least partially reversible and include glomerular thickening and epithelial proliferation, cortical tubular atrophy with necrosis, degeneration and thickening of tubular epithelium, and intratubular and intersitial calcification. The clinical laboratory manifestions of these changes will include proteinuria, increase in blood urea nitrogen, decrease in renal concentrating ability, renal tubular acidosis, decrease in renal blood flow and glomerular filtration rate, and hypokalemia. The hypokalemia probably results from defective tubular reabsorption of potassium and may cause lethargy, severe muscular weakness, or paralysis. The impending hypokalemia may be reflected in typical electrocardiographic findings prior to clinical manifestations.

Prophylactic Premedication. The side effects of amphotericin administration may be eliminated or diminished by careful preparation with antipyretics and/or antihistaminics. Salicylate is offered as oral aspirin or intravenous sodium salicylate.

Promethazine (Phenergan) or chlorpromazine (Thorazine) in combination with aspirin may be given 30 minutes before the first dose of amphotericin B.

Administration

Intravenous Administration. The daily dose of amphotericin B should be administered intravenously over a period of 6 hours to the hospitalized patient for whom adequate medical supervision and nursing care are available. The drug is very irritating, and care must be taken to be certain that the needle is securely within the vein and that no perivascular leakage occurs. The antibiotic should be administered in a concentration of 0.1 mg/ml (1 mg/10 ml) or less in 5% dextrose in water. Patients may vary in their tolerance to amphotericin B and in the rate at which it may be administered. Although the total dosage for treatment of systemic fungal infections has not been well established, it has been my custom to administer 40 mg/kg of the antibiotic over a 6–8 week period. Initially, a test dose of 0.1 mg/kg should be given over a period of 6 hours. Subsequently, the drug should be gradually increased in daily increments over a period of 5–7 days until a total daily dose of 1 or 1.5 mg/kg is reached. The larger dose is commonly tolerated by infants and younger children.

Since the excretion of the drug is slow and since renal toxicity manifested by increasing blood urea nitrogen invariably occurs, it is usually possible after 1 week of therapy to maintain good levels of amphotericin B by administering the drug 2 out of every 3 days.

Other Antifungal Agents

Although amphotericin B is the treatment of choice for most systemic mycoses, there are two additional agents that may be considered in special circumstances.

Flucytosine. Flucytosine may be used in the treatment of cryptococcosis (in combination with amphotericin B) or in systemic candidiasis. Sensitivities should be obtained before administration of the drug. If not present initially, resistance may develop during therapy. The dosage is 50–150 mg/kg/day given in four divided doses. Bone marrow suppression, nausea, vomiting, and hepatotoxicty may occur. The dosage should be reduced if there is an increasing blood urea nitrogen or abnormal creatinine clearance.

Miconazole. Miconazole* may also be used as an adjuvant to amphotericin B for treatment of candidiasis or cryptococcosis. The dosage is 20–40 mg/kg/day, which must be administered intravenously in three divided doses. The complications include phlebitis, pruritus, rash, arrhythmias, nausea, vomiting, hyperlipidemia, and hyponatremia.

Histoplasmosis

CYNTHIA BLACK-PAYNE, M.D., *and* JOSEPH A. BOCCHINI, JR., M.D.

The majority of childhood infections with *Histoplasma capsulatum* are benign and self-limited. Amphotericin B is the most effective drug available for the patients who do require therapy. Since

---

* Manufacturer's warning: Safety and efficacy for use in children under 1 year of age have not been established.

amphotericin B is commonly associated with uncomfortable side effects and a high incidence of renal and hematologic toxicities, prudence in patient selection is mandatory. The drug should be reserved for those with serious and life-threatening histoplasmal infections. These include children found to have disseminated histoplasmosis, children with acute symptomatic disease complicated by underlying immunosuppression or immunodeficiency, and children with histoplasmal lymphadenitis resulting in compression of vital organs. Infants experiencing acute progressive primary histoplasmosis and children with severe pulmonary symptoms should also be considered as candidates for therapy.

The polyene antibiotic amphotericin B is available as a bile salt and buffer complex that forms a colloidal suspension upon hydration. The marketed product contains 50 mg of amphotericin B that is dissolved in 10 ml of sterile water and then further diluted in 5% dextrose to the optimal concentration of 0.1 mg per 1.0 ml. The final diluting solution should be free of electrolytes to avoid aggregation of the colloid. This combination is stable for 24 hours and does not need to be protected from light. Administration of amphotericin B should extend over a period of 4 to 6 hours to avoid cardiotoxicity and diminish infusion side effects.

Therapy is initiated with a test dose of 0.1 mg/kg of amphotericin B (not to exceed a total dose of 1.0 mg) to monitor for side effects and to exclude hypersensitivity. The following day, 0.25 mg/kg is administered; on the third 0.5 mg/kg; and on the fourth and subsequent days 1.0 mg/kg as tolerated. Accelerated dosing schedules, including giving the first dose immediately following the test dose, should be considered in the critically ill patient. Toxic symptoms, such as chills and fever, are often experienced during the infusion. These can be minimized by giving acetaminophen before the dose and adding 10–15 mg of hydrocortisone to the intravenous fluid. If nausea and vomiting occur, premedication with oral Benadryl is helpful. Fortunately, some tolerance to these side effects usually develops with time, allowing these drugs to be discontinued. One unit of heparin per milliliter is combined with the suspension to decrease the incidence of thrombophlebitis.

Prior to therapy a complete blood count, serum potassium, blood urea nitrogen (BUN), and serum creatinine levels should be obtained. These are followed biweekly for the first four weeks and weekly thereafter. Significant renal toxicity in children is rarely a problem; however, the BUN should not be allowed to exceed 40 mg/dl nor the creatinine 3.0 mg/dl. In case of rising values, the amphotericin dosage should be decreased or the treatment schedule varied. Significant urinary potassium wasting often occurs during therapy and can usually be treated with oral replacement. A mild anemia also develops, which rarely requires intervention.

A universally accepted treatment schedule for histoplasmosis with amphotericin B does not exist. In fulminating cases and in the immunosuppressed host, therapy should extend for a minimum of 4 weeks at 1 mg/kg/day. Cessation of treatment is based on clinical improvement, hematologic values that normalize and, if feasible, negative cultures. Established signs of clinical improvement in pediatric patients with disseminated histoplasmosis are improved appetite, playfulness, weight gain, defervescence, and lessening hepatosplenomegaly.

Relapses are uncommon; but when they occur, retreatment with amphotericin B for a longer course is necessary. Relapses are less common in adults if the total cumulative dose of amphotericin B is at least 30 mg/kg.

In 1981, ketoconazole, a comparatively safe oral antifungal agent, was licensed for use in several mycotic diseases and has been used to a limited extent in children. Experience to date with ketoconazole indicates that it has a place in the treatment of systemic histoplasmosis but sufficient controlled trials are lacking. Its use for infected children should be reserved for those in whom an observation period for response will not be hazardous.

Surgery is rarely required for the diagnosis or therapy of childhood histoplasmosis. Surgical intervention may become necessary in rare cases when sclerosing mediastinitis results in obstruction of the vena cava, pulmonary vessels, esophagus, or tracheobronchial tree. In general, only children with concomitant neoplastic diseases require amphotericin B in addition to the surgery.

Coccidioidomycosis

H. ROBERT HARRISON, Ph.D., M.D., M.P.H.

Most human coccidioidal infection is either asymptomatic or mildly symptomatic, is self-limited, goes undiagnosed, and by definition is thus not treated. This article deals with the types of pediatric coccidioidal infection that require therapy, which I classify as follows: (1) chronic nonresolving or progressive pulmonary infection in "normal" children, (2) acute pulmonary infection (either primary or relapse) in children whose immune function is compromised (by illness and/or therapy), (3) acute pulmonary infection in infants, and (4) disseminated infection (outside the lungs), including skin, bone, mediastinal mass, and meningitis.

There are two basic options with regard to medical therapy: amphotericin B and ketoconazole. The former is parenteral, fungicidal, and unpleasant and has a host of serious side effects but acts relatively rapidly on the fungus. Ketoconazole is given orally, is probably primarily fungistatic, is relatively well-tolerated, and appears in children to have relatively few side effects. Thus amphotericin B should be used in overwhelming, rapidly progressive coccidioidal disease in which quick action is desired and the side effects are justified by the life-threatening nature of the illness. Such cases include *all infants* with category 3 disease and selected cases in categories 1 and 2 (note that coccidioidal meninigitis is not included).

Specific Therapy

Categories 1, 2, and 3: Pulmonary Disease. Most patients except infants can be treated with oral doses of ketoconazole. Although experience is limited, we have successfully treated pneumonia in a few children and adolescents with Hodgkin's disease, systemic lupus erythematosus, and renal transplants on immunosuppressive therapy.

We aim for a maintenance dose of 10–20 mg/kg/day in one dose, higher than that used for adults. Each tablet is scored and contains 200 mg of drug. The parent is instructed to cut the tablet with a razor blade *perpendicular* to the score, and then, if necessary, break each half in two again along the score. This allows dosing in 50-mg quarter-tablet increments.

Therapy is started at as close as possible to 5 mg/kg once daily 1–2 hours before breakfast. In young children the pieces of tablet can be crushed into applesauce or juice. The dose is doubled after 1 week (to approximately 10 mg/kg) and can, if necessary, be further increased after another week.

We have not yet encountered in children a therapeutic failure or progressive disease on treatment. Such cases, as well as infants and those with immediate life-threatening illness (overwhelming pneumonia) require amphotericin B. This drug is administered, if necessary, intravenously beginning at 0.25 mg/kg/day and is increased by 0.3 mg/kg/day to a maximum of 1 mg/kg/day. It is usually administered daily for 10–14 days and then gradually decreased in frequency to once weekly or less depending upon the patient's clinical response and the degree of renal and hematologic toxicity present. The drug is diluted 1 mg to 10 ml of 5% glucose in water and infused over 4 to 6 hours.

In the earlier literature surgical excision of localized granulomas has been recommended. We have not found this to be necessary in children, although it is conceivable that in refractory or localized cavitary disease that is not improving, excision may be desirable.

Category 4: Disseminated Infection. SKIN AND BONE. Such disease may be treated with high-dose ketoconazole as already described. Response of bone disease has been more variable than other types of disease in the few children whom we have treated. Amphotericin B and surgical excision are alternatives to be considered in unresponsive cases.

MEDIASTINAL MASSES. We have seen two children presenting with chronic fever, weight loss, fatigue, cough, supraclavicular node enlargement, and mediastinal mass on radiography in whom the presumptive diagnosis was lymphoma until biopsy confirmed massive lymphadenopathy with coccidioidal granulomata. Both were successfully treated with ketoconazole at 10–20 mg/kg/day.

MENINGITIS. The life-threatening aspect of this illness is hydrocephalus due to blockage of cerebrospinal fluid flow and/or resorption and brain stem herniation due to increased intracranial pressure. The infection itself is chronic and *not* acutely lethal.

Emergency therapy requires placement of a ventriculoperitoneal shunt with relief of excess pressure. It is important that the diagnosis be suspected prior to the neurosurgical procedure so that an occluder reservoir and on-off valve device can be placed subcutaneously on the skull in the shunt line. This device is essential for disease monitoring and therapy. We have had great success with the Heyer-Schulte assembly (V. Meuller, distributor, Chicago, Illinois), but others are available.

Ongoing therapy is long-term, usually years, and both patient and physician must become adjusted to a close relationship. The most frequent long-term life-threatening complications encountered are shunt obstruction and infection. Thus the pediatrician caring for the child and administering medical therapy must be alert and responsive to signs of either disorder and must develop a close working relationship with a pediatric neurosurgeon. Any combination of headache, fever, vomiting, change in mental status, gait disturbance, and abdominal pain with peritoneal findings should prompt an immediate shunt tap through the reservoir, assessment of shunt hydrodynamics, with cell count, Gram's stain, and culture of the fluid. Pediatric neurosurgical care must be easily and quickly available. Shunt obstructions occur most commonly in the first 6 months of therapy due to the ventriculitis of the disease. The ventriculitis produces high protein, cell count, and general debris, all of which can clog the valve mechanism.

Medical therapy consists of intraventricular therapy with miconazole plus oral ketoconazole. No cisternal or intrathecal drug administration is necessary. Intraventricular therapy is performed with the rigor of a surgical procedure. The on-off valve is closed, preventing drainage of ventricular fluid, gloves and mask are put on, and the skin site over the device is shaved, prepped three times with povidone-iodine, and cleaned with alcohol. The subcutaneous reservoir is then punctured with a 27-gauge "butterfly"-type needle and 2–5 cc of cerebrospinal fluid withdrawn. Next, 3–5 mg (depending on the age of the patient) of miconazole in 2 cc of 5% glucose in water is injected into the reservoir, and followed with 1 cc of glucose water "flush." The valve is left closed for 1 hour following instillation, or until headache occurs, whichever occurs first. Intraventricular therapy is given initially on a daily basis, usually for 2–3 weeks, and is gradually tapered, over months, to once weekly or less often depending on the child's clinical and laboratory response.

This is an essentially painless, well-tolerated procedure. Even children as young as 2 years old rapidly learn to climb upon the examining table and lie quietly without restraint throughout the procedure, which normally requires 5–10 minutes. Parents are taught to open the shunt valve themselves, eliminating the necessity to "hang around" for an hour. The shunt reservoirs in our experience will last for 2–3 years without leakage if a small gauge needle is used. In 7 years of experience involving seven children and hundreds of ventricular injections, we have encountered only one documented iatrogenic shunt infection.

Oral therapy employs ketoconazole at a maintenance dose of 20 mg/kg/day. This is reached as discussed above. Pathologic evidence based on tissue obtained from our patients at the time of neurosurgical procedures indicates that, at this dosage, effective levels of drug penetrate into tissue.

Side Effects

The hematologic and renal toxicity of amphotericin B is well-known. This toxicity must be monitored carefully as therapy progresses. Infusions of drug are often associated with fever, chills, and vomiting. These have been treated with various combinations of preinfusion aspirin, diphenhydramine, promethazine hydrochloride, and, if necessary, intravenous meperidine.

We have observed no side effects with the intraventricular administration of miconazole. The most common side effects of oral doses of ketoconazole have been abdominal pain and emesis 1 to 6 hours after administration. These symptoms resolved within 6 months of initiation of therapy in all patients. We have advised parents to repeat the dose if vomiting occurs within 1 hour of ingestion. Mild urticarial reactions occurred in one patient after 1 month of treatment; these resolved when the drug dose was split and given twice daily. Two months later she was returned to her once daily dose without recurrence of urticaria. No patient has had clinical hepatitis, elevation in liver function tests, or decreased serum cholesterol levels. The long-term side effects of ketoconazole and

miconazole in children are unknown. Ketoconazole has been found to suppress ACTH-induced cortisol release and to block testosterone synthesis, although the clinical consequences of these actions are not clear.

Disease Monitoring

Almost all patients requiring therapy will have positive serum complement fixation (CF) titers at ≥1:16 and negative skin tests. Patients with progressive pulmonary disease and meningitis tend to have very high serum titers. Patients with meningitis most often have positive ventricular fluid fungal cultures, elevated protein and cell count, decreased sugar, and positive ventricular fluid CF titers.

The best way to monitor disease activity in nonmeningeal disease is to follow the appearance of the lesions (chest or bone radiographs, observation of the skin) and the CF titer. Both disease activity and titer change slowly, so that we usually use monthly CF titers for the first 3 months and then every 2 or 3 months thereafter. A skin test with 1:100 coccidioidin is performed every 6 months. It is of utmost importance to perform the CF test *consistently;* that is, always in the same laboratory and in one that is proven and reliable. The error in the test itself is generally thought to be one twofold dilution. Thus, wildly varying titers from month to month should make one question the competence of the laboratory. Another serologic test that is of use, particularly if sera are anticomplementary, is quantitative immunodiffusion. Titers are generally similar to those obtained with the CF test.

In meningitis, the above parameters plus the ventricular fluid cell count, sugar, protein, bacterial and fungal culture, and CF titer are followed on the same schedule.

Duration of Therapy

Duration of treatment is unclear for ketoconazole and is generally limited by toxicity for amphotericin B. Relapses of disease have been observed in adults following cessation of ketoconazole therapy.

Our results with ketoconazole have been so favorable, and the medication has been so well tolerated, that we have treated patients until their clinical disease has disappeared, serum CF titers were <1:16, and skin tests were positive. For meningitis cases, we continue miconazole intraventricularly until the ventricular fluid culture, if initially positive, is negative for 1 year *and* the ventricular fluid CF titer is 1:2 or less. These guidelines have resulted in courses of ketoconazole therapy as short as 3 months in some pneumonia patients to 1–2 years in other more severe cases and over 4 years in meningitis cases. Miconazole has been discontinued successfully in several of the meningitis cases without ventricular relapse, and our first meningitis case, diagnosed in 1976, now has a positive skin test. All patients have had steady decline in ventricular and serum CF titers.

Cysticercosis

JAMES SANTIAGO GRISOLIA, M.D.

The cysticercus causes more central nervous system disease than any other parasite. It is common throughout the third world, including South America, China, India, Southeast Asia, and parts of Africa. In Mexico, at least 2% of the entire population carries this infection, and due to immigration, many physicians in the United States are being called upon to treat it.

The clinical manifestations depend largely on the anatomic localization of the parasites, overall number of parasites, and host immune factors. Cysts localized to muscle usually cause no symptoms, although a painful myositis can result. Lesions in cerebral cortex may produce seizures or focal neurologic deficits or both. Lesions in the cerebral ventricles may result in a noncommunicating hydrocephalus, occasionally with a ball valve mechanism causing sudden complete blockage and syncope. Cysts in the basilar cisterns cause a reactive meningitis, communicating hydrocephalus, cranial nerve palsies, or dementia. True strokes may result if this inflammation thromboses a cerebral vessel.

Radiologic studies include, most importantly, the computerized tomographic scan, which is sensitive in detecting isolated cysts, either with or without calcification, as well as hydrocephalus and edema. CT scanning may be normal in up to 30–40% of infected patients. Skull films may reveal brain calcification or soft tissue films of the thighs may reveal calcified muscular cysts, but these techniques rarely produce positive results. Other studies available in the United States, including angiography, myelography, etc., may be helpful in selected patients. The place of magnetic resonance imaging is yet to be determined. The technique's sensitivity to edema and insensitivity to calcification should provide a very different, complementary view of parenchymal cysts.

Lumbar puncture may be normal or present any combination of abnormalities, mimicking acute purulent meningitis or a mild aseptic process. The degree of abnormality depends on the extent of cisternal involvement, chronicity of the lesions and host response. A low CSF glucose is said to carry a poor prognosis. CSF eosinophilia may be searched for by Wright's or eosinophil stain. The presence of any eosinophils is abnormal and is seen in up to 40% of cases. This finding is fairly specific for CNS parasitosis but may also be seen in CNS foreign body reactions and occasionally in other brain infections.

Serological studies may be performed on CSF or serum, but are generally more sensitive on serum. The most reliable test that is widely available in the United States is indirect hemagglutination test (IHA), best performed at the Centers for Disease Control (CDC) in Atlanta, Georgia. The specificity is rather high, with most false positives occurring in other parasitic diseases. The echinococcus and cysticercus IHAs cross-react extensively, for example. Up to 40% of cysticercotic patients may have negative serologies. Other promising serological tests are being developed.

Until recently, the only available treatment has been symptomatic. Anticonvulsants, steroids for hydrocephalus or brain swelling, and ventriculoperitoneal shunting for hydrocephalus have formed the mainstays of therapy. Now, several drugs have been developed that cross the blood-brain barrier to effectively kill encysted larvae in the brain. Of these, praziquantel is available in the United States and is the best studied.

Praziquantel effectively kills cysticerci in vitro and in vivo, and significantly reduced clinical and radiologic manifestations in two prospective studies. Some spectacular anecdotal responses have been recorded. In a disease where the natural history is often benign and where the most severe effects apparently occur after the cyst has died, the impact of effective larval killing is hard to assess. The benign seizure disorder caused by an isolated parenchymal lesion will probably not be altered by Praziquantel. The progressive scarring and hydrocephalus caused by meningeal involvement will probably not be altered by praziquantel. A better candidate is the acute encephalitic form, which appears to respond well to a combination of praziquantel and steroids.

Although experience with praziquantel* in children is not extensive, the dose of 50 mg/kg/day, given in three divided doses for a period of 15 days, appears successful in adults and children for treatment of cerebral lesions.† Decadron, 1–3 mg/kg/day should be given in divided doses for at least the first 3–5 days with a rapid taper. Steroid coverage helps to reduce inflammation and edema resulting from death of many larvae at once.

Surgical indications include most importantly hydrocephalus, which generally responds well to standard shunting techniques. Occasionally, if ventriculitis is present, repeated shunt occlusions may

---

* Manufacturer's warning: Safety in children under 4 years of age has not been established.

† This use of praziquantel is not listed in the manufacturer's directive.

occur with significant morbidity and mortality. This process of ventricular scarring may be minimized or averted by surgical removal of any intraventricular cysts, which is technically easiest before cicatrization reduces cyst mobility. This approach to cyst removal should offer the greatest advantage in children, who have the least prior scarring and the longest future course. After initial shunting, intraventricular contrast may be introduced by shunt puncture under sterile conditions and CT scanning performed. If intraventricular cysts are localized, elective removal may then be accomplished, occasionally by simple ventriculostomy and pipette extraction. Resection of isolated lesions in the brain substance itself appears to be completely unnecessary unless seizures are uncontrollable despite sustained, rational anticonvulsant therapy. Adhesions in the basilar cisterns should not be surgically lysed, unless the optic nerve tracts or chiasm are involved with progressive blindness. Cysts in the cisterns may be removed if mass effect is significant, generally preceded by ventriculostomy or shunting from above. Spinal adhesions may cause progressive myelopathy and are said to respond well to surgical lysis.

This disease continues to present challenges because of its varied clinical manifestations and variable course. Its increasing frequency in the United States, as well as major advances in diagnosis and treatment, demand the attention of pediatricians throughout the United States.

Mucormycosis

JOHN F. BROWN, JR., M.D.

Mucormycosis is a disease caused by saprophytic fungi. It almost always occurs in a compromised host. Broad nonseptate hyphae are found in the tissues, usually growing into the arteries, producing thrombosis, infarction, and necrosis, and resulting in the most rapidly progressive fungal disease known.

The portal of entry of the fungus and the type of previous debility of the patient largely determine whether the form of infection will be rhinocerebral, pulmonary, gastrointestinal, disseminated, cutaneous, or focal. Rhinocerebral and focal infections are more often associated with the acidosis of uncontrolled diabetes. Pulmonary and disseminated forms occur more often in patients with blood diseases, particularly leukemia and lymphoma.

Unfortunately many cases of mucormycosis are diagnosed after death. Although mucormycosis is rare, the diagnosis must be considered in patients who are immunosuppressed or in those with diabetic acidosis. It is most urgent that scrapings and tissue biopsies of suspicious lesions be obtained and examined.

The general management is determined by the extent of the associated disease and the pattern of organ involvement. General measures include the prompt and vigorous control of the diabetes if present and the treatment of any dehydration or acidosis. One must consider reducing or temporarily withholding immunosuppressive therapy.

Surgery plays a vital role. The drainage of sinuses or abscesses, the removal of devitalized tissue, and/or the débridement of infected tissues must not be delayed.

When there is destruction of the hard palate, a prosthesis should be fitted immediately so that the patient will be able to swallow and satisfy nutritional needs. Later plastic repair of residual defects in the mucous membranes, bone, and craniofacial structures may be required.

Baseline studies should be obtained before amphotericin B therapy, the antibiotic of choice, is started. These studies are hemaglobin, hematocrit, serum potassium and creatine, and creatinine clearance. They should be monitored three times a week until stable. There should then be weekly follow-ups of serum creatinine and potassium plus hematocrit.

Premedications such as oral acetaminophen (10–15 mg/kg) and diphenhydramine hydrochloride (1.25 mg/kg) given 30 minutes prior to the amphotericin B infusion often reduces or eliminates the toxic effects, which include fever, chills, headache, nausea, and vomiting. If toxic symptoms persist, 10–15 mg of intravenous hydrocortisone may be given at the same time. Extreme chills usually can be stopped immediately with intravenous meperidine.

Amphotericin B should be prepared according to the package insert. The concentration infused should be no more than 0.1 mg/ml in 5% dextrose in water (never saline). The infusion does not need to be protected from light. The experience of many clinicians has been that there are less side effects if the infusion is given within 1 to 3 hours instead of usual 6 hours.

In this rapidly progressive disease one cannot take 7 to 10 days to reach a 1 mg/kg daily dose. A more reasonable program is an initial dose of 0.25 mg/kg followed by a 0.25 mg/kg increase daily until 1.0 mg/kg daily is reached. It may be necessary to hold the same dosage level or resort to alternate-day therapy until the patient develops tolerance to a given dose. When the clinical picture improves, the dosage may dropped to 3 times a week and later to twice a week. The total dose is dependent on the clinical improvement and the toxic effects of the amphotericin B; 35–40 mg/kg will be the average total dose required.

The amphotericin B dose should be cut in half

or the dose schedule reduced to two or three times a week if the hematocrit drops to 25% or the creatinine rises to 3.0 mg/dl (or 1.5 mg/dl when the child is less than 10 years of age). Daily oral potassium supplementation usually prevents the hypokalemia that develops with daily amphotericin therapy.

Wound infections may be treated with 3% topical amphotericin B ointment and débrided bony lesions may be irrigated with 10% amphotericin B solution.

Toxocara Canis Infections (Including Visceral Larva Migrans)

GORDON WORLEY, M.D.

Toxocara canis is a dog round worm (ascarid) which infects almost all puppies and many dogs in the United States and elswhere. Human infection is acquired by ingesting embryonated eggs. Three clinical forms of infection are recognized: visceral larva migrans (VLM), ocular toxocariasis, and asymptomatic infection.

VLM is a clinical syndrome usually occurring in toddlers (children ages one to four years) characterized by fever, hepatosplenomegaly, pulmonary symptoms (asthma, pneumonia), and occasionally encephalitis accompanied by a peripheral eosinophilia, which may be marked. Any organ may be involved. There is frequently a history of pica and puppy ownership. The syndrome is self-limited and rarely lethal. Although by some definitions VLM must be caused by those parasites for which man is a paratenic host (for instance, *Toxocara canis*, *Toxacara cati*, *Ascaris suum*, and other animal ascarids), the same signs and symptoms can however also be caused by migrating larvae of parasites for which man is the natural host (for instance, *Ascaris lumbricoides*, hookworm, and *Strongyloides stercoralis*). Children with VLM should be checked for lead poisoning, since the two conditions have been reported to occur concomitantly, probably, since pica is a mode of acquisition for both. Siblings of children with VLM may also have the syndrome and should be evaluated.

Ocular toxocariasis usually presents with strabismus, leukocoria, diminished visual acuity, and/or pain. The disease occurs in older children (school age) who are otherwise asymptomatic. Patients should be referred to a pediatric ophthalmologist for diagnosis, since the clinical differentiation between ocular toxocariasis and retinoblastoma may be difficult.

Most *Toxocara canis* infections are unrecognized and are probably either asymptomatic or produce only mild complaints; seropositivity is widely prevalent in some sections of the United States but infection is rarely diagnosed.

Definitive diagnosis of *Toxocara canis* infection can be made only by identification of larvae in tissue. In cases of VLM, if a tissue diagnosis is felt necessary, an open liver biopsy is preferable to a closed needle biopsy, which may miss granulomata. Antibodies appear in serum soon after infection, and titers can be measured using an enzyme-linked immunosorbent assay (ELISA) employing the second-stage larval secretory piece as the antigen. An antibody titer of 1:32 or greater is presumptive evidence of *Toxocara canis* infection in cases with symptoms compatible with VLM. The diagnosis of ocular toxocariasis should not depend upon the ELISA because of the wide prevalence of seropositivity in asymptomatic children and the report of a seronegative case of *Toxocara canis* disease. The Parasitic Diseases Division of the Centers for Disease Control, Atlanta, Georgia, will perform antibody titer determinations on serum from suspected cases of *Toxocara canis* infection using the ELISA. The diagnosis of *Toxocara canis* infection cannot be made by examination of the stool for ova and parasites because the parasite does not complete its life cycle in man. However, since the VLM syndrome can also be caused by parasites for which man is the natural host, microscopic examination of sputum for larvae and of the stool for ova should be done periodically during the course of symptoms.

Recommendations about the treatment of visceral larva migrans caused by *Toxocara canis* are necessarily arbitrary, since no adequate clinical trial of any drug has been published. For patients with encephalitis, cardiac involvement, or severe pulmonary symptoms, the current treatment of choice is diethylcarbamazine* at 2–4 mg/kg three times daily for two to three weeks. In experimental animals, it is larvicidal and has better tissue penetration into brain and muscle than the alternate, thiabendazole. Death of the larvae releases antigens that can provoke a Mazzotti reaction, a complex immunologic phenomenon manifest by pruritus, hives and other rashes, lymphadenopathy, fever, arthritis, and occasionally hypotension. The immediate hypersensitivity component of the reaction may begin shortly after diethylcarbamazine is given. For this reason, steroids in an antiinflammatory dose (20–40 mg of prednisone) and an antihistamine should be given several hours prior to treatment and for 3 or 4 days, or as long as symptoms persist. Steroids alone should not be given to patients with visceral larva migrans, since

---

* Diethylcarbamazine is no longer available commercially. Apply to the Centers for Disease Control, Atlanta, Georgia, if this drug is required.

compromise of the host's ability to limit the infection may result.

Thiabendazole has been reported to reduce the severity and shorten the duration of the symptoms in cases of visceral larvae migrans caused by *Toxocara canis*. In experimental animals, the drug is not larvacidal but acts by inhibiting migration, allowing for larvae contained in the liver to be eliminated there through immunologic mechanisms. Also in experimental animals, the drug is ineffective in eliminating larvae in brain and muscle. Thiabendazole is given at 25 mg/kg after meals twice daily for 5 to 7 days. The FDA considers both drugs to be investigational for the treatment of *Toxocara canis* infection.

The treatment of ocular toxocariasis should be directed by a pediatric ophthalmologist. Since much of the ocular damage is caused by inflammation associated with *Toxocara canis* infection, steroids are the mainstay of treatment and may be given systemically or by injection into or behind the eye, depending upon the site and severity of involvement. There are reports of successful treatment of ocular toxocariasis by diethylcarbamazine* and thiabendazole, but their use is controversial, since death of larvae in the eye may provoke a severe inflammatory response, worsening the outcome.

All dogs and puppies of the families of children with visceral larva migrans or ocular toxocariasis should be dewormed. Prevention of *Toxocara canis* disease in man is possible if puppies and nursing bitches are given an appropriate antihelmintic once a week for three weeks, beginning two weeks postpartum and then once every six months. There are many effective veterinary preparations, and some available over the counter.

Malaria

PARVIN H. AZIMI, M.D.

Malaria is a major infectious disease and public health hazard in many parts of the world, being responsible for some two million deaths annually in endemic areas. A definite worldwide resurgence of this infection has been noted during the past two decades, which has been reflected in the United States by an increasing number of cases reported to Centers for Disease Control. Among several complex reasons offered in explanation for this extensive resurgence is the development of resistance on the part of the *Anopheles* mosquito vector to dichlorodiphenyltrichloroethane (DDT). Until recently this insecticide was regarded as a mainstay in the control of the vector population. In addition, a number of strains of *Plasmodium falciparum*, the cause of malignant tertian malaria,

have now become resistant to chloroquine, a drug universally regarded as one of the most effective antimalarial agents. This resistance is becoming increasingly evident in malarial endemic areas of Asia, Latin America, Africa, and Oceana, particularly so in the Southeast Asian strains.

Although malaria is no longer endemic in the United States, widespread travel by its citizens to affected areas has resulted in an increased incidence of the disease in this country. Further contribution to the number of affected individuals has been made more recently by the influx of immigrants, especially from Southeast Asia, and also by transfusions of malaria-contaminated blood. The occurrence of congenital malaria has been reported as well in the United States on several occasions.

If clinically suspected, an effort should be made to confirm the diagnosis of malaria by identifying the particular species of parasite in appropriate blood smears. This often requires the experience of expert laboratory personnel. Identification of the species is important, since the strains of *P. falciparum* causing the malignant tertian variety of the disease are the ones among which resistance to chloroquine is becoming especially manifest. Although recently described in vitro studies could possibly detect the drug sensitivity of the *P. falciparum*, the patient usually requires urgent treatment before the results of these tests become available. This emphasizes that knowledge of the particular area wherein the infection was acquired could be important and helpful in the choice of the antimalarial drug to be used.

Prevention

Malaria risk by country is reported annually in "Health Information for International Travel" published by the United States Public Health Service and available from the Centers for Disease Control, Atlanta, Georgia.

If at all possible, prevention should include avoidance of travel in endemic areas, minimizing mosquito contact through the use of insect repellants, mosquito nets, and adequate clothing. Chemoprophylaxis with chloroquine is the mainstay of prevention. Fortunately all species of *Plasmodium* with the exception of some strains of *P. falciparum* have remained sensitive to chloroquine.

For adults, 300 mg chloroquine base (500 mg chloroquine phosphate) is taken once a week, commencing one week before travel to the endemic areas and continuing for 6 weeks after termination of exposure in the endemic areas. For children of less than 50 kg weight, 5 mg chloroquine base/kg is taken once a week, starting before travel to the endemic areas and continuing for 6 weeks after termination of exposure in the endemic areas.

Chloroquine-Resistant *P. falciparum*. Prophylaxis against chloroquine-resistant *P. falciparum* is becoming a major problem in the endemic areas already mentioned. For these strains a combination of sulfonamide and pyrimethamine in a fixed ratio tablet containing 500 mg sulfadoxine and 25 mg pyrimethamine is used. This drug is marketed by Hoffmann-La Roche under the name of Fansidar.* This is effective for both prevention and treatment of chloroquine-resistant *P. falciparum*. For adults one Fansidar tablet per week should be taken on the same day of the week from one week before to 6 weeks after exposure to the endemic areas. For children the following dosage is recommended; 6–11 months: $\frac{1}{8}$ tablet; 1–3 years: $\frac{1}{4}$ tablet; 4–8 years: $\frac{1}{2}$ tablet; 9–14 years: $\frac{3}{4}$ tablet, once weekly from one week before until 6 weeks after exposure to endemic areas. Chloroquine should be added if *P. vivax* exposure is also likely. *P. falciparum* resistant to Fansidar has been reported in many areas of Asia and East Africa. In these cases *Medical Letter* recommends the use of quinine for prophylaxis. Prevention of attack after departure from endemic areas of *P. vivax* and *P. ovale* is achieved by the use of primaquine (dosage given below) for 14 days, along with the last 2 weeks of chloroquine prophylaxis.

Treatment

The following schedule is recommended for the treatment of malaria due to all species except chloroquine-resistant *P. falciparum*.

In adults chloroquine base 600 mg (1 gm) is given followed by 300 mg base (500 mg) in 6 hours and then 300 mg base (500 mg) per day for two days. For children 10 mg base/kg (max. 600 mg base) followed by 5 mg base/kg 6 hours later and then 5 mg base/kg per day for two days. For prevention of relapses in adults with *P. vivax* and *P. ovale* infection, primaquine phosphate is given in a dose of 15 mg base (26.3 mg) per day for 14 days, and in children in a dose of 0.3 mg base/kg per day for 14 days. Oral chloroquine phosphate is the drug of choice for the treatment of all forms of malaria not due to chloroquine-resistant *P. falciparum*. Most patients do not need hospitalization and can be treated on an out-patient basis, but severe cases and chronically ill patients may require hospitalization. Chloroquine phosphate is effective in prompt control of fever and rapid eradication of parasites from the blood. Both chloroquine and quinine are effective against intraeryrhocytic parasites and have no effect on extraerythrocytic liver forms, which are responsible for relapses in *P. vivax* and *P. ovale* malaria. The drug of choice for treatment of the extra-erythrocytic liver forms is primaquine, this drug

* Manufacturer's warning: Do not give Fansidar to infants less than 2 months of age.

having no effect on blood forms. For this purpose primaquine is given after a course of chloroquine and when the patient has become afebrile. Caucasian patients with G6PD deficiency should not receive primaquine since severe hemolysis could occur. In these patients chloroquine is generally used for each relapse. The black population with G6PD deficiency can generally tolerate primaquine without severe hemolysis.

Primaquine is necessary for elimination of liver forms of the parasite in mosquito-acquired malaria but not in transfusion malaria or congenital malaria, in which these liver forms do not exist. During treatment patients should be monitored clinically and by blood smears. Failure to clear parasitemia while on chloroquine implies that the patient may have chloroquine-resistant *P. falciparum* malaria.

Chloroquine-Resistant *P. falciparum*. For adults three Fansidar tablets in a single dose are curative in approximately 80 to 90% of immune individuals. However, the *Medical Letter* recommends a regimen of quinine sulfate, 650 mg three times a day for 3 days, plus pyrimethamine, 25 mg two times a day for 3 days, plus sulfadiazine, 500 mg four times a day for 5 days. For children a combination of quinine sulfate, pyrimethamine, and sulfadiazine in the following dosages is recommended: quinine sulfate, 25 mg/kg/day in 3 doses for 3 days; pyrimethamine, 6.25 mg/day for 3 days (for children less than 10 kg); 12.5 mg/day for 3 days (for children 10–20 kg); and 25 mg/day for 3 days (for children 20–40 kg); and sulfadiazine, 100–200 mg/kg/day in 4 doses for 5 days (max. 2 gm/day).

An alternative regimen includes a combination of quinine sulfate plus tetracycline or clindamycin. Tetracycline is used in a dosage of 250 mg four times a day for 7 days for adults and 5 mg/kg four times a day for 7 days for children. Clindamycin is used in a dosage of 900 mg three times a day for 3 days for adults and 20–40 mg/kg/day in 3 doses for 3 days for children.

Cerebral Malaria. Treatment of cerebral malaria requires hospitalization and parenteral therapy. Quinine dihydrochloride administered intravenously is the drug of choice for the treatment of cerebral malaria in children. The dose is 12.5 mg/kg dissolved in saline solution, and half of the dose is infused intravenously over one hour. The other half can be given in 6 hours if the patient remains unable to take oral treatment.

Infection During Pregnancy. During pregnancy chloroquine is used for prophylaxis and treatment of malaria caused by susceptible strains. The use of chloroquine in pregnancy appears to be safe, although defects in offspring have been noted when large doses of chloroquine have been used for the treatment of connective tissue disease during pregnancy. The drugs used to treat chloroquine-resistant *P. falciparum* infection may produce fetal malformations if used during pregnancy. Quinine can cause abortion, premature labor, and optic nerve defects; tetracycline can cause defective bone and tooth development. Pyrimethamine has been shown to be teratogenic in laboratory animals. It is therefore quite obvious that the treatment of chloroquine-resistant *P. falciparum* during pregnancy remains an unresolved problem. When confronted with this situation, treatment should not be withheld, but the least toxic agents should be used. Folinic acid supplementation should be used whenever pyrimethamine is used during pregnancy.

Congenital Malaria. Since transplacental transmission of erythrocytes has been shown to occur before or during birth, congenital malaria can result if the transmitted erythrocytes harbor the malarial parasite. Since this transmission can occur before or during delivery, it is difficult to distinguish between actual congenital and perinatal acquisition of malaria. When malaria is acquired congenitally or perinatally, the drug of choice for treatment would be chloroquine phosphate, since passage of the sporozoite forms does not occur and the exoerythrocytic cycle does not exist.

Babesiosis

GEORGE A. JACOBY, M.D.

Babesiosis is a usually self-limited, malaria-like disease caused in the United States by infection of human red blood cells with the protozoan parasite *Babesia microti*. Most infections are subclinical and are detected only by serologic surveys. Severe infections with fever, hemolytic anemia, hemoglobinuria, and renal failure have occurred in splenectomized adults. Symptomatic infection in the pediatric age group is rare.

The illness usually resolves spontaneously and requires only symptomatic treatment. Severe infections in adults have been successfully treated by exchange transfusion. Chloroquine and other antimalarials, diminazene aceturate, and pentamidine isethionate have been administered without clear benefit. Recently, a premature infant with transfusion babesiosis was cured with clindamycin plus quinine, a combination also shown to be effective against *B. microti* infection in hamsters.

Therefore, an ill or immunocompromised patient with babesiosis should be treated with clindamycin, 20 mg/kg/day, PO, IV, or IM, divided, four times a day (maximum: 600 mg every 6 hours), and quinine sulfate, 25 mg/kg/day orally, divided, three times a day (maximum 650 mg tid), both for 7 to 10 days.

Drugs for Parasitic Infections*

Parasitic infections are now encountered throughout the world. With increasing travel, and especially with the recent large emigration from Southeast Asia, the Caribbean, and Central and South America, physicians anywhere may see infections caused by previously unfamiliar parasites. The table that begins on page 607 lists first-choice and alternative drugs with recommended dosages for most parasitic infections. In every case, the need for treatment must be weighed against toxicity of the drug. A decision to withhold therapy may often be correct, particularly when the drugs can cause severe adverse effects. When the first-choice drug is initially ineffective and the alternative is more hazardous, it may be prudent to try a second course of treatment with the first drug before using the alternative. Several drugs recommended in the table have not been approved by the U.S. Food and Drug Administration. When a physician prescribes an unapproved drug, or an approved drug for an unapproved indication, it may be advisable to inform the patient of the investigational status and adverse effects of the drug. A second table on page 615 lists adverse effects of some antiparasitic drugs.

PARTIAL LIST OF GENERIC AND BRAND NAMES

albendazole—Zentel (SKF)
amphotericin B—Fungizone (Squibb)
benzyl benzoate—Scabanca (Canada); others
*bithionol—Bitin (Tanabe, Japan)
chloroquine—Aralen (Winthrop); others
copper oleate—Cuprex (Beecham)
crotamiton—Eurax (Westwood)
*dehydroemetine—(Hoffmann-LaRoche, Switzerland)
diethylcarbamazine—Hetrazan (Lederle)
*diloxanide furoate—Furamide (Boots, England)
furazolidone—Furoxone (Norwich Eaton)
iodoquinol (diiodohydroxyquin)—Yodoxin (Glenwood)
lindane (gamma benzene hexachloride)—Kwell (Reed and Carnrick); others
malathion—Prioderm Lotion (Purdue Frederick)
mebendazole—Vermox (Janssen)
*melarsoprol—Arsobal (Rhône Poulenc, France)
**metrifonate—Bilarcil (Bayer, Germany)
metronidazole—Flagyl (Searle); others
niclosamide—Niclocide (Miles)
*nifurtimox—Lampit (Bayer, Germany)

---

* Available from the Parasitic Diseases Division, Center for Infectious Diseases, Centers for Disease Control, Atlanta, Georgia 30333; 404-329-3670
** Not available in the USA

**niridazole—Ambilhar (Ciba-Geigy, Switzerland)
oxamniquine—Vansil (Pfizer)
paromomycin—Humatin (Parke, Davis)
*pentamidine isethionate—(May & Baker, England)
piperazine—Antepar (Burroughs Wellcome); others
praziquantel—Biltricide (Miles)
primaquine phosphate—Primaquine (Winthrop)
pyrantel pamoate—Antiminth (Pfipharmecs)
pyrethrins and piperonyl butoxide—Rid (Pfipharmecs); others
pyrimethamine—Daraprim (Burroughs Wellcome)
pyrimethamine and sulfadoxine—Fansidar (Roche)

quinacrine—Atabrine (Winthrop)
*quinine dihydrochloride
**spiramycin—Rovamycin (Poulenc, Canada)
*stibogluconate sodium (antimony sodium gluconate)—Pentostam (Burroughs Wellcome, England)
*suramin—Germanin (Bayer, Germany)
tetrachloroethylene—NEMA Worm Capsules, Vet (Parke, Davis)
thiabendazole—Mintezol (Merck Sharp & Dohme)
trimethoprim-sulfamethoxazole—Bactrim (Roche); Septra (Burroughs Wellcome); others
**tryparsamide

DRUGS FOR TREATMENT OF PARASITIC INFECTIONS

Infection	Drug	Adult Dose*	Pediatric Dose*
AMEBIASIS (Entamoeba histolytica)			
asymptomatic			
Drug of choice:	Iodoquinol[1]	650 mg tid × 20d	30–40 mg/kg/d in 3 doses × 20d
Alternatives:	Diloxanide furoate[2]	500 mg tid × 10d	20 mg/kg/d in 3 doses × 10d
	Paromomycin	25–30 mg/kg/d in 3 doses × 7d	25–30 mg/kg/d in 3 doses × 7d
mild to moderate intestinal disease			
Drug of choice:	Metronidazole[3]	750 mg tid × 5–10d	35–50 mg/kg/d in 3 doses × 10d
	plus iodoquinol[1]	650 mg tid × 20d	30–40 mg/kg/d in 3 doses × 20d
Alternative:	Paromomycin	25–30 mg/kg/d in 3 doses × 7d	25–30 mg/kg/d in 3 doses × 7d
severe intestinal disease			
Drug of choice:	Metronidazole[3]	750 mg tid × 5–10d	35–50 mg/kg/d in 3 doses × 10d
	plus iodoquinol[1]	650 mg tid × 20d	30–40 mg/kg/d in 3 doses × 20d
Alternatives:	Dehydroemetine[2,4] **plus**	1 to 1.5 mg/kg/d IM (max. 90 mg/d) for up to 5d	1 to 1.5 mg/kg/d (max. 90 mg/d) IM in 2 doses for up to 5d
	iodoquinol[1]	650 mg tid × 20d	30–40 mg/kg/d in 3 doses × 20d
OR	Emetine[4] **plus**	1 mg/kg/d (max. 60 mg/d) IM for up to 5d	1 mg/kg/d in 2 doses (max. 60 mg/d) IM for up to 5d
	iodoquinol[1]	650 mg tid × 20d	30–40 mg/kg/d in 3 doses × 20d
hepatic abscess			
Drug of choice:	Metronidazole[3]	750 mg tid ×5–10d	35–50 mg/kg/d in 3 doses × 10d
	plus iodoquinol[1]	650 mg tid × 20d	30–40 mg/kg/d in 3 doses × 20d
Alternatives:	Dehydroemetine[2,4] **followed by**	1 to 1.5 mg/kg/d (max. 90 mg/d) IM for up to 5d	1 to 1.5 mg/kg/d (max. 90 mg/d) IM in 2 doses for up to 5d
	chloroquine phosphate **plus**	600 mg base (1 gram) daily × 2d, then 300 mg base (500 mg) daily × 2–3 wks	10 mg base/kg (max. 300 mg base)/d × 2–3 wks
	iodoquinol[1]	650 mg tid × 20d	30–40 mg/kg/d in 3 doses × 20d

* The letter d indicates day.

Table continued on following page

DRUGS FOR TREATMENT OF PARASITIC INFECTIONS (*continued*)

Infection	Drug	Adult Dose*	Pediatric Dose*
OR	Emetine[4] **followed by** chloroquine phosphate **plus** iodoquinol[1]	1 mg/kg/d (max. 60 mg/d) IM for up to 5d 600 mg base (1 gram) daily × 2d, then 300 mg base (500 mg) daily × 2–3 wks 650 mg tid × 20d	1 mg/kg/d in 2 doses (max. 60 mg/d) IM for up to 5d 10 mg base/kg/d (max. 300 mg base/d) × 2–3 wks 30–40 mg/kg/d in 3 doses × 20d

AMEBIC MENINGOENCEPHALITIS, PRIMARY (Naegleria sp; Acanthamoeba sp)

Drug of choice[5]:	Amphotericin B[6]	1 mg/kg/d IV, uncertain duration	1 mg/kg/d IV, uncertain duration

Ancylostoma duodenale, see HOOKWORM

ANGIOSTRONGYLUS cantonensis

Drug of choice:	Thiabendazole[6,7]	25 mg/kg bid × 3d	25 mg/kg bid × 3d
OR	Mebendazole[7]	100 mg bid × 5d	100 mg bid × 5d for children >2 years

ANISAKIASIS (Anisakis sp)

Treatment of choice:	Surgical removal		
Alternative:	Thiabendazole[6,7]	25 mg/kg bid × 3d	25 mg/kg bid × 3d

ASCARIS lumbricoides (roundworm)

Drug of choice:	Mebendazole	100 mg bid × 3d	100 mg bid × 3d for children >2 years
OR	Pyrantel pamoate	11 mg/kg once (max. 1 gram)	11 mg/kg once (max. 1 gram)
Alternative:	Piperazine citrate	75 mg/kg (max 3.5 grams)/d × 2d	75 mg/kg (max. 3.5 grams)/d × 2d

BABESIA

Drug of choice:	Clindamycin[6] **plus** quinine	1.2 grams bid parenteral or 600 mg tid oral × 7d 650 mg tid oral × 7d	20–40 mg/kg/d in 3 doses × 7d 25 mg/kg/d in 3 doses × 7d

BALANTIDIUM coli

Drug of choice:	Tetracycline[6]	500 mg qid × 10d	10 mg/kg qid × 10d (max. 2 grams/d)
Alternative:	Iodoquinol[1,6]	650 mg tid × 20d	40 mg/kg/d in 3 doses × 20d

CAPILLARIA philippinensis

Drug of choice:	Mebendazole[6]	200 mg bid × 20d	200 mg bid × 20d
Alternative:	Thiabendazole[6]	25 mg/kg/d × 30d	25 mg/kg/d × 30d

Chagas' disease, see TRYPANOSOMIASIS

Clonorchis sinensis, see FLUKES

CUTANEOUS LARVA MIGRANS (creeping eruption)

Drug of choice:	Thiabendazole	Topically and/or 25 mg/kg bid (max. 3 grams/d) × 2–5d	Topically and/or 25 mg/kg bid (max. 3 grams/d) × 2–5d

DIENTAMOEBA fragilis

Drug of choice:	Iodoquinol[1]	650 mg tid × 20d	40 mg/kg/d in 3 doses × 20d
OR	Tetracycline[6]	500 mg qid × 10d	10 mg/kg qid × 10d (max. 2 grams/d)

Diphyllobothrium latum, see TAPEWORMS

DRACUNCULUS medinensis (guinea worm)

Drug of choice:	Niridazole[8]	25 mg/kg (max. 1.5 grams)/d × 10d	Same as adult, divided into 2 doses
Alternative:	Metronidazole[3,6]	250 mg tid × 10d	25 mg/kg/d (max. 750 mg/d) in 3 doses × 10d

* The letter d indicates day.

Table continued on opposite page

DRUGS FOR TREATMENT OF PARASITIC INFECTIONS (*continued*)

Infection	Drug	Adult Dose*	Pediatric Dose*
Echinococcus, see TAPEWORMS			
Entamoeba histolytica, see AMEBIASIS			
ENTEROBIUS vermicularis (pinworm)			
Drug of choice:	Pyrantel pamoate	A single dose of 11 mg/kg (max. 1 gram); repeat after 2 weeks	A single dose of 11 mg/kg (max. 1 gram); repeat after 2 weeks
OR	Mebendazole	A single dose of 100 mg; repeat after 2 weeks	A single dose of 100 mg for children >2 years; repeat after 2 weeks
Fasciola hepatica, see FLUKES			
FILARIASIS			
Wuchereria bancrofti, Brugia (W.) malayi, Acanthocheilonema perstans, Loa loa			
Drug of choice:	Diethylcarbamazine[9]	Day 1: 50 mg Day 2: 50 mg tid Day 3: 100 mg tid Days 4 through 21: 2 mg/kg tid	Day 1: 25–50 mg Day 2: 25–50 mg tid Day 3: 50–100 mg tid Days 4 through 21: 2 mg/kg tid
Tropical eosinophilia			
Drug of choice:	Diethylcarbamazine[9]	2 mg/kg tid × 7–10d	2 mg/kg tid × 7–10d
Onchocerca volvulus			
Drug of choice:	Diethylcarbamazine[9]	25 mg/d × 3d, then 50 mg/d × 5d, then 100 mg/d × 3d, then 150 mg/d × 12d	0.5 mg/kg tid × 3d (max. 25 mg/d), then 1.0 mg/kg tid × 3–4d (max. 50 mg/d), then 1.5 mg/kg tid × 3–4d (max. 100 mg/d), then 2.0 mg/kg tid × 2–3 wks (max. 150 mg/d)
	followed by suramin[2,10]	100–200 mg (test dose) IV, then 1 gram IV at weekly intervals × 5 wks	10–20 mg (test dose) IV, then 20 mg/kg IV at weekly intervals × 5 wks
Alternative:	Mebendazole[11]	1 gram bid × 28d	
FLUKES, hermaphroditic			
Clonorchis sinensis (Chinese liver fluke)			
Drug of choice:	Praziquantel[6]	25 mg/kg tid × 1d	25 mg/kg tid × 1d
Fasciola hepatica (sheep liver fluke)			
Drug of choice:	Praziquantel[6,12]	25 mg/kg tid × 1d	25 mg/kg tid × 1d
Alternative:	Bithionol[2]	30–50 mg/kg on alternate days × 10–15 doses	30–50 mg/kg on alternate days × 10–15 doses
Fasciolopsis buski (intestinal fluke)			
Drug of choice:	Praziquantel[6]	25 mg/kg tid × 1d	25 mg/kg tid × 1d
Alternative:	Tetrachloroethylene[13]	0.1 ml/kg (max. 5 ml)	0.1 ml/kg (max. 5 ml)
Heterophyes heterophyes (intestinal fluke)			
Drug of choice:	Praziquantel[6]	25 mg/kg tid × 1d	25 mg/kg tid × 1d
Alternative:	Tetrachloroethylene[13]	0.1 ml/kg (max. 5 ml)	0.1 ml/kg (max. 5 ml)
Metagonimus yokogawai (intestinal fluke)			
Drug of choice:	Praziquantel[6]	25 mg/kg tid × 1d	25 mg/kg tid × 1d
Alternative:	Tetrachloroethylene[13]	0.1 ml/kg (max. 5 ml)	0.1 ml/kg (max. 5 ml)
Opisthorchis viverrini (liver fluke)			
Drug of choice:	Praziquantel[6]	25 mg/kg tid × 1d	25 mg/kg tid × 1d
Paragonimus westermani (lung fluke)			
Drug of choice:	Praziquantel[6]	25 mg/kg tid × 1–2d	25 mg/kg tid × 1–2d
Alternative:	Bithionol[2]	30–50 mg/kg on alternate days × 10–15d	30–50 mg/kg on alternate days × 10–15d
GIARDIASIS (Giardia lamblia)			
Drug of choice:	Quinacrine HCl	100 mg tid p.c. × 5d	2 mg/kg tid p.c. × 5d (max. 300 mg/d)
Alternatives:	Metronidazole[3,6]	250 mg tid × 5d	5 mg/kg tid × 5d
	Furazolidone	100 mg qid × 7–10d	1.25 mg/kg qid × 7–10d

* The letter d indicates day.

Table continued on following page

DRUGS FOR TREATMENT OF PARASITIC INFECTIONS (*continued*)

Infection	Drug	Adult Dose*	Pediatric Dose*
GNATHOSTOMIASIS (Gnathostoma spinigerum)			
Drug of choice:	Surgical removal		
OR	Mebendazole	200 mg PO q3h × 6d	
HOOKWORM (Ancylostoma duodenale, Necator americanus)			
Drug of choice:	Mebendazole	100 mg bid × 3d	100 mg bid × 3d for children >2 years
OR	Pyrantel pamoate[6]	11 mg/kg once (max. 1 gram)	11 mg/kg once (max. 1 gram)
Hymenolepis nana, see TAPEWORMS			
ISOSPORIASIS (Isospora belli)			
Drug of choice:	Trimethoprimsulfamethoxazole	160 mg TMP, 800 mg SMX qid × 10d, then bid × 3 wks	
LEISHMANIASIS			
L. braziliensis (American mucocutaneous leishmaniasis) and L. mexicana (Ameridan cutaneous leishmaniasis)			
Drug of choice:	Stibogluconate sodium[2]	10 mg/kg/d (max. 600 mg/d) IM or IV × 10d (may be repeated)	10 mg/kg/d IM or IV (max. 600 mg/d) × 10d
Alternative:	Amphotericin B	0.25 to 1 mg/kg by slow infusion daily or every 2d for up to 8 wks	0.25 to 1 mg/kg by slow infusion daily or every 2d for up to 8 wks
L. donovani (kala azar, visceral leishmaniasis)			
Drug of choice:	Stibogluconate sodium[2,14]	10 mg/kg/d (max. 600 mg/d) IM or IV × 6–10d (may be repeated)	10 mg/kg/d IM or IV (max. 600 mg/d) × 6–10d
Alternative:	Pentamidine isethionate[2]	2–4 mg/kg/d IM for up to 15 doses	2–4 mg/kg/d IM for up to 15 doses
L. tropica (oriental sore, cutaneous leishmaniasis)			
Drug of choice:	Stibogluconate sodium[2]	10 mg/kg/d (max. 600 mg/d) IM or IV × 6–10d (may be repeated)	10 mg/kg/d IM or IV (max. 600 mg/d) × 6–10d
Alternatives:	Topical treatment[15]		
LICE (Pediculus humanus, capitis, Phthirus pubis)[16]			
Drug of choice:	Pyrethrins with piperonyl butoxide	Topically[17]	Topically[17]
Alternatives:	Malathion lotion 0.5%	Topically[18]	Topically[18]
	Lindane	Topically[17]	Topically[17]
	0.03% Copper oleate	Topically	Topically
Loa loa, see FILARIASIS			
MALARIA (Plasmodium falciparum, P. ovale, P. vivax and P. malariae)			
PROPHYLAXIS			
suppression or chemoprophylaxis of disease while in endemic area (all Plasmodium except chloroquine-resistant P. falciparum)			
Drug of choice:	Chloroquine phosphate[19]	300 mg base (500 mg) once weekly beginning 1 week before and continued for 6 wks after last exposure in endemic area	**<50kg:** 5 mg base/kg once weekly beginning 1 week before and continued for 6 wks after last exposure in endemic area
suppression or chemoprophylaxis (chloroquine-resistant P. falciparum)[20,21]			
Drug of choice:	Pyrimethamine **plus** sulfadoxine[22,23]	1 tablet (25 mg pyrimethamine, 500 mg sulfadoxine) once weekly from one week before until 6 weeks after exposure	**6–11 mos:** $\frac{1}{8}$ tablet; **1–3 yrs:** $\frac{1}{4}$ tablet; **4–8 yrs:** $\frac{1}{2}$ tablet; **9–14:** $\frac{3}{4}$ tablet once weekly from one week before until 6 weeks after exposure
prevention of attack after departure from areas where P. vivax and P. ovale are endemic[24]			
Drug of choice:	Primaquine phosphate[25]	15 mg base (26.3 mg)/d × 14d (with last 2 wks of chloroquine prophylaxis)	0.3 mg base/kg/d × 14d (with last 2 wks of chloroquine prophylaxis)

* The letter d indicates day.

Table continued on opposite page

DRUGS FOR TREATMENT OF PARASITIC INFECTIONS (*continued*)

Infection	Drug	Adult Dose*	Pediatric Dose*
TREATMENT			
treatment of uncomplicated attack (all Plasmodium except chloroquine-resistant P. falciparum)			
Drug of choice:	Chloroquine phosphate[19,20]	600 mg base (1 gram), then 300 mg base (500 mg) in 6 hrs, then 300 mg base (500 mg)/d × 2d	10 mg base/kg (max. 600 mg base), then 5 mg base/kg 6 hrs later, then 5 mg base/kg/d × 2d
treatment of uncomplicated attack[26] (chloroquine-resistant P. falciparum)			
Drug of choice:	Quinine sulfate	650 mg tid × 3d	25 mg/kg/d in 3 doses × 3d
	plus pyrimethamine	25 mg bid × 3d	**<10 kg**: 6.25 mg/d; **10–20 kg**: 12.5 mg/d; **20–40 kg**: 25 mg/d × 3d
	plus sulfadiazine	500 mg qid × 5d	100–200 mg/kg/d in 4 doses × 5d (max. 2 grams/d)
Alternative:	Quinine sulfate	650 mg tid × 3d	25 mg/kg/d in 3 doses × 3d
	plus tetracycline[6]	250 mg qid × 7d	5 mg/kg qid × 7d
OR	**plus** clindamycin	900 mg tid × 3d	20–40 mg/kg/d in 3 doses × 3d
treatment of severe illness, parenteral dosage—only if oral dose cannot be administered (regardless of severity) (all Plasmodium except chloroquine-resistant P. falciparum)			
Drug of choice:	Quinine dihydrochloride[2,27]	600 mg in 300 ml normal saline IV over at least 1 hr; repeat in 6–8 hrs if oral therapy still cannot be started (max. 1800 mg/d)	25 mg/kg/d; administer half of dose in 1-hr infusion, then other half 6–8 hrs later if oral therapy still cannot be started (max. 1800 mg/d)
OR	Chloroquine HCl[20]	200 mg base (250 mg) IM q6h	Not recommended
treatment of severe illness, parenteral dosage (chloroquine-resistant P. falciparum)			
Drug of choice:	Quinine dihydrochloride[2,26,27]	600 mg in 300 ml normal saline IV over at least 1 hr; repeat in 6–8 hrs if oral therapy still cannot be started (max. 1800 mg/d)	25 mg/kg/d; administer half of dose in 1-hr infusion, then other half 6–8 hrs later if oral therapy still cannot be started (max. 1800 mg/d)
prevention of relapses ("radical" cure after "clinical" cure) (P. vivax and P. ovale only)			
Drug of choice:	Primaquine phosphate[25]	15 mg base (26.3 mg)/d × 14d or 45 mg base (79 mg)/wk × 8 wks	0.3 mg base kg/d × 14d
MITES (Sarcoptes scabiei)			
Drug of choice:	10% Crotamiton	Topically	Topically
Alternative:	Lindane	Apply topically once	Apply topically once
	Benzyl benzoate	Topically	Topically
	Sulfur in petrolatum	Topically	Topically
Naegleria species, see AMEBIC MENINGOENCEPHALITIS, PRIMARY			
Necator americanus, see HOOKWORM			
Onchocerca volvulus, see FILARIASIS			
Opisthorchis viverrini, see FLUKES			
Paragonimus westermani, see FLUKES			
Pediculus capitis, humanus, Phthirus pubis, see LICE			
Pinworm, see ENTEROBIUS			
PNEUMOCYSTIS carinii			
Drug of choice:	Trimethoprim-sulfamethoxazole	TMP 20 mg/kg/d, SMX 100 mg/kg/d oral or IV in 4 doses × 14d	TMP 20 mg/kg/d, SMX 100 mg/kg/d oral or IV in 4 doses × 14d
Alternative:	Pentamidine isethionate[2]	4 mg/kg/d IM × 12–14d	4 mg/kg/d IM × 12–14d
Roundworm, see ASCARIS			
Scabies, see MITES			

* The letter d indicates day.

Table continued on following page

DRUGS FOR TREATMENT OF PARASITIC INFECTIONS (*continued*)

Infection	Drug	Adult Dose*	Pediatric Dose*
SCHISTOSOMIASIS			
S. haematobium			
Drug of choice:	Praziquantel	40 mg/kg once	40 mg/kg once
Alternative:	Metrifonate	10 mg/kg every other wk × 3 doses	10 mg/kg every other week × 3 doses
S. japonicum			
Drug of choice:	Praziquantel	20 mg/kg three times in one day	20 mg/kg three times in one day
S. mansoni			
Drug of choice:	Praziquantel	40 mg/kg once	40 mg/kg once
Alternative:	Oxamniquine	15 mg/kg once[28]	15 mg/kg once[28]
S. mekongi			
Drug of choice:	Praziquantel	20 mg/kg three times in one day	20 mg/kg three times in one day
Sleeping sickness, see TRYPANOSOMIASIS			
STRONGYLOIDES stercoralis			
Drug of choice:	Thiabendazole	25 mg/kg bid (max. 3 grams/d) × 2d[29]	25 mg/kg bid (max. 3 grams/d) × 2d[29]
TAPEWORMS—Adult or intestinal stage			
Diphyllobothrium latum (fish), Taenia saginata (beef), Taenia solium (pork),[30] Dipylidium caninum (dog)			
Drug of choice:	Niclosamide	A single dose of 4 tablets (2 grams) chewed thoroughly	**11–34 kg**: a single dose of 2 tablets (1 gram); **>34 kg**: a single dose of 3 tablets (1.5 grams)
OR	Praziquantel[6]	10–20 mg/kg once	10–20 mg/kg once
Alternative:	Paromomycin[6]	1 gram q 15 min × 4 doses	11 mg/kg q 15 min × 4 doses
Hymenolepis nana (dwarf tapeworm)			
Drug of choice:	Niclosamide	A single daily dose of 4 tablets (2 grams) chewed thoroughly × 5d	**11–34 kg**: a single dose of 2 tablets (1 gram) × 5d; **> 34 kg**: a single dose of 3 tablets (1.5 grams) × 5d
OR	Praziquantel[6]	15–20 mg/kg once	15–20 mg/kg once
Alternative:	Paromomycin[6]	45 mg/kg once/d × 5–7d	45 mg/kg once/d × 5–7d
Larval or tissue stage			
Echinococcus granulosus (sheep, cattle, human, deer Hydatid cysts)			
Drug of choice:	See footnote[31]		
Cysticercus cellulosae			
Drug of choice:	Praziquantel	50 mg/kg/d in 3 divided doses × 14d	50 mg/kg/d in 3 divided doses × 14d
Alternative:	Surgery		
Toxocariasis, see VISCERAL LARVA MIGRANS			
TOXOPLASMOSIS (Toxoplasma gondii)[32]			
Drug of choice:	Pyrimethamine[33]	25 mg/d × 3–4 wks	2 mg/kg/d × 3d (max. 25 mg/d), then 1 mg/kg/d[34] × 4 wks
	plus		
	trisulfapyrimidines	2–6 grams/d × 3–4 wks	100–200 mg/kg/d × 3–4 wks
Alternative:	Spiramycin	2–4 grams/d × 3–4 wks	50–100 mg/kg/d × 3–4 wks
TRICHINOSIS (Trichinella spiralis)			
Drug of choice:	Steroids for severe symptoms **plus** thiabendazole[35]	25 mg/kg bid × 5d	25 mg/kg bid × 5d
Alternative:	Mebendazole[6]	200–400 mg tid × 3d, then 400–500 mg tid × 10d	
TRICHOMONIASIS (trichomonas vaginalis)[36]			
Drug of choice:	Metronidazole[3]	2 grams once or 250 mg tid orally × 7d	15 mg/kg/d orally in 3 doses × 7d

* The letter d indicates day.

Table continued on opposite page

DRUGS FOR TREATMENT OF PARASITIC INFECTIONS (*continued*)

Infection	Drug	Adult Dose*	Pediatric Dose*
TRICHOSTRONGYLUS species			
Drug of choice:	Thiabendazole[6]	25 mg/kg bid × 2d	25 mg/kg bid × 2d
Alternative:	Pyrantel pamoate[6]	11 mg/kg once (max. 1 gram)	11 mg/kg once (max. 1 gram)
TRICHURIS trichiura (whipworm)			
Drug of choice:	Mebendazole	100 mg bid × 3d	100 mg bid × 3d
TRYPANOSOMIASIS			
T. cruzi (South American trypanosomiasis, Chagas' disease)			
Drug of choice:	Nifurtimox[2]	5 mg/kg/d orally in 4 divided doses, increasing by 2 mg/kg/d every 2 wks until dose reaches 15–17 mg/kg/d	
T. gambiense; T. rhodesiense (African trypanosomiasis, sleeping sickness) hemolymphatic stage			
Drug of choice:	Suramin[2]	100–200 mg (test dose) IV, then 1 gram IV on days 1, 3, 7, 14, 21	20 mg/kg on days 1, 3, 7, 14 and 21
Alternative:	Pentamidine isethionate[2]	4 mg/kg/d IM × 10d	4 mg/kg/d IM × 10d
late disease with CNS involvement			
Drug of choice:	Melarsoprol[2,37]	2–3.6 mg/kg/d IV × 3 doses; after 1 wk 3.6 mg/kg/d IV × 3 doses; repeat again after 10–21 days	18–25 mg/kg total over 1 mo. Initial dose of 0.36 mg/kg IV, increasing gradually to max. 3.6 mg/kg at intervals of 1–5d for total of 9–10 doses
Alternative:	Tryparsamide	One injection of 30 mg/kg IV every 5d to total of 12 injections; may be repeated after 1 mo.	Unknown
	plus suramin[2]	One injection of 10 mg/kg IV every 5d to total of 12 injections; may be repeated after 1 mo.	Unknown
VISCERAL LARVA MIGRANS[38]			
Drug of choice:	Diethylcarbamazine[6]	2 mg/kg tid × 7–10d	2 mg/kg tid × 7–10d
OR	Thiabendazole[6]	25 mg/kg bid × 5d	25 mg/kg bid × 5d

Whipworm, see TRICHURIS

Wuchereria bancrofti, see FILARIASIS

* The letter d indicates day.

1. Dosage and duration of administration should not be exceeded because of possibility of causing optic neuritis. Maximum dosade is 2 grams/day.

2. In the USA, this drug is available from the Parasitic Diseases Division, Center for Infectious Diseases, Centers for Disease Control, Atlanta, Georgia 30333; telephone: 404-329-3670.

3. Metronidazole is carcinogenic in rodents and mutagenic in bacteria; it should generally not be given to pregnant women, particularly in the first trimester.

4. Dehydroemetine is probably as effective and probably less toxic than emetine. Because of the toxic effects on the heart, patients receiving emetine should have electrocardiographic monitoring and should remain sedentary during therapy.

5. One patient with a Naegleria infection was successfully treated with amphotericin B, miconazole, and rifampin (JS Seidel et al, N Engl J Med, 306:346, 1982). Experimental infections with Acanthamoeba have been reported to respond to sulfadiazine.

6. Considered an investigational drug for this condition by the U.S. Food and Drug Administration.

7. Effectiveness documented only in animals.

8. Niridazole is absolutely contraindicated in the presence of hepatocellular disease, portal hypertension, or a history of mental disorders or seizures.

9. Diethylcarbamazine should be administered with special caution in heavy infections with Loa loa because it can provoke encephalopathy. Antihistamines or corticosteroids may be required to reduce allergic reactions due to disintegration of microfilariae in treatment of all filarial infections, especially those caused by Onchocerca and Loa loa. Surgical excision of subcutaneous Onchocerca nodules is recommended by some authorities before starting drug therapy.

10. Some Medical Letter consultants use suramin only if microfilariae persist after diethylcarbamazine therapy and nodulectomy.

11. Limited data (AR Rivas-Alcala et al, Lancet, 2:485, 1981; 2:1043, 1981).

12. Limited data available on use of praziquantel for this indication.

Table continued on following page

13. Given on empty stomach. Although approved for human use, it is available currently only as a veterinary product. No alcoholic beverage should be consumed before or 12 hours after therapy.

14. For the African form of visceral leishmaniasis, therapy may have to be extended to at least 30 days and may have to be repeated; for children, some authorities recommend 20 mg/kg/d for 2–4 weeks.

15. Application of heat 39–42°C directly to the lesion for 20 to 32 hours over a period of 10 to 12 days has been reported to be effective in L. tropica minor.

16. For infestation of eyelashes with crab lice, use ophthalmic ointment containing 0.25% physostigmine or ophthalmic ointment of yellow oxide of mercury.

17. Some consultants recommend a second application 5 to 7 days later to kill hatching progeny.

18. Effective against head and body lice. No data for pubic lice.

19. Dosage is oral unless otherwise stated. If chloroquine phosphate is not available, hydroxychloroquine sulfate is as effective; 400 mg of hydroxychloroquine sulfate is equivalent to 500 mg of chloroquine phosphate.

20. In P. falciparum malaria if the patient has not shown a response to conventional doses of chloroquine in 48–72 hours, parasitic resistance to this drug should be considered.

21. Chloroquine-resistant strains of P. falciparum have been reported from **America**: Bolivia, Brazil, Colombia, Ecuador, French Guiana, Guyana, Panama (South), Peru, Surinam, Venezuela; **Asia and Oceania**: Bangladesh, Burma, China (South), India (East), Indonesia, Kampuchea, Laos, Malaysia, Papua New Guinea, Philippines, Solomon Islands, Thailand, Timor (East), Vanuatu, Vietnam; **Africa**: Burundi, Comoro Islands, Madagascar, Rwanda, Sudan (Central), Tanzania, Uganda, Zaire (Northeast), Zambia.

22. Chloroquine should be taken simultaneously because exposure to other species of malaria may also occur. Pyrimethamine plus sulfadoxine is available in a fixed-dose combination as *Fansidar* (Roche). Pyrimethamine is teratogenic in animals.

23. P. falciparum resistant to *Fansidar* has been reported in many areas of Southeast Asia (Thailand, Kampuchea), in Indonesia, Papua New Guinea, Brazil, Colombia, and East Africa. In these areas quinine 325 mg bid may be useful prophylaxis for selected patients.

24. For prevention of attack after departure from areas where P. vivax and P. ovale are endemic, which includes almost all areas where malaria is found, many experts prescribe primaquine phosphate. Others prefer to avoid the toxicity of primaquine and rely on surveillance to detect cases when they occur, particularly when exposure was limited or doubtful.

25. Primaquine phosphate can cause hemolytic anemia, especially in patients whose red cells are deficient in glucose-6-phosphate dehydrogenase. This deficiency is most common in Blacks, Asians, and Mediterranean peoples. Patients should be screened for G-6-PD deficiency before treatment. Primaquine should not be used during pregnancy.

26. Quinine alone will usually control an attack of resistant P. falciparum but, in a substantial number of infections, particularly with strains from Southeast Asia, it fails to prevent recurrence. Addition of pyrimethamine and sulfadiazine lowers the rate of recurrence. Quinine is an abortifacient in early pregnancy and can cause premature labor in later gestation.

27. P. falciparum infections from Southeast Asia may require a loading dose of 20 mg/kg (NJ White et al, Am J Trop Med Hyg, 32:1, 1983). IV administration of quinine dihydrochloride can be hazardous and it must be given slowly. Constant monitoring of the pulse and blood pressure is necessary to detect arrhythmia or hypotension. Oral drugs should be substituted as soon as possible. If quinine dihydrochloride is unavailable, quinidine gluconate can be used; 800 mg is diluted in 250 ml or 5% dextrose and given *very slowly* IV under ECG monitoring; widening of the QRS inverval requires stopping the drug.

28. In East Africa, the dose should be increased to 30 mg/kg/d, and in Egypt and South Africa, 30 mg/kg/d × 2d.

29. In disseminated strongyloidiasis, thiabendazole therapy should be continued for at least five days.

30. Niclosamide and paromomycin are effective for the treatment of T. solium but, since they cause disintegration of segments and release of viable eggs, their use creates a theoretical risk of causing cysticercosis. They should therefore be followed in 3 or 4 hours by a purge. Quinacrine is preferred by some clinicians because it expels T. solium intact.

31. Surgical resection of cysts is the treatment of choice. When surgery is contraindicated, or cysts rupture spontaneously during surgery, mebendazole (experimental for this purpose in the USA) can be tried (JF Wilson and RL Rausch, Ann Trop Med Parasitol, 76:165, 1982; ADM Bryceson et al, Trans Roy Soc Trop Med Hyg, 76:510, 1982). Recently albendazole has been reported to be effective (DL Morris et al, Br Med J, 286:103, 1983; AG Saimot et al, Lancet, 2:652, 1983).

32. In ocular toxoplasmosis, corticosteroids should also be used for anti-inflammatory effect on the eyes.

33. To prevent hematological toxicity from pyrimethamine, it is advisable to administer leucovorin (folinic acid), about 10 mg/day, either by injection or orally. Pyrimethamine is teratogenic in animals.

34. Every two to three days for infants.

35. The efficacy of thiabendazole for trichinosis is not clearly established; it appears to be effective during the intestinal phase but its effect on larvae that have migrated is questionable.

36. Sexual partners should be treated simultaneously. Outside the USA ornidazole and tinidazole have been used for this condition. Metronidazole-resistant strains have been reported; higher doses of metronidazole for longer periods of time are sometimes effective against these strains.

37. In frail patients, begin with as little as 18 mg and increase the dose progressively. Pretreatment with suramin has been advocated for debilitated patients.

38. For severe symptoms or eye involvement, corticosteroids can be used in addition.

ADVERSE EFFECTS OF SOME ANTIPARASITIC DRUGS

BITHIONOL (*Bitin*)
Frequent: photosensitivity skin reactions; vomiting; diarrhea; abdominal pain; urticaria

CHLOROQUINE HCI and CHLORO-QUINE PHOSPHATE USP (*Aralen; and others*)
Occasional: pruritus; vomiting; headache; confusion; depigmentation of hair; skin eruptions; corneal opacity; weight loss; partial lopecia; extraocular muscle palsies; exacerbation of psoriasis, eczema and other exfoliative dermatoses; myalgias
Rare: irreversible retinal injury (especially when total dosage exceeds 100 grams); discoloration of nails and mucous membranes; nerve-type deafness; blood dyscrasias; photophobia

CROTAMITON (*Eurax*)
Occasional: skin rash; conjunctivitis

DEHYDROEMETINE - similar to emetine, but possibly less severe

DIETHYLCARBAMAZINE CITRATE USP (*Hetrazan*)
Frequent: severe allergic or febrile reactions due to the filarial infection; GI disturbances
Rare: encephalopathy; loss of vision in onchocerciasis

DILOXANIDE FUROATE (*Furamide*)
Frequent: flatulence
Occasional: nausea; vomiting; diarrhea; urticaria; pruritus

EMETINE HCI USP
Frequent: cardiac arrhythmias; precordial pain; muscle weakness; cellulitis at site of injection
Occasional: diarrhea; vomiting; peripheral neuropathy; heart failure

FURAZOLIDONE (*Furoxone*)
Frequent: nausea, vomiting
Occasional: allergic reactions, including pulmonary infiltration; headache; orthostatic hypotension; hypoglycemia; polyneuritis; urticaria; fever; vesicular rash
Rare: hemolytic anemia in G-6-PD deficiency and neonates; disulfiram-like reaction with alcohol; MAO inhibitor interactions

IODOQUINOL (*Yodoxin*)
Occasional: rash; acne; slight enlargement of the thyroid gland; nausea; diarrhea; cramps; anal pruritus
Rare: optic atrophy and loss of vision after prolonged use in high dosage (for months)

LINDANE (*Kwell; Gamene*)
Occasional: eczematous skin rash; conjunctivitis
Rare: convulsions; aplastic anemia

MEBENDAZOLE (*Vermox*)
Occasional: diarrhea; abdominal pain
Rare: leukopenia

MELARSOPROL (*Mel B; Arsobal*)
Frequent: myocardial damage; albuminuria; hypertension; colic; Herxheimer-type reaction; encephalopathy; vomiting; peripheral neuropathy
Rare: shock

METRIFONATE (*Bilarcil*)
Frequent: reversible plasma cholinesterase inhibition
Occasional: nausea; vomiting; abdominal pain; headache; vertigo

NIRIDAZOLE (*Ambilhar*)
Frequent: immunosuppression; vomiting; cramps; dizziness; headache
Occasional: diarrhea; slight ECG changes; rash; insomnia; paresthesia
Rare: psychosis; hemolytic anemia in G-6-PD deficiency; convulsions

OXAMNIQUINE (*Vansil*)
Occasional: headache; fever; dizziness; somnolence; nausea; diarrhea; rash; insomnia; hepatic enzyme changes; ECG changes; EEG changes
Rare: convulsions

PAROMOMYCIN (*Humatin*)
Frequent: GI disturbance
Rare: eighth-nerve damage (mainly auditory); renal damage

PENTAMIDINE ISETHIONATE
Frequent: hypotension; hypoglycemia often followed by diabetes mellitus; vomiting; blood dyscrasias; renal damage; pain at injection site; GI symptoms
Occasional: may aggravate diabetes; shock; liver damage; cardiotoxicity; delirium
Rare: Herxheimer-type reaction; anaphylaxis; acute pancreatitis

PIPERAZINE CITRATE USP (*Antepar; others*)
Occasional: dizziness; urticaria; GI disturbances
Rare: exacerbation of epilepsy; visual disturbances; ataxia; hypotonia

PRAZIQUANTEL (*Bitricide*)
Occasional: sedation; abdominal discomfort; fever; sweating; nausea; eosinophilia; headache; dizziness

PRIMAQUINE PHOSPHATE USP
Frequent: hemolytic anemia in G-6-PD deficiency
Occasional: neutropenia; GI disturbances; methemoglobinemia in G-6-PD deficiency
Rare: CNS symptoms; hypertension; arrhythmias

PYRANTEL PAMOATE (*Antiminth*)
Occasional: GI disturbances; headache; dizziness; rash; fever

PYRETHRINS and PIPERONYL BUTOXIDE (*Rid; others*)
Occasional: allergic reactions

PYRIMETHAMINE USP (*Daraprim*)
Occasional: blood dyscrasias; folic acid deficiency
Rare: rash; vomiting; convulsions; shock

QUINACRINE HCI USP (*Atabrine*)
Frequent: dizziness; headache; vomiting; diarrhea
Occasional: yellow staining of skin; toxic psychosis; insomnia; bizarre dreams; blood dyscrasias; urticaria; blue and black nail pigmentation; psoriasis-like rash
Rare: acute hepatic necrosis; convulsions; severe exfoliative dermatitis; ocular effects similar to those caused by chloroquine

QUININE DIHYDROCHLORIDE and SULFATE
Frequent: cinchonism (tinnitus, headache, nausea, abdominal pain, visual disturbance)
Occasional: hemolytic anemia; other blood dyscrasias; photosensitivity reactions; arrhythmias; hypotension
Rare: blindness; sudden death if injected too rapidly

SPIRAMYCIN (*Rovamycin*)
Occasional: GI disturbance
Rare: allergic reactions

STIBOGLUCONATE SODIUM (*Pentostam*)
Frequent: muscle pain and joint stiffness; bradycardia
Occasional: colic; diarrhea; rash; pruritus; myocardial damage
Rare: liver damage; hemolytic anemia; renal damage; shock; sudden death

SURAMIN SODIUM (*Germanin*)
Frequent: vomiting; pruritus; urticaria; paresthesia; hyperesthesia of hands and feet; photophobia; peripheral neuropathy
Occasional: kidney damage; blood dyscrasias; shock; optic atrophy

* Reproduced, with permission from The Medical Letter, Vol. 26 (Issue 657), March 16, 1984.

Continued on following page

TETRACHLOROETHYLENE (*NEMA Worm Capsules, Vet*)
 Frequent: epigastric burning; dizziness; headache
 Occasional: drowsiness; disulfiram-like effect with alcohol
 Rare: hepatic necrosis

THIABENDAZOLE (*Mintezol*)
 Frequent: nausea; vomiting; vertigo
 Occasional: leukopenial; crystalluria; rash; hallucinations; olfactory distur-

bance; Stevens-Johnson syndrome
 Rare: shock; tinnitus; intrahepatic cholestasis; convulsions

TRIMETHOPRIM-SULFAMETHOXA-ZOLE (*Bactrim; Septra;* and others)
 Frequent: rash; nausea and vomiting
 Occasional: hemolysis in G-6-PD deficiency; acute megaloblastic anemia; granulocytopenia; thrombocytopenia; pseudomembranous colitis; kernicterus in newborn

Rare: agranulocytosis; aplastic anemia; hepatotoxicity; Stevens-Johnson syndrome; aseptic meningitis; fever; confusion; depression; hallucinations; deterioration in renal disease; intrahepatic cholestasis; methemoglobinemia

TRYPARSAMIDE
 Frequent: nausea; vomiting
 Occasional: impaired vision; optic atrophy; fever; exfoliative dermatitis; allergic reactions; tinnitus

---

* Reproduced, with permission from The Medical Letter, Vol. 26 (Issue 657), March 16, 1984.

Toxoplasmosis

JAMES W. BASS, M.D.*

Pyrimethamine (Daraprim), an antimalarial drug, is highly effective in destroying the proliferative forms (tachyzoites) of toxoplasmosis, but it is not effective in eradicating the intracellular or encysted form of the parasite. Although both pyrimethamine and sulfonamides are individually active against toxoplasmosis, an eightfold synergistic activity is achieved when pyrimethamine is given in combination with a sulfonamide drug. Sulfadiazine and triple sulfonamide (trisulfapyrimadines) are both highly effective, while other sulfonamide drugs, including sulfisoxazole, are much less effective. Since renal toxicity is less with triple sulfa, this may be the sulfonamide of choice to use with pyrimethamine in the treatment of toxoplasmosis. Successful treatment depends on functional humoral immunity to maintain suppression of parasitemia and functional cell-mediated immunity to keep the encysted forms in an inactive or latent state. In fact, asymptomatic primary acquired infection followed by lifelong asymptomatic latent infection is the usual response in the immunocompetent host. Symptomatic infection with progressive disease occurs most commonly in individuals with congenital or acquired defects in these immune systems. Examples are the pregnant female, the congenitally infected infant, individuals who have primary immunodeficiency diseases with defects in humoral or cell-mediated immunity, or more commonly in both systems.

Normal individuals with latent infection who develop cancer, particularly lymphoma, and those who receive chemotherapy, which further compromises cell-mediated immunity, frequently have problems with reactivated toxoplasmosis with progressive disease. Patients with the acquired immune deficiency syndrome (AIDS) who have a severe acquired defect in cell-mediated immunity and a defect in ability to produce specific humoral antibodies to new antigens develop progressive local (cerebral toxoplasmosis) and systemic toxoplasmosis. Individuals with ocular and central nervous system infection may have locally progressive disease, as humoral antibodies do not permeate these tissues well. These infections are particularly more prone to progression when the host experiences transient or persistent impairment of cell-mediated immunity, as may be caused by other infections, such as hepatitis B, herpes, and cytomegalovirus, or due to other host factors such as malnutrition. These facts must be taken into consideration in the treatment of patients with toxoplasmosis. The mature immunocompetent host may require no specific treatment, while aggressive chemotherapy for extended periods is nearly always required to control infection in immunocompromised individuals. Treatment in these individuals is aimed at controlling the infection with specific chemotherapy as well as treating the underlying defect in immunity.

Specific Therapy

The recommended dosage of pyrimethamine for treatment of toxoplasmosis in infants and children is 1 mg/kg/day orally, divided into two equal doses; after 2 to 4 days, this dose may be reduced by one half and continued for one month. Some authorities recommend higher dosages, with loading doses of 2 mg/kg/day† for one to two days followed by a continued dosage of 1 mg/kg/day for periods varying from only 21 days to as long as a year, depending on the type of infection and the presence or absence of immune defects in the host. The total daily dose of pyrimethamine should not exceed 25 mg/day.

A sulfonamide should always be used in conjunction with pyrimethamine for maximal effectiveness. Triple sulfa or sulfadiazine, 100–120 mg/kg/day, orally in four equally divided doses is recommended.

---

* The opinions or assertions contained herein are the private views of the author and are not to be construed as official or as reflecting the views of the Department of the Army or the Department of Defense.

† The dosage of 2 mg/kg/day is higher than that recommended by the manufacturer.

Both pyrimethamine and sulfonamide are potentially toxic drugs, so patients receiving these drugs should be monitored for untoward reactions associated with each. Crystalluria, hematuria, and hypersensitivity skin rashes are associated with sulfonamide toxicity, and a dose-related reversible bone marrow depression occurs frequently with the relatively high dosages of pyrimethamine that are required for treatment of toxoplasmosis compared with the smaller dosages used for the treatment of malaria. Additionally, absorption of pyrimethamine varies, so that toxicity may occur in some patients on relatively small dosages, and favorable treatment response may fail to occur in others receiving relatively large dosages. All patients who are treated with pyrimethamine should have blood cell counts and platelet counts twice a week. Severe thrombocytopenia, leukopenia, or anemia may require a downward adjustment in the pyrimethamine dosage or temporary discontinuance of the drug. Bone marrow depression by pyrimethamine may be prevented or minimized by the daily administration of folinic acid (leucovorin calcium injection), which may be given parenterally or by ingestion. Leucovorin will not interfere with the antiparasitic activity of pyrimethamine, but it will counteract its hemotologic effects. The dosage recommended for children and adults is 5–10 mg daily or every other day. There are no data to establish the optimal dosage of folinic acid in newborns or very young infants, but 1 mg along with 100 mg of fresh bakers' yeast daily, has been recommended by some authorities.

Other drugs that are effective in the treatment of toxoplasmosis are spiramycin, clindamycin, and trimethoprim-sulfamethoxazole, but they are less active than pyrimethamine-sulfa combination therapy. Spiramycin has been shown to be effective in the treatment of pregnant women with toxoplasmosis. It is less toxic than pyrimethamine-sulfa therapy, and it has not been shown to be teratogenic, a problem that has caused concern with the use of pyrimethamine, particularly during the first trimester before organogenesis is completed. Spiramycin can be used in this circumstance as soon as the diagnosis is made. Unfortunately, it is not available in the United States. Clindamycin is concentrated in the ocular choroid, and encouraging results have been reported with the use of this drug in the treatment of ocular toxoplasmosis, but comparative studies are needed to establish if it is as effective as or more effective than pyrimethamine-sulfa treatment of ocular toxoplasmosis. Although trimethoprim-sulfmethoxazole is effective in the treatment of toxoplasmosis, it is significantly less effective than pyrimethamine-sulfa, so it is not recommended for treatment of this disease.

Corticosteroid treatment is recommended only in conjunction with antitoxoplasmosis chemotherapy in patients with active inflammatory lesions such as central nervous system infection with marked elevation of the cerebrospinal fluid protein or progressive choroidoretinitis, particularly with involvement of the macula or the optic nerve. The dosage recommended is 1 to 2 mg/kg/day (maximum 80 mg/kg/day) of prednisone or the equivalent dosage of another corticosteroid. Corticosteroid therapy should be continued until signs of the abatement of acute inflammation, such as a significant decrease of cerebrospinal fluid protein levels, or evidence of arrest of choroidoretinitis lesions, occurs. The dosage should then be tapered and the drug discontinued.

Congenital Toxoplasmosis

All infants suspected of having congenital toxoplasmosis should be treated immediately pending confirmation of the diagnosis. Asymptomatic normally appearing infants may suffer further serious neurologic damage if treatment is delayed. Immediate treatment of infants with obvious far-advanced disease may arrest progression of the infection and minimize further tissue injury and neurologic damage. Optimal duration of treatment is not known. A minimum of 21 days is recommended, but some authorities recommend treatment be continued for one year.

Acquired Toxoplasmosis

Acquired toxoplasmosis in immunocompetent individuals is most often asymptomatic. A mild transient infectious mononucleosis–like illness is seen most often in patients who have symptomatic infections, and these patients rarely require treatment except in exceptional instances in which symptoms are severe and persistent. Rarely, a severe life-threatening fulminating disease occurs, and these patients frequently have meningoencephalitis pneumonia and a florid typhus-like skin rash. Early diagnosis and treatment of these patients may be lifesaving.

Ocular Toxoplasmosis

Hypersensitivity to products of the toxoplasma organism appears to be responsible for most of the inflammatory reaction that occurs with relapse or reactivation of ocular toxoplasmosis. For this reason, corticosteroids have been used and shown to be beneficial as adjunctive therapy along with antitoxoplasmosis chemotherapy. Duration of treatment is determined by clinical response and tolerance of therapy.

Congenital or Acquired Immunodeficiency

Treatment of patients with congenital or acquired immunodeficiency who develop acquired toxoplasmosis or reactivation of latent toxoplasmosis often requires long-term antitoxoplasmosis chemotherapy. Duration of therapy is usually determined by response to treatment directed at restoring or treating the underlying immunodeficiency disease.

Cholera

DAVID A. SACK, M.D.

Cholera is an acute diarrheal disease associated with profuse watery stools and is caused by the bacteria *Vibrio cholerae* serogroup 01. Among diarrheal diseases, this disease is unique in two respects. It tends to strike in epidemic fashion; and secondly, the purging rates may be exceptionally high, leading to life-threatening dehydration within a matter of hours. Mortality in epidemics without medical care can be as high as 40%. Fortunately, simple therapy is available that will save nearly all patients.

During the disease, *V. cholerae* 01 colonizes the small intestine and elaborates a potent enterotoxin that binds to the surface of the enterocyte. Through stimulation of adenylate cyclase the toxin evokes intestinal hypersecretion of salts and water, which leads to diarrhea. Because of the loss of large amounts of salt, water, and base, patients develop isotonic dehydration and metabolic acidosis.

The traditional home of cholera is the Gangetic Delta of the Indian subcontinent. Currently, however, the disease is occurring in Southeast Asia, India, Middle East, and many countries in Africa. It is also endemic on the Gulf Coast of the United States, where contaminated sea food is the usual vehicle for transmission. In other areas of the world, contaminated water and/or food is implicated. Although cases in the United States have been in adults, in other areas, children under age 5 have the highest incidence rates.

Clinical Presentation

The outstanding feature of cholera is the severe watery diarrhea, usually associated with vomiting but not fever or evidence of sepsis. Because of the high volume of secretion in the small intestine, the stool loses its fecal characteristics. Instead it has the appearance of "rice water," i.e., a clear or pale watery fluid with flecks of mucus. Generally the diarrhea is painless, without severe abdominal cramps or tenesmus. Other symptoms relate to the effects of dehydration—weakness, thirst, and absence of urine production.

Examination of the patient shows evidence of dehydration with sunken eyes, poor skin turgor, dry mucous membranes, "washerwoman's" fingers, and a thready rapid pulse. Severely dehydrated cases may have no detectable radial pulse,

depressed mental status or coma, and rapid deep breathing caused by acidosis.

Treatment

Treatment includes rapid correction of dehydration by using intravenous and/or oral rehydration (depending on the severity of dehydration), maintenance of hydration as long as diarrhea continues, and antibiotics.

To rehydrate patients, one must first assess the degree of dehydration on the basis of a rapid clinical evaluation. Patients who are severely dehydrated or in shock require immediate intravenous fluids while patients with mild or moderate dehydration should receive oral rehydration solution (ORS). A summary of the clinical parameters used to determine severity of dehydration are shown in Table 1. The patient should be weighed on admission to determine fluid requirements for rehydration and to provide a baseline for comparison with later weight measurements when assessing hydration status.

Intravenous Rehydration. If intravenous (IV) therapy is needed, an isotonic solution that approximately matches the electrolyte composition of the cholera stool should be used. Cholera stool contains high concentrations of sodium, potassium, and bicarbonate; hence, similar levels of these salts are needed in the IV solution. "Dhaka solution" provides the appropriate concentration of salts and has been used extensively in Bangladesh. "Diarrhoea Treatment Solution" (DTS) has also been formulated specifically for severe diarrhea and is similar to Dhaka solution. Of the commercially available fluids, Ringer's lactate most closely approximates the ideal except for the low potassium concentration. Potassium can be supplemented by giving ORS as soon as possible or by giving other forms of oral potassium.

Isotonic saline has been used in emergency situations; however, without potassium or base, patients will frequently have complications related to continuing acidosis and hypokalemia.

For correction of severe dehydration, the fluids should be given rapidly with complete replacement of the deficit within about 2 hours. This means that a 10-kg child with severe dehydration would receive 1 liter (100 ml/kg) of IV fluid in about 2 hours. This rate of IV administration is higher than pediatricians usually employ for other conditions, but cholera dehydration is best treated by rapid replacment.

Oral Rehydration. Patients with mild or moderate dehydration can generally be rehydrated with oral rehydration alone. Even though the intestine is hypersecreting fluid, the intestine can absorb fluid if it has glucose to transport sodium and water into the cell. The WHO/UNICEF packet is the most convenient and reliable form for pre-

Table 1. ASSESSMENT OF DEHYDRATION AND FLUID REQUIREMENTS IN CHOLERA

Signs/Symptoms	Degree of Dehydration		
	Mild	*Moderate*	*Severe*
General	Thirsty	Weakness	Drowsy to coma
Radial pulse	Normal	Rapid and weak	Rapid, very weak, or absent
Respiration	Normal	May be deep	Deep and rapid
Systolic blood pressure	Normal	Normal to low	Usually < 80 mm Hg
Skin elasticity	Slight decrease	Pinch retracts slowly	Pinch retracts very slowly (>2 sec)
Eyes	Normal	Sunken	Deeply sunken
Mucous membranes	Moist	Dry	Dry
Urine flow	Normal	Minimal	Usually done
Percent body weight loss	4–5%	6–9%	≥ 10%
Estimated fluid deficit (ml/kg)	40–50	60–90	100

paring ORS, though hospitals and clinics can prepare their own solution.

The principles of rehydration with ORS are similar to IV rehydration. One should first estimate the degree of dehydration, calculate the deficit, and then administer that volume to the patient. A 10-kg child with mild dehydration would therefore require 500 ml (50 ml/kg) ORS for rehydration. This should be given over a 2- to 4-hour period (or more rapidly if the child will accept it).

Hydration Maintenance. In cholera severe purging may continue for 1 or 2 days (longer without antibiotics) and one should anticipate administering ORS to replace these losses until the diarrhea stops. If possible, the stool volume should be measured by placing the patient on a cholera cot with a bucket beneath a central hole where the stool is collected. The stool volume can then be measured and recorded on an intake-output worksheet. These stool volumes should approximately match the intake of ORS (Table 2). Deficits or surpluses should be adjusted in the subsequent time period. Occasional patients, especially those whose purging rate is >10 ml/kg/hr, will again become dehydrated while receiving ORS. These patients will again need to be rehydrated with IV solution and then placed back on ORS for maintenance.

In addition to ORS, which replaces stool losses, patients should receive plain water or other hypotonic fluids, such as breast milk for nursing children, to replace normal physiologic losses.

Antibiotics. Oral doses of antibiotics are indicated in cholera to decrease the duration and volume of purging, to decrease the hydration fluid requirements, and to decrease the hospitalization time. The antibiotic rapidly kills the vibrio organisms in the lumen, thus preventing further production of cholera enterotoxin. Tetracycline is the antibiotic of choice for cholera (50 mg/kg/day in 4 divided doses for 3 days). Though tetracycline is not commonly used in pediatric practice because

Table 2. COMPARISON OF ELECTROLYTE COMPOSITION OF CHOLERA STOOL AND REHYDRATION SOLUTIONS (mmole/liter)

Solution	Cation		Anion		Glucose
	Na	*K*	*Cl*	*Base*	
Diarrhea treatment solution	117	13	82	48*	51
Dhaka solution	133	13	98	48*	
Ringer's lactate	130	4	109	28†	
Oral rehydration solution (WHO/UNICEF)	90	20	80	30‡	111
Cholera Stool (approximate values)					
Adult	135	15	90	30	
Children	100	25	90	30	

* Acetate.

† Lactate.

‡ Bicarbonate. Plans are being made to use trisodium citrate dehydrate (2.9 grams per liter) in place of the current sodium bicarbonate (2.5 grams per liter).

Table 3. INGREDIENTS FOR PREPARING ONE LITER OF HOMEMADE ORAL REHYDRATION SOLUTION

	Carbohydrate		NaCl		HCO_3*		KCl†	
	Grams	(tablespoon)‡	Grams	(teaspoon)‡	Grams	(teaspoon)	Grams	(teaspoon)
Glucose ORS	20	(2)	3.5	(½)	2.5	(½)	1.5	(¼)
Sucrose ORS	40	(4)			same electrolytes			
Rice ORS§	50	(6)			same electrolytes			

* Bicarbonate should be included in ORS to treat cholera if at all possible. For mild diarrhea, more commonly associated with other etiologic agents, bicarbonate is sometimes omitted.

† If potassium chloride is not available, provide potassium with foods high in potassium.

‡ Tablespoon and teaspoon measurements are approximate but assume a level measuring spoon. Many household spoons are not accurate.

§ Rice powder (50 grams) should be mixed with water, boiled for 5 minutes, and cooled. The electrolytes are added. Consistency is that of a thin gruel.

it accumulates in developing teeth and bones, it is used in cholera because of its marked beneficial effect and because the short course of therapy used in cholera is not associated with dental staining.

Epidemics have occurred with tetracycline-resistant strains in East Africa and Bangladesh. In this situation, the alternative antibiotic is furazolidone (5 mg/kg/day in 4 divided doses for 3 days). Chloramphenicol and trimethoprim-sulfamethoxazole are also effective but are used infrequently.

Complications During Cholera Therapy

Vomiting occurs frequently with cholera and makes administration of ORS more difficult. Even with vomiting, ORS can be given, but it needs to be given in frequent small amounts, e.g., with a spoon. Vomiting generally stops as soon as the patient is rehydrated and the acidosis is corrected.

Edema may occur after rehydration and indicates that excess rehydration fluid has been given. It does not indicate hypernatremia. One need only stop giving ORS until puffiness disappears.

Hypoglycemia, usually presenting as seizures, occurs rarely in children with cholera. If seizures do occur, blood should be obtained for glucose determination, and IV glucose should be given immediately.

Public Health Concerns

Because of cholera's potential for epidemic spread and high mortality rates, suspected cholera should be reported immediately to appropriate health authorities. In certain situations, prophylactic tetracycline has been given to family members of infected individuals, but this is not generally recommended. Prophylactic tetracycline administration to populations should not be given because it may cause selection for tetracycline-resistant strains.

Vaccination with the currently available injectable vaccine is also not recommended because it provides relatively low protection rates (50%) for only 6 months. Efforts to provide rehydration therapy are more cost effective in controlling the consequences of an epidemic than is a vaccination campaign.

Treating Cholera with Minimal Resources. While cases of cholera do occur in the United States, most cases occur in developing countries where supplies of IV fluids, ORS packets, and logistic support are minimal. Even in these settings effective therapy can be provided using readily available ingredients found in the home or market. Here, oral rehydration fluids must be used maximally to conserve whatever few IV fluids are available. Although glucose is used in the WHO/UNICEF packet, table sugar (sucrose) can also be used, since glucose (and fructose) is released in the intestine from the hydrolysis of sucrose. Rice powder (and perhaps other food starches) can also be used as an alternative to glucose, since this is also digested to glucose in the intestine. Ingredients for making these homemade solutions are shown in Table 3.

During a cholera epidemic in a setting with minimal resources establishment of a temporary diarrhea treatment center is an efficient way for handling the large number of very ill patients who require treatment. Family members and other local nonmedical people can be trained to prepare and administer ORS. Mortality rates for cholera in such treatment centers have been about 3%, which, though higher than in centers with IV fluids, is a marked improvement over the 40% found in untreated cholera.

The Management of Septic Shock

D. H. SHAFFNER, JR., M.D.
and S. C. ARONOFF, M.D.

Septic shock is a state of generalized hypoperfusion that accompanies systemic infection. Although gram-negative bacteria are most frequently implicated etiologically, other bacteria, fungi, protozoa, and viruses may give rise to the syndrome.

The early stage of septic shock is characterized by vasodilation. The child appears flushed and febrile. The reduction in peripheral vascular resistance coupled with increased metabolic demand results in tachycardia and a subsequent increase in cardiac output. Blood pressure is frequently low owing to a relative hypovolemia. This stage has been labeled "warm shock."

With the release of endogenous catecholamines, blood pressure may normalize; however, with intense vasoconstriction, tissue hypoperfusion results. The patient appears cold and clammy and has a decrease in capillary refill. The complications of septic shock relate to multiple organ system failure following prolonged hypoxia.

The management of the child with septic shock requires aggressive monitoring, antimicrobial therapy, and support of the cardiovascular, respiratory, and renal systems. Successful management of these patients is accomplished best in an intensive care setting.

Monitoring

Since therapy needs to be individualized, constant monitoring of cardiovascular, respiratory, and renal function is necessary. Frequent periodic evaluation of neurologic status, cardiac rhythm, and peripheral perfusion is needed in all cases.

The placement of an intra-arterial catheter allows for continuous measurement of systolic, diastolic, and mean arterial pressures. This line also provides a sampling port for arterial blood gas determinations, electrolytes, and other necessary parameters.

Measurement of preload (ventricular filling pressure) is accomplished with a central venous catheter or a Swan-Ganz catheter. In most cases, the former is adequate and safer. Frequent measurement of central venous pressure allows for precision in fluid management. Calculation of cardiac output from arterial oxygen saturation and mixed venous oxygen saturation provides a guide in the use of cardiotonic agents and vasodilators.

An indwelling urinary bladder catheter allows for the collection of urine cultures initially and monitoring of urine output. Collections of urine for creatinine determination over 4- to 8-hour intervals provide an estimate of glomerular filtration rate.

Anti-infective Therapy

Anti-infective therapy can be applied most specifically when the invading organism is identified and the source of the infection is known. Identification of the organism is accomplished by bacterial cultures of available body fluids. Additional information can be gained by Gram-stained smears of material from petechiae, wounds, sputum, urine, and buffy coats. Indirect determinations of bacterial antigens also provide useful information in identifying the causative pathogen.

The goal of anti-infective therapy is elimination of the pathogen and is accomplished by the removal of contaminated foreign bodies, incision and drainage of abscesses, and antibiotic administration. Without sterilization, hemodynamic stabilization may not be possible.

Antibiotic administration is based on the clinical setting and the suspected pathogens (Tables 1 and 2). Failure of effective antibiotic therapy to clear the pathogen results from bacterial drug tolerance, inadequate dosage, or inadequate drainage of a localized site of infection. Since renal impairment is common in septic shock, close monitoring of serum aminoglycoside concentrations and alteration of dosing schedules are often needed.

Fluid Therapy

Septic shock is associated with hypovolemia caused by extravasation of intravascular fluid and peripheral vasodilation. Fluid is required to meet maintenance requirements, to correct the deficit, and to replace ongoing fluid losses. The goal of therapy is to maximize tissue perfusion without producing pulmonary edema or hyperviscosity.

The fluids available for replacement therapy include crystalloids (lactated Ringer's solution and normal saline), colloids (albumin and hetastarch), and blood components. Crystalloid solutions have the advantages of being less expensive, easier to store, and more readily available. Lactated Ringer's and normal saline are equally effective. The disadvantages of these solutions are the need for larger volumes to restore hemodynamic stabilization and the possibility of producing pulmonary edema.

Colloid administration requires less volume for hemodynamic stabilization than crystalloids and maintains intravascular oncotic pressure. The disadvantages of colloids include an increase in extravascular extravasation seen with severe capillary leak and decreased perfusion due to hyperviscosity.

Blood component therapy should be used as clinically indicated. Packed red cells are given to maintain a hematocrit of 35 to 45%, a range that minimizes the risk of hyperviscosity in the microvasculature. Platelets, fresh frozen plasma, cryoprecipitate, and vitamin K should be administered as needed to maintain normal coagulation.

Careful replacement of fluid deficit is necessary to maintain tissue perfusion without fluid overload. The fluid challenge is a technique used to determine fluid requirements. A volume of fluid (10 ml/kg) is given over a brief period of time and measurement of left ventricular filling pressure

Table 1. BACTERIAL PATHOGENS ASSOCIATED WITH SEPTIC SHOCK BASED ON CLINICAL SETTINGS

Setting	Pathogens	Therapy
Neonatal period	Group B streptococci	Ampicillin and gentamicin
	Enterobacteriaceae	Ampicillin and cefotaxime if CNS
	Listeria monocytogenes	involved
	Staphylococci (with invasive monitoring)	Oxacillin or vancomycin and gentamicin if suspect line colonization
Older children	*Haemophilus influenzae*	Oxacillin and chloramphenicol
With source from community setting	*Streptococcus pneumoniae*	
	Neisseria meningitidis	
	Staphylococcus aureus	
With suspected GU tract source	*Enterobacteriaceae*	Ampicillin and gentamicin
	Enterococcus	
With suspected respiratory tract source	Gram-positive organisms	Cefuroxime
	H. influenzae	
With suspected abdominal source	*Enterobacteriaceae*	Aminoglycoside and clindamycin
	Anaerobic organisms	
With immune compromise	*S. aureus*	Ticarcillin, nafcillin and gentamicin
	Enterobacteriaceae	
	Pseudomonas species	

(CVP or pulmonary artery wedge pressure) is monitored. In the face of a large deficit, the increase in filling pressure will be minimal or transient. When the deficit is small or absent, sustained elevations of filling pressure will occur. Further information can be gained by including serial assessments of cardiac output. A fluid challenge producing a decrease in cardiac output suggests that the left ventricle is maximally dilated, and diuretics or vasodilatory therapy may be more appropriate than additional fluid. A fluid challenge that produces a rise in cardiac output indicates that additional volume may be given safely.

The major complication of fluid administration is overload, which results in increased hydrostatic pressure and pulmonary edema. Pulmonary edema is best avoided by adequate monitoring of blood pressure, central venous pressure, cardiac output, renal output, and arterial oxygen saturation.

Acid-Base Status. The metabolic acidosis that occurs with septic shock is caused by tissue hypoperfusion and lactic acid production. When acidosis is severe (pH < 7.2) and metabolic in nature, parenteral sodium bicarbonate (1–2 meq/kg/dose) will improve cardiac function. Only partial correction of the acidosis should be attempted, since the complications of overcorrection include hyperna-

Table 2. ANTIMICROBIAL DOSAGES (INTRAVENOUS)

Ampicillin	Neonate	<7 day	100–200 mg/kg/day given q 12 hr
		>7 day	given q 8 hr
	Child		200–400 mg/kg/day given q 4–6 hr
Gentamicin	Neonate	<7 day	5 mg/kg/day given q 12 hr
		>7 day	7.5 mg/kg/day given q 8 hr
	Child		5–7.5 mg/kg/day given q 8 hr
Cefotaxime		<7 day	100 mg/kg/day given q 12 hr
		>7 day	150 mg/kg/day given q 8 hr
Oxacillin	Neonate	<7 day	40 mg/kg/day given jq 12 hr
		> day	60 mg/kg/day given q 8 hr
	Child		100 mg/kg/day given q 4–6 hr
Vancomycin		<7 day	30 mg/kg/day given q 12 hr
		>7 day	60 mg/kg/day given q 6 hr
Chloramphenicol			50–100 mg/kg/day given q 6 hr
Cefuroxime			100–200 mg/kg/day given q 6–8 hr
Clindamycin			15–40 mg/kg/day given q 6–8 hr
Ticarcillin			200–300 mg/kg/day given q 4–6 hr
Nafcillin	Neonate	<7 day	40 mg/kg/day given q 12 hr
		>7 day	60 mg/kg/day given q 8 hr
	Child		150–200 mg/kg/day given q 4 hr

tremia, hyperosmolarity, hypokalemia, hypocalcemia, alkalosis, and resultant decreased oxygen delivery to the tissues, paradoxical CNS acidosis, and worsening respiratory acidosis.

Cardiovascular Pharmacotherapy

Tissue oxygen delivery can be maximized by improving cardiac output. Cardiac output is dependent on heart rate, preload, peripheral vascular resistance, and myocardial contractility. Each of these factors needs to be considered individually.

Heart rate is usually elevated in septic shock. A 50% elevation in heart rate is well tolerated in children. If the heart rate is not elevated or bradycardia exists, isoproterenol or atropine can be used to augment cardiac output.

Preload augmentation is discussed under fluid therapy.

Afterload has many components, although peripheral vascular resistance to left ventricular outflow is the most important. In the early stages of septic shock, peripheral vascular resistance is low. Blood flow is often maldistributed and needs to be redirected. Dopamine* (< 5 µg/kg/min) increases cerebral, coronary, splanchnic, and renal blood flow. In late septic shock, vasoconstriction occurs and may be reversed with vasodilatory therapy (see below).

Myocardial contractility, which is decreased in septic shock, may be improved pharmacologically. Because of the rapid onset of action, ease of titration, short half-life, and readily reversible toxicities, sympathomimetic amines are more useful in this situation than cardiac glycosides. These agents should be used cautiously to avoid arrhythmias, vasoconstriction, and increased myocardial oxygen consumption.

The use of individual drugs needs to be tailored to each patient. For example, when adequate perfusion is established, it may be better to accept a slightly low blood pressure than to push pressor therapy further. High dosages of many of these agents cause vasconstriction, which increases blood pressure at the expense of perfusion.

Dopamine is a sympathomimetic amine that has different effects at different dosages. Low dosages (2–4 µg/kg/min) yield a dopaminergic response with increased flow to cerebral, coronary, splanchnic, and renal vascular beds. At higher dosages (4–8 µg/kg/min), chronotropic and inotropic responses result in an increased cardiac output. Even higher doses (> 10 µg/kg/min) give an alpha-adrenergic response and peripheral vasoconstriction.

Dobutamine, in dosages ranging from 2 to 20 µg/

kg/min, is a beta agonist, which improves cardiac output by increasing contractility without raising the heart rate in older children. Dobutamine and low-dose dopamine may be used in combination to increase cardiac output and direct flow to important tissues while avoiding vasoconstriction.

Isoproterenol is used at dosages of 0.05–0.4 µg/kg/min, is a pure beta-adrenergic agonist, and causes more tachycardia and vasodilation than dobutamine. Because of the vasodilation, additional fluid administration may be required to maintain adequate preload during drug administration. Isoproterenol is used in situations in which augmentation of heart rate or further vasodilation is desired. Drug-associated complications include increased myocardial oxygen demands, arrhythmias, and dilatation of skeletal vasculature ("splanchnic steal"). To avoid this last problem, isoproterenol should be used in conjunction with low-dose dopamine.

Epinephrine and norepinephrine are less useful in septic shock, since they augment cardiac output by increasing heart rate and because of the associated alpha agony (vasoconstriction). In situations in which vasoconstriction is required, these agents should be used briefly to avoid further decreases in tissue perfusion.

Vasodilators are useful when left ventricular filling pressure is high, blood pressure is adequate, and the patient is peripherally vasoconstricted. Vasodilators increase cardiac output and tissue perfusion by decreasing afterload. Nitroprusside (0.5–10 µg/kg/min) is titrated to achieve maximal tissue perfusion and urine output without inducing hypotension.

Respiratory Support

Oxygen delivery can be addressed in terms of respiratory, cardiac, and hematologic factors. Early intervention with mechanical ventilation is required to decrease metabolic demands. Additionally, the early application of positive end-expiratory pressure has been advocated as a means of reducing adult respiratory distress syndrome.

Pulmonary edema is one of the major respiratory complications seen in septic shock and results from one of three mechanisms. First, left ventricular dysfunction with its incumbent increase in pulmonary capillary hydrostatic pressure drives fluid into the alveolar space. Second, capillary leakage caused by damaged endothelium allows the escape of proteinaceous fluid into the pulmonary interstitium. Finally, over-aggressive fluid therapy causes increased intravascular pressure and adds to pulmonary fluid accumulation.

The other major pulmonary complication of septic shock is adult respiratory distress syndrome. In this disease, type II alveolar cells are damaged; decreased surfactant production results in atelec-

---

* Safety and efficacy of dopamine in children have not been established.

tasis, hypoxemia, and diffuse alveolar infiltrates. Since treatment is difficult and mortality is high, adequate ventilatory pressures are required to distend alveoli yet must be balanced against compromising cardiac output and the risk of barotrauma.

Ventilatory support in septic shock should include supplemental oxygen delivered under pressure to keep alveoli open. Pulmonary physiotherapy and drainage may be used to avoid secretion accumulation and atelectasis. Careful attention to fluid therapy and appropriate monitoring are needed to control pulmonary edema.

Renal Support

Acute renal failure is a frequent complication of septic shock. Oliguria is defined as a urine output of less than 0.5 cc/kg/hour. Determination of the cause of oliguria requires measurement of serum and urinary creatinine, urea nitrogen, electrolytes, and osmolalities. A low fractional excretion of sodium (<1%) is suggestive of a prerenal cause of oliguria (hypovolemia). A high fractional excretion of sodium indicates oliguria of renal origin.

Therapy is designed to convert renal insufficiency from oliguria to nonoliguric failure in order to reduce morbidity and decrease the need for dialysis. Treatment with furosemide or mannitol is usually the first step. Diuretic therapy also causes compartmental fluid shifts, volume loss, and electrolyte abnormalities. Patients resistant to diuretics should receive a trial of low-dose dopamine to increase renal perfusion.

The indications for dialysis include excesses of fluid, sodium, potassium, or acid that cannot be managed medically. Hemodialysis has a theoretical advantage over peritoneal dialysis, since splanchnic perfusion in septic shock is often inadequate to produce good fluid or solute clearance. When indicated, dialysis should be implemented promptly. A complication of dialysis is removal of dialyzable drugs needed in management.

Additional Modalities

Recent studies suggest that the morbidity of septic shock may be reduced with *steroid therapy.* Steroids should be used early in high doses (methylprednisolone, 30 mg/kg/dose, administered every 4 to 6 hours for 3 to 5 days). The proposed mechanisms of action include the stabilization of white cells and platelets, preventing their release of vasoactive and destructive substances as well as preventing their aggregation and resultant microembolization. Steroids should be stopped as soon as signs of shock disappear.

Naloxone is used to treat hypotension secondary to the release of beta endorphin. The effects of naloxone infusion are immediate and last for several hours. The efficacy of naloxone has not been proved.

Immunization Practice
SAMUEL P. GOTOFF, M.D.

Active and passive immunization provides an opportunity to prevent or modify a number of infectious diseases. The benefits of various immunization techniques are apparent from descriptions of the morbidity and mortality associated with diseases when these methods were unavailable or as they now occur in countries where immunization is not practiced. Unfortunately, there are some risks associated with all immunizations, and those who carry out these procedures should share that information with parents. Printed discussions of the benefits and risks of immunizations are provided in the public sector and in many private practices.

Recommendations or guidelines for immunization are developed by the Committee on Infectious Diseases of the American Academy of Pediatrics (AAP), which prepares reports every few years ("Red Book"), and the Advisory Committee on Immunization Practice (ACIP) of the U.S. Public Health Service, whose reports are published in *Morbidity and Mortality Weekly Report.* Recommendations are frequently based on the best available studies, which may be incomplete. Hence, there may be controversy among the experts and occasional revisions of guidelines. Additional information from the AAP "Red Book" Committee appears in "News and Comment" and bulletins from the AAP.

ROUTINE IMMUNIZATION SCHEDULE

The recommended schedule for active immunization of normal healthy children is given in Table 1. Delays are permissible, and concomitant administration of all nine antigens is appropriate in some circumstances, such as when the patient may not return.

Haemophilus influenzae Type b Polysaccharide Vaccine

A highly purified polymer of ribose, ribitol, and phosphate has been prepared from the capsule of *Haemophilus influenzae* type b (Hib). Since the cumulative risk of a child's developing invasive Hib disease is estimated at one in 200, this vaccine is a valuable new contribution. Unfortunately, children under 18 months of age respond poorly to this vaccine, and the antibody response in children 18–23 months of age is not as good as that in older children. Approximately 75% of children 18–23 months of age (and 90% of children 24

Table 1. RECOMMENDED SCHEDULE FOR ACTIVE IMMUNIZATION OF NORMAL INFANTS AND CHILDREN

Age		
2 mo	DTP*	TOPV†
4 mo	DTP	TOPV‡
6 mo	DTP	
1 yr		Tuberculin test§
15 mo	Measles, mumps, rubella vaccine	
18 mo	DTP	TOPV
18–24 mo	*Haemophilus influenzae* type b vaccine	
4–6 yr	DTP	TOPV
14–16 yr	Td‖—repeat every 10 years	

* Diphtheria and tetanus toxoids combined with pertussis vaccine.

† Trivalent oral poliovirus vaccine.

‡ A third dose of TOPV is optional but may be given in areas of high endemicity of poliomyelitis.

§ Test should be done at the time of, or preceding, the measles immunization.

‖ Combined tetanus and diphtheria toxoids (adult type) for those more than 6 years of age, in contrast to diphtheria and tetanus (DT) toxoids which contain a larger amount of diphtheria antigen. Tetanus toxoid at time of injury: For clean minor wounds, no booster dose is needed by a fully immunized child unless more than 10 years have elapsed since the last dose. For contaminated wounds, a booster dose should be given if more than 5 years have elapsed since the last dose.

months of age and older) have levels ≥ 1 µgm/ml 3 weeks postvaccination, levels that correlate with protection. While efficacy data from Finland suggested protection in children older than 18 months of age, the difference in the attack rate in vaccinated and control populations between 18 and 23 months of age was not significant. Thus, there are no convincing data on efficacy in this age group.

The vaccine is recommended for all children between 24 and 71 months of age. There is disagreement regarding its administration in children between 18 and 23 months of age, a group accounting for approximately 12% of all invasive Hib disease in children under 5 years of age. Physicians may choose to immunize children of this age, particularly those in high-risk groups (e.g., children in day care centers), while recognizing that efficacy has not been demonstrated and that immunogenicity is less than optimal. Immunization at this age does not produce tolerance, and a second dose of vaccine at 24–36 months of age may be necessary to insure protection. Second-generation vaccines, which should be immunogenic in the younger child, are being developed. Administering Hib vaccine along with diphtheria tetanus pertussis (DTP) and trivalent oral polio vaccine (TOPV) at 18 months of age is attractive logistically. The polysaccharide vaccines rarely produce complications. Despite the limitations discussed, I favor administration of the Hib vaccine at the 18-month visit.

Risks, Contraindications, and Exceptions. Risks associated with the use of vaccines vary from trivial to severe. Reactions may be classified into relatively common side effects and infrequent severe complications. In some cases, such as paralytic poliomyelitis following administration of live oral poliovirus vaccine, the pathogenesis of the complication is demonstrated by isolation of the attenuated virus from cerebrospinal fluid. In other cases, such as encephalopathy in association with pertussis vaccine, one cannot attribute the reaction to the immunization with certainty, but the temporal association occurs more often than in unvaccinated populations.

Contraindications to immunization may be relative or firm. In general, fever, immunodeficiency, and pregnancy are contraindications. Live virus vaccines may replicate excessively in children with certain congenital or acquired immunodeficiency diseases, whether primary or secondary. Because of the potential for transmission by the fecal-oral route, oral poliovirus vaccine should not be given to contacts of immunodeficient children. In contrast, household contacts may receive measles-mumps-rubella (MMR) vaccine, since these parenterally administered attenuated viruses are not transmissible.

Allergy and Hypersensitivity Reactions. Antigens prepared in eggs (measles, mumps, influenza, yellow-fever) may cause reactions in children who have had anaphylactic reactions to egg protein in the past. In such patients, I prefer to see a negative scratch test before proceeding with vaccination.

Pertussis Vaccine. The major controversy in routine immunization practice concerns pertussis vaccine. This is the most reactogenic agent currently in routine use, and it should be replaced by a safer vaccine in the future. At present, under ordinary circumstances, the benefits of the vaccine outweigh the risks. However, children who have had previous significant reactions should not be given further pertussis vaccine. These reactions include temperature greater than 40° C, seizures, excessive somnolence, screaming spells lasting 3 hours or more, a hypotensive shock-like state, and an allergic reaction to the vaccine. Moreover, I would defer pertussis vaccination in a child with any history of seizures or with a neurologic condition that might predispose to seizures. Since the risk of pertussis is currently small in most communities in the United States, it seems prudent to delay pertussis vaccination in infants who are more likely to have seizures until their neurologic status is well defined.

Measles in the Community. Exceptions should be made to the schedule in Table 1 under certain epidemiologic conditions. If exposure to measles

626   IMMUNIZATION PRACTICE

is likely in a given community, infants 6–11 months old may be immunized with measles vaccine and reimmunized at 15 months of age with MMR.

Gamma Globulin. Live virus vaccines should not be given to children who have received gamma globulin within the previous 3 months, except for rabies vaccine and rabies immune globulin for postexposure prophylaxis.

Poliomyelitis. Live oral vaccine (OPV) should be avoided in families in which there are patients with impaired T-cell or B-cell immunity. It is generally not recommended for use in persons over 18 years of age since adults seem to be at somewhat greater risk of developing vaccine-associated paralysis, which occurs at a rate of one in 3–4 million vaccinees. Concern for parents who may be susceptible when their infant is due for polio immunization has led to the administration of inactivated polio vaccine (IPV). Two injections of IPV should be given to the parent prior to immunizing the child with OPV. Other pediatricians may recommend no immunization for the parents since they are very likely to be immune from inapparent exposure and the risk is extremely low. In any case, it is advisable to discuss the problem with the parents and obtain consensus on the plan for immunization.

Boosters. Since waning immunity to measles, mumps, and rubella has not been recognized, booster immunization is not recommended. However, there is no evidence that a second injection of MMR is harmful, and this vaccine may be given if proof of initial immunization is lost.

Routine administration of tetanus toxoid is recommended every 10 years after the last DPT given at the time of school entrance or as part of wound management. Children older than 7 years should be given adult-type tetanus and diphtheria toxoids (Td).

SPECIAL SITUATIONS AND NONROUTINE IMMUNIZATIONS

A number of vaccines and immune globulins are available for use in special situations (Table 2). Children in institutions may be at risk from influenza, varicella, and the hepatitides and should be considered for active or passive immunization.

Children over 6 months of age with chronic cardiopulmonary disorders who are more susceptible to complications of influenza should be immunized. Epidemiologic variations of influenza may occur yearly, so attention should be paid to the current ACIP recommendation. Subvirion ("split") preparations are used for children under 13 years of age to minimize side effects. Two doses, 4 weeks apart, are required.

Patients at increased risk of serious pneumococcal disease (e.g., those with anatomic or functional

Table 2. IMMUNIZATION PRACTICES FOR SPECIAL SITUATIONS

Exposure	Immunization
Hepatitis A	ISG
Hepatitis B	Hepatitis B vaccine and/or HBIG
Measles	Measles vaccine or ISG
Meningococcus	Group A and C vaccines*
Rabies	Rabies vaccine and rabies immune globulin
Tetanus	Td and/or tetanus immune globulin
Tuberculosis	BCG*
Varicella	VZIG (vaccine in clinical trials)

* Chemoprophylaxis may be preferred.

asplenia or nephrotic syndrome) should receive the 23-valent pneumococcal vaccine if they are 18 months of age or older.

At this time, meningococcal polysaccharide vaccines for group A and C meningococci are recommended for use in epidemic situations and after close exposure in conjunction with antibiotic prophylaxis. Group A vaccine is effective in children over 6 months of age; group C vaccine is effective in children over 2 years of age.

BCG vaccine is available for use in limited situations but is infrequently given in the United States. It may be considered for infants who will be repeatedly exposed to untreated patients with sputum-positive pulmonary tuberculosis when the usual surveillance and treatment programs are not feasible.

Hepatitis B vaccine should be considered for members of high-risk groups such as users of illicit injectable drugs, frequent recipients of blood or blood products, and household and sexual contacts of hepatitis B carriers. Newborns of women who are hepatitis B carriers should be given a single dose of 0.5 ml of hepatitis B immune globulin and 10 μgm of hepatitis B vaccine at birth and 1 and 6 months later. These infants should be tested for antibody at 9 months of age.

Immune serum globulin (ISG) should be used for pre- or postexposure prophylaxis against hepatitis A, measles, and poliomyelitis. Specific immune globulins are available for hepatitis B, rabies, tetanus, and varicella (VZIG). VZIG is available through the American Red Cross and is recommended for high-risk susceptible individuals who are exposed to varicella, such as immunocompromised patients, newborn infants whose mothers develop varicella 5 days before to 2 days after delivery, and pregnant women, although one cannot insure that the fetus will be protected. A varicella vaccine is currently undergoing clinical trials and should be available soon for prophylaxis in immunocompromised patients.

Foreign Travel

Epidemiologic conditions or local health regulations may mandate special immunizations. The best source of information is "Health Information for International Travel," which is available from the Superintendant of Documents, U.S. Government Printing Office, Washington, D.C. 20402. Several vaccines may be considered.

Cholera. While the vaccine is not very effective, certain countries require a vaccination certificate. A single dose of vaccine is sufficient to satisfy requirements, but a full primary series is recommended for high-risk groups (persons living under unsanitary conditions or with compromised gastrointestinal defense mechanisms).

Plague. Vaccination is recommended for travelers who may have contact with wild rodents or rabbits in rural areas of South America, Africa, and Southeast Asia where plague is enzootic.

Rabies. The vaccine should be considered if a child will visit a country where rabies is a constant threat. While pre-exposure prophylaxis may provide protection to children with inapparent exposure, it does not eliminate the need for additional therapy after a known rabies exposure. Acquisition of rabies antibodies should be demonstrated 2–3 weeks after pre-exposure vaccination.

Yellow Fever. Certain countries in South America and Africa have requirements for immunization. The vaccine must be administered at a designated yellow fever vaccination center.

19

Allergy

Allergic Rhinitis

MICHAEL KALINER, M.D.,
and JAY SLATER, M.D.

Allergic rhinitis is a common and complex pediatric disease, affecting approximately 7 to 10 per cent of children. The seasonal variety consists of rhinorrhea, nasal itching, sneezing and congestion occurring during well-defined seasons due to inhalation of pollen allergens, while the perennial form results from the inhalation of year-round allergens. In both cases, the underlying pathophysiologic event is allergen-induced degranulation of tissue mast cells.

The therapy of allergic rhinitis, which must be sensible and empathetic, should be firmly grounded in an understanding of nasal physiology, immunology, aerobiology, and pharmacology. Since the condition is likely to be lifelong, it is especially important that the therapeutic program be based upon the informed and reasoned expectations of the patient or parents with regard to the promise and limitations of each form of therapy. Antihistamines and decongestants have continued to be the mainstays of treatment. However, environmental and physiologic control may in some cases be adequate therapy without incurring the risks of polypharmacy, and the recent availability of intranasal steroids and cromolyn may offer safe chronic therapy without adversely affecting alertness and school performance. A reasoned and stepwise approach offers patients the best chance of effective relief with minimal side effects.

Environment. Control of the environment will usually be suggested by history and skin testing. Certain allergens are eliminatable, such as pets, kapok-stuffed furniture, and down comforters and pillows. When the complete elimination of the offending agents is not possible or feasible, attention should be paid to those spaces where the patient spends the most time, especially the bedroom. Dust control entails daily damp-mopping and the elimination of dust-trapping items such as rugs, drapes, upholstery, and stuffed toys. Mattresses and pillows should be sealed in dust-proof covers with tape over the zippers. Particular attention should be paid to filtering the air from forced hot air furnaces and/or using effective high-efficiency particulate air (HEPA) filter units. Pets should be removed from the household of allergic individuals, after which an extensive (perhaps professional) house cleaning should be performed. Cockroach-derived allergens may be a serious problem for some inner-city patients, and an aggressive attempt at pest control should be undertaken for such children. Molds grow in damp environments, and dehumidification along with judicious use of commercial mold cleaners will usually be helpful. Relocation to avoid pollen antigens is unlikely to be worthwhile; air conditioning, air filters, and closed windows are more likely to have a beneficial effect. Occupational or school exposure to environmental allergens should also be explored.

Supportive Measures. Physiologic measures are often overlooked. Saline nose drops or sprays relieve discomfort and may facilitate mucociliary flow and allergen removal. Air humidification may also be useful in heated buildings or dry climates when mold sensitivity is not a problem. Exercise is known to cause nasal vasoconstriction, and a regimen of morning exercise has been suggested in the care of patients with allergic rhinitis.

Antihistamines. The antihistamines used for allergic rhinitis are oral agents that reversibly block H1 receptors in the nasal mucosa. Most are substituted ethylamines that fall into one of six classes, depending upon the substitutions. The basic ethylamine group is shared by anticholinergics, ganglionic and adrenergic blocking agents, local anesthetics, and antispasmodics; it is not surprising, therefore, that antihistamines exhibit some of these properties. Central nervous system alterations are the most common side effects. Most patients experience sedation, but some children may experience paradoxical stimulation. Gastrointestinal effects, including oral dryness, epigastric distress, nausea, vomiting, diarrhea, and constipation are also reported frequently. The various classes differ in their pharmacologic effects, and an adverse response to one agent should lead to the selection of a drug in another class.

Antihistamines will effectively reduce nasal pruritus, secretions, and episodic sneezing. By themselves, however, antihistamines are not effective for congestion. The alkylamines, such as chlorpheniramine, are effective with the fewest undesirable side effects. Patients who are prone to somnolence may be started on a low dose at bedtime and slowly advanced until an effective dose is obtained. Terfenadine, a nonsedating antihistamine, has recently become available in the United States and appears to be therapeutically effective without central nervous system side effects.

Decongestants. TOPICAL. Topically administered decongestants such as phenylephrine and oxymetazoline are predominantly α-adrenergic agonists that cause local vasoconstriction. They are available in several different concentrations, some of which are appropriate for use in children as young as two years. They should be used with care in infants, as there have been several reports of complications due to overdosage. In no case should they be used continuously for more than 3 days each week, as rebound congestion and rhinitis medicamentosa are well-known complications of prolonged use. Despite these limitations, they can be useful as short-term therapy while other modalities are initiated.

ORAL. Oral decongestants such as pseudoephedrine are sympathomimetic agents that stimulate α- and, to a lesser extent, β-adrenergic receptors. They also act indirectly by causing the release of norepinephrine from sympathetic nerve endings. Unlike the topical agents, oral decongestants do not cause rebound congestion and rhinitis medicamentosa. However, tachyphylaxis may occur with frequent use, and systemic side effects are common. Special care must be taken when administering these agents to infants. In addition, patients with hyperthyroidism, hypertension, or diabetes mellitus, or those taking monoamine oxidase inhibitors, should be given these drugs only with great caution; alternative modalities should be used if at all possible.

Steroids. TOPICAL. Topical nasal steroids for use in allergic rhinitis have recently become available. These agents act by reducing late-phase allergic reactions and mucus secretion, inhibiting vascular permeability, and preventing eicosanoid formation. Beclomethasone dipropionate (Beconase, Vancenase) and flunisolide (Nasalide) are potent topical glucocorticoids that have been approved for children over six (flunisolide) or twelve (beclomethasone) years of age. Both are absorbed in small amounts, but no adrenal suppression or systemic actions have been noted with the usual doses. Side effects are entirely local, the most common of which is nasal burning (flunisolide), which lasts for a few seconds. Nasal dryness is more common with beclomethasone. Nasal mucosa biopsies in patients using intranasal steroids for up to 6 years have failed to show evidence of mucosal damage. Nonetheless, since long-term and pediatric studies are lacking and because of recent isolated reports of nasal septal perforations associated with intranasal steroids, every effort should be made to titrate to the minimum effective dose, and long-term continuous use should be avoided. It is also important to stress that, unlike the other drugs mentioned here, intranasal steroids may take from several days to 2 weeks to have effect, and short-acting agents may be needed in the interim. Furthermore, while ocular symptoms may be partially relieved by a reduction in the nasolacrimal reflex, most patients will need additional therapy for these symptoms.

Experience has shown a striking synergism between antihistamines and topical nasal steroids. Our practice is to initiate flunisolide, two sprays in each nostril twice daily plus chlorpheniramine to control symptoms and then to titrate each agent to the lowest effective dose. If possible, medications are started before the pollen season and adjusted as needed during the course of the season. It is not uncommon to find patients well controlled on a single spray of flunisolide every day or every other day, along with a single, low dose of antihistamine.

SYSTEMIC. Steroids administered systemically effectively relieve allergic rhinitis, but their well-known risks generally outweigh potential benefits. Brief courses (less than 2 weeks) may be required in extraordinary cases as other treatments are initiated or during the height of a pollen season.

Cromolyn Sodium. Cromolyn sodium prevents mast cell degranulation by stabilizing the mast cell membrane. It has no intrinsic antihistaminic or anticholinergic properties, nor does it interfere with the binding of IgE to the mast cell membrane or the binding of antigen to surface-bound IgE. A hand-powered topical nasal spray (Nasalcrom) is approved for use in children over 6 years old. It is remarkably devoid of side effects and is clearly effective in allergic rhinitis. However, it may be necessary in some patients to use the drug as much as six times a day, which may cause a compliance problem. In seasonal allergic rhinitis, best results are obtained if administration precedes the onset of the season by 1 or 2 weeks.

Anticholinergics. The nasal mucosa secretory apparatus is predominantly under cholinergic control, hence anticholinergics such as atropine and related drugs are effective in rhinorrhea and nasal congestion. Major side effects are frequently seen with systemically administered preparations, but topical agents that avoid these problems may soon become available.

Desensitization. Immunotherapy (desensitization) with the specific offending allergens may be highly effective in reducing the symptoms of allergic rhinitis. A successful course of therapy will be accompanied by a reduction in antigen-specific IgE, a rise in IgG-blocking antibodies, reduced mast cell reactivity, and an increase in antigen-specific suppressor T cells. However, because of expense, inconvenience, and the possibility of severe, even life-threatening adverse reactions, it should be reserved for patients in whom other measures either fail to adequately control symptoms or do so only with unacceptable side effects or alterations in life style. We generally try to control the patient's symptoms with medications for two seasons and then, if unsuccessful, discuss immunotherapy.

It can be anticipated that in response to appropriate immunotherapy, approximately 85 percent of the subjects allergic to pollens or dust will experience a reduction in both their symptoms and the need for medication. This entails the weekly or semiweekly subcutaneous injection of progressively increasing doses of a minimal number of appropriate inhalant allergens. After an adequate maintenance dose is achieved, injections are given biweekly or monthly for at least 1 to 2 years and, if effective, for 3 or 4 years. At that time, therapy is discontinued on a trial basis for at least one season.

Surgery. Surgery may be appropriate to correct other conditions—such as nasal polyps or a severely deviated nasal septum—that exacerbate the patient's nasal congestion. However, other procedures such as turbinectomy or submucosal resection have no role in the therapy of allergic rhinitis.

Future developments may include the use of cyclooxygenase or lipoxygenase inhibitors and intranasal immunotherapy as well as the development of safer and more potent allergen extracts.

Asthma

R. MICHAEL SLY, M.D.

Asthma is a chronic pulmonary disease characterized by increased irritability of the airways and manifested by recurrent episodes of generalized airway obstruction that is usually reversible. One

can prevent or interrupt the chain of events that leads to allergic asthma by elimination of allergens, prevention or modification of release of mediators, inhibition of the actions of mediators, or reversal of their actions. Cromolyn prevents movement of calcium ions into the cell, inhibits both immediate and late phase asthmatic responses to challenge with inhaled allergen, and can reduce bronchial hyperreactivity. Cholinergic agents such as acetylcholine or methacholine increase the formation of cyclic guanosine monophosphate from guanosine triphosphate, enhancing antigen-induced mediator release. Cholinergic agents also cause bronchoconstriction by direct action on smooth muscle. Thus, an anticholinergic agent such as atropine or ipratropium bromide can cause inhibition of mediator release and bronchodilation.

Beta-adrenergic stimulation with an agent such as isoproterenol increases formation of cyclic adenosine monophosphate from adenosine triphosphate through interaction with adenylate cyclase. An increase in the concentration of cyclic AMP before allergen challenge of the mast cell inhibits release of mediators, and increased cyclic AMP concentrations in smooth muscle cause bronchodilation by augmenting sequestration of calcium.

The chief mode of action of theophylline is unknown, but it enhances contractility of fatigued diaphragm and can inhibit the bronchoconstrictive effect of inhaled adenosine, which is released by allergenic challenge. Therapeutic doses of theophylline cause only 10% inhibition of phosphodiesterase, insufficient to ascribe the beneficial effect of theophylline to an increase in cyclic AMP due to inhibition of the phosphodiesterase responsible for its degradation.

One of the chief beneficial effects of adrenal corticosteroids is probably induction of plasma proteins that inhibit activation of phospholipase A_2, one of the enzymes responsible for liberation of arachidonic acid from membrane phospholipids. Corticosteroids can also prevent and reverse the beta-adrenergic receptor uncoupling from the adenylate cyclase system that can follow continual treatment with beta-adrenergic agonists and is partly responsible for the tolerance or subsensitivity that ensues. Corticosteroids also have many other potentially beneficial effects, including a decrease in vascular permeability and inhibition of resynthesis of histamine. Corticosteroids inhibit the late asthmatic response to allergen inhalation but are much less effective in inhibiting the immediate response.

Elimination of Allergens and Irritants

The most effective treatment for allergy is elimination of exposure to the allergen. House dust mites and other components of house dust are the allergens identified most commonly in patients with allergy to inhalants. Precautions that limit

Table 1. PREPARATION OF A DUST-FREE BEDROOM*

1. Remove all carpet, rugs, curtains, and venetian blinds. Use only a plain, wooden floor or tile. Small cotton throw rugs may be acceptable if washed at least weekly in a washing machine. Use permanent press curtains that can be laundered weekly or no curtains at all. Shades are acceptable at the windows.
2. Clean the room and closet thoroughly and wax the floor.
3. Close and seal hot air vents unless there is a central high-efficiency particulate air (HEPA) filter or an electronic air filter. As an alternative, fiber glass or cheesecloth filters may be placed over the air vents, but do not place flammable material in contact with metal that may become hot.
4. Encase all mattresses, box springs, and pillows in air tight, dustproof covers, sealing with adhesive tape where the zipper ends. Durable covers are available from Allergen-Proof Encasings, Inc., 1450 East 363rd St., Eastlake, Ohio 44094, and Allergy Control Products, 28 High Ridge Avenue, Ridgefield, Ct. 06877.
5. Use comforters, quilts, mattress pads, and pillows filled only with dacron or polyester. Replace pillows each year unless encased in allergen-proof covers. Launder blankets and bedspreads at least monthly.
6. Permit use of stuffed toys only if filled with polyester or other synthetic stuffing.
7. Minimize furniture and eliminate upholstered furniture.
8. Dust the room daily and clean thoroughly at least weekly, including window sills, tops of window frames, and tops of doors. Vacuum the covered mattress at least weekly.
9. Air the room thoroughly during and after cleaning; otherwise keep doors and windows closed. Keep the allergic patient out of the room for at least 1 hour after vacuuming or cleaning.
10. Keep only clothing currently in use in the closet, and keep the closet door closed.

* Modified from Sly, R. M.: Textbook of Pediatric Allergy. New Hyde Park, New York, Medical Examination Publishing Co., 1985, p. 307.

exposure to these allergens can help control asthma in such patients (Table 1). Cats and dogs are sources of potent allergens and should be eliminated completely from the houses of patients with allergy to them.

Exposure to allergenic fungi can occur both outdoors and indoors. Patients with allergy to fungi should avoid dead leaves, mulch, hay, and ensilage. Fastidious cleaning of bathrooms, kitchens, and laundry rooms is necessary, with special attention to shower curtains, sinks, refrigerator drip trays, and garbage pails. Use of a dehumidifier may be required to prevent growth of fungi in a damp basement or a damp room.

Complete avoidance of allergenic pollens is impossible, and there is virtually no habitable region where some do not abound. Air conditioning can reduce exposure to pollens and other inhalant allergens substantially, and central HEPA filters or electronic air filters are even more effective.

Irritants can cause bronchoconstriction in asthmatics whether there is also allergy or not. Cigarette smoking is the most common source of local air pollution. Both active and passive smoking can cause airway obstruction. Maternal smoking in-

creases the frequency as well as the severity of asthma among children. Cigarette, cigar, and pipe smoking should be prohibited in the house of an asthmatic patient.

Wood-burning stoves, gas ranges, kerosene heaters, and fireplaces can be sources of irritants. Proper venting and adjustment are essential when exposure to these is unavoidable. Use of an exhaust fan during cooking can minimize inhalation of irritating cooking fumes.

During periods of intense air pollution from industry or motor vehicles asthmatic patients should avoid strenuous exercise and if possible should remain indoors, breathing filtered air.

Pharmacologic Treatment

Theophylline. Although the major mode of action of theophylline is still unknown, extensive investigation has established a sound basis for safe and effective use of this drug. There is a log linear relationship between bronchodilation and serum theophylline concentration over the range of 5–20 μg/ml. Most children require serum concentrations of at least 10 μg/ml to approach optimal response, but most experience adverse side effects at concentrations that exceed 20 μg/ml. Furthermore, there is substantial variation in rates of metabolism and elimination of theophylline from patient to patient, with serum half-lives ranging from 1–10 hours. Serum half-life in a healthy, young adult can vary by as much as 55% within 3 to 4 days.

Ninety per cent of the drug is usually eliminated by metabolism in the liver by cytochrome P450 enzymes. Accordingly liver disease can substantially reduce clearance of the drug, increasing serum concentrations from a given dose. Other factors that can decrease theophylline clearance include heart failure, viral respiratory diseases, and concurrent treatment with erythromycin, troleandomycin, oral contraceptives, allopurinol, and cimetidine (but not ranitidine). Propranolol also decreases theophylline clearance, but its use is generally contraindicated in asthmatics. Dietary xanthines found in chocolate, coffee, tea, and colas can cause modest decreases in clearance, and so can high carbohydrate diets and administration of influenza vaccine. Renal failure has a negligible effect because only 10% of the drug is excreted without prior biotransformation.

Factors that can increase clearance of theophylline, decreasing the serum concentration, include smoking tobacco or marijuana, ingestion of charcoal-broiled beef, high protein diets, and treatment with phenobarbital, phenytoin, or intravenous isoproterenol.

Rates of elimination also vary with age. Average doses are shown in Table 2, but because of individual variations in rates of clearance and varia-

Table 2. AVERAGE DOSES OF THEOPHYLLINE BY AGE

<1 year old	0.3 × age (weeks) + 8 mg/kg/day
1–9 years old	24 mg/kg/day
9–12 years old	20 mg/kg/day
12–18 years old	16 mg/kg/day
>18 years old	12 mg/kg/day

tions in the serum concentration at which adverse effects occur from patient to patient, I recommend starting at approximately $\frac{2}{3}$ the average dose and later increasing the dose gradually if necessary to the average dose. Factors known to alter theophylline clearance require modification of the dosage, and signs or symptoms of possible theophylline toxicity may necessitate a reduction in dosage. Maintenance dosage should be based upon ideal body weight for obese patients.

Determination of serum theophylline concentrations is often necessary to assure optimal therapy. Peak concentrations are most helpful in assuring administration of safe doses. Peak concentrations usually occur $\frac{1}{2}$ to $1\frac{1}{2}$ hours after administration of liquid theophylline preparations and $1\frac{1}{2}$ to $2\frac{1}{2}$ hours after administration of a plain tablet or capsule. Peak concentrations that follow administration of a sustained-release preparation are more difficult to predict but usually occur 4 to 8 hours after administration of most products and 6 to 10 hours after Theo-Dur, Sustaire, or Uniphyl. Absorption of sustained-release preparations is delayed at night, possibly due to the recumbent position, and the peak concentration may not occur until the following morning. Administration of a sustained-release preparation with a meal usually delays attainment of the peak concentration by 1 to 2 hours but causes much more extreme delays for products such as Theolair-SR with pH-dependent dissolution. Administration of Theo-Dur Sprinkle (but not Theo-Dur tablets) with meals not only delays the peak but also substantially reduces bioavailability. Theo-Dur Sprinkle should be administered at least 1 hour before or 2 hours after meals. Sustained-release preparations are helpful even in children too young to swallow capsules because the beads from the capsule can be sprinkled on a teaspoonful of applesauce and swallowed without alteration in the sustained-release properties. The child must not chew the beads, however, and sustained-release tablets must be broken only where scored. Decreasing the number of doses required daily enhances compliance. Capsules cannot be divided accurately because many beads may contain no theophylline.

Table 3 shows recommended changes in dosage for various peak serum theophylline concentrations at steady state after 5 half-lives of the drug (usually within 20–36 hours after regular dosing has started) for patients in whom inadequate con-

Table 3. THEOPHYLLINE DOSAGE ADJUSTMENTS RECOMMENDED FOR VARIOUS PEAK SERUM CONCENTRATIONS*

Serum Concentration (μg/ml)	Adjustment in Total Daily Dosage
<5	100% increase in 2–4 equal increments at intervals of 2 days
5–7.5	50% increase in 2 equal increments at intervals of 2 days
8–10	20% increase
11–13	10% increase if necessary for control of symptoms
14–20	10% decrease if side effects present
21–25	10% decrease
26–30	25% decrease after omitting next dose
31–35	33% decrease after omitting next dose
>35	50% decrease or more after omitting next 2 doses

* From Hendeles, L., et al.: Am. J. Dis. Child. 132:876, 1978; and Sly, R. M.: Textbook of Pediatric Allergy. New Hyde Park, New York, Medical Examination Publishing Co., 1985, p. 115.

trol of symptoms suggests a need for an increase in dosage. Changes in dosage should be cautious near concentrations of 10–20 μg/ml, because a change of 10% in dosage may cause a greater change in the serum concentration.

Signs and symptoms of theophylline toxicity include restlessness, nausea, vomiting, irritability, headache, abdominal pain, hematemesis, twitching, convulsions, pallor, fever, and coma. Most children have adverse side effects if the serum concentration exceeds 20 μg/ml, but some have side effects at concentrations as low as 15 μg/ml, and rare children cannot tolerate concentrations of 10 μg/ml. Convulsions are rare at concentrations less than 30 μg/ml.

Treatment of serious toxicity from oral administration of the drug includes induction of vomiting or gastric lavage followed by administration of a slurry of 30 gm activated charcoal. If ipecac has been administered to induce vomiting, one should delay administration of the charcoal until after emesis because charcoal adsorbs ipecac. Administration of charcoal several times at intervals of 2 hours or less can be of further benefit, especially after ingestion of a sustained-release preparation. The charcoal can even remove theophylline that has already been absorbed. A saline cathartic is also indicated. Hemoperfusion with resin or activated charcoal cartridges may be indicated for concentrations of 60 μg/ml or more 4 hours after ingestion and may merit consideration for serum concentrations of 40–60 μg/ml if clearance is unusually slow or if there are symptoms of toxicity.

Beta-Adrenergic Agonists. Although isoproterenol is one of the most effective bronchodilators, it has a short duration of action of only 1–2 hours. Another limitation is the decrease in arterial P_{O_2}

of a few torr that can follow its inhalation despite lessening of airway obstruction. This phenomenon, also observed after subcutaneous administration of epinephrine or treatment with intravenous aminophylline, is probably due to aggravation of the ventilation-perfusion imbalance typical of acute asthma. It can be prevented by simultaneous administration of supplemental oxygen.

Efforts to develop safer drugs with longer durations of action have led to the introduction of metaproterenol, bitolterol mesylate, terbutaline, albuterol, and fenoterol, which elicit longer lasting bronchodilation than isoproterenol (5–6 hours or more after inhalation for the last three; 6–8 hours for bitolterol) and most are effective after oral administration. Inhalation is the route of choice for their administration because of rapid bronchodilation after very small doses that cause minimal side effects, including very little cardiac stimulation at doses usually recommended. Oral or intravenous administration does cause cardiac stimulation.

Metered-dose inhalers usually deliver drugs as effectively as powered nebulizers, which may require 6–8 times as much drug for the same bronchodilating effect. The bronchodilator is best delivered from a metered-dose inhaler during a slow inhalation from functional residual capacity (the end of a quiet exhalation) to total lung capacity followed by breathholding for 10 seconds. Intervals of several minutes between inhalations enhance response to two or three inhalations. Use of a spacer tube or cone can increase pulmonary deposition of aerosol by permitting evaporation of the large propellant particle that surrounds the bronchodilator particle, reducing the particle size to one more consistent with delivery to the lower airway, and by allowing a decrease in the speed of the particles before they reach the patient, reducing deposition in the pharynx by impaction. Use of a chamber such as the Inhal-Aid or Aerochamber obviates the need for synchronization of inhalation with actuation of the canister, enabling children as young as three years of age to receive effective treatment with metered-dose inhalers.

Continual treatment with either inhaled or oral beta agonist drugs can elicit tolerance or subsensitivity manifested by some decrease in the peak and duration of bronchodilation that follows each dose. Regular treatment with terbutaline, albuterol, or fenoterol for 12–13 weeks may reduce peak improvement in parameters of airway obstruction and duration of bronchodilation after a given dose by 30–60%. When tolerance occurs, it has usually become maximal within the first two weeks of continual treatment and may apply to all beta-adrenergic drugs, not just the drug that induced the tolerance. Adrenal corticosteroids administered by intravenous injection can restore beta-adrenergic responsiveness within one hour in such patients, however, and oral or inhaled corticosteroids can minimize tolerance induced by concurrent treatment with a beta agonist. Continual treatment with a beta agonist can induce tolerance to tachycardia and tremor as well as to bronchodilation.

Beta-adrenergic agonists and theophylline can have additive effects on bronchodilation when used together. Combined therapy can sometimes minimize adverse side effects by reducing the dose of each drug required for the same bronchodilating effect. Administration of bronchodilators concurrently by both inhaled and systemic routes may also enhance bronchodilation.

Concurrent treatment with theophylline and an oral beta agonist has caused chest pain with electrocardiographic changes in a few asthmatic children in whom symptoms and electrocardiographic abnormalities resolved after discontinuation of the beta agaonist. Orally administered beta agonists can cause premature ventricular contractions in susceptible adults with chronic obstructive pulmonary disease. Administration even by inhalation can cause chest pain with electrocardiographic changes in rare asthmatic adults with cardiovascular disease. In general these drugs seem quite safe at recommended doses, however. The chief potential hazard of their use may be overdependence in a patient who may use larger and larger doses at shorter and shorter intervals, not recognizing the loss of effectiveness of the drug and the need for other therapy. Tolerance is less likely to remain unrecognized with the more recent drugs than with isoproterenol because of their longer duration of action. When it occurs, however, the patient must know whom to contact for adjunctive therapy. Accordingly, completely unsupervised use of these drugs may be dangerous.

Cromolyn. Cromolyn is a prophylactic drug that can inhibit both immediate and late bronchoconstrictive effects of allergen, exercise-induced asthma, bronchoconstriction induced by inhalation of ultrasonically nebulized distilled water, and the decrease in tracheal mucus velocity induced by allergen challenge in asthmatics. It can also inhibit bronchoconstriction induced by toluene diisocyanate, sulfur dioxide, and methacholine or histamine in some patients. It may prevent seasonal increases in bronchial reactivity or may reduce bronchial reactivity within 8 weeks of treatment.

Improvement has occurred in 60–89% of asthmatics treated with cromolyn. Improvement is sometimes dramatic, but treatment for 12 weeks may be necessary for maximal response at times. The usual initial dose is 20 mg four times a day. After improvement this can usually be decreased to 20 mg three times a day without loss of control. If response is inadequate, a larger dose of 40 mg three or four times a day may be helpful. Adequate bronchodilation to permit satisfactory delivery to the lower airways is necessary and may require an initial increase in use of bronchodilators or even adrenal corticosteroids to assure an adequate trial of cromolyn.

Children less than 5 years old are usually unable to inhale cromolyn effectively from the Spinhaler, but the cromolyn nebulizer solution permits treatment of these young children as well as the few older children in whom inhalation of cromolyn powder may trigger coughing or wheezing. The solution can be nebulized by an air compressor such as the DeVilbiss #561 compressor and nebulizer. The nebulizer solution is compatible with both metaproterenol inhalant solution and terbutaline solution, and both cromolyn and the bronchodilators are stable in such solutions for at least 1 hour. Thus the cromolyn and bronchodilator can be nebulized simultaneously for patients who need both. Coughing and wheezing after inhalation of cromolyn powder are often inhibited by pretreatment with an inhaled bronchodilator.

Significant adverse reactions are extremely rare, occurring in only 1–2% of patients treated. The commonest minor side effect is throat irritation due to deposition of the powder. Swallowing a liquid after treatment prevents this annoyance.

Adrenal Corticosteroids. Adrenal corticosteroids are very effective in the treatment of asthma, but their use is limited by numerous possible adverse side effects. Suppression of linear growth and the most common side effect, suppression of the hypothalamic-pituitary-adrenal axis, depend upon dose, the duration of treatment, and the corticosteroid selected. Some adrenal suppression can follow even a single dose, and as little as 2.5 mg daily of prednisone can maintain adrenal suppression.

Adrenal function has usually returned to normal within 9 months after discontinuation of continual therapy, and plasma cortisol concentrations may become normal within 2 weeks after discontinuation of daily prednisone in children. Children at risk for adrenal insufficiency who encounter stress, such as the stress of a severe asthmatic episode unresponsive to usual therapy with bronchodilators, should receive parenteral corticosteroids.

Use of the smallest dose necessary for the shortest time possible can minimize adverse effects. Prednisone, prednisolone, or methylprednisolone, 2 mg/kg/day divided into 3 or 4 equal doses (total daily dose 20–80 mg), usually controls asthma adequately within three days. One can then discontinue the corticosteroid, or it can be tapered over several days. When a corticosteroid is necessary, the dose should be adequate to control symptoms, and occasionally treatment for more than three days may be necessary.

If continual treatment with a corticosteroid is necessary, inhaled beclomethasone, triamcinolone acetonide, or flunisolide is least likely to cause adverse side effects. The recommended dose of inhaled beclomethasone is 100 μg three or four times a day (maximum total daily dose 500 μg for children). Inhaled beclomethasone probably induces adrenal suppression only at doses that exceed 14 μg/kg/day. The recommended dose of triamcinolone acetonide aerosol for children 6–12 years old is 100–200 μg three or four times a day (maximum 1200 μg/day for children or 1600 μg/day for adults). An advantage of this preparation over other inhaled corticosteroids is the delivery device, which includes a spacer tube that minimizes deposition of drug in the pharynx and may thus minimize the side effect of pharyngeal or laryngeal candidiasis. This has not been a frequent or serious side effect of inhaled corticosteroids, however. The dose of flunisolide recommended for children 6–15 years old is 500 μg twice daily (maximum daily dose for adults is 2 mg). The small risk of pharyngeal candidiasis can be minimized by rinsing the mouth after inhalation of beclomethasone or flunisolide.

If continual treatment with an oral corticosteroid becomes necessary, use of prednisone, prednisolone, or methylprednisolone as a single morning dose on alternate days reduces the risk of adrenal suppression, at least at small or modest doses. Dexamethasone is not a suitable choice for therapy on alternate days because of its longer biologic half-life.

Immunotherapy

At least 15 published, placebo-controlled studies attest to the beneficial effect of immunotherapy in patients with allergic asthma due to allergy to inhalant allergens, including ragweed pollen, grass pollen, mountain cedar pollen, cat allergen, house dust, and *Dermatophagoides pteronyssimus*. Immunotherapy induces specific IgG blocking antibody; suppresses the usual seasonal increase in specific IgE antibody that follows environmental exposure and decreases specific IgE concentrations in the serum over several years; reduces basophil reactivity and sensitivity to allergen; induces increases in specific IgG and IgA antibodies in secretions; and reduces in vitro lymphocyte responses to allergen. Immunotherapy may inhibit late-phase asthmatic responses to inhaled allergen.

Response to therapy is specific for allergens included in the allergy extract and dependent upon the dose administered. Small doses are ineffective, but treatment must begin with small doses to avoid systemic reactions to the injections of the extract. The dose is gradually increased over several weeks or months with weekly or more frequent injections to the maximal dose tolerated. The interval between injections can then often be increased to 4 weeks, and therapy is continued until the patient has been free of significant symptoms or substantially improved for 1 to 1½ years. Periodic renewal of the extract is necessary to maintain potency. Symptoms may recur a few months or a few years after discontinuation of therapy. Improvement usually occurs in 80–90% of patients appropriately treated for allergy to unavoidable inhalant allergens such as pollens or mites. That improvement usually occurs during the first year of therapy, but some who do not improve during the first year improve during the second year.

Immunotherapy can induce hypersensitivity where previously there was none; accordingly treatment extracts should contain only allergens to which the patient has demonstrable allergy. Results of skin testing should correlate with the clinical history.

Immunotherapy with bacterial vaccines is not of demonstrable benefit.

Immunotherapy is indicated for most patients with allergic asthma and allergy to unavoidable inhalant allergens. It is not appropriate for those who have recently failed to respond to an adequate trial of immunotherapy with large doses of potent extracts that have included all relevant allergens.

Intermittent Asthma

Most patients with asthma experience episodes of mild or moderate airway obstruction fewer than six times each year. These patients need treatment that will afford rapid relief of symptoms. An inhaled beta-adrenergic agonist is most rapidly effective. The best choice is albuterol or fenoterol because of sustained bronchodilation and long lasting inhibition of exercise-induced asthma. Dosage is indicated in Table 4. For children 3–6 years old an Inhal-Aid or Aerochamber permits effective delivery of the drug from the metered-dose inhaler. Such a chamber is also helpful for older children unable to coordinate actuation of the canister with inhalation. Children younger than three years old and older children unable to use the metered-dose inhaler with the chamber during moderately severe airway obstruction require nebulization of the beta-adrenergic agonist by an air compressor. Both metaproterenol inhalant solution and terbutaline are available for nebulization. Terbutaline and unit-dose metaproterenol inhalant solution are free of sulfites, which can provoke bronchoconstriction in some asthmatics.

Because airway obstruction is likely to persist for several days after relief of symptoms, the patient should receive treatment with a bronchodilator for 4 or 5 days after resolution of coughing or wheezing. A sustained-release theophylline preparation is most convenient because of the possibility of dosing at intervals of 8 or 12 hours. I prefer Theo-Dur tablets (200 or 300 mg) for children who can swallow tablets. The 100-mg

Table 4. BETA–ADRENERGIC AGONIST DRUGS

Drug	Route	Dose
Albuterol	Inh	180 µg q 4–6 h (MDI)
	Oral	2–4 mg tid-qid (>12 years old)
Bitolterol mesylate*	Inh	740–1110 µg q 8 hr (MDI)
Ephedrine	Oral	0.5–1 mg/kg q 4–6 h
Epinephrine, 1:1000, aqueous	SC	0.01 ml/kg (max. 0.3 ml) q 20 min × 3 if necessary; may repeat in 4 hr
Epinephrine, 1:200, aqueous suspension (Sus-Phrine)	SC	0.005 ml/kg (max. 0.3 ml); may repeat in 8 hr
Ethylnorepinephrine (Bronkephrine)	SC	0.01–0.02 ml/kg (max. 0.5 ml); may repeat in 20 minutes
Fenoterol†	Inh	160–320 µg q 4–6 h (MDI)
Metaproterenol‡	Inh	0.1–0.3 ml q 4–6 h (inhalant solution, 5%, diluted in 3 ml saline and nebulized)
	Inh	1.3–1.95 mg q 4–6 h (MDI)
	Oral	0.5 mg/kg q 6–8 h (max. 20 mg qid)
Terbutaline§	Inh	400 µg q 4–6 h (MDI)
	Inh	0.1 mg/kg q 4–6 h (max 6 mg, nebulized)
	SC	0.01 mg/kg (max. 0.25 mg); may repeat in 20 min (max. 0.5 mg in 4 h)
	Oral	0.075 mg/kg or 2.5 mg q 6 h tid (max. 5 mg q 6 h tid)

Inh = by inhalation; SC = by subcutaneous injection; MDI = metered-dose inhaler.

* Bitolterol mesylate is not recommended for children under 12 years of age.

† Fenoterol is an experimental drug and is not yet approved for use by the FDA. It is not recommended for children under 12 years of age.

‡ Inhaler dose of metaproterenol is not recommended for use in children under 12 years of age.

§ Terbutaline is not recommended for children under 12 years of age.

tablets do not have quite the same sustained release as the larger tablets. For younger children who cannot swallow tablets, I recommend sprinkling the sustained release beads from a capsule such as Slo-bid Gyrocaps or Somophylline-CRT on applesauce every 8 hours. Both the initial dose of the inhaled beta-adrenergic drug and the sustained-release theophylline are started at the first sign of symptoms, but the theophylline is continued for 4 to 5 days after resolution of symptoms. Administration of theophylline once daily in a preparation such as Uniphyl tablets may be appropriate for children at least 12 years of age, and use of this convenient preparation may further enhance compliance, but meals can enhance its bioavailability.

Infants and toddlers who will not swallow sustained-release beads require liquid preparations of theophylline or metaproterenol or both at intervals of 6 hours.

Frequent Asthma

Patients with airway obstruction several times each month or somewhat less frequently if episodes are severe require continual drug therapy when avoidance of allergens is impossible or insufficient. Use of a sustained-release theophylline preparation is most practical. Such a patient also requires treatment of acute asthma that may recur despite continual treatment with theophylline, and an inhaled beta agonist is most appropriate for this purpose.

If continual treatment with theophylline at optimal doses does not afford adequate control of symptoms and restoration of pulmonary function to normal, a trial of cromolyn is indicated. Some recommend a trial of cromolyn before continual treatment with theophylline because of the remarkable paucity of side effects from cromolyn.

When even the combination of bronchodilators and cromolyn afford inadequate control, one should add inhaled beclomethasone, triamcinolone acetonide, or flunisolide. Both cromolyn and inhaled corticosteroids are effective only when delivered adequately to the lower airways. Airway obstruction should be controlled if necessary with oral corticosteroids when one initiates therapy with these inhaled drugs. If attempts to discontinue the oral corticosteroid are unsuccessful, it may be necessary to continue treatment with prednisone, prednisolone, or methylprednisolone as single doses in the morning on alternate days.

Exercise-Induced Asthma

Nasal breathing or use of a muffler or scarf wrapped around the nose and mouth or a cold weather mask can minimize the airway obstruction induced by strenuous exercise. When these measures are inadequate, pretreatment with inhaled albuterol or fenoterol can inhibit exercise-induced asthma for 4–6 hours. Cromolyn is most effective in inhibiting exercise-induced asthma only during the first hour after treatment, although it has some effect for four hours. A sustained-release theophylline preparation may be most convenient for inhibition of this abnormal response to exercise in a youngster who may be exercising unpredictably at any time of day, but optimal effectiveness would require continual treatment or administration of an unusually large dose to maintain the serum concentration at 15–20 µg/ml if tolerated. When a single drug does not afford adequate protection, combinations of an inhaled beta agonist with cromolyn or theophylline or all three may be more effective.

A warm-up period before strenuous exercise may be helpful by causing brief, exercise-induced asthma that is followed by a refractory period that may persist 60–90 minutes.

For asthmatic children in whom 1 to 2 minutes of strenuous exercise causes bronchodilation while exercise for 5 to 6 minutes causes airway obstruction, activities that require only intermittent, brief intervals of exercise may be more tolerable than

Table 5. TREATMENT OF STATUS ASTHMATICUS

1. Intravenous fluids: 360–400 ml/M^2 during first hour; then 1500–3000 ml/m^2/24 hours when dehydration is present.
2. Aminophylline: 5 mg/kg diluted and infused intravenously over 20 minutes; follow with constant infusion of 0.5–1.1 mg/kg/hr to maintain serum concentration of 10–20 µg/ml (preferably 14–18 µg/ml if necessary and tolerated).
3. Oxygen. Maintain arterial PO$_2$ > 65 torr and <100 torr.
4. Sodium bicarbonate: 1.5–2.0 mEq/kg diluted and infused intravenously over 10–20 minutes when there is metabolic acidosis. Repeat same dose over next 45 minutes and every hour if arterial pH remains less than 7.25 and serum sodium less than 145 mEq/liter.
5. Metaproterenol* inhalant solution or terbutaline* by inhalation after nebulization q 4 hours (see Table 4).
6. Adrenal corticosteroids: hydrocortisone, 4 mg/kg, or methylprednisolone, 1 mg/kg, q 4 hours by intravenous injection.
7. SEDATIVES, TRANQUILIZERS, MORPHINE, and ANTIHISTAMINES CONTRAINDICATED.
8. Endotracheal intubation and controlled ventilation for progression to respiratory failure despite these measures.

* Metaproterenol and terbutaline are not recommended for children under 12 years of age.

those that require more prolonged exercise. Swimming is usually tolerated especially well, partly because of inhibition of exercise-induced asthma by ventilation with air fully saturated with water. Appropriate pretreatment with medication enables most children with asthma to tolerate whatever activities they choose, however.

Prophylaxis

Pretreatment with cromolyn is the method of choice for prevention of asthma due to unavoidable exposure to allergen when this is predictable.

Status Asthmaticus

The treatment for acute, severe asthma administered most frequently at emergency rooms in the United States has been 1:1000 aqueous epinephrine by subcutaneous injection followed by epinephrine 1:200 (Sus-Phrine) when there has been a satisfactory response (Table 4). Terbutaline by subcutaneous injection is at least equally effective and often reduces the number of injections required. An inhaled beta agonist is also as effective as injected epinephrine but may require somewhat more prolonged observation for possible recurrence of airway obstruction. Administration by nebulization may deliver the drug to the lower airways better than use of a metered-dose inhaler during severe airway obstruction.

Failure of adequate response to the beta agonist establishes the diagnosis of status asthmaticus. Some also require failure of response to intravenous theophylline or aminophylline for this diagnosis.

The indicated treatment is summarized in Table 5. Correct dehydration with 5 or 10% glucose in ⅓ normal saline or 5% glucose in saline followed after establishment of renal flow by a polyionic, hypotonic solution containing potassium, but do not overhydrate when there is no dehydration.

Intravenous theophylline (Travenol Laboratories) is the drug of choice, which avoids the risk of rare allergic reactions to the ethylenediamine of aminophylline and obviates the need for calculating the theophylline equivalence of aminophylline, which is only 78.9% anhydrous theophylline when assayed as the dihydrate. Nevertheless, aminophylline is still used more widely than intravenous theophylline in the United States.

The initial infusion of aminophylline, 5 mg/kg, is safe for patients with serum theophylline concentrations expected to be less than 3 μg/ml (Table 5). Each dose of 1 mg/kg increases the serum concentration by approximately 2 μg/ml, but the rate at which the concentration then falls depends upon the rate of clearance for the particular patient. Determination of the serum concentration one half hour after completion of infusion of the loading dose indicates whether an additional small bolus may be required to obtain a serum concentration of 14–18 μg/ml. Determination of another serum concentration approximately 6 hours after completion of the infusion of the initial loading dose indicates whether the rate of constant infusion of theophylline is adequate or excessive, and any required correction can be made. Subsequent determinations of theophylline concentrations 12 hours later and then at intervals of 12–24 hours assure continued safe, effective therapy. Some patients cannot tolerate concentrations of 14 μg/ml without adverse side effects and should be maintained at lower concentrations that do not cause side effects. Lower concentrations are satisfactory whether or not there are side effects if airway obstruction has been relieved adequately.

If the patient has already received theophylline within the previous 24 hours (36 hours for Theo-24 or Uniphyl), it is safest to determine the serum concentration before administration of the initial loading dose. That concentration must be interpreted with consideration of the type of preparation administered and the anticipated time and duration of peak response to avoid overdosing a patient who may still be absorbing a sustained-release preparation.

If necessary the inhaled beta agonist can be administered more frequently than at intervals of 4 hours with continual cardiac monitoring for arrhythmias or electrocardiographic signs of ischemia. Tachycardia and other adverse effects of beta agonist drugs are more frequent with intravenous administration than with inhalation, and response to intravenous treatment is no better than to inhalation therapy.

Inhalation of nebulized atropine sulfate (0.01

Table 6. CLINICAL SCORING SYSTEM FOR CHILDREN WITH STATUS ASTHMATICUS*

	Score†		
	0	*1*	*2*
Po2	70–110 in air	≤70 in air	≤70 in 40% O2
or			
Cyanosis	None	In air	In 40% O2
Inspiratory breath sounds	Normal	Unequal	Decreased or absent
Use of accessory muscles of respiration	None	Moderate	Maximal
Expiratory wheezing	None	Moderate	Extreme or none because of poor air exchange
Cerebral function	Normal	Depressed or agitated	Coma

* From Wood, D. W., et al.: Am. J. Dis. Child. 123:227, 1972.
† Total score of 5 suggests impending respiratory failure. Score of 7 with arterial Pco2 ≥ 65 torr indicates respiratory failure.

mg/kg, maximum 1 mg, diluted to 3 ml in normal saline) can cause further bronchodilation and can be given at intervals of 4 hours alternating with inhalation of the beta agonist at intervals of 4 hours. Use of inhaled atropine has not been studied extensively in children, however.

Progression to respiratory failure despite the measures listed in Table 5 indicates a need for intubation and mechanical ventilation. Use of a clinical scoring system facilitates diagnosis of respiratory failure (Table 6).

Allergic Rhinitis

Control of allergic rhinitis to facilitate filtration and conditioning of inspired air is especially important in patients with asthma. Antihistamines are helpful for most patients with allergic rhinitis but may cause bronchoconstriction in a small proportion of asthmatics and are contraindicated in status asthmaticus. Nasalcrom or intranasal beclomethasone or flunisolide is often effective.

Unlabeled Use of Approved Drugs

Many of the drugs safest and most effective in the treatment of asthma are not labeled for use in children. The United States Food and Drug Administration regulates industry rather than physicians, however. Lack of approval does not indicate disapproval. Choice of therapy should be determined by all information available regarding safety and effectiveness in children. Use of a drug not labeled for use in children, however, must be distinguished from use of a drug contraindicated in children because investigation has shown it to be unsafe or ineffective in children.

Serum Sickness

LEONARD BIELORY, M.D.

Serum sickness as classically described in 1905 by von Pirquet and Schick consisted of a spectrum of clinical findings that included fever, malaise, cutaneous eruptions, primarily urticaria, arthralgias, lymphadenopathy, edema, and albuminuria. Their patients consisted mainly of children who developed one or a combination of these symptoms 6–10 days after their first exposure to heterologous antisera for the treatment of various infectious diseases. The administration of heterologous antisera remained the major cause of serum sickness until the advent of modern drug therapy. Presently the most frequently encountered medications producing serum sickness include the penicillins, streptomycin, cephalosporins, sulfonamides, thiouracils, and hydantoins. Penicillin-induced serum sickness is most common, but it is unusual with dosages under 2 g/day. The medications producing serum sickness with the highest frequency are still the heterologous proteins that are presently being used for crotalid and arachnid envenomation, specific clostridial infections, and rabies and as immunosuppressant agents for organ allograft rejection or preconditioning agents for organ transplantation.

The treatment of serum sickness is either prophylactic or symptomatic. Prophylactically, all physicians should maintain up-to-date vaccinations of their patients as recommended by the American College of Physicians Committee's Guide for Adult Immunization and the Red Book of the American Academy of Pediatrics in order to immunize their patients against those diseases still treated with heterologous antisera. Heterologous antisera is still in use in several underdeveloped countries for acute infections such as diphtheria. All individuals traveling to underdeveloped countries should be vaccinated for endemic infectious agents as recommended by the Centers for Disease Control in their Morbidity and Mortality Weekly Reports. Most cases of serum sickness are probably never seen by the physician, since the clinical spectrum of complaints are very similar to what the public perceives as the 'flu' and patients are apt to treat themselves with fluids, aspirin, and bedrest. It is only the unusual circumstance of a frightening cutaneous eruption or severe arthralgias that usually brings a person to the attention of a physician for medical treatment.

Symptomatic treatment of serum sickness is based upon the severity and extent of the patient's complaints. First, if possible, the offending antigen should be eliminated. It is known from animal models that elimination of antigen will lead to rapid resolution of immunopathologic damage.

Symptomatic treatment usually involves the use of combinations of antipyretics, analgesics, antihistamines, and glucocorticosteroids.

Antipyretic medications such as the salicylates, as noted by von Pirquet and Schick, are of some benefit in ameliorating the febrile response but have relatively little effect on the arthralgias or the various cutaneous eruptions. In addition, the use of salicylates must be considered in the light of their effect on platelet function, since some serum sickness patients develop thrombocytopenia. Acetaminophen (Tylenol) as an antipyretic is a better choice in thrombocytopenic individuals.

Other symptoms, particularly those associated with proteinuria or arthralgias, usually warrant treatment with a "burst" of glucocorticosteroids. "Burst" glucocorticoid therapy involves the use of 1–2 mg/kg/day of prednisone in divided doses for 7–10 days. This is followed by consolidation to once a day doses coinciding with the normal diurnal variation of cortisol levels and then tapering the drug by 10 mg decrements to 30 mg and then 5 mg decrements to 10 mg and then by 2.5 mg decrements until the prednisone is discontinued within a period of about 3–4 weeks.

Antihistamines have proved to be of value in the treatment of generalized urticaria and pruritus with such medications as diphenhydramine (Benadryl) 50 mg every 4 hours (1 mg/kg in children) or alternatively hydroxyzine (Atarax, Vistaril) 25 mg every 4 hours (0.3 mg/kg in children). The prophylactic value of antihistamines in serum sickness has not been proved, but these drugs may be useful. Doses of diphenhydramine or cyproheptadine are started four days prior to the expected onset of serum sickness and continued for a period of 1–2 weeks. Marked urticarial eruptions or angioedema is usually treated with aqueous epinephrine, 1:1000, 0.01 ml/kg subcutaneously with a maximum of 0.3–0.5 ml every 15 minutes for 3 doses. If attacks of angioedema recur after using the preceding treatment, intramuscular aqueous epinephrine suspension (Sus-Phrine) can be used at a dose of 1:200, 0.005 ml/kg with a maximum of 0.2 ml every 6 hours.

In the event that large amounts of heterologous antisera are required over a course of days the usual precautions as recommended by the pharmaceutical company for its administration should be strictly followed. Skin testing with the antigen and appropriate controls should be done prior to the administration of the heterologous protein. If there is an immediate hypersensitivity reaction, desensitization may be required to prevent anaphylaxis. This will not prevent the occurrence of serum sickness.

Glucocorticosteroids in the form of prednisone (or intravenous methylprednisolone) at a dose of 1 mg/kg/day in 3 or 4 divided doses should be started concomitantly with the first dose of heterologous antisera. This dose should be increased to 1.5 mg/kg/day at the first sign of serum sickness, maintained for 3 or 4 days or as long as the heterologous protein must be given and then tapered by 10-mg decrements every 2 or 3 days to 30 mg and then tapered by 5-mg decrements every 2 or 3 days to 10 mg and then tapered using 2.5-mg decrements over the course of a week. If the antigen persists longer than expected and the patient has a breakthrough of symptoms while glucocorticosteroids are being tapered, the dose at which the symptoms reappeared (usually between 10 and 20 mg prednisone) should be doubled. The glucocorticosteroids may then be decreased on alternate days rather than daily in 10-mg decrements every 2 or 3 cycles until a dose of 30 mg is reached and then tapered by 5-mg decrements every 2 or 3 cycles until 20 mg and then tapered by 2.5-mg decrements every 2 or 3 cycles until the alternate-day dose has been discontinued. If exacerbations occur on the off days one should increase the dose to a previous level that controlled the symptoms and then taper even more slowly. When the alternate-day therapy is achieved, it is maintained for 2–4 weeks to permit the hypothalamic-pituitary-adrenal (HPA) axis to recover and then tapered 5 mg a week. The alternate-day regimen has been shown to cause far less HPA axis suppression and to result in fewer opportunistic infections.

In cases requiring the readministration of heterologous antisera where the 'accelerated' form of serum sickness is expected within 24–72 hours after administration, the concomitant use of glucocorticoids as described above is recommended. One should also be extremely careful of the possibility of anaphylaxis, since the patient has had a previous exposure to the heterologous protein.

Local reactions at the site of intramuscular injections of heterologous antisera during the course of serum sickness can range from a mild urticarial eruption to a severely indurated granulomatous lesion. Treatment usually involves the use of oral antihistamines for the mild reaction and systemic "burst" of glucocorticosteroids for the severe reaction.

Allergic Gastrointestinal Disorders

C. WARREN BIERMAN, M.D.,
and JANE TODARO, M.D.

In 1980 the Food Allergy Committee of the American Academy of Allergy was renamed "Committee on Adverse Reactions to Foods" in recognition of the fact that an individual's reaction to food and food additives is complex and often variable. These reactions sometimes have an immune basis, sometimes are secondary to other illnesses, and sometimes may be manifestations of inborn metabolic errors. Often combinations of several factors are present.

The treatment of food allergy or intolerance is the removal of the offending food or foods from the diet. This can be done by prescribing an elemental diet or a diet composed of simple foods selected from grains, fruits, vegetables, meats, and milk substitutes or from a rotating diet. In order to recommend a limited diet intelligently, the pediatrician must know the composition of various foods, particularly formulas (Table 1). Specific attention must be paid to the protein source, the carbohydrate source, and the fat source. Patients with cow's milk protein intolerance may also become allergic to soy milk, and goat's milk has at least 9 antigens that cross-react with cow's milk. In the elimination of solid foods in the diet, the physician must be aware of cross-reacting food groups and be certain of the nutritional adequacy of the diet.

Once symptoms are controlled, patients may be rechallenged periodically, both to be certain that the particular food needs to be excluded and to see if the patient can now tolerate that food. Food allergies are often outgrown when they show up in the first year of life. Of those children diagnosed as food allergic during the first year or two of life, fully 44% will outgrow their allergies.

If there continues to be confusion about sensitivity to a food, a double-blind challenge is useful in identifying the reaction. This should be done in a setting that is equipped to treat a medical emergency.

Drug Treatment. While avoidance of offending food remains the cornerstone of therapy for food allergy, certain medications may be useful in suppressing secondary manifestations. Cromolyn sodium is used widely in Europe for "food allergy." However, it is not approved for this use in the United States and cromolyn capsules are not appropriate, since each 20-mg capsule contains 20 mg of lactose. Oral prednisone in small doses (2–4 mg/day) is useful in eosinophilic gastroenteritis, but not in other food allergies. H_1 and H_2 antihistamines have no proven role in preventing allergic reactions to food, but the H_1 antihistamines may be used in treating some of the resulting clinical reactions, such as urticaria.

Referral. Consultation with a subspecialist should be sought when there is continuing failure to thrive in a younger child, particularly if there is laboratory and clinical evidence of malabsorption or unexplained weight loss. Severe diseases, such as glucose-galactose malabsorption and celiac disease, are complicated lifelong diseases requiring

Table 1. MAJOR INGREDIENTS OF COMMONLY USED INFANT FORMULAS

Product	Protein Source	Carbohydrate Source	Fat Source
Human milk	40% casein 60% lactalbumin	Lactose	Human milk fat
Cow's milk	80% casein 20% lactalbumin	Lactose	Butterfat
Similac	82% casein 18% lactalbumin	Lactose	Coconut, corn
Enfamil	40% casein 60% lactalbumin	Lactose	Soy, coconut
Isomil	Soy protein isolate	Corn, sucrose	Corn, coconut, soy
ProSobee	Soy protein isolate	Glucose polymers	Soy, coconut
Meat Base Formula	Beef hearts	Sucrose, tapioca starch	Sesame
Portagen	Sodium caseinate	Corn, sucrose	88% MCT, corn
Nutramigen	Casein hydrolyzate	Sucrose, tapioca	corn
Pregestimil	Enzymatically hydrolyzed milk protein	Corn, tapioca	corn, MCT (coconut)
Vivonex	Purified amino acids	Glucose, oligosaccharides	Soy, coconut safflower

consistent evaluation and follow-up. Patients with severe unremitting eczema, rhinitis with recurrent otitis media with effusion, or asthma should also be referred. Such a referral should provide the patient and parents with a team approach, and the consultants should communicate regularly with the referring physician about the patient's course.

Adverse Reactions to Drugs

H. JAMES WEDNER, M.D.

Adverse reactions to drugs may be classified into three broad groups: dose-related toxic effects, idiosyncratic reactions, and hypersensitivity reactions. The toxic reactions are unwanted pharmacologic effects of the drug in question. They will occur, to a greater or lesser extent, in all patients if sufficient quantities of the drug are given. They are "normal" properties of the drug.

Side Effects

Toxic reactions may be subdivided into those that occur within the therapeutic dose range, commonly referred to as side effects, and those that occur when doses of the drugs produce blood or tissue concentrations in excess of therapeutic levels. In some cases these two classifications will merge, since the sensitivity of individuals to side effects varies widely and one individual can tol-

erate high levels of a given drug without observable side effects while another is unable to tolerate the drug at all. Patient perception is also of great significance. The same degree of a given symptom, nausea for example, may be severely compromising to one patient and largely overlooked by another. This phenomenon is seen with many drug side effects, including the somnolence associated with antihistaminics. This is a true side effect, since many individuals become sleepy within the true therapeutic dose range. With the same blood level the somnolence may be mild or it may be overwhelming and necessitate discontinuance of the drug.

With antihistaminics, as is the case with a number of drug groups, switching from one chemical class of drug to another may allow one to maximize the therapeutic potential while minimizing the side effect. Another approach to side effects is to simply continue the drug. The undesirable side effects may disappear, and therapeutic potential is maintained. It is also possible to minimize side effects by starting at relatively low doses of a drug and increasing the dose gradually over a period of time. This is effective not only with antihistaminics but also with such diverse groups as beta-adrenergic agonists or antihypersensitive agents. It is important in all cases to explain to patients that there is a potential for an undesirable side effect and that this effect may indeed disappear if they will persevere in taking the drug.

Toxic Effects

In contrast to undesirable side effects, toxic reactions to drugs occur at dosages that yield blood levels in excess of the therapeutic range. Toxic reactions are still, however, intimately related to the chemical nature of the agent and amount of drug that is given. Examples of this type of reaction include cardiac toxicity with digitalis; postural hypotension with antihypertensive agents; and nausea, vomiting, and, if sufficient drug is given, convulsions with theophylline or its salts. It is important to remember that the gap between therapeutic and toxic levels of a given drug varies greatly with the type of pharmacologic agent. It may be quite broad, giving the physician a great deal of latitude in prescribing the drug, or narrow, requiring careful monitoring of blood levels to assure maximum benefit with minimum chance for a toxic side effect. A notable example of this phenomenon occurs in the use of theophylline for the treatment of asthma. With theophylline, the therapeutic range is generally considered to be 10 to 20 µg/ml, while the toxic range, beginning with mild anorexia and progressing through nausea and vomiting, generally starts between 18 and 20 µg/ml. The toxic effects become progressively worse at higher blood levels. Because the ability to transform theophylline biologically varies widely from patient to patient, it is impossible to predict with any degree of certainty the blood level that will be achieved by a given dose. Therefore, it is recommended that measuring the exact blood level is the only way to achieve maximum therapeutic benefit while minimizing side effects. It should also be noted that with theophylline, as with a number of other drugs, some patients may experience a degree of discomfort at blood levels that are in the relatively low range and that may be as low as 10 to 15 µg/ml in a small percentage of patients. In this instance one can still achieve therapeutic benefit by carefully adjusting the dose to achieve a blood level that reduces the majority of unwanted toxic effects while remaining in the low end of the therapeutic range. Similar considerations should be taken into account with any drug for which the toxic and therapeutic ranges approximate one another.

It is also important to remember that with some classes of drugs the toxic effects are related to the total amount of drug given and not to the absolute blood level achieved. In these instances one must keep in mind the progressive amount of drug (dose × duration) and discontinue use of that particular agent prior to reaching a level that is associated with toxic side effects. Excellent examples of this phenomenon are found with gold salts and a number of antibiotics. The aminoglycoside antibiotics cause renal and ototoxicity based on the total amount of drug given; chloramphenicol also has a toxic effect, bone marrow depression, which is related to the total cumulative dose.

Idiosyncratic Reactions

In contrast to dose-related toxic side effects, idiosyncratic reactions to drugs bear no relation to the amount or duration of therapy. They may occur with the initial introduction of the drug or may occur after long periods of time on an adequate therapeutic dose. They are impossible to predict, with the exception that a patient who has had one idiosyncratic reaction to a drug is likely to have a second if the drug is reinstituted. It is also important to remember that some idiosyncratic reactions to drugs are relatively benign while others are life threatening. Fortunately the majority of idiosyncratic reactions, to a greater or lesser extent, fall into the former category. One must always be aware of the potential for an idiosyncratic reaction. In those instances in which the idiosyncratic reaction may be life threatening, the physician must balance the potential for idiosyncratic reactions with the potential therapeutic benefit. This should take into account the frequency at which idiosyncratic reactions occur and the severity of those reactions. For example, although the aplastic anemia seen with chloramphenicol is disastrous, the percentage of treated patients actually experiencing this idiosyncratic reaction is significantly less, for example, than the chance of a penicillin reaction. For this reason it would be inappropriate to withhold this drug in cases in which it would life saving for fear of an idiosyncratic reaction. On the other hand the use of this drug in instances in which another antibiotic with significantly less potential toxicity is available would be inappropriate.

Toxic effects of drugs and idiosyncratic reactions to drugs most probably have different underlying biochemical bases. However, in some instances toxic effects and idiosyncratic effects are very similar. And when an adverse effect occurs, such as bone marrow depression with chloramphenicol, it is important to differentiate the dose-related toxic effects from the idiosyncratic reactions. A patient who has had an idiosyncratic reaction to a drug should not be given the drug again unless one is faced with dire consequences. On the other hand, in instances in which overdosages occur, the toxic effects can be prevented with appropriate dose regimens, and this does not prevent the patient from receiving that drug or a drug of the same class again.

Hypersensitivity Reactions

Hypersensitivity reactions can occur with virtually any drug in the pharmacopeia. These reactions can be differentiated into 3 basic types: immediate hypersensitivity (Type I), delayed antibody mediated of the Arthus type (IgG Type II and III), and cell mediated (Type IV). Immediate type reactions may be further subdivided into anaphylactic and anaphylactoid reactions. *Anaphylactic* reactions refer to those in which the drug induces the production of IgE antibody directed against the drug or more appropriately against a drug-protein complex; the reaction occurs on subsequent administration of the drug following interaction of the agent with specific IgE molecules bound to tissue mast cells or circulating basophils. In contrast, *anaphylactoid* reactions refer to those instances in which release of mast cell mediators is accomplished through a non–IgE-mediated mechanism. This may be the result of direct interaction of a drug with the mast cell membrane, with the release of chemical mediators by the drug polymyxin B; or it may occur secondarily, as with interaction of a drug with the complement system, generating the anaphylatoxins C5a and C3a. These anaphylatoxins are capable of inducing the release of mediators from mast cells and or basophils. In either case the net result is the same, since the mediators released are identical.

A complete discussion of the chemical mediators of anaphylaxis is beyond the scope of this review. Suffice it to say that there are a diverse number of chemical entities, including (1) biogenic amines, histamine, and to a lesser extent serotonin; (2) lipoxygenase products of arachidonic acid, leukotrienes C, D, and E (also called slow-reacting substance of anaphylaxis, SRSA); (3) cyclooxygenase products of arachidonic acid, largely prostaglandin D_2; (4) platelet-activating factor (acetyl glyceral ether phosphorylcholine); (5) a number of enzymes, including a trypsin-like enzyme; (6) *chemoattractants* for both eosinophils and polymorphonuclear leukocytes; (7) the matrix component heparin. These factors, alone or in combination, are responsible for the symptoms of immediate hypersensitivity reactions, skin pruritus, urticaria, angioedema, laryngeal edema, wheezing, and hypotension. The severity of the reaction will depend on the location of the activated mast cells and the number of mast cells activated. Hypersensitivity reactions may be extremely mild, (mild pruritus or hives) or may be an overwhelming, life-threatening, severe systemic allergic reaction (anaphylaxis).

Since anaphylactoid reactions do not require the production of IgE antibody they may occur on the initial use of a given drug, although in some instances they do occur after prolonged exposure. An example of this type of hypersensitivity is the severe reaction seen with various radiocontrast dyes. In this instance current evidence would suggest that, in susceptible individuals, injection of radiocontrast media results in the activation of complement with release of anaphlotoxins and subsequent stimulation of mediator release from mast cells. The reactions that are seen to radiocontrast material suggest two other major points concerning anaphylactoid reactions. First, not all individuals will experience this type of reaction when presented with the drug. In the majority of cases the factors that determine those patients who will react to a given drug are at the present time unknown. Secondly, although not all individuals will have a reaction on their initial exposure to the drug, in general, patients who have one anaphylactoid reaction to a given agent will continue to have anaphylactoid reactions unless some intervention is taken. In the case of radiocontrast materials, pretreatment of patients with corticosteroids and an H_1 type antihistaminic as well as an H_2 antihistaminic is sufficient to decrease the severity of or completely abrogate the reaction in more than 90% of the cases. The protocol we utilize at Washington University is shown in Table 1.

Another group of agents that frequently cause anaphylactoid-type reactions, either local or systemic, are local anesthetics. Although a small minority of reactions to local anesthetics represent true anaphylactic sensitivity, in the majority of cases it would appear that mediator release is the result of direct interaction of the drug with the plasma membrane of mast cells. As in many other reactions, the reaction to local anesthetics is highly class-specific. Thus, it is possible, using appropriate skin testing and provocative dose challenge protocols to find a local anesthetic to which the patient does not react. At Washington University School of Medicine we generally test to three non-cross reacting local anesthetics: lidocaine, carbocaine and tetracain. We use 1% or 2% solutions diluted 1:100 and 1:10. Scratch or prick tests are done starting with the most dilute concentration. If the patient does not react, intradermal skin tests are performed, again starting with the lowest concentration. Of the three local anesthetics, the one that caused no reaction is selected and 0.1 cc followed by 0.5 cc is given subcutaneously. If no local or systemic reaction is seen in 20 to 30 minutes, the agent can be utilized.

Another point that must be considered when dealing with local anesthetics and many other drugs is the fact that in some instances the patient may not be reacting to the drug per se but rather to a constituent of the drug preparation. This is particularly true with preservatives such as metabisulfites or parabens. Indeed, several patients seen by the author for sensitivity to local anesthetics turned out in fact to be highly sensitive to sodium metabisulfite and methyl paraben and had no reaction when tested with a metabisulfite- and paraben-free preparation of a number of local

Table 1. PROTOCOL FOR PRETREATMENT OF PATIENTS WITH RADIO-CONTRAST MEDIA SENSITIVITY

Time Before Procedure	Drug	Dose*	Route
25 hr	Cimetidine†	300 mg	PO/IV or I.M.‡
19 hr	Cimetidine	300 mg	PO/IV or I.M.‡
13 hr	Cimetidine	300 mg	PO/IV or I.M.‡
	Prednisone	50 mg	PO/IV§
7 hr	Cimetidine	300 mg	PO/IV‡
	Prednisone	50 mg	PO/IV
1 hr	Cimetidine	300 mg	PO/IV or I.M.‡
	Prednisone	50 mg	PO/IV§
	Diphenhydramine	50 mg	PO/IV‡

* Usual adult dosage. Equivalent pediatric dosage:
    Cimetidine 5–10 mg/kg.
    Prednisone 0.8–1.75 mg/kg.
    Diphenhydramine 1.25 mg/kg.
† Not recommended for patients under 16 years of age. If protocol without cimetidine has failed, then cimetidine 5–10 mg/kg may be added.
‡ Oral route is preferred unless patient is unable to take oral medication.
§ For intravenous route give 40 mg methyl prednisolone.

anesthetics. This patient was subsequently able to undergo extensive dental work under local anesthesia using a preservative-free preparation.

A number of drugs cause immediate hypersensitivity reactions by mechanisms that do not involve IgE formation or direct or indirect mediator release. The classic example is aspirin and all of the large group of nonsteroidal anti-inflammatory agents (NSAI). These compounds have been studied extensively; however, the mechanism for reactions to aspirin and NSAI, either aspirin-sensitive asthma or rhinitis, remains obscure. Neither IgE-mediated nor direct mast cell activation seems to be present. Since aspirin is a potent inhibitor of the enzyme fatty acid cyclooxygenase, it inhibits prostaglandin synthesis and it has been suggested that individuals sensitive to aspirin may have a marked inhibition of a necessary prostaglandin such as PGE_2 or enhanced secretion of detrimental lipoxygenase products such as the leukotrienes. However, efforts to identify these metabolites have proved unsuccessful to date. Aspirin and NSAI are not unique, and there are many other drugs in which the differentiation between anaphylactic and anaphylactoid reactions is difficult.

Anaphylactic reactions, as pointed out above, are the result of the generation of IgE (and perhaps IgG_4) type antibodies. As such, the drug must serve as a hapten and be conjugated to tissue proteins to be immunogenic. For this reason the ability of any drug to induce anaphylactic-type reactions is related to its ability to bind covalently (or in some cases noncovalently) to appropriate tissue proteins. The classic example of this type of reaction is seen in penicillin-allergic individuals.

In the majority of patients penicillin is coupled to protein via an amide bond, forming a penicilloyl protein derivative. In some patients penicillin couples by other means such as disulfide formation between penicillenic acid and cysteine or methionine. These derivatives, in susceptible individuals, are highly immunogenic. The great ability of penicillin to interact with protein most probably accounts for the large number of patients sensitive to penicillin or its semisynthetic derivatives. It is important to remember that in the case of penicillin the major offending agent is not penicillin itself but rather the penicilloyl moiety, which is generated by cleavage of the beta-lactam ring.

A significant percentage of individuals (15–18%) do not react to the penicilloyl moiety; rather, they react to a group of "minor determinants," the result of other types of penicillin-protein conjugations, which can be detected by skin testing using penicilloic acid or penicillin G itself. In these instances the exact immunogen is not known, and one relies on rapid conjugation of penicillin G or penicilloic acid to tissue proteins, which then interact with cell-bound IgE. It is important to remember that antibodies to penicillin are directed against the core of the molecule, i.e., the sulfur-containing thiozolidone (5-membered) and the beta-lactam (4-membered) rings. For this reason a patient sensitive to one penicillin should be considered sensitive to any penicillin derivative. Indeed, even the newer, highly modified semisynthetic penicillins and cephalosporins cannot be excluded, as evidenced by recent reports of allergic reactions to piperacillin and moxalactam. There are some rare exceptions to this rule. At Washington University we have seen three patients sensitive to carbenicillin but no other penicillin, but this is exceedingly unusual (also see below). In addition to penicillin, the cephalosporins are also potential problems: a small proportion of individuals produce a true anti-cephalosporin IgE. A much larger percentage, between 5 and 15% of penicillin-allergic patients, have an anti-penicillin IgE that crossreacts with cephalosporins. Thus, although some authors consider cephalosporins to be a suitable alternative in penicillin-sensitive individuals, we do not, and due care, such as provocative dose challenge (see below), must be taken when treating penicillin-sensitive individuals with cephalosporins.

Because the appropriate immunogens have been elucidated, patients with suspected penicillin allergy can be skin tested. Studies by our group, and others have shown that penicillin skin testing can determine with a high degree of confidence whether a patient is or is not at risk for a severe systemic reaction upon receiving the drug. Unfortunately only the major determinant is available commercially at present (penicilloyl-polylysine, Pre-Pen, Kremers Urban). This will still identify 85% or more of patients at risk for anaphylaxis to penicillins. We strongly recommend that skin testing be preformed in all patients with suspected penicillin allergy when penicillin or cephalosporins are the drug of choice. Moreover, as demonstrated by our group, it is possible to desensitize highly sensitive individuals with penicillin, using a protocol of increasing amounts of oral penicillin followed by parenteral penicillin and subsequent administration of the drug in full therapeutic doses. This procedure is of significant benefit and allows acutely ill patients who require penicillin for a life-threatening illness to be treated appropriately. In general, similar studies on desensitization have not been carried out with other drugs, with the exception of insulin, for which desensitization is also of great value.

In the case of penicillin the exact chemistry of the immunogen has been elegantly described. However, with the majority of drugs, the exact chemistry of the immunogen is largely unknown; although evidence would suggest that an IgE antibody directed against the drug is present. As a result, in contrast to penicillin, one must rely almost solely on the historical evaluation of the patient to determine that a drug-related immediate hypersensitivity reaction is present, since adequate skin test reagents are not available and simple skin testing with the drug in question may yield spurious results.

Recently, allergic sensitivity to trimethoprim-sulfamethoxazole (Bactrim/Septra) has become an increasing problem, particularly in patients with the acquired immune deficiency syndrome (AIDS) and other states in which immunity is compromised. This is most likely due to the widespread use of this combination as a prophylactic measure, particularly for pneumocystis. We have skin tested several of these patients and have seen positive skin reactivity at concentrations that do not cause a wheal and flare reaction in normal individuals. This suggests that this is a true IgE-mediated reaction. In addition we have desensitized two patients without difficulty, one to sulfonamide alone and the other to the combination drug. We do not, however, recommend this procedure at the present time, as adequate studies have not been performed to indicate the efficacy of the skin testing or the effectiveness of the oral desensitization procedure.

In instances in which one suspects, from historical evaluation, that the patient does have a true allergy two procedures are available. Obviously, the most logical is to find an alternative therapeutic modality. In the majority of instances it is possible to find an alternative noncrossreacting drug. If a noncrossreacting drug is unavailable or would not provide sufficient therapeutic benefit because of the severity of the patient's illness, a procedure similar to that which has been described for penicillin can be utilized. Begin with extremely small doses and administer increasingly larger amounts of the drug until therapeutic levels are obtained. The patient should be monitored closely for signs of allergic reactions and the protocol either modified or discontinued if these occur. We suggest that if possible the initial stages of the desensitization should be done orally to reduce the chance of a severe reaction.

When there is some degree of doubt as to the allergic nature of the patient's reaction, one can use the "provocative dose challenge" technique. In this technique a subtherapeutic dose of the drug is given, preferably by the oral route, and the patient is observed for allergic symptoms for 20 to 60 minutes. If no reaction occurs, a second and perhaps third and fourth challenge with increasingly larger doses can be given; if no adverse reaction occurs, the drug can be given in full therapeutic doses.

It is important to remember that these techniques, either progressive desensitization or provocative dose challenge, are designed merely to circumvent or prevent a severe systemic allergic reaction (anaphylaxis). They are not designed to prevent any allergic reaction at all, and once desensitized, patients are still capable of exhibiting mild allergic reactions, usually evidenced by generalized pruritus or hives. These patients should be maintained on the drug as long as is necessary and the minor allergic manifestations treated with an appropriate antihistamine in adequate doses. Once a patient with proven drug hypersensitivity has been adequately desensitized it is important that the drug be maintained for as long as is necessary. It is not clear at present how long the desensitized state remains. In some instances it may be as long as several days; on the other hand, it may be relatively short, on the order of 6 to 12 hours. In this case stopping therapy would necessitate reinstitution of the desensitization protocol, which could be difficult since the patients tend to be somewhat hyperreactive for a period of time after the desensitized state is lost.

In addition to inducing IgE-type antibodies, drugs are also capable of inducing IgG-type antibodies. In many instances IgG-type antibodies are relatively innocuous and neither effect the bioavailability of the drug nor cause any significant side reaction. For example, greater than 90% of patients who receive parenteral penicillin will develop IgG antipenicillin antibodies. This, however, does not mean that they will have any subsequent difficulties when penicillin therapy is reinstituted. On the other hand, IgG antibodies may lead to significant drug reactions. Several types of reactions have been recognized. All are the result of antibodies that are directed against the drug itself and haptenized on tissue proteins or antibodies that are directed against tissue proteins that are altered by interaction with the drug and are thus recognized as foreign. Drug-protein conjugates may interreact with antibody in the fluid phase, yielding significant amounts of antigen-antibody complexes. This then results in a serum sickness–like picture. In addition, if the complex is of the appropriate size, specific organs may be affected, for example, kidneys in drug-induced lupus erythematosus or Henoch-Schönlein purpura. In addition, drugs may be bound only to a specific organ, yielding diseases that are organ specific. Perhaps the best example of such a drug reaction is the production of antibodies that react with quinine (quinidine) bound to platelets, resulting in quinine-induced severe thrombocytopenia. Similarly drugs may bind to the liver, yielding a drug-induced hepatitis, or to a variety of other specific organs. Although these diseases may in many ways mimic autoimmune type phenomena, they are generally self-limited and respond well simply to removal of the drug. The use of corticosteroids in these types of drug reactions is controversial and in the majority of instances there is rapid clearing of drug and drug-protein conjugates by antibody, and the use of steroids neither hinders nor helps.

A variety of drugs are also associated with the development of cell-mediated immunity or delayed-type hypersensitivity. In this instance the drug-protein conjugate results in the production of "effector" or cytotoxic T cells. Delayed sensitivity has been associated with a large number of drugs. Whether given orally or parenterally or applied to the skin, the major organ affected is the skin. When the drug is applied locally, the classic picture is a pruritic papulopustular eruption limited to the areas of application. In cases of a systemic reaction the most common reaction is a generalized eczematoid dermatitis. Other forms include erythema multiforme and in rare cases erythema nodosum. Although many drugs have been implicated in Type IV reactions, in many instances actual proof has been lacking. Reapplication of a drug to the skin (patch testing) can be done to identify reactions; on the other hand, drugs given parenterally or orally may require more sophisticated studies, such as in vitro blast transformation. In this instance simple incubation of the drug with white cells in vitro may be inappropriate, since, as already discussed for Type I reactions, the true immunogen is a drug-protein conjugate. In the case of a "fixed drug eruption" (a skin reaction that occurs in the same limited area of the skin each time the drug is introduced) a serum factor has been described that transforms lymphocytes, suggesting that this is a Type IV reaction. Although patch testing or other laboratory studies can be performed in most instances, sophisticated laboratory studies are not necessary and sufficient information can be obtained from a careful history.

For all of the hypersensitivity states it is important to remember that immunogenicity or lack thereof, or the type of response that is stimulated, is related not only to the drug and its chemical properties but also to the route of administration. For example, many drugs are much less immunogenic when given orally than when given parenterally. A drug applied to the skin may induce a Type IV reaction while the same drug in oral or parenteral form may be relatively nonimmunogenic. A case in point is the antihistaminics, which are infrequent producers of hypersensitivity unless applied topically, when they commonly produce delayed hypersensitivity reactions. These considerations are not without practical benefit. Selection of the appropriate dosage form, avoiding those associated with the induction of hypersensitivity states, may help to prevent hypersensitivity reactions.

While by no means complete, the list of drug-related adverse effects presented here does indicate the broad diversity of such reactions. Drugs may have side effects that represent pharmacologic actions other than those that are actually desired. These toxic effects may occur at blood levels within the therapeutic range or at supratherapeutic blood levels or may be related to the cumulative dose given. The adverse reaction may be idiosyncratic in nature or may result from a hypersensitivity state. Hypersensitivity reactions of the anaphylactoid type may represent a pharmacological effect of the drug on an unknown enzyme system (e.g., aspirin), interaction with complement system, or direct action of the drug on the surface of the mast cell or basophil. In addition, those drugs capable of conjugating with tissue proteins may generate an immune response against the drug-protein complex. The immune response may be a

Type I anaphylactic-type reaction by production of specific IgE, a Type II or III response due to the production of IgG and subsequent formation of either antigen-antibody complexes or cytotoxic antibodies, or a Type IV cell-mediated response.

Finally, one must always remember that a single drug can be associated with all three types of adverse reactions noted above. And, it may be as critically important to differentiate the type of adverse reaction as to recognize the reaction itself. For example, thrombocytopenia may be seen with certain semisynthetic penicillins as a toxic effect or on an immunologic basis. Similarly, nephritis in patients treated with semisynthetic penicillins may be part of a serum sickness reaction or may be the interstitial nephritis associated with several semisynthetic penicillins; the most recently described being mezlocillin and piperacillin. The differentiation of immunologic from a nonimmunologic basis may allow the use of an alternative beta-lactam antibiotic in the latter case while an immunologically based reaction precludes further use of this class of antibiotic. Similar considerations are important for many other classes of drug. Thus, when possible, the type of adverse reaction—toxic, idiosyncratic or immunologic—should be determined.

It is imperative that the physician be aware of the broad diversity of adverse reactions to drugs that can occur. In the majority of cases a detailed drug history will be sufficient to alert the physician to the potential of an adverse reaction to a drug and this can then be handled either by use of an alternative therapeutic modality, by appropriate treatment of the patient to block the effects of mediator release, or by appropriate desensitization procedures. It is also important that the patient as well as the physician be apprised of the potential for side effects, the nature of these side effects, and the methods that will be utilized to decrease or circumvent them. In this way the problem of drug-related adverse reactions can be minimized, and when the occur, they can be treated appropriately. No drug is free of adverse effects and as long as physicians continue to utilize drug therapy adverse reactions will continue to be a major problem. This should not lead to therapeutic nihilism but rather to the utilization of measures to minimize or circumvent these reactions.

Physical Allergy

JOHN A. ANDERSON, M.D.

Physical factors, such as mechanical pressure, light, heat, cold, water, and exercise, may result in urticaria, angioedema, or systemic signs and symptoms usually associated with allergic reactions. As a group, these reactions are referred to as physical allergies. The exact incidence of physical factors resulting in "allergic" reactions in children is unknown, but urticaria caused by physical factors accounts for approximately 3% of all patients with urticaria and 10% of patients with chronic urticaria (mostly adults). Cold-induced urticaria followed by cholinergic urticaria is the most common physical urticaria seen in children.

The therapy used in physical allergy involves either avoidance of the physical agent or pharmacologic therapy designed to combat the effects of chemical mediators released by exposure to these agents.

GENERAL PRINCIPLES OF PHARMACOTHERAPY

Table 1 lists the antihistamines used for the treatment of physical allergy and the usual doses for children, beginning with the most commonly used drug. Table 2 lists the emergency and adjuvant drugs used in the treatment of these conditions.

The prime drug used in the emergency treatment of urticaria and angioedema is Adrenalin. In the usual case of urticaria/angioedema and exercise-induced anaphylaxis seen in the emergency situation, a systemically administered antihistamine, such as IM Benadryl, is also given. Follow-up treatment could include Sus-Phrine, a long-acting form of epinephrine (4–6 hours), and antihistamines to be taken at home, such as Benadryl, 25 mg three times daily, or Chlor-Trimeton, 4 to 8 mg three times daily.

For prophylactic treatment of any of the physical urticaria/angioedema conditions or exercise-induced anaphylaxis, the use of a single antihistamine listed in Table 1 might be tried, but hydroxyzine (Atarax) usually is most effective. Because Benadryl and Atarax are likely to produce drowsiness, other antihistamines, such as either the chlorpheniramines or brompheniramines, might be tried. Cyproheptadine (Periactin) is most efficacious in the treatment of cold urticaria. In resistant cases of cold urticaria/angioedema, various combinations of antihistamines might be tried, including Benadryl, Atarax, or Chlor-Trimeton during the day, plus Phenergan or PBZ at night. Azatadine (Optimine*) and clemastine fumarate (Tavist†), and terfenadine (Seldane‡) are newer, longer-acting antihistamines usually used for the treatment of allergic rhinitis. Terfenadine has the least effect on the central nervous system. How-

---

* Manufacturer's Precaution: Clinical experience in children is limited. Drug cannot be recommended below age 16 years.
† Manufacturer's Precaution: Safety and efficacy in children have not been established.
‡ Manufacturer's Precaution: Not recommended for children below the age of 12 years.

Table 1. ANTIHISTAMINES FOR TREATMENT OF PHYSICAL ALLERGY

Antihistamine Class (*Histamine Receptor*)	Drug (*Trade Name*)	Usual Dose, 27-KG Child (*Dose by Weight*)
Ethanolamine (H-1)	Diphenhydramine (Benadryl) (more sedative)	12.5–50 mg 3 × daily (5 mg/kg/24 hr—not to exceed 300 mg/24 hr)
Ataractic (H-1)	Hydroxyzine (Atarax, Vistaril) (more sedative)	10–25 mg 3 × daily
Alkylamine (H-1)	1. Chlorpheniramine (Chlor-Trimeton, Teldrin) 2. Brompheniramine (Dimetane) (less sedative)	2–8 mg 3 × daily
Piperidine (H-1)	1. Cyproheptadine (Periactin)	2–4 mg 3–4 × daily (0.25 mg/kg/24 hr)
	2. Azatadine (Optimine)	1–2 mg 2 × daily; not recommended under 12 yr of age
Phenothiazine (H-1)	Promethazine (Phenergan)	6.25–12.5 mg 3 × daily
Ethylenediamine (H-1)	Tripelennamine (PBZ)	25–50 mg 3 × daily (5 mg/kg/24 hr—not to exceed 300 mg/24 hr)
Benzhydryl ether (H-1)	Clemastine fumarate (Tavist)	1.34 mg 2 × daily; not recommended under 12 yr of age
Piperidinebutanol (H-1)	Terfenadine (Seldane) (less sedative)	60 mg 2 × daily for 12 yr of age or older; not recommended below this age
Thioguanidine (H-2)	Cimetidine (Tagamet)	20–40 mg/kg/24 hr; very limited experience in children under 16 yr of age
Ethenediamine (H-2)	Ranitidine (Zantac)	Dosage not established in children; see manufacturer's recommendations
Ataractics (H-1, H-2?)	Doxepin (Sinequan)	10–25 mg 2 × daily for 12 yr of age or older as a single drug; not to exceed 75 mg/24 hr; not recommended below this age

Table 2. EMERGENCY AND ADJUVANT DRUGS FOR TREATMENT OF PHYSICAL ALLERGY

Drug Type	Drug (*Trade Name*)	Usual Children's Dosage
Sympathomimetics and Beta Agonists	Epinephrine HCL 1:1000 (Adrenalin)	0.1–0.3 ml/dose subQ (0.005–0.01 ml/kg/dose)
	Epinephrine 1:200 in thioglycolate (Sus-Phrine)	0.05–0.15 ml/dose subQ (0.005 ml/kg/dose)
	Epinephrine HCL 1:1000 (Adrenalin) in Ana-Kit (Hollister-Stier Labs.)	0.3 ml/dose; 2 doses possible
	Epinephrine HCL 1:1000 (Adrenalin) in Epi-Pen and Epi-Pen Jr. (Center Labs.)	0.3 ml and 0.15 ml (Epi-Pen and Epi-Pen Jr., respectively) in automatic doser
	Metaproterenol (Alupent, Metaprel)	1–3 puffs by inhalation; not recommended under 12 yr of age
	Terbutaline (Bricanyl, Brethine)	2.5–5.0 mg 3 × daily; not recommended under 12 yr of age
	Albuterol (Proventil, Ventoline)	1–2 puffs by inhalation 3 × daily or 2–4 mg 3 × daily; not recommended under 12 yr of age
Methylxanthine	Theophylline (Slo-Phyllin 60, 125, 250 mg) (Theo-Dur 100, 200, 300 mg)	Therapeutic blood levels, 10–20 µg/ml
Corticosteroid	Prednisone (Prednisone 5 mg)	As needed
Other	Cromolyn Sodium (Intal)	20-mg powder by inhalation per dose; not recommended under 5 yr of age

ever, in some cases of pruritus-urticaria/angioedema, these drugs might be tried if other antihistamines have failed to control the condition.

Recently, there have been reports of successful use of the combination of an H-2 histamine receptor drug, cimetidine (Tagamet*) or ranitidine (Zantac*), with one of the H-1 antihistamines, such as hydroxyzine, in the treatment of chronic urticaria. Experience has shown the effect to be variable among patients. In some resistant cases of chronic urticaria, doxepin (Sinequan†), which has been shown to exhibit some H-2 and H-2 antihistamine-like activity, has been used as a single drug. The experience in children is limited, and any drug trial should be cautious in nature.

In addition, terbutaline (Bricanyl) and theophylline compounds have been shown to decrease histamine release in hypersensitivity states. Both drugs decreased chronic urticaria/angioedema in some studies, in spite of the fact that neither drug has been shown to significantly alter the antigen-induced immediate-reacting skin test. From experience, we have found that some resistant cases of chronic urticaria/angioedema (physically induced or idiopathic) respond to the addition of either terbutaline† (2.5 mg three times a day) or a theophylline compound (enough Slo-Phyllin given three times a day to maintain a theophylline level between 10 and 20 µg/ml) to one of the single or multiple antihistamine regimens.

Corticosteroids may be used in the treatment of severe emergency urticaria/angioedema or anaphylaxis. These drugs may be helpful on a short-term basis for exacerbation of the problem but are not a substitute for the antihistamines. Corticosteroids have not been helpful on a long-term basis in the routine treatment of physical allergies.

SPECIFIC THERAPY

Dermographia. Treatment of dermographia consists of avoiding trauma and, when necessary, the use of an antihistamine. Hydroxyzine (Atarax) is the most likely drug to be helpful in this condition (on an as-needed basis), although other antihistamines and drug combinations may be tried.

Pressure Urticaria/Angioedema. Treatment consists of avoiding sustained pressures as much as possible. Antihistamines, and even corticosteroids, can be tried but are usually not helpful.

Vibratory Angioedema. Treatment consists of avoiding vibrating stimuli. Usually the condition is mild and does not require medications. However, prophylactic antihistamines and corticosteroids

have been used successfully—in one case—in which the condition was serious and avoidance was not possible (e.g., dental work).

Urticaria/Angioedema Secondary to Light Exposure. Drug ingestion combined with sunlight exposure may result in either a direct toxic rash (phototoxic reaction) or an immunologic contact dermatitis (photoallergic reaction). Drugs implicated in causing a phototoxic reaction include psoralens, topical coal tar, and dimethylchlortetracycline. Drugs implicated in photoallergic reactions include phenothiazines, sulfonamides, and griseofulvin. Bacteriostatic agents like bithionol and halogenated salicylamides, used in soaps and topical medications, can also induce reactions.

Light can also produce sunburn and exacerbate primary dermatologic and systemic diseases, including the polymorphic light eruption and systemic lupus erythematosus.

Management of this condition is often difficult and consists primarily of avoiding the reaction-producing light wavelength. In the case of drug sensitivity, the treatment consists of correctly identifying and then avoiding the causative drug or chemical.

Repeated exposure to small, increasing doses of sunlight may induce tolerance in some patients. It is advisable to wear protective garments whenever possible. Sunscreens or sun-blocking agents can be used to help protect skin exposed to sun in susceptible individuals.

Chemical sunscreens act by absorbing a specific portion of the ultraviolet light spectrum. Chemical sunscreens include agents such as para-aminobenzoic acid (PABA), esters of PABA, the benzophenones, digalloyl trioleate, the cinnamates, the anthranilates, the pyrones, and the salicylates. For an agent to be effective, it must have the ability to absorb ultraviolet light in the 290- to 320-nm range—the range at which virtually all sunburns occur. Five per cent PABA in 50 to 70% ethanol provides an excellent protection against sunburn. The benzophenones, unlike the other sunscreens, also absorb long-wave ultraviolet light in the 320- to 400-nm range.

Recently, criteria for sun protection have been established. Sun protective factors (SPF)—the ratio of the amount of exposure necessary to produce a minimal erythematous response with a sunscreen in place divided by the amount of exposure needed to produce the same reaction without the sunscreen—now serves as a measure of the sunscreen's protection. Any commercial sunscreen with an SPF value of 15 should be an excellent protective agent. Examples include Pre-Sun 15, Pabanol, Supershade 15, Total Eclipse, Sundown 15, Ti Screen, and Piz Buin 8.

Sensitivity to wavelengths of light above 320 nanometers may be avoided by the use of physical

---

* Manufacturer's Precaution: Safety and efficacy in children have not been established.

† Manufacturer's Precaution: Not recommended for use in children under 12 years of age.

sunscreens or sun-blocking agents, even though they are less cosmetically acceptable than the chemical sunscreens. Some available agents include zinc oxide paste (RVPaque), titanium dioxide (A-Fil Cream or Solar Cream), and red veterinary petrolatum (RVP Cream or RV Plus).

The 280- to 320-nm UV light (sunburn range) is filtered by window glass. The higher wavelengths, which can still produce light sensitivity in some patients, are not filtered by ordinary glass.

Antihistamines and corticosteroids given orally may reduce the reactions to light. Although the antimalarial drug chloroquine has been used in resistant cases of light sensitivity, the results are disappointing.

Cholinergic Urticaria. "Keeping cool" is a good rule when one is considering the management of cholinergic urticaria. Antihistamines are usually helpful, beginning with hydroxyzine (Atarax) or diphenhydramine (Benadryl), and progressing to combination therapies. A trial on anticholinergic medications has been advised, but this type of treatment has not been helpful in this condition in our experience.

Another method, that of deliberately producing the rash (such as taking a warm shower) in order to produce a short refractory period, is also not a helpful treatment method in our opinion.

Localized Heat Urticaria. This rare disorder can be confirmed by placing a carefully heated Erlenmeyer flask of water on an area of skin. The hive reaction usually occurs within minutes. Antihistamines have been reported to block the heat challenge.

Cold-Induced Urticaria/Angioedema. The mainstay of treatment in cold-induced conditions is to avoid chilling the body. During the summer, one should be careful about sudden changes in temperature, especially swimming in cold water. During the winter, one should be certain to wear good gloves and warm footgear since the skin of the extremities is already at a lower ambient temperature. A hat is important since the head is a major source of heat loss from the body. A mask can be helpful for protecting the exposed area of the face.

In one study, cyproheptadine (Periactin) was the superior antihistamine in preventing cold reactions, but hydroxyzine (Atarax) and other antihistamines and antihistamine-theophylline or -terbutaline combinations should be tried in stubborn cases.

Gradual "desensitization" to cold by taking serial baths with increasingly cold water has been advocated as a therapy for this condition. In our opinion, the therapy is generally unsuccessful.

Exercise- and Cold-Induced Asthma. Most children with asthma have some degree of bronchoconstriction when they exercise; in some asthmatics, exercise is the major reason for wheezing. Children may also wheeze when exposed to cold air. Running is the exercise most likely to produce wheezing, and swimming is the exercise least likely to do so. The therapy in exercise-induced asthma involves avoidance of that type of exercise and the degree of exercise that produces significant difficulty—when possible. To restrict otherwise normal children, however, from all exercise, especially running, is not practical in our society.

In some cases, children can "run through" their exercise-induced asthma. Breathing through the nose rather than the mouth while exercising, thus allowing the inhaled air to become properly heated and humidified, reduces exercise-induced asthma. Recently, the use of an inexpensive, disposable, hard-paper surgical mask that fits over the nose and mouth has been found to reduce exercise-induced asthma significantly. The mask works by allowing the patient to "rebreathe" a reservoir of warm, humidified air when exercising.

Medication also can be used to reduce or prevent an exercise-induced asthma (Table 2). Cromolyn sodium* (Intal) by inhalation one half hour before exercise provides significant help in 60% of children up to 2 to 4 hours. Sympathomimetics and beta-agonists taken immediately before exercising, such as albuterol (Proventil, Ventolin), terbutaline (Bricanyl, Brethine), and metaproterenol† (Alupent, Metaprel), are most efficacious in reducing the incidence of exercise-induced asthma, but there are some potential cardiovascular side effects with these drugs, as opposed to essentially no side effects with cromolyn sodium. Oral sympathomimetic agents and oral theophylline agents are helpful but not as efficacious as metaproterenol, albuterol, or cromolyn sodium. Inhaled atropine-like compounds are helpful in this condition in about one third of the cases.

The treatment of cold-induced asthma is similar to that of exercise-induced asthma.

Exercise-Induced Anaphylaxis. Recently, a group of young adults have been described who develop symptoms of anaphylaxis, including pruritus, generalized urticaria, angioedema, nasal stuffiness, and, on occasion, abdominal colic, dizziness, and collapse while exercising, particularly jogging. These patients were found not to have exercise-induced asthma or cholinergic urticaria. The mechanism of action in this condition is not clear, although some patients are atopic and may be experiencing increased exposure during jogging to environmental allergens, such as pollen. Case

---

* Cromolyn sodium is not recommended for children under 5 years of age.

† Inhalation form is not recommended for children under 5 years of age.

reports have also described patients who only have anaphylaxis after exercising following a meal of shrimp or celery or—in one patient—following any meal.

The therapy for this condition involves the avoidance of strenuous exercises like jogging. In some instances, this is not acceptable to the patient. The use of antihistamines, such as hydroxyzine (Atarax), or other drug combinations prior to exercise may be helpful. On an emergency basis, Adrenalin is the prime mode of therapy for anaphylaxis. Since some patients may have a history of a potential life-threatening episode of exercise-induced anaphylaxis and may refuse to discontinue the practice of strenuous exercise, they should be supplied with Adrenalin in a loaded syringe and taught to use this drug in an emergency situation. Ana-Kit (supplied primarily for patients allergic to stinging insects) contains such a conveniently loaded syringe of Adrenalin. The dose may be varied but usually is 0.3 ml, which is suitable for an older teenager and adult but not a young child. An automatically administered Adrenalin device that will penetrate clothing (i.e., of the thigh) is also available (Epi-Pen and Epi-Pen Jr.). The doses are fixed at 0.3 ml and 0.15 ml respectively and are suitable for different age children. See Table 2 for recommended pediatric doses of epinephrine.

Anaphylaxis

IRVING W. BAILIT, M.D.

Anaphylaxis is the most frightening and potentially life-threatening allergic reaction in man. Clinical manifestations usually appear in 1 to 30 minutes. The rapidity of the reaction is directly related to its intensity. Deaths result from acute laryngeal edema, acute pulmonary emphysema, and cardiovascular collapse. Manifestations may affect different organ systems, which include skin (urticaria, angioedema), respiratory (acute wheezing, laryngeal stridor), cardiovascular (hypotension, shock), gastrointestinal (cramps, vomiting, diarrhea), and central nervous (seizures, loss of consciousness).

Atopic persons are more susceptible to anaphylaxis. Deaths are less common in children and are mostly caused by laryngeal edema. Classic anaphylaxis is the result of IgE mediated release of chemical mediators (histamine, leukotrienes, ECF-A, kinins, and prostaglandins) in previously sensitized individuals. Anaphylactoid reactions are similar nonimmunologic responses resulting from direct release of mediators from tissue mast cells and basophils.

Numerous diverse agents can trigger anaphylactic reactions. The most common are drugs, especially penicillin and aspirin, and the stinging insects (yellow jacket, honeybee, hornet, wasp, and fire ant). Foods most likely to provoke an immediate allergic reaction include nuts, milk, egg, fish, shellfish, legumes, berries, and seeds. Radiographic contrast media will cause anaphylactoid reactions in 1 to 2% of those tested. Other causes are hormones, antisera, enzymes, exercise, and immunotherapy for venoms and environmental allergens.

TREATMENT

Anaphylactic reactions are sudden in onset and require immediate treatment. All medical personnel should be trained in the proper management of such reactions and have the needed medication and equipment readily available. They should also be trained in basic cardiopulmonary resuscitation. Initial management should be started in the office. Severe, unresponsive patients should be transferred to hospital intensive care units when transfer is feasible.

The most important drug is aqueous epinephrine (Adrenalin), 1:1000 (0.01 ml/kg). The usual pediatric dose is 0.3 ml (range 0.1–0.5 ml) given subcutaneously for mild reactions and intramuscularly for moderate reactions. Dose may be repeated three times at 15 to 20-minute intervals. Blood pressure should be monitored. In cases of cardiovascular collapse, epinephrine dose may be diluted in 10 ml of saline and given slowly over several minutes by intravenous injection.

If the antigen is introduced by an injection or sting on an extremity, apply a tourniquet proximal to the site and inject epinephrine 1:1000 (0.1–0.2 ml) subcutaneously at the injection/sting site to prevent antigen absorption.

Follow epinephrine therapy with diphenhydramine (Benadryl) given orally or IM (25–50 mg). Severe reactions should be treated intravenously (2 mg/kg) up to 50 mg per dose over 3 minutes. Continue this drug orally for 48 hours (5 mg/kg/24 hours).

In the presence of acute wheezing, administer aminophylline (5–7 mg/kg) in IV solution slowly over a 20-minute period. If necessary maintain by constant infusion (0.6–1.0 mg/kg/hr) and monitor theophylline levels.

Hypotensive patients should be placed in a recumbent position with the lower extremities elevated. Give IV normal saline rapidly (2000–3000 ml/m²/24 hrs). Use volume expanders for hypovolemia. If IV saline and epinephrine do not maintain adequate blood pressure, use vasopressor drugs.

1. Metaraminol bitartrate (Aramine): Give 0.4 mg/kg in 500 ml of 5% D/W or saline slowly while monitoring the rate of infusion with the blood

pressure response and possible cardiac arrhythmias.

2. Levarterenol bitartrate (Levophed) may be used as an alternative drug. Add 4 mg (4 ml) to 1000 ml of 5% D/W at a rate of 1 to 2 ml/min while monitoring the blood pressure. In children give 1 mg (1 ml) in 250 ml of 5% D/W at 0.5 ml/min.

Corticosteroids may be useful for control of persistent or recurrent symptoms. Since these drugs take up to several hours for significant effect they are not first line therapy for the acute episode. Start with 7 mg/kg of hydrocortisone (Solu-Cortef), 100 to 300 mg, followed by 7 ml/kg/24 hr at 4- to 6-hour intervals. Methylprednisolone (Solu-Medrol), 2 mg/kg/stat and 2 mg/kg/24 hr may also be used. Milder reactions can be treated with oral steroids.

Monitor vital signs and maintain a patent oral airway. Oxygen should be available and administered when there is evidence of hypoxia. In the presence of laryngeal edema a cricothyrotomy tube or a large (#12 or #14) needle should be available to establish a temporary airway until facilities and personnel are available to insert an endotracheal tube or perform a tracheostomy.

Measurement of central venous pressure and arterial blood gases, and electrocardiogram may be necessary for optimum management.

In addition to the above medications, necessary equipment includes a tourniquet, needles and syringes, parenteral fluids with intravenous tubing, oral airway, suction bulb, Ambu bag, and a cricothyrotomy tube or large needle (#12 or #14).

PREVENTION

Many anaphylactic reactions can be prevented by taking a comprehensive history of previous reactions to drugs, foods, immunizations, insect stings, and diagnostic agents. Avoid when possible drugs that have caused previous allergic responses.

A history of penicillin sensitivity is an indication to avoid penicillin and its analogs and the cephalothins to which they may cross react. Testing for reaction to penicillin using both the major and minor antigen determinants is a reliable method of determining the presence of penicillin hypersensitivity. Avoid penicillin positive skin test reactors and give penicillin orally in preference to parenteral administration. For life-threatening situations requiring penicillin (i.e., subacute bacterial endocarditis) in proven penicillin-sensitive patients, consider the newer methods of oral desensitization.

Remember that allergic children are more likely to develop hypersensitivity to foods, drugs, and radiocontrast agents. Questionable food reactions may be skin tested by the scratch or prick method or by RAST testing. While many foods are tolerated with increasing age, some food anaphylaxis (nuts and fish) may persist for a lifetime.

Patients with previous anaphylactoid reactions to radiocontrast media in whom repeat study is mandatory should be pretreated with prednisone 50 mg orally every 6 hours for three doses prior to study and diphenhydramine (Benadryl) 50 mg IM 1 hr before the procedure.

Children who have had serious anaphylactic reactions to stinging insects and positive venom skin tests should be given protective immunotherapy to the offending venoms.

Known egg-sensitive children should be tested for reaction to vaccines grown from chick embryo tissue prior to administration of the vaccine.

Physicians who administer programs of immunotherapy for venoms or inhalant allergens must be prepared to treat systemic reactions. Local reactions can be used as a guideline in determining antigen dose. Seasonal allergens should be decreased during the active pollen season. Observe patients for at least 20 minutes after injection.

Children with a history of an anaphylactic reaction should have an emergency kit containing a loaded epinephrine syringe (AnaKit, EpiPen). Patient or parent must be instructed on the indications and technique for its use. A bracelet that identifies the patient and his hypersensitivity reaction may prove useful (MedicAlert Foundation, Turlock, California).

20

Accidents and Emergencies

Botulinal Food Poisoning

BARRY H. RUMACK, M.D.

Botulism is most frequently due to improperly home-processed foods such as vegetables, meats, fruits, pickles, and seafood. Rarely, commercial products are involved and recently these have been fish and meat products, especially in soups. Simple cooking for 6 to 10 minutes is capable of destroying the formed toxin.

Treatment. Empty the stomach, being careful to protect the airway. Administer activated charcoal and a cathartic. Hospitalize if there are *any* symptoms (paralysis, ptosis, blurred vision, diplopia, sore throat, other). Administration of antitoxin should be done under the supervision of the Centers for Disease Control or state health department. Guanidine therapy has been used in some cases, as has penicillin. The value of either of these drugs is questionable. Treatment consists primarily of antitoxin and respiratory support. Patients with minimal findings, usually mild neurologic, that do not progress will not require therapy. Treatment for the supportive and other needs of the patient is similar to treatment of any serious neurologic problem. Recovery is the rule with modern therapy.

Acute Poisoning

BARRY H. RUMACK, M.D.

The epidemiology of poisonings has been difficult to determine until recently because of previous poor case finding. The Rocky Mountain Poison Center, for example, reported 7545 cases in 1972 and 73,700 cases in 1982. This increase is well above the increase in population in the region served over this time and is probably due to increased visibility of the poison center and better case finding. Mortality had been reported at 1 or 2 cases a year since the poison center was opened in 1956 and jumped rapidly with modern data-collecting methods. A decline in mortality rate over the past 5 years is due to a number of factors, including advent of container closure safety laws; tremendous improvement in quality and availability of emergency physicians; earlier awareness of potential toxicity by parents and relatives; and rapidly available, high quality information concerning poison treatment. The American Association of Poison Control Centers reported over 251,000 cases in 1983 and about 750,000 cases in 1984.

Categories in which cases occur are presented in Table 1. The percentages have been rounded off and undoubtedly vary somewhat from community to community. Local poison centers should be consulted for area statistics and specific local problems.

While there are many poison prevention activities, one of the most effective is distribution of a poison checklist and a discussion of the problem by the pediatrician, nurse practitioner, or health associate at the 6-month checkup. Giving the mother a bottle of syrup of ipecac is probably the only way to make sure it actually will get into a home. Table 2 provides the checklist, which should be reproduced and distributed to parents.

MANAGEMENT OF THE INITIAL EVENT
Telephone

Most cases will initially come to attention over the telephone. If the parent or patient calls the physician rather than a poison information center,

Table 1. FORMS OF POISONING

	Per Cent
Drugs—Miscellaneous	15.4
Life Forms and Products	13.5
Central Nervous System Drugs	11.9
Household Products	11.8
CNS Drugs—Analgesics	9.5
Personal Products	8.4
Pesticides	6.3
Petroleum Products	5.7
Over-the-Counter Drugs	5.2
Dietary Supplements	2.8
Autonomic Drugs	1.9
Antiseptics	1.6
Local-Acting Agents	1.6
Gastrointestinal Products	1.5
Antimicrobials	1.1
Hormones	1.0
Cardiovascular Drugs	0.9

Table 2. CHECK LIST FOR POISON-PROOFING THE HOME

KITCHEN	☐ No household products under the sink ☐ No medicines on counters or open areas, refrigerator top, or window sills ☐ All cleaners, household products, and medications out of reach ☐ All cleaners, household products, and medications in original, safety top containers
BATHROOM	☐ Medicine chest cleaned out regularly ☐ Old medications flushed down toilet ☐ All medicines in original safety top containers ☐ All medicines, sprays, powders, cosmetics, fingernail preparations, hair care products, mouthwash, and so on out of reach
BEDROOM	☐ No medicines in or on dresser or bedside table ☐ All perfumes, cosmetics, powders, and sachets out of reach
LAUNDRY AREA	☐ All bleaches, soaps, detergents, fabric softeners, bluing agents, and sprays out of reach ☐ All products in original containers
GARAGE, BASEMENT	☐ Insect spray and weed killers in locked area ☐ Gasoline and car products in locked area ☐ Turpentine, paints, and paint products in locked area ☐ All in original containers
GENERAL HOUSEHOLD	☐ Alcoholic beverages out of reach ☐ Ashtrays empty and out of reach ☐ Plants out of reach ☐ Painted surfaces in good repair ☐ All household and personal products out of reach

certain factors become imperative for providing quality care.

History Records. All poison calls must be noted, with time, name, address, phone number, substance, and amount ingested. Any advice provided should be written down. Some patients will become hysterical or comatose on the phone and will require the dispatch of emergency equipment. Follow-up calls may be necessary to change initial advice. In fact, it is considered inappropriate to manage a patient over the telephone without calling back at intervals (usually 1, 2, 4, and 24 hours) to make sure instructions have been followed and patients are responding appropriately.

Severity. Determination of the degree of the problem is important in order to make recommendations for care. No Danger—e.g., a patient who has eaten a crayon or sucked on a ball point pen. Potential Danger—e.g., a patient who has consumed a bottle of adult aspirins. Clearly the patient will have to be seen within a short time; the decision to be made is whether this should be at the office or hospital. Immediate Danger—e.g., a child who has ingested some strychnine-base rat poison. An emergency vehicle should usually be sent to the scene, since it will have trained personnel, suction, and medications.

Prevention of Absorption

Eye. Rapid dilution with copious quantities of water is imperative. Any source of clean water should be used as gently as possible after an episode. A common error is to communicate to patients that they should go immediately to the emergency department. This should be done *after* initial dilution.

Skin. Many agents, such as organophosphate insecticides, are absorbed well through the skin. Warm soapy water with a soft cloth or sponge should be used to cleanse the skin following any chemical contact. Many patients have developed delayed symptoms because contaminated clothing was left in place. Medical personnel who come in contact with these chemicals also should clean off affected areas so they do not become patients.

Oral. The use of dilution should be reserved for the times and chemicals when a lowered concentration of the substance would decrease toxicity. Medication, for example, should not be diluted, since this might serve to enhance absorption. Water or milk is the safest agent for use. The use of dilution in such situations as caustic ingestion is particularly important within 30 seconds after ingestion if burns are to be prevented.

Emesis. Syrup of ipecac in appropriate doses (30 ml for adult dose; 10 to 15 ml for pediatric dose) has been shown to be a safe and effective means of producing emesis. While apomorphine has a more rapid onset of action than ipecac syrup has, the average percentage of recovery is the same. Apomorphine is notoriously toxic in children because of its narcotic depressant effects, which may persist past the reversal effects of naloxone administered to counteract the toxicity of this emetic. In addition, apomorphine may result in protracted vomiting, which is often unresponsive to narcotic antagonist intervention. Emesis 60 minutes after ingestion produces recovery of 30 per cent of gastric contents.

Emesis is generally contraindicated when the patient is comatose, convulsing, or without the gag reflex. Strong acid or base ingestion is another reason for not inducing emesis since this will reexpose the patient's esophagus to these agents, thus contributing to further damage.

Lavage. Gastric lavage with a large-bore tube is a rapid and effective way to empty the stomach. While there has been criticism in the past of this technique, most comparative studies were performed with ipecac emesis and a small-bore (No. 16 French) lavage tube. Proper lavage with large (No. 36 to 40 French) tubes utilizing 10 to 20 liters of warm tap water in an adult or 5 to 10 liters of warm saline in a child is the method of choice to empty the stomach if a contraindication to emesis exists, if the patient is symptomatic, or if an adult has ingested an unusually large or toxic amount of agent.

Cathartics. The rationale for the administration of cathartics in the poisoned patient is to hasten the toxin through the gastrointestinal tract to minimize its absorption. Although no controlled data are available for the use of cathartic agents, they are indicated in several situations: ingestion of enteric-coated tablets, when the lag time following ingestion is greater than 1 hour, and with hydrocarbons. Preferred agents are the saline cathartics (sodium sulfate, magnesium sulfate, citrate, or phosphates), which have a relatively prompt onset of action and lower toxicity than the oil-based cathartics, which have attendant aspiration risks.

Charcoal. It has been demonstrated that sufficient quantities of charcoal will bind many toxins that have not been removed by emesis or lavage. Charcoal can "catch up" with drugs and other agents once they have passed through the pylorus. Ample evidence shows that administration of charcoal following methods to empty the stomach will result in lower plasma levels than if emesis or lavage alone is used. Concomitant administration of activated charcoal with syrup of ipecac renders the ipecac ineffective. Hence, charcoal should not be administered until after emesis has occurred.

Enhancement of Excretion

Urinary excretion of a few toxins can be hastened by forced alkaline diuresis or by dialysis (hemodialysis or peritoneal dialysis).

Diuresis. Forced diuresis is rarely useful in serious poisonings if the drug is excreted in the urine in active form. The technique should not be used unless it is specifically indicated, as it may increase the likelihood of cerebral edema, a common cause of death in poisonings. Acid diuresis has been largely abandoned due to exacerbation of associated renal problems related to rhabdomyolysis. Some new evidence indicates that with salicylates urine pH is more important than urine flow.

Excretion of the following can be hastened by forced diuresis: jequirity beans (alkaline diuresis), phenobarbital (alkaline diuresis), and salicylates (alkaline diuresis). Hypertonic or pharmacologic diuretics should be given, along with adequate fluids. The usual urine flow is 0.5 to 2 ml/kg/hr; with forced diuresis, urine flow should increase to 3 to 6 ml/kg/hr. Alkaline diuresis should be chosen on the basis of the pK_a of the toxin, so that ionized drug will be trapped in the tubular lumen and not reabsorbed. (See Table 3.) Thus, if the pK_a is less than 7.0, alkaline diuresis is appropriate. Osmotic load is also important, and either type of diuretic should be given at intervals.

Alkaline Diuresis. This can usually be accomplished with bicarbonate. It is well to observe for potassium depletion, in which case it is necessary to administer potassium chloride or potassium citrate, which has both potassium and considerable alkalinizing ability. It is also available orally as K-Lyte effervescent tablets ("fizzies"), which are a quite palatable form. Follow serum K^+ deficiency carefully.

Dialysis. Hemodialysis (or peritoneal dialysis if hemodialysis is unavailable) is useful in the poisonings listed below. Dialysis should be considered part of supportive care if the patient satisfies any of the following criteria:

1. Clinical criteria
   a. Stage 3 or 4 coma or hyperactivity caused by a dialyzable drug that cannot be treated by conservative means.
   b. Hypotension threatening renal or hepatic function that cannot be corrected by adjusting circulating volume.
   c. Apnea in a patient who cannot be ventilated.
   d. Marked hyperosmolality that is not due to easily corrected fluid problems.
   e. Severe acid-base disturbance not responding to therapy.
   f. Severe electrolyte disturbance not responding to therapy.
   g. Marked hypothermia or hyperthermia.
2. Immediate dialysis may be considered in ethylene glycol and methanol poisoning only if acidosis is refractory and blood levels of methanol of 100 mg/dl are consistently maintained.
3. Dialysis is indicated on basis of condition of

Table 3.   TOXICOKINETIC DATA OF DRUGS AND TOXINS (NUMBERS EXPRESSED AS A MEAN OR AS A RANGE)

Agent	pK$_a$	Vd (1/kg)	Ther. T$\frac{1}{2}$ (hrs)	O.D. T$\frac{1}{2}$ (hrs)	Diuresis	Dialysis	Specific Therapy
Acetaminophen	9.5	0.75	2	4	No	No	N-Acetylcysteine
Amitriptyline	9.4	40+	36	72	No	No	Physostigmine
Amobarbital	7.9	2.4	16	36+	No	No	
Amphetamine	9.8	0.60	8–12	18–24	No	Yes	Chlorpromazine/ Diazepam
Bromide	—	40+	300	300	Yes	Yes	
Caffeine	13	0.75	3.5	4–120	No	No	
Chloral hydrate	—	0.75	8	10–18	No	No	
Chlorpromazine	9.3	40+	16–24	24–36	No	No	
Codeine	8.2	3	2	2	No	No	Naloxone
Coumadin	5.7	0.1	36–48	36–48	No	No	Vitamin K
Desipramine	10.2	50+	18	72	No	No	Physostigmine
Diazepam	3.3	1–2	36–72	48–144	No	No	
Digoxin	—	7–10	36	13	No	No	
Diphenhydramine	8.3	—	4–6	4–8	No	No	Physostigmine
Ethanol	—	0.6	2–4	—	No	No	
Ethchlorvynol	8.7	3–4	1–2	36–48	No	No	
Glutethimide	4.5	20–25	8–12	24+	No	No	
Isoniazid	3.5	0.60	2–4	6+	Alkaline	Yes	
Methadone	8.3	6–10	12–18	12–18	No	No	Naloxone
Methicillin	2.8	0.60	2–4	2–4	Yes	Yes	
Pentobarbital	8.11	2.0	10–20	50+	No	No	
Phencyclidine	8.5	—	—	12–48	No	Yes	
Phenobarbital	7.4	0.75	36–48	72–120	Alkaline	Yes	
Phenytoin	8.3	0.60	24–30	36–72	No	No	
Quinidine	4.3, 8.4	3	7–8	10	No	No	
Salicylate	3.2	0.1–0.3	2–4	25–30	Alkaline	Yes	
Tetracycline	7.7	3	6–10	6–10	No	No	
Theophylline	0.7	0.46	4.5	6+	No	Yes	

patient—in general, dialyze if patient is in a coma deeper than level 3 or has other major toxicity unresponsive to standard care.

Ammonia	Iodides
Amphetamines	Isoniazid
Anilines	Meprobamate
Antibiotics	Paraldehyde
Barbiturates (long-acting)	Potassium
Boric acid	Quinidine
Bromides	Quinine
Calcium	Salicylates
Chloral hydrate	Strychnine
Fluorides	Theophylline
	Thiocyanates

(Other drugs may be dialyzable, but the information should be verified prior to institution of dialysis therapy.)

4. Dialysis not indicated except for support—therapy consists of intensive care.

Antidepressants (tricyclics and MAO inhibitors also)	Heroin and other opiates
Antihistamines	Methaqualone (Quaalude)
Barbiturates (short-acting)	Methyprylon (Noludar)
Chlordiazepoxide (Librium)	Oxazepam (Serax)
	Phenothiazines
Diazepam (Valium)	Phenytoin (Dilantin)
Digitalis and related drugs	Synthetic anticholinergics and belladonna compounds
Diphenoxylate with atropine (Lomotil)	

While the long-acting barbiturates (cleared by the kidneys) are more readily dialyzable than the short-acting ones (cleared by the liver), dialysis may be helpful if the patient satisfies criteria for supportive dialysis needs as outlined above. Salicylate poisoning generally responds very well to intensive alkaline diuretic therapy, but, if complications such as renal failure or pulmonary edema develop hemodialysis is indicated.

Peritoneal dialysis and exchange transfusion may be more useful in small children than hemodialysis. This technique is usually so slow as to be useless. Most major centers can dialyze even infants, making the peritoneal route obsolete for acute cases. Again, the main purpose of these procedures may not be removal of the poison but restoration of fluid or acid-base balance. The infant who has been poisoned and whose serum sodium is rising because of excess bicarbonate administration may be helped considerably by an exchange transfusion even if little poison is removed.

Dialysis should *not* be performed as initial therapy but only when the criteria listed above are met.

Hemoperfusion

Perfusion of blood through charcoal- or resin-filled devices is gradually becoming more widely available in many centers. These techniques will probably allow rapid removal of many substances previously considered dialyzable but will not be likely to remove large quantities of agents with large volumes of distribution.

SPECIFIC POISONS OF MAJOR CONCERN TO PEDIATRICIANS

Acids

Products. Toilet bowl cleaners (such as bisulfate, which becomes sulfuric acid on contact with water), automobile batteries, swimming pool pH adjustment solutions, and acids in concentrated forms at hardware and paint stores.

Treatment. Emesis and lavage should be avoided to prevent re-exposure of mucous membranes. Dilution with simple solutions such as water or milk within the first 30 to 60 seconds may prevent or decrease future scarring and stricture formation. Unfortunately, most patients arrive in medical facilities at much longer intervals from ingestion, and dilution is probaby ineffective. Dilution in the amount of 15 ml/kg to a maximum of 250 ml orally is adequate. For example, 150 ml of water in a 1 year old child who has swallowed some 28% acetic acid photographic stop bath will reduce the acid to a concentration well under that of vinegar used for salad dressing. Caution must be used with dilution to make sure that it is safe to give oral fluids. Steroids can be given in pharmacologic doses, although their value is unknown. Esophagoscopy should be reserved for concentrated acid ingestions or for those children salivating due to pain on swallowing. All children should be followed after 10 days to 3 weeks to be sure that pyloric stricture has not occurred.

Alkalies

Products. Contained in Clinitest tablets, drain cleaning crystals, and dishwasher soaps. Many new liquid drain cleaners contain little or no caustic agent. Those with less than 4% sodium or potassium hydroxide do not produce strictures, although they may produce burns. Industrial cleaners brought home in unlabeled containers may pose a significant hazard. Household bleaches (usually 5.4% sodium hypochloride) are not considered significant caustics.

Treatment. Immediate dilution with water or milk is the key treatment. All other therapy after the first 30 seconds simply treats sequelae. Vomiting should *not* be induced. Acid "neutralizers" (lemon juice, vinegar, and so on) should be avoided since they simply add to injury. A steroid in pharmacologic doses should be begun immediately and continued for 3 weeks if esophageal burns are discovered. Esophagoscopy is indicated in all patients with exposure to strong caustics, even in the absence of mouth burns. It is best performed 12 to 24 hours after exposure. This permits burns to develop to the point that they are readily seen but not to the point of necrosis. Patients are placed NPO immediately after dilution and observed for signs of mediastinitis (usually fever). Antibiotics are usually not given prophylactically. Dilatation of stricture may be attempted, but severe circumferential strictures may require surgical replacement of the esophagus.

Amphetamines and Related Drugs

Product. Numerous street drugs, such as "speed," STP, MDA, or DMT. While more closely regulated now, "diet pills" containing a variety of amphetamines and analogs are still found.

Treatment. In most cases nothing more is required than simple observation. Chlorpromazine has been used extensively to treat hyperactivity but should be avoided in the case of street drugs as it may result in synergistic hypotension. Diazepam is a safer choice.

Anticholinergics

Products. Examples of medications: amitriptyline (Elavil, Triavil), anisotropine (Valpin), atropine, belladonna, benactyzine (Deprol), chlorpheniramine (Ornade, Teldrin, etc.), cyclopentolate (Cyclogel), desipramine (Norpramin, Pertofrane), dicyclomine (Bentyl), diphenhydramine (Benadryl), doxepin (Sinequan), homatropine, hyoscine, hyoscyamus, imipramine (Tofranil, Presamine), isopropamide (Darbid), mepenzolate (Cantil), methantheline (Banthine), methapyrilene (Sominex, Compoz, Cope), nortriptyline (Aventyl), pipenzolate (Piptal), propantheline (Probanthine), protriptyline (Vivactil), pyrilamine, scopolamine, stramonium (Asthmador).

Examples of plants: *Amanita muscaria* (although muscarine is present in minute amounts, major toxic effects are anticholinergic), bittersweet (*Solanum dulcamara*), black henbane (*Hyoscyamus niger*), black nightshade (*Solanum nigrum*), *Lantana camara* (also known as red sage, wild sage), potato leaves, sprouts, tubers (*Solanum tuberosum*), wild tomato (*Solanum carolinense*).

Many antihistamines, antispasmodics, sleep aids, decongestants, analgesics, antiparkinsonism agents, and miscellaneous drugs, chemicals, and plants may produce clinically recognizable anticholinergic findings.

Treatment. In severe states, treatment will be necessary.

Convulsions	Diazepam
Myoclonic jerking	Physostigmine
Hallucinations	Physostigmine
Coma	Physostigmine
Hypertension	Physostigmine
Arrhythmias	Alkalinize blood to pH 7.50 and use physostigmine, lidocaine, or phenytoin

Physostigmine is a potentially dangerous drug and must be used with caution in asthmatics, diabetics, or those with gangrene. It must be given slowly (no more than 1 mg/min IV) or cholinergic overdrive may occur.

Benzodiazepines

Products. Valium, Librium, Dalmane, and a variety of minor tranquilizers.

Treatment. Patients with pure benzodiazepine overdoses rarely require more than observation. The use of naloxone, while not harmful, is probably not helpful. Physostigmine should not be used.

Cyanide

Products. Pesticides, metal polishes, photographic solutions, fumigating products, and some poisons. It is rarely seen and usually catastrophic.

Treatment. Creation of methemoglobin so as to provide an overwhelming supply of Fe^{+++} allows competition of the hemoglobin for cyanide with the cytochromes. TREATMENT CAN KILL. Pediatricians must be aware that the vial of sodium nitrite in the cyanide antidote kit is enough to kill most 1 to 2 year old children. Dosage of sodium nitrite in children is 0.3 ml/kg to a maximum of one vial.

Digitalis Glycosides

Products. Oleander, foxglove, digoxin, and digitoxin.

Treatment. Potassium must not be given unless depletion can be documented by measurements. Atropine may be useful initially. Phenytoin at low doses (1 mg/kg/dose) may be helpful. Cholestyramine orally may help lower levels. Kayexalate may be necessary to treat hyperkalemia. Pacemaker wires may be necessary. Specific antibodies—FAB fragments—are extremely effective but virtually unobtainable.

Ethanol

Products. Alcoholic beverages, cold remedies, perfumes, aftershave lotions, and fondue fuel.

Treatment. Intensive supportive care and correction of hypoglycemia. As numbers of young chronic alcoholics (ages 11 to 13 and older) increase, signs of withdrawal (delirium tremens, convulsions) must be expected and treated, usually with benzodiazepines. Extracorporeal techniques are not helpful in removing ethanol.

Hydrocarbons—Petroleum Distillates

Products. A wide variety of products contain natural (e.g., turpentine) and mineral (e.g., gasoline from petroleum cracking) hydrocarbons. The following divides these substances into toxicologic groups.

Group I—Heavy greases, oils, and petroleum jellies

Aspiration hazard	Slight
Systemic toxicity	Unusual

Group II—Gasoline, kerosene, and naphthas

Aspiration hazard	Moderate
Systemic toxicity	Moderate, and usually dependent upon aromatic content

Group III—Petroleum ether, benzine, and rapidly evaporating solvents

Aspiration hazard	Slight
Systemic toxicity	High, and usually due to anesthetic capacity

Group IV—Mineral seal oils (furniture polishes)

Aspiration hazard	High
Systemic toxicity	High, but only on secondary basis to aspiration since agents usually are not absorbed

Group V—Solvents containing toxic constituents or halogenated solvents

Aspiration hazard	Moderate
Systemic toxicity	Very high, and dependent upon the toxic constituent Most commonly pesticides heavy metals, benzene, 1,1,1-trichloroethane

Treatment. Recommended treatment, while considered controversial in the middle 1970s, is straightforward if each group is considered for its own toxicity rather than lumping all hydrocarbons together. Induction of emesis was the most controversial recommendation. Recent data indicate rare need for emesis, with 6-hour observation being the most important treatment. This is because most patients who have aspirated have done so in the act of swallowing rather than vomiting.

Induction of emesis should, however, be reserved for those situations when large quantities of hydrocarbons with risk of systemic toxicity have been consumed. Estimates of volume consumed are extremely difficult in children.

Examples of agents which may be useful to vomit are cleaning solvents with 1,1,1-trichloroethane, benzene, and pesticides with hydrocarbon solvents.

Examples of agents which do not need to be vomited are mineral seal oils, heavy greases, and petroleum jellies.

Steroids should not be administered, as they decrease the mononuclear cell response, and simultaneous antibiotics do not protect from an enhanced infection rate. Antibiotics should be used only on indication, such as increasing infiltrate size or positive tracheal aspirate. Fever per se is not an indicator for antibiotics. Administration of oils to "thicken" the hydrocarbons is no longer considered appropriate as lipoid pneumonitis may occur. Lavage should be avoided because of the increased risk of emesis and lack of control of the emetic stream with a tube in the pharynx. Generally, most children will have a benign course and do not need hospitalization. Observation for 24 hours or until cessation of symptoms is necessary in 2 to 5% of cases.

Iron

Products. As a medication in various concentrations, as an additive to multiple vitamins, and in soluble form in garden supplies. Elemental iron does not equal the weight of the tablet and must be calculated for each preparation as a percentage of weight after subtraction of other elements and rates of hydration. The usual 300-mg tablet contains about 60 mg of elemental iron.

Treatment. If the patient is not yet vomiting, then induction of emesis or lavage with a large-bore tube should be performed. Lavage is generally performed with 5% sodium bicarbonate or a similar solution. The use of oral or lavage deferoxamine has been abandoned because of the poor stoichiometry and expense. Production of iron carbonate or iron phosphate is most likely equally effective. Fleet's phosphate solution diluted 1:4 has the dual advantage of a cathartic effect. When used in excess, this solution has resulted in the death of a child.

Total iron and total iron binding capacity together will provide an accurate estimate of free (unbound) iron. Treatment with deferoxamine intravenously is usually instituted if free iron is greater than 50 or total iron is in excess of 500. Stage I is best treated without regard to the iron poisoning but rather with an eye toward correction of hypotension and acidosis. Severe Stage III may not respond to standard treatment because of iron deposition in vascular structures. Exchange trans-

fusion has been used from time to time in this situation with some good response. Extracorporeal techniques such as dialysis are of no benefit.

Lomotil, Imodium

A combination of opiate and atropine is particularly toxic even in "therapeutic" doses to children. The drug is contraindicated under all circumstances under age 6.

Treatment. Naloxone (Narcan) is an effective antidote for the diphenoxylate and should be used in sufficient doses. Discharge from care should not occur until the patient has been symptom-free for 12 to 24 hours without naloxone administration.

Should arrest or hypoxia occur, the standard treatment for such a state, with the addition of naloxone, is appropriate.

Metals—Arsenic, Lead, and Mercury

Products. A wide variety of products ranging from old paint and plaster to ant poisons may contain these metals. Frequently the source of the metal is unknown, and because of some neurologic or other problem, the physician wishes to "rule out" this possibility.

Treatment. Dilution is the major therapeutic step for all these metals. Arsenic and mercury can be effectively removed with British anti-lewisite (BAL) (dimercaprol). BAL, unfortunately, is painful and produces a serum-like reaction in 70 to 80% of patients. BAL, therefore, should be used only in patients unable to take oral drugs or who are acutely ill. D-penicillamine is the drug of choice in these patients if they can take it orally and are not penicillin-allergic. For diagnostic and therapeutic purposes, a D-penicillamine mobilization test should be done. It allows significantly greater accuracy than a single urine test for heavy metals. The test and followup treatment are performed as follows:

Day 1—Collect a 24-hour urine specimen.

Day 2—250 mg of D-penicillamine at 0, 6, 12, and 18 hours and collect a 24-hour urine specimen. Comparison of these two urine specimens will indicate whether there are significant body burdens of lead, arsenic, or mercury. If the result of day 2 is more than three times that of day 1 (in μg per 24 hours total) and over 150 μg, it is considered a positive test.

Days 3–7—250 mg D-penicillamine qid.

Days 8–12—No drug.

Day 13—Begin cycle again and continue until the initial 2-day mobilization is normal. If more than three cycles are needed, then pause for 1 month after day 7.

Children under 10 kg should have 100 mg/kg periodically in four divided doses (to a maximum of 1 gm per day) rather than 250 mg qid.

Organophosphate and Carbamate Insecticides

Products. Chlorthion, Co-Ral, DFP, Diazinon, Malathion, Para-oxon, Parathion, Phosdrin, TEPP, Thio-TEPP, Carbaryl.

Treatment. Atropine plus a cholinesterase reactivator, pralidoxime (Protopam), is a chemical antidote for organophosphate insecticide poisoning. After establishing a clear airway and eliminating any cyanosis, large doses of atropine should be given and repeated every few minutes until signs of atropinism are present. An appropriate starting dose of atropine is 2 to 4 mg intravenously in an adult and 0.05 mg/kg in a child. The patient should receive enough atropine to stop secretions (approximately 10 times the normal dose). As much as 1 gm of atropine per 24 hours may be needed in an adult.

Because atropine antagonizes the parasympathetic effects of the organophosphates but does not alter the muscular weakness, pralidoxime should also be given immediately in more severe cases and repeated every 8 to 12 hours as needed (1 gm IV for older children and 250 mg intravenously for infants at a rate of no more than 500 mg/min). Pralidoxime should be used in addition to—not in place of—atropine if red cell cholinesterase is less than 25% of normal. Pralidoxime is probably not useful later than 36 hours after the exposure. Morphine, theophylline, aminophylline, succinylcholine, and tranquilizers of the reserpine and phenothiazine types are contraindicated. Hyperglycemia is common.

Decontamination of the skin (including nails and hair) and clothing with soapy water is extremely important. Decontamination of the skin must be done carefully to avoid abrasions, which increase organophosphate absorption significantly.

Phencyclidine

Products. Sold only as an illicit drug, e.g., angel dust, PCP, and "PeaCe Pill."

Treatment. An adequate supportive environment is all that is required in most instances. Serious cases may require haloperidol to control behavior. Forced acid diuresis should not be used. Recent reports of rhabdomyolysis and renal failure indicate care should be taken before diuresis is induced.

Narcotics and Synthetic Congeners

Products. Propoxyphene (Darvon), heroin, Talwin, Demerol, codeine, and so on.

Treatment. Children receiving an overdose of opiates can develop respiratory depression, stridor, coma, increased oropharyngeal secretions, sinus bradycardia, and urinary retention. Methadone is less likely to cause miosis than other narcotics. Pulmonary edema rarely occurs in children; deaths usually result from respiratory arrest and cerebral edema. Convulsions may occur with propoxyphene overdosage. Patients are usually in a coma on admission. If seizures are seen, then Darvon must be considered. Small pupils, absent bowel sounds, and bradycardia are common.

The treatment of choice is naloxone (Narcan), 0.4 mg intravenously, which rapidly produces a marked improvement without causing respiratory depression. The dose can be safely repeated and increased as needed. Before concluding that naloxone is ineffective, a minimum of 1 mg should be given push IV to children less than 6 months and 2 mg should be given to children older than 6 months. Nalorphine (Nalline) is an older drug with a respiratory depressant effect of its own. It should no longer be used. An improvement in respiratory status may be followed by respiratory depression, since the depressant action of narcotics may last 24 to 48 hours while the antagonist's duration of action is only 2 to 3 hours. Give intravenous fluids cautiously, since narcotics exert an antidiuretic effect and may precipitate cerebral or pulmonary edema.

Withdrawal in the Addict. The severity of withdrawal signs should be evaluated as explained in Table 4. Diazepam (Valium), 10 mg every 6 hours orally, has been recommended for the treatment of mild narcotic withdrawal in ambulatory adolescents. Ambulatory or hospitalized patients with moderate or severe withdrawal signs can be given the same dose of diazepam intramuscularly. Diazepam is recommended because it is nonhepatotoxic and nonmutagenic, is not known to affect the fetus when given to pregnant women, and is a good anticonvulsant. Diazepam therapy can be discontinued when the withdrawal score falls below 2. Diphenoxylate with atropine (Lomotil) is used to treat severe diarrhea and abdominal cramps.

Methadone maintenance is not usually recommended for adolescents, although it may be used for withdrawal purposes. One method of administration is to give methadone orally every 12 hours, starting with a 25-mg dose and decreasing the amounts by 5 mg every 12 hours. When the dose of methadone is 10 mg, add 3 tablets of diphenoxylate with atropine (Lomotil) three times daily for 1 day, followed by 2 tablets three times daily for 2 days. If signs of withdrawal recur, 10 mg of methadone orally or diazepam (orally or intramuscularly) is given.

The abrupt discontinuation of narcotics (cold turkey method) is not recommended and may cause severe physical withdrawal signs.

Withdrawal in the Neonate. A newborn infant in narcotic withdrawal is small for gestational age and demonstrates yawning, sneezing, decreased Moro reflex, hunger but uncoordinated sucking action, jitteriness, tremor, constant movement, a

Table 4. SCORING SYSTEMS FOR COMA, HYPERACTIVITY, AND WITHDRAWAL

Classification of Coma
0   Asleep, but can be aroused and can answer questions.
1   Comatose, does withdraw from painful stimuli, reflexes intact.
2   Comatose, does not withdraw from painful stimuli, most reflexes intact, no respiratory or circulatory depression.
3   Comatose, most or all reflexes are absent but without depression of respiration or circulation.
4   Comatose, reflexes absent, respiratory depression with cyanosis, circulatory failure, or shock.

Classification of Hyperactivity
1+   Restlessness, irritability, insomnia, tremor, hyperreflexia, sweating, mydriasis, flushing.
2+   Confusion, hyperactivity, hypertension, tachypnea, tachycardia, extrasystoles, sweating, mydriasis, flushing, mild hyperpyrexia.
3+   Delirium, mania, self-injury, marked hypertension, tachycardia, arrhythmias, hyperpyrexia.
4+   Above plus: convulsions, coma, circulatory collapse.

Classification of Withdrawal
Score the following finding on a 0-, 1-, 2-point basis:

Diarrhea	Hypertension	Restlessness
Dilated pupils	Insomnia	Tachycardia
Gooseflesh	Lacrimation	Yawning
Hyperactive bowel sounds	Muscle cramps	

1 to 5	mild
6 to 10	moderate
11 to 15	severe

Seizures indicate severe withdrawal regardless of the rest of the score.

(From Frederick H. Lovejoy, Jr., M.D., in Gellis and Kagan, Current Pediatric Therapy 9, W. B. Saunders Co., 1980.)

shrill and protracted cry, increased tendon reflexes, convulsions, vomiting, fever, watery diarrhea, cyanosis, dehydration, vasomotor instability, and collapse. The onset of symptoms commonly begins in the first 48 hours but may be delayed as long as 8 days, depending upon the timing of the mother's last "fix" and her predelivery medication. The diagnosis can be easily confirmed by identifying the narcotic in the urine of the mother and baby.

Several methods of treatment have been suggested for narcotic withdrawal in the neonate. Phenobarbital, 8 mg/kg/24 hr intramuscularly or orally in four doses for 4 days and then reduced by one third every 2 days as signs decrease, may be continued for as long as 3 weeks. Methadone may be necessary in those infants with congenital methadone addiction who are not controlled in their withdrawal by large doses of phenobarbital. Dosage should be 0.5 mg/kg/24 hr in two divided doses but can be gradually increased as needed. Slow tapering off may be necessary over 4 weeks for methadone addiction.

It is not clear whether prophylactic treatment with these drugs decreases the complication rate. The mortality rate of untreated narcotic withdrawal in the neonate may be as high as 45%.

Nitrites

Products. Nitrite and nitrate compounds found in the home include amyl nitrite, nitroglycerin, pentaerythritol tetranitrate (Peritrate), sodium nitrite, nitrobenzene, and pyridium. High concentrations of nitrites in water or spinach have been the most common cause of nitrite-induced methemoglobinemia.

Treatment. After administering activated charcoal, induce vomiting and follow with a saline cathartic. Decontaminate any affected skin with soap and water. Oxygen and artificial respiration may be needed. If the blood methemoglobin level exceeds 40% or if levels cannot be obtained, give 0.2 ml/kg of 1% solution of methylene blue intravenously over 5 to 10 minutes. Avoid perivascular infiltration, since it causes necrosis of the skin and subcutaneous tissues. A dramatic change in the degree of cyanosis should occur. Transfusion is occasionally necessary. Epinephrine and other vasoconstrictors, are contraindicated. If reflex bradycardia occurs, atropine can be used to block it.

Phenothiazines

Products. Chlorpromazine (Thorazine), prochlorperazine (Compazine), trifluoperazine (Stelazine), and so on.

Treatment. Extrapyramidal signs are dramatically alleviated within minutes by the slow intravenous administration of 1 to 5 mg/kg of diphenhydramine (Benadryl). No other treatment is usually indicated. Dialysis is contraindicated. Patients with overdoses should be treated conservatively. An attempt should be made to induce vomiting with apomorphine after administration of activated charcoal. Charcoal absorbs chlorpromazine and probably other phenothiazines very well. Emetics are often unsuccessful in this situation because phenothiazines are potent antiemetics; gastric lavage, therefore, may be the only practical way to remove gastric contents. A large amount of intravenous fluid without vasopressor agents is the preferred method of treating tranquilizer-induced neurogenic hypotension. If a pressor agent is required, norepinephrine (levarterenol) should be used. Epinephrine should not be used because phenothiazines reverse epinephrine's effects.

Plants

Many common ornamental, garden, and wild plants are potentially toxic. Small amounts of a plant that are ingested may cause severe illness or death. These effects usually involve the cardiovascular, gastrointestinal, and central nervous systems and the skin.

Autumn Crocus (Colchicine). Monitor fluids and electrolytes. Abdominal cramps may be relieved with meperidine or atropine.

Caladium (Arum Family) (Dieffenbachia, Calla Lily, Dumb Cane) (Oxalic Acid). Accessible areas should be washed thoroughly. Corticosteroids relieve airway obstruction. Apply cold packs to affected mucous membranes.

Castor Bean Plant (Ricin-a Toxalbumin). Fluid and electrolyte monitoring. Saline cathartic. Forced alkaline diuresis will prevent complications due to hemagglutination and hemolysis.

Foxglove and Cardiac Glycosides. If vomiting has not occurred, induce emesis or provide lavage followed by charcoal cathartics. Potassium should not be given in acute overdosage unless there is laboratory evidence of hypokalemia. In acute overdosage, hyperkalemia is more common.

The patient must be monitored carefully for electrocardiographic changes. The correction of acidosis will better demonstrate the degree of potassium deficiency present. In some cases, phenytoin (Dilantin), beta-adrenergic blocking agents such as propranolol (Inderal), or procainamide (Pronestyl) is necessary to correct arrhythmias. A pacemaker may be needed.

It has recently been noted that digoxin has an enterophepatic circulation. The use of oral binding agents such as cholestyramine resin (Cuemid, Questran) has been suggested in massive digitalis overdoses.

Jequirity Bean (Abrin-a Toxalbumin). Symptomatic. Renal failure can be prevented by alkalinizing the urine. Gastric lavage or emetics are contraindicated because the toxin is necrotizing. Saline cathartics are indicated.

Jimsonweed. Emesis or lavage should be followed by activated charcoal and cathartics. Physostigmine, 0.5 to 2 mg intravenously (can be repeated every 30 minutes as needed) dramatically reverses the central and peripheral signs of atropinism. Neostigmine is ineffective because it does not enter the central nervous system. High fever must be controlled. Catheterization may be needed if the patient cannot void.

Larkspur (*Delphinium ajacine*, Delphinine). Symptomatic. Atropine may be helpful.

Monkshood (Aconite). Activated charcoal, oxygen. Atropine is probably helpful.

Oleander (Dogbane Family) (Oleandrin). If vomiting has not occurred, induce emesis or provide lavage followed by charcoal cathartics. Potassium should not be given in acute overdosage unless there is laboratory evidence of hypokalemia. In acute overdosage, hyperkalemia is more common.

The patient must be monitored carefully for electrocardiographic changes. The correction of acidosis will better demonstrate the degree of potassium deficiency present. In some cases, phenytoin (Dilantin), beta-adrenergic blocking agents such as propranolol (Inderal), or procainamide (Pronestyl) is necessary to correct arrhythmias. A pacemaker may be needed.

Poison Hemlock (Coniine). Symptomatic treatment. Oxygen and cardiac monitoring equipment are desirable. Assisted respiration is often necessary. Give anticonvulsants if needed.

Rhododendron (Andromedotoxin). Atropine can prevent bradycardia. Epinephrine is contraindicated. Antihypertensives may be needed.

Yellow Jessamine. (The active ingredient, gelsemine, is related to strychnine.) Symptomatic treatment. Because of the relation to strychnine, forced acid diuresis and diazepam (Valium) for seizures would be worth trying.

Strychnine

Products. Rodenticides, tonics, and cathartics. It is also occasionally added to hallucinogenic drugs.

Treatment. If the patient is seen before the onset of symptoms, vomiting should be induced, followed by administration of activated charcoal, which is a very efficient adsorber of strychnine. Since ipecac is also adsorbed by activated charcoal emesis must be induced before charcoal is given. Convulsions can be controlled with diazepam (Valium), 0.1 to 0.3 mg/kg to a maximum of 10 mg. External stimulation should be minimized. Forced acid diuresis is very helpful, since strychnine is not significantly protein-bound and is present in large concentration in the serum. It is rapidly cleared in the urine. The hyperacute nature of strychnine intoxication makes hemodialysis impractical.

Tricyclic Antidepressants

Products. Amitriptyline, imipramine, doxepin, trimipramine, nortriptyline, desipramine, protriptyline, and so on.

Treatment. Treatment of the five major problems of arrhythmias, coma, convulsions, hypertension (and, later, hypotension), and hallucinations consists of intensive supportive measures followed by administration of physostigmine in the following doses; child under 12 years of age—0.5 mg intravenously over 60 seconds. If there is no effect, the dose may be repeated at 5-minute intervals to a maximum of 2 mg. Repeat as necessary only for life-threatening situations. Adult and adolescent—2 mg intravenously over 60 seconds. If there is no effect, repeat in 10 minutes to a maximum dose of 4 mg. Repeat for life-threatening situations.

Physostigmine is a dangerous drug that must be given slowly to avoid iatrogenic convulsions. It is contraindicated in asthma, vascular gangrene, or

Text continued on page 665

Table 5. DRUG FORMULARY IN TOXICOLOGY

Substance	Indications	Adolescent Dose	Pediatric Dose
Activated charcoal	Gastrointestinal decontamination	5 to 10 times the estimated amount ingested or 15 to 30 gm in 60 to 120 ml of water. Mix well before use. Give orally or by nasogastric tube	5 to 10 times the estimated amount ingested or 0.5 to 1 gm/kg mixed with 30 to 60 ml of water mixed with 5 to 10 ml of cherry syrup before use. Mix well before use. Given orally or by nasogastric tube
Amyl nitrite pearls (kit from Eli Lilly and Company)	Cyanide poisoning	Inhalation for 30 seconds out of every min. New ampule every 3 mins	Same as adolescent dose
Atropine sulfate	Organophosphate and carbamate insecticides	2 to 3 mg/dose of IV solution (0.4 mg/ml) every 2 to 5 min until fully atropinized and then as necessary to maintain atropinization	0.05 mg/kg of IV solution (0.4 mg/ml) every 2 to 5 min until fully atropinized and then as necessary to maintain atropinization
Calcium disodium ethylene diamine tetra-acetate (calcium disodium versenate) (CaEDTA)	Heavy metal (lead) poisoning	1 gm IM or IV over 1 hour twice a day for 5 to 7 days. Repeat course after rest period. Add procaine for IM use	50 to 75 mg/kg/24 hr IM or IV divided into 2 to 3 doses for 5 to 7 days. Repeat course at 50 mg/kg/24 hr after rest period. Add procaine for IM use
Chlorpromazine (Thorazine)	Amphetamine-induced hyperactivity and psychosis	25 mg/dose IV every 6 hours. Reduce dose if barbiturate ingested. Titrate subsequent doses to desired response	1 mg/kg/dose every 6 hours. Reduce dose if barbiturate ingested. Titrate subsequent doses to desired response
Deferoxamine (Desferal)	Iron poisoning	1 to 2 gm IM every 6 to 8 hours. For severe intoxication IV dose at a rate not to exceed 15 mg/kg/hr. Do not exceed 6 gm in 24 hours	50 mg/kg not to exceed 1 to 2 gm IM every 6 hours. For severe intoxication IV dose at a rate not to exceed 15 mg/kg/hr. Do not exceed 6 gm in 24 hours
Dexamethasone (Decadron)	Cerebral edema	10 mg IV as an initial dose followed by 4 mg every 6 hours IV	0.4 mg/kg IV as an initial dose followed by 0.1 mg/kg/dose IV every 4 to 6 hours
Diazepam (Valium)	Control of seizures	5 to 10 mg/dose IV titrated to control seizures	0.1 to 0.25 mg/kg/dose IV titrated to control seizures*
Dimercaprol (BAL)	Heavy metal (arsenic, mercury, lead, gold) poisoning	3 mg/kg/dose IM at 4- to 6-hour intervals for first 5 days, then 3 mg/kg/dose every 12 hours for next 5 to 9 days	3 to 4 mg/kg/dose IM at 4- to 6-hour intervals for first 5 days, then 3 to 4 mg/kg every 12 hours for next 5 to 9 days
Diphenhydramine (Benadryl)	Phenothiazine extrapyramidal reaction	25 to 50 mg/dose IV slowly, then every 6 hours orally or IV for maintenance	1 to 2 mg/kg/dose IV slowly, then every 6 hours orally or IV for maintenance
Ethacrynic acid (Edecrin)	Enhanced urinary excretion	50 mg/dose or 0.5 to 1.0 mg/kg/dose IV every 8 hours	0.5 to 1.0 mg/kg/dose IV every 8 hours†

Drug	Indication	Adolescent Dose	Child Dose
Ethanol	Methanol and ethylene glycol poisoning	Ethanol given as a 50 per cent solution IV at a dose of 0.5 to 1.5 ml/kg every 2 to 4 hours to maintain a blood level between 100 and 150 mg/dl. In mild cases, 3 to 4 ounces of whiskey every 4 hours orally	Same as adolescent dose.
Furosemide (Lasix)	Enhanced urinary excretion	20 to 40 mg/dose IM or slowly IV (over 1 to 2 minutes) every 8 to 12 hours	1 to 3 mg/kg/dose IM or slowly IV (over 1 to 2 minutes) every 8 to 12 hours
Glycerol	Cerebral edema	2 gm/kg/24 hr in 4 divided doses orally	3 gm/kg/24 hr in 4 divided doses orally
Ipecac syrup	Induction of emesis	30 ml orally with fluids followed by motion	15 ml orally repeated in 15 min if not effective. Given with fluids followed by motion
Isoproterenol (Isuprel)	Hypotension	2 mg in 1000 ml of 5 per cent dextrose in water (conc. of 2 μg/ml), IV at rate of 0.1 μg/kg/min and increased slowly as needed	Same as adolescent dose.
Levarterenol (Levophed)	Hypotension	4 ml vial added to 1000 ml of 5 per cent dextrose in water (conc. of 4 μg/ml), IV at rate of 0.1 to 0.2 μg/kg/min and increased slowly as needed	Same as adolescent dose.
Magnesium sulfate (Epsom salt)	Gastrointestinal catharsis	5 gm or 50 ml of a 10 per cent solution orally and repeat every 4 hours until productive of stool	250 mg/kg/dose orally and repeat every 3 hours until productive of stool.
Mannitol	Enhanced urinary excretion Cerebral edema	25 to 50 gm in a 20 per cent solution IV over 30 min every 4 to 6 hours (max. 200 gm/24 hr)	1 to 2 mg/kg in 20 per cent solution IV over 30 min every 4 to 6 hours (max. 100 mg/24 hr)‡
Metaraminol (Aramine)	Hypotension	10 mg/ml in a 10-ml vial. Add 100 mg to 1000 ml of 5 per cent dextrose in water (conc. of 100 μg/ml). Given IV at rate of 5 μg/kg/min and increased slowly as needed	Same as adolescent dose.
Methylene blue	Methemoglobinemia	1 per cent solution given IV slowly over 5 to 10 min at a dose of 10 mg, repeated in 4 hours if needed	1 per cent solution at a dose of 1 to 2 mg/kg given IV slowly over 5 to 10 min, repeated in 4 hours if needed
Naloxone hydrochloride (Narcan)	Reversal of narcotic depression	0.4 mg IV repeated every 2 to 3 min for 2 or 3 doses for initial effect. Continue therapy until narcotic effect no longer present	0.01 mg/kg/dose IV repeated every 2 to 3 min for 2 or 3 doses for initial effect. Continue therapy until narcotic effect no longer present
Oxygen	Carbon monoxide poisoning	100 per cent oxygen by inhalation	Same as adolescent dose.

Table continued on following page

Table 5. DRUG FORMULARY IN TOXICOLOGY *(continued)*

Substance	Indications	Adolescent Dose	Pediatric Dose
D-Penicillamine (Cuprimine)	Heavy metal (lead, mercury) poisoning	250 to 500 mg orally every 6 to 8 hours, depending on severity	For acute therapy 25 to 50 mg/kg/24 hr in 4 divided doses orally for 5 days. For chronic therapy 25 mg/kg/24 hr in 4 divided doses orally (max. 1 gm/24 hr)
Physostigmine salicylate (Antilirium)	Anticholinergic poisoning	2 mg slowly over 2 to 3 min IV with repeat in 2 to 5 min if no effect. Once effect accomplished, give lowest effective dose slowly every 30 to 60 min with recurrence of symptoms	0.5 mg slowly over 2 to 3 min IV with repeat in 2 to 5 min if no effect. Once effect accomplished, give lowest effective dose slowly every 30 to 60 min with recurrence of symptoms
Pralidoxime chloride (2PAM)	Organophosphate insecticide	0.5 to 1.0 gm IV after initial treatment with atropine, given slowly at a rate of 500 mg/min and repeated every 8 to 12 hours as needed	250 mg/dose given slowly IV after initial treatment with atropine and repeated every 8 to 12 hours as needed
Prednisone	Caustic injury to esophagus	10 to 20 mg/dose IV, IM, or orally every 6 hours for 2 to 3 weeks with dosage tapering at end of therapy	2 to 3 mg/kg/24 hr IM, IV, or orally every 6 hours for 3 weeks with dosage tapering at end of therapy
Sodium bicarbonate	Enhanced urinary excretion of acid compounds by alkalinization of urine	2 meq/kg/dose IV during first hour followed by sufficient NaHCO₃ to keep urinary pH > 7.5 (generally 2 meq/kg every 6 to 8 hours). Additional potassium necessary to accomplish alkalinization	2 to 4 meq/kg/dose IV during hour followed by sufficient NaHCO₃ to keep urinary pH > 7.5 (generally 2 meq/kg every 6 hours). Additional potassium (3 to 4 meq/kg day) necessary to accomplish alkalinization
Sodium thiosulfate (kit from Eli Lilly and Company)	Cyanide poisoning	50 ml of 25 per cent solution at a rate of 2.5 to 5.0 ml/min IV 15 min after sodium nitrite. May be repeated once	1.65 ml/kg of 25 per cent solution at a rate of 2.5 to 5.0 ml/min IV 15 min after sodium nitrite. May be repeated once
Sodium nitrite (kit from Eli Lilly and Company)	Cyanide poisoning	10 to 20 ml of 3 per cent solution at a rate of 2.5 to 5.0 ml/min IV. May be repeated once with persistence or recurrence of symptoms	0.33 ml/kg of 3 per cent solution at a rate of 2.5 to 5.0 ml/min IV. May be repeated once with persistence or recurrence of symptoms
Vitamin K₁	Hypoprothrombinemia	5 mg/dose IV	2 to 5 mg/dose IV

* Manufacturer's Warning: Safety not established in the neonate.
† Manufacturer's Precaution: Until further experience in infants is accumulated, therapy with ethacrynic acid is contraindicated.
‡ Manufacturer's Warning: Dosage requirements for patients 12 years of age and under have not been established.

urinary tract obstruction. Propranolol or pheny-toin may be used if physostigmine is ineffective for treatment of arrhythmias. Alkalinization with sodium bicarbonate, 0.5 meq/kg intravenously, may dramatically reverse ventricular arrhythmias. Bicarbonate should be administered with physo-stigmine to all patients with significant arrhythmias to achieve a plasma pH of 7.5 to 7.6. Forced diuresis is contraindicated. A QRS interval greater than 100 milliseconds specifically identifies pa-tients with major tricyclic antidepressant overdo-sage.

Hypotension is a major problem, since tricyclic antidepressants block the reuptake of catechola-mines. This may produce a rebound hypotension following initial hypertension. Treatment with physostigmine is not effective. Infusion of sodium bicarbonate, 0.5 meq/kg, to produce a plasma pH of 7.5 or 7.6 will help avert hypotension. Vaso-pressors are generally ineffective, and the mortal-ity rate is 60% in patients with hypotension who prove unresponsive to initial fluids. Orogastric charcoal, 0.5 gm/kg every 4 to 6 hours during the first 24 hours following ingestion, appears to in-terrupt an enterohepatic recirculation of tricyclics and shorten the plasma half-life.

DRUG FORMULARY

Table 5 lists the most commonly used drugs for treatment of poisoned patients. These drugs all should be available in a hospital intending to treat poisoned patients.

Salicylate Poisoning

FRANK A. SIMON, M.D.

Salicylate intoxication may result from the inges-tion of a single excessive dose or may follow the more delayed accumulation of toxic levels of med-ication. Chronic intoxication may result from the repeated administration of too large a dose of aspirin or by the simultaneous ingestion of several medications all of which contain unrecognized amounts of salicylate. These episodes are the result of the nonlinear, saturable kinetics of salicylate elimination.

The management of salicylate intoxication re-quires a knowledge of the basic principles of the treatment of poisonings. Initial therapy is to pro-vide adequate supportive care. Once the patient is stabilized, specific measures directed against the intoxication should be started. The stomach should be emptied to decrease the chance of further absorption of the drug, and activated charcoal should be given to absorb drug that remains in the gastrointestinal tract. Attempts should be made to decrease the level of drug already absorbed.

Intravenous fluid administration is essential for symptomatic patients with salicylism in whom there are major disturbances in fluid, electrolyte, and acid-base balances. If there is evidence of de-creased perfusion or hypotension, the child should be given an infusion of an isotonic solution, normal saline, with at least 5% glucose at a rate of 20 ml/kg/hr for 1 hour. Repeated administration of this therapy should be based on the patient's response. If there is no resolution of the symptoms of volume depletion, the infusion should be repeated.

Gastric emptying is best accomplished by emesis, induced by syrup of ipecac. If the patient is not profoundly lethargic or seizing, 15 ml of syrup of ipecac should be given followed by at least 8 oz of fluid other than milk. If vomiting does not occur within 20 minutes, the dose should be repeated. If vomiting is contraindicated, the stomach can be emptied by lavage with 0.5 normal saline. A large-bore tube must be used to permit the passage of intact tablets.

Once the stomach has been emptied, activated charcoal in an amount 10 times the estimated dose of salicylate should be given. An approximation of 1 cup of activated charcoal mixed with water to produce a slurry may be substituted. The charcoal will help to decrease absorption of salicylate re-maining in the gastrointestinal tract and will serve as a marker of when the drug has cleared the large intestine. Additional efforts to reduce ab-sorption by the administration of cathartics is controversial and not necessary.

Further specific therapy must be directed at correcting the existing metabolic disturbances. The degree of dehydration must be estimated, and appropriate volumes of fluid must be provided intravenously. This solution should contain ap-proximately 75 mEq/l of Na, up to 75 mEq/l HCO_3, and 5 gm/l of glucose. Once urine output is established, 40 mEq/l of KCl must be added to the solution to help correct the anticipated hypokale-mia.

In the presence of a continuing acidosis, sodium bicarbonate can be used in place of sodium chlo-ride in maintenance fluids. This would be a con-centration of 30 mEq/l. Supplemental potassium at 40 mEq/l must be continued. Correction of the acidosis will reduce tissue and CNS levels of sali-cylate by trapping the drug in the blood. If the metabolic acidosis is corrected and the urine pH is maintained in excess of 7.5, the urine excretion of salicylate can be increased fivefold. The alka-linization of the urine will be impossible in the presence of hypokalemia. Excess sodium bicarbo-nate or drugs such as acetazolamide should be avoided. Their use is associated with additional complications.

Hemodialysis, peritoneal dialysis, and exchange transfusions are all effective methods of reducing serum salicylate levels. These methods are rarely needed. They should be used only in severe cases, in those not responding to adequate conventional therapy, or in those with renal failure. These techniques should be used by experienced physicians.

In chronic poisonings, the severity of the symptoms does not correlate with the blood level. Levels over 20 mg/100 ml are in the toxic range. Therapy must be based on the occurrence of symptoms. The same therapeutic approach outlined for acute ingestion is applicable. Gastric emptying will probably not be required. Activated charcoal may be helpful, and the correction of the metabolic abnormalities is essential. Adequate glucose must be given to correct any hypoglycemia.

Acetaminophen Poisoning

SUSAN S. FISH, Pharm.D.,
and
FREDERICK H. LOVEJOY, JR., M.D.

First reports of hepatotoxicity from acetaminophen overdose in animals appeared in 1964, and in 1966 case reports of liver damage in humans began to appear. Today it is well accepted that acute ingestions of excessive amounts of acetaminophen may lead to hepatic necrosis. Acetaminophen poisonings occur commonly. Nationally, in 1983, acetaminophen alone or in combination accounted for 5.8% of calls to poison centers, but only 13% of those were of sufficient severity to require antidotal treatment. Acetaminophen overdoses outnumber those from all other drugs. However, only about 8% of untreated patients with toxic acetaminophen ingestions develop severe alterations in liver function, and 1–2% die in hepatic failure.

Hepatotoxicity is the major effect of massive ingestion of acetaminophen. It is thought that in this situation a larger amount of the reactive metabolite is formed via P-450 metabolism. Hepatic glutathione is rapidly depleted. When glutathione levels drop by 70%, the electrophilic metabolite instead binds covalently and irreversibly to amino acids of hepatic proteins, resulting in cell damage and liver necrosis. This hepatic necrosis is directly related to the extent of glutathione depletion.

Therapy is therefore aimed at supplying glutathione or another sulfhydryl donor. Exogenous glutathione is not taken up by the liver, so a glutathione precursor or glutathione surrogate must be used. Three such sulfhydryl compounds have been evaluated. Cysteamine has been useful for preventing hepatotoxicity in humans, if used within 10 to 12 hours of the ingestion, but produces severe nausea and vomiting. Methionine protects animals against the hepatotoxic effects of acetaminophen but appears less useful in humans. N-acetylcysteine, already available in the United States as Mucomyst, a mucolytic agent, has been shown to be protective both orally and intravenously in animals and humans if used within 10 to 12 hours after ingestion. N-acetylcysteine reacts directly with the toxic acetaminophen metabolite and also stimulates glutathione synthesis in vitro.

The treatment of an acetaminophen overdose begins with gastrointestinal decontamination using emesis or lavage. Emesis may be accomplished using syrup of ipecac, 15 ml in children and 30 ml in adults, with copious amounts of fluids. If vomiting does not occur within 20 to 30 minutes, this procedure should be repeated. In the event that emesis is contraindicated, lavage should be performed using a large-bore orogastric or nasogastric tube. Care should be taken to protect the airway against possible aspiration, especially with concomitant ingestion of central nervous system depressant drugs. Activated charcoal with a cathartic can be useful in adsorbing acetaminophen remaining in the gastrointestinal tract but may also adsorb the oral antidote. For this reason, charcoal should only be used within the first 4 to 6 hours after ingestion and prior to beginning antidotal therapy.

When a potentially toxic dose has been ingested (greater than 140 mg/kg, or greater than 7.5 gm in adults), or when a serum acetaminophen level is greater than 200 mcg/ml at 4 hours, 100 mcg/ml at 8 hours, or 50 mcg/ml at 12 hours, N-acetylcysteine (Mucomyst) should be administered within 10 to 12 hours of the ingestion. Treatment beginning more than 24 hours postexposure is ineffective. A loading dose of 140 mg/kg of N-acetylcysteine orally is followed by 70 mg/kg every 4 hours for 17 additional doses. Mucomyst is available as a 10% or 20% solution and should be diluted to a 5% solution using cola, grapefruit juice, orange juice, or other suitable beverage. Because of its sulfurlike odor, the use of a covered cup with a straw aids compliance. If a dose is vomited within 1 hour, it should be repeated. A slow nasogastric infusion of N-acetylcysteine has been useful when oral administration is not tolerated. Antiemetic medications may also be helpful.

Liver function tests should be monitored daily for 4 days. If they remain within normal limits during this time, liver damage has probably been avoided.

Other treatment is supportive. Fluid and electrolyte balance must be maintained in the face of protracted vomiting. Complications of hepatic or renal failure are treated as they arise. Coagulopathy is treated with vitamin K and clotting factor concentrates or fresh frozen plasma, as needed.

Acetaminophen is removed by both hemodialysis and hemoperfusion, with clearances of 50–150 ml/min and 70–200 ml/min, respectively. However, the clinical utility of these procedures is still being debated. Delay in preparing the patient and equipment for hemodialysis or hemoperfusion is inevitable, and the additional amount of acetaminophen removed may not justify the risk of the procedure except in enormous ingestions when endogenous elimination processes are overwhelmed. This has not been studied in a controlled manner.

Drugs that induce hepatic microsomal enzymes can raise the risk of acetaminophen-induced liver damage by increasing the amount of reactive acetaminophen metabolite formed. For this reason, patients chronically taking phenobarbital, ethanol, or other enzyme inducers may be at higher risk from large doses of acetaminophen. Patients with pre-existing liver disease also appear at higher risk of hepatic damage from toxic ingestions of acetaminophen.

Glutathione depletion may occur more rapidly in fasting or protein-deficient patients. This has been shown in animals, but the clinical relevance is unknown.

Children appear to be relatively resistant to the toxic effects of acetaminophen. Although both severe and fatal liver damage have been reported in children, these occur less often than would be expected from the children's serum acetaminophen levels. Children have a higher capacity than adults for sulfation of acetaminophen and probably form less of the toxic metabolite. Until conclusive evidence is achieved, treatment recommendations for children are identical to those for adults.

Although chronic administration of acetaminophen has been reported to result in hepatic and renal toxicity, treatment is directed at discontinuing acetaminophen and supporting the patient.

Increased Lead Absorption and Acute Lead Poisoning

J. JULIAN CHISOLM, JR., M.D.

The vast majority of children with increased lead absorption now referred to pediatricians by screening clinics are asymptomatic. Acute lead encephalopathy is now rare. Increased lead absorption (with or without symptoms) is a reportable condition. The Centers for Disease Control 1985 guidelines list four risk categories according to the following blood lead groups: class 1 ("normal"), blood lead values (PbB)* found in healthy populations without undue exposure to lead, PbB <25 μg; class II (moderate risk), PbB = 25–49 μg, class III (high risk), PbB = 50–69 μg; class IV (urgent risk), PbB $\geq$ 70 μg.

When based on a confirmatory venous sample for PbB, this classification is useful as an initial guide to therapy; however, the trend of PbB and free erythrocyte protoporphyrin (FEP)† values is far more important than single values in the long-term management of this chronic condition. In classes III and IV the risk of symptoms and impairment of central nervous system (CNS) function is distinctly increased, particularly if venous PbB in excess of 45–50 μg is long sustained.

In all cases, first priority is given to identification of the important source of excess lead in the child's environment and to prompt separation of the child from the source. Chelating agents are useful in children in classes III and IV, the higher risk categories.

These agents should be used in the asymptomatic phase of lead poisoning, as institution of chelation therapy *after* the onset of acute encephalopathy does not reduce the incidence of severe CNS sequelae. A team approach involving public health personnel, physician, pediatric nurse-practitioner, medical-social worker, and behavioral psychologist is likely to be the most effective. If possible, children should be referred to a special lead clinic for long-term follow-up.

Identification and Abatement of Lead Sources

A thorough history can facilitate the identification and abatement of the most important sources of lead. This crucial part of therapy is usually performed by health department personnel, to whom all information should be reported. Environmental history should include a list of all dwellings visited by the child: primary residence, homes of relatives and babysitters, schools, and day care centers and the age and state of repair of each building. In the United States virtually all such buildings built before 1950 have lead-bearing paints on exposed exterior and/or interior surfaces. Structures in poor repair often have lead-containing chips or pulverized fragments in the household dust. Play areas, especially dirt playgrounds and dirt yards, painted metal fences and walls, and vacant lots formerly containing lead-painted structures should be identified.

Occupational histories for all adults in the various dwellings should be taken to ascertain whether any are exposed to lead-bearing dusts. "Dusty" lead trades include, but are not limited to, the following occupations: secondary lead smelting

---

* PbB = μg lead/dl of whole blood.

† FEP = μg "free" protoporphyrin/dl erythrocytes. Analogous terms include zinc protoporphyrin (ZnP) and erythrocyte protoporphyrin (EP). Values are sometimes stated as concentration in whole blood rather than in erythrocytes.)

(recovery of lead from old storage batteries), lead scrap smelting, storage battery manufacturing and repair, metal founding, ship breaking, automobile assembly and body radiator repair, demolition of painted metal structures (bridges), and demolition and renovation of old housing and other structures. In the renovation and maintenance of older housing, the grinding, sanding, and burning of old paint poses an extremely serious hazard. If such workers wear their work clothing home, they contaminate their vehicles and the floors, carpets, and furniture of their homes with fine lead-bearing dusts. When such clothing is mixed with other clothing in the washing machine, lead may be transferred to the uncontaminated clothing. Workers should change their shoes and clothing and leave them for proper cleaning at their place of employment and should shower before coming home.

It is now recognized that exposure to lead-contaminated household dust and soil in outside play areas can account for most cases in which PbB is sustained in a range of 25–50 μg and that normal hand-to-mouth activity is the major route of entry of lead into the body. In old housing areas, weekly or more frequent scrubbing of not only floors but also of all woodwork (windows, doors, porches), as well as daily damp dusting of all surfaces a child can touch, is often effective in lowering a young child's PbB. Vacuuming, particularly wet vacuuming, is also helpful, but dry sweeping should be avoided, as it does not remove fine particulates. When lead in paint is found in the dwelling, many local ordinances require its removal. Although this is commonly done by burning with a gas torch and mechanical sanding, these procedures are contraindicated because they generate much dust, thus presenting an acute and potentially serious hazard not only to the worker but also to any infant or young child remaining in the house during the process. Under such conditions, it is not uncommon for a child's PbB to rise within a short time from <30 μg to >90 μg. Removal of lead paint with hot air guns, scrapers, and, wherever feasible, chemical removers presents a lesser hazard and is preferable. Even so, all infants and young children and pregnant and nursing women should find temporary "safe" residence elsewhere *day and night* until the entire "deleading" process is completed, the debris thoroughly removed by repeated wet cleaning, and the areas repainted with "lead-free" paint. All scaling old paint should also be removed. PbB should be determined frequently in the exposed child until the hazard is abated, since incomplete abatement, a common occurrence, is detected most often by a rise in the child's PbB. It is sometimes appropriate to determine PbB in all family members; if it is elevated in all, a common source, such as contamination of food, should be suspected.

In addition to ingestion of lead-bearing paint, severe symptomatic lead poisoning has been associated with the following: ingestion and retention in the stomach of metallic lead (fishing weights, curtain weights, shot); contamination of acidic foods and beverages from improperly lead-glazed ceramic pitchers, pots, and cups; burning of battery casings or lead-painted wood in the home; Asiatic cosmetics (Surma, Al Kohl); oriental folk medicines; Mexican folk remedies (azarcon, greta). Inhalation of fumes of leaded gasoline, which has been reported in American Indians, can cause a potentially fatal acute toxic encephalopathy.

Dietary Factors

Deficient dietary intake of calcium, magnesium, zinc, iron, and copper, as well as excessive dietary fat, increases the absorption, retention, and toxicity of lead. A diet adequate in these minerals and limited in fat should be assured. For those intolerant of cow's milk (sensitivity, intestinal lactase deficiency), "lactose-free" milk products or an alternative source is necessary to ensure adequate calcium intake. The use of low fat milk and the avoidance of fried foods and fatback should limit excessive dietary fat. Acidic foods such as fruits, fruit juices, tomatoes, sodas, and cola drinks may leach lead from the lead-soldered seams of cans. Dietary lead intake may be reduced if the above items are purchased fresh, frozen, or packaged in aluminum cans, other metal cans with welded seams, or glass, cardboard, or plastic containers. These dietary recommendations are used in all children with increased lead absorption (classes II, III, and IV). *Despite regulation of dietary factors, dust control is of much greater importance.* Children with sickle cell disease (hemoglobin SS) may have secondary zinc deficiency; in such cases, transfer to a safe housing area is likely to be the only effective measure.

Precautions in the Use of Chelating Agents

Edetate (EDTA) is not metabolized in the body but rather is excreted unchanged exclusively by glomerular filtration in the kidney. Calcium (Ca) EDTA but not dimercaprol (BAL) must be withheld during periods of anuria. Administration of CaEDTA at the dosage levels given (Table 1) must not exceed 5 successive days. Dosage should be reduced when glomerular filtration rate (GFR) is reduced, and the drug should probably be withheld in non–life-threatening situations when acute renal disease not due to lead is present. Untoward reactions to CaEDTA include the following: local reactions at injection site, hypercalcemia, elevated BUN, proteinuria, microscopic hematuria, and fever. If pretreatment serum chemistries show

Table 1. DOSAGE SCHEDULE FOR CHELATING AGENTS IN CHILDREN

BAL-CaEDTA in Combination

Dosage: BAL* 83 mg/m² of body surface area/dose (IM)
CaEDTA† 250 mg/m² of body surface area/dose (IM)

Administration: For the first dose, inject BAL (IM) only; beginning 4 hours later and every 4 hours thereafter for 5 days, inject BAL and CaEDTA simultaneously at separate and deep IM sites; rotate injection sites.

CaEDTA Only

Dosage: 500 mg/m² of body surface/dose q12hr (IM)

Administration: IM injection simpler in young children, but if IV route preferred, as in adults, infuse each dose over a 6-hour period; allow 1 week between each 5-day course of therapy.

D-Penicillamine‡

Dosage: 500 mg/m² of body surface area/day for long-term oral therapy

Administration: Give entire daily dose on empty stomach 2 hours before breakfast; contents of capsule may be mixed in a small amount of chilled fruit or fruit juice immediately prior to administration. Give 25 mg pyridoxine daily concurrently.

---

* BAL. The dosage recommended for adults by the FDA is 2.5 mg/kg of body weight/dose every 4 hours, which in "standard man" (70 kg, 1.73 m²) is equivalent to approximately 100 mg/m² of body surface area/dose, or about 20% higher than the dose recommended here for children.

† CaEDTA. Edathamil calcium-disodium (Versenate) is available in 20% solution. For IM use, add sufficient procaine to yield a final concentration of 0.5% procaine. IM injection is more convenient in children and permits better control of IV fluids, a vital consideration in cases of encephalopathy. It has been used in this clinic for 35 years without untoward incident. If given IV in combination with BAL, infuse the total daily dose (1500 mg/m² of body surface area) over 24 hours and monitor ECG continuously.

‡ D-Penicillamine. β, β-dimethylcysteine is available as Cuprimine in 125- and 250-mg capsules. It is approved for several uses, but is not approved for use in lead poisoning; see recommendations of AMA Council on Drugs.

---

evidence of hepatocellular injury (elevated SGPT, SGOT) or impaired renal function (elevated serum creatinine, urea nitrogen), chelation therapy should probably be withheld in asymptomatic cases. Carry out pretreatment and on the fifth day monitor serum creatinine, serum urea nitrogen, serum calcium, serum phosphorus, morning fasting plasma zinc and copper, and routine urinalysis. If any abnormalities are found, repeat this 2 and 3 days after a 5-day course of CaEDTA. Patients receiving CaEDTA IV should also be monitored by ECG for irregularities of cardiac rhythm. CaEDTA causes a substantial diuresis of zinc. If morning fasting plasma zinc has not rebounded to the normal range 3 days after therapy, consider oral zinc supplementation.

D-Penicillamine is contraindicated in children with renal disease and in those with a history of sensitivity to penicillin. Reactions to this drug can be minimized if oral dosage is restricted to ≤500 mg/m² of body surface/day. Patients who react to D-penicillamine usually do so within the first

month. Neutropenia, proteinuria, and hypersensitivity reactions (angioneurotic edema, Stevens-Johnson syndrome, thrombocytopenia, acute hemolysis) as well as erythematous rashes are contraindications to its further use. Since it also causes a modest diuresis of iron, zinc, and copper, these metals should be replaced by oral supplements not exceeding the recommended daily dietary allowances for these metals. Pyridoxine (25 mg/day) should be given concurrently.

BAL, which is limited to the treatment of acute encephalopathy and to those patients with PbB >100 μg, should not be given in the presence of severe hepatocellular injury. It is judicious to place patients receiving BAL on parenteral fluids, at least during the first 24 to 48 hours, and then advance them cautiously to clear oral liquids, in order to minimize vomiting, one of the troublesome side-effects of BAL. BAL may induce moderate to severe intravascular hemolysis in children with glucose-6-phosphate dehydrogenase (G6PD) deficiency. BAL may not be given concurrently with medicinal iron. Medicinal iron may be given concurrently with CaEDTA and D-penicillamine.

Management of Asymptomatic Cases with Increased Lead Absorption

Before treatment PbB and FEP values should be confirmed on a sample of venous blood, as 10% or more of fingerprick screening samples may be seriously contaminated by exogenous lead. For children in class II, dietary correction, vigorous treatment of iron deficiency, stringent dust control, separation of the child from circumscribed environmental lead sources, and close follow-up will suffice. Chelating agents are rarely used to treat this group. PbB and FEP are measured serially every 3 months for at least 18 months to determine responses to medicinal iron and whether the level of lead absorption is increasing, stable, or decreasing.

Indications for chelation therapy in children in class III are not firmly established. We have limited chelation therapy to children in this group who meet one or more of the following criteria: PbB ≥45–50 μg; 24-hr CaEDTA mobilization test ≥0.75 μg Pb excreted/1 mg CaEDTA administered; daily urinary output of coproporphyrin >250 μg/day, urinary δ-aminolevulinic acid output ≥3 mg/m²/day; or behavioral changes and mild nonspecific symptoms suggestive of early clinical plumbism. FEP is of no value in making decisions regarding chelation therapy. The initial 5-day course of CaEDTA only (Table 1) is given in a hospital or a convalescent pediatric facility, followed by either oral D-penicillamine or one to three additional 5-day courses of CaEDTA only. Discharge from the pediatric convalescent facility is keyed to the availability of "safe" housing for the child. PbB and FEP are always checked 2 to 3 weeks following discharge, and at 1- to 3-month intervals during the next 18 months or longer, including at least one summer during which PbB remains <30 µg or declines to the normal range. Administration of chelating agents to out-patients is rarely appropriate. It will not counteract the effects of continued excessive intake of lead and indeed may increase the absorption and retention of lead.

For children in class IV, the risk of serious acute toxicity is unacceptable. As the administration of the diagnostic CaEDTA mobilization test may be hazardous in these children, they are always treated with CaEDTA only (Table 1) for 5 days, and the first day's urinary output is used to determine the chelatable lead (µg Pb excreted/mg CaEDTA administered/day). BAL is not given to such patients unless symptoms are clearly evident or PbB is >100 µg. In such cases, BAL during the first 72 hours only should suffice. Further chelation therapy in this group is the same as that described for children in class III.

Treatment of Symptomatic Cases

Children with one or more of the following: persistent vomiting, ataxic gait, gross irritability, severe anemia, seizures, and alterations in the state of consciousness are treated as potential cases of acute encephalopathy. Symptomatic patients are maintained on parenteral fluids until symptoms abate.

Chelation therapy is started as soon as adequate urine flow is established. Initially, 10% dextrose in water (10–20 ml/kg of body weight) is given over a period of 1 to 2 hours). If this fails to initiate urination, mannitol* (1–2 gm/kg body weight) is infused IV in 20% solution at a rate of 1 ml/min. As soon as urine flow is established, further IV fluid therapy is restricted to basal water and electrolyte requirements, to a minimal estimate of the quantities required for replacement of deficits due to vomiting and dehydration and to increased requirements resulting from convulsive activity or intercurrent fever. Proper fluid therapy is vital to survival in encephalopathy and is best monitored by placing an indwelling catheter and measuring the rate of urine flow. The rate of infusion is adjusted hourly until a rate is found that maintains the rate of urine flow within basal metabolic limits (0.35 to 0.5 ml urine secreted/calorie metabolized/24 hr). This is equivalent to a daily urinary output of 350–500 ml/m²/day. Seizures are controlled initially with diazepam (Val-

ium)† and thereafter with running doses of paraldehyde during the first few days. Long-term anticonvulsive drugs, such as phenytoin sodium (Dilantin) and barbiturates, are begun toward the end of the first week of therapy while paraldehyde is being reduced. During the acute phase, one should not await the development of frank seizures; better control can be achieved if doses of paraldehyde are given whenever there is a palpable increase in muscle tone or muscle twitching. Body temperature is maintained at normal but not at hypothermic levels.

Chelation therapy with BAL and CaEDTA is given according to the dosage schedule for combined therapy in Table 1. The usual 5-day course may be cautiously extended to 7 days if clinical evidence of encephalopathy persists beyond 4 days. Serial PbB measurements should be made after the last doses of BAL and CaEDTA and at 7, 14, and 21 days thereafter, as PbB generally rebounds following brief courses of chelation therapy. If PbB rebounds to >40 µg Pb, one or more additional 5-day course of CaEDTA only is indicated. If a convalescent pediatric facility is available, rebound may sometimes be minimized if the initial course of BAL and CaEDTA is followed by oral D-penicillamine.

In symptomatic cases, no time is wasted in attempts to evacuate residual lead from the bowel by enema, as enemas are often ineffectual, and the attendant delay may further jeopardize the child's life. Surgical decompression for relief of increased intracranial pressure is contraindicated. The role of steroids in combating cerebral edema in acute lead encephalopathy is not clear. Asymptomatic cases with PbB ≤100 µg are treated for the first 3 days with a BAL-CaEDTA combination, after which BAL is dropped, and CaEDTA only is continued in reduced dosage (500 mg/m² of body surface q 12 h 1M) for an additional 2 days. For those with PbB <100 µg and mild or questionable symptoms, treatment with CaEDTA only (Table 1) should suffice.

Long-term Management

At the outset of treatment a long-term plan of management is developed to meet the needs of each specific child. Age, the intensity of hand-to-mouth activity, pica, and family composition and resources, as well as environmental exposure and laboratory data, are taken into account in developing such a plan. The aim is to minimize recurrences, to curb pica, and if paint is the major problem, to find a safe dwelling for the family.

---

* Manufacturer's precaution: Use of mannitol in pediatric patients has not been studied comprehensively.

† Manufacturer's precaution: The safety and efficacy of injectable diazepam in children under 12 years of age have not been established. Oral diazepam is not to be used in children under 6 months of age.

When the child's principal guardian is highly motivated and has the time, the behavioral psychologist may be able to devise a plan that will minimize pica and other highly repetitive hand-to-mouth activity. All pediatric housemates of index cases should be examined. Class III and IV cases should be reported to the medical-social service for assistance in the housing, financial, and emotional problems that such families usually have. Ideally, the level of lead absorption should be reduced so that PbB falls within a few months to 25 μg Pb. In old, dilapidated housing areas in the United States this is beyond the practical realm. Very poor families simply cannot afford "safe" housing. At the very least, PbB should be maintained at <45 to 50 μg Pb to reduce the degree of impairment that subsequently may impede the child's progress in school.

For children with long-sustained PbB in excess of 50 μg Pb or recurrent episodes of clinical plumbism, and survivors of encephalopathy, prolonged follow-up for at least 6 years is mandatory. Phenobarbital and phenytoin are generally adequate for control of seizures; recurrence of seizures without recurrent excess lead ingestion is usually indicative of a lapse in medication or failure to increase the dose in accordance with growth. For children in classes III and IV, follow-up psychometric evaluation should be carried out between 4 and 6 years of age to facilitate appropriate school placement for those in whom learning impediments are identified. When clinical evaluation and follow-up psychometric testing indicate no significant long-lasting impediments, parents should be reassured.

Iron Poisoning

ARNOLD H. EINHORN, M.D.

Childhood poisonings due to the accidental ingestion of iron-containing hematinics or vitamin preparations remain common despite increased public awareness and improved safety packaging. Such medications are widely used and readily available without prescription, not only at pharmacies but also at food and discount stores. Many are marketed in the form of brightly colored and dangerously attractive pills or tablets suggesting candies.

The toxicity of any medicinal iron-containing compound is directly related to its elemental iron composition, which may differ widely among various products. Ferrous sulfate, the salt most widely prescribed and the ingredient most often involved in childhood poisonings, contains 20% of elemental iron; preparations with gluconate (12% of elemental iron) or fumarate (33% of elemental

iron) salts are also used frequently. Ferric salts (phosphate, pyrophosphate, ammonium citrate) are less commonly prescribed and are less dangerous.

Toxicity

Normally the mucosal cells of the small intestine effectively control both the absorption and the elimination of dietary iron or small excesses of iron intake. Incorporated into ferritin, modest iron surpluses are either eliminated in the stools or absorbed after conversion from ferrous (divalent) to ferric (trivalent) iron that combines with apoferritin to form ferritin. This physiologic regulatory mechanism is inoperative when overwhelmed by excessive amounts of iron. The massive ingestion of iron may be fatal in untreated patients, and in survivors may cause both early and delayed morbidity that is primarily gastrointestinal, circulatory, hepatic, cerebral, and metabolic. Minimal toxic dose and minimal lethal dose of iron overdose for a child have not been clearly determined. The mean lethal dose has been estimated at 300 mg per kg of elemental iron, but toddlers have died after ingesting as little as 200 mg of elemental iron (less than 5 tablets of ferrous sulfate); on the other hand, recoveries have been reported in children from as much as 15 gm (3000 of elemental iron). However both mortality and morbidity have considerably been reduced in the last two decades as a result of the institution of improved therapy.

The clinical manifestations that may be fatal, albeit rarely, characteristically progress in three phases:

The first phase of hemorrhagic gastroenteritis and acidemia usually begins within 30 to 60 minutes after ingestion, with emesis frequently bloody and diarrhea also often hemorrhagic. Hemoconcentration with blood hyperviscosity, metabolic acidemia, dehydration, circulatory collapse may develop concurrently or may follow the hemorrhagic gastroenteritis within 4 to 6 hours. The patient with severe clinical toxicity who receives no specific treatment and who survives may improve either spontaneously or in response to supportive therapy.

If no symptoms appear within the first 6 to 12 hours after toxic iron ingestion or are limited to very mild gastrointestinal disturbances, it is unlikely that the course will progress further and such patients may be discharged.

The second "asymptomatic" phase is one of relative improvement, which is frequently misleading, lasting for 6 to 24 hours, during which symptoms subside or are minimal.

A critical third phase may develop about 24 to 48 hours after ingestion, characterized by progressive or rapid onset of shock, jaundice, and hepatic failure, bleeding diathesis, coma, or convulsions. Appropriate supportive and specific treatment during the first phase may prevent this delayed third phase, which may be fatal.

There may be a fourth phase of delayed gastrointestinal complication with pyloric stenosis or obstruction secondary to gastric scarring, which may develop within 1 to 2 months after recovery from the acute illness. Postintoxication liver cirrhosis is not seen in children.

Treatment

Treatment includes prompt emptying of gastric contents and measures minimizing further absorption of ingested iron; supportive therapy for preventing and correcting shock, dehydration, acidemia, and blood loss; maintaining airway ventilation and oxygenation; sustaining renal function; and chelation with deferoxamine (DFO) in severe intoxications.

Gastric Evacuation and Neutralization. Pharmacologic induction of vomiting with 15 ml of Ipecac Syrup should be limited to the first 30 minutes after ingestion provided the child has had no bloody vomitus and should be followed by gastric lavage through a large-bore orogastric tube of sufficient size to permit passage of any undissolved tablets. Beyond the first 30 minutes after ingestion, induction of emesis may be dangerous because of the corrosive effects of iron on the gastrointestinal mucosa; lavage without emesis is then preferable using a 1% sodium bicarbonate solution.

Gastric lavage should be followed by a radiographic examination of the abdomen to ascertain whether the procedure has been successful in removing the tablets. In exceptional instances where repeated gastric lavages proved fruitless to remove clumps of imbedded tablets gastrostomy has been necessary. Alkalinization of the gastric contents binds the iron salt into a noncorrosive, insoluble nonabsorbable ferrous carbonate precipitate. After the lavage is completed, 150 ml of 1% sodium bicarbonate should be left in the stomach to neutralize any residual iron. Iron salts are not absorbed effectively by activated charcoal. In the past, intragastric instillation of disodium phosphate dihydrate (Fleet phosphate) solution diluted 1:4 was recommended to bind the iron salt. Because of the potential danger of hyperphosphatemic convulsions, hypocalcemia, hyperosmolar dehydration, hypokalemia, and central nervous system disturbances secondary to treatment with undiluted solution, the use of sodium diphosphate solution is no longer recommended.

If there is profuse diarrhea, rectal lavage with the bicarbonate solution may prevent further damage to the rectal sigmoid mucosa by the iron fragments.

Supportive Therapy. Whether the patient is symptomatic or not, if the number of tablets ingested is five or more, or unknown, intravenous fluids should be started to prevent or correct acidemia and dehydration and to maintain renal function. The hydrating solution should contain at least 1 to 2 mEq/kg of sodium bicarbonate. Colloid solutions, plasma analogs, blood, and catecholamines may be required to combat peripheral vascular collapse. Fresh frozen plasma or plasma components, platelets, and vitamin K may be essential in the presence of disseminated intravascular coagulopathy. If there are any nervous system manifestation or threat thereof, measures to ensure airway patency and maintain ventilation and oxygenation must be instituted at once. Excretion of ferrioxamine, the end product of chelated iron depends upon maintenance of a satisfactory urine output, which will not take place without adequate correction of the hypovolemia and the acidemia.

Chelation. Deferoxamine (DFO) is a highly effective iron-binding compound that has been used with good results in severe iron intoxication. The chelating agent, specific for iron, is a siderochrome of microbial origin. In vitro its iron-binding capacity exceeds that of transferrin. Deferoxamine combines with iron to form ferrioxamine, which is excreted largely in the urine except for a small proportion that is metabolized in the body. The soluble DFO hydrochloride or mesylate salt binds 9.3 mg of trivalent iron per 100 mg of chelate. Whereas iron salts do not dialyse well, extracorporeal hemodialysis will remove effectively ferrioxamine in the presence of inadequate renal function.

Parenteral treatment with DFO should be restricted to subjects with severe iron intoxication because of the potential toxicity of the iron complex ferrioxamine. The iron toxicity should be regarded as severe if the amount of ingested iron is known to exceed 25 mg per kilo of elemental iron, that is, five tablets or more of ferrous sulfate tablets by a toddler, or the serum iron concentration (normally 65–75 μg/dl) exceeds 350 μg/dl within four to six hours after the ingestion or exceeds the total iron-binding capacity by 50 μg. Serum iron levels tend to decline from 4 to 6 hours after ingestion regardless of the amount taken; a serum iron level less than 300 μg/dl in a sample obtained beyond this time interval does not rule out serious intoxication.

An intravenous DFO challenge of 15 mg/kg/hr administered over one hour in 50 ml of 5% dextrose in water should be administered to all patients who have ingested either an unknown quantity of iron salts or are known to have ingested five tablets of the ferrous salt or more, have been symptomatic in the first 6 hours of ingestion or are either seen after 6 hours of ingestion or in a situation in which iron levels and total iron-binding capacity are not readily available. After fluids are given to ensure adequate renal function, the passage of a urine of rosé, orange, or reddish brown color signals the presence of iron as ferrioxamine in the urine and is an indication for instituting parenteral DFO therapy at once.

Other clinical and laboratory clues that indicate severity of intoxication include severe or bloody emesis, bloody diarrhea, persistence of radiographic opacities after emesis and lavage, fever and leukocytosis exceeding 15,000, hemoconcentration, hypotension and hypoperfusion, hematologic evidence of coagulopathy, clinical and laboratory evidence of liver failure, including jaundice, hypoglycemia and normal liver function tests, and evidence of obtundation or convulsions. All patients who manifest features reflecting potential severity within the first six hours after ingestions require gross monitoring of the circulatory, neurologic, hepatic, renal, hematologic, and acid base status based on clinical and laboratory parameters.

The recommended intravenous dose of DFO is 15 mg/kg/hr to be given for 6 hours in a solution of 200 ml of 5% dextrose in water. As long as the color of the urine continues to be vin rosé, orange, or reddish brown, additional intravenous courses of 15 mg/kg of DFO are to be given, usually in 6-hour courses separated by an interval of several hours. The DFO is not to be administered more rapidly than 15 mg/kg/hr; adverse reactions from the drug such as hypotension, irritability, and convulsions were reported in the past when the drug was given rapidly or in combination with large amounts of oral deferoxamine. These untoward effects virtually disappeared when both the oral therapy and the rapid infusion of the chelating agents were discontinued. In less severe poisoning the intramuscular route is also effective, provided the patient is normotensive and presents only mild manifestations of poisoning. The recommended IM dose of DFO is 10 mg/kg/hr up to a total of 1.0 gm every 4 to 6 hours for a total of 4 gm/24 hr. Oral therapy with deferoxamine is contraindicated except when the serum iron level exceeds several thousand micrograms and the need to remove with extreme speed all residual iron from the stomach outweighs by far the inherent toxicity of oral DFO. When given orally, DFO does not prevent the absorption of iron from the intestinal tract; toxicity may result from the passage into the circulation of large quantities of the chelate complex ferrioxamine. However, when serum iron levels exceed several thousand μg/dl, gastric lavage has been recommended with a solution containing 2 gm of DFO mesylate per liter of water and sufficient sodium bicarbonate to alkalinize the gastric contents and increase the DFO complexation of iron. We do not recommend, however, that after lavage DFO be left in the stomach. In the patient with oliguria and anuria secondary to hypotension and circulatory collapse hemodialysis or exchange transfusion may be required to remove the chelated iron complex ferrioxamine.

Prevention

The most effective means of reducing the needless morbidity and potential fatalities from iron poisoning is prevention rather than treatment. Iron preparations often find their way into the home, as prenatal therapy, as a mineral supplement of an elderly member of the household, or as incorporated in vitamin preparations, some of which are fruit flavored, animal shaped, and chewable. Especially attractive to small children are chewable vitamin wafers that represent popular cartoon characters. Marketed in bottles containing as many as 250 tablets and available without prescription and without a danger warning, they are usually considered safe by parents. Proper labeling and educational measures directed to physicians, pharmacists, and parents are necessary to counteract the problem created by the attractive formulation and accessibility of iron-containing medications, which combined with the natural curiosity of children, are the major factors that create this serious problem. As has been emphasized by Robotham and Lietman (1980) "an ounce of prevention is worth more than a pound of deferoxamine."

Insect Stings

DAVID F. GRAFT, M.D.

Systemic anaphylaxis resulting from the stings of insects of the order Hymenoptera (honeybees, yellow jackets, hornets, and wasps) affects 1% of children and may be mild, with only cutaneous symptoms (pruritus, urticaria, angioedema), or severe, with potentially life-threatening symptoms (laryngeal edema, bronchospasm, hypotension). Of the 40 deaths per year in this country attributed to insect stings, only one or two occur in children. A large local reaction may occur in up to 10% of individuals and consists of swelling greater than 2 inches (5 cm) in diameter that persists for longer than 1 day.

Acute Management. Individuals presenting with anaphylaxis require careful observation. A subcutaneous injection of aqueous epinephrine (1:1000) at a dose of 0.01 ml/kg (maximum 0.3 ml) is the cornerstone of management and often will be sufficient to terminate a reaction. This may be repeated in 10 to 15 minutes if necessary. Oral antihistamines such as diphenhydramine hydrochloride (Benadryl, 1–2 mg/kg) or chlorpheniramine (2–4 mg/kg) are also usually given. They

Table 1. EPINEPHRINE INJECTION KITS FOR EMERGENCY SELF-TREATMENT OF SYSTEMIC REACTIONS TO INSECT STINGS

Injection Kit	Dosage
EpiPen*	Delivers 0.3 ml 1:1000 (0.3 mg epinephrine)
EpiPen Jr.*	Delivers 0.3 ml 1:2000 (0.15 mg epinephrine)
Ana-Kit†	Delivers up to 0.6 ml 1:1000 (0.3 ml at one time, total 0.6 mg epinephrine)

* The EpiPen and EpiPen Jr. are spring-loaded automatic injectors and are distributed by Center Laboratories, Port Washington, New York.

† Ana-Kit is capable of delivering fractional doses and is distributed by Hollister-Stier Laboratories, Spokane, Washington.

may lessen urticaria or other cutaneous symptoms, but in more serious or progressive reactions, their use should not retard the administration of epinephrine.

Inhaled sympathomimetic agents such as isoproterenol may decrease bronchoconstriction but will not address other systemic manifestations such as shock. Aminophylline is the drug of choice if bronchoconstriction persists following epinephrine. Severe reactions may require treatment with oxygen, volume expanders, and pressor agents. Corticosteroids such as prednisone (0.5–1 mg/kg/day) are often used, but their delayed onset of action (4–6 hr) limits their effectiveness in the early stages of treatment.

Systemic reactions commencing more than several hours after a sting usually manifest only cutaneous symptoms. Most are easily managed with oral antihistamines and observation. Treatment recommendations for large local reactions include ice, elevation, and antihistamines. A short course of prednisone (0.5–1 mg/kg/day for 5 days), especially if initiated immediately after the sting, may be the best treatment for massive large local reactions. Controlled studies in progress will help to resolve this issue.

Decreasing Future Reactions

Preventing Stings. Since many stings occur when a child steps on a bee, shoes should always be worn when outside. Hives and nests around the home should be exterminated. Good sanitation should be practiced, since garbage and outdoor food, especially canned drinks, will attract yellow jackets. Brightly colored clothing and perfumes should be avoided.

Emergency Epinephrine. To encourage prompt treatment, epinephrine is available in emergency kits for self-administration (Table 1). These are used immediately after the sting to allow the patient the time to get to a medical facility. The Ana-Kit contains a preloaded syringe that can deliver two 0.3-ml doses of epinephrine. Smaller doses may also be given. The physician who prescribes this kit must provide thorough instruction and must be confident that the patient can perform the injection procedure. These kits can be confusing to nonmedical personnel, and some patients have a tremendous fear of needles. A practice self-injection with saline will resolve this question. The newer EpiPen (0.3 mg epinephrine) and EpiPen Jr. (equivalent of 0.15 mg epinephrine, 1:1000) offer a concealed needle and a pressure-sensitive spring-loaded injection device that make them suited for children and families who are uncomfortable with the injection process.

In general, a child who is stung should receive an antihistamine and be watched for 1 hour. If any signs of a generalized (systemic) reaction occur, epinephrine should be administered, and the child should be seen by a physician. If no systemic signs occur in the first hour, the child may resume regular activities. Children who are receiving maintenance injections of venom immunotherapy (see the following) are advised that emergency self-treatment will probably not be required; however, they should have the kit available if they are far from medical facilities.

Venom Immunotherapy (Table 2). A child who has experienced a sting-induced systemic reaction should be referred to an allergist, who will perform skin tests with dilute solutions of honeybee, yellow jacket, yellow hornet, white-faced hornet, and *Polistes* wasp venoms. Radioallergosorbent testing (RAST) cannot replace venom skin testing but may provide additional information. If the reaction was severe (life-threatening—bronchospasm, laryngeal edema, shock) and the venom testing is positive, immunotherapy with the appropriate venoms is commenced. Increasing amounts of venom are given weekly for several months until a 100-mcg dose (equals two stings) is reached. Maintenance injections are given every 6 weeks after the first year of treatment. Venom therapy is highly effective, protecting 97% of patients from reactions to in-hospital challenge stings.

The disadvantages of venom treatment include high cost, systemic and local reactions to injections, and the unknown length of therapy. No long-term side effects have been reported. About 25% of patients develop negative skin tests after 3 to 5 years of treatment and may be candidates for discontinuing therapy. Prior to the mid-1970's, nearly all insect-allergic individuals were treated with mixed whole-body extract (WBE). However, this therapy has been shown to be only as effective as placebo, and consequently it should not be used.

Recently, children with milder cutaneous systemic reactions were studied prospectively for 4 years. Since only 10% of untreated children had systemic reactions (all of which were again mild in

Table 2. SELECTION OF PATIENTS FOR VENOM IMMUNOTHERAPY

Sting Reaction	Skin test/RAST	Venom Immunother- apy
1. Systemic, non-life-threatening (child): immediate, generalized, confined to skin (urticaria, angioedema, erythema, pruritis)	+ or −	No
2. Systemic, life-threatening (child): immediate, generalized, may involve cutaneous symptoms but also has respiratory (laryngeal edema or bronchospasm) or cardiovascular symptoms (hypotension/shock)	+	Yes
3. Systemic (adult)	+	Yes
4. Systemic	−	No

5. Large local
    >2 inches (5 cm) in diameter
    >24 hours
	+ or −	No

6. Normal <2 inches (5 cm) in diameter <24 hours	+ or −	No

severity) when they were restung, the authors concluded that venom immunotherapy was not routinely indicated for this group. Children with large local reactions or negative skin tests are not candidates for venom treatment.

Arthropod Bites and Stings

BERNARD A. COHEN, M.D.

Arthropod bites and stings are a major cause of morbidity in infants and children and account for 65% of all deaths from venomous animals in this country. These ubiquitous organisms are elongated invertebrates with segmented bodies, true appendages, and chitinous exoskeletons. Arthropods of importance to physicians include millipedes and centipedes, the eight-legged arachnids (scorpions, spiders, ticks, and mites), and five-legged insects (lice, blister beetles, bed bugs, bees, wasps, ants, fleas, moths, butterflies, flies, and mosquitoes).

MILLIPEDES (DIPLOPODA) AND CENTIPEDES (CHILOPODA)

Although superficially similar, millipedes are vegetarian feeders and centipedes are carnivorous. When handled, millipedes exude a defensive fluid, which may produce immediate burning, erythema, and edema that progresses to vesicles, bullae, and erosions.

Although all centipedes contain poison glands, and some bites result in severe systemic symptoms, in the United States reactions to envenomation are limited to a transient sharp pain at the site. *Treatment*: Irritant reactions and bites can be treated with cool tap water compresses or topical steroids. In severe reactions, prednisone 1 mg/kg/day tapered over 10–14 days, can be used.

ARACHNIDS

Arthropods of this class are recognized by their fused cephalothorax and four pairs of legs. Medically important orders include scorpions, spiders, ticks, and mites.

Scorpions. Scorpions are nocturnal tropical arachnids and are readily identified by their stout pinching claws, elongated abdomen, and narrow tail, which ends in a conspicuous bulblike stinger that it swings over the head to attack prey. Poisonous species in North America are restricted to the deserts of the American Southwest and Mexico. They remain hidden in garages, basements, closets, crevices, and gravel. When accidentally provoked, they will bite, producing a hemolytic reaction consisting of localized burning, swelling, purpura, necrosis, and lymphadenitis. Occasionally a more severe neurotoxic reaction results in nausea, lacrimation, diaphoresis, abdominal cramps, restlessness, and rarely, in small children shock, seizures, and death. Children under 3 years of age account for 75% of all deaths from scorpion stings.

TREATMENT. In mild reactions, cool compresses, topical steroids, and anithistamines will provide symptomatic relief. In severe reactions, local measures, including the application of ice to the bite and a tourniquet proximal to the sting may be helpful until a specific antiserum can be administered. In infested areas, creosote or other repellents may be applied to basements, garages, and out buildings; and shoes, boots, and clothing should be inspected carefully before dressing.

Spiders (Araneae). Spiders are distinguished from other anthropods by their compact cephalothorax and large baglike abdomen. The majority of encounters in North American occur with the black widow (*Latrodectus mactans*), a web spinner that prepares its trap across privy seats and cool dark sites in vacant buildings. The female is very aggressive, attacking humans with little provocation, and may be recognized by her red ventral hourglass markings. Local reactions to bites may be painful but are often unnoticed and sometimes followed within 30 minutes by dizziness, nausea, diaphoresis, lacrimation, muscular rigidity, tremors, paresthesias, and headaches. The number of bites is estimated at 500 each year, with a mortality rate of 1% overall and approaching 5% in small children. Symptoms in nonfatal cases increase in severity for several hours, perhaps a day, and slowly dissipate in 2–3 days.

TREATMENT. Prompt treatment with specific antiserum is required for relief of symptoms, especially in children (Antivenin, Merck Sharp & Dohme). After a skin or conjunctival test for horse serum sensitivity, one vial of antivenom reconstituted in 2.5 cc of diluent is administered intramuscularly, or the antivenom may be given intravenously in 10–50 cc of saline over 15 minutes.

Other supportive measures include warm baths, intravenous injections of 10 cc of 10% calcium gluconate, morphine, and barbiturates as needed for control of muscle pain and cramps. In healthy adults and older children antivenom may be deferred pending results of therapy with muscle relaxants and analgesics. Methocarbamol* (Robaxin injectable and tablets), is a useful alternative muscle relaxant, and 10 cc should be administered over 5 minutes followed by 10 cc in 250 cc of 5% dextrose water at 1 cc a minute. When the patient is improved or if the reaction is mild, methocarbamol, 800 mg every 6 hours, may be given orally.

Brown Recluse (*Loxosceles reclusa*). Slightly smaller than the black widow, the brown recluse spans an overall diameter of 3–4 cm with a body 10–12 mm long and 4 mm wide. It abounds in the south central United States, where it can be distinguished from other brown spiders by its characteristic dark brown violin-shaped band extending from the eyes to the end of the cephalothorax. Although occasionally producing a fatal systemic reaction in young children, loxoscelism is characterized by a gangrenous slough at the bite site. Local pain appears 2–8 hours after the attack followed by an area of erythema, which develops a necrotic central bulla surrounded by an irregular area of purpura. Over 7–14 days necrosis progresses from a well-demarcated eschar to ulceration up to 20 cm in diameter.

TREATMENT. No specific antivenom is available in the United States for treatment of brown recluse spider bites. Antihistamines should be used to treat urticarial reactions, and antibiotics may be initiated if secondary infection develops. The use of steroids is controversial, but some experts recommend immediate administration of systemic corticosteroids as soon as the diagnosis is entertained. Intralesional steroids (4 mg of dexamethasone) may be helpful and can be repeated if the lesion continues to increase in size. Large ulcers usually require excision and skin grafting. Semipermeable or occlusive dressings (Duoderm, Vigilon, Opsite) may be applied to facilitate healing.

Ticks (Acari). Ticks are blood-sucking arachnids with short legs and a leathery integument. They are important vectors for a number of rickettsial and viral disorders and erythema chronicum migrans. Tick bite pyrexia and tick paralysis are produced by a toxin elaborated by the female tick and are promptly relieved by removal of the tick.

Typically tick bites go unnoticed for several days until a pruritic red papule with a red halo develops at the site. These lesions may resolve in several weeks unless the tick mouth parts are left in place, resulting in a foreign body reaction, which may persist for months. Erythema chronicum migrans is a peculiar eruption produced by a spirochete transmitted by the bite of the *Ixodes dammini* tick. Three to 20 days after a bite from an infected tick, an expanding indurated annular red plaque with central clearing up to 20 cm in diameter appears at the site. The rash occurs most commonly in children and may be associated with a rhematoid factor–negative oligoarticular arthritis (Lyme arthritis), meningoencephalitis, and myocarditis.

TREATMENT. Individuals who have spent time in infested wooded and grassy areas should be carefully inspected daily and all ticks removed immediately. Once the ticks have become embedded in the skin, techniques for removal include application of a hot unlighted match, petrolatum, liquid nitrogen, chloroform, nail polish remover, ethyl chloride spray, and mineral oil. Residual mouth parts are readily removed by skin punch biopsy.

Persistent symptomatic bite reactions will improve with intralesional steroid injections of triamcinolone 0.1 cc of 5–10 mg/cc. Erythema chronicum migrans and its associated symptoms may be aborted with oral penicillin or tetracycline,† 250 mg four times daily for two weeks.

Mites (Acari). Infestations with the human *Sarcoptes scabiei* mite has reached epidemic proportions in some communities. It spares no age or socioeconomic group and has been identified as a significant medical problem in schools and day care centers and among promiscuous teenagers and adults. The eruption is asymptomatic for weeks to months until the individual becomes sensitized to the mite or its waste products. Papules, vesicles, pustules, and burrows are characteristically found on the wrists, finger webs, axillae,

---

* Safety and efficacy for use in children under 12 years of age have not been established except in tetanus.

† Use of tetracycline in children less than 8 years of age may cause discoloration of permanent teeth.

genitals, breasts, and buttocks. The scalp, palms, and soles are also involved in infants and toddlers. A generalized eczematous eruption may occur in sensitized individuals and overshadow the characteristic lesion, making diagnosis difficult. Diagnosis requires demonstration of mites, eggs, or fecal material from skin scrapings.

TREATMENT. The treatment of choice is 1% gamma benzene hexachloride (Scabene, Kwell), but its use in young children is controversial. Percutaneous absorption of the drug can be reduced by restricting therapy to a single 6–8-hour application without a preceding bath and followed by thorough cleansing. Therapy should be repeated in one week only if live mites can still be demonstrated. All members of the household should be treated, but prescriptions must be limited to 1 ounce per person per treatment. Alternative therapies for pregnant individuals and infants include 6% precipitated sulfur in petrolatum and 10% crotamiton (Eurax) cream or lotion applied daily for three days.

Clothing and bedsheets should be laundered in hot water, but extensive treatment of fomites is not necessary, because the mites are dormant at room temperature.

Pruritus, which may last for weeks despite adequate therapy, should be treated with cool baths, emollients, and antihistamines such as hydroxyzine 2–5 mg/kg/day divided every 6 hours or diphenhydramine 5 mg/kg/day divided every 6 hours.

Other Mites. Children are also commonly infested with animal mites from dogs, cats, mice, and birds. A self-limited itchy papular eruption appears on exposed areas of the arms, legs, and trunk. Harvest mites (red bugs, chiggers) are frequently encountered in parks and grassy areas. Pruritic red papules and nodules with central hemorrhagic puncta appear at sites where the mite larvae are caught in clothing, such as at the waist band, sock bands, and underwear. The larvae are removed inadvertently by scratching, and pruritus wanes over 5–7 days.

TREATMENT. Symptomatic therapy includes topical corticosteroids, shake lotions (calamine), cool compresses, antihistamines, and in severe cases systemic corticosteroids (prednisone 0.5–1 mg/kg/day tapered over 10–14 days).

Effective prophylaxis can be achieved with insect repellants sprayed onto clothing, including diethyltoluamide (DEET), ethyl hexanediol, dimethyl phthalate, dimethyl carbate, and benzyl benzoate.

INSECTS

Insects are ubiquitous six-legged arthropods with well-defined body segments, including a head, thorax, and abdomen. Organisms of medical significance include bees, wasps, and ants (Hymenoptera, see page 673), lice (Anoplura), blister beetles (Coleoptera), bed bugs and kissing bugs (Heteroptera), fleas (Siphonaptera), moths and butterflies (Lepidoptera), and flies and mosquitoes (Diptera).

Pediculosis. Human lice are a major public health problem, especially in areas of overcrowding or where facilities are inadequate for keeping people and clothing clean. Pediculosis occurs in three clinical forms: head and body lice infestations produced by two interbreeding varieties of *Pediculus humanus* with characteristic elongated abdomens, and pubic lice caused by *Phthirus pubis* or the crab louse, which has a short hairy abdomen and two pairs of crablike claws anteriorly. Lice are acquired through close contact with infested individuals or fomites.

PEDICULUS HUMANUS CAPITIS. Head lice are seen almost exclusively in girls and women. Lice may be identified on the scalp, and nits are seen about 1 inch from the surface, particularly in the postauricular and occipital areas. Pruritus is intense, and secondary infection is common.

Treatment. Patients should be instructed to vigorously lather the scalp and adjacent hairy areas with 1% gamabenzene hexachloride (Kwell) shampoo for 5 minutes and then rinse thoroughly. Remaining nits may be removed with a fine tooth comb. The nits may be loosened by application of a solution of equal parts white vinegar and water. Retreatment may be necessary in one week because some nits may survive the initial application. Pyrethrins (Rid, R & C shampoo) are effective alternatives, and generally retreatment is not required.

PEDICULUS HUMANUS HUMANUS. The body louse hides in the seams of clothing and produces tiny itchy papules and wheals, particularly in the interscapular, shoulder, and wrist regions.

Treatment. Infestation is effectively treated by laundering of clothing and bedding with hot water.

PHTHIRUS PUBIS. Crab louse infestation has become epidemic among promiscuous teenagers and adults. The insects are readily identified as grayish spots clinging to the skin in the genital area. Lice and nits may also spread to other hair-bearing areas, including the chest, axillae, and eyelashes. Maculae caeruleae are greenish blue patches produced by bites on the chest, abdomen, and thighs of infested individuals.

Treatment. A 1% gamabenzene hexacholoride lotion should be applied to involved areas, except for the eyelashes, left on for 8–12 hours, and then thoroughly rinsed. Pyrethrin lotions should be massaged onto infested areas and then rinsed after 10 minutes. Pediculosis of the eyelashes can be safely treated with petrolatum applied twice daily for 7–10 days followed by mechanical removal of nits.

Blister Beetles (Meloidae). Blister beetles contain cantharidin, a volatile substance that produces an intraepidermal vesicle when the insects alight on the skin or are inadvertently crushed. Blister beetle dermatosis consisting of a linear vesicular eruption is common during the summer months when the insects are most plentiful.

TREATMENT. Lesions should be left intact to heal spontaneously in 3–4 days. Large lesions (greater than 1 cm) may be drained and compressed with aluminum acetate (Burow's, Blueboro) solution.

Bed Bugs (Cimex lectularius). Bedbugs are reddish-brown blood-sucking insects that hide in crevices in floors and walls and feed on unsuspecting victims at night. Although they are a disappearing nuisance, they are still seen occasionally in older, less affluent areas. Although most individuals sleep through the attack, sensitive victims awaken during the bloodmeal, which lasts 5–10 minutes. The bite is followed by an urticarial plaque, which may persist for weeks and become reactivated by subsequent bites at other sites. Lesions appear most commonly on the face and other areas not protected by clothing.

TREATMENT. The bugs are effectively eradicated from the home with insecticides such as chlordane, gamabenzene hexachloride, or hexachlorocyclohexane. Symptomatic relief may be obtained from cool compresses, topical corticosteroids, and oral antihistamines.

Kissing Bugs (Reduviidae). Although most of these insects prey upon other insects, earning them the name "assassin bug," 75 species attack man. Bites occur frequently on the face particularly at a mucocutaneous juncture and result in various reactions, including red papules, giant urticaria, grouped vesicles, and hemorrhagic nodular lesions.

TREATMENT. Treatment is symptomatic. Insecticides and repellents are not effective.

Fleas (Siphonaptera). Fleas are a common nuisance for humans and animals. Although there are only two parasites that are consistently associated with man, *Pulex irritans* and *Tunga penetrans*, fleas are only partially host specific, and cat and dog ectoparasites commonly attack man. The bite may go unnnoticed, but sensitized individuals may discover pruritic urticarial wheals with a central hemorrhagic punctum. Multiple lesions in a linear or roseate pattern are typical.

Papular urticaria, a pruritic urticarial eruption at sites of fresh and old reactivated flea bites, occurs almost exclusively in children. Individual papules persist for 1–2 weeks and are found on exposed areas of the arms, legs, and trunk, sparing the buttocks and genitals. Lesions tend to recur in spring and summer but may persist year round for 3–4 years.

TREATMENT. Acute reactions are relieved with shake lotions (calamine), topical steroids, cool tap water compresses, and oral antihistamines. Impe-

tiginized lesions should be treated with topical or oral antibiotics if necessary. Fleas may be eliminated by the removal or treatment of infested pets and vacuuming and spraying of carpets, floors, and other infested areas with 5% malathion powder or 1% lindane dust. Despite these measures fleas may survive in the household for months.

Moths and Butterflies (Lepidoptera). Contact with the hairs of the brown tail moth indigenous to the Northeastern United States and the puss caterpillar found in the Southeastern states from Virginia to the Gulf of Mexico may produce a burning papular eruption and occasionally a severe systemic reaction.

TREATMENT. Tape stripping to remove embedded hair reduces local reactions. Systemic reactions such as muscle cramps, headache, tachycardia, restlessness, and rarely shock and seizures require supportive therapy with antihistamines, systemic steroids, and parenteral calcium gluconate.

Flies and Mosquitoes (Diptera). These ubiquitous insects are important vectors in the transmission of viral and parasitic diseases. Mosquitoes (Culicidae) attack exposed sites on the face and extremities, producing pruritic urticarial plaques that persist for hours. Sandflies, moth flies, or owl flies (Psychodidae) bite silently, seeking out the ankles, wrist, knees, and elbows, and produce white wheals, which resolve over several days. Black flies (Simuliidae) horseflies (Tabanidae), and houseflies (Muscidae) attack silently and inflict a painful bite.

TREATMENT. Bite reactions are relieved with antihistamines, cool tap water compresses, and topical steroids. Sensitive individuals should wear protective clothing and insect repellents (Cutter, 6-12, Off).

Animal and Human Bites and Bite-Related Infections

WILLIS A. WINGERT, M.D.

NONVENOMOUS ANIMAL BITES

Domestic and Wild Animal Bites

Dogs are responsible for 85% of all reported animal bites. About 50% of dog and cat bites are provoked or occur following teasing, feeding, or playing with the animal.

In the management of domestic or wild animal bites, there are three major considerations: (1) the care of lacerations, puncture wounds, scratches, or crushed necrotic tissue; (2) the inoculation of infectious bacterial organisms from the animal's mouth; and (3) the risk of transmission of rabies virus from animal to man.

Carry out the following steps:

1. Anesthetize the wound appropriately.

2. Wash all lacerations and puncture wounds for at least 15 minutes with 20% soap solution. Benzalkonium chloride (Zephiran), aqueous solution, is an alternative.
3. Since dog bites tend to produce crushing injuries (the jaws exert a pressure of 400 lb/sq inch during a bite), meticulously and aseptically debride all traumatized or potentially nonviable tissue, making sure to remove all foreign particles.
4. Obtain complete hemostasis.
5. Irrigate the wounds thoroughly with at least 1000 ml normal saline solution. This is a major deterrent to secondary infection.
6. Large lacerations and facial wounds may require sutures. If so, provide adequate drainage. Do not suture puncture wounds, which are difficult to irrigate thoroughly and which have a high incidence of secondary infection.
7. If the wound is on the hand or arm or if the animal's teeth penetrated to the bone or to a tendon sheath, administer prophylactic penicillin G or a cephalosporin. Initial cultures are not helpful; they rarely correlate well with subsequent infection.
8. Observe all wounds, especially those caused by cats, for secondary or generalized infection. Recheck the wound no later than 48 hours, and sooner if the area becomes painful or inflamed. The most common secondary infections from dog and cat bites result from the gram-negative organism *Pasteurella multocida* and from gram-positive *Staphylococcus aureus* and *S. epidermidis*. *P. multocida* characteristically causes local pain, swelling, inflammation, local abscesses, and lymphangitis, with regional lymphadenopathy manifested as early as 4 hours and as late as 48 hours after the bite.
9. Observe selected patients for at least 21 days. Bites by rats, mice, and cats may transmit two pathogenic organisms causing systemic disease: *Spirillum minus*: After an incubation period of 14 to 18 days, an indurated lesion appears at the bite site, accompanied by marked regional adenopathy, a purple or red macular body rash, prolonged relapsing fever, and myalgia. *Streptobacillus moniliformis*: After an incubation period of 7 to 10 days, fever, chills, and severe headache occur, followed by a dull red maculopapular rash on the extremities and a persistent polyarthritis. Both organisms are susceptible to penicillin. If symptoms develop, hospitalize the patient, obtain a blood culture, and administer vigorous penicillin therapy (200,000 U/kg/day) IV or IM. Tetracycline 50 mg/kg/day PO (maximum 2 gm/day) is effective in penicillin-allergic patients. Notify parents of children under 8 years of age of possible dental defects if tetracycline is required.

Cat bites and scratches also may transmit tularemia, either in ulceroglandular or typhoidal form, and cat-scratch disease, the causative agent of which has not been isolated.

Monkey bites may transmit *Herpesvirus simiae*, which causes a potentially fatal encephalitis or myelitis in humans after a 1- to 3-week incubation period.

10. Splint extremities that are extensively lacerated until the wounds have healed—7 to 10 days.
11. Capture, isolate, and observe domestic animals for 10 days. Determine the vaccination status of the animal if possible. If the animal does not become ill or die during this period, rabies prophylaxis is unnecessary. Animals that have received rabies immunization within 2 years are unlikely to transmit rabies but require observation.

    If the animal becomes ill during the period of observation, a veterinarian should evaluate the animal and may sacrifice it and ship the head under refrigeration to a qualified laboratory for examination of the brain by fluorescent antibody technique.
12. Immunize all patients meeting the following criteria:
    a. Bitten by an escaped wild animal, whether the animal appears sick or well. This is especially important if the animal was behaving aberrantly. The prevalence of rabies in wild animals has doubled in the past 3 years. The major animals involved are skunks, foxes, bats, and raccoons. These species should be considered rabid until proved otherwise. A normally shy and nocturnal wild animal that appears aberrantly near human habitation in the daytime and displays aggressive behavior or partial paralysis must be considered rabid. Rabies in small rodents and lagomorphs (rabbits and hares) is extremely rare, and bites by these animals usually do not require prophylactic treatment.
    b. Bitten by a domestic animal that is ill or behaving aberrantly. Rabies is manifested by two types of aberrant behavior: "Furious," i.e., highly excitable; unpredictable; unusually aggressive, anorexic, or displaying pica; drooling. "Paralytic": Dogs and cats may run away and hide in secluded places, and cattle may stand immobile and drooling as though a foreign body were lodged in their throat. In some geographic areas, rabies may occur more frequently in cats than in dogs, possibly due to ex-

posure to rabid skunks (feral cats) and to lack of rabies immunization.

   c. Bitten by a stray domestic animal that is not captured in a community in which the incidence of rabies is high, either in that domestic species or in the local wild fauna. Contact the local public health department for information. A captured stray animal should be evaluated by a veterinarian and held for examination or killed immediately for examination of the brain.

   d. Bitten by a wild animal, sick or well, that is kept as a pet. Rabies virus may be present in saliva for a variable period before the onset of clinical symptoms. The duration of this period depends upon the species. Asymptomatic rabid dogs may secrete the virus up to 3 days, cats for 2 days. However, asymptomatic skunks may secrete the virus for 18 days and bats for several months.

13. Prophylactic treatment:

    Administer human rabies immune globulin (RIG), 20 IU/kg as a single dose, for rapid passive immune protection (half-life about 21 days). Infiltrate half the dose around the wound site if such infiltration does not compromise circulation to the area (e.g., finger or toe).

    Administer human diploid cell strain (HDVC) rabies vaccine, (Merieux Institute or Wyeth), 1 ml intramuscularly immediately and repeat on days 3, 7, 14, and 28 after the first dose. (The World Health Organization currently recommends a sixth dose 90 days after the first).

    Do not mix the vaccine and the serum together in the same syringe and do not inject at the same site.

    RIG is administered once, at the beginning of prophylaxis, but may be administered up to the eighth day after the first dose of HDVC. Thereafter an active antibody response to HDVC has occurred, and RIG is not necessary.

    In patients who are receiving corticosteroids and immunosuppressive agents, measure the rabies serum antibody titer at least by day 28, since response may be inadequate. If the titer is less than 1:20, give additional booster doses at 14-day intervals until repeat antibody testing indicates a titer of > 1:20. State or local health departments may be contacted for serological testing.

14. Prevent tetanus by administering a tetanus toxoid booster or 250 units of human immune tetanus globulin if unimmunized.

15. Educate parents regarding suitability of pets for children.

   a. Use judgment in timing, purchase, and choice of a pet: Large breeds and guard dogs (e.g., German shepherds) are more dangerous than small breeds and working dogs (e.g., beagles, spaniels). Children under 5 years of age seldom exercise good judgment around pets and often provoke animals to bite.

   b. Always supervise small children when around dogs and cats, either strange animals or family pets.

   c. Keep aggressive animals under strict control, especially guard dogs.

   d. Completely immunize all pets, both dogs and cats, and keep immunizations current.

   e. Wild animals are dangerous, unpredictable pets.

16. Pre-exposure rabies treatment: For those likely to be exposed to rabies, by occupation or recreation (e.g., veterinarians or spelunkers), consider pre-exposure immunization. Three 1 ml doses of rabies HDCV at 0, 7, and 28 days are required, with booster doses or antibody determinations at 2-year intervals thereafter.

HUMAN BITES

Human dental plaques and gingivae harbor at least 42 different species of organisms, and human saliva contains 10^8 bacteria per ml. Pathogenic organisms include *Staphylococcus aureus* (frequently penicillinase-producing strains), group A and viridans streptococci, *Eikenella corrodens* (which causes indolent ulceration), *Bacteroides melaninogenicus*, *Proteus* spp., *Escherichia coli*, *Neisseria* spp., *Klebsiella* spp., *Aerobacter* spp., *Mycobacterium tuberculosis*, *Actinomyces* spp., spirochetes, and hepatitis B virus. Atypical strains of *Pasteurella multocida* have been isolated from human bite wounds.

A blow by the clenched fist with stretched extensor tendons may strike the incisor teeth of an adversary, resulting in a serious penetrating wound. As the hand opens, the tendons retract, lie proximally to the laceration, and tend to seal pathogenic bacteria within a closed tendon sheath. The infection then spreads through various compartments of the hand, resulting in tenosynovitis, septic arthritis, osteomyelitis, and immobile joints.

Treatment

1. Culture the wound for both aerobes and anaerobes, even though the results are seldom helpful in guiding early therapy.

2. Anesthetize the area appropriately. For extensive wounds, a general anesthetic may be required.

3. Irrigate the area with at least 1000 ml normal saline solution.

4. Debride meticulously, removing crushed, devitalized tissue, and visible foreign bodies.

5. X-ray the area for foreign bodies not grossly visible.

6. Except for facial wounds, do not suture. Apply dry sterile dressings daily.

7. Immobilize extremities that have sustained lacerations.

8. Administer tetanus prophylaxis either by a tetanus toxoid booster or by human tetanus antitoxin, 250 units IM.

9. Administer a broad spectrum antibiotic: cephalexin, 50 mg/kg/day, or cefalor, 40 mg/kg/day PO.

10. Suture facial wounds: Eliminate dead space by closing with absorbable 3-0 or 4-0 suture. Close facial skin with 4-0 or 6-0 nylon sutures. Examine the wound at 24 and 48 hours for infection or inflammation.

11. Hospitalize all patients with extensive wounds, wounds that involve joints and bones (fractures), lacerations involving the hand or foot, or inflammation developing a minor wound. Administer penicillin G, 200,000 U/kg/day (or ampicillin, 100–150 mg/kg/day), and methicillin, 250 mg/kg/day, intravenously. If the patient is allergic to penicillin, administer cefuroxime, 150 mg/kg/day or cefazoline 100 mg/kg/day. Evaluate the wound daily and obtain appropriate cultures to identify specific organisms. The type and duration of further intravenous therapy are guided by the clinical response. Continue all antibiotic therapy for at least 10 days.

12. If seen 12 hours after the bite, 60% of all wounds will be seriously secondarily infected by *S. aureus*, *E. corrodens*, or related bacteria. Hospitalize the patient. Administer penicillin G or ampicillin plus methicillin plus an aminoglycoside (Amikacin, 20 mg/kg/day or gentamicin, 5 mg/kg/day), intravenously until a pathogen is isolated by culture. Vancomycin or a cephalosporin is an alternative drug for penicillin-sensitive patients.

13. Inspect all wounds at least 12-hour intervals for the first 48 hours. Suppurative tenosynovitis is a surgical emergency.

14. Biting is a common form of child abuse. If the child is less than 5 years of age or if circumstances of the trauma are uncertain, photograph the bitten areas. Consult a forensic pathologist for identification of the assailant either by pattern and measurement of the tooth marks or by three-dimensional scanning electron microscopy. Examine the patient carefully for other signs of injury or neglect, including x-rays of long bones and chest for old or new fractures. Report suspected cases promptly to local authorities as required by state law.

VENOMOUS ANIMAL BITES
Poisonous Snakes

Nineteen species of venomous snakes occur in the United States: Seventeen species of the family Crotalidae, or pit vipers, including rattlesnakes (genera *Crotalus* and *Sistrurus*) and the copperheads and moccasins or cottonmouths (*Agkistrodon*); and two species of the family Elapidae, or coral snakes, which are limited to southern and southwestern states.

Pit viper venoms are complex poisons containing, depending on species, 3 to 12 small lethal proteins and peptides and 5 to 15 digestive enzymes. The pharmacologic actions of these components include the following:

1. Local tissue necrosis.

2. Capillary endothelial cell injury resulting in altered permeability and transudation of erythrocytes and plasma into tissues and pulmonary alveoli.

3. Local progressive swelling.

4. Hypovolemia progressing to shock.

5. Pulmonary edema.

6. Coagulation defects.

7. Hemolysis.

8. Renal shutdown.

9. Disturbance in neuromuscular transmission by venoms of the coral snakes and the Mojave rattlesnake (*C. scutulatus*), leading to curarelike muscle paralysis.

10. Probable liberation of histamine, bradykinin, adenosine, and prostaglandins with specific pharmacologic actions.

Envenomation, therefore, produces complex poisoning involving almost all organ systems either primarily or secondarily.

Management

First Aid in the Field

1. Avoid panic. Studies on experimental animals indicate that the median lethal dose (LD_{50}) of venom is decreased significantly by increasing muscular activity.

2. Identify the species and size of the snake, if possible. If not possible, using a long stick, kill the snake with sharp blows on the neck. Do not mutilate the head, since the scale pattern is a major method of species identification. Transport the dead snake in a cloth bag or at the end of a long stick to the closest person capable of identifying the species. Never handle an allegedly dead snake.

3. Immobilize the extremity by splinting as if for a fracture.

4. Transport the victim to the nearest medical facility without delay.

5. *Do not*: a) excise the bitten area; b) apply a tourniquet; c) use cryotherapy; d) make incisions

over the fang marks and apply suction. These measures have *never* been demonstrated to be effective in humans and both traumatize the envenomated areas with introduction of secondary infection and interfere with subsequent clinical estimation of severity of envenomation.

Hospital Management

1. Establish a physiologic baseline:
   a. Verify that the snake was poisonous. Pit vipers: indentation or pit between but below level of eye and nostril on each side of head; vertical elliptical pupils; triangular head with definite neck area; moveable maxillary fangs; single row of subcaudal plates just below anal plate at tail (harmless snakes have a double row); rattles (*Crotalus* species). Coral snakes: round pupils; small, fixed maxillary fangs; a black snout; a species-specific sequential pattern of color bands completely encircling the body—red-yellow (or white)-black (mimics have other sequences).
   b. Record vital signs.
   c. Rapidly evaluate signs and symptoms: One or more distinct fang punctures, usually somewhat irregular; local progressive swelling; ecchymosis; hemorrhagic blebs at or near bite site; fasciculations of face and extremities; paresthesias of face, mouth, and tongue: numbness, tingling, metallic taste; history of known sensitivity to horse serum and antibiotics.
   d. Obtain blood for the following determinations: complete blood count and erythrocyte morphology; platelet count; type and cross-match; coagulation screen—prothrombin time, PTT, fibrinogen level, fibrin split products (if available), bleeding time (template). If severely envenomated, BUN, serum electrolytes, serum protein, blood gases, and pH.
   e. Urinalysis with particular attention to hematuria.
   f. Measure and record the circumference of the injured extremity at proximal point of edema and approximately 4 inches (10 cm) proximal to this level.
2. In case of pit viper bites, determine the severity of envenomation. Grade the reaction as follows:
   No envenomation: No local or systemic reaction although fang marks are present.*
   Minimal: Local swelling but no systemic reaction.

Moderate: Swelling that progresses beyond the site of the bite with a systemic reaction, paresthesias, and/or laboratory changes such as a decrease in platelets or fibrinogen level, fall in hematocrit, or hematuria.
Severe: Marked local swelling and ecchymosis, progressing rapidly up the extremity; severe general symptoms such as bleeding or shock; marked laboratory changes.

3. Perform a skin test for sensitivity to horse serum.
   Inject intradermally 0.02 ml of 1:10 dilution of horse serum (included in the antivenin package).
   Inject 0.02 ml normal saline at another site as a control.
   Note: This skin test is neither highly reliable nor sensitive.
4. Start intravenous infusions in two extremities: One line for life support, if needed, administration of blood, plasma, epinephrine, or measurement of central venous pressure. A second line to administer antivenin.
5. Administer an adequate amount of antivenin intravenously: Antivenin (*Crotalidae*) Polyvalent, North and South American antisnake serum (Wyeth Laboratories). Initial dose, based on grade of envenomation:
   No envenomation: 0 antivenin
   Minimal: 5 vials (50 ml)
   Moderate: 10 vials (100 ml)
   Severe: 15 vials (150 ml)

Exceptions: Small children require 1½ times the recommended dose. Patients known to be bitten by *C. scutulatus* should receive an initial dose of 10 vials.

Dilute the antivenin in 250 ml 0.25 normal saline and administer intravenously as rapidly as possible, preferably over 2 hours. Rate of administration depends upon the child's weight (20 ml/kg/hr) and the appearance of a systemic allergic reaction to the antivenin.

   a. Every 20 minutes, measure the circumference of the affected extremity and compare with the initial determinations. Mark the progress of swelling with a time line. Note development of any systemic reactions (e.g., shock, hemorrhages).
   b. Repeat the initial dose of antivenin intravenously every 2 hours until no further progression of swelling occurs and general symptoms abate.

Verified bites by coral snakes require five vials of *Micrurus fulvius* antivenin (Wyeth) administered intravenously in 250 ml 0.25 normal saline as rapidly as possible, preferably within 2 hours.
6. Monitor and support the physiological status

---

* Bites by the Mojave rattlesnake (*C. scutulatus*) require careful evaluation, since the venom, while very lethal neurologically, may cause only slight local reaction.

of the circulatory, respiratory, and renal systems.

   a. Monitor the vital signs, especially the blood pressure. Insert a central venous catheter in severely envenomated patients. Treat hypovolemic shock by administering 10 to 20 ml/kg of a plasma expander (*not* a crystalloid solution).

   b. Repeat hemoglobin, hematocrit, and platelet levels every 4 hours until stable. Transfuse with 10 ml/kg packed red cells or whole blood if levels are falling.

   c. Obtain serial electrolyte determinations and correct abnormalities in fluid and electrolyte balance as indicated.

   d. Monitor intake and output of urine as an index of renal function. Repeat the urinalysis periodically for evidence of hematuria or proteinuria.

   e. Administer oxygen by mask as needed. In case of coral snake or Mojave rattlesnake envenomation, prepare to insert an endotracheal tube and ventilate mechanically. Appearance of dysphagia (drooling), diplopia or ptosis, slurred speech, or hoarseness (cranial nerve palsies) is an indication for intensive care monitoring.

7. If envenomation is severe or if incision and suction has been applied, administer a broad spectrum antibiotic (ampicillin or amoxicillin) prophylactically for secondary infection for 7 to 10 days. Later cultures of the wound will guide the choice of antibiotic.

8. Prevent tetanus by administering tetanus toxoid as a booster for previously immunized patients or 250 units of human immune tetanus globulin if the patient is unimmunized.

9. Immobilize the extremity in a position of function on a well-padded splint. Maintain at or slightly below heart level. Debride hemorrhagic blebs, vesicles, and superficial necrotic tissue aseptically between the third and fifth days, provided coagulation studies are within normal limits. Cleanse daily and cover with dry sterile dressings.

10. Begin rehabilitation therapy within 5 days to prevent contractures and deformities.

11. Observe for serum sickness developing after 7 to 14 days. Administer prednisone 2 mg/kg day in four divided doses or an equivalent amount of dexamethasone. Continue until all signs and symptoms have subsided. Antihistamines are of little value except for sedation or to alleviate pruritus.

12. Notify the police or the State Department of Fish and Game if the patient was bitten by a captive venomous snake. Most states require a license to collect or to maintain a venomous animal.

ARTHROPODS

Spiders

Spider venoms cause two major types of reactions: neurotoxic reactions due to black widow (*Latrodectus mactans*) bites; and local tissue necrosis due to bites of at least 24 species, including the notorious brown recluse (*Loxosceles* spp.), jumping spiders (*Phidippus*), wolf spiders (*Lycosa* spp.), orb weavers (*Argiope* and *Neascona* spp.), and others. Tarantulas inflict painful but rarely toxic bites.

Latrodectus venom blocks neuromuscular transmission, probably due to excess release of transmitter substance (acetylcholine) from nerve terminals, with subsequent depolarization and exhaustion.

Other spider venoms cause necrosis of the dermis by several mechanisms: Cellular damage to the endothelium of capillaries and venules, with subsequent thrombosis and infarction; and interaction with complement, causing localized lysis of polymorphonuclear leukocytes and mast cells and releasing kinins and other proteolytic enzymes and histamine.

Black Widow (*Latrodectus mactans*) Envenomation

1. Identify the offending spider, if possible:

   a. *L. mactans* female is shiny, coal black, with a 1 to 1.5 cm-long body and a leg span up to 5 cm. A red marking, characteristically shaped like an hourglass *but* with several variations, is present on the ventral abdomen. Note: In southern states, this genus also has red and brown species.

   b. Determine the situation in which the bite occurred: *Latrodectus* builds disorganized webs in dark recesses, cracks in walls, and outdoor privies, rarely in open areas.

   c. The bite is usually moderately painful.

   d. Examine the bite site with a magnifying lens for fang marks—two small puncture wounds about 1 mm apart.

2. Hospitalize all children who develop symptoms or signs, usually within 2 hours after the bite. These include severe local and radiating pain; muscle fasciculation, spasm, or rigidity; and hypertension.

3. Relieve muscle spasm by careful intravenous administration of diazepam (Valium), 0.3 mg/kg.

4. In severe envenomation (severe muscle spasm, hypertension, or in children under 5 years of age) administer one ampule (2.5 ml) of *Latrodectus mactans* antivenin IV diluted in 60 ml of 0.5 normal saline after appropriate skin tests for horse serum sensitivity slowly, over at least 30 minutes.

5. Serially monitor vital signs and symptoms for 48 hours. Control hypertension with appropriate medication (propranolol) as required.

6. A second dose of antivenin may be administered if symptoms persist. This is very unusual.

All Other Spider Bites

1. Identify the etiology of the bite, if possible.

   a. Spider bites usually cause little or no initial pain and often are not felt by the patient. Severe pain would indicate some other offender.

b. Spiders rarely bite more than once. Multiple lesions rule out arachnidism.

c. The appearance of the bite varies from local erythema and edema to a wheal or a vesicle, which may ulcerate. Severe envenomation, especially by *Loxosceles*, results in a "target lesion": A small bleb surrounded by an ischemic ring, later outlined by an erythematous ring of extravasated erythrocytes.

2. Identify the offending spider if possible. The highly poisonous recluse spiders live indoors in closets, trunks, and attics and outdoors in woodpiles and under rocks. The web is irregular. *Loxosceles* sp. range from 9 to 12 mm in size and are fawn or brown in color, with a dark brown mark on the dorsal cephalothorax (often resembling a violin). Using a magnifying glass, count the eyes: small, black dots on head. *Loxosceles* sp. have six eyes (all others have eight).

3. Hospitalize the patient if a typical target lesion appears or if a lesion increases rapidly in size within 12 hours.

4. Treatment of choice is dapsone* PO 50 mg bid (1.25 mg/kg/day) until the lesion has regressed. This method, while very effective in human adults and verified in experimental animals, has not been used extensively in young children. Mild hemolysis is the only common side effect, although other rare side effects involve bone marrow and liver toxicity.

5. Alternate treatment (usually effective in about 50% of envenomations) is dexamethasone 0.10 mg/kg IM every 6 hours. When the lesion no longer progresses, give dexamethasone 0.05 mg/kg or prednisone 0.25 mg/kg orally every 6 hours for 5 days.

6. Administer a systemic antibiotic to all patients with ulcerating lesions or lymphangitis. Drugs of choice are dicloxacillin 25 mg/kg/day or a cephalosporin (cephradine) 50 mg/kg/day intravenously or cefaclor 40 mg/kg/day by mouth.

7. Administer appropriate tetanus prophylaxis.

8. Cleanse ulcerating lesions daily with an antiseptic solution (e.g., betadine) and cover with a dry sterile dressing. After the eschar sloughs, surgically debride the entire area and repair by plastic surgery.

9. For a minor envenomation that shows no vesiculation, target lesions, or evidence of progression, apply a potent topical steroid ointment such as triamcinolone, 0.1% ointment qid. However, observe the lesion at 24-hour intervals for secondary infection.

Scorpion Stings

Two lethal scorpions, *Centruroides sculpturatus* and *C. gertschii*, are found in the Southwest from Arizona to California and in Texas and northern Mexico. Other scorpion stings produce a painful local but not severe systemic reaction, probably by local release of kinins.

Centruroides venom increases release of acetylcholine at the presynaptic terminal of the neuromuscular junction, causing depolarization and subsequent muscle twitching, fibrillation, and excessive continuous muscular activity. The venom stimulates sympathetic nerves directly and may cause a "sympathetic storm," with marked central nervous system stimulation leading to convulsions and to hypertension. Direct cardiotoxicity with myocardial edema and necrosis has been observed.

Treatment

1. Identify the offending scorpion. The potentially dangerous *C. sculpturatus* is a small (2 to 7.5 cm), uniformly yellow scorpion without stripes and with few tactile hairs. Examine the stinger with a magnifying glass (handle the animal with tweezers). A small tubercle (spine or tooth) occurs on the last segment of the tail, just below the sting. Observe and tap the area that has been stung. Since *Centruroides* venom is low in digestive enzymes, swelling and bleeding are rare. However, the area is extremely sensitive to touch and tapping may cause excruciating pain.

2. Stings by scorpions other than *Centruroides* require only relief of pain: Cold compresses over the wound, injection of a local anesthetic, e.g., lidocaine directly into the wound site, or acetaminophen orally. *Do not* administer narcotics. These drugs potentiate the action of scorpion venom.

3. Administer tetanus prophylaxis as indicated.

4. Hospitalize patients stung by *C. sculpturatus*. Monitor vital signs, especially blood pressure. Obtain an electrocardiogram. Control CNS symptoms by sedation with phenobarbital, 5 to 10 mg/kg IM, repeated every 6 to 8 hours, as required. Administer propranolol as a sympathetic blocking agent for marked hypertension not responding to sedation.

Scorpion antivenin is available only in Arizona from the Poisonous Animals Research Laboratory, Arizona State University, Tempe. Call the Regional Poison Control Center: 602-253-3334.

This antivenin has not yet been approved by the Food and Drug Administration.

Other Arthropods

Centipede bites cause pain, local swelling and tenderness, lymphangitis, lymphadenopathy, and rarely local necrosis. Treatment consists of relief of pain by analgesics, cold compresses, or injection of local anesthetic such as lidocaine.

Triatoma protracta, the western cone-nose, kissing or assassin bug, is 10 to 20 mm long and black or dark brown in color. The bug's long proboscis breaks the skin of children (often around the lips), injects a lytic saliva, and ingests the victim's blood. An unidentified protein component in the saliva causes an allergic response in children. The area swells and itches, and the patient may develop nausea, faintness, chills, or anaphylactic shock.

If the reaction is mild, apply a topical steroid and administer an antihistamine by mouth, such

---

* This use of dapsone is not listed in the manufacturer's directive.

as chlorpheniramine maleate (Chlor-Trimeton), 2 to 4 mg, every 6 hours.

For severe reactions, administer prednisone 2 mg/kg/day PO in four divided doses until the reaction subsides.

Burns

LAURIE S. AHLGREN, M.D.

Each year one million Americans are burned. One third of these burn victims are children less than 15 years of age. Although many of the burns children sustain require minimal medical attention, over 30,000 of these injuries require hospitalization, and 3000 are fatal. Scald injury is the most prevalent burn in childhood, and accounts for 45% of burn admissions in children under four years of age. While clothing ignition is now a rare cause of death in childhood, it is responsible for 10% of all nonfatal hospital burn admissions. Seventy-five percent of pediatric burn fatalities occur in housefires in which the child is unable to escape.

The ABC's of life support are of utmost importance to burn victims. If inhalation injury is suspected, humidified oxygen should be administered immediately by mask or nasal prongs. An adequate airway must be established. Early nasotracheal intubation is indicated for progressive airway edema or unmanageable secretions. Intubation is also indicated if hypoxemia persists despite supplemental oxygen therapy. This is seen most commonly in inhalation injuries and full-thickness burns of the chest.

Children with burns greater than 20% of the body surface area (BSA) and infants with burns greater than 15% of the BSA require intravenous fluids to maintain adequate perfusion. Less extensive burns associated with inhalation injury or burns resulting from chemicals or electricity also require venous access. These patients must have a large-bore IV placed in an unburned area and maintenance Ringer's lactate solution infused until proper fluid replacement can be calculated. Cutdown and central venous cannulation, which have higher rates of septic and technical complications, should be avoided unless percutaneous venous access is impossible or central venous pressure monitoring is imperative.

Fluid Resuscitation

Estimates of fluid needs for the first 24 hours after the burn are based on the depth and extent of body surface area injured. Lund and Bowder charts, which allow for the inversely changing proportionate size of children's heads and extremities, aid in estimating the percentage of surface area burned to the second and third degree. Areas of first degree burn are not used in fluid therapy calculations.

For most children the Parkland formula, infusing 4 ml of Ringer's lactate/kg/% BSA burned, offers the best fluid resuscitation. One half of the calculated fluid is given over the first 8 hours of therapy. The patient's response to therapy, however, determines the rate of infusion. Pulse and blood pressure must be restored. Once vital signs, acid-base balance, and mental status are within normal limits, urine output becomes a sensitive indicator of adequate perfusion. Fluid therapy is modified to maintain the patient's urine output at 1–2 ml/kg/hr. This modification usually results in older children receiving 3 ml/kg/% BSA burned and in infants receiving 5 ml/kg/% BSA burned for the first 24 hours.

During the second 24 hours after the burn, the patient will begin to resorb edema fluid and diurese. Consequently, only one half to three fourths of the first day's fluid requirement is infused as 5% dextrose in 0.5 normal saline. Colloid, in the form of albumin or fresh frozen plasma, is administered at a rate of 0.5 ml/kg/% BSA burned. After 48 hours the evaporative fluid loss is 85% free water and is replaced with 1–2 ml/kg/% BSA burned with 5% dextrose in 0.25 normal saline. Potassium supplementation and red blood cell transfusion may also be needed.

Patients with burns less than 20% BSA can be managed by increasing their oral fluid intake an average of 1% for each percent BSA burned. Care must be taken to prevent the child from preferentially imbibing excess free water, since this can rapidly lead to hyponatremia. Infants should continue their regular formula. Older children should be offered full liquids or dietary supplements that provide calories as well as salt and water. A return to a normal diet in 1 to 2 days is advisable, with continued surveillance of excessive free water intake. Teenagers especially have become hyponatremic after water and soft drinks are allowed ad lib.

Wound Care and Triage

Emergency room physicians must triage burns into one of three groups: minor, major, critical.

Minor Burns. Minor burns are those covering less than 10% BSA and involving less than 2% full-thickness injury. They are generally treated on an out-patient basis. First aid to minor burns includes cooling the burn with water or ice. The burn is then gently cleaned with saline. Blebs and blisters are left intact. Closed bulky dressings are applied after a thin coating of silver sulfadiazine. Tetanus prophylaxis is given if needed, but no antibiotics are prescribed. Parents are instructed to return the child for a dressing change in 2 days or immediately if the dressing falls off or if the child's temperature rises above 39°C (102°F).

Major Burns. Patients with major burns encompassing greater than 10% BSA or more than 2% third-degree injury require inpatient care. Hospitalization should also be considered in children less than 2 years of age and in children with burns to the hands, feet, face, or perineum, flame burns, electrical burns, and in children who are suspected victims of child abuse. It is often desirable to admit children with lesser burns who come from questionable social situations and observe parental care of the wound for 1 to 2 days before beginning out-patient treatment.

Initial care to major burns differs from minor burn care in that the wound is débrided of all loose skin and blisters using strict sterile technique. Analgesia, using 0.05 mg/kg morphine sulfate or 0.5 mg/kg meperidine hydrochloride IV push, can be given during wound débridement.

Escharotomies may be needed to enhance blood flow to extremities with circumferential burns or to allow ventilation in extensive chest burns. Loss of Doppler flow pulsations in digital arteries is a reliable indication for performing escharotomies. Incisions are made through the entire thickness of the burn on the lateral aspects of the extremity. Escharotomies to the chest are along the lower costal margin. Since the burns that necessitate escharotomies are full-thickness burns, local anesthesia is not needed.

Following burn débridement, the application of silver sulfadiazine is quite soothing. Occlusive bulky dressings complete the initial wound care. Baseline weights, serum electrolytes, glucose and osmolality, CBC, arterial blood gas levels, and nasopharyngeal cultures are obtained. Carbon monoxide levels are determined if the child was burned in an enclosed space. Tetanus prophylaxis is given as needed. Penicillin is administered prophylactically only if the patient has a known cardiac anomaly or a concomitant streptococcal infection.

Critical Burns. Critical burns are those that cover more than 30% BSA or involve electrical "crush" type injuries or inhalation injuries. These children should be transferred to regional burn centers. Prior to transport, the airway must be assured, a reliable intravenous line must be established, fluid resuscitation must be instituted, and a nasogastric tube and a bladder catheter must be placed. The burn should be wrapped in dry sterile dressings, and if vital signs allow, the patient may have mild IV sedation.

Special Problems

Ileus. Ileus following extensive burns is not uncommon, and gastric dilatation with vomiting and aspiration may occur. The subsequent chemical pneumonitis superimposed on the pulmonary response to burn injury may be lethal. Nasogastric decompression is, therefore, mandatory until the intestinal tract is known to be working.

Fever. Fevers up to 39°C (102°F) are routinely seen in burn victims, especially in burned children. This febrile response is not completely understood but is thought to represent pyrogens released during the body's natural inflammatory response to injury. The fevers often persist until the eschar is removed. Antipyretics are usually not efficacious. Tympanic membranes, throats, and burn wounds should be inspected, but extensive septic work-ups are not indicated unless the temperature exceeds 40°C (104°F).

Sepsis. Sepsis is the major cause of death in critically burned patients who survive to hospitalization. *Pseudomonas aeruginosa* is now the main lethal bacterial invader. Topical burn therapy is geared toward local control. One-half percent silver nitrate solution, the original topical antibiotic, is not used in children because of the hyponatremia that can occur, sometimes within hours. Mafenide acetate 10% cream (Sulfamylon) penetrates eschar well and kills *Pseudomonas*. Unfortunately, because of its carbonic anhydrase inhibition, it causes a metabolic acidosis that makes it unsuitable for use in children. Silver sulfadiazine 1% cream penetrates eschar moderately well and kills *Pseudomonas*. Unlike both silver nitrate and mafenide acetate, it is not painful when applied. Although leukopenia following silver sulfadiazine therapy has been seen, the clinical significance of this side effect has not been well established. It is, therefore, the topical antibiotic of choice in children.

Despite topical therapy, wound surveillance is imperative to ensure early recognition of burn wound sepsis. Quantitative wound cultures growing more than 10^6 organisms/cm^2 demand additional wound débridement and appropriate systemic antibiotic administration. Antistreptococcal prophylaxis (penicillin) is recommended only for patients with valvular heart disease, patients with concomitant or recent streptococcal infection, and patients whose admission throat cultures are positive for hemolytic streptococcus. Tetanus prophylaxis is indicated if the patient has not been adequately immunized.

Inhalation Injuries. Inhalation injuries may not be readily apparent. Burns on the face, singed nasal hairs, and carbonaceous sputum all suggest inhalation injury, but just as their presence does not confirm inhalation injury, neither does their absence exclude it. Early flexible bronchoscopy may be necessary to establish the diagnosis. Once established, the treatment consists of the administration of 100% oxygen and the observation for one of the following clinical phases.

The first phase occurs 1 to 12 hours after the burn and is characterized by laryngeal edema, bronchospasm, or acute lung consolidation. Laryngeal edema produces a prolonged inspiratory phase and is best treated by endotracheal intubation. Bronchospasm has a prolonged expiratory phase with wheezing and is best treated by a croup tent and a single large intravenous dose of corticosteroids. Acute lung consolidation is characterized by progressive hypoxemia, and its fulminant course is rarely moderated by full ventilatory support.

Phase two occurs 6 to 72 hours after the burn and manifests as pulmonary edema. Leaky pulmonary capillaries and fluid overload account for this clinical picture. Standard medical management of pulmonary edema, including fluid restriction and diuretics, is effective in most cases.

Phase three occurs in children with severe inhalation injuries who manage to survive 3 days after the burn. They almost universally acquire a staphylococcal or gram-negative bronchopneumonia. Good pulmonary toilet and bacteria-specific systemic antibiotics give the best chance of survival for this third clinical phase of inhalation injuries.

Nutrition. Nutrition is a common problem in children with burns greater than 30% BSA. Burn ileus, fever, and pain reduce appetite. The hypermetabolic state associated with large burns may require up to four times basal caloric needs. In addition, heat calories are lost through evaporation unless the ambient temperature is near 34°C (101°F) with high humidity. It may be physically impossible for the child to eat enough to supply the necessary calories. Supplemental enteral nutrition via nocturnal nasogastric tube feeding remedies this problem with minimal patient discomfort. Rarely, total parenteral nutrition is necessary to provide adequate calories, but it is recommended that the total parenteral nutrition catheter be changed every 3 days over a guide wire to reduce the risk of catheter sepsis.

Facial Burns. Facial burns in children fortunately are rarely full-thickness burns. Because it is difficult to dress the face occlusively, the burns are gently cleansed, débrided, thinly coated with an antibiotic ointment, and left open. The ointment should be reapplied as needed to keep the wound covered. The eyes should be examined by an ophthalmologist before soft-tissue swelling obscures the view. Occasionally, full-thickness burns to the eyelids require tarsorrhaphy to protect the eyes during healing.

Near-Drowning

J. MICHAEL DEAN, M.D.

Drowning is a leading cause of death in children, and near-drowning is associated with significant morbidity. Near-drowning is strictly defined as an immersion accident in which the victim does not die within 24 hours. For our purposes here, however, the term near-drowning will be used for all patients who survive the accident long enough to reach the hospital.

Emergency management consists of immediate ventilation and restoration, if necessary, of circulation. The airway should be cleared of debris and vomitus, and mouth-to-mouth ventilation should be started as quickly as possible (even while the patient is still in the water). If cardiac arrest has occurred, it is secondary to respiratory arrest, and ventilation and oxygenation may restore spontaneous cardiac activity. If the child requires cardiopulmonary resuscitation, he should be transported to a hospital, and resuscitation should be continued (i.e., he should not be pronounced dead at the scene under any circumstances). If the child is hypothermic, the resuscitation efforts must continue until the child's temperature exceeds 30–31°C (86–87.8°F); with temperatures below this level, cardiac resuscitation may be impossible. In addition, profound hypothermia (under 31°C or 87.8°F) will depress the neurologic system, and the child may have an examination incorrectly suggestive of brain death. Thus, unless it is known that the child was under water for an extremely long time (several hours), resuscitation efforts must continue until the temperature is relatively normal. Following restoration of the heart beat, hypothermia should be corrected slowly, at a rate not to exceed 1°C (1.8°F) per hour.

Respiratory failure often occurs in these victims. Children who are breathing should be placed on 100% oxygen by mask, and after stabilization, they may be weaned according to arterial blood gas measurements. If the P_{O_2} cannot be maintained above 100 mm Hg in 50% or less oxygen, then continuous positive airway pressure should be employed, which requires endotracheal intubation. Children who cannot maintain normal carbon dioxide tension (35–40 mm Hg) should also be intubated and must be mechanically ventilated. While setting up for intubation, the physician must ventilate the child with a bag and mask and maintain the patency of the airway. If mask ventilation is used, this will increase gastric distension, and the risk of aspiration is increased. Therefore, nasogastric tubes should be placed in these children early in their management to prevent the potentially disastrous complications of aspiration pneumonia.

By far the most difficult problem in near-drowning is the insult to the central nervous system. An estimate of the severity of injury is possible from the first hospital evaluation of the Glasgow coma scale (Table 1).

Children who have *initial* Glasgow scores under 8 are at high risk of neurologic sequelae and

Table 1. THE GLASGOW COMA SCALE

Eye Opening	Points
No response	1
Response to pain	2
Response to voice	3
Spontaneously	4
Verbal Response	
No response	1
Incomprehensible sounds	2
Inappropriate words	3
Disoriented conversation	4
Oriented and appropriate	5
Motor Response	
No response	1
Decerebrate posturing	2
Decorticate posturing	3
Flexion withdrawal	4
Localizes pain	5
Obeys commands	6
Maximum Score	15

intracranial hypertension; children who have a better Glasgow coma score at the first hospital have a uniformly good outcome. Children with Glasgow coma scores of 7 or less should be monitored for intracranial hypertension and treated appropriately if it occurs. Children in this category (Glasgow score < 8) should be intubated, hyperventilated moderately (carbon dioxide 25–35 mm Hg), and kept on a fluid restricted diet. The head should be elevated 30° and kept in the midline (to avoid jugular venous obstruction). Endotracheal suctioning should be minimized if there is intracranial hypertension.

Intracranial pressure monitoring is accomplished with a subarachnoid bolt or an intraventricular drain, which is inserted by a neurosurgeon. Cerebral perfusion pressure is maintained above 50 mm Hg and is calculated as mean arterial pressure minus the mean intracranial pressure. In order to do this calculation, the transducers must be referenced to the same level (i.e., the heart). If the intracranial pressure exceeds 20 mm Hg or if the cerebral perfusion pressure drops below 50 mm Hg, mannitol 0.25 gm/kg is administered to lower intracranial pressure. Hyperventilation may be increased (decreasing P_{CO_2} to 20 mm Hg). Fever should be aggressively prevented, but hypothermia is dangerous and without proven benefit. If seizures occur, they should be very aggressively treated, since seizure activity will exacerbate the primary neuronal injury. If an intraventricular drain has been used for monitoring pressure, cerebrospinal fluid may be drained, thus lowering

intracranial pressure. If intracranial pressure continues to be elevated despite normothermia, absence of seizures, hyperventilation, and mannitol therapy, then barbiturate coma may be instituted. This is accomplished with a loading dose of 5 mg/kg pentobarbital, followed by 1–5 mg/kg/hr continuous intravenous infusion. This therapy will lead to cardiac depression, often requires sophisticated hemodynamic support, and should not be attempted in the absence of a Swan-Ganz catheter. While barbiturates are often effective in lowering intracranial pressure, their benefit on long-term outcome is doubtful.

The prognosis of children who arrive at the hospital awake is excellent, and careful attention to pulmonary disease will result in normal survival. Children who are comatose on presentation have a poor outcome if they do not start to awaken within 6 hours. Children who present at the first hospital with a Glasgow coma score less than 8 are at high risk of neurologic sequelae or death. Children in this category who survive with normal outcomes generally have not suffered persistent intracranial hypertension at any time in their hospital course; the occurrence of refractory intracranial hypertension is an extremely grim prognostic sign. The origin of sufficient cerebral edema to lead to intracranial hypertension is primarily cytotoxic, owing to neuronal death, and it is doubtful that any measures will salvage children with this degree of injury. Intracranial pressure monitoring *may* be of value in two respects. One, efforts can be made to avoid the development of intracranial hypertension, and an increase of intracranial pressure can alert the clinician to take further steps in its treatment. Two, if the child develops persistent intracranial hypertension (above 20–30 mm Hg despite treatment), consideration may be given to limiting further resuscitative efforts.

In contrast to earlier reports, near-drowning is a lethal disease in cold or warm water, and severely brain-injured children have a grim prognosis. With all these limitations, however, one can expect to salvage (with good neurologic outcome) about 10 to 15% of all children who present to the hospital without any neurologic function (Glasgow coma score = 3) in full cardiac arrest. This is similar to the other populations of children who have suffered cardiac arrest outside the hospital. Intracranial pressure monitoring or other brain resuscitative measures appear to have had minimal impact on this survival rate. However, 15% salvage justifies continued recommendations to resuscitate all children involved in immersion accidents.

21

Unclassified Diseases

The Histiocytosis Syndromes

KENNETH A. STARLING, M.D.

Except for infants with the newly described "congenital self-healing histiocytosis syndrome," virtually all patients with histiocytosis require some form of therapy. In the child with a single granuloma of bone, surgical biopsy or curettage usually induces healing. No further therapy may be needed, although frequent observation of the lesion and examinations for other lesions are obligatory. Usually there is complete healing, and grafting is not necessary. If the lesion is in the skull, a CAT scan of the brain, with and without enhancement, is indicated. Enhancing masses in the parasellar region have been observed in a number of children with skull lesions, and additional therapy is indicated in these children. If the lesion occurs in a long bone or in the vertebral bodies, low-dose radiation therapy (250–750 rads) may enhance healing and thereby prevent pathologic fractures. Radiotherapy is also indicated in those children who are found to have intracerebral masses, since the presence of such a mass is often associated with the development of diabetes insipidus.

Younger children with multiple bone lesions and all children with visceral involvement, particularly those with visceral dysfunction, should be given chemotherapy. Despite numerous trials by the pediatric cooperative groups and individual institutions, no single drug seems to be clearly superior to the other antineoplastic agents. Nor have combinations of antineoplastic agents produced superior results; in fact, they have had deleterious effects in children younger than 1 year of age. It has been demonstrated clearly that failure to respond to one drug does not mean that the disease will not respond to another agent. Therapy is usually given for 3–4 months before it is determined to have failed. There may be im-

provement in some areas and progression of disease in others. A general trend toward improvement suggests continuation of the same drug. If there is rapid progression of disease, a change of therapy might be considered after 4–6 weeks.

The use of corticosteroids at the beginning of drug therapy is controversial; however, their long-term use is not advisable. A trial of 4 weeks is recommended, in combination with another agent, and the corticosteroid is then tapered over 6–7 days. The dose of prednisone most commonly used is 60 mg/m^2/day in three or four divided doses.

The drugs most commonly recommended for the initiation of single-agent therapy, with or without corticosteroids, are vinblastine, methotrexate, and chlorambucil. Other drugs that have been shown to be effective are vincristine, 6-mercaptopurine, and cyclophosphamide.

The recommended doses of these drugs used as single agents are as follows:

1. Vinblastine: 6.5 mg/m^2/week. The principal side effect of vinblastine is myelosuppression.

2. Methotrexate: (a) 60–120 mg/m^2/every 2 weeks, if given intravenously. (b) 20–25 mg/m^2/week, if given by mouth. The principal side effects of methotrexate are ulceration of the mucous membranes and myelosuppression. Liver and lung damage have been reported with long-term usage of methotrexate.

3. Chlorambucil: 5–6 mg/m^2/day. The principal side effect of chlorambucil is myelosuppression.

4. Vincristine: 1.5–2 mg/m^2/week (maximum dose, 2.0 mg). The principal side effect of vincristine is neurotoxicity.

5. 6-Mercaptopurine: 50 mg/m^2/day. The principal side effect of 6-mercaptopurine is myelosuppression; however, hepatic toxicity is reported with long-term use.

6. Cyclophosphamide: 90–150 mg/m^2/day. The principal side effect of cyclophosphamide is mye-

losuppression; however, long-term use can result in bladder irritation and eventual scarring.

The dosage of all these drugs should be adjusted for toxicity; if the toxicity is not tolerable, a change of drugs is indicated. In addition, long-term side effects of the alkylating agents chlorambucil and cyclophosphamide have not been well documented in children.

In the past few years a number of children who were thought to have histiocytosis have been found instead to have specific immunologic defects. While a number of different immunologic changes have been described in children with histiocytosis, there have been no consistent findings. Immunotherapy with crude bovine thymic extract has achieved some success, but it is still in the investigative stages.

Sarcoidosis

EDWIN L. KENDIG, JR., M.D.

Sarcoidosis is a multisystem granulomatous disease of unknown cause. It is relatively rare in children. Since the disease process displaces normal tissue by sarcoid tissue, symptoms and signs depend on the organ or tissue involved. Most commonly affected are the lungs, lymph nodes, eyes, skin, liver, and spleen. Bones may also be involved, although this occurs less often; indeed, any organ or tissue may be affected.

Since the causative agent of sarcoidosis is not known, there is no recognized specific therapy. Adrenocorticosteroids are the only agents currently available that can suppress the acute manifestations of the disease. These agents are utilized only during acute and dangerous episodes.

Adrenocorticosteroid therapy is indicated in patients with intrinsic ocular disease, diffuse pulmonary lesions, central nervous system lesions, myocardial involvement, hypersplenism, and persistent hypercalcemia. Relative indications include progressive or symptomatic pulmonary disease, constitutional symptoms, joint involvement, disfiguring skin and lymph node lesions, persistent facial nerve palsy, and lesions of the nasal, laryngeal, and bronchial mucosa.

Fresh lesions appear to be more responsive to adrenocorticosteroid therapy than older ones. Although the suppressive action is often temporary, it is beneficial when the unremitting course of the disease will result in loss of organ function. For example, adrenocorticosteroid therapy can reduce the level of serum calcium and may thus help prevent nephrocalcinosis, renal insufficiency, and, possibly, band keratitis. The use of adrenocorticosteroids in the treatment of patients with only asymptomatic miliary nodules or bronchopneumonic patches in the lung fields is debatable.

Prednisone or prednisolone, 1 mg/kg/day in three or four divided doses, is continued until clinical manifestations of the disease disappear. A maintenance dose (15 mg every other day) is then given until a course of at least 6 months' treatment has been carried out.

Temporary relapse may occur following the discontinuation of adrenocorticosteroid treatment, but improvement usually follows without resumption of therapy. In the management of ocular disease, adrenocorticosteroids in the form of either ointment or drops (0.5–1%) are utilized in conjunction with systemic treatment. During the course of local therapy, the pupils are continuously dilated by use of an atropine ointment (1%).

Adrenocorticosteroid ointment may also be used in the treatment of cutaneous lesions, but only in conjunction with systemic therapy; better results are obtained with the latter.

Other drugs occasionally used in the treatment of sarcoidosis in adults (oxyphenbutazone, chloroquine, potassium para-aminobenzoate, azathioprine, and chlorambucil), as well as transfer factor, have seldom been used in children.

Familial Mediterranean Fever

THOMAS J. A. LEHMAN, M.D.

The emphasis of current therapy for familial Mediterranean fever is on prophylactic colchicine administration to suppress the febrile attacks and possibly prevent amyloidosis. Children with familial Mediterranean fever who are of Sephardic Jewish or Arab origin or who have a family history of amyloidosis should receive continuous colchicine therapy. However, the physician caring for a child with familial Mediterranean fever who is of some other ethnic background must carefully weigh the benefits of ongoing colchicine administration against the knowledge that the febrile paroxysms are transitory and resolve without sequelae. Therapy should be restricted to those who are experiencing an unacceptable level of absenteeism from school or whose lives are otherwise significantly disrupted by the disease.

Colchicine* is administered in 0.6-mg tablets. A dosage of 0.6 mg bid is usually required to suppress the attacks in children 4–12 years of age, while 0.6 mg tid is often required for older children. These dosages have been utilized without toxicity in a large number of children. Transient diarrhea is often reported at the initiation of therapy but

---

* This use of colchicine is not listed by the manufacturer.

resolves spontaneously in most cases. Families in which the patient is young or in which there are young siblings should be specifically warned about the risk of accidental ingestion. Ingestion of as few as 8 mg (14 pills) of colchicine has led to death.

Patients at risk for the development of amyloidosis should receive colchicine continuously. The necessary duration of colchicine therapy for others is unclear. Although the disease is inherited, there are marked variations in the frequency of attacks without treatment. Once the attacks are initially controlled, colchicine may be gradually withdrawn. However, the episodes often recur when the dosage is decreased, and most patients require continuing therapy.

There is no specific therapy for the acute febrile attack once it has begun. A large hourly dose of colchicine at the first indication of an attack has been recommended for adults who are not receiving ongoing colchicine therapy, but this has not proven satisfactory in children. The fever and pleuritis or peritonitis will resolve spontaneously within 72 hours and should be treated with conservative measures of bed rest and hydration. Aspirin or acetaminophen may provide mild relief. Routine usage of narcotics should be avoided because of the recurrent nature of the attacks and the resultant potential for addiction. If the patient presents with peritonitis and primarily right lower quadrant pain, it may be impossible to exclude the possibility of appendicitis; appropriate surgery should be performed.

The arthritis of familial Mediterranean fever may be treated with appropriate dosages of nonsteroidal anti-inflammatory drugs. It is usually self-limited and ceases when the paroxysmal attacks are controlled. The chronic arthritis of the hip or sacroiliac joints that occurs may be treated symptomatically with anti-inflammatory drugs but does not respond well. Prophylactic colchicine administration is of uncertain benefit for these patients, who may ultimately require joint replacement.

22

Special Problems in the Fetus and Neonate

Disturbances of Intrauterine Growth

JOSEPH L. KENNEDY, JR., M.D.

Infants with birth weights more than two standard deviations from the mean for gestational age are arbitrarily defined as having disturbances of growth. Overnutrition of the fetus (large for dates), while classically associated with large parents or with diabetic mothers, is also seen with transposition of the great vessels and in some syndromes (cerebral gigantism, Beckwith's syndrome). Some of these infants are susceptible to hypoglycemia; screening tests for glucose should be done early.

Infants with birth weights two standard deviations below the mean for gestational age or those less than the tenth percentile have intrauterine growth retardation. Various factors can affect birth weight. Maternal size, family stature, and altitude should be taken into account when assessing the infant.

There are two types of intrauterine growth retardation. In the first there is an altered growth potential with an infant who is small throughout the pregnancy. Small size associated with small maternal or familial stature and some infants with syndromes or multiple congenital anomalies are found in this type.

A second type is associated with impaired support for growth due to placental, maternal, or environmental factors. This type includes infants with intrauterine infection, placental insufficiency secondary to hypertension, chronic abruption or placental infarct and fetal crowding associated with intrauterine anomalies, oligohydramnios, or multiple gestation. Maternal illness, substance abuse,

and perhaps socioeconomic factors affect growth support. Infants with impaired growth generally fall further below the norm as pregnancy progresses and are often said to have third trimester growth retardation.

Management of intrauterine growth retardation should begin during the pregnancy with screening for poor growth, frequent examinations, and ultrasound evaluation of fetal size and amount of amniotic fluid. Non-stress testing should begin at 26 weeks and contraction stress testing should be done as indicated together with evaluation of the biophysical profile (ultrasound evaluation of fetal movement, amount of amniotic fluid, and fetal breathing movements together with fetal heart rate and posture/tone).

During the pregnancy, bed rest on the left side may be effective when it is thought that there may be impaired placental blood flow, as with hypertensive disorders. Diuretics should be avoided, since they tend to diminish placental blood flow. A mother thought to be at risk of delivering an infant with severe growth retardation or chronic asphyxia should be transferred to a high risk center. Early delivery may be indicated to remove the infant from a less than optimal environment. During labor and delivery, problems with hypoxia may be minimized by careful fetal monitoring. Asphyxia, if it occurs, should be promptly treated with effective resuscitation. Meconium aspiration should be prevented by aspirating the nasopharynx or trachea as indicated.

In the newborn nursery, the infant should be observed for birth defects and signs and symptoms of chronic or acute hypoxia: seizures, brain edema, irritability, altered consciousness, diminished urine output, respiratory failure, persistent fetal circulation, and cardiac dilatation with mitral insufficiency. Early feedings should be begun by mouth or by gavage, or if the infant has been seriously hypoxic or is also immature or otherwise impaired, by the intravenous administration of glucose.

The infant is examined for minor anomalies that lead to the diagnosis of unsuspected major anomalies. Examination of the placenta is important and often helpful in ruling out intrauterine infection. TORCH screening of cord blood serum is often unrewarding. If intrauterine infection is strongly suspected, viral culture of the urine for CMV and examination of the spinal fluid for protein and cells may be helpful.

Because the infant is small and often hypoxic, heat loss and heat production may be impaired and temperature control defective. Careful attention should be paid to thermal environment, particularly when the infant is wet or exposed for examination or procedures.

Metabolic complications such as hypocalcemia and hypoglycemia should be watched for and treated.

Some infants with chronic in utero hypoxia have a high hematocrit level and blood flow to various organs may be diminished because of increased blood viscosity. These infants are particularly susceptible to hypoglycemia. Plasma reduction exchange transfusion may be useful in infants with central hematocrits over 65%, especially if clinical manifestations suggest hyperviscosity syndrome.

Early postnatal weight gain and early head growth may be indicators that an infant will do well. The ultimate prognosis for infants with extreme intrauterine growth retardation must be guarded, particularly when the cause is unknown. The infant need not be kept in the hospital until a particular weight is achieved. When he is gaining well, feeding well, and can obtain heat balance, he may be discharged home.

Birth Injuries

JOSEPH L. KENNEDY, JR., M.D.

The introduction of fetal monitoring techniques and the more common use of cesarean section, particularly in breech birth, have combined in recent years to make serious birth injury less common. The new techniques have in themselves contributed some problems. Pediatricians must be intimately familiar with the marks of the normal birth process so that they may offer a worried parent justified reassurance. Attempts at treatment of minor birth injuries are often interfering and may in fact foster undue parental concern.

Superficial Injuries. *Caput succedaneum and molding* are to be expected in most deliveries. The shape of the infant's head is often of deep concern to the parents. Molding may be marked when the infant is large, the labor long, the mother primigravid, or the membranes ruptured prior to the onset of labor. Parents should be reassured that the head will look normal in a matter of days and that molding is normal and not associated with brain damage. The edema, suffusion, and localized intradermal hemorrhage of the presenting part begins to regress within 12 to 24 hours. Within the caput may be found localized abrasions, lacerations from intrauterine scalp sampling, and the puncture marks, sometimes with localized hemorrhage, of the monitoring electrode. These breaks in the skin represent a potential portal of entry for bacteria, particularly when there has been premature rupture of membranes or a long labor. Local treatment with a topical antibiotic cream or powder may prevent abscess or cellulitis.

The caput associated with the use of vacuum extraction may be more marked. Lesions similar to the caput occur not uncommonly with breech delivery. Bruising and edema of the genitalia worry parents; reassurance is usually warranted. Severe intratesticular hemorrhage may, however, produce late fibrotic changes. Hemorrhagic necrosis of portions of the labial or perianal areas results in localized sloughing with healing in 10 to 14 days. No treatment is needed other than careful cleaning of the affected areas. Unusual presentations such as that of face, arm, or leg result in similar localized changes. Extensive enclosed hemorrhage, particularly in the premature infant, may be a significant extravascular source of bilirubin and, rarely, a significant source of blood loss. Muscle crush injury with shock, disseminated intravascular coagulation, and renal damage has been described.

Lacerations may be caused by amniotomy, episiotomy, fetal blood sampling, fetal incision at cesarean section, or by the edge of a forceps blade. Sutures are sometimes required. Topical antibiotic cream or powder may be used to prevent infection. These wounds do well without a dressing.

Superficial forceps injury consisting of erythema with abrasion, superficial drainage, and crusting will heal rapidly and without scarring. Dressings are contraindicated. *Deep forceps injury* (subcutaneous fat necrosis) becomes evident between the fourth and eighth days. It heals spontaneously in a matter of weeks. Progression to an abscess is seen rarely. As with other neonatal skin injuries, warm soaks are contraindicated because of the susceptibility of the neonate to waterborne bacterial infection and of the newborn skin to thermal injury. Subcutaneous fat necrosis presumably from trauma attendant to delivery is occasionally seen elsewhere on the body, where it may be confused with a local cellulitis.

Scalp abscess occurs in 5% of infants who have

had intrauterine monitoring. Most lesions are small and self-limited. A few have required incision and drainage. Careful cultures always reveal bacteria, usually those of the vaginal flora. Systemic antibiotics are not indicated unless signs of septicemia are present, nor is continued hospitalization required. Large or enlarging lesions should be followed weekly until resolution begins, because there have been a few reports of osteomyelitis and subgaleal abscess. Biparietal scalp necrosis with abscess formation occurs when the widest part of a large fetal head is pressed against the ischial spines during labor. Management is similar.

Tight nuchal cord causes localized cyanosis, edema, suffusion, and petechiae above the neck. Similar changes may be seen with face presentation, nuchal encirclement during breech delivery or during vertex delivery with shoulder dystocia, or when ergotrate has been given to the mother before the trunk has been delivered. Localized facial cyanosis alone may be seen in severe congenital hypothyroidism, and in a rare infant who responds to a cold environment primarily by vasoconstriction of the face. The soft tissue lesions require no treatment. Infants with nuchal cord should be watched for respiratory distress, which may occur because of nasal mucosal edema in an infant who is an obligate nasal breather. Nasal obstruction is relieved with an oral airway. Some infants born after partial cord compression become hypovolemic because of sequestration of the infant's blood in the placenta, when flow in the umbilical vein is impeded. Serial monitoring of blood pressure, pulse, respiratory rate, and hematocrit should be done in infants with a history of cord compression.

Cephalhematoma is usually unilateral and parietal in location. It is initiated during the birth process and hence is rarely demonstrable within the first few hours of life. Associated linear skull fractures are not rare, but skull radiographs are unnecessary since depressed fractures do not occur in the absence of other trauma, and since the expectant treatment is the same whether or not a linear fracture is present. Resolution of the lesion may take 4 to 10 weeks. It is sometimes accompanied by calcification of the lesion, new bone formation, and occasionally, a partial collapse of the swelling. Initially the periosteal stretching may produce local tenderness; it has become customary for this reason to lay the infant's head on the unaffected side. Parents are often very anxious and need a great deal of reassurance that healing will occur without untoward effects. The breakdown of hemoglobin in a large cephalhematoma may cause the serum bilirubin to rise by 3 to 5 mg/dl but can never be the sole explanation for marked neonatal jaundice. Cephalhematoma should never be aspirated because of the danger of introducing infection.

Subaponeurotic hemorrhage occurs rarely after difficult deliveries and vacuum extraction. The premature infant is somewhat more susceptible. Diagnosis is made by the appearance of increasing scalp swelling crossing suture lines, often fluctuant or crepitant, associated with pitting edema. Hemorrhage may be severe enough to cause death in hypovolemic shock. Prompt diagnosis and treatment with blood and plasma expanders may be lifesaving. The milder lesions will regress spontaneously, but, like other enclosed hemorrhages in the neonate, may be associated with some rise in serum bilirubin, and rarely with disseminated intravascular coagulation.

Intracranial Hemorrhage. The exact diagnosis of a neonatal intracranial hemorrhage (*subdural hemorrhage, intraventricular hemorrhage, intracerebral hemorrhage,* or *subarachnoid hemorrhage*) is less important than the immediate management of the affected infant. Diagnosis of hemorrhage is suspected when there is lethargy, hypotonia, seizures, focal neurologic signs, irregular respiration, apnea, fall in hematocrit, metabolic acidosis, bloody spinal fluid, full fontanel, or irritability. The maternal history is usually one of abnormal presentation, prolonged second stage of labor, or difficult delivery, often with oxytocin augmentation. Intraventricular hemorrhage, common in the small sick premature infant in whom it may not represent a true birth injury, can occur also in the term infant. Computer tomography (CT scan) is the best way of ascertaining the location and extent of the hemorrhage, but echoventriculography offers a more convenient way of obtaining almost as much information.

Routine tapping of the subdural space in an infant without skull fracture, localizing signs, or evidence of increased intracranial pressure is contraindicated since it may in itself cause subdural bleeding. Neurosurgical consultation is advisable if the diagnosis is suspected. In most infants, careful observation and symptomatic treatment are preferable to overvigorous diagnostic measures.

Seizures should be controlled with phenobarbital, 10 mg/kg IV or IM followed by 6 mg/kg/24 hr parenterally in two divided doses. The initial 10 mg/kg dose may be repeated if necessary. Serum phenobarbital levels should be kept in the range of 10 to 25 μg/ml. Phenytoin (10 mg/kg IV) is of little additional help and has a 24-hour delayed onset of action. It should be used only when seizures are severe, prolonged, and refractory to treatment. Intravenous diazepam* is synergistic with the barbiturates, and the combination of the two drugs has been reported to cause severe respiratory depression. Diazepam should not be

---

* Manufacturer's warning: Safety of parenteral diazepam in the neonate has not been established.

used unless artificial ventilatory support is immediately available. Hypoglycemia, hypocalcemia and hyponatremia are common in these infants; a search for these metabolic abnormalities should be made in every infant and appropriate treatment undertaken.

Supportive therapy of the infant with intracranial hemorrhage should include IV nutrition, treatment of associated hypoglycemia, monitoring for hypovolemia and appropriate replacement of blood or plasma, and careful attention to fluid balance to prevent aggravation of a seizure disorder by overhydration.

As recovery ensues, electroencephalography may sometimes give helpful prognostic information. CT scan, serial echoventriculograms, and monitoring of head circumference daily for 10 days, then twice weekly, will give early indication of the need for neurosurgical intervention for hydrocephalus.

Skeletal Injuries. *Clavicular fracture* occurs with shoulder dystocia, particularly with large infants and with breech delivery. Diagnosis is made by the obstetric history and by finding pain, crepitus, or angulation on palpation. There is usually only little displacement; healing with palpable callus is evident at 2 to 3 weeks. A figure-eight bandage is unnecessary; simple pinning of the shirtsleeve to the shirt with gentle handling suffices. A follow-up examination should be done at 2 to 6 weeks to identify the rare fracture that goes on to nonunion.

Fractures of the humerus, femur, or other long bones are usually associated with difficult breech delivery. Simple fractures of the humerus in good alignment require only immobilization and splinting, and the arm adducted and the forearm flexed at 90°. Poor alignment will require casting. Fractures of the femur do best with immobilization by splint or cast, together with traction. Prognosis for birth fractures is good.

Separation of an epiphysis of the humerus (usually proximal) or *femur* (usually distal) is suspected when there is pain and lack of movement of the affected extremity after a difficult delivery. Diagnosis is confirmed by x-ray studies at 10 to 14 days, when callus formation will be evident. Treatment is similar to that for fracture. Brachial plexus injury can be associated and should be looked for.

Neuromuscular Injuries. Although *brachial plexus injury* is usually caused by lateral traction of the neck during difficult breech extraction or vertex delivery with shoulder dystocia it may occur spontaneously in utero. When injury is severe or extensive, chest fluoroscopy (or inspiratory and expiratory films) should be done to identify diaphragmatic paralysis. Immediate treatment consists of pinning the arm in abduction, external rotation and supination for 10 to 14 days. After this time physiotherapy is begun with careful pas-sive exercising several times daily. Careful neurologic follow-up is mandatory. The prognosis is generally good except when the damage extends to the lower nerve roots. Diaphragmatic paralysis requires chest physiotherapy during the immediate neonatal period, follow-up x-ray films, and careful observation during any intercurrent respiratory infection.

Facial palsy, sometimes associated with brachial palsy but more commonly an isolated finding, is usually resolved in several weeks. It requires no treatment except when the eye is involved. In this instance instillation of 0.5% methylcellulose drops should be made four times daily to prevent corneal ulceration.

Paralysis of the radial, obturator, or external popliteal nerves is uncommon, requires no treatment, and resolves spontaneously.

Sixth nerve palsy, usually unilateral, is found not uncommonly at birth. Its cause is unknown and it disappears spontaneously by age 1 month.

Spinal cord injury occurs with severe anoxia or with difficult breech deliveries, particularly when the fetal neck is hyperextended. Cesarean section will prevent most such injuries. Early diagnosis and supportive care should help minimize problems in the infant who is to survive. Diagnosis is suggested by flaccid paralysis with areflexia of arms and legs, diaphragmatic breathing, and urinary retention. Four-hourly Credé maneuver of the bladder will help prevent bladder damage and urinary tract infection. Chest physiotherapy and positioning is useful in the infant with thoracic involvement to prevent atelectasis and pneumonia. X-ray films of the spine will occasionally show a fracture or dislocation. The prognosis in general is poor, but an occasional, severely affected infant has survived with only minimal residual damage.

Internal Thoracic Injuries. Attempt at amniocentesis may puncture the lung causing *pneumothorax* and sometimes subcutaneous emphysema after birth. Treatment is immediate tube thoracostomy with underwater drainage. Prognosis is good. Some cases of *chylothorax* are thought to be due to injury to the thoracic duct during delivery. Treatment of chylothorax causing respiratory embarrassment consists of repeated needle aspirations or tube thoracostomy.

Internal Abdominal Injuries. Intra-abdominal bleeding may occur from rupture of the liver or spleen, the latter usually only when it is enlarged, as with erythroblastosis. Shock, abdominal distention, and occasionally a bluish discoloration of the abdomen warrant immediate surgical intervention, with concurrent replacement of intravascular volume with blood, plasma, or albumin. More commonly rupture of the liver results in a *subcapsular hematoma* with gradual deterioration over several days. Infants at risk because of birth history should have careful monitoring of pulse, blood pressure, and hematocrit, together with daily gentle palpation of the surface of the liver. The liver or spleen also may be injured by amniocentesis, intrauterine blood transfusion, or vigorous resuscitative efforts at birth.

Injury of the adrenal glands may be hypoxic rather than traumatic in origin. Blood transfusion to restore volume together with prompt surgical intervention may be lifesaving in the infant with massive hemorrhage. Milder lesions may be followed carefully. There is no need to administer corticosteroids.

Rupture of the bladder at delivery, presenting as ascites, is almost totally confined to male infants with bladder neck obstruction. Treatment is of the underlying condition.

Other Birth Injuries. Serious eye injuries are rare. Subconjunctival and retinal hemorrhages are common, unassociated with other bleeding, and require no treatment. Skull fractures are rare and are usually of little clinical significance. Small linear fractures are not uncommonly found when multiple serial x-ray films are done on infants with cephalhematoma (cf. supra). Linear fractures require no treatment; followup should be done at 2 months, however, to rule out the development of a leptomeningeal cyst. Depressed "fractures" are usually intrauterine spontaneous skull depressions. Neurosurgical repair is indicated for cosmetic reasons since many do not resolve spontaneously. Attempts to elevate the depressed area by applying pressure or suction are contraindicated since further damage may result.

Management of the Newborn Infant at Delivery

DAVID BATEMAN, M.D.,
JEN WUNG, M.D.,
and L. STANLEY JAMES, M.D.

Infants who begin breathing normally at birth require no more assistance than gentle suctioning of the mouth and nose with a bulb syringe to remove secretions, mucus, and amniotic fluid. They should be wiped dry, wrapped in a warm towel, and returned to their mothers under the watchful eye of an experienced nurse.

RESUSCITATION OF THE NEWBORN INFANT

Intrapartum asphyxia is the most important reason for a newborn infant to require resuscitation. In its most dangerous form, intrapartum asphyxia is superimposed upon chronic intrauterine asphyxia. The correct management of birth asphyxia aims at its prevention or, at least, anticipation, by the surveillance of fetal well-being dur-

ing the antenatal period and through labor. This involves identifying such predisposing conditions as hypertension, diabetes, intrauterine growth retardation, and oligohydramnios. Attention must be paid to the progress of labor, the quality of amniotic fluid, the fetal heart rate and, when appropriate, the heart rate pattern and the pH of fetal scalp blood. Unfortunately, the tools of obstetric surveillance remain imperfect; approximately half of the deliveries in which newborn resuscitation is needed cannot be identified by high-risk screening during the prenatal period.

Personnel. Preparation for the delivery of an asphyxiated infant requires that the resuscitation staff be armed with important details of the maternal and intrapartum history. At least two experienced persons are needed at the delivery of an asphyxiated infant. One person attends to the infant's airway, performs suctioning, and administers positive pressure oxygen via bag and endotracheal tube or bag and mask. The second person monitors the heart rate and pulse pressure and administers cardiac massage when needed. In rare situations additional persons must be available for drawing up emergency medications or blood and fluids, or assisting in umbilical catheterization.

Equipment. Basic resuscitation equipment must be instantly available in the delivery area. This includes a suction apparatus (a de Lee trap is most reliable), a source of oxygen with regulator and tubing, a self-inflating infant ventilation bag capable of delivering 100% oxygen, face masks to fit both preterm and term infants, laryngoscope with size "0" blade, and endotracheal tubes of sizes 2.5 mm, 3.0 mm, and 3.5 mm, fitted with flexible stylettes and adaptors for the ventilation bag. (We prefer "Cole"-type endotracheal tubes for use in the delivery room because these are designed with shoulders that prevent selective intubation of the right mainstem bronchus.)

The examination table must permit ease of access to the infant for resuscitation procedures. The table should be equipped with an overhead radiant heater and a good procedure lamp.

A comprehensive list of additional resuscitation equipment and medications has been provided by the American Academy of Pediatrics and American College of Obstetricians and Gynecologists in "Guidelines for Perinatal Care," 1983, Appendix B. Much of this equipment is needed only in special situations and may be kept in a crash cart in the delivery area.

Apgar Score. The Apgar scoring system (Table 1) is a valuable tool for quickly assessing an infant's ability to negotiate the transition from intrauterine to extrauterine life. It is also a general index of the asphyxiated infant's need for resuscitation. Traditionally, Apgar scores are assigned at 1 minute and 5 minutes of age. Infants whose low scores

Table 1. CLINICAL EVALUATION OF NEWBORN INFANT IN DELIVERY ROOM BY APGAR SCORING METHOD*

Sign	0	1	2
Heart rate	Absent	Slow (below 100)	Over 100
Respiratory effort	Absent	Weak cry; hypoventilation	Good; strong cry
Muscle tone	Limp	Some flexion of extremities	Active motion; extremities well flexed
Reflex irritability (response to stimulation of sole of foot)	No response	Grimace	Cry
Color	Pale	Blue	Completely pink

* The score is the sum of the numerical evaluation given for each sign. Maximum score = 10; minimum score = 0.

fail to rise to at least 7 by 5 minutes should have the score repeated at 10-minute intervals until their condition improves or stabilizes. In general, the lower the score and the longer it persists despite resuscitory efforts, the longer and more severe the asphyxiating insult has been and the more likely it is to be associated with poor outcome. Significant birth asphyxia is commonly defined as a 5-minute Apgar score of 5 or less. Analogy with the fetal animal model of acute total asphyxia allows interpretation of the physiologic variables composing the Apgar score of the asphyxiated human infant. Four stages of asphyxia are described by the infant's pattern of respiratory effort at the time of birth: hyperpnea, primary apnea, gasping, and terminal apnea.

Normal labor is invariably accompanied by at least mild asphyxia. This has the effect of raising heart rate and blood pressure above fetal baseline levels, increasing muscle tone, and stimulating respiratory effort (hyperpnea). The infant is born with an Apgar score in the 7–9 range and needs no resuscitation (1 or 2 points for color are usually deducted from the 1-minute score due to normally low intrauterine P_{O_2}).

With more severe intrauterine asphyxia an infant may be born in the stage of primary apnea. The 1-minute Apgar score ranges from 4 to 6 and the infant may require sensory stimulation, oxygen by mask, or brief positive-pressure ventilation to recover. (Stimulation may consist of drying the infant with a towel—which serves a double purpose—or a gentle jostling, to remind him to breathe.) Ordinarily these maneuvers are rapidly successful, and the infant's 5-minute score rises to 7 to 10.

Gasping at birth suggests more profound or prolonged asphyxia. Heart rate has usually fallen to less than 100 beats per minute. The infant is flaccid and reflex response is poor. The 1-minute score rarely exceeds 3. Oxygen must be delivered intermittently under positive pressure to expand and ventilate the lungs and achieve a successful resuscitation. The infant's 5-minute Apgar score depends not only upon the duration of the intrauterine asphyxia but upon the skill of the pediatrician in resuscitation.

Infants born in the stage of terminal apnea are completely lacking in muscle tone and reflex activity. The color is pallid, reflecting peripheral vasoconstriction, severe acidosis, hypotension, and profound bradycardia. Without a full-scale resuscitation these infants may fail to survive.

Occasionally, terminal apnea may be difficult to distinguish from primary apnea. This is especially true when primary apnea is prolonged as a result of maternal medication or is accompanied by vagally mediated reflex bradycardia, which commonly occurs when the infant's hypopharynx is stimulated by thick secretions or vigorous suctioning. Effective resuscitation in primary apnea may consist of stimulation and gentle suctioning alone. By contrast, heart rate and respiration in an infant with terminal apnea are also depressed, but the depression is accompanied by a profound absence of muscle tone, reflex activity, and pulse pressure. An apneic infant who does not improve promptly with stimulation should be ventilated with oxygen by an endotracheal tube or a bag and mask.

RESUSCITATION OF THE SEVERELY ASPHYXIATED INFANT

The objective of resuscitation is to establish efficient cardiopulmonary function as soon as possible in order to prevent or ameliorate the adverse consequences of asphyxia. Evidence of a successful resuscitation is seen first in an increase in heart rate followed by a rise in blood pressure; color will then improve, and then the infant will start to gasp. The establishment of normal rhythmical breathing takes several minutes longer. Although oxygenation is achieved promptly, the P_{CO_2} falls more gradually, and the metabolic acidosis is corrected even more slowly, over a period of 2–3 hours.

It must be emphasized that the overwhelming majority of asphyxiated infants, even those who have reached the phase of terminal apnea, can be resuscitated simply by ventilating the lungs with oxygen. In this sense infants differ markedly from adults, who usually require pharmacologic or electrical stimulation of the heart.

Ventilation cannot succeed until obstructing mucus and fluid are removed from the airway. Suctioning must be quick and gentle; it is best accomplished using a bulb syringe or de Lee catheter. The infant's head should be turned to one side to allow drainage away from the glottal area. Thick secretions may be partially removed with a gauze pad. After the airway is suctioned, the infant's head is turned to a neutral position with the neck only slightly extended. Positive pressure ventilation is best delivered by a properly positioned endotracheal tube. It is essential that the person responsible for resuscitation be properly trained in this technique, which can be dangerous in inexperienced hands. The correct use of a laryngoscope and endotracheal tube is best learned on a cat anesthetized with ketamine as well as on stillborn or newly dead infants. This procedure should not be used until the physician or nurse has achieved this necessary skill. Common mistakes leading to failure of intubation include overly deep positioning of the laryngoscope blade and hyperextension of the neck, making it impossible to visualize the airway. Hypopharyngeal structures are fragile and may be injured by blind probing with a tube containing a stylette.

Once the tube is in place, positive pressure is applied with the bag while the nurse or assistant listens to the chest. Chest movement and the sound of air entering the lungs indicate correct placement. Selective intubation of the right mainstem bronchus is a common error, which can be corrected by slowly pulling back the tube until breath sounds in the right and left chest are equal. In very low birth weight infants it may be difficult to localize breath sounds by auscultation; inflation of the stomach may mimic inflation of the chest. When an intubated infant remains cyanotic and bradycardic after a brief period of apparently adequate ventilation, one must suspect that the endotracheal tube is either plugged or malpositioned. The infant should be reintubated or, if this proves difficult, bagged using a face mask. Rarely, if an infant has been first resuscitated unsuccessfully with a bag and mask, a pneumothorax may be present. This acts as a space-occupying lesion and must be evacuated before ventilation can be effective.

If a person skilled in intubation is not available, resuscitation may be accomplished with a bag and mask. Effective positive pressure ventilation depends upon the choice of a face mask able to provide an air-tight seal. An assortment of masks in sizes to fit small premature infants, normal term infants, and extremely large infants must be available. (Usually these sizes are numbered 0, 1, and 2, respectively.) We prefer to use soft rubber masks with a contoured, cushioned edge. However, it should be emphasized that while the use of the bag and mask is more simple than intubation, it is less effective and more difficult to achieve good and prompt lung expansion. In the infant who is hypotonic and apneic, the inflating gas goes pref-

erentially to the stomach, which then acts as a splint to prevent movement and descent of the diaphragm.

The bag should be squeezed gently but firmly enough to produce visible inflation of the lungs. Usually a rate of about 40 breaths per minute is sufficient to correct respiratory acidosis and abolish cyanosis. The rate may be reduced as spontaneous respiration and movements appear. Overly vigorous squeezing may lead to pneumomediastinum or pneumothorax; although most self-inflating bags have a pressure release valve set at 30–40 cm H_2O, the valve orifice is usually small and with rapid, vigorous squeezing, pressures twice these can easily be generated. (Some institutions attach a pressure gauge to the bag so that overventilation may be avoided. We have found this device to be cumbersome and distracting during actual resuscitations, but we highly recommend its use during training sessions.)

If the heart rate cannot be heard or does not increase within the first minutes of resuscitation, cardiac massage should be promptly instituted. This is achieved by compression of the lower third of the sternum by three quarters to one inch in 6–8 vigorous bursts at a rate of 120/minute. Cardiac massage should be interspersed with 2 or 3 lung inflations. These two maneuvers must not be done simultaneously, as this increases the danger of pneumomediastinum and pneumothorax. Two to three episodes of cardiac massage are usually sufficient to restore the heart beat or correct the bradycardia. If, on ausculation, this has not taken place, a second episode of cardiac massage should be commenced and the same procedure followed. We do not recommend that cardiac massage be continued for longer than 5 minutes because of the risk of salvaging a severely brain-damaged infant.

Severely asphyxiated infants requiring cardiac massage will usually benefit from administration of sodium bicarbonate to assist in the correction of their metabolic acidosis. This should be given intravenously, usually through the umbilical vein, in a dose of 2–3 meq/kg (1 mg/cc diluted with an equal quantity of distilled water to reduce the hypertonicity). The administration of hypertonic solutions of glucose and sodium bicarbonate to premature infants is controversial because these solutions may potentiate the dangers of intraventricular hemorrhage. Paradoxical acidosis may also occur if the infants' lungs have not been first expanded and ventilation established. Because of this latter potential complication, we do not recommend administration of alkali until after the first 5 minutes of resuscitation.

Naloxone may be useful if an infant's respiratory depression is caused by a high level of transplacentally acquired narcotic, but one must never attempt to use naloxone as a substitute for needed resuscitation and ventilation. In contrast to treatment of the adult, cardiotonic drugs are rarely indicated during the resuscitation of the newborn.

Blood or blood products may be life-saving in the event of profound blood loss due to vasa previa or abruptio placenta involving the fetal vessels or for severe anemia resulting from Rh isoimmunization. Unless there is evidence of blood loss, however, most severely asphyxiated infants, even those in a state of vascular collapse, are hypervolemic rather than hypovolemic. The administration of fluid and colloid merely adds to the burden of their circulating intravascular volume, predisposing them to congestive heart failure and pulmonary edema. We do not recommend the routine administration of blood, colloid, or other fluids during resuscitation unless there is clear evidence of blood loss. (An exceptional situation in which hypovolemia may occur is with the asphyxia caused by acute compression of the cord shortly before delivery, i.e., a tight nuchal cord or prolapse of the cord.)

MECONIUM ASPIRATION

Meconium may be passed in utero by an asphyxiated infant and then aspirated into the trachea during intrauterine gasping. At birth, the infant's first breath will drive the tenacious meconium into the small airways, producing a severe obstruction to ventilation. Rational management of the meconium-stained infant consists of timely and thorough suctioning. The obstetrician must suction the mouth and nares of the infant before the thorax is delivered, reducing the volume of meconium that can be forced into the distal airways by the first breath. After delivery, unless the infant is extremely vigorous and breathing well, the trachea should be quickly intubated to remove meconium. The person resuscitating should suck directly on the endotracheal tube, extubate, then blow out through the tube to clear it of meconium. This process should be repeated until the trachea is cleared. Occasionally, meconium is so viscous that additional tubes are required. Persons well-trained in the resuscitation of meconium-stained infants should be able to perform intubation for suctioning 2 to 3 times per minute; ventilation (which, in any case, would be ineffective until the meconium is removed) is therefore delayed in these infants by 1 to 2 minutes.

The consequences of meconium aspiration may be grave. Infants with severe pneumonitis often require high pressure/high FIO_2 ventilator settings. Pneumothorax and pneumomediastinum are common. Mortality becomes extremely high when meconium aspiration is superimposed upon pulmonary vascular hypertension caused by chronic intrauterine hypoxia (persistent fetal circulation syndrome).

The value of tracheal suctioning to remove meconium prior to ventilation must not be underestimated. At Babies Hospital, meconium-stained amniotic fluid is the indication for 25% of the calls for a pediatrician to attend a delivery. In a 12-month period with 3900 births, there were 450 requests because of significant meconium. All of these infants required intubation and suctioning in the delivery room. Thirty-nine subsequently required admission to the NICU, some for indications other than meconium. Only 10 of these infants required additional support of ventilation, 9 by CPAP and one by intermittent mandatory ventilatory assistance because of persistence of the fetal circulation. Thus with prompt and effective delivery room care only 2% of infants with significant meconium require ventilatory support (approximately 0.25% of all deliveries).

MANAGEMENT OF THE VERY LOW BIRTH WEIGHT INFANT

Whatever their eventual outcome (e.g., severe hyaline membrane disease or intraventricular hemorrhage), tiny infants, when asphyxiated at delivery, almost always respond quickly to ventilation with oxygen. Meconium aspiration rarely occurs unless the infant is severely growth retarded.

For reasons related to the development of bronchopulmonary dysplasia, routine or prophylactic intubation and ventilation of small premature infants is to be avoided. Many small infants are quite vigorous at birth; their mild respiratory distress can be managed using continuous positive airway pressure (CPAP) delivered by nasal prongs. However, infants with respiratory distress or apnea who develop significant acidosis and hypotension are vulnerable to intraventricular hemorrhage, and they should be intubated until their blood pH and circulatory status become stable.

HEAT LOSS IN THE DELIVERY ROOM

The temperature of the delivery area, though comfortable for adults, may be cold enough to impose a significant metabolic stress upon a newborn infant. When the infant is wet, evaporation magnifies the heat loss. An infant's response to cold increases oxygen demand, making the stress worse for an infant who is hypoxic.

Newborn infants must be kept warm and dry. Simple measures suffice for the normal infant, who may be wrapped in warm dry sheets or cuddled by his mother after drying. An infant who requires the attention of a physician, or who is premature, is best cared for after drying under an overhead radiant warmer until the temperature stabilizes. Infants should be transferred to the nursery in a warm transport incubator.

Respiratory Distress Syndrome

WILLIAM OH, M.D.

The management of respiratory distress syndrome (RDS) will be divided into three components: prevention, supportive therapy, and assisted ventilation.

PREVENTION OR AMELIORATION OF RDS

Since RDS is primarily a disease of developmental delay in lung maturation, the most logical way of preventing or minimizing the severity of this disease is to prevent premature onset of labor and delivery of a premature infant. However, the state of the art is such that while some premature labors are secondary to complications of pregnancy, such as premature rupture of membrane, multiple pregnancy, incompetent cervix, and so on, a large proportion of premature labors are still unexplained. Therefore, the approach to prevention of RDS is twofold: (1) to delay the delivery of a premature infant as long as possible until the incidence of RDS would be the lowest. This goal can be achieved by the use of a tocolytic agent to stop premature uterine contraction and by identification of the risk of RDS by amniocentesis and assessment of surfactant levels in the amniotic fluid; and (2) when the delivery of a premature infant is inevitable because of the maternal and fetal risks involved in prolonging the pregnancy, pharmacologic intervention to reduce the incidence and severity of RDS is feasible under certain circumstances.

In regard to the use of tocolytic agents, several drugs have been tried clinically with variable degrees of success. The currently approved tocolytic agent (by the Food and Drug Administration) is ritodrine hydrochloride, a beta-mimetic agent. This drug is given intravenously at first until the uterine contractions are successfully stopped; thereafter it can be continued in the oral form. As with other tocolytic agents that have been tried previously (intravenous alcohol, diazoxide, terbutaline), the effectiveness of this drug is variable, but it is most effective under the following circumstances: intact membranes, early stage of labor, and absence of complications such as third trimeter bleeding and chorioamnionitis. Ritodrine hydrochloride is also not without potential risk both to the mother and to the infant. In the mother, pulmonary edema may occur when a large fluid load is given along with ritodrine hydrochloride. In the infant, hyperglycemia during the first hours of life also has been documented as a result of the maternal transfer of ritodrine hydrochloride into the fetus prior to delivery. These potential complications should be considered whenever this drug is used.

Several pharmacologic agents or hormones have been shown to accelerate fetal pulmonary surfactant production. These include glucocorticoid, thyroxine, xanthine derivatives (aminophylline, theophylline), tocolytic agents (intravenous alcohol), heroin, estrogen, prolactin, and epidermal growth factor. To date, administration of glucocorticoid to the mother has been found to be beneficial in several clinical trials. However, this drug is not without potential maternal and fetal risks; therefore, its usage should be individually justified and the risk-benefit ratio carefully assessed. The known risks for glucocorticoid include potential increase in the incidence and severity of maternal and neonatal infections, particularly in the presence of high-risk factors such as prolonged rupture of amniotic membranes with chorioamnionitis. It has also been shown that administration of glucocorticoid to a severity toxemic mother may increase the risk of intrauterine fetal death. Since chorioamnionitis, along with prolonged rupture of membranes, and toxemia of pregnancy concurrent with intrauterine growth retardation are associated with advancement of fetal lung maturity, these two maternal complications would generally preclude the administration of glucocorticoid for the purpose of preventing RDS.

Another important factor that should be considered in the issue of antenatal prevention of RDS with glucocorticoid administration to the mother is the fact that it would require a minimum of 24 hours of treatment time for significant clinical effectiveness. On this basis, it is important to point out that unless there are adequate clinical parameters to assure that the delay in the delivery of the fetus for at least 24 hours is achievable, glucocorticoid should not be administered to the mother.

The two most commonly used synthetic glucocorticoids for maternal administration are betamethasone (6 mg/dose for 2 doses IM at 12-hour intervals) and dexamethasone at the same dose. Once again, it is emphasized that the indication for maternal glucocorticoid administration to prevent RDS should be individually determined, with careful assessment of the risk-benefit ratio. Although a number of obstetricians from various perinatal centers still frown on the use of maternal glucocorticoid therapy for the prevention of RDS, the consensus is that with proper clinical determinations of indications, this drug may be used under the following circumstances: (1) when fetal lung immaturity is evident by a low lecithin:sphingomyelin ratio (less than 2:1) in the amniotic fluid, or a negative foam stability test (a semi-quantitative test for the presence of surfactant in the amniotic fluid), (2) in the absence of clinical complications such as severe toxemia and maternal infections, and (3) if there are assurances that the delivery can be delayed for at least 24 hours following the administration of the glucocorticoid to the mother.

Currently, a number of clinical trials are in progress to evaluate the potential beneficial effects of artificial surfactant in the prevention and amelioration of hyaline membrane disease. Although this agent appears promising, it is still in the experimental stage and should be considered as such.

SUPPORTIVE THERAPY FOR RDS

It is well known that RDS is a self-limiting disease, starting generally at birth and lasting for 3 to 5 days. The duration and severity of the disease as well as the occurrence of complications depend on the effectiveness of the supportive therapy. It is also known that the recovery from RDS depends on the ability of the neonatal lung to generate adequate surfactant during the first 3 to 5 days of life. The ability to generate surfactant in turn depends on the level of lung maturity, the cellular injury that may occur during the course of therapy, and the maintenance of optimal oxygenation, perfusion, acid-base balance, fluid and electrolyte balance, and thermal control. The goals of supportive therapy are to maintain these physiologic conditions without iatrogenic complications.

Oxygen Therapy

Oxygen treatment is one of the most important components of the supportive therapy for RDS. The goal of oxygen therapy is to achieve adequate tissue oxygenation without producing oxygen toxicity in the retina (retrolental fibroplasia) and in the lung (bronchopulmonary dysplasia or chronic lung disease). To achieve adequate tissue oxygenation, the following parameters must be attained: arterial blood Po_2 between 50 and 70 mm Hg, hemoglobin oxygen saturation of $\geq 95\%$, and an adequate perfusion to assure delivery of a normal amount of oxygen into the tissue. The latter can be achieved by maintaining normal hemoglobin mass as well as arterial blood pressure and blood flow.

The oxygen can be administered to infants placed in the incubator. If a higher concentration is desirable without frequent fluctuation, a plastic hood may be used as a chamber in which the infant's head can be placed and oxygen administered into it. This method of oxygen delivery is particularly helpful and desirable when nursing procedures require frequent entry into the incubator. It is also essential that the oxygen be delivered in a warm and humidified form to prevent

local damage to the mucous membranes of the respiratory tract. The ambient oxygen concentration should be monitored at frequent intervals and recorded; the oxygen tension should be monitored in the arterial blood or by the use of a transcutaneous Po_2 monitor. The latter is a noninvasive instrument that has been developed recently to continuously record the cutaneous oxygen tension; the accuracy has been verified by a good correlation with the simultaneously obtained arterial blood Po_2. The frequency of its use is increasing in various perinatal centers, particularly in the management of very severely ill infants with respiratory distress.

The source of arterial blood samples and the frequency of the monitoring of arterial Po_2 will depend on the severity of the disease and the risk of oxygen toxicity in the infants being treated. In general, infants with higher gestational age and larger birth weight having lower risk for retrolental fibroplasia, and having less severe disease probably require less intensive arterial blood Po_2 monitoring. In these circumstances, it may be feasible to monitor the oxygen therapy by sampling from a peripheral artery (temporal, radial, or brachial arteries), at 4- to 6-hour intervals. In these circumstances one is often tempted to use arterialized capillary samples for Po_2 measurement; however, it is emphasized that this manner of Po_2 measurement is notoriously difficult to rely upon, particularly in acutely ill, hypoperfused, and young infants.

In severely ill infants, samples obtained from an indwelling umbilical arterial catheter placed in the descending aorta are preferred, and the frequency of blood sampling can be adjusted according to the clinical severity of the disease. Utilizing infants' color as a way of monitoring the adequacy of oxygenation may carry a significant risk of oxygen toxicity since a "clinically pink" infant may have a Pao_2 in the range that may result in retrolental fibroplasia. Therefore, in those infants who are at high risk for retrolental fibroplasia, the Pao_2 should be monitored while oxygen is being administered under whatever concentration the infant may require.

Acid-Base Balance

RDS is associated with respiratory and metabolic acidosis. The respiratory acidosis is due to retention of CO_2, while the metabolic acidosis is a result of anaerobic metabolism with accumulation of lactic acid. The respiratory acidosis can be monitored closely with periodic blood gas analysis, as previously described; intervention with assisted ventilation is necessary if the CO_2 retention is significant enough to cause secondary apnea or impending apnea. That level is generally in the range of 60 to 70 mm Hg of Pa_{CO_2}, which is generally associated with a pH of less than 7.20.

Infants with RDS often may have fetal distress prior to delivery, which in turn may be associated with significant metabolic acidosis at birth. If the degree of metabolic acidosis is significant (pH $\leq$ 7.20), sodium bicarbonate may be given in an appropriate manner to correct the acidosis. Since inappropriately large doses of sodium bicarbonate administration may increase the incidence of intracranial hemorrhage, it is important that the dosage, form, and route, as well as the speed of administration, are correct. It is mandatory that an acid-base determination be done prior to the use of alkali so that the actual base deficit as well as the degree of acidosis can be estimated and the appropriate dose of bicarbonate calculated. The formula used is: Dose of sodium bicarbonate (meq/kg body weight) = base deficit $\times$ 0.3 $\times$ body weight. The sodium bicarbonate should be given in the form of half-strength sodium bicarbonate solution (0.9 M sodium bicarbonate mixed with sterile water in a 1:1 proportion), and the drug may be given intravenously (not by umbilical vein) over a period of 1 meq per 3 to 5 minutes.

The subsequent development of metabolic acidosis indicates that the infant's treatment in regard to correction of hypoxemia is not optimal. Therefore, when the clinician has to repeatedly utilize sodium bicarbonate to treat metabolic acidosis, the oxygen therapy and maintenance of tissue perfusion should be reassessed.

Treatment of Hypotension and Hypovolemia

Hypotension may occur during the course of treatment of RDS. This complication can be detected by continuous monitoring of the arterial blood pressure, either by direct measurement of arterial blood pressure through an indwelling umbilical arterial catheter or by use of the noninvasive ultrasound blood pressure device DINAMAP* if the direct measurement of blood pressure is not feasible. A nomogram for normal arterial blood pressure for neonates of various birth weights and postnatal ages should be available in the intensive care nursery, and the diagnosis of hypotension can be made if the blood pressure of the infant falls below two standard deviations of the mean. The initial approach to treatment of hypotension is to provide intravascular infusion of a volume expander in the form of Plasmanate at a dose of 10 ml per kilogram body weight. If the volume depletion and shock are associated with anemia, suggesting hemorrhage, blood transfusion should

be given at the dose appropriate to correct the estimated amount of blood loss.

If hypotension persists following volume expansion, one may use vasoactive drugs such as dopamine.† The dose is 5 to 10 μg/kg/min initially, and the dose should be titrated subsequently according to the infant's arterial blood pressure.

Temperature Control

It is well known that temperature control in very small infants, particularly those with RDS, is of prime importance for optimal survival. The goal of temperature management is to maintain the normal core body temperature of the sick infant at an ambient thermal environment that will entail the lowest metabolic rate. This ambient temperature is defined as neutral thermal environment and is variable depending on the infant's body weight and postnatal age. Such a nomogram has been devised, and it should be made available to the clinicians caring for infants with RDS in the nursery. As noted, another important maneuver for maintaining normal body temperature is to assure that the oxygen delivered to the infant is properly warmed and humidified to minimize heat loss via the respiratory tract.

Fluid and Electrolyte Management

During the course of management of RDS, appropriate maintenance of fluid and electrolyte balance is important to assure a normal metabolic milieu and prevent cardiopulmonary complications. It has been shown that fluid overload in low birth weight infants, and particularly those with RDS, may lead to increased incidence of symptomatic patent ductus arteriosus. Therefore, the amount of fluid given to these infants should be limited to what is required for maintenance, which amounts to approximately 90 to 120 ml/kg/24 hr for infants weighing between 1000 and 1500 grams; in infants weighing below 1000 grams, the fluid requirement is higher, but the amount should be individually determined because of variability in their requirements, particularly in the area of normal fluid loss via the route of insensible water loss. Sodium requirement of these infants is 2 meq/kg/24 hr. A system of monitoring the fluid and electrolyte balance should also be instituted by measuring the urine volume, urine specific gravity or osmolarity, changes in body weight, and serum electrolytes. These parameters should be determined and recorded on a daily basis; the status of fluid and electrolyte balance can be interpreted on the basis of these data.

---

* DINAMAP (No. 847), manufactured by Applied Medical Research, 5041 West Cypress Street, Tampa, Florida 33607.

† Manufacturer's Warning: Safety and efficacy of dopamine in children have not been established.

Application of Continuous Positive Airway Pressure

Continuous positive airway pressure (CPAP) is a useful mode of treatment for moderately severe RDS. This mode of treatment is based on the principle that by applying a certain amount of positive pressure (2 to 6 mm Hg) during the expiratory phase of a spontaneously breathing infant, one can mechanically maintain alveolar stability, thus improving ventilation. It is necessary to determine the arterial blood gases for proper institution of this treatment. In general, during the first 24 hours of life, infants with RDS requiring oxygen up to 60% maintain a PaO_2 of 50 mm Hg would be appropriate candidates for the institution of CPAP. It has been shown that by starting CPAP early (not waiting for the oxygen concentration to reach 100% to maintain PaO_2 at 50 mm Hg), the clinical course of RDS can be modified to a less severe form. The institution of CPAP can be done noninvasively by nasal prongs to avoid intubation.

ASSISTED VENTILATION

In infants with severe RDS, assisted ventilation is necessary to increase the survival rate. The usual indications for the use of respirators are as follows: (1) $PaO_2 \leq 50$ mm Hg at an FIO_2 of 1.0; (2) $PaCO_2 \geq 70$ mm Hg; (3) pH ≤ 7.20; and (4) persistent apnea. Positive pressure respirators are used, which require intubation. The endotracheal tube is introduced through either the nasal cavity or the oral cavity. The choice of respirator and route of intubation depends on the expertise of the medical, nursing, and respiratory therapy personnel in the intensive care unit. The amount of peak inspiratory pressure applied initially depends on the size of the infant and the compliance of the lung. One may start with an arbitrary number of pressures and judge the effectiveness of ventilation by the chest expansion, breath sounds, and color of the infant. It is essential that blood gas determinations be done to judge the effectiveness of ventilation. The inspiratory-expiratory ratio (IE ratio) of the respirator setting should be maintained at approximately 1 to 1.5. The frequency of blood gas determinations will depend on the severity of the disease and the progress of therapy. Positive end expiratory pressure (PEEP) is generally used to improve the alveolar stability. Complications such as extrapulmonary air leak, infection, and symptomatic patent ductus arteriosus should be watched for and promptly treated.

When the infant's condition improves, the weaning process may begin by lowering the peak inspiratory pressure, followed by lowering the oxygen concentration. The weaning process should always

be monitored closely by the blood gas determinations, either by arterial blood sampling through the umbilical arterial catheter or by the use of a transcutaneous PO_2 monitoring device.

Neonatal Pneumothorax and Pneumomediastinum

HENRY L. DORKIN, M.D.

Neonatal pneumothorax and pneumomediastinum are defined as extra-alveolar air accumulations in the pleural space and mediastinum, respectively. Such air collections (1) may occur spontaneously in normal newborns, (2) can result from congenital renal/pulmonary malformations, and (3) often complicate underlying respiratory disease and its therapy. The last group includes but is not limited to cystic fibrosis, hyaline membrane disease, esophageal perforation, meconium aspiration, bronchiolitis, asthma, and positive pressure ventilation with or without constant distending pressure. Presenting symptoms may be subtle (mild tachypnea, irritability) or absent, the event being diagnosed only after a screening chest roentgenogram is obtained in a high-risk patient. Alternatively, presentation may be a medical emergency in the form of vascular collapse and respiratory failure.

Air leak begins with alveolar overdistention and rupture. If the air vents directly into the pleural space, either through normal pleura or congenital bleb, a pneumothorax forms. If the air vents into the perivascular interstitium and dissects along the bronchovascular bundle supplying the alveoli, air may eventually enter the mediastinum. Such a pneumomediastinum may be the maximum extension of the leak, or it can lead to cervical, subcutaneous, or retroperitoneal soft tissue emphysema, even pneumopericardium. Sometimes, the mediasternal leak will penetrate the pleural space by this less direct route, resulting in both pneumomediastinum and pneumothorax.

Therapy for pneumothorax is a function of resultant respiratory compromise. If the diagnosis of pneumothorax is made in a relatively asymptomatic patient, observation is acceptable. Serial vital sign determinations, cardiorespiratory monitoring, careful physical exams, and sequential light transillumination and/or chest roentgenograms should be used for observation while treating any other underlying disease. If air accumulates under tension and the patient is in impending vascular collapse and respiratory failure, immediate needle aspiration of the air pocket (preferably under sterile conditions using a large syringe, three-way stopcock, and needle/catheter) may be lifesaving.

The needle should be passed just above the upper rib margin of the chosen interspace, thus avoiding the neurovascular bundle that runs along the lower rib margin. Care should be taken to avoid large internal structures such as heart, spleen, and kidney by using axillary or anterolateral sites. A clamp placed on the needle will prevent deeper penetration after the pleural cavity is entered. If the patient is not in extremis but has enough pleural air to be symptomatic, needle evacuation of the pleural space can be attempted in a less hurried fashion. In many cases of pneumothorax, however, unsuccessful needle aspiration or rapid reaccumulation leads to surgical placement of a thoracostomy tube for water seal or vacuum (-5 to -15 cm H_2O) drainage. Placement must be careful, especially if the air is loculated, in order to assure communication between tube and gas collection. After instilling local anesthesia, the method of tube placement varies among institutions, some using a trocar and others a curved clamp mode of insertion. If the pneumothorax has resolved after 48–72 hours and no longer exhibits an air leak, the tube may be removed in standard fashion.

Therapy for pneumomediastinum is usually unnecessary, as such air accumulations do not often compromise ventilation. However, if tension develops and causes cardiac tamponade, decompression may be required. Careful needle aspiration from the subxiphoid approach is recommended, with care being taken to avoid liver and heart. If necessary, a mediastinal thoractostomy tube can be placed under water seal or suction.

Some physicians advocate accelerated gas resorption techniques for treating extra-alveolar air, especially pneumothorax. The physiologic pressure gradient that keeps the pleural space evacuated may be increased 7- to 9-fold by administering 100% oxygen until all nitrogen has been replaced in the extra-alveolar location. This approach works best in pneumothorax but is contraindicated in severe distress or tension pneumothorax/pneumomediastinum. One must carefully consider the risks of exposing premature and term infants to 100% oxygen before taking this approach.

Alveolar rupture during artificial ventilation can be difficult to treat because continuous distending and intermittent high positive pressures may be required for survival. Obviously, all efforts should be made to lower these pressures as quickly as possible. Spontaneous resolution is less likely in these cases.

Known medical complications of air leak in infants include hypotension, hypertension, tachycardia, bradycardia, systemic air embolism, intraventricular hemorrhage, and inappropriate antidiuretic hormone secretion. Therapeutic complications include both laceration of the lung

parenchyma during aspiration or chest tube insertion and perforation of viscus.

It should be reiterated that similar clinical presentations may occur with lobar emphysema and lung pseudocyst. Careful radiographic differentiation should prevent the severe complications that often occur when these structures are confused with pneumothoraces and treated as such.

Bronchopulmonary Dysplasia

JOAN E. HODGMAN, M.D.

A syndrome of chronic respiratory distress and oxygen dependency accompanied by changes in the chest radiograph commonly follows assisted ventilation of the infant of very low birth weight.

Sensible management of ventilated infants involves control of oxygen levels and respirator pressures and early weaning from endotracheal tubes. Relative fluid restriction during the first week of intensive care will decrease the incidence of bronchopulmonary dysplasia (BPD) in surviving infants. Physiotherapy and tracheal toilet are particularly important, considering the decrease in cilial function and the increase in mucus secretion characteristic of the condition. Caloric intake should be pushed as soon as tolerated because BPD is accompanied by a 25% increase in metabolic rate, presumably due to increased work of breathing. Growth failure is prominent in the first year, with improvement in pulmonary function occurring with acceleration of physical growth.

There is a compulsion to decrease oxygen levels as rapidly as possible in order to facilitate discharge of the infant. This is probably an error that contributes to increased pulmonary vascular resistance and cor pulmonale. Ambient oxygen should be given to maintain a Pao_2 of 55 mm Hg and a RPEP/RVET below 0.35. These levels can be readily attained in home programs with the use of nasal catheters.

Diuretics have a beneficial effect on pulmonary mechanics and are recommended to control the increase in interstitial fluid that occurs in BPD. Furosemide is the drug of choice for initiation of treatment in doses of 1–2 mg/kg/day. Electrolytes must be followed to minimize the complications of hyponatremia, hypokalemia, and metabolic acidosis. Renal calcification associated with calciuria has been reported after 12 days of furosemide therapy; this was reversed when treatment was changed to oral diuretics. In infants who respond to furosemide, substitution of chlorothiazide (Diuril) at 20 mg/kg/bid should be made as soon as possible.

The characteristic smooth muscle hypertrophy present in BPD suggests that bronchodilators should have a place in therapy. Theophylline in doses recommended for apnea of prematurity improves pulmonary mechanics and may shorten the length of time ventilation is needed when used early in the course of the disease before the development of significant fibrosis. Isoproterenol also decreases airway resistance and increases conductance. Before chest physiotherapy and airway suction, brief inhalation of a 0.1% solution is recommended, especially for infants who wheeze.

The place of steroids in the management of BPD has not been settled. Recent controlled studies have shown good results from short courses of dexamethasone in ventilator-fast infants. Weaning from the ventilator was possible in all treated infants, but long-term outcome was not influenced. Rate of complicating infections was high in one study but not in the most recent. A 2- to 3-week trial of dexamethasone at beginning doses of 2–3 mg/kg/day, which are tapered after the first week, is indicated in the ventilator-dependent infant early in the disease course. The place of long-term treatment has not been established, and the effects of steroids on both susceptibility to infection and growth must be considered.

Although administration of vitamin E showed apparent early promise in prevention of BPD, studies, including one by the original proponents of this therapy, have failed to confirm a protective effect.

Infants do not need to remain hospitalized for their full convalescence. Oxygen therapy and chest physiotherapy are feasible at home, with proper patient selection and a program for parental support. Early discharge will decrease both the expense of intensive care and the emotional deprivation associated with the treatment of the infant with BPD.

Neonatal Atelectasis

JOAN E. HODGMAN, M.D.

Neonatal atelectasis is not present at birth, as infants are born with lungs partially expanded by lung fluid. Postnatal collapse of portions of the lung resulting in nonaerated parenchyma or atelectasis is always secondary to some other disease process. Treatment of atelectasis involves diagnosis and correction of the primary problem.

Extrinsic pressure occurs most frequently from pneumothorax during positive pressure ventilation but may appear spontaneously in a term infant following meconium aspiration. Removal of the pleural air by thoracentesis, followed by placement of a chest tube if the air is under tension, will correct the atelectasis. Accumulation of blood or other fluid, such as in chylothorax large enough to cause collapse of the lung, must also be removed by thoracentesis. Rarely, such an accumulation may be present at birth. Under these circumstances usual resuscitative measures will be ineffective, and the physician must be prepared to tap the chest as a part of the resuscitation without waiting for a diagnostic radiograph.

Masses in the chest that may cause extrinsic pressure on the lung are usually obvious on the chest radiograph. Aberrant vessels causing tracheobronchial obstruction are usually much less obvious and must be searched for by ultrasonography and appropriate contrast studies.

Lung collapse resulting from intrinsic endobronchial occlusion is usually the result of inflammatory disease. Copious secretions and decreased ciliary action are expected accompaniments to elevated ambient oxygen and mechanical ventilation, especially in the small preterm infant. Recurrent migrating atelectasis is a regular feature of bronchopulmonary dysplasia. Early meticulous attention to bronchial toilet will help to alleviate the problem. The infant should be intubated with the largest possible tube. Diameters less than 3.5 mm cannot be adequately suctioned, and we find smaller tubes unnecessary even in the smallest infant. The air or oxygen administered must be humidified and warmed to about 32°C (89.6°F). A program for regular position changes needs to be instituted early. Chest physiotherapy and suctioning must also be started early on a schedule adjusted to the needs of each infant. Bronchodilators will temporarily improve lung function and their use before suctioning will facilitate drainage from the lung. Isoproterenol 0.5% or isoetharine 0.25% can be instilled as an aerosol for 5 to 6 breaths before each regular suctioning session. When atelectasis is present, successful weaning from the ventilator is unlikely. It is particularly important, therefore, to atend carefully to the details of clearing bronchial secretions in order to alleviate intrinsic atelectasis in the infant on assisted ventilation.

Development of atelectasis after extubation occurs with some frequency, especially in the right upper lobe. Every reasonable effort should be made to avoid reinstitution of assisted ventilation, which will increase the risk for chronic lung disease. Intermittent laryngoscopy for tracheal suctioning has worked well in our hands. This should be preceded by administration of bronchodilators. Although most intrinsic atelectasis is the result of pulmonary changes inherent in ventilatory treatment, the presence of underlying disease such as mucoviscidosis should be considered in the resistant patient.

Lobar Emphysema

HENRY L. DORKIN, M.D.

Lobar emphysema may be defined as marked over-distention of a lung subunit, usually a segment or lobe, with anatomic and/or physiologic consequences to other intrathoracic structures. This entity may present acutely or subacutely as a cause of neonatal respiratory distress. Acutely, symptoms are usually present in the first days of life and include dyspnea, compression of normal ipsilateral and contralateral lung tissue, ventilation-perfusion mismatch, and vascular compromise. Clearly this is an emergency. Subacute cases have milder but often progressive respiratory distress and are usually diagnosed by 4 months of age. Alternatively, lobar emphysema can present more subtly in older patients with intermittent symptoms of cough, wheeze, tachypnea, or recurrent chest infection.

Both congenital and acquired forms of the disease are seen. Congenital or infantile lobar emphysema is more common in males and usually affects the upper or middle lobes. The etiology is uncertain, but it has been attributed to localized abnormalities of both the bronchi and parenchyma. Bronchial obstruction may occur from various causes, such as bronchomalacia, bronchial stenosis/atresia, extrinsic compression, or intraluminal secretions. Parenchymal involvement may be in the form of either abnormally developed alveoli or a polyalveolar lobe. Acquired lobar emphysema is seen in patients with bronchopulmonary dysplasia or pulmonary interstitial emphysema and is thought to be a consequence of the underlying lung disease or its therapy. The lesion is seen predominantly in the middle and lower lobes, more often involving the right lung. Endobronchial damage from repetitive tracheal suctioning, especially suctioning after the catheter tip has adhered to the mucosa, has been proposed as an iatrogenic factor.

Therapy is in part a function of the presenting clinical scenario and requires an early team approach coordinating the pediatrician, surgeon, radiologist, and anesthesiologist. Clinical and laboratory signs of respiratory failure or vascular compromise require aggressive management. Patients modestly distressed may deteriorate rapidly and, therefore, all should be closely watched by experienced personnel using frequent vital sign checks and cardiorespiratory monitors.

Respiratory care of the distressed neonate includes frequent assessment of respiratory effort and gas exchange efficacy. Nasal flaring, cyanosis, increasing tachypnea, retractions, paradoxical respiratory motion of the lower rib margin or abdominal wall, asymmetric breath sounds or percussion, and shift of the cardiac impulse towards or across the midline are objective signs of increasing respiratory embarrassment. Careful, sequential use of chest roentgenography helps to confirm the diagnosis, illustrates rapidity of progression, and may prevent confusion with tension pneumothorax (which is treated quite differently). An arterial line (umbilical or radial) should be established for frequent blood gas determination and continuous arterial pressure monitoring. Transcutaneous O_2/CO_2 monitors and oximetry complement the arterial line data but will not give direct hemodynamic information.

Medical management should include humidified oxygen sufficient to assure adequate oxygen delivery to vital organs and the periphery. It should be remembered that addition of oxygen will diminish the usefulness of cyanosis as an indicator of respiratory insufficiency. When possible, the patient should be placed in the lateral decubitus position with the affected lobe dependent. Intubation may be necessary for good pulmonary toilet and ventilatory support. Positive pressure ventilation may be necessary but should be used carefully. Such ventilation, especially when used with positive end expiratory pressure, may cause increased air trapping with deterioration. Sometimes selective intubation of the nonemphysematous lung may improve gas exchange with concomitant partial deflation of the diseased lobe. This may be more successful with the acquired form.

Nonrespiratory medical management should include the evaluation of electrolytes, glucose, urea nitrogen, and hematologic data. A secure venous line should be placed with fluids appropriate to replete and maintain fluid/electrolyte balance. A peripheral IV is often adequate, although a central line also provides data on central venous pressure. Urine output should reflect good renal perfusion. A nasogastric tube should be placed and the child given nothing by mouth because of feeding-related stress, possible aspiration, and preoperative precaution. The significant incidence of associated cardiac defect (patent ductus, ventricular septal defect) warrants preoperative evaluation if time permits.

For neonates with severe distress, definitive therapy is surgical excision of the affected lung tissue. Preoperative blood typing and clotting studies are needed and careful anesthesia induction performed such that the patient does not struggle and develop respiratory deterioration. The surgeon may elect bronchoscopy prior to thoracotomy if it is thought that an obstruction amenable to an airway approach is present. Otherwise, relief of mediastinal compression does not occur until the emphysematous lobe is removed.

Nonoperative management may be appropriate for infants growing well with minimal symptoms, particularly those detected beyond 4 months of age. Acute decompensation during viral respiratory tract infection can occur as a result of progressive air trapping during tachypnea. Such patients should be monitored accordingly. If the population for nonoperative management is carefully selected, follow-up comparison between conservatively and surgically treated patients with similar degrees of disease suggests similar results.

Meconium Aspiration Syndrome

DAVID R. BROWN, M.D.

Meconium aspiration is a cause of respiratory distress in term neonates. It occurs when meconium that has been released prenatally is aspirated into the lower airways. Respiratory distress occurs because the meconium obstructs the small airways either directly or by causing airway swelling and lumen closure in response to chemical irritation.

Prenatal meconium release happens in approximately 10% of all deliveries. The development of meconium aspiration syndrome occurs in less than 5% of these neonates. Aspiration usually occurs postnatally, with the neonate's first breaths. Since most neonates do not aspirate before delivery and cannot breathe during delivery until the thorax is delivered, aspiration can be prevented in most patients by suctioning the upper airway between the time the head is delivered and the time the thorax is delivered. Suctioning is accomplished using a DeLee suction catheter and trap, and the procedure can be performed equally effectively at vaginal or operative deliveries in which the head is delivered first.

This early suctioning of the upper airway should be all that is required to prevent the aspiration of any meconium. However, when meconium can still be suctioned from the upper airway after the neonate has been delivered, laryngoscopy should be performed and, if meconium is visible at the vocal cords, endotracheal suctioning should be performed using a mouth-to-endotracheal-tube technique. When a badly asphyxiated meconium-stained baby requires endotracheal intubation as part of a resuscitation procedure, the trachea should be suctioned after intubation but before positive pressure ventilation is begun. If meconium is present in the trachea, the child should be reintubated after the meconium has been completely cleared. In circumstances in which endotracheal suctioning is performed, it is absolutely essential that this procedure do no harm. In the case of the vigorous neonate with meconium visualized at the vocal cords, care must be taken to avoid causing bradycardia or respiratory arrest. In the case of the badly asphyxiated neonate, initiation of resuscitation with mechanically assisted respiration should not be delayed more than 30–60 seconds just to suction meconium.

These suggested procedures should prevent meconium aspiration syndrome in almost all except the rare cases in which aspiration has occurred prenatally. When aspiration has occurred, the patient should be managed in a neonatal intensive care unit. The most common clinical problems associated with meconium aspiration syndrome are pneumothorax and respiratory failure. Pneumothorax should be managed by inserting a chest tube and evacuating the air through a water trap using negative pressure. Respiratory failure should be confirmed by measuring pH, P_{CO_2}, and P_{O_2}. Treatment is dictated by the severity and character of the respiratory failure and may include added oxygen and mechanically assisted respiration. Endotracheal lavage with saline and treatment with steroids are not indicated in the management of meconium aspiration syndrome. Since meconium is sterile, antibiotic therapy is also unnecessary unless there is some other indication that sepsis may be a problem.

For the neonate with meconium staining but no signs of aspiration, as well as for the neonate with meconium aspiration whose acute respiratory failure has been treated, there are additional problems that require careful management. These include hypoglycemia, hypocalcemia, polycythemia, anuria, seizures, and persistent fetal circulation (PFC). All these problems can develop as a result of acute or chronic asphyxia. Since prenatal meconium release can be a result of intrauterine asphyxia, all meconium-stained neonates are at risk for developing any or all of these medical problems. Adequate management of these additional problems requires that frequent Dextrostix tests be done to assure that the blood glucose is normal, that the hematocrit be checked, and that experienced nursing personnel be available to observe the baby closely and to record voiding frequency and report to a physician any respiratory distress, cyanosis, or suspected seizure activity.

Any clinical or biochemical abnormalities that develop should be treated in an intensive care nursery. Hypoglycemia can occur as late as 24–48 hours after delivery if the patient is growth retarded. It should be treated initially with 6–8 mg/kg/min glucose intravenously; the amount of glucose should be adjusted to achieve a blood glucose of 50–70 mg/dl. Until the neonate has voided once following admission to the nursery, a low fluid administration rate (40–50 ml/kg/day) should be used. This expectant therapy is all that is usually required until diuresis occurs. If polycythemia (hematocrit > 70%) is associated with any clinical signs of distress, it can be treated with a partial exchange transfusion, exchanging the baby's blood for normal saline, lactated Ringer's solution, or plasma. Seizures can occur any time within the first 48–72 hours of life but occur earlier in more severely brain-injured neonates. They can be treated with phenobarbital and phenytoin as needed after specific causes not related to asphyxia are ruled out. Hypocalcemia may occur, especially if sodium bicarbonate has been used to resuscitate the neonate. However, unless the serum calcium concentration is exceptionally low (< 6.0 mg/dl) or unless seizures develop, intravenous calcium therapy is not necessary. The most serious potential complication of asphyxia is PFC. This clinical syndrome occurs when the neonate's blood circulation bypasses the lungs. It is thought to be caused either by mechanical obstruction due to embolization of the smaller pulmonary arteries or by pulmonary arterial hypertrophy and spasm. Special attention should be paid to any signs of respiratory distress or cyanosis in a formerly asymptomatic neonate or to any acute deterioration in respiratory status in a patient with an aspiration syndrome. If the chest X-ray view shows a pneumothorax, this should be treated with an indwelling chest tube, and any blood gas abnormalities should be promptly corrected. PFC can be a very serious problem requiring vigorous mechanically assisted respiration, paralysis (with curare or pancuronium), and tolazoline therapy.

Meconium aspiration syndrome is thus a largely preventable cause of respiratory distress that occurs in less than 1% of term babies. Prevention requires suctioning of the upper airway during the time between delivery of the head and delivery of the thorax. Postnatal management requires treatment of respiratory failure in babies who have the aspiration syndrome and attention to a number of post asphyxia problems in all meconium-stained babies.

Disorders of the Umbilicus

JEFFREY J. POMERANCE, M.D., M.P.H.

There once was a baby named Jane
Whose umbilicus had two arteries and a vein
Someone slipped in a small catheter
In just looking after her
Her navel will ne'er be the same!

During fetal life the umbilical cord (together with the placenta) is an extremely vital organ, serving as lungs, kidneys, and gastrointestinal tract for the fetus. Once the fetus is born, however, the umbilical cord becomes a vestigial organ and serves no specific function save as a repository for catheters inserted by ever-aggressive neonatologists. The umbilicus, although no longer serving a useful function, may still pose problems for the newborn

infant. Infections, hemorrhage, delay in separation of the cord, and congenital anomalies constitute these entities.

INFECTIONS/HEMORRHAGE/DELAY IN SEPARATION OF CORD

Omphalitis. In its severe form, omphalitis or infection of the umbilicus is rare in the United States today, but when it does occur, it is a potentially life-threatening disease because of its proximity to major blood vessels, which may act as conduits and very quickly release large numbers of bacteria directly into the blood stream (*septic umbilical arteritis*).

Diagnosis of omphalitis is dependent upon finding serous to sanguinous to purulent discharge from the umbilical stump. At times, the discharge may be foul smelling, but this does not imply a more serious infection, only the presence of anaerobic organisms. Most commonly, infection remains restricted to the cord but may spread to the surrounding skin.

Treatment for mild omphalitis (that not involving periumbilical spread) generally requires only local measures of cleansing and antibiotic ointment. A vigilant watch must always be kept for evidence of spread of infection. Omphalitis that has shown evidence of periumbilical spread should be treated locally as in the mild form, but in addition the infant should receive oral or parenteral antibiotics. Oral antibiotics may be used when the periumbilical spread is very limited. In these cases, very careful attention should be paid to evidence of further spread or to the presence of systemic symptoms. Marking the border of periumbilical erythema may be helpful in decision making, as it will then be easy to determine if the margin of the erythema is advancing. Final selection of systemic antibiotics should be made by culture and sensitivity results. Initial antibiotic therapy should include broad-spectrum coverage (e.g., methicillin and gentamicin) and may be further guided by local hospital experience. Many hospital nurseries across the country are now experiencing invasive infections with a type of *Staphylococcus epidermidis* resistant to most antibiotics but sensitive to vancomycin.

Granuloma of the Umbilicus. Usually the umbilical cord separates by the sixth to eighth day of life. When separation is delayed or infection is present, granulation tissue may be formed at the base of the umbilicus. A serous or serosanguineous discharge from the umbilical stump suggests this diagnosis. The granuloma should be directly visualized. It may appear as a small red mass within the deepest part of the umbilicus, although larger ones may protrude from the umbilicus. Granulomas should be differentiated from everted intestinal (or even gastric) mucosa or an *umbilical* *polyp*. Mucosa is purported to feel velvety and moist, whereas a granuloma should feel more like dry velvet. It seems likely that unless there are some additional visual clues such as unusual size or fecal discharge that allow the examiner to suspect bladder or intestinal mucosa, this rare anomaly will frequently be misdiagnosed. (See Patent Urachus and Enteroumbilical Fistula).

Treatment consists of cauterization with a silver nitrate stick. Care must be taken to avoid touching normal skin, which can be burned by silver nitrate as well. This treatment may be repeated as necessary every 3 to 4 days until the base is dry.

Hemorrhage. Hemorrhage from the umbilical cord may be due to inadequate ligation of the cord, trauma, failure of thrombosis of the cord vessels, or premature separation of the umbilical stump. Additionally, systemic bleeding disorders such as hemorrhagic disease of the newborn and disseminated intravascular coagulation may be associated with umbilical cord hemorrhage. Treatment consists of pressure dressings and correction of the bleeding diathesis, if present.

Delay in Separation of Cord. Delayed separation of the umbilical cord for more than 10 days has been associated with a defect in neutrophil mobility, which in turn leads to increased incidence of serious life-threatening infections. However, it is fairly common at our hospital to have parents report delayed umbilical cord separation of 14 days or more. Perhaps some parents use emollients, which prevent drying and/or bacterial invasion, which normally hasten cord separation.

CONGENITAL ANOMALIES

Single Umbilical Artery. A single umbilical artery occurs in about 1 of every 100 live singleton births and in about 5–7 of every 100 twin births. There is an association between the presence of a single umbilical artery (in singleton births) and the presence of other anomalies. After much back and forth discussion in the literature, most authorities now agree to examine carefully for other defects. The great majority of infants with significant additional defects have at least one other defect that can be recognized on physical examination. If none is found, further invasive studies are not warranted. If an additional defect is recognized, further assessment of other systems (especially the genitourinary tract) is indicated.

Umbilical Hernia. Umbilical hernia differs from omphalocele in that it is always covered by skin. Diastasis of the rectus muscle persists. This defect is generally small and can easily be reduced through the umbilical ring. Umbilical hernia occurs more frequently in premature infants and black infants.

Small umbilical hernias will almost always close spontaneously by one year of age. Large ones (5

cm or more) may require surgical closure, but unless it persists beyond age 3 to 5 years, becomes strangulated (very rare), is symptomatic, or enlarges in size after 1 year of age, surgery should be postponed, as closure may be spontaneous. Although there has been much controversy over the years, most authorities do not advocate taping or "strapping" of umbilical hernias, as it does not appear to accelerate or increase the chances of closure. Additionally, if done improperly it may cause strangulation.

Omphalocele. Omphalocele is a congenital defect of the abdominal wall occurring in about 1 out of 5,000 to 10,000 deliveries. The defect always includes the insertion of the umbilical cord. When small, it may cover an area only slightly larger than the umbilicus itself (*umbilical cord hernia*), but when large, it may include the entire midline area from the umbilicus to the xiphoid process. The protruding mass is covered by peritoneum, which is subject to rupture at the time of delivery. At times the amnion may be adherent to the peritoneal sac as well, making rupture almost a certainty. Omphalocele is frequently (30%–70%) associated with other anomalies (chromosomal anomalies, cardiac anomalies, and so on), which may well be the deciding factor in survival.

Historically, the diagnosis of omphalocele has been made at the time of birth. Today, however, with increasing frequency the diagnosis is made antepartum by the use of ultrasound examination. This has led to heated discussion about the optimal mode of delivery, vaginal versus cesarean section. At present the majority opinion seems to favor surgical delivery, especially when the defect is large, although controlled studies have not as yet been done. Such a study would of necessity require a multicenter cooperative effort that extended over a significant time period.

At the time of delivery, special care must be taken by both obstetric and pediatric teams to avoid rupture of the sac. The sac should be kept moist with sterile towels saturated with warm sterile saline. In order to avoid excessive heat and water loss, clear plastic refrigerator wrap should be placed over the moist towels. Immediate surgical consultation should be sought (antenatally if possible) to determine the timing and type of repair. Frequently, the abdominal cavity is undersized owing to the absence of the usual stimulus to grow, ordinarily supplied by the mass effect of appropriately located abdominal contents. Small lesions may be closed directly, but larger ones may require a staged approach. A synthetic plastic material such as Silastic or Mersilene is sewn to the margins of the defect and pulled together at the top forming a "chimney." Steady pressure over a course of days is applied to the protruding abdominal mass, thus gradually enlarging the intra-abdominal space in order that it may accommodate the intestinal contents.

If it is deemed best to postpone surgical closure, the sac may be painted with 0.5% Mercurochrome applied three times a day. Epithelialization progresses from the periphery inwards and may take as long as 6 weeks or more. Final surgical closure of the resultant ventral hernia is generally completed at 6 to 12 months of age.

The prognosis for small lesions is generally excellent. The only infants that do not do well are those who have other associated serious anomalies. Large defects, especially those that encompass the liver, have less positive prognoses. Respiratory embarrassment is the rule, rather than the exception, and prolonged assisted ventilation is required. Intercurrent infection is constantly a threat. Survival in these infants varies greatly (depending on associated anomalies as well) but may be as low as 50%. Survival rates with both small and large defects taken together is about 75–80%.

Patent Urachus. Patent urachus is a rare anomaly. It results from a failure of the allantoic duct to close. Usually the umbilicus appears entirely normal, although additional tissue may be present. The clue to the correct diagnosis is the fluid (urine) discharge. Analysis of the fluid for urea or creatinine should confirm the diagnosis. Radiographic evaluation of the anatomy should probably be performed as well.

Treatment consists of surgical excision. Outcome is generally excellent.

Enteroumbilical Fistula. Enteroumbilical fistula should be suspected whenever meconium or fecal material extrudes from the umbilical stump. Direct inspection with or without the aid of a magnifying glass generally will locate the orifice. Radiographic evaluation should confirm the fistula's connection with the small bowel. The greatest danger of enteroumbilical fistula is that of inversion of the intestine through the fistula. If this complication occurs, at the very least morbidity will be greatly increased. Therefore, surgical excision should be performed soon after diagnosis.

Neonatal Ascites

TIMOS VALAES, M.D.

The emphasis in this chapter will be on the management of isolated neonatal ascites in contrast to generalized edema and fluid accumulation in all the body cavities (hydrops fetalis). Nevertheless, there is considerable overlap in the causes of the two conditions, and often ascites predominates in the clinical picture of hydrops and requires immediate paracentesis to relieve the respiratory embarrassment. In the great majority of the cases the ascites is present at birth, i.e., the onset is in the intrauterine life. Ultrasonography has considerably facilitated the etiologic diagnosis of ascites and, even more importantly, has shifted the diagnosis and often the treatment to the intrauterine life.

Management of Fetal Ascites

Distention of the fetal abdomen by free fluid is relatively easy to detect and differentiate from dilatation of abdominal hollow organs such as the gastrointestinal tract, the urinary collecting system, the female genital tract, and the bile ducts and the gall bladder. The presence or absence of generalized fetal edema and of hepatosplenomegaly provides key information in the etiologic diagnosis of fetal ascites. Appropriate laboratory investigations should be undertaken whenever the sonographic information does not provide a definite etiology. Because of the frequency of urinary ascites and the possibility of intrauterine intervention to relieve the underlying obstructive uropathy, it is important in the sonographic investigation of fetal ascites to visualize the kidneys, the ureters and the bladder, and to estimate the volume of amniotic fluid as an indicator of renal function. A further refinement involves the real-time assessment of bladder filling and emptying, particularly after administration of furosemide to the mother. In the absence of a definite cause for early fetal ascites, continuous sonographic monitoring is indicated because spontaneous resolution has been well documented. This is more likely to happen if cryptogenic fetal ascites is associated with polyhydramnios. Following spontaneous resolution of fetal ascites, laxity of abdominal wall with, as an extreme, the "prune belly" appearance is the tale-telling finding at birth. Resolution of fetal ascites accompanied by oligohydramnios indicates progressive renal failure as a result of retrograde pressure from urinary obstruction. In this event renal dysplasia and pulmonary hypoplasia incompatible with survival are already present.

Intrauterine drainage of early fetal ascites either by repeated paracentesis or by placement of a special shunt catheter from the fetal abdomen to the amniotic cavity should be undertaken in order to avoid the effects on pulmonary development of the elevation of diaphragm and in cases of urinary ascites in order to decompress the obstructed urinary tract, avoid renal dysplasia, and maintain an adequate volume of amniotic fluid, thus preventing the development of Potter's syndrome.

It should be emphasized that both in utero and after birth only a small percentage of the cases with obstructive uropathy are complicated by urinary ascites. In the majority of the cases megacystis megaureters and hydronephrosis are present, and decompression in utero requires the placement of a shunt catheter from the dilated bladder to the amniotic cavity. Theoretically, preterm delivery with extrauterine decompression of the urinary tract offers an alternative solution. Nevertheless, it appears that by 30–32 weeks of gestation, when the risk of prematurity is acceptable, the majority of the cases have suffered irreparable renal damage and pulmonary hypoplasia, while those who have escaped this fate can safely be left to be delivered spontaneously, provided they are closely monitored sonographically.

Ascites and, more commonly, hydrops can result from fetal paroxysmal supraventricular tachycardia, which is relatively easily diagnosed with fetal heart monitoring or fetal EKG. Correction of tachycardia and heart failure has followed digitalization by administering digitalis to the mother. Resolution of the tachycardia and of the ascites and hydrops may take 1 to 2 weeks, and digitalization should continue up to the delivery. Whether transplacental digitalization or diuretics will be helpful in the management of fetal ascites or hydrops due to cardiac malformations or congenital heart block has not been well documented but may be worth trying.

Fetal ascites of other than renal or cardiac etiology is not amenable to intrauterine treatment, and fetal paracentesis for diagnostic purposes is rarely justified. (The treatment of immunologic hydrops fetalis with intrauterine transfusion is outside the scope of this chapter.) Occasionally fetal abdominal paracentesis during early labor will be necessary to allow for vaginal delivery and to prevent respiratory difficulties after birth.

Management of Neonatal Ascites

A long list of diseases and conditions is associated with ascites in the newborn and small infant. Obviously, the treatment of the underlying condition, if available, leads to the permanent resolution of ascites. Irrespective of the etiology of ascites, aspiration of the ascitic fluid is often indicated for diagnostic purposes and to relieve the respiratory embarrassment caused by the increased intra-abdominal pressure and the resultant elevation of the diaphragm.

Technique of Abdominal Paracentesis. The newborn is placed in supine position and the extremities restrained. The right or left lower abdominal quadrant is prepared with an antiseptic solution, such as povidone-iodine complex (Betadine), and draped. A 20 or 22 gauge "Intracath" needle and catheter are introduced just below the umbilicus and outside the lateral border of the rectus muscle. When the peritoneal cavity is entered, as indicated by the feeling of "give," the catheter is advanced and the needle removed while suction is applied with a syringe. Enough fluid is removed to relieve the respiratory embarrassment.

Complete removal of the ascitic fluid should be avoided for fear of abrupt shift of intravascular fluid and circulatory collapse. A sterile dressing is placed after withdrawal of the catheter. Some leakage of ascitic fluid through the puncture site is likely to occur. Vital signs should be followed closely after the paracentesis. The fluid should be sent for chemical analysis (total protein, electrolytes, urea, creatinine, and triglycerides, if milky in appearance), cell count, Gram's stain, and culture. The chemical analysis of the ascitic fluid, particularly in cases of urinary ascites, when high urea and creatinine are expected, can be misleading, as the fluid rapidly equilibrates with the rest of the extracellular fluid and loses its diagnostic characteristics. This is not likely to occur with meconium or infectious peritonitis or with bilious or chylous ascites. In the latter the characteristic appearance and chemistry develop only after milk feedings have been given.

Specific Treatment. The etiology determines the specific medical or surgical treatment of neonatal ascites. Thus, laparotomy and the appropriate surgical closure, anastomosis, or "-ostomy" are the treatments used for bilious ascites and ascites associated with the generalized type of meconium peritonitis. Similarly, relief of the obstruction leads to resolution of the ascites associated with hydrometrocolpus from imperforate hymen or atresia of the vagina.

The treatment of urinary and chylous ascites and the ascites associated with liver disease will be discussed separately.

Management of Neonatal Urinary Ascites

Whether present at birth or developing in the first few days of life, the leakage of the urine in the peritoneal cavity is the result of obstructive uropathy, and the principles of treatment are the same irrespective of the level of obstruction. The site of leakage or perforation is not always apparent, and its localization is not essential for treatment. Decompression of the urinary tract, initially by catheterization, should be attempted. If the cause of obstructive uropathy is posterior urethral valves or bladder neck obstruction, catheter drainage is often sufficient. Prolonged adequate drainage, necessary for recovery of renal function, is achieved by suprapubic vesicostomy. This achieves adequate drainage and allows for the recovery of renal function. If the initial ultrasonographic assessment and the cystourethrogram demonstrate unilateral or bilateral obstruction proximal to the bladder, nephrostomy or ureterostomy is necessary. Nephrostomy is also necessary when, in spite of vesicostomy, urinary ascites persists and the upper urinary tract remains dilated. Very rarely will it be necessary to localize the site of perforation and close it surgically. Even when urinary ascites results from transection of a persistent urachus, during umbilical artery cutdown, catheter drainage of the bladder proves sufficient to seal the perforation.

In spite of its dramatic clinical presentation, urinary ascites from obstructive uropathy has good prognosis. Ascites indicates that there is good urine production and renal function. The initial impression of severe renal failure is misleading. Anuria or oliguria is due to the escape of the urine in the peritoneal cavity, while the grossly elevated BUN, creatinine, and often potassium do not reflect the functional status of the kidneys but the fact that the urine in the peritoneal cavity equilibrates with the plasma—reverse peritoneal dialysis. Occasionally, life-threatening hyperkalemia will need to be treated with Kayexalate retention enema (1 gm of resin per kg of body weight every 2–6 hours) and/or glucose-insulin infusion (1 unit of insulin per 3 gm of glucose). Initially fluid administration should be restricted to insensible water loss (400 ml per square meter of body surface per day) and liberalized as soon as adequate drainage and decreasing ascites are demonstrated. The effectiveness of the treatment is monitored by following closely the changes in body weight, abdominal girth, and sonographic appearance of the urinary tract and by the improvement in urine output, blood electrolytes, BUN, and creatinine.

The surgical techniques used to correct the various types of urinary tract obstruction are beyond the scope of this chapter.

Management of Neonatal Chylous Ascites

A variety of malformations of the intestinal lymphatics have been described in isolated congenital chylous ascites as well as in chylous ascites associated with sporadic or hereditary congenital lymphedema. Chylothorax often coexists. The diagnosis is based on the characteristic milky appearance and high triglyceride content and lymphocyte count of the fluid after milk feeding has been started. Chylous ascites associated with lymphedema is often complicated by protein-losing enteropathy with severe malnutrition as an additional problem. Surgical exploration, in an effort to localize the site of the leakage of lymph, is seldom rewarding. Success has been reported with formulas containing only medium-chain triglycerides ("Portagen"), which are transported directly by the portal system without chylomicron formation, which increases the intestinal lymph flow. When this fails, a trial of complete bowel rest, achieved by total parenteral nutrition—including lipid infusion—for a period of several weeks, has resulted in permanent sealing of the leaking lymphatics.

Surgical efforts to excise the malformed cisterna chyli, resection of the loops with the most extensive lymphangiectasia, and finally, peritoneovenous shunts should be considered in intractable chylous ascites but offer few chances of success.

Management of Neonatal Ascites Due to Liver Failure

The treatment of ascites due to liver failure and cirrhosis is similar in all pediatric age groups and, with few exceptions, independent of the primary cause of liver failure. The predominant liver diseases of early infancy, extrahepatic biliary atresia and cryptogenic "neonatal hepatitis," do not produce liver failure and ascites early in the neonatal period. Fetal and neonatal ascites or hydrops have been described as an early manifestation of several hereditary storage diseases, such as Wolman's and Gaucher's, gangliosidoses, mucopolysaccharidoses, and sialidosis. Other metabolic diseases that can result in a rapidly evolving liver failure and ascites include galactosemia and fructose intolerance. The latter is unlikely to manifest in the neonatal period, as modern infant formulas do not contain cane sugar, and fruit juices are not introduced in the diet of infants before several weeks of age. Early recognition and special diets lacking the offending monosaccharide result in reversal of the liver failure and ascites.

Of the transplacentally transmitted agents, toxoplasma, treponema, and the cylomegalovirus can cause fulminant hepatic failure. The hepatitis B virus is usually transmitted perinatally, and the rare acute yellow atrophy develops after the first month of life. Similarly, cholestasis and ascites in sick, very low birth weight infants on parenteral nutrition develop slowly and after at least 3 weeks of total parenteral nutrition.

The ill-defined familial, fatal neonatal hepatitis offers the most dramatic example of acute liver failure and ascites in early life. Cholestatic jaundice, coagulopathy, and hyperammonemia with convulsions and coma develop within the first week of life, leading rapidly to death in spite of supportive treatment. The histology of the liver is that of "giant cell hepatitis" with extensive hepatocellular necrosis. The search for an infectious agent or metabolic disorder has been unrewarding. Specifically, extensive search for the markers of hepatitis viruses, including the non-A, non-B virus(es), in both the patients and their mothers has been negative. The author has treated two infants in two families with exchange transfusions to correct the coagulopathy and ameliorate the hyperammonemia. Immediate improvement of the general status followed the procedure, with gradual resolution of jaundice, hepatosplenomegaly, and ascites in the next several months. At follow-up at 7 and 12 years of age there was no evidence of liver or other metabolic disease, and growth and development were normal. It is difficult to explain this experience and to argue that exchange transfusion is the specific treatment for this condition. Nevertheless, with the excuse of using an effective method to correct the coagulopathy, exchange transfusion should be tried in neonatal acute liver failure of unknown etiology and should be used definitely in familial cases.

The symptomatic management of ascites accompanying liver disease includes (a) sodium restriction to 1–2 mEq/kg/day and (b) diuretics. Spironolactone, 3–5 mg/kg/day with a maximum dose of 10 mg/kg/day, is the agent of choice, since ascites from liver disease is associated with secondary hyperaldosteronism. If there is no response after treatment with increasing doses for 6–8 days, furosemide or ethacrynic acid* (1–2 mg/kg/day) is added. Electrolytes should be closely monitored and deviations corrected. (c) Correction of hypoproteinemia and reduced intravascular volume is carried out by administration of either 1 gm/kg salt-poor human albumin or 10 ml/kg of fresh frozen plasma over 2–3 hours followed by furosemide or ethacrynic acid. Success with this symptomatic treatment will be transient if the underlying process is irreversible.

Infants of Drug-Dependent Mothers

ROSITA S. PILDES, M.D.,
and GOPAL SRINIVASAN, M.D.

Drug withdrawal is the final insult to the neonate who has been exposed in utero to pharmacologic agents that may adversely affect total development as well as development of individual organ systems. Treatment, therefore, should be instituted as early in pregnancy as possible.

INTRAPARTUM CARE

A detailed history of drug intake should be taken on all pregnant women at the time of admission, keeping in mind that not all neonatal withdrawal syndromes are due to narcotics and not all women taking drugs are drug dependent. This information must then be relayed to the pediatrician to facilitate therapeutic intervention in the neonate without excessive investigation because of inadequate information. Drugs that have been reported to cause neonatal withdrawal symptoms are listed in Table 1.

The intrapartum period is the most inopportune time for withdrawal of drugs from the mother, who is already undergoing the additional stress from labor and delivery. Methadone and meperi-

---

* Manufacturer's warning: Do not treat infants with ethacrynic acid.

Table 1. DRUGS ASSOCIATED WITH NEONATAL WITHDRAWAL SYNDROME

Narcotics
  Heroin
  Methadone
  Codeine
Barbiturates
Analgesics
  Pentazocine (Talwin)
  Propoxyphene hydrochloride (Darvon)
Tranquilizers and Sedatives
  Bromides
  Chlordiazepoxide (Librium)
  Desipramine hydrochloride (Pertofrane)
  Diazepam (Valium)
  Ethchlorvynol (Placidyl)
  Glutethimide (Doriden)
  Hydroxyzine hydrochloride (Atarax)
Combination of Drugs
  Ts and blues [Talwin and tripelennamine (Pyribenzamine)]
Alcohol
Sympathomimetics
  Amphetamines
Phencyclidine (PCP)

dine are commonly used to prevent intrapartum withdrawal. Excessive fetal movements and increased oxygen requirements secondary to withdrawal may cause fetal distress; fetal monitoring is therefore essential, and a physician well versed in resuscitation should be present in the delivery room. Respiratory depression at birth may result from excessive use of drugs prior to delivery but can usually be overcome by prompt attention to the airway. Naloxone (Narcan) is not recommended because the drug may precipitate acute withdrawal symptoms, including seizures.

Most drug-dependent mothers do not take a single drug, and the presence of other drugs may alter or potentiate the withdrawal response of the infant. A very careful history of additional drugs must be obtained, and a toxicology screening of cord blood and urine collected during the first day of postnatal life should be performed.

NEONATAL CARE

Treatment in the neonatal period is directed not only at therapy of the withdrawal syndrome but also at problems secondary to prematurity and intrauterine growth retardation. Supportive therapy includes correction of hypoxemia, hypoglycemia, and polycythemia and provision of adequate fluid and calories. Respiratory alkalosis secondary to tachypnea rarely requires therapy. The increased incidence of syphilis, gonorrhea, and hepatitis in drug-dependent mothers must be kept in mind and the infant checked accordingly.

Therapeutic intervention is not always necessary, since symptoms, when present, are often self-limited. A quiet, comforting environment with gentle handling, swaddling, and frequent feedings

Table 2. DRUGS USED FOR TREATMENT OF NEONATAL WITHDRAWAL SYNDROME

	Dose/kg	Route	Interval Between Doses
Phenobarbital	1–2 mg	IM or PO	q 6 hr
Chlorpromazine	0.5–0.7 mg	IM or PO	q 6 hr
Paregoric	0.05–0.1 ml	PO	q 4–6 hr
Diazepam	0.3–0.5 mg	IM or PO	q 8 hr

may be sufficient. Therapy is indicated when the symptoms interfere with adequate weight gain and well being. These include vomiting or diarrhea, marked irritability and tremors that interfere with sleep or feeding, and seizures.

Therapeutic regimens vary considerably among centers, and a number of scoring systems have been developed in an attempt to standardize evaluation of symptoms and treatment responses. Most of the pharmacologic agents used have been successful in controlling the acute withdrawal syndrome. Although narcotic withdrawal symptoms are relieved most specifically by use of a narcotic, most pediatricians are reluctant to use a narcotic in the infant for fear of promoting drug dependence.

The various pharmacologic agents that have been used for therapy of drug withdrawal are outlined in Table 2. The choice of drugs is arbitrary; we prefer phenobarbital or chlorpromazine, but paregoric is often used in infants with diarrhea. In general, the drug is titrated starting with the smallest recommended dose until the desired effect is achieved. Once the infant is asymptomatic for 2 to 3 days, the drug is tapered until it is completely discontinued. Infants whose symptoms are controlled for only short periods of time may need more frequent administration. Tapering should be started by first gradually lowering the dose and then increasing the length of time between administrations. The tapering process may proceed every 48 hours as long as withdrawal symptoms do not reappear. Tremors, however, may persist for months.

Phenobarbital has been used extensively since 1947 and appears to provide adequate control of symptoms. Suppression of withdrawal signs is accomplished by a generalized, nonspecific central nervous system depression. Side effects include excessive sedation, which may lead to inadequate fluid and caloric intake. Diarrhea may remain uncontrolled. The duration of phenobarbital therapy ranges from 4 to 14 days in our nursery. The potential for withdrawal symptoms from phenobarbital therapy must be kept in mind; usually, infants requiring treatment for 2 weeks or less have not shown signs of barbiturate dependence.

Chlorpromazine was introduced in 1959 and is effective in controlling symptoms within hours after it has been initiated. The drug may be given orally or intramuscularly if vomiting or diarrhea is present. Side effects include extrapyramidal signs in infants who have received more than 2.8 mg/kg/24 hr. In our nursery, the mean duration of therapy with chlorpromazine has been 9 days, with a range of 3 to 17 days.

Paregoric (camphorated tincture of opium) has been used since the nineteenth century. Paregoric appears to control symptoms, with restoration of normal central nervous system function as measured by sucking behavior, whereas central nervous system depression may be observed with phenobarbital or diazepam therapy. The usual dose of paregoric is 0.05 to 0.1 ml/kg every 4 hours before feeding. If at the end of the 4-hour period symptoms have not decreased, the dose may be increased. Once the symptoms are controlled for at least 48 hours, tapering may begin. One of the drawbacks in the use of paregoric is the prolonged period often required for the tapering process (20 to 45 days). In addition, paregoric contains camphor, a known central nervous system stimulant. Camphor is absorbed rapidly and excreted slowly in the urine because it is lipid soluble and requires glucuronide conjugation. For this reason, tincture of opium (laudanum) is preferable whenever a narcotic is used. Care must be exercised in using the correct dilution, since laudanum comes in a 10% solution equivalent to 1% morphine, whereas paregoric contains 0.04% morphine. Laudanum must be diluted 25-fold to obtain the same dilution and can then be used similarly to paregoric.

Diazepam is effective in suppressing withdrawal signs but does not appear to offer any advantages over the other drugs. Diazepam is usually given intramuscularly at the onset but may be continued orally. Once symptoms are controlled, the initial dose is cut in half; the time interval between doses is then increased to 12 hours, then the dose is cut in half again. The drug is usually administered for only a few days, since it is poorly metabolized and excreted and has a prolonged half-life. Moreover, the parenteral preparation contains sodium benzoate, which competes with bilirubin for albumin-binding sites.

Methadone has been introduced more recently because of its wide use in the therapy of heroin addiction in adults. Theoretically, methadone is the drug of choice in infants of methadone-dependent mothers.* However, methadone is not easily available, the dose is not standardized, and there is greater difficulty in weaning the infant. Moreover, withdrawal symptoms from methadone

---

*The use of methadone in infants is not listed by the manufacturer.

respond to the same drugs used for heroin withdrawal.

The variety in therapeutic approaches indicates that the optimal regimen has yet to be demonstrated. Further studies based on clinical as well as biochemical observations are necessary to compare the effects of the various drugs. Unfortunately, long-term effects are difficult to obtain, since follow-up of infants of addicted mothers is fraught with numerous problems.

Management of the neonate also requires sensitivity toward the needs of the mother. Support, encouragement, and teaching are necessary to improve the mother's self-esteem. The infant should not be transferred to the high-risk nursery except when therapeutic intervention is necessary. Since the mother will frequently be discharged prior to the infant, these hours of early contact may be the most important in promoting maternal-infant bonding and possibly preventing the high incidence of child abuse.

Breast feeding by drug-addicted mothers should be undertaken cautiously, with careful monitoring of the infant. The advantage of promoting maternal-infant bonding must be weighed against the potential risk to the neonate. For example, methadone is excreted in breast milk; yet, breast feeding should be encouraged in mothers enrolled in methadone programs, and the dose of methadone cut down to minimum levels. Drugs such as heroin have been known for years to be excreted in breast milk, and at one time withdrawal symptoms were treated by breast feeding with gradual weaning. Almost all analgesics (codeine, meperidine, propoxyphene hydrochloride, pentazocine, diazepam, and barbiturates) appear in breast milk in low levels but may accumulate in the neonate. Individual variation in drug excretion will determine whether the neonate will be sleepy, hypotonic, or depressed or have poor sucking. Thus, breast feeding recommendations must be individualized and should be based on the risk to benefit ratio to the infant.

POSTNEONATAL CARE

Exacerbation or recurrence of withdrawal symptoms may be present for 3 to 6 months after birth and include restlessness, agitation, tremors, and brief periods of sleep. Medication should be avoided if at all possible. Additional problems that arise after discharge are thrombocytosis and an increased incidence of sudden infant death syndrome.

DISCHARGE PLANNING

The social service department should be involved with the family, and the infant can be discharged to the mother if there are adequate support systems in the home. Many addicted mothers appear anxious to keep their babies but do not have a realistic view of their own ability to care for the infant. Good prognostic signs include a stable marital relationship, successful raising of other children, addiction to a single drug, enrollment in a drug program, and a short duration of addiction. The caretakers should be aware of the expected behavior of the infant, such as increased sensitivity to auditory stimuli, decreased visual orientation, excessive crying, and increased sucking needs. The infants often respond to a soft soothing voice, gentle rocking, holding, and use of a pacifier. Follow-up visits by a visiting nurse, social worker, or ex-addict counselor may be helpful. A great deal of time and energy is invested in each case to insure supervision of the child's care, but despite all efforts, approximately 15 to 20% of the infants require placement in foster homes.

LONG-TERM PROGNOSIS

Early withdrawal symptoms of irritability, hyperactivity, sleep, feeding problems, and hypertonicity may persist for several months. Longitudinal studies are scarce because a large percentage of the patients are lost to follow-up. In one study behavioral disturbances, brief attention span, and temper tantrums were identified in 7 of 14 infants of mothers addicted to heroin. Children of mothers maintained on methadone who were followed up to 18 months of age were noted to have a higher incidence of otitis media, head circumference below the third percentile, neurologic findings of tone discrepancies, developmental delays, poor fine motor coordination, and lower scores on Bayley mental and motor developmental indices. High correlation has been reported between the hyperexcitable state in the neonate and neurologic and behavioral dysfunction at 1.5 to 4 years of age.

Acquired immune deficiency syndrome (AIDS) has been reported in infants born to drug-addicted mothers who are sexually promiscuous. Intrauterine growth retardation, failure to thrive, lymphadenopathy, hepatosplenomegaly, parotitis, interstial pneumonia, profound cell-mediated immunodeficiency with reversed T_4/T_8 ratios, and hypergammaglobulinemia have been observed in children with AIDS. The mode of transmission is unclear, but clinical histories strongly suggest vertical transmission.

Maternal Alcohol Ingestion Effects on the Developing Child

N. PAUL ROSMAN, M.D.,
and EDGAR Y. OPPENHEIMER, M.D.

Because the effects of prenatal exposure to alcohol are not reversible postnatally, management is confined to *prevention* and *remediation*.

Prevention

It seems clear that maternal alcohol consumption during pregnancy may adversely affect the developing fetus. While a safe level of alcohol consumption during pregnancy has not been firmly established, women consuming five or more drinks on an occasion should be told that such intake is potentially damaging to their unborn child. These women should be advised to stop drinking. Women consuming three to four drinks on an occasion should be told that this may pose a small risk to the fetus, and here, too, discontinuance of drinking should be recommended. Light drinking (intake of less than 1 oz of absolute alcohol per day) has not been demonstrated to be injurious to the unborn child; nonetheless, consumption of even small amounts of alcohol in pregnancy is probably best not encouraged. In addition to providing information about the risks of different levels of alcohol consumption, drinking women should also be given ongoing medical care and supportive counseling.

Remediation

Although the adverse effects of prenatal alcohol consumption cannot be undone postnatally, it is essential to help affected children reach their full potential. Thus, such children must be provided all necessary remedial services. Illustrative medical, surgical, and educational assistances in the overall management of the child and the family are outlined below.

Medical Management. It is important to identify affected infants in an attempt to prevent fetal alcohol effects in subsequent pregnancies. Such identification will also avoid unnecessary diagnostic tests. Other problems that call for medical management include the following: (1) undernutrition and growth failure, (2) developmental disabilities, (3) jitteriness in the newborn and attention deficit disorder and hyperactivity in the older child, (4) visual refractive errors and strabismus, (5) hearing problems, (6) infections and immunologic deficiencies, and (7) cardiac, urogenital, and hepatic disorders.

Surgical Management. Associated abnormalities in which surgical intervention may play a role include the following: (1) atrial and ventricular septal defects and tetralogy of Fallot; (2) cleft lip and cleft palate; (3) strabismus and ptosis; (4) hypospadias, uteropelvic junction obstruction, and other urinary tract abnormalities; (5) skeletal deformities, hip dislocation, and scoliosis; (6) inguinal and umbilical hernias; (7) myelomeningocele; and (8) accompanying tumors.

Educational and Other Remedial Services. The following therapies are beneficial: (1) infant stimulation programs, (2) remedial services at school, (3) physical therapy, including special gymnastic programs, (4) occupational therapy, (5) speech and language therapies, (6) behavioral modification, and (7) psychological support and family counseling.

Excessive alcohol ingestion by pregnant women has been referred to as the most frequent known teratogenic cause of mental deficiency in the Western World. While such a claim very likely overestimates alcohol's true teratogenic potential, the need to prevent new cases and to intervene therapeutically in those so identified is clear.

Preparation of the Neonate for Transfer

JEFFREY B. GOULD, M.D., M.P.H.

Successful infant *transport* is dependent upon (1) anticipating the need for transport before the infant critically deteriorates, (2) stabilizing the infant to minimize stress and hypoxemia, and (3) preparing the parents.

When to Transport

The decision to transfer an infant to a more specialized facility is ideally made when the patient's diagnostic and therapeutic requirements are expected to exceed those available in the hospital of birth. The key to success is to initiate transfer before the patient's condition seriously deteriorates, thus avoiding many possible complications and greatly improving the outcome. Lists of conditions "requiring transport" usually include such categories as very low birth weight (<1500 gm), severe asphyxia, respiratory distress, sepsis/meningitis, metabolic abnormality, multiple congenital anomalies, and surgical emergencies. As hospitals become more experienced members of perinatal transport networks, there has been local refinement of these lists by multidisciplinary newborn committees consisting of physicians, nurses, and administration and technical staff. This local refinement based on an assessment of the local facilities, medical, nursing, and support capabilities; past experience caring for "transport infants"; and past experience with the time and difficulties of transports serves to "fine tune" the transport decision. It is often difficult to decide if an infant really needs transport or should be observed for "a few more hours." When in doubt, a call to the senior transport physician on call will be useful.

The Initial Transport Call

The initial transport call sets into motion a course of collaborative care that begins in the local hospital (stabilization phase), continues in the tertiary care center (intensive care phase), and often terminates with transport of the infant back to the local hospital (growth and preparation for discharge to home phase). This initial call must contain information that will identify the patient's immediate and projected needs. Such factors as perinatal history, condition at birth, subsequent course, and current status are critical, as they allow the transport consultant to evaluate the working diagnosis, assess the ongoing treatment, and suggest steps to further stabilize the infant. The initial call also helps the team set their operational priorities; establish the composition of the transport team (need for respiratory therapist, senior neonatologist, etc.); assess the need for special or extra equipment (e.g., extra heat devices for a very small premature, extra supplies of saline for a large gastroschisis), and in some cases recommend the tertiary care facility that can best meet the infant's specific needs.

Another important aspect is the determination not to transport an infant. Such decisions are usually reserved for moribund infants whose likelihood for survival would not be improved by transport to a more specialized facility. It is often helpful to make this decision in consultation with the "transport neonatologist."

Stabilization Prior to Transport

Regardless of the illness, the more stable the infant at the time of transport, the greater is the likelihood of a favorable outcome. The stabilized infant has 1) a normal temperature (37°C rectal, 36.3°–36.5°C skin); 2) an arterial oxygen level that is neither brain damaging (<40 mm Hg) or eye damaging (>80 mm Hg); 3) a pH that is not severely acidotic (<7.3); 4) a hematocrit and blood volume that provide for good tissue perfusion; 5) fluid status that avoids dehydration and water intoxication; and 6) no metabolic derangement such as hypoglycemia or hypocalcemia.

Temperature. Infants who are hypothermic have increased oxygen consumption, a tendency toward acidosis and hypoglycemia, and tolerate stress poorly. One of the most important aspects of stabilization is to keep the patient from getting hypothermic. The typical transport infant is a premature who has required extensive resuscitation in the delivery room. These infants are usually cold when they reach the nursery. While their physiologic needs are being attended to (e.g., intubation, starting IV, placing catheters) their temperature and chances for intact survival will continue to fall unless special equipment (such as radiant warmers) is used and special precautions taken. Even though a small premature is on a radiant heat bed, a prolonged period under sterile drapes while a catheter is being placed can lead to a serious drop in temperature. Also, an infant will rapidly cool when removed from a warm incubator

for emergency intubation. An adequate number of devices to supply heat to exposed infants is a sound investment for even the smallest nursery. A hypothermic infant's temperature should be checked every 15 minutes until normal.

Oxygenation. Central cyanosis, and an oxygen level below 50 to 60 mm of Hg should be treated by increasing the percent oxygen. The persistence of poor color, low oxygen levels, and high levels of CO_2 (>60 mm Hg) suggests that ventilation is inadequate, especially when the cardiac rate falls to less than 100. The patient should be treated with artificial ventilation by bag and mask or bag and endotracheal tube. The adequacy of ventilation and the specific treatment of a persistently low heart rate may be treated using the guidelines for neonatal resuscitation (see section on Resuscitation).

Acidosis. The Ph may be determined from a warmed heel stick or even a venous sample. When the pH is <7.3, acidosis should be treated. If the CO_2 is >50, this respiratory acidosis should be treated by increasing the depth (watch the chest for adequate movement) or rate of ventilation. If the base deficit is greater than 10, correct this metabolic acidosis by giving a slow infusion of sodium bicarbonate (as described in section on Resuscitation).

Hypovolemic Shock. Shock due to low blood volume may present as pallor, cool skin, poor capillary filling, poor urine output, and persistence of low oxygen and a metabolic acidosis. This should be treated with whole blood or blood products as described in section on Resuscitation.

Dehydration. The signs of dehydration are similar to those of hypovolemic shock. While the hematocrit is usually low in hypovolemia, it is often high in dehydration. Treatment involves expansion of the blood volume with 10 ml/kg of fresh frozen plasma or 5% albumin followed by the infusion of D-5-W.

Metabolic Considerations. The blood sugar should be followed with Dextrostix. Hypoglycemia may be treated with 2 to 4 ml/kg of D-25-W IV stat followed by an infusion of D-10-W. Be sure to continue following Dextrostix.

In addition to the major steps to stabilize infants, some acute processes will require medical intervention prior to the arrival of the transport team. Suspected sepsis as evidenced by hypo- or hyperthermia, lethargy or irritability, vomiting, unexplained deterioration, or pneumonia, especially in an infant born to a mother with prolonged rupture of membranes or a temperature, must be immediately treated using standard guidelines. A gastric aspirate for smear and culture, blood culture, L. P., suprapubic tap, one surface culture, and a culture of the placenta should be obtained. In many instances these specimens are sent with the infant to the tertiary center.

Seizures will also require immediate treatment following standard guidelines.

A pneumothorax is often diagnosed following sudden and unexplained pulmonary deterioration. This must be immediately aspirated if symptomatic. However, one need not use a chest tube as the introduction of "Intracath" type needle at the anterior axillary line at the level of the nipple will often suffice as a temporary measure. The needle should be attached to a syringe or vacuum and water trap set up for continuous evacuation.

Intestinal obstruction at esophageal, duodenal, or lower levels should always be treated with an indwelling catheter attached to an intermittent suction device. Intermittent suctioning by staff using a syringe is usually not very effective and poses a serious risk of aspiration.

Certain surgical conditions also require immediate therapy. Myelomeningocele, gastroschisis, and omphaloceles should be kept moist and clean by covering with moist, warm saline packs. The infant must be positioned to take the stress off the mass, and evaporative heat loss must be avoided.

There are two common pitfalls to be avoided in caring for a critically ill infant prior to transport: 1) not giving standard neonatal care such as eye prophylaxis, vitamin K, or identification prints and 2) not recording the time and quantity of all medications and fluids given the infant and all urine and stool output.

While it is impossible to discuss all the problems and their immediate treatments here, this is precisely the goal of the initial transport call—to assess the patient's needs and to develop therapies to be followed prior to the arrival of the transport team.

Preparation of Parents

To most parents transport of their infant is devastating. The period of maternal-infant separation increases their anxiety and despair. It is helpful to explain to both parents the reason for transport and the greatly improved outlook for the majority of transported infants. Prior to transport, the transport physician should also speak with the parents. The father or another central family member should be encouraged to visit the infant as soon after admission as possible. Firsthand experience with the neonatal intensive care unit (NICU) and its staff can then be carried back and serve as a source of support to the mother. The NICU should contact the referring hospital several hours after admission so that a report of the infant's current status and prognosis can be relayed to the mother.

Although a great deal of time may have been spent with the mother or parents prior to transport, during this initial shock period it is unlikely that many of the details will be remembered. It is helpful to meet with the mother or parents 12 hours after transport. I have found the question, "Things were pretty hectic after the birth of your baby. I wonder if you could tell me what you understand about his/her condition and its treatment?" to be extremely useful.

Final Preparation for Transport

Prior to the arrival of the transport team one should collect copies of the mother's and infant's charts, 10 ml of clotted maternal blood, 10 ml of clotted cord blood, copies of x-rays and EKG's, culture specimens, and the placenta. With the arrival of the transport team, the status of the patient's stabilization will be re-evaluated, as will the need to institute further therapy prior to transport. Attempts will be made to ensure optimal stabilization and decisions will be made as to whether the infant should have a more stable peripheral IV, an umbilical artery catheter, or perhaps intubation for marginal respiratory status, if these were not already required during the period of pretransport stabilization; as a last step the team will contact the tertiary center for a final consultation. The patient's course, needs, and expected time of arrival will be discussed. At this point it is important that the route from nursery to ambulance be cleared by holding elevators, clearing corridors, and positioning the vehicle.

Breast-Feeding

MARIANNE R. NEIFERT, M.D., *and*
K. MICHAEL HAMBIDGE, M.D.

Infant feeding experts universally agree that breast milk represents optimal nutrition during the early months of life. Breast-feeding confers protection against gastrointestinal and upper respiratory infections, which has profound significance in underdeveloped countries and lesser but real importance in developed settings. The relationship developed through breast-feeding can be an important part of early maternal-infant interaction and provides a source of security and comfort for the infant apart from the provision of nutrients.

PREPARATION

The majority of women have made a decision about infant feeding by the third trimester. The physician should inquire early in the prenatal period about the intended feeding method. If bottle feeding has been selected, one should inquire how the decision was made, since many women decline to breast-feed because of misinformation rather than a true preference for bottle feeding. If breast-feeding is intended, the physician should support the decision, convey the advantages of breast-feeding, and perform a physical examination of the breasts. Breast enlargement during pregnancy is a good prognostic sign, implying glandular development. The nipples should be inspected for inversion by grasping between the thumb and forefinger. The normal nipple will protrude, while an inverted nipple retracts inward. Inverted nipples should be treated prenatally by Hoffman's exercises, performed by gently pulling at the areolar margins with the index fingers, vertically then horizontally, to help make the nipples more protractile. Milk cups, or breast shields, worn over inverted nipples during the later months of pregnancy can help draw them out.

"First do no harm" should guide prenatal breast and nipple preparation, since vigorous nipple manipulation may be traumatic and harmful. Soap should be avoided on the breasts in the last trimester because of its drying effect. Exposing the nipples to air by letting down the flaps of a maternity bra may help condition them for nursing. Gentle rolling or pulling the nipples is thought to enhance elasticity, but no proof exists that breast manipulation actually fosters breast-feeding success. A positive attitude and knowledge about how the breasts work, acquired through reading materials and classes, probably does more to guarantee success than physical manipulation of the breasts. Mothers can be referred to local La Leche League groups, in which knowledgeable leaders offer accurate information, and a variety of mother-infant couples provide firsthand observations of successful breast-feeding.

INITIATION OF BREAST-FEEDING

As soon as both mother and baby are stable after delivery, the infant may be put to the breast. In the absence of complications, nursing can occur in the delivery room or recovery room within the first hour after birth. Correct positioning and proper breast-feeding technique are crucial to assure effective nursing and minimize sore nipples. To nurse while sitting, the infant should be elevated to the height of the breast and turned completely to face the mother, so their abdomens are touching. The mother's arm supporting the infant should be held tight at her side, bringing the baby's head in line with her breast. The breast should be supported by the lower portion of the free hand while the nipple is pinched by the thumb and index fingers to make it more protractile. The infant's initial licking, mouthing, and rooting help make the nipple erect. When the infant opens his or her mouth, as much nipple and areola as possible should be inserted.

Time restrictions should not be imposed, but nursing guidelines are 5 minutes per breast at each feeding the first day, 10 minutes on each side at each feeding the second day, and 15 minutes or more per side thereafter. It is preferable to have the infant nurse at both breasts at each feeding, even if this means limiting the sucking time at the first breast to 5 to 7 minutes. Following the let-down reflex, a vigorous infant can empty the breast in approximately 5 minutes, but additional suckling assures complete breast emptying, stimulates more milk production, and satisfies the infant's sucking urge. The mother should alternate the breast on which she begins feedings so that the breast last suckled is the one first nursed at the next feeding. In order to prevent nipple trauma, the mother should be careful to break suction gently after feedings by inserting her finger between the baby's gums.

COMMON MINOR PROBLEMS

Sore Nipples. Many women experience transient, mild nipple tenderness during the early days of breast-feeding. Tenderness usually begins to resolve once milk is in and the let-down reflex is well conditioned. Assuring proper nursing position and technique, removing the infant correctly from the breast, nursing for shorter periods more frequently, beginning feedings on the least sore side, air drying the nipples well after feedings, and applying lanolin cream after nursing will all help minimize tenderness. Mismanagement of sore nipples can lead to chronic, painful open cracks or blisters. *Monilia* infection, often introduced by oral thrush in the infant, can be a cause of late-onset sore nipples. Treating the infant's thrush and applying nystatin cream to the mother's nipples often resolve the condition.

Engorgement. Lactogenesis, or the onset of copious milk secretion, occurs on the second to fifth post-partum day and is associated with marked engorgement, or swelling, of the breast. The engorgement can make the nipple-areola junction convex and difficult for the infant to grasp. Hand expression of milk prior to nursing will soften the areola. Unrelieved engorgement can lead to involution of mammary glandular tissue and rapid diminution of milk supply. Thus, separation of mother from infant, occurring with premature birth, routine phototherapy, or maternal post-partum complications, can be associated with unrelieved engorgement and subsequent difficulty establishing lactation. An efficient electric breast pump such as the Medela or Egnell can be pivotal in maintaining milk supply during these times.

Nipple Confusion. It is still the rare infant who does not receive bottle supplement during the nursery stay. In some instances, routine supplementation causes an infant to prefer bottle feeding, with its different tongue and mouth action and the rapid, easy flow of fluid. When put to the breast, such an infant may act as though he or she does not know what to do with the mother's nipple. This can be a most frustrating problem, since milk supply will rapidly diminish in the absence of effective and regular infant suckling. The use of a nipple shield over the maternal nipple should be discouraged, since this practice simply reinforces the artificial nipple and prevents direct infant contact with the mother's nipple. Prevention of nipple confusion should be emphasized by early introduction to the breast and the avoidance of bottle nipples until the infant can nurse well.

MANAGEMENT OF BREAST-FEEDING

Normal Routines. An important role of the physician is to establish for new mothers the norms for breast-fed infants. A mother should expect her infant to nurse as often as every 2 to 3 hours for the first several weeks. During this period, it is critical that the mother be allowed sufficient rest. Guidelines for minimizing outside activities, household chores, and other duties will prove more helpful than prolonging the normal feeding interval by pacifiers, water, or formula. Breast-fed infants usually pass a stool with every feeding during the early weeks. After the first or second month, the stooling pattern usually diminishes, so that the older breast-fed infant may pass a stool once every several days. It is quite common for breast-fed infants to awaken to nurse at night for several months, and many parents find that taking the infant into their own bed to nurse is a harmless method of making nighttime feedings less disruptive to the parents' sleep.

Maternal Diet. Nursing mothers should eat a well-balanced, nutritious diet, with increased calcium and fluids. Dieting to reduce weight is contraindicated during lactation. Prepregnancy weight will usually be attained by 6 months post partum without dieting. Vitamin supplements, though frequently used, are not usually necessary, provided the maternal diet is adequate. Iron supplements should be taken only if a specific indication exists. No dietary restrictions are necessary for the nursing mother unless she observes reactions in the infant following ingestion of specific foods. Common offenders are cow's milk, eggs, chocolate, citrus, nuts, and other known allergens.

Poor Weight Gain. Poor weight gain among breast-fed infants is a common, frustrating problem that is best prevented by appropriate anticipatory guidance and early follow-up. An initial visit earlier than 2 weeks is suggested for breast-fed infants of primiparous mothers to establish that the infant is nursing with appropriate technique at frequent intervals and is stooling and voiding normally. Established infant weight gain should be evident by the return to birth weight no later than 2 weeks of age. A breast-fed infant who has not demonstrated a satisfactory pattern of weight gain by 2 weeks of age should be seen frequently until adequate weight gain of approximately an ounce per day is verified. A careful history and observation of a feeding may reveal inappropriate nursing technique or feeding intervals. When such problems are identified within the first few weeks, breast-feeding can usually be enhanced, and appropriate weight gain can be demonstrated within a few days by simple modifications in the nursing schedule. When milk supply has been inadequate for more than several weeks, improving lactational performance is much more difficult because mammary alveolar tissue may have involuted markedly.

If an infant is failing to thrive at the breast, supplementation with formula is usually warranted to assure the nutritional well-being of the infant at the same time the breast-feeding schedule is improved. The use of the Lact-Aid Nursing Trainer is the best method of supplementing the breast-fed infant (P.O. Box 1066, Athens, TN 37303). This device allows the infant to receive supplemental formula simultaneously while breast-feeding. The baby suckles both the mother's nipple and a thin tube connected to a bag of formula. Modest declines in growth percentiles after 3 months may provide an indication for introduction of beikost.

Working and Nursing. Specific recommendations are necessary for the large population of women who elect to breast-feed but out of necessity or choice return to work before the infant is weaned. Only recently has it been acknowledged that working and nursing can be compatible and not necessarily mutually exclusive. Returning to work after 16 weeks post partum interferes less with long-term breast-feeding than earlier returns. Part-time work is associated with longer duration of nursing than full-time employment, and mothers who express milk when away from the baby tend to nurse longer than those who do not.

When a mother must return to work, she should arrange "lactation breaks" to privately express milk at regular intervals in order to maintain a generous milk supply and to provide milk for feeding the infant in her absence. Expressed milk should be refrigerated and used within 48 hours. Frozen milk can be stored up to 4 weeks in a refrigerator-top freezer and up to 4 months in a deep freezer at −20°C (−4°F). Some work places now have "pumping lounges" with electric pump facilities for lactating employees. Other creative options include nearby or on-site child care so that the mother might go to the babysitter during her lunch hour or have the infant brought to the work place to nurse. It is clear that both public institutions and private industry must be willing to provide options for nursing to continue among working mothers if broad infant feeding recommendations can become reality for the large proportion of women who return to work during their infant's first year.

Breast-Feeding the Premature or Sick Newborn. When infant illness, prematurity, or a birth defect precludes direct nursing at the breast, specialized information and support are necessary for these unique circumstances. The mother should have access to an effective breast pump to empty her breasts at regular intervals and maintain an adequate milk supply. Although hand expression is always available, and a variety of hand pumps are readily accessible, a piston-type electric breast pump, such as the Medela or Egnell, is the most effective method of maintaining a generous, long-term milk supply. Such pumps can be rented from surgical supply shops and pharmacies. As soon as the infant is stable, he or she should be introduced to the breast so that actual breast-feeding can eventually be achieved.

Mastitis. A small percentage of nursing mothers experience mastitis during the course of breast-feeding. Weaning is *not* necessary with mastitis, and in fact, failure to empty the affected breast has been demonstrated to predispose it to abscess formation. Mastitis should be suspected whenever a nursing mother complains of a "flulike" illness, with local breast tenderness. Associated symptoms include malaise, chills, fever, and erythema and pain in the affected breast. Antibiotic therapy should be initiated promptly and continued for 10 days. A sterilely collected milk sample can be used to guide antibiotic choice, but in general adequate coverage against *Staphylococcus aureus* should be provided. Analgesics may be necessary for several days to control discomfort.

Mothers may find it more comfortable to initiate nursing on the unaffected side, and then move the infant to the affected breast only after the let-down reflex has occurred. Since good emptying of the breast is such an important part of treatment, nasal oxytocin to enhance the let-down reflex or an electric pump to facilitate milk expression may be helpful adjunctive therapy.

Breast Milk Jaundice. In a small percentage of breast-fed infants, an unidentified property of the milk inhibits conjugation of bilirubin and leads to persistent unconjugated hyperbilirubinemia, which peaks in the second week of life and may persist for several weeks. Breast milk jaundice should *not* be diagnosed unless other causes of hyperbilirubinemia have been ruled out, a normal conjugated bilirubin has been documented, and the infant is clearly thriving and gaining on breast milk. Persistent hyperbilirubinemia in undernourished infants might more accurately be labeled "lack of breast milk jaundice." Breast milk jaundice can be treated by a 24- to 36-hour trial off breast milk, during which the bilirubin level falls several mg/dl. It is important to instruct the mother on the maintenance of milk supply by pumping during the interval the infant is formula fed and to aid her in getting the baby back to breast feeding.

Vitamins. The content of vitamins A, C, and B in breast milk are adequate among well-nourished mothers, although vitamin content of milk declines among malnourished women. The content of vitamin D has been controversial. Recommendations vary, but vitamin D supplements, often given as vitamin ADC drops, are frequently advised for breast-fed infants, especially dark-skinned children or those having infrequent sun exposure. Fluoride content of milk is little affected by fluoridation of the maternal water supply, although a fluoride supplement is usually recommended for breast-fed infants only when the water supply contains less than 1 ppm of fluoride. Breast milk contains adequate iron to meet the needs of healthy, term infants for the first 4 to 6 months. Supplemental iron is usually recommended after the infant doubles the birth weight.

Maternal Drug Therapy. Many factors play a role in determining the effect of maternal drug therapy on the nursing infant, including the route of administration, the dosage, the molecular weight of the drug, ionization, fat solubility, and protein binding. For most drugs, the dosage delivered to the nursing infant is subtherapeutic, except for drugs concentrated in milk. In general, any drug that is prescribed therapeutically for newborns can be consumed via breast milk without ill effect. Very few drugs are absolutely contraindicated; they include radioactive compounds, antimetabolites, and lithium. Many drugs, although contraindicated in the past, have subsequently been shown to pose no real hazard to the breast-fed infant. All drugs delivered to the infant via breast milk should be viewed with a risk/benefit assessment. For example, it might be preferable to nurse and take low-dose birth control pills than to deny the infant the benefits of breast milk or to become pregnant while nursing. It should be recognized that the knowledge base about drugs in breast milk is rapidly changing, so recommendations may be modified as new information becomes available. A regional drug center, such as Rocky Mountain Drug Consultation Center (303-893-DRUG), can serve as a valuable source of knowledge about drugs in breast milk.

Weaning. Infant weaning has evolved from the predominatly mother-led process observed during the last several decades to the more baby-led process now being witnessed. More women are nursing their infants longer in a society in which late nursing is generally uncommon. Clinicians need to recognize the legitimate psychological needs of infants and toddlers that can be met by nursing, apart from the nutritional role of breast-feeding. Weaning gradually, by allowing the baby to outgrow the need to nurse, is preferred to abrupt, imposed weaning.

CONCLUSION

An important role for clinicians working with mothers and infants is to offer breast-feeding information, support, and appropriate anticipatory guidance. When a woman successfully achieves her own goal in breast-feeding, she experiences competency in her early mothering, which may set the tone for her subsequent parenting.

Feeding the Low Birth Weight Infant

EKHARD E. ZIEGLER, M.D.

In recent years there has been a much expanded use of parenteral nutrition in low birth weight infants. This has been associated with increased sophistication in the formulation of parenteral regimens. A major impetus for the expanded use of parenteral nutrition has been the tendency to delay introduction of enteral feedings in the belief that this will reduce the risk of necrotizing enterocolitis. Feeding protocols in use today call for withholding of enteral feedings for up to 2 weeks in infants considered at high risk of necrotizing enterocolitis. This approach is feasible only because safe methods of parenteral nutrition using peripheral veins are available.

Nutritional support of low birth weight infants typically proceeds in three phases: a *parenteral phase*, during which enteral feedings are not provided at all; a *transition phase*, during which enteral feedings are gradually introduced, and parenteral nutrition is reduced; and a final *enteral phase*, during which all feedings are enteral. Typically, infants do not grow during the parenteral phase but begin to grow during the transition phase and grow rapidly (catch-up growth) during the enteral phase.

THE PARENTERAL PHASE

Administration of fluids intravenously is begun shortly after birth, providing energy in the form of glucose. Electrolytes are frequently omitted for the first 24 hours. A decision to provide amino acids and minerals as well as glucose—referred to subsequently as parenteral nutrition—should be made as early as possible and not later than 48 hours of age. Factors entering into the decision include birth weight, perinatal risk factors with regard to necrotizing enterocolitis, the severity of postnatal illness, and any other factors that may delay introduction of enteral feedings. As a general rule, infants with birth weights less than 1500 gm should receive parenteral nutritional support. The

Table 1. PERIPHERAL VENOUS NUTRITION SOLUTION FOR LOW BIRTH WEIGHT INFANTS*

Nutrient	Amount per 100 ml
Amino acids	1.4 gm
Glucose	2.5–15.0† gm
Acetate	3.1 meq
Sodium	3.0 meq
Potassium	0.0–3.0† meq
Chloride	0.56‡ meq
Calcium	20.0 mg
Phosphorus	18.6 mg
Magnesium	3.6 mg
Zinc	0.12 mg
Copper	24.0 µg
Manganese	6.0 µg
Chromium	0.26 µg

* 3 ml of M.V.I.-12 (Multi-Vitamin Infusion) (Armour Pharmaceutical Co.) are added to each 24-hour supply.

† Desired concentration to be specified by prescribing physician; K >3.0 meq/100 ml available on request.

‡ Cl will vary depending on concentration of K^+, which is added as KCl.

major exception concerns infants with birth weights above 1250 gm who are considered likely to tolerate enteral feedings by 3 days of age. Larger infants may tolerate somewhat longer periods with only glucose and electrolytes, but even term infants should usually be given parenteral nutrition if enteral feedings cannot be initiated by 4 days of age.

The immediate postnatal period is often quite stormy, and it is unlikely that true growth will occur even if sufficient nutrients are provided. Therefore, nutritional support should be based on the limited objective of preventing nutritional depletion by replacement of ongoing losses, including expenditures of energy. A variety of parenteral nutrition regimens for high risk infants are currently employed in nurseries across the country, testifying to a certain lack of consensus regarding optimal composition. The composition of the peripheral venous nutrition (PVN) solution used at the author's institution is indicated in Table 1.

The solution is designed to provide adequate, but not excessive, intakes of amino acids, minerals, and vitamins when used as the primary source of intravenous fluids. It has the advantage of providing flexibility with regard to concentrations of glucose and potassium. On a special request basis, amino acid and sodium concentrations other than those specified are available. In order to avoid administration of excessive amounts of amino acids and, perhaps, of other nutrients, the PVN solution is not administered in amounts exceeding 200 ml/kg/day. In the occasional premature infant requiring fluid intake greater than 200 ml/kg/day, the additional fluids are generally administered as a

5% glucose solution. It must be emphasized that the amino acid concentration of 1.4 gm/dl is not sufficient for growing infants. If and when energy intakes exceed 80 kcal/kg/day, it is advisable to increase the amino acid concentration to 2.0–2.4 gm/dl.

Because biochemical evidence of essential fatty acid deficiency may develop in small premature infants within a few days of birth, parenteral administration of lipid emulsions should be initiated between 4 and 6 days of age unless enteral feedings have been initiated. The dose of lipid required to prevent essential fatty acid deficiency is about 0.5 gm/kg/day. When infused slowly (0.05 gm/kg/hr), intravenous lipid emulsions at this dosage rarely give rise to hyperlipidemia and are probably safe even in the presence of moderate hyperbilirubinemia. Monitoring for hyperlipidemia is mandatory, however, and should be performed by determination of serum triglyceride concentration at the end of the daily infusion period. Triglyceride concentrations should be kept below 150 mg/dl. To avoid exceeding this value, it may be necessary to reduce the rate of infusion or the total amount infused. Inspection of a spun hemotocrit tube for serum lactescence is frequently used instead of triglyceride determination, but it must be cautioned that this method does not reliably detect hyperlipidemia of a mild to moderate degree. If the amount of intravenous lipids is increased beyond 0.5 gm/kg/day in order to increase energy intake, monitoring of serum triglyceride concentrations is particularly important. Most neonatologists prefer not to exceed doses of 2.5–3.0 gm/kg/day.

THE TRANSITION PHASE

An important initial role of enteral feedings is to test the functional maturity of the gastrointestinal tract and to provide a stimulus for morphologic, functional, and endocrine maturation of the gut. Thus, there may be major beneficial effects of enteral feedings even during the period in which most of the intake of energy and specific nutrients is provided by the parenteral route.

There are two decisions to be made: what to feed and by what method. Expressed milk from the infant's own mother is the feeding of choice. It is important that the milk collected by the mother is fed in the order in which it was collected. In this way the infant receives initially colostrum, followed by transitional milk, and eventually mature milk. Donated breast milk, when available, is the second choice, especially when it is mature milk. Since some form of heat treatment is required to prevent transmission of infectious agents, cellular elements of the milk are lost and some loss of protective factors is inevitable. If formula is to be used, it should be one of the premature infant

formulas (see the section Feedings). Most neonatologists prefer to start milk or formula at energy concentrations less than 67 kcal/dl. However, the scientific basis for this practice is not established.

The second decision is whether to feed by continuous intragastric infusion or by bolus. Continuous infusion is associated with fewer cardiovascular and pulmonary effects and is the preferred method for very small infants. At the author's institution a regimen of cycles consisting of 3 hours of infusion followed by 1 hour without infusion has been used for years and has worked satisfactorily. Gastric contents are aspirated before the next cycle, and the physician is notified if the volume aspirated exceeds 20% of the volume infused.

Transpyloric feeding, i.e., introduction of feedings into the duodenum or jejunum, has the advantage that the often sluggish rate of gastric emptying does not limit the volume of milk or formula that can be administered. However, many neonatologists believe that the disadvantages (e.g., impaired nutrient absorption) and risks (e.g., intestinal perforation) outweigh the advantages, and transpyloric feeding is not widely used today.

THE ENTERAL PHASE

During the transition phase just described the objective of nutritional management was the replacement of ongoing losses. With the onset of growth, greater intakes of energy and nutrients are needed for the formation of new body tissues. If energy or protein intake is inadequate, growth rate will be limited. When sufficient energy and protein but too little calcium and phosphorus are provided, the infant will develop rickets. It is apparent that nutritional management of the growing premature infant must be based on an understanding of nutrient requirements.

Nutrient Requirements. Until requirements can be established for all nutrients by appropriately designed feeding studies, estimates of nutrient requirements obtained by the factorial method serve as interim guidelines. These estimates represent for each nutrient the sum of tissue accretion plus losses via feces, urine, and skin. Use of the fetus as a model for the growing premature infant has the major advantage that body composition of the human fetus is known. No more satisfactory model is available.

Estimates of nutrient requirements obtained by the factorial method form the basis for the advisable intakes presented in Table 2. Because of variability among infants, the requirement, which is based on average values, has been increased by 10% to give an advisable intake. A margin of only 10% above requirements has been used because premature infants have very limited tolerance to excessive intakes. Advisable intakes of nutrients

Table 2. ADVISABLE NUTRIENT INTAKES AND COMPOSITION OF HUMAN MILK AND OF FORMULAS FOR LOW BIRTH WEIGHT INFANTS (per 100 kcal)

Nutrient	Advisable Intake		Human Milk*	Similac Special Care	Enfamil Premature	"Preemie" SMA Ready-to-Feed
	700–1000 gm	*1000–1500 gm*				
Protein (gm)	3.25	3.20	2.30	2.70	3.00	2.50
Calcium (mg)	165.00	160.00	36.00	178.00	117.00	93.00
Phosphorous (mg)	115.00	110.00	19.00	89.00	59.00	49.00
Magnesium (mg)	6.50	6.00	4.80	12.30	10.50	8.60
Sodium (meq)	3.20	2.80	1.70	1.90	1.70	1.70
Potassium (meq)	2.20	2.00	2.10	3.20	2.80	2.40
Chloride (meq)	2.90	2.40	1.90	2.30	2.40	1.80
Iron (mg)	2.40	2.20	0.20	0.37	0.16	0.37
Zinc (mg)	1.50	1.30	0.50	1.50	1.00	0.62
Copper (mg)	0.17	0.16	0.08	0.25	0.09	0.09

* Preterm, 14 days post partum

have been stated in relation to energy requirements (i.e., are expressed per 100 kcal) because for most nutrients it is more important that they be provided in the correct proportions to each other than that they be directly related to body weight.

It is evident from the values presented in Table 2 that advisable intakes of nutrients decrease somewhat with increasing body weight. At still higher body weights (not shown) they gradually approach those of the full-term infant.

Feedings. As mentioned previously, the feeding of choice is milk from the infant's own mother. The mother should be encouraged to attempt lactation and every effort should be made to aid her in this effort. The success rate is likely to be a direct function of the support provided. Milk should be placed in suitably small containers that should be dated so as to enable subsequent use of the milk in sequence. Usually, milk will need to be frozen, although refrigeration is adequate if storage is required for only a few days. By feeding the milk in sequence the infant receives initially colostrum, with its high concentration of anti-infectious substances, followed by transitional and eventually mature milk. Because of the small volumes of milk consumed, the time scale is expanded compared with the time over which the milk was collected.

Even preterm milk, with its somewhat higher protein content compared with term milk, provides a number of nutrients in inadequate amounts; i.e., amounts that do not meet the needs of the growing low birth weight infant. From a comparison of advisable intakes of the low birth weight infant with the nutrient content of preterm milk (Table 2), it is evident that per unit of energy lesser amounts of protein and of most minerals are provided than are presumed to be advisable.

In essentially every feeding study of preterm infants in which human milk has been compared with formulas designed for low birth weight in-fants, weight gain has been found to be less rapid with human milk than with formula. The difference is greatest when pooled donor milk is used, but even with milk from the infant's own mother there is slower growth than with formula. In addition, undermineralization of the skeleton is more pronounced with human milk than with formula. There seems to be little dispute about these facts. There is dispute, however, about what should be done about the problem. One school of thought holds that somewhat slower growth is of no particular consequence and is therefore an acceptable price for the benefits mother's milk confers on the infant. Similarly, undermineralization of the skeleton may have no long-term consequences. The opposing view, to which the author subscribes, holds that from a physiological point of view a diet that permits less than full realization of the subject's growth potential cannot be considered optimal. In addition, slowed growth exposes the infant to the risks of extra days or weeks of hospitalization. Although skeletal undermineralization does not generally progress to such an extent, in some infants spontaneous fractures occur.

We therefore recommend the supplementation of human milk with protein and minerals. Such supplementation corrects the nutritional inadequacies without diminishing the advantages of human milk. Supplementation should be initiated when the infant begins to gain weight. Supplements specifically designed for the purpose are preferable to use of concentrated infant formula. Table 3 indicates the composition of two such supplements. The Enfamil Human Milk Fortifier is supplied in packets containing 0.95 gm and is added to 25 ml of human milk. The Iowa Supplement (which is not commercially available) is provided in units of 0.4 gm and is added to 15 ml of milk. Although the two supplements differ somewhat in composition, protein and minerals are the

Table 3. SUPPLEMENTS FOR HUMAN MILK (amounts added to each 100 ml of milk)

Nutrient	Enfamil Human Milk Fortifier	Iowa Human Milk Supplement
Energy (kcal)	14.00	9.00
Protein (gm)	0.70	0.90
Carbohydrate (gm)	2.70	1.25
Sodium (meq)	0.30	0.80
Potassium (meq)	0.40	0.33
Chloride (meq)	0.50	0.67
Calcium (mg)	60.00	90.00
Phosphorus (mg)	33.00	66.00
Magnesium (mg)	4.00	1.30
Zinc (mg)	0.80	0.70
Copper (mg)	0.04	0.07

main ingredients and are supplied in amounts calculated to raise intakes of these nutrients to levels that approximately meet requirements.

When the infant's mother does not provide milk, and there is no other source of human milk available, three formulas specifically designed to meet the nutritional needs of low birth weight infants are available. As may be seen in Table 2, these formulas vary somewhat in the amounts of nutrients provided (relative to energy). On the whole these formulas meet nutrient requirements of the low birth weight infant more closely than formulas designed for term infants. All three formulas contain as their source of protein a blend of bovine whey proteins and casein in a ratio of 60:40. All three formulas provide half the amount of carbohydrate in the form of lactose. The fat blend of each formula contains at least some medium-chain triglycerides to capitalize on the ease and efficiency with which this fat is absorbed. The content of polyunsaturated fatty acids (PUFA) is higher in the formulas than in human milk, but sufficient vitamin E is present to provide a satisfactory E:PUFA ratio. It should be noted that all formulas are low in iron content (Table 2), reflecting the widely held belief that iron has adverse effects on small preterm infants and should therefore be withheld, despite the recognized need for an exogenous source of iron. At the author's institution, however, supplemental iron (2–3 mg/kg/day) is provided beginning at about 2 to 3 weeks of age, provided the infant is receiving full enteral feedings.

Various approaches to vitamin supplementation are currently in use, reflecting the lack of agreement with regard to necessary intakes of several vitamins and the lack of a commercially available vitamin supplement designed for premature infants. At the author's institution, all low birth weight infants receive a specially formulated vitamin supplement providing 12 vitamins, including (per day) 1500 IU of vitamin A, 400 IU of vitamin D, 15 IU of vitamin E, 60 μg of folic acid, 20 μg of biotin, and 60 mg of ascorbic acid (infants fed Similac Special Care, with greater vitamin concentratons than the other formulas, receive half the dose).

Neonatal Intestinal Obstruction

ROBERT M. FILLER, M.D.

Neonates with bilious vomiting, abdominal distention, and failure to pass meconium within 24 hours have intestinal obstruction until proved otherwise. The four most common causes include intestinal atresia, malrotation, meconium ileus, and Hirschsprung's disease. The diagnosis of intestinal obstruction is usually made on flat and upright radiographs of the abdomen. Barium enema is used to better define the specific type of obstruction and to rule out an unsuspected colonic atresia.

To prevent aspiration and progressive intestinal distention, nasogastric intubation and suction should be instituted in all patients prior to diagnostic studies and transport of the patient. In most cases, a No. 10 French nasogastric catheter can be used. Smaller tubes often fail to achieve the desired result. Infants should be nursed in a thermoneutral environment, and care must be taken to avoid hypothermia during radiologic studies. Correction of fluid and electrolyte abnormalities may be necessary before surgery when the diagnosis is delayed; but when the diagnosis is made early, dehydration and electrolyte imbalance are not usually problems. Ampicillin (200 mg/kg/day) and gentamicin (5–7.5 mg/kg/day) are given intravenously just prior to surgery and continued for 24 hours in uncomplicated cases. In patients with significant peritoneal contamination antibiotics are continued for 1 week and clindamycin (50 mg/kg/day) is added to the regimen.

Intestinal Atresia

The principle of surgical treatment for intestinal atresia is to excise the atretic area of intestine and join the ends to establish continuity. However, for atresias at certain sites, resection and end-to-end anastomosis are technically dangerous or not feasible, and alternative measures are necessary. For example, it is often easier to bypass an atresia in the second portion of the duodenum by means of a duodenojejunostomy rather than to excise an atretic segment near the common bile duct. Similarly, an end-to-end anastomosis may be technically impossible in those with high jejunal atresia because of the marked discrepency in size between the dilated proximal bowel and the ribbonlike distal bowel. In these cases, a side-to-side jejunostomy becomes the best solution even though a small percentage of patients develop a blind loop syndrome that needs later correction. It has been known for many years that a grossly dilated intestine just proximal to an atresia has ineffective peristalsis even after the obstruction has been relieved. This may result in partial intestinal obstruction. In addition, the overdistended loop tends to become a stagnant pool of intestinal fluid, with bacterial overgrowth that can produce a blind loop syndrome. To prevent this problem, enormously dilated intestine is excised with the atretic segment. However, when this is not feasible because of overall short intestinal length or duodenal involvement, the diameter of the dilated segment is narrowed by plication or tapering.

Intestinal Malrotation

Malrotation of the intestine is associated with intestinal obstruction when the duodenum is compressed by bands that run from the cecum to the posterior parietes (Ladd's bands) or when midgut volvulus occurs. The latter event is an extreme emergency, since the viability of all of the small intestine and half of the colon is in jeopardy. When midgut volvulus is suspected, immediate operation is necessary even if fluid and electrolyte resuscitation is incomplete. At surgery, the intestines are eviscerated, and volvulus is corrected by counterclockwise rotation of bowel around the axis of the superior mesenteric artery. Ladd's bands are divided in all cases, and the duodenum is freed so that it descends in a straight line into the abdomen to the right of the spine. The cecum ends up in the left upper quadrant. If the bowel is viable, an incidental appendectomy is performed. Intestinal resection for localized areas of bowel necrosis is necessary. When the viability of the entire midgut is in doubt after reduction of a volvulus, the intestines are replaced in the abdomen, and the wound is closed. The abdomen is re-explored 24 hours later and intestine that is definitely necrotic is excised. In general, it is wiser to exteriorize the cut ends of potentially ischemic intestine rather than perform an end-to-end anastamosis.

Meconium Ileus

Meconium ileus is caused by inspissated meconium in the lumen of the distal small bowel and almost always is associated with cystic fibrosis. In 50% of cases meconium ileus is complicated by intestinal atresia, volvulus, intestinal infarction, and meconium peritonitis.

In cases of simple meconium ileus attempts at disimpacting the obstructing meconium by enema techniques are preferable to immediate surgical therapy. Various enema preparations have been used. Gastrografin, a hypertonic iodine solution combined with a wetting agent, has received the most attention in the literature. Its high osmolarity draws fluid into the bowel lumen and separates the meconium from the intestinal wall. However, because of this high osmolarity, Gastrografin can produce hypovolemic shock when large fluid shifts into the intestine occur. Therefore, we prefer to employ an enema solution of 25% diatrizoate sodium (Hypaque) with 5% acetylcysteine (Mucomyst), which has an osmolarity less than half that of Gastrografin and yet appears to be as effective. Intravenous fluid therapy during the Hypaque enema is not necessary in the well-hydrated neonate. Care must be taken to avoid intestinal perforation during the procedure, which usually requires several instillations of irrigating fluid until it passes into the dilated intestine above the obstruction.

Operative treatment is required for all infants with complicated meconium ileus as well as for those in whom enema therapy has failed. Many surgical methods have been used to relieve the obstruction. We prefer to relieve the obstruction by enterotomy and irrigations with 5% acetylcysteine. If irrigation fails to relieve the obstruction (less than 10% of cases), an intestinal stoma is created proximal to the point of obstruction.

In infants with complicated meconium ileus, the atretic, infarcted, or perforated intestine is excised. It is usually unwise to attempt intraoperative irrigations and end-to-end anastomoses in these patients because of the likelihood of anastomotic complications. Creation of a double-barreled ileostomy is preferable.

Hirschsprung's Disease

When x-ray evaluation suggests that intestinal obstruction is due to Hirschsprung's disease, a punch biopsy of the rectal mucosa 1.5 cm above the dentate line is performed at the bedside. If this indicates the absence of ganglion cells, a right transverse loop colostomy is performed. The colostomy is also biopsied to confirm the presence of ganglion cells at the stoma. A definitive operation to correct Hirschsprung's disease is performed when the child is 6 to 12 months of age.

The postoperative management of infants who require surgery for intestinal obstruction is similar regardless of the type of corrective procedure employed. Nasogastric suction is maintained until bowel movements begin and nasogastric tube output is minimal. Oral feedings are then started with breast feeding or with infant formula except in those patients with cystic fibrosis in whom Pregestimil, a protein hydrolysate formula with medium chain triglycerides and added amino acids, is used. Postoperative antibiotic therapy is maintained as previously noted.

A significant number of infants with short intestinal length or complicated surgical problems have prolonged malabsorption after surgery.

Often they do not tolerate a full diet for several weeks (or even years) after surgery. Nutrition must be maintained intravenously in these infants while dietary manipulations and intestinal regeneration are proceeding.

Hemolytic Diseases of the Neonate

ROBERT R. CHILCOTE, M.D.,
and LAWRENCE M. GARTNER, M.D.

When presented with evidence of hemolysis, the clinician must rapidly consider the possible causes of red cell destruction and the impact of anemia on oxygen delivery, and anticipate the consequences of increased bilirubin production. Should hemolysis continue at a rate that threatens the neonate, the clinician must rapidly institute measures to alleviate this process—most often by exchange transfusion.

CLINICAL PRESENTATION

A carefully taken family history of an expectant mother may warn of impending fetal and neonatal hemolysis and allow the obstetrician and pediatrician to formulate a plan to monitor the fetus and consider amniocentesis. Particular attention should be given to previous obstetrical events and transfusions that could have sensitized the mother to Rh or other blood group antigens. A history of familial icterus, early gallbladder disease, or splenectomy should alert the physician to inquire further about inherited red cell abnormalities. If the fetus is at risk, appropriate consultation should be obtained well before the time of delivery. This allows time to confirm questionable diagnoses and, if necessary, obtain diagnostic studies on affected family members. Narrowing the range of diagnostic possibilities may allow the team to obtain definitive studies on infant cord blood.

Conditions that shorten fetal red cell life-span increase red cell synthesis; anemia develops when production fails to compensate for destruction. Severe anemia causes a hydropic fetus, a condition attended by high fetal and neonatal mortality and characterized by pallor, edema, hepatomegaly, and anemia at birth. The birth of a hydropic infant without diagnosis is an indication for further hematologic investigation, even if the infant is born dead. Small amounts of fetal or neonatal blood can be examined and used to classify the abnormalities so that the family may be counseled about the risk of recurrence, prevention, and management of future pregnancies.

Toxic levels of indirect bilirubin are not found in utero, since the placenta transfers unconjugated bilirubin into the maternal circulation. However, after birth, hemolytic rates that may reduce the hemoglobin concentration by only a few grams per deciliter and thereby escape detection on routine hematologic screening may produce bilirubin loads that quickly exceed the newborn's capacity to conjugate the newly formed bilirubin and excrete it into bile. In the presence of severe hemolysis, the pale, anicteric neonate may become visibly yellow within 30 minutes after delivery. Unconjugated bilirubin is a lipophilic substance that may, under circumstances as yet incompletely understood, cross the blood-brain barrier and poison neuronal cells. When the concentration of indirect bilirubin rises above 20 mg/dl in the healthy full-term infant, the infant becomes at risk for bilirubin encephalopathy. This risk is markedly increased even at much lower serum bilirubin concentrations when there is or has been poor tissue perfusion, acidosis, hypoxemia, hypoalbuminemia, bacterial infection, or hypoglycemia, especially in the preterm infant.

Newborns with significant hemolysis will usually become icteric in the first 24 hours of life, often within 6 hours of birth. Destruction of less than 10% of circulating red cells may not necessarily lead to a clinically detectable change in hemoglobin concentration, hematocrit, or reticulocyte count, but may raise the bilirubin concentration to a level greater than expected for physiologic jaundice of the newborn. An indirect bilirubin in excess of 12 to 14 mg/dl in the full-term infant suggests that hemolysis is contributing to the bilirubin load; if the child is anemic, an elevated bilirubin value is even more significant. The role of anemia becomes more understandable when one recognizes that in the absence of sequestered extravascular blood the source of bilirubin is dependent on the circulating red cell mass. Thus, a child with a hematocrit of 30% as opposed to 60% will produce only half as much bilirubin and have a lower serum concentration. On the other hand, enhanced enteric bilirubin absorption due to intestinal obstruction, absence of feeding, or caloric deprivation may increase serum bilirubin concentrations without increase in red cell destruction. Although the factors that control serum bilirubin levels are complex, changes in indirect bilirubin concentrations provide a better clinical guide to changes in the rate of red cell destruction than changes in hemoglobin or reticulocyte levels.

Severe and persistent hemolysis rarely elevates the direct-reacting serum bilirubin concentrations. An exception is seen in infants with severe Rh erythroblastosis requiring multiple intrauterine transfusions. In these cases, elevation of the direct fraction may be seen in the cord blood, reflecting the inability of the placenta to transfer the water-soluble conjugated (direct-reacting) pigment. Transient elevations of the direct fraction may also be seen during recovery from severe hemolytic

Table 1. HEMOLYSIS IN THE NEONATE

Extrinsic abnormalities
  Rh(D) erythroblastosis
  ABO incompatibility (generally blood group O mothers)
  Minor blood group incompatibilities
  "DIC" (secondary to poor tissue perfusion, hemorrhagic shock, infection, cavernous hemangioma, etc)
  Large hematomas, swallowed blood
  Congenital infection (herpes, toxoplasmosis, CMV, rubella, syphilis, malaria)
  Bacterial sepsis

Intrinsic abnormalities of red cell
  Heritable spherocytosis (HS), elliptocytosis, pyropoikilocytosis
  Hexose shunt abnormality (G6PD deficiency)
  Glycolytic enzyme deficiency (deficiency of PK, GPI, TPI, PGK, HK)
  Galactosemia
  Hereditary 5' nucleotidase deficiency
  Stomatocytosis
  Abnormal fetal hemoglobin (alpha or gamma chain)

disease. Cholestasis resulting from severe hemolysis in the neonate has been proposed as a cause for the "inspissated bile" syndromes, although this diagnosis is difficult to substantiate. The initial workup of infants with hemolysis depends heavily on laboratory parameters. Serial hemoglobin levels, bilirubin values, and determinations of the proportion of reticulocytes and nucleated red cells in cord blood help separate infants with clinically significant brisk hemolysis from those with less severe hemolysis. A cord blood hemoglobin concentration of less than 14 gm/dl is evidence of anemia. It should be noted that anemia, even when severe, does not appreciably change the neonatal heart rate, respiratory pattern, or blood gases; one must follow the hemoglobin level.

DIFFERENTIAL DIAGNOSIS

Diseases that destroy the red cell can be either intrinsic, such as abnormalities of red cell metabolism, membrane function, or hemoglobin, or extrinsic, such as isoimmunization. A list of causes of hemolysis in the neonate is given in Table 1.

Rh-negative mothers sensitized to the Rh antigen by a previous pregnancy, abortion, or transfusion of Rh-positive red cells or blood products containing Rh-positive cells will, when the conceptus is Rh-positive, develop anti-Rh titers that rise during pregnancy. Polyclonal anti-D antibodies belonging to the IgG fraction cross the placenta and attach to fetal red cells, causing their destruction. Anemia may develop and when severe may cause hydrops fetalis. The direct Coombs' test is positive and erythrocyte precursors as immature as erythroblasts are released into the circulation.

ABO blood group and other minor antigens may also induce hemolysis but the impact is generally less severe than in Rh disease—though there

are occasional dramatic exceptions. Mild to moderate hyperbilirubinemia develops more often in ABO incompatibility but does not require exchange transfusion. The hemoglobin may fall in the first weeks of life, occasionally to levels as low as 5 to 6 gm/dl. Although these infants should be followed closely for the development of feeding difficulties (the neonatal equivalent of exercise intolerance), transfusion is rarely necessary. "Spherocytes" are present on the peripheral smear, a result of membrane loss to reticuloendothelial cells. The osmotic fragility test is positive and it may be difficult to distinguish this disorder from hereditary spherocytosis. However, with ABO incompatibility, the Coombs' test is positive and with time becomes negative. In congenital spherocytosis the abnormally fragile cells persist and family screening with the osmotic fragility test will often diagnose an affected but asymptomatic parent.

Mothers who have autoimmune diseases with IgG antibodies against the red cell may, even though splenectomized, give birth to infants with immune hemolytic anemia. In these situations, the infant's Coombs' test is positive but evidence of blood group incompatibility is lacking.

As the incidence of Rh disease declines, intrinsic abnormalities of red cell function are becoming increasingly important causes of hyperbilirubinemia and anemia. Heritable spherocytosis ("congenital icterus"), an autosomal dominant disorder, is one of the more common hemolytic anemias of man and can present with severe hemolysis in the neonatal period; this may occur even if other affected family members have not experienced this complication, since the severity of the clinical disease may differ dramatically among those with the same genotype. In this disorder and several others to be discussed below, an experienced laboratory can make the diagnosis on cord blood. Knowledge of the diagnosis alerts the pediatrician to potential problems in the first months of life, such as life-threatening anemic crisis. Failure to obtain samples for study before transfusion may unnecessarily delay diagnosis.

Recently, an extremely severe type of spherocytosis with bizarre poikilocytes due to unstable red cell membrane structure has been described. The red cells are characterized by deficiencies of cytoskeletal membrane proteins and thermal instability occasioning the name "pyro"poikilocytosis.

Abnormalities of alpha or gamma chain structure are probably underdiagnosed in the newborn, but in non-Oriental populations do not cause hydrops or severe neonatal hemolytic anemia. Beta thalassemias and sickle cell disease, beta chain abnormalities, do not cause anemia or hemolysis until 4 to 6 months of age.

Metabolic abnormalities of the red cell such as deficiencies of hexose monophosphate shunt enzymes (e.g., G6PD) lead to susceptibility to oxidative stresses, especially those generated by infection or certain chemicals. Most medications used in the neonatal period can be administered to children with deficiency of G6PD without inducing hemolysis; there is no evidence that the usual dose of 1 mg of vitamin K-₁ oxide is hazardous.

Glycolytic enzymopathies (e.g., deficiency of pyruvate kinase, glucose phosphate isomerase, triose phosphate isomerase) cause small, spherical-appearing, "crenated" or "echinocytic" red cells shaped like sea urchins and may result in serious hemolytic anemia in the newborn period. It is especially important to recognize the latter deficiency, since it is accompanied by severe neuromuscular deterioration in the first year of life that may lead to respiratory failure.

Galactosemia is frequently accompanied by hemolysis, and the child may develop additional problems with the institution of milk feeding.

Congenital erythropoietic porphyria is a very rare cause of severe hemolysis in the newborn and should be recognized promptly, since severe cutaneous blistering, necrosis, and scarring may result from exposure of these infants to phototherapy (and sunlight). The diagnosis may be made dramatically by exposing urine and stool to ultraviolet light (Woods Lamp), producing a brilliant orange fluorescence.

Routine pregnancy screening should include determination of maternal blood group (ABO) and Rh type, as well as a hemantigen screen. All Rh-negative mothers should be further studied for the presence of RH(D) antibodies. Regardless of maternal blood group and type, all cord bloods should be sent for ABO and Rh typing as well as for direct Coombs' testing. Positive Coombs' tests should be reported to the attending physician immediately and the nature of the antibody on the red cells determined. In these cases, hematocrit, reticulocyte, nucleated red cell, and platelet counts and blood smear should be examined immediately. Total and direct serum bilirubin and albumin concentrations should also be determined. A similar work-up is indicated in all cases of neonatal anemia, even when the Coombs' test is negative and there is no maternal-infant red cell immunoincompatibility.

If congenital infection is suspected, appropriate serum IgM and antibody titers should be obtained. Intrinsic red cell abnormalities can be diagnosed on cord blood and both heparinized and EDTA anticoagulated tubes should be stored for further study if necessary; many of these disorders can be diagnosed on blood retained for several weeks or longer. Peripheral smears of newborns are normally replete with unusually shaped red cells and red cell inclusions. However, after careful study of the peripheral smear, experienced observers can generally help guide diagnostic tests.

THERAPY

Although therapy for these disorders is based on experience accumulated over the last 30 years, many of the recommendations have not been carefully evaluated in well-designed trials; some aspects of management are necessarily controversial, especially in children who present with marginal hemolysis, anemia, and indirect bilirubinemia. The therapeutic options available include intrauterine transfusion, postnatal exchange transfusion, and phototherapy.

Intrauterine Transfusion. A discussion of intrauterine exchange transfusion is beyond the scope of this presentation. Mothers who appear to be at risk for Rh sensitization should be followed with serologic studies and, when appropriate, referred for amniocentesis to determine the rate of hemolysis in the fetus.

Resuscitation and Immediate Exchange Transfusion. The severely hydropic infant, with a cord blood hemacrit less than 5 to 8 gm/dl, whose condition is due to Rh sensitization, may require intensive resuscitative measures in the delivery room and transfusion of plasma and red cells to correct shock and restore oxygen transport. The team may also have to support ventilation and correct acidemia. Immediately following stabilization of the infant, an exchange transfusion should be performed. Preparation for such catastrophic intervention improves the infant's chance for survival.

While some authorities have proposed a variety of additional bilirubin and hematologic parameters for exchange transfusion immediately following delivery, modern neonatal intensive care units are equipped to monitor biochemical, physiologic and hematologic parameters, and the stable, asymptomatic erthyroblastosis infant with moderate anemia and mild to moderate hyperbilirubinemia can be observed over the first few hours to determine whether the rate of rise of the serum bilirubin or the rate of fall in the hematocrit require intervention. The infant with falling hematocrit but only a modestly increasing serum bilirubin concentration may require only simple transfusion, at least initially. There is no evidence that performance of an exchange transfusion immediately after delivery reduces the need for subsequent exchange transfusions. In fact, exchange transfusions performed during this early period of life when major cardiovascular and pulmonary adjustments are occurring may well place the infant at undue risk.

Criteria for Therapy. Within the first 4 hours after delivery, the team should establish a maximum allowable serum bilirubin level. If it appears that the infant's bilirubin will exceed that level, efforts should then be made to use phenobarbital (see below), phototherapy, appropriate nutritional and general health management and, finally if these measures fail, exchange transfusion to prevent the serum bilirubin from exceeding that level. The total bilirubin rather than indirect bilirubin levels is generally used for these criteria. Only when the direct bilirubin fraction exceeds 20% of the total bilirubin is it appropriate to subtract it from the total and use the net indirect-bilirubin concentration. It should also be recognized that laboratories differ on the accuracy of bilirubin determinations; neonatal bilirubin values should be subjected to regular quality control studies.

We recommend that phototherapy be instituted in *full-term* infants with hemolytic disease when the total serum bilirubin exceeds 10 mg/dl, in infants weighing *1500 to 2500 grams* (32 to 38 weeks) when the serum bilirubin exceeds 8 mg/dl, and in infants weighing less than 1500 grams as soon after birth as possible regardless of serum bilirubin concentration. Phototherapy units should be equipped with an equal mixture of "Special Blue" lamps and "Daylight" lamps to obtain optimal photodegradation of bilirubin and the energy output should be checked once daily. Energy output of fluorescent lamps falls significantly after 2000 to 4000 hours of use.

Phototherapy should be continued until serum bilirubin levels have fallen to one half of the exchange transfusion indication level or stabilized at that level for a minimum of 12 hours. After stabilization of serum bilirubin levels, it is essential that they be monitored for an additional 48 hours, longer in some cases.

Should serum bilirubin levels rise despite phototherapy, exchange transfusion should be performed in a timely manner to prevent the bilirubin value from exceeding the predetermined maximum allowable level. This can best be predicted by graphing serum bilirubin concentrations. If the projected maximum allowable level will be reached within 4 hours of the last determination, the transfusion blood should be prepared and the exchange transfusion started without waiting for another bilirubin result. If laboratory data have been erratic, preparations for the exchange can be made while the serum bilirubin determination is repeated. If bilirubin values are still rising, the procedure can be initiated without further delay.

While there continues to be some controversy over maximum allowable levels and the use or nonuse of albumin-bilirubin binding data, it has been our policy to use the serum bilirubin criteria indicated in Table 2, based on birth weight and infant condition. In our hands, this has resulted in a significant reduction in the incidence of autopsy-proven kernicterus.

In the past 10 years, with the use of photo-

Table 2. INDICATIONS FOR NEONATAL EXCHANGE TRANSFUSION (mg/dl)

	<1000	1000–1500	1500–2500	>2500
Healthy	10	14	18	20
High risk*	10	12	16	18

* Infants with hemolysis or asphyxia, hypoxia, acidosis, hypoalbuminemia, hypothermia, and septicemia.

therapy and prevention of Rh erythroblastosis with Rhogam, many pediatricians have become less experienced in the techniques of exchange transfusion. Since mortality due to exchange transfusion may be less than 0.5% in highly experienced hands and up to 10 times higher when performed by inexperienced physicians, the need for exchange transfusion should be anticipated and the infant transferred to an appropriate neonatal intensive care center with ample lead time.

Technique for Exchange Transfusion. The goal of exchange transfusion is to remove a substantial proportion of antibody-coated or intrinsically abnormal red cells without subjecting the neonate to undue cardiovascular stress. Exchanges are less effective in removing circulating antibody or bilirubin than in removing red cells. CPD anticoagulated Rh negative red cells, preferably drawn less than 2 days before, are cross-matched against the mother's serum for infants with Rh erythroblastosis. The blood should match the infant's ABO type as well. For infants with ABO erythroblastosis, type O blood should be utilized. Type- and Rh-specific blood compatible with the infant should be utilized and cross-matched against maternal blood for all other hemolytic disorders. The cells should be sedimented and plasma removed to bring the hematocrit above 45%. In some centers, stored blood is supplemented with adenine to increase shelf life. There is a suggestion that blood donated by individuals with sickle trait or HbSC may compromise the hypoxic acidotic infant and, until more is known about this phenomenon, it is prudent to screen all donors with a test for sickling. Feedings are changed to clear liquids, and the blood is warmed, using a thermostatically controlled blood warmer. If none is available, allow blood to slowly warm to room temperature but never place the bag in hot water.

An umbilical venous catheter is passed through the ductus venosus into the inferior vena cava, avoiding, if possible, the portal circulation. Respiratory status, perfusion, and cardiovascular dynamics are closely monitored by electronic devices. Though early studies suggested that the hydropic infant was often volume overloaded, more recent studies indicate that this is unusual. The decision to decrease the infant's blood volume should be individualized and made only when there is evidence of cardiac overload as shown, for example, by a venous pressure exceeding 10 to 12 cm of water. In addition to obtaining necessary hematologic and bilirubin baseline studies, remaining portions of the first 10 to 20 ml exchange aliquot should be retained in anticoagulated tubes (heparin "green top" and ACD "yellow top") for additional studies should intrinsic causes of hemolysis be suspected. Using 5 to 10 ml aliquots for small infants, and 20 ml for larger infants, the blood is exchanged to a total of 160 to 180 ml/kg body weight. "Pushes" and "pulls" of blood should be slow and gentle, but intentional delays to allow "equilibration" are of little or no value and may prolong the procedure, increasing the risk of complications. The umbilical catheter should be removed at completion of the procedure. Phototherapy is instituted when the exchange is finished to help keep the bilirubin from rising. Antibiotic therapy is not indicated following exchange transfusion unless clinical or laboratory data suggest the presence of infection.

After exchange transfusion, glucose is continued through a separate peripheral intravenous line and bilirubin determinations and serum potassium and sodium levels repeated every 4 to 8 hours until stable. If bleeding and thrombocytopenia develop, 1 unit of platelets is given; thrombocytepenia without bleeding is not treated prophylactically unless the platelet count falls to less than 10,000 to 20,000/mm^3. Serum ionized calcium can be monitored but supplementation is generally not necessary.

Whole blood, blood products, and even washed red cells contain considerable numbers of viable mononuclear cells. These cells are capable of immunologic reactivity and may carry viruses. Though there are currently no guidelines, further study of the use of frozen and/or irradiated cells may ultimately prove them to be safer; at the present time they are not recommended unless the infant is suspected of having congenital immunodeficiency.

Over a period of several days and occasionally over a period of several weeks, especially in infants with Rh erythroblastosis, the hemoglobin level may fall to values that require additional small, simple transfusions. Weekly hematocrit determinations are indicated for at least the first 6 weeks following birth, even when no exchange transfusion has been performed.

Phenobarbital. This antiepileptic sedative barbiturate also stimulates synthesis of microsomal drug metabolizing enzymes. The most important clinically is hepatic bilirubin glucuronosyl transferase, the major catalyst for bilirubin conjugation. Administration of this agent for at least 1 week prior to delivery will increase hepatic bilirubin conjugating capacity in near-term and term fetuses and neonates. This increased activity will persist if the drug is administered to the newborn. In this short-term situation, phenobarbital has little or no effect on prematures but can be useful in modestly reducing serum bilirubin levels and the frequency of exchange transfusions in full-term infants with hemolytic disease.

While we do not recommend the use of phenobarbital for general use in the prevention of physiologic jaundice because of its potential addicting effect, we start selected patients such as the mother carrying a fetus with proven Rh hemolytic disease with a daily dose of 60 mg per day at 34 weeks' gestation. The newborn should receive a dose of 5 mg per kg per day starting on the first day of life.

PREVENTION AND GENERAL MEASURES

It is now possible to dramatically reduce Rh sensitization in Rh-negative females by administering anti-Rh immunoglobulin following each exposure to Rh-positive red cells. Anti-Rh immunoglobulin should be given to all Rh-negative women as soon as possible and preferably within 72 hours after birth, abortion, amniocentesis, ruptured ectopic pregnancy, manual version, or transfusion or injection of blood products from an Rh-positive donor. Women who have had very complicated deliveries with possible fetal to maternal bleeding should be studied for fetal red cell contamination by the Kleinhauer-Betke method. If significant fetal cells are seen, a double dose of anti-Rh immunoglobulin should be given to prevent sensitization.

Hyperviscosity Syndromes

VIRGINIA D. BLACK, M.D.

Infants with an elevated venous hematocrit may demonstrate a variety of symptoms that suggest a reduction in cardiac output or poor peripheral blood flow. Cyanosis, peripheral pallor, and cardiopulmonary symptoms may be present. Less severely affected infants may be ruddy or have no obvious abnormalities.

The syndromes producing these disorders may be divided into two general categories: those associated with an elevated venous hematocrit and those associated with an elevated whole blood viscosity. The great majority of affected infants have both polycythemia and hyperviscosity. In most institutions, determination of whole blood viscosity is not readily available, hence infants with a venous hematocrit of 70% or more can safely be regarded as having hyperviscosity. Infants with hematocrits as low as 55%, however, may also have an abnormal whole blood viscosity. Polycythemia is defined as a venous hematocrit of 65% or greater.

The treatment of these syndromes should be directed toward improving blood flow. This is best achieved by reducing the venous hematocrit and monitoring central venous pressure when indicated. An umbilical venous catheter should be inserted under sterile technique to a level just above the diaphragm. Central venous pressure can then be obtained and a partial plasma exchange transfusion can be carried out. Equal volumes of blood are exchanged for Plasmanate. Electrolyte and water solutions should not be used. Recent studies suggest that the use of fresh frozen plasma may increase gastrointestinal complications.

The usual volume for exchange is determined by the following equation:

$$\frac{C \; Hct^* - D \; Hct\dagger}{C \; Hct} \times weight \; (kg) \; (80 \; ml/kg)$$

An arbitrary hematocrit of 50% is desired at the end of the exchange. This figure has been selected because it reduces the likelihood of continued hyperviscosity and yet should prevent later anemia. The procedure should be performed before 24 hours of age and preferably within 12 to 15 hours after birth. If the syndrome is not identified until after the first day of life, the procedure should be performed only for serious symptoms.

The risks of partial plasma exchange are the same risks as an exchange transfusion: bleeding, vessel injury, infection, and clots; these occur in fewer than 1 in 100 patients. In addition, some institutions have had a high incidence of postexchange abdominal symptoms, including necrotizing enterocolitis. Infants with hyperviscosity may already have diminished flow to the gastrointestinal tract. The additional manipulation of blood

---

*C Hct = current hematocrit
†D Hct = desired hematocrit or 50%

flow during the exchange may further reduce flow to a compromised bowel.

Following the partial plasma exchange the infant's vital signs should be monitored for several hours. Feedings are held for 2 to 4 hours and then resumed. The hematocrit can be monitored immediately following the exchange and several hours later. It is uncommon for a second exchange to be needed if the volume exchanged is determined correctly. Although seizures and hyperbilirubinemia are frequently attributed to these syndromes, neither is common. Hypoglycemia is usually improved after the partial exchange.

A two-year follow-up of infants randomized to either partial plasma exchange or symptomatic treatment has been completed. Data from this study suggest that partial plasma exchange will not prevent sequelae. Small but significant differences were seen in infants treated with exchange. Exchanged infants, however, had more immediate gastrointestinal symptoms, including necrotizing enterocolitis.

There is no good evidence that the sequelae of hyperviscosity persist into school age. Hence, it may be reasonable to observe or treat symptomatically the child who does not have serious symptoms. If feedings are not tolerated or the infant's alertness changes, the decision to withhold treatment must be re-evaluated. Frequent changes in sleep states and difficulty alerting are classically associated with this syndrome.

Long-term follow-up studies of infants with neonatal hyperviscosity suggest significant motor and neurologic sequelae at an early age. The sequelae have not been limited to symptomatic infants and are not eliminated by early partial plasma exchange transfusion. Infants with these syndromes should be followed closely for both fine and gross motor as well as language development. These sequelae are frequently subtle and often missed in the first year of life. The relationship between neonatal hyperviscosity and perceptual-motor handicaps remains to be elucidated.

23

Special Problems in the Adolescent

The Children of Divorcing Parents

DANE G. PRUGH, M.D.

In recent years in all socioeconomic groups in this country and in many parts of the world, the growing complexity of society is reflected in a significant rise in the rate of divorce. In the United States the rate is now about 5.0 per 1000 population, an increase of more than 100% over the past 20 years. Divorce is more common in couples whose parents were divorced. Teenage marriages and premarital pregnancies in themselves increase the likelihood of divorce. Three quarters of all divorces occur in marriages with children, frequently young children. Although the divorce rate has recently shown some evidence of leveling off (a slight drop has even occurred in a few areas), it has been estimated that by 1990 11% of all children under 18 will be living with a divorced parent and that 32% will have done so sometime during childhood.

THE DIVORCE PROCESS

Until recently the public, as well as concerned specialists, tended to see divorce as a unified episode. Now, we realize that divorce is in fact a series of changes, a process consisting of related phases: the initial phase of family stress, the phase culminating in legal separation, and the phase of postdivorce restabilization. During the first year after a divorce, both parents experience the emotional distress and anxiety related to the disorganization in their lives, the loss of self-esteem and social support, and the necessary role adjustments each must make. The degree of success the non-custodial parent has in adjusting to his or her new life has far-reaching social, emotional, and financial implications for the eventual stabilization of the rest of the family. Some estimates suggest that most families do not become stable following divorce for at least 2 years.

For any child of divorce, mourning is inevitable. The child must come to terms with the loss of one parent and the necessarily more limited relationship with that parent. The child must also mourn the loss of the family constellation as he or she had always known it; many children wish somehow to reunite the family. During their mourning, children may become embroiled in parental arguments about custody and then feel guilty and suffer conflicts over loyalty. Parents' hurt feelings over a child's resentment or seeming disinterest may exacerbate the course of the child's mourning. Almost inevitably children of divorce feel devalued and suffer from lowered self-esteem; adolescents often become conflicted in attempting to deal with their feelings of divided loyalty and love.

Although many parents show concern for their children's feelings about the divorce, some, in their bitterness and anger, may unconsciously use the children as pawns in continuing conflicts with the former spouse. Other parents, experiencing the social and emotional isolation that follows the disruption of the family, are overly dependent on their children for solace. Individual parents may try to turn a child against the other parent; this can be particularly confusing and conflict provoking to a child. During and following a divorce, sibling relationships may become realigned, and grandparents may become newly involved in the family dynamics, contributing sometimes positively, sometimes negatively, to the family's eventual adjustment. Although some have observed that divorce is neither more nor less stressful for children than an unhappy marriage, Rutter believes that particularly if parental conflict persists after a divorce, children can have more difficulty with divorce than with the death of a parent.

Until relatively recently, most divorce courts have awarded custody of young children to the mother and have let adolescents themselves make the decision, difficult at best, as to which parent they prefer to live with. Now, however, judges may award custody to either the father or mother, depending on what seems in their opinion best for the children; visitation arrangements are adapted to suit the ages of the children. Custodial fathers are still the exception in the majority of divorce settlements, however. The recently developed concept of joint custody calls for at best especially mature and objective parents. At worst, joint custody can result in far-reaching, destructive consequences. On the positive side, "no fault" divorces tend to moderate those adversarial aspects of the legal process that so often intensify the difficulties both parents and children are facing. The importance of the father's role in a divorce situation has only recently been adequately recognized; fathers suffer upon being separated from their children, and children in turn suffer upon being deprived of their fathers. In general, divorced fathers, as well as mothers, and the children do better after divorce when there is as much continuity, regularity, and predictability in parent-child contact as possible.

CHILDREN'S REACTIONS TO DIVORCE

The impact of divorce upon the child is related to his level of emotional development, to his capacity for understanding, to his particular temperament, and to the overall quality of his psychological adjustment. In addition, the nature of the parent-child relationship and the circumstances of the divorce and postdivorce events all affect the child's ability to cope with the stresses of his parents' separation. The "prelogical" thinking of preschool children often makes them believe their "badness" was the cause of the divorce; older children and adolescents are more realistic in their thinking but still have feelings of guilt and uncertainty. Wallerstein and Kelly have described typical behavioral reactions at differing levels of development. Regression to more infantile behavior, clinging, bewilderment and confusion, and fear of abandonment are common reactions in young preschool children. Older preschool children typically respond with anxiety, sadness, self-blame, and diminished self-esteem; often they have temper tantrums. Younger school age children show fear and sadness and may experience difficulties with their schoolwork and with peer group relationships. Older school age children react by show-

ing sadness; they are often angry with the noncustodial parent. Early adolescents may experience both a profound sense of loss and intense anger; they often also exhibit social and academic problems. Older adolescents may become withdrawn or depressed and exhibit anger toward one or another parent.

Many of these behavioral responses are transitory, although a child's mourning usually lasts at least several months. Some responses may, however, continue for many months, even for years if the child's grief is unresolved. In some predisposed children, divorce or postdivorce problems may precipitate more serious neurotic, antisocial, or even psychotic disorders. Although approximately one third of Wallerstein's and Kelly's subjects coped fairly well with divorce, over half of the preschool and one quarter of the school age group were found in 1-year follow-ups to have worsened significantly. In another study, severe parental conflict that continues after divorce has been shown to be predictive of poor adult adjustment for the children involved. The general impression is that the majority of children can, over time, cope adequately with divorce; the risk of difficulty in adaptation is high, however.

THE PEDIATRICIAN AND DIVORCE

A wide variety of services exist to help couples who are contemplating divorce: marital counselors and various social services, including family agencies and legal aid; mental health centers and individual social workers, psychiatrists, psychologists; and, more recently, specially trained divorce counselors. Sometimes, thanks to help from such sources, a solution to the domestic conflict is found, and court action is avoided. In fact, as divorce is becoming increasingly easy, some lawyers and judges now earnestly encourage couples to explore one or another of the above avenues for help before court action is begun.

In addition to these approaches to help for families contemplating or actually in the process of divorce, health care professionals—and the pediatrician especially—can also play an important role. Clearly, the pediatrician cannot act as a marriage counselor, but he or she is particularly well placed to help couples recognize serious marital discord in its early stages as it surfaces in parental disagreement over child management. Divorce may even be avoided if the pediatrician is successful in encouraging such a couple to seek help at this early stage.

Once a divorce is under way, the pediatrician finds himself in a particularly sensitive and challenging position with the parents as well as with the children who have been his patients. The most important aspect of the pediatrician's role in helping families in divorce involves his awareness of the divorce process and the attendant problems that can be anticipated. With this knowledge the pediatrician either can provide parent guidance and counseling of children and adolescents himself or may refer children or parents to appropriately trained specialists or agencies. In line with this new demand on the pediatrician, the Task Force on Pediatric Education recommended in 1978 that pediatric residents have training in a psychosocial approach to the management of family crises, including separation and divorce, as part of an increase in training in the biosocial and development aspects of pediatrics.

The most likely time for a pediatrician to become involved in the divorce process is when parents express their concern about their children's reactions to an impending or actual divorce. Parents often want and need support and advice about how to discuss the divorce with their children and how to deal with the children's feelings. During the phase of family stress, the pediatrician should wisely be alert to the tendency of parents to spend less time than usual with their children and to be inconsistent in their discipline; parents can be helped with such problems if the pediatrician is supportive and nonjudgmental. As the divorce process unfolds, both parents may need help in anticipating and then accepting their children's reactions. Although the pediatrician ought always to take a neutral position about the reasons for the divorce, he can still listen sympathetically to the single parent's often pervasive feelings of loneliness or depression. At this stage, suggesting further help from a mental health specialist or a mental health facility may well be appropriate.

In dealing with divorced or divorcing parents, the pediatrician can suitably help custodial parents understand a child's need to see the noncustodial parent regularly. When appropriate, the pediatrician can counsel one parent not to try to turn a child against the other parent. Finally, the pediatrician can direct single parents to community facilities such as well-staffed day care centers, homemaker services, and support systems such as Parents Without Partners, Grandparents Anonymous, and other self-help groups.

The pediatrician can be a singularly effective sounding board for children of divorce who, as one study shows, almost always want some sympathetic adult to ask about and *listen sympathetically* to their feelings of anger, fear, guilt, or depression. They may also need to be helped to understand that their behavior has not been the cause of the divorce. A book about divorce can be helpful, but it is no substitute for a chance to talk with the pediatrician whom the child already knows and trusts. A 50-minute hour is not necessary; 10 or 15 minutes, with return appointments if indicated, can be most helpful. With his awareness of the current domestic situation and his knowledge of the child's past history, the pediatrician, as he talks with the child, is in the advantageous position of being able to help either directly or indirectly by suggesting further outside counseling. In complicated situations, he may help parents accept the need for direct consultation with a child psychiatrist or psychologist or a mental health facility. If uncertain about the next step, he may employ telephone consultation with a child psychiatrist, in order to gain specialized advice to supplement his own insights.

In considering outside sources of help for the child, the pediatrician should also be informed about the discussion groups for children of divorced parents, which are now being developed in many schools, churches, mental health centers, and other community settings. Child mental health specialists should know of these.

It is not easy for the busy pediatrician to meet the needs of families going through a divorce; even with maximum and optimum help from other professionals and from appropriate social agencies, the task is difficult. When the pediatrician is aware, however, of problems that can be anticipated and sees the value and appropriateness of a psychosocial approach to their solution, this new demand on the pediatrician can become one more satisfying challenge to his skill and expertise.

Obesity

MARJORIE A. BOECK, Ph.D., M.D.

Obesity is the most common nutritional disorder in the developed countries of the world. A variety of treatment approaches to obesity exist, including diet counseling, very low calorie diets, behavior modification, exercise, pharmacotherapy, and surgery. Unfortunately, none of these approaches has proved to be particularly successful either for weight loss or for maintenance of weight loss if it has been achieved. As with other illnesses with a poor prognosis for complete cure, the statistical probability of a poor outcome in obesity should not be used as a rationale to avoid treating the patient. Once it has been determined that the obesity is exogenous, the general pediatrician is in an excellent position to design and monitor a weight reduction program.

Obesity is usually arbitrarily defined as a weight that is 20% greater than ideal for height, and morbid obesity as a weight 50% greater than ideal weight. When the child or adolescent presents himself or herself to the physician for help in weight reduction it is important to determine whether the patient is actually obese. Usually this determination can be made by simply looking at

Table 1. OBESITY STANDARDS (CAUCASIAN NORTH AMERICANS): INITIAL LEVEL OF TRICEPS SKINFOLD THICKNESS INDICATING OBESITY

Age	Males (mm)	Females (mm)
5	12	14
6	12	15
7	13	16
8	14	17
9	15	18
10	16	20
11	17	21
12	18	22
13	18	23
14	17	23
15	16	24
16	15	25
17	14	26
18	15	27
19	15	27
20	16	28
21	17	28

(From Selzer and Mayer: A single criterion of obesity. Postgrad Med 38:A101, 1965. Courtesy of McGraw-Hill, Inc.)

the patient. The current emphasis on excessive slimness as beauty, however, leads many normal weight teenage girls to caloric restriction. As many as 60% of teenage girls diet at some point during their adolescence, while only 12–15% are even mildly overweight. Some of these girls may go on to develop an eating disorder such as anorexia nervosa or bulimia.

It is useful for both diagnosis and treatment planning to have a simple method for determining ideal body weight. The method most commonly used in an office setting is the nomogram, which relates weight to age, sex, and height. The shortcomings of this method include failure to take into account ethnic differences and variations in "body frame" and inability to distinguish weight due to muscle from that due to fat. Another easily utilized method for calculating ideal weight assumes a baseline of 100 pounds for a 5 foot female, adding 5 pounds for each inch over 5 feet and subtracting 10% for a "small" frame or adding 10% for a "heavy" frame. Similarly, ideal weight for a male utilizes a baseline of 106 pounds for the first 5 feet plus 6 pounds for each additional inch. The correction factor for body frame is the same. The method is not very accurate for individuals much shorter than 5 feet. The most reliable office measure of body fat is the triceps skinfold thickness. Triceps skinfold measurements are taken using constant tension calipers placed at the midpoint between the olecranon and acromial processes of the nondominant arm of a standing subject and are compared to standards for age and sex (Table 1).

Only a small fraction of obese children and adolescents have endogenous obesity secondary to genetic or endocrine abnormalities. Many parents, however, feel their child must have a "glandular problem." The great majority of individuals have exogenous obesity, a poorly understood syndrome with multiple etiologies. Those few patients with endogenous obesity can usually be readily identified by history and physical examination, since nearly all of the causes of endogenous obesity are characterized by growth failure. Such patients are usually at less than the fifth percentile for height and their bone age is delayed. The exogenously obese child is almost always at the fiftieth percentile or greater in height and has a bone age that is normal or advanced. Causes of endogenous obesity include hypothyroidism, Cushing's syndrome, Froehlich's syndrome, and the genetic Laurence-Moon-Biedl and Prader-Willi syndromes. Patients with hypothyroidism can be plump with myxedema, a dull facial expression, dry skin, constipation, short stature, and retarded bone age. Hypothyroidism by itself seldom causes massive obesity. Patients with Cushing's syndrome are short, with truncal obesity, moon facies, and buffalo hump. They may have characteristic purplish rather than pink-red striae of the skin resulting from thinning of dermal connective tissue, and they may be hypertensive. Genetic syndromes that include obesity are the Laurence-Moon-Biedl syndrome and the Prader-Willi syndrome. Patients with both syndromes are short, with mental deficiency and hypogonadism. Froehlich's syndrome is a rarely encountered condition in which a hypothalamic tumor results in polyphagia, obesity, and hypogonadism.

Both the initial assessment of the obese child or adolescent and the patient's eventual management require attention to historical information, physical findings, and laboratory results. A comprehensive history should include information as to the age of onset of excessive weight gain, maximum weight attained, and any identifiable precipitating events or circumstances. Note should be made of the presence of chronic or earlier serious health problems, previous starvation, abdominal surgery, or prolonged bed rest, all of which have been associated with the onset of excessive weight gain. The family pattern of weight gain and history of obesity-related conditions such as diabetes, high blood pressure, and heart disease should be elicited. Further questioning about the family's attitude toward obesity and any perceived relationship between eating and various moods and life stresses will be important in gaining a perspective on which therapeutic strategies have the best probabilities for success. It is important to assess the child's or adolescent's motivation to lose weight. Is he or she self-motivated or, alternatively, coerced by parents or school authorities into seeking treatment? Why is the individual choosing to address the problem at this particular time? Patterns of eating should be investigated, including the number of meals and snacks per day, the rate of eating, food preferences, the degree of hunger and satiety, and the occurrence of bingeing and nocturnal eating. The patient should be questioned regarding previous efforts at weight loss, including the type of weight reduction program employed, the duration of the effort, the amount of weight lost, and the reason for terminating the attempt. The impact of obesity upon social functioning, including peer relationships, leisure activities, school performance, and employment, should be assessed. An estimate of the patient's energy expenditure can be made by reconstructing the pattern of a typical weekday and weekend day.

The physical examination should include careful measurement of height and weight, with plotting of these values on a growth chart. Triceps skinfold measurements should be made with standardized calipers. Vital signs including blood pressure, measured with a thigh cuff if necessary, should be obtained. One should take note of the distribution of body fat, hirsutism, acne, and color of striae if present. Special attention should be paid to examination of the thyroid gland, back, and weight-bearing joints. It is often very difficult to detect organomegaly or masses on the abdominal exam. There is an increased incidence of certain orthopedic disorders, including slipped capital femoral epiphysis and tibia vara, in the obese. An assessment of pubertal development should be made. Patients with exogenous obesity have normal or slightly advanced sexual development. Male patients with exogenous obesity should have a normal sized phallus. The buried phallus in obese patients often gives the misleading impression of being small. Size can be determined by measuring from the phallic base.

Obesity in the child or adolescent may be associated with abnormal glucose tolerance, hyperinsulinemia, hypercholesterolemia, and hypertriglyceridemia. Therefore, fasting levels of glucose, cholesterol, and triglycerides should be obtained. Other laboratory tests are not indicated unless the patient is hypertensive, is of short stature, or has other clinical evidence of an endocrinologic disorder. Because decreased thyroid function can have a subtle presentation, the short obese child or teenager should be screened with serum thyroxine (T_4) and thyroid-stimulating hormone (TSH) levels. Because patients with Cushing's disease have been described who had growth failure and obesity without other signs of excessive cortisol secretion, children who are short and obese should

be given an overnight dexamethasone suppression test.

ROLE OF PARENTS

Parents exert a powerful influence on the eating and physical activity patterns of their children. In the case of younger children, parents are the focus of much of the nutrition counseling. Although teenagers are usually seen alone, it is inadvisable to exclude other family members from the treatment process totally. They are frequently responsible for both food purchase and preparation. Parents may help their child or teenager by purchasing special sugar-free drinks or by having the entire family alter cooking habits, e.g., baking rather than frying chicken. Alternatively, the family may appear to sabotage the dieting efforts deliberately. For example, freshly baked cakes may be left on the kitchen counter instead of being stored away as usual. Well-intentioned parents may make adhering to a diet more difficult by constantly nagging their youngsters.

DIET COUNSELING

The treatment for obesity most frequently employed by individuals with or without the advice of a physician is dieting. Low calorie diets should not be used by teenagers until completion of the growth spurt (Tanner Stage 4). The purpose of a diet for most children who have not yet completed their growth spurt is to promote the growth of the child's lean mass while holding his or her adipose mass constant. This can usually be achieved by following a diet of usual foods from the four basic food groups in normal proportions. In general, we do not prescribe any diet on our first encounter with an obese individual. We obtain a 24-hour diet recall and ask the patient to complete a diet diary during the next week and bring it to the second visit. Diets are highly individualized depending on current eating patterns, degree of motivation, intellect, amount of family support, and monetary considerations. For a teenage boy currently consuming over 2 liters of regular soda or fruit punch daily, the initial plan might be simply to alter the nature of his fluid intake. A teenage girl who snacks constantly on soda and candy while studying after dinner might initially substitute a cup of unbuttered popcorn. Many teenagers do not exhibit an orderly pattern of eating. A common pattern is to skip both breakfast and lunch and then eat rather continuously from after school until bedtime. The diet is frequently high in fat and concentrated sweets and low in fruits and vegetables. Many teenagers claim they eat very little. They are often correct that the quantity they consume is small, but their choices are very high

Table 2. LIST OF "FREE" FOODS*

Artichokes	Greens	Diet soda/seltzer
Asparagus	Lettuce	Mineral water
Broccolli	Mushrooms	Tea
Brussels sprouts	Peppers	Coffee
Cabbage	Radishes	Broth
Cauliflower	Spinach	Mustard
Celery	Sprouts	Herbs
Cucumbers	Summer squash	Spices
Eggplant	Tomatoes	Lemon
Green beans	Zucchini	Vinegar
Green onions	Water	Soy sauce
		Sour pickles

*Vegetables are served raw.

in calories. For such individuals a list of "free" foods, which essentially provide no calories, is invaluable (Table 2). Some adolescents prefer to be given food exchange lists or calorie counters so they can devise their own diets. Others want to be given a diet plan that details the foods and portions to be eaten at each meal. No matter what procedures are used, dieting is a painful, slow process that requires sacrifice on a daily basis.

Vitamin and mineral supplementation should be used with diets providing fewer than 1200 calories per day. Before the diet program begins, it is very important that the teenager have a realistic expectation about the rate of weight loss. It takes an energy deficit of 3500 to 3600 kcal to lose 1 pound. In other words, the teenager needs to take in 500 calories per day less than he or she utilizes in order to lose 1 pound per week. Compliance with these new dietary habits for a prolonged period in order to attain and maintain weight losses is a major difficulty. Individuals should be encouraged to use the concept of "calorie banking," i.e., planning ahead and saving some calories in advance to be used at a later date for special parties or holidays. Weigh-in and counseling sessions on a weekly basis are essential initially. Individuals will differ as to when they can reasonably be followed at biweekly intervals.

We favor a dietary approach utilizing food exchanges such as those devised by the American Diabetic Association. This allows the child or teenager flexibility in the choice of foods eaten without counting calories. Foods are divided into six categories: milk, vegetable, fruit, meat, fat, and bread (Table 3). Each food in a given category has an equal amount of carbohydrate, protein, fat, and calories and thus may be substituted for any other food in the same category. The distribution of protein, fat, and carbohydrate is important in order to lose the maximum amount of adipose tissue with a minimum loss of nitrogen. The number of food exchanges is determined such that 15–20% of the calories are from protein, 30–35% from fat, and the remaining 45–50% from carbohydrates, preferably ones that supply vitamins and minerals and are high in fiber. The distribution of food exchanges for different caloric level diets is given in Table 4.

Table 3. FOOD EXCHANGES: EXAMPLES OF TYPES AND AMOUNTS

Milk Exchange		*Meat Exchange*	
Whole milk*	1 cup	Beef, lamb, chicken, fish	1 oz
Evaporated milk	½ cup	Frankfurter	1
Skim milk	1 cup	Egg	1
Yogurt, plain	1 cup	Tuna	¼ oz
		Shrimp	5 small
Vegetable Exchange		Smooth peanut butter	2 T
Broccoli	1 cup	Cottage cheese	¼ cup
Green beans	1 cup	Cheddar, American	1 slice
Mushrooms	1 cup		
Summer squash	1 cup	*Fat Exchange*	
Tomato	1	Butter, margarine	1 t
Beets	½ cup	Mayonnaise, oil	1 t
Carrots	½ cup	Almonds	6 small
Peas, green	½ cup		
Winter squash	½ cup	*Bread Exchange*	
		Muffin	1
Fruit Exchange		Cereal, dry	¾ cup
Apple	1 small	Rice, cooked	½ cup
Banana	½ small	Noodles, cooked	½ cup
Grapes	12	Saltine crackers	5
Orange	1 small	Corn, sweet	⅓ cup
Raisins	2 T	Popcorn	1 cup
Strawberries	1 cup	Ice cream*	½ cup
Apple juice	½ cup	Potato chips*	½ cup
Orange juice	½ cup	Vegetable soup	½ cup

*Add two fat exchanges if used.

Table 4. DISTRIBUTION OF FOOD EXCHANGES FOR DIFFERENT CALORIE LEVELS

1000 Calories	1500 Calories
8 oz skim milk or skim milk yogurt	16 oz skim milk or skim milk yogurt
2 vegetable	3 vegetable
4 fruit	5 fruit
5 bread	8 bread
5 meat	5 meat
2 fat	5 fat
57 gm protein, 137 gm carbohydrate, 25 gm fat	73 gm protein, 209 gm carbohydrate, 40 gm fat
1200 Calories	**1800 Calories**
16 oz skim milk or skim milk yogurt	16 oz skim milk or skim milk yogurt
3 vegetable	3 vegetable
4 fruit	5 fruit
6 bread	10 bread
5 meat	7 meat
3 fat	6 fat
69 gm protein, 169 gm carbohydrate, 30 gm fat	91 gm protein, 237 gm carbohydrate, 51 gm fat

VERY LOW CALORIE DIETS

Very low calorie diets are defined as diets providing fewer than 800 kcal/day. These diets provide up to 70 gm of high-quality protein as well as vitamin and mineral supplements. They are not to be confused with the low calorie "liquid protein" diets that were associated with sudden death in physically healthy individuals owing to myocardial atrophy. Although primarily used with adults, these diets have been used successfully in children and adolescents in an inpatient setting. There have been no diet-related deaths in over 10,000 cases with the very low calorie diet limited to 3 months under careful medical supervision. Weight loss is more rapid, with losses of 20 kg in 12 weeks, but the dropout rate is very high. Side effects include postural hypotension, constipation, and cold intolerance. Most individuals, however, can maintain their normal activity level. Unfortunately, losses have been poorly maintained in follow-up despite special maintenance strategies. Further research is needed to ascertain the characteristics of persons who can achieve nitrogen balance on very low calorie diets. We recommend that diets providing fewer than 900 calories per day be restricted to research centers.

BEHAVIORAL TREATMENT

Behavioral programs focus on "how to eat" on the assumption that eating habits must change if the patient is to maintain weight loss. The child or teenager is asked to keep a diary of all food eaten and the circumstances surrounding its consumption: time, place, activity, and mood. This identifies specific behaviors to be targeted for change. The child or teenager may be asked to focus on slowing down the rate at which food is eaten, using smaller plates, eating mainly in certain areas, and avoiding other activities while eating (e.g., watching television, reading a book). Various studies on the effectiveness of behavioral treatment indicate that its advantage is not in the amount of weight lost but, rather, in the maintenance of weight once loss has occurred.

EXERCISE

An exercise program should be a part of every weight reduction plan. In fact, weight loss following exercise is generally greater than would be expected through the direct expenditure of energy alone. There is some evidence that increased activity in the obese may decrease appetite while it increases the metabolic rate. Within 24–48 hours after caloric restriction, both obese and lean individuals experience a 15–30% decrease in basal metabolic rate. Thus, caloric restriction without an increase in physical activity may not result in continued weight loss. Compliance with exercise programs in this age group is poor, however, with various studies reporting a 25–75% dropout rate. Reasons for this poor compliance include embarrassment, lack of transportation or money, and time pressures. Buddy systems and rewards for attendance at exercise sessions may be of help. It is important to recommend kinds of exercise, such as walking and climbing stairs, that do not require elaborate, expensive facilities. Obese individuals might benefit from special physical education classes within the school curriculum in which they could participate with less embarrassment with others who have similar skills and stamina.

PHARMACOTHERAPY

Anorexic drugs have resulted in rapid weight loss in adults, alone and in combination with behavior therapy. Studies indicate, however, that the loss is no greater than when behavior therapy is used alone and that when the drugs are stopped, the weight is more rapidly regained. Anorexic drugs are rarely used in children, primarily because of their side effects and the fear that they might cause growth retardation. In teenagers, they are seldom used because of the potential for abuse. In those instances in which they have been used, they seemed to be less effective than in adults. This has been attributed to poor compliance. Anorexic drugs represent a heterogeneous cluster of compounds. It may be possible in the future to tailor drug treatment to the individual's pattern of eating, but at present there is little role for pharmacotherapy in the treatment of child and adolescent obesity.

SURGERY

The surgical method of choice for weight reduction since 1966 has been gastric plication or bypass. Although primarily used as a treatment of last resort in adults who are more than twice the ideal weight for their height, it has been used in highly selected groups of morbidly obese older adolescents and with somewhat less success in patients with Prader-Willi syndrome. After gastric bypass, patients decrease their food intake to avoid the intense discomfort and vomiting that occur when small additional amounts of food are eaten. There is no diarrhea. Patients also report a change in eating patterns, consuming fewer fats, sweets, milk, and milk products. There has been less depression, anxiety, irritability, and preoccupation with food during weight loss subsequent to gastric bypass procedures than had occurred during previous nonsurgical attempts at weight reduction. In the largest reported series of adolescents who underwent gastric bypass, all but one lost weight. There was no interruption of growth in height, no metabolic problems, and no mortality. Gastric bypass is a safe and successful procedure in carefully selected adolescents.

SUMMARY

In summary, the greatest likelihood of success in treating mild to moderate obesity is a program including diet, behavior modification strategies, and exercise individually tailored to each patient. Long-term monitoring of progress in a group or individual setting is of great importance. The physician should pay special attention to dieting teenage girls who are only mildly overweight; this may signal the onset of anorexia nervosa. Surgery is an option for carefully selected, morbidly obese late adolescents who have failed to lose weight using other treatment modalities. While current therapeutic modalities fall far short of success, it is hoped that results of basic and clinical research will lead to more promising strategies for the future.

Homosexual Behavior

LAWRENCE S. NEINSTEIN, M.D.

DEFINITION

Homosexuality is one of the most emotionally charged issues for the adolescent and his or her family and physician. A homosexual can be defined as a person with a persistent, erotic attraction as an adult to members of the same sex, and who usually, but not always, engages in sexual relationships with them. In 1974, the American Psychiatric Association ended its classification of homosexuality as a mental disorder and labeled it as an alternative choice of sexual expression. Several points are important in applying the above definition to an individual, and in particular to teenagers.

1. Sexuality is a continuum—Kinsey developed a seven-point scale (0–6) for rating sexual behavior based on psychological reactions and overt sexual practices. A "0" is a person who is exclusively heterosexual, while a "6" is a person who is exclusively homosexual. The other numbers represent people on a continuum of degrees of homosexual and heterosexual fantasy and behavior.

2. Some homosexual experimental behavior is common for many adolescents. For most adolescents, this genital play apears to be part of a developmental process leading to a heterosexual identity. However, this type of incident can lead to confusion and panic in many teenagers.

3. Some heterosexual adolescents will engage in homosexual behavior under certain circumstances. This may include noncoed boarding schools, the armed services, or prison settings. Most of these individuals have heterosexual behavior after leaving such an environment.

In distinction from homosexuals, a transvestite is an individual who derives pleasure by dressing in the clothing of the opposite sex. A transexual is an individual who believes that the body he or she was born with does not match the sex he or she prefers to be.

PREVALENCE

As many as 50% of males and 30% of females engage in some homosexual experimentation during adolescence. Approximately 10% of males are exclusively homosexual during at least 3 years of their lives, and 5% of males for their entire lives. The prevalence in females has been more difficult to obtain but is about half that of males.

ETIOLOGY

While there is controversy over the factors involved in homosexual and heterosexual identity, the cause is unknown. The influence of genetics, of prenatal hormone levels, and of environment have all been postulated. While compelling evidence for any one of these factors is lacking, it seems likely that sexual identity is well-formed during childhood—even before adolescence. Several myths exist regarding homosexuality:

1. Homosexuality is a mental disorder. Homosexuality is *not* a mental disorder but a sexual preference. Homosexual adolescents may have problems identifying or adjusting to their sexual preference, leading to other fears and anxieties. The exposure of most homosexual adolescents to a societal environment of negative attitudes, lack of positive role models, and lack of family contacts can lead to problems with self-esteem and sexual behavior.

2. Homosexuals are child molesters. Most child molestation acts are committed by heterosexual males, not homosexual males.

3. Homosexual males are effeminate and wish to be female. The majority of homosexual males cannot be differentiated from heterosexual males and have no desire to be female.

COUNSELING

Physicians should be able to deal with the anxieties of adolescents with strong homosexual tendencies and the fears of heterosexual adolescents involved with homosexual experimentation. If the physician finds it impossible, because of moral or religious convictions, to be objective in counseling and in taking care of a teenager with homosexual behavior, it is important to offer the teenager a referral to another professional.

The goals of the physician in counseling a young person or parent concerned about homosexuality should be to understand the feelings of all involved, to identify what their concerns are, to provide factual information, and to provide practical suggestions to help reduce the concerns and/ or frictions.

To achieve any of these goals the concern of homosexuality must be discovered. Most adolescents are reluctant to discuss sexual issues, let alone homosexual concerns. In helping the teenager to discuss sexuality, it is helpful to first build rapport by asking less threatening questions about their medical concerns, school, hobbies, and friends. It is also essential to ensure confidentiality regarding sexual issues. There are different approaches in finding out about sexual identity or concerns. The physician can ask questions about dating and sexual activity and then later ask about sexual preference. It is often helpful to preface this with a reason for the inquiry (e.g., special medical problems). Alternatively, one can ask if there are any concerns or questions regarding the body, sexual activity, or sexual identity. Another approach is to state that many teenagers have concerns or questions about homosexuality and ask if there is anything that the individual would like to ask.

If a concern is raised, it is helpful to explore several areas. What is the teenager actually concerned about? If a homosexual encounter occurred, what actually happened? Is this a single encounter or one of many? Has the teen had sexual experiences with other people? Is there an interest in heterosexual sex? What are the teen's sexual fantasies? What does it mean to the teenager to be homosexual? What makes the teen think he or she is homosexual? What does it mean to the parent to have a homosexual son or daughter?

After these areas are explored, it is important to provide the teen and/or parents with factual information. This includes the prevalence of adolescent homosexual experimentation, the continuum of sexual behavior, and the fact that many teenagers worry about their sexual identity. The adolescent and his or her family must be aware that it is often difficult to assess and predict adult sexual behavior based on adolescent sexual behavior. However, the physician can help clarify the issues and keep the teen intregrated into his or her family and social system regardless of sexual preference. The physician should encourage family ties, as acceptance from the family is extremely important to the adolescent. The physician should discourage blame and guilt if homosexuality is discovered. The sexual aspects should be de-emphasized. The adolescent is a son or daughter who is homosexual, and not a homosexual who is a son or daughter.

Psychosocial areas need to be explored, as the social consequences of homosexual behavior can include peer rejection, family rejection, and harassment at school and job. For those adolescents who have a homosexual orientation, the evaluation should also include an assessment of their desire to remain homosexual or to try and alter their current sexual preference. However, adolescents should not be forced into therapy to change their sexual identity.

MEDICAL CONCERNS

The major medical concerns for physicians caring for adolescents with homosexual behavior include sexually transmitted diseases, gay bowel syndrome, and acquired immune deficiency syndrome (AIDS). Because of multiple partners, the high prevalence of asymptomatic carriers, and anonymity among patients, there is an epidemic of sexually transmitted diseases among the homosexual population. These problems are predominantly in homosexual males.

Anorectal and pharyngeal gonorrhea are fairly common in homosexual males. The majority of infections are asymptomatic. Symptoms include rectal burning, tenesmus, and mucopurulent discharge. Complications include fissures, abscesses, fistulas, and strictures. The preferred therapy for rectal and pharyngeal gonorrhea is 4.8 million units of aqueous penicillin G plus 1 gm of probenecid. Spectinomycin can be used for rectal gonorrhea in patients allergic to penicillin but is not recommended for pharyngeal gonorrhea. Sulfamethoxazole/trimethoprim, 9 tablets daily as a single dose for 5 days, can be used for pharyngeal gonorrhea in patients allergic to penicillin and in those with pencillinase-producing gonococcal pharyngeal infections. Gonorrhea cultures from the rectum, urethra, and pharynx are recommended every 3 to 6 months in homosexual males with multiple partners.

Syphilis is more common in homosexual males than in heterosexual males. About 50% of syphilis cases in the United States are among homosexual males. The primary lesion may be missed if present in the rectum. Syphilis serology is also recommended every 6 months in homosexuals with multiple partners.

Hepatitis B infections are prevalent in homosexual males, occurring in 37 to 51% of these individuals. A successful vaccine is now available for hepatitis B and should be used in homosexual males with multiple partners.

The gay bowel syndrome can include proctitis, colitis, and gastroenteritis. Infecting agents include *Neisseria gonorrhoeae*, *Treponema pallidum*, *Chlamydia trachomatis*, herpes simplex virus, human papilloma virus (condylomata acuminata), *Entamoeba histolytica*, *Giardia lamblia*, *Shigella*, *Salmonella*, and *Campylobacter jejuni/fetus*. The evaluation of an adolescent with rectal complaints and a history of rectal intercourse should include proctoscopy, routine and gonococcal cultures of stools, culture of stools for ova and parasites, and a syphilis serology.

Venereal warts are common in the rectal area in individuals having rectal intercourse. External warts can be treated with podophyllum resin (podophyllin). Internal warts can be treated with electrocautery. However, patients with internal warts are best referred to physicians familiar with their treatment, as overly aggressive therapy can lead to strictures. Examining serology for syphilis is essential.

The acquired immune deficiency syndrome (AIDS) is the disease causing the most concern among homosexual males. The most common problems are *Pneumocystis carinii* pneumonia and Karposi's sarcoma. Other opportunistic infecting agents include herpes simplex virus, cytomegalovirus, *Candida albicans*, *Cryptococcus neoformans*, *Toxoplasma gondii*, and *Mycobacterium tuberculosis*. The cause is most likely a human T-lymphotropic retrovirus. Because of the long incubation period, most cases fall out of the adolescent age group. The youngest homosexual patient with AIDS has been 15, and 95% are older than 25. However, young homosexual males may present with generalized lymphadenopathy. The prognosis of these patients is still unclear; therefore these individuals must have careful follow-up. Special clinics to follow patients with generalized lymphadenopathy or suspected AIDS are available in larger urban areas.

Sex Education

JOHN W. KULIG, M.D.

Sex education should be incorporated into anticipatory guidance provided from birth through late adolescence. Health providers have a unique opportunity to facilitate communication about sexuality between parents and their children as well as to provide specific factual information. Although comprehensive sex education should ideally occur within the home, most teenagers report receiving such information from peers. Parents often believe that sex education is being taught at school, yet only about one third of all schools provide specific courses in sex education, and only 10% are truly comprehensive in nature. Teenagers in particular are often eager to discuss sexuality-related concerns with both parents and health providers yet are often inhibited by the obvious discomfort generated by their questioning. In addition, parents of teenagers still commonly believe the myth that withholding information about sexuality may delay the onset of sexual activity.

Health providers can encourage and support parents in their role as sex educators in the family, provide age-appropriate guidance during the course of primary care visits, and assume an advocacy role on behalf of formal sex education programs in the community. Even in the absence of formal discussions about sexuality at home, children learn much from observing parental attitudes, vocabulary, and interactions. Parents of infants and toddlers should be advised to use proper terms when referring to body parts and to react calmly to the genital manipulation that commonly occurs with increased body awareness. Questions from preschoolers should be answered accurately in a simple, straightforward manner and in language appropriate to age. The concept of privacy should be reinforced at this time and proper names should continue to be used for both body parts and functions.

An important component of sex education at this age is the introduction of specific warnings aimed at reducing the risk of sexual misuse by an older child or adult. School age children who have not requested information on their own may be provided with specific data during "teachable moments," such as the birth of a sibling, the experience of "playing doctor," or the chance exposure to sexually explicit magazines or films. A parent's reaction to each of these events in a calm, nonpunitive manner will do much to avert feelings of guilt or discomfort on the part of the child. When explicit questions are posed, the parent should respond promptly with a simple factual answer rather than deferring the question to a later age or to the other parent.

With the onset of puberty, body image and physical development assume paramount importance to the young teenager. At this point it is essential that the adolescent be provided an opportunity for a confidential interview with the health provider as well as privacy during the physical examination. Emphasis on the normalcy of the examination can do much to alleviate the anxieties of an early adolescent faced with a rapidly changing body. At this stage, females should be provided with specific information about breast asymmetry, menarche, menstrual hygiene, and the management of menstrual cramps, while males should be advised about pubertal gynecomastia, erections, and nocturnal emissions. Masturbation should be acknowledged as a normal means of sexual expression in both sexes. The teaching of both breast self-examination and testicular self-examination should be considered an integral component of primary care for the early adolescent. In addition, adolescent females should be carefully prepared for their first pelvic examination, which should always be conducted in a gentle, sensitive manner.

Sexual history taking in adolescence is best accomplished through the use of "informative questions," which provide normative data and solicit a broader response than "yes or no" questions. Questioning should vary according to developmental stage, level of anxiety, presenting concern, and mode of sexual expression. Sexual history taking may also be facilitated by asking about the patient's relationship with a best friend, which in a dating relationship may lead to explicit information about sexual activity. A history of sexual activity in an adolescent should lead both to careful questioning about the character of the relationship as well as to a contraceptive history and the provision of contraceptive counseling, as appropriate. Questioning with use of "reality testing" may counter the magical thinking and feelings of invulnerability and denial that often characterize adolescent sexual behavior. For example, one might point out that a teenager who is sexually active without the use of contraception has, in fact, made a decision either to become pregnant or to father a child. Few teenagers have considered their response to an unplanned pregnancy. Health professionals who choose not to provide contraceptive counseling services should become aware of community agencies that serve adolescents.

Parents should be encouraged to maintain a dialogue with their adolescents and to express their beliefs openly and honestly. Parents should be cautioned, however, that teenagers do not need their approval to become sexually active and that the provision of contraceptive advice and services may reduce the risk of consequences of this activity. There is no evidence that such information stimulates sexual activity but rather may do just the opposite by satisfying curiosity without the need for experimentation. Numerous contemporary pamphlets, texts, and audiovisual materials on the topic of sex education are available for use by health providers, educators, and parents. A bibliography of low-cost resources on sex education for adolescents was recently published by the Committee on Adolescence of the American Academy of Pediatrics (Publications Department, American Academy of Pediatrics, P.O. Box 927, Elk Grove Village, Illinois 60007).

Adolescent Sexuality, Contraception, Pregnancy, and Abortion

JOHN W. KULIG, M.D.

Adolescents' health concerns about sexuality include a broad range of issues ranging from questions about the normalcy of their pubertal growth and development to dealing with the consequences of early sexual activity. Sexual expression among teenagers often reflects a developmental sequence that begins with self-exploration during puberty, followed by group dating, and then individual dating, which may initially be exploitative in nature. By high school graduation, approximately two thirds of all American teenagers have experienced at least one episode of sexual intercourse. Health providers must recognize both the medical and social consequences of early sexual activity, including not only sexually transmitted disease and pregnancy but also anxiety, depression, and multiple somatic complaints. Sexual history taking should include the asking of "informative questions" in a nonjudgmental fashion, with an assurance of confidentiality. Counseling should deal not only with the anatomy and physiology of reproduction and contraception but should also address decision making, positive options, and the denial of consequences that is so commonly seen in midadolescence.

The health provider must assure the adolescent that he or she is comfortable in addressing these concerns in a forthright manner. Questions should be age-appropriate, should not presume sexual preference, and should explicitly address the possibility of sexual abuse if suspected. Physical assessment during adolescence should include specific statements about the normalcy of pubertal development, and health education during this period should incorporate the teaching of breast and testicular self-examination. An annual pelvic examination with Papanicolaou smear and endocervical cultures is indicated in all sexually active adolescent females in order to detect cervical dysplasia and asymptomatic gonococcal and chlamydial infection. Pelvic examination is also indicated in the evaluation of menstrual disorders, lower abdominal pain, vaginal discharge, DES exposure in utero, and in the confirmation of pregnancy and the prescription of contraception.

CONTRACEPTION

Contraceptive counseling is an essential component of health education for the adolescent and may be conducted by the health provider or ancillary personnel and reinforced with the use of free or low-cost handouts and films. Surveys have consistently shown that maintenance of confidentiality is the most important factor in the provision of contraceptive care for teenagers. Counseling should be individualized, should be provided in a nonjudgmental manner for both males and females, and should address choices regarding sexual activity as well as the specific contraceptive methods available. Adolescents who choose to remain abstinent should be supported in this decision and encouraged to resist peer pressure.

Contraceptive Pill. The oral contraceptive pill remains the most popular choice among adolescent females. If indicated, the pill may be started as early as 6 to 12 months postmenarche after ovulatory cycles have been established. Among the medical contraindications to oral contraception, those that are most likely to affect adolescents include pregnancy, migraine headaches, hypertension, cyanotic heart disease, active liver disease, collagen vascular disease, diabetes mellitus, lipid disorders, severe depression, and a history of thromboembolic disease. Counseling should emphasize the noncontraceptive benefits of the pill, such as the resolution of dysmenorrhea and the reduced risk of pelvic inflammatory disease, iron deficiency anemia, benign breast disease, and certain forms of cancer. Serious complications of pill usage are exceedingly uncommon among teenagers; however, smoking should be discouraged in hopes of further reducing this risk.

A fixed-dose combination pill containing 1 mg of norethindrone and 35 mcg of ethinyl estradiol is a low-dose formulation suitable for the vast majority of adolescent women. Lower dose pills and those containing progestin only should be avoided owing to an unacceptable incidence of breakthrough bleeding, which is likely to markedly reduce compliance. The newly released triphasic formulations may possibly lead to confusion due to the presence of multicolored pills reflecting the difference in dosages. A 28-day pill packet is preferred to a 21-day packet, since the patient can simply be advised to take one pill each day at the same time of day, rather than remembering to stop for one week prior to beginning a new packet. A complete physical examination including breast and pelvic examination with Papanicolaou smear and cultures should first be performed. The pill should be started on the fifth day of menses or on the Sunday after menses in order to avoid administration during an unsuspected pregnancy. Patients should be scheduled to return to the physician 6 weeks after starting the pill, then at 3-month intervals for the first year and at 6-month intervals thereafter. Weight, blood pressure, and side effects are monitored at the interval visits, and the complete physical examination is repeated annually. Minor side effects such as breast tenderness, weight gain, and spotting often resolve after two or three cycles of use; thus, a change in pill formulation should generally not be instituted until after the 3-month follow-up visit. Drug interactions, particularly with anticonvulsants, may require an adjustment in dosage of both medications. The pill should be discontinued prior to surgery or orthopedic immobilization, but periodic "pill holidays" are not recommended.

Intrauterine Device. The intrauterine device (IUD) is not commonly used among nulliparous adolescents due to a relatively high expulsion rate, increased cramping, and an increased risk of pelvic inflammatory disease, with potential for subsequent infertility. The IUD might be considered in patients with a history of prior pregnancy or failure with oral contraception or barrier methods due to poor compliance and in sexually active adolescents with mild mental retardation. Copper or progesterone-containing devices should be inserted during menses in selected adolescents with no prior history of pelvic infection or multiple sexual partners.

Barrier Methods. Barrier methods would be ideal for adolescents if compliance could be assured. These methods are reversible, have few side effects, and reduce the risk of sexually transmitted infection. Condom use is the only method that allows the male to directly share in the responsibility for contraception. Condoms are available over the counter to minors, do not require a prescription, and do not require visits to a health provider. Condoms with a spermicidal lubricant and reservoir tip are advocated for use by adolescent males, and explicit instructions on proper storage and use should be provided. Spermicidal foams and creams are also available over the counter for adolescent females and, when used with condoms, provide a very high level of efficacy. Spermicidal suppositories may be less acceptable due to the need to wait for dissolution, which may produce an unpleasant burning sensation in the vagina. The vaginal contraceptive sponge is another inexpensive, nonprescription method that acts to absorb semen, block the cervical os, and release a spermicide. The sponge is effective for 24 hours after insertion but must be left in place for 6 hours after intercourse. Some patients have experienced difficulty with removal of the sponge. The diaphragm has been successfully used by motivated older adolescents, especially those who are comfortable with tampon insertion. The diaphragm is used in conjunction with a spermicidal cream or jelly and must initially be fitted by a health provider. Patients are asked to return in 1 week with the diaphragm in place to assure proper size and insertion. Diaphragms should be replaced annually or earlier if a significant change in weight occurs. The cervical cap, which is currently undergoing evaluation and modification, is not FDA approved and appears to have unacceptable failure rates and side effects.

Other Methods. Postcoital contraception has recently been demonstrated to be highly effective with the administration of only four Ovral oral contraceptive pills. Two pills are taken at each dose, 12 hours apart, within 48 to 72 hours of intercourse. The emetic doses of estrogen prescribed for 5 days in the past are no longer necessary for this indication.

Depo-medroxyprogesterone acetate given in a dose of 150 mg IM every 3 months will induce a secondary amenorrhea in a majority of patients. While not FDA approved for use as a contraceptive, this drug appears to be safe and effective for use in patients with moderate to severe mental retardation or mental illness as well as in selected patients with conditions such as sickle cell disease or severe congenital heart disease, in whom alternate methods are contraindicated yet the risk of pregnancy may be life threatening. The most troublesome side effects include irregular menstrual spotting or bleeding and weight gain.

"Natural family planning" is of limited usefulness among adolescents owing to unpredictable ovulation, the prolonged period of abstinence required each month, and the need to monitor the calendar, basal body temperature, and cervical mucus for optimal results. Withdrawal or coitus interruptus is also ineffective owing to poor control on the part of the adolescent male and the possible presence of sperm in the preejaculate fluid. Despite the lack of efficacy, either of these two methods is preferable to no attempt at contraception. Except in the event of a life-threatening emergency, surgical sterilization is not an option in an adolescent without involvement of the courts. Finally, abstinence should be emphasized as a positive choice, without risks, side effects, or cost.

PREGNANCY

Health providers caring for adolescents are very likely to face the issue of pregnancy diagnosis and referral, since approximately 1,300,000 teenage pregnancies occur each year. Common presentations include physical symptoms such as amenorrhea, nausea, breast tenderness, back pain, and urinary tract symptoms; behavioral presentations may include personality changes, truancy, and decline in school performance and general signs of anxiety, depression, or even suicidal behavior. A high index of suspicion will result in the correct diagnosis even in the absence of a confirmatory menstrual history. A 2-minute urinary slide pregnancy test is usually positive within 2 to 4 weeks after conception or 4 or 6 weeks since the last normal menstrual period. A negative test should be followed by contraceptive counseling and a repeat urinary pregnancy test in 1 to 2 weeks if menses have not resumed. Positive tests should be confirmed by pelvic examination to estimate uterine size and to confirm length of gestation. Serum pregnancy testing and pelvic ultrasound may be helpful in cases of suspected ectopic pregnancy.

Pregnancy counseling should then be conducted to assess the patient's response to the diagnosis and to discuss all options. With the patient's permission, parents and partners should be involved in helping the patient reach a decision. Although patients often express fear of parental reaction to pregnancy, most younger teenagers eventually consent to parental involvement, and their response is usually quite supportive. Options include terminating the pregnancy by therapeutic abortion or continuing the pregnancy, with subsequent adoption of the infant or raising the infant alone or with the assistance of a parent or partner. Early referral for therapeutic abortion or prenatal care is indicated in either case, preferably to a local agency that provides special services for pregnant adolescents and their partners. The medical complications of adolescent pregnancy are most common in patients younger than age 16, but the social consequences impact throughout adolescence. Prenatal programs that attempt to keep the pregnant adolescent in school and to teach parenting skills are aimed at averting the serious psychosocial sequelae, including a high risk of repeat pregnancy, child abuse, and neglect.

ABORTION

Since laws governing therapeutic abortion in minors vary by state, each health provider should become familiar with local law as well as area resources. Early referral is indicated to reduce the risk of medical complications. First trimester abortions are performed by suction curettage on an outpatient basis, while second trimester abortions often require an inpatient stay for induction of labor with hypertonic saline or prostaglandin instillation. Medical complications of therapeutic abortion are rare, and future child-bearing is not compromised. Follow-up should include the selection of an appropriate method of contraception.

Management of a Drug-Using Adolescent

RICHARD H. SCHWARTZ, M.D.

Adolescents of any socioeconomic group anywhere may be affected by the disease of alcohol/ drug (chemical) dependency, the symptoms or social consequences of which include adolescent turmoil, unpredictable explosive temper, conduct disorder (chronic lying, thievery, aggression, and/or promiscuity), bizarre behavior, venereal disease, truancy, serious academic underachievement, depression, involvement in motor vehicle accidents, running away, personality disorders, chronic argumentativeness and disrespect for others, amotivation, low sense of goal direction, and suicidal tendencies. It appears that drug use is the Great Imitator during adolescence and must be considered as a primary cause of, and not merely a secondary effect of, such mood disturbances and behaviors. Because endogenous depression, serious non–drug-related mental illness, and life with a physically or sexually abusive parent may lead to some of the same symptoms as found with drug abuse, pediatricians or their consultants must carefully evaluate each adolescent who exhibits these symptoms in order to reach the correct diagnosis. However, drug use should be a primary consideration.

EVALUATION

The first step in evaluating a teenage patient with any of the above symptoms is to obtain a comprehensive history, preferably during a counseling session. To elicit information about possible drug abuse the physician should ask the patient a few nonthreatening questions about school, family relationships, jobs, friends, and recreational activities, academic performance subject by subject, vocational aspirations, frequency of conflicts with parents, attendance at hard rock concerts, if any close friends are hassled by their parents for drinking a little beer, participation in drinking games at parties, if any close friend has ever been drunk or high, how many cans of beer the adolescent who drinks alcohol may consume before he or she "catches a buzz."

Drug-using adolescents often become proficient in techniques of denial or minimization of their own role, blaming others, selective muteness, and overt hostility when threatened by references to drug use. Therefore, a more thorough drug and alcohol assessment, if the pediatrician's suspicions are aroused, should be done by a professional with expertise and experience in the field of substance abuse, rather than by a well-meaning but naive pediatrician who may easily be manipulated and misled ("conned") by a drug-using adolescent.

The physical examination is unlikely to provide any hard evidence regarding drug use, although some indications of the adolescent's sympathy with the drug culture may be provided by his or her attitude toward the physician and attire. Lack of sustained eye contact, lack of spontaneity, a flattened affect, and an attitude of hostility, secretiveness, or persistent evasiveness should alert the physician to the possibility of drug use, especially

when combined with a preference for the hairstyles and clothing favored by drug users. These are "soft signs" and require correlation with the history and laboratory findings as in the diagnosis of any other disease. It is usually more fruitful to concentrate on the adverse social consequences of drug use and avoid threatening direct questions about such use. Intoxicated behavior or concrete evidence of drug use is not often witnessed by parents or a drug-using adolescent until fairly late in the progressive stages of the drug use syndrome.

LABORATORY DIAGNOSIS

Because it is so difficult to diagnose drug use, any array of factors in the history combined with any of the attitudes just described should raise the suspicion that an adolescent has this disorder. And because of the potentially life-threatening consequences of continued drug use, the physician should order laboratory tests to assist in further evaluation of such a patient.

Marijuana Use. Metabolites of marijuana (cannabis) and phencyclidine persist in the body for several days after last use of those drugs and may be detected by laboratory analysis of a urine specimen. The half-life of marijuana is 72 hours, and if the adolescent is using cannabis every day, evidence will be detectable in the urine up to several weeks after the beginning of a period of complete abstinence. Casual or infrequent users of marijuana will have a negative (clean) urine by immunoassay methods 48–72 hours after abstinence.

A urine specimen collected for analysis of these substances should be obtained from a first voiding on a Monday morning (because most adolescents use drugs on Friday and Saturday evenings), preferably under direct surveillance to avoid possible deliberate substitution or adulteration of the urine specimen by the adolescent. Most frequent users of illicit drugs are well aware of procedures for adulterating a specimen for laboratory analysis of such use, including substituting urine of a non–drug-using friend, diluting the specimen with tap water, drinking large quantities of water before voiding, and purposely adding blood, household bleach, salt, or an acidic substance. Thus, when direct observation is not possible, the urine specimen should be checked for color, pH, specific gravity, and freshness (warmth of the specimen when obtained in the physician's office or at home).

Testing urine specimens serially (consecutive Monday morning urine specimens), for the presence of cannabinoids is more informative than a single test for such substances. If cannabinoids are present in two mid-week urine specimens obtained several days apart, or if three weekly spot-checked Monday-morning specimens are positive, it is likely that the adolescent is using marijuana frequently enough to warrant a more complete drug evaluation. Such an adolescent may well need immediate intervention and treatment of his or her drug abuse disorder.

Alcohol Use. Frequent use of alcohol is more difficult to detect than marijuana use, but the patient should be questioned carefully about citations for driving while intoxicated, what he or she does with friends for relaxation, and how often the adolescent or his or her close friends have been incapacitated by alcohol. If alcohol use has been heavy, damage to the parenchyma of the liver may be present and detected as elevation of the hepatic enzyme gamma glutamyl transpeptidase. This test, however, is relatively nonsensitive and nonspecific for adolescent alcoholism.

Acute alcohol ingestion may be detected by administration of a Breathalyzer test or immunoassay of a urine specimen obtained within 6 hours of ingestion. Such use may also be detected, even as late as 12 hours postingestion, by sophisticated urine toxicology methods such as gas chromatology, but such means are much more expensive and the results are not available for some time after the sample is drawn.

CHEMICAL DEPENDENCY

Chemical dependency is the increasingly preferred term for compulsive drug use. Either persistent, frequent use of mood-altering, pleasure-producing drugs or indulgence in prolonged binges of such drug use characterize the adolescent who has lost control of his or her use of drugs. Such an individual has a preoccupation with a self-perceived need to obtain a euphoric "high" not reached by other means, usually in the company of peers who have the same mind-set. These adolescents may develop a tolerance to their drug(s) of choice, so that they require ever increasing quantities of the drug to achieve the same degree of euphoria. Because the chemically dependent young person obtains much of his or her pleasure in life from the social use of drugs, he or she cannot or will not stop using these substances. Thus, even though the adolescent may have tried one or more times to remain abstinent, and despite being apprised of the many adverse consequences of drug use (academic underachievement, family conflicts, internalized shame and guilt, legal complications, acute toxic reactions), it must be recognized that the chemically dependent adolescent usually cannot break free of his or her disease without intensive and prolonged professional help.

Outpatient Management. After the adolescent has been evaluated by a pediatrician or consultant who is an expert in chemical dependency, a time must be chosen when the patient is not under the influence of drugs to bring the entire family together (excluding young children) for treatment.

At this initial session the goal is for every family member present to agree to a drug-free lifestyle for him- or herself and for the parents to state unequivocally that they are prepared to do anything and everything to accomplish that goal. Behavioral changes that will be necessary for the drug user include (1) total abstinence from all drugs (including alcohol), (2) complete and immediate dissociation from drug-using friends, (3) cooperation in the provision of periodic urine specimens to monitor compliance with the plan, and (4) participation in family meetings each week.

Other activities in which the drug-user must participate include attendance at a peer-support group such as Alcoholics Anonymous or Narcotics Anonymous two or three times a week for the first month, two times a week for the second month, and once weekly for the next three months. A sponsor from the support group should be assigned to act as role model for the drug-using adolescent and to monitor attendance and participation at meetings. The adolescent and family may need psychotherapeutic or pastoral counseling, which should be done by someone expert in managing individuals with alcohol- or drug-related problems.

It is important for the adolescent and professionals who are helping him or her to manage the drug problem to communicate on a regular basis with school guidance counselors, teachers, the pediatrician, group therapy sponsor, and interested others. Further, the teenager must comply with a mutually agreed upon list of house rules, the breaking of which will have fair but definite and clear consequences. The adolescent's parents would do well to attend a parent support group such as Al-Anon or Toughlove. Parents of drug-using teenagers often feel embarrased, guilty, insecure, and alienated from parents of "successful" teenagers. Lastly, if the drug which the adolescent has heavily abused is alcohol, a medically supervised trial of disulfiram (Antabuse) (250 mg/day in a single dose for two to three months) should be considered. Antabuse requires an intensive education as to the reasons for use and its effects if alcohol is ingested, and it should not be prescribed unless it is part of a comprehensive plan of management including regular attendance at AA meetings.

If this necessarily authoritarian plan of therapy is unsuccessful, the young person dependent on drugs (including alcohol) should be admitted to an adolescent-oriented drug rehabilitation program or therapeutic community with or without his or her consent unless the age of majority had been reached.

Inpatient Management. The basic principles of managing drug abuse are the same, regardless of which of the following drugs is abused: alcohol, marijuana, cocaine, stimulants, depressants, hallucinogens, PCP, or inhalants. Methadone may be included in the regimen for management of opiate abuse, Antabuse has been found to be helpful in the treatment of some alcoholics, and phenothiazine or trifluoperazine may be required to treat subacute or chronic drug-related PCP or LSD psychosis as part of the overall treatment plan. Antidepressant medication may be a necesary adjunct in the management of selected severely endogenously depressed and chemically dependent adolescents.

Detoxification is almost always unnecessary for adolescent drug users unless the dependence is on an opiate, barbiturate, or diazepam, or unless the patient had attempted to withdraw from alcohol dependence previously and had shown severe acute symptoms. When necessary, such detoxification can usually be accomplished in three to seven days (unless the drug is diazepam).

Drug rehabilitation programs for adolescent drug users should meet six criteria. (1) No drugs whatever should be permitted in the program, including alcohol, mood-altering drugs, and tranquilizers. (2) Peer-group support should be encouraged. (3) Some staff members should be ex-drug users or alcoholics. (4) Intense family participation should be mandatory. (5) The chemically dependent patient should be separated from friends and/or parents for a minimum of one to two months. (6) The program must have an aftercare program that includes a large enough group of graduates close enough geographically to the patient that they form an easily accessible peer group of drug-free supporters.

Pediatricians play a crucial role in the identification and treatment of drug-dependent adolescents. By familiarizing themselves with the symptoms of chemical dependency, the techniques of the assessment of a drug-using adolescent, and the resources in their areas to help rehabilitate drug users they will be much better able to serve their adolescent patients and their families.

24

Miscellaneous

Primary Immunodeficiency Disease

JAMES G. McNAMARA, M.D., *and* JOHN M. DWYER, M.D., Ph.D.

DEFICIENCIES OF ANTIBODY PRODUCTION

The development of commercially available intravenously administered immune globulin preparations (Gamimune [Cutter Laboratories] and Sandoglobulin [Sandoz Pharmaceuticals]) has revolutionized the treatment of patients with immunodeficiencies principally affecting the B cell system. We have completely abandoned the intramuscular use of immunoglobulin in the treatment of antibody deficiency states in favor of the intravenous products, which are equally safe and capable of providing a greater degree of passive antibody protection. Immune globulin intravenous (IGIV) is used in a dose of 100–400 mg/kg, with most patients requiring therapy in the 200 mg/kg dose range. As with any immune globulin preparation, anaphylactoid reactions may occur rarely. It is judicious therefore to give the first infusion at a very slow rate and double that rate every half hour until the desired infusion rate is achieved.

IgG Deficiencies. The spectrum of syndromes featuring hypogammaglobulinemia in childhood is quite large, and not all of these conditions require replacement therapy. Two such examples are the physiological hypogammaglobulinemia of prematurity and transient hypogammaglobulinemia of infancy (THI). Extremely premature infants are born with only a fraction of the transplacentally derived IgG that would have been present had they been born at term, and it may be many months before they reach the corrected gestational age at which they will begin to produce adequate immunoglobulin. Until that time these infants may have very low IgG levels. Trials are currently

underway to determine whether the prophylactic use of IGIV reduces the incidence of infections in these high-risk neonates. Currently, we recommend IGIV for sick neonates with an IgG < 200 mg/dl but will hold treatment in the otherwise healthy neonate. Similarly, THI is seen in term infants who have a delay in their production of IgG. This delay is probably due to a T cell defect. Again, we do not generally infuse those patients prophylactically unless they have a serious infection and an IgG < 200 mg/dl. Most children outgrow this problem at age 3.

Patients with congenital syndromes characterized by low IgG, such as x-linked agammaglobulinemia (SLA) and hypogammaglobulinemia with IgM, clearly benefit from the regular prophylactic administration of gammaglobulin as part of their treatment regimens. There have been no clear studies published that address how much of the IGIV preparation is needed to prevent infections. Using the guidelines mentioned earlier, we try to keep the patient's monthly preinfusion nadir in the 300–400 mg/dl range. We are quite pleased with the reduction of serious infections achieved by maintaining this level. When these patients or any others, become ill, they have an increased catabolic rate. Patients receiving IGIV will catabolize this glycoprotein much more rapidly than usual and require more frequent IGIV to maintain adequate IgG levels. One of the most serious infectious complications of SLA is the development of encephalitis from enteroviruses, which usually leads to progressive neurologic deterioration. We have successfully treated one such patient with the IGIV preparation given intrathecally* via an Ommaya reservoir (total = 5.6 gm over a 2-week period).

Patients with IgG subclass deficiencies may benefit from IGIV therapy. IgG subclass 2 deficiencies

---

* Intrathecal administration is not mentioned in the manufacturer's directive.

are being reported more frequently in patients with ataxia-telangiectasia, diabetes, and systemic lupus erythematosus, and as an isolated, sometimes familial defect. Many patients with IgA deficiency also lack IgG$_2$. Those patients in the IgA deficiency group with anti-IgA antibodies are not candidates for this treatment modality, since the trace amount of IgA in the IGIV may trigger an anaphylactic reaction. Since IgG$_3$ has a much shorter half-life than the other subclasses (approximately 7 days versus 26 to 28 days), deficiencies of this subclass may require more frequent replacement therapy.

IgA Deficiencies. The IgA deficiencies are a heterogenous group. Selective IgA deficiency is defined as a serum IgA of < 5 mg/dl and may be seen in association with recurrent infections, allergic phenomenon, autoimmune diseases, or signs of mild T cell abnormalities. Secretory IgA is usually very low in these patients but may be an isolated deficiency in itself. Secretory piece deficiency has also been reported as a clinical syndrome. Currently, there is no effective replacement therapy for these patients. In some patients with chronic draining otitis media we have used fresh colostrum ear drops (rich in secretory IgA) as an adjunct to routine medical treatment with excellent results. As with any immunodeficient patient we use aggressive bacteriocidal antibiotic treatment when indicated. When patients with IgA deficiency need blood products, several strategies are available to avoid the risk of anaphylaxis. For elective surgery, autologous blood transfusions can be considered as well as the use of IgA deficient donors, who are available through many blood banks. At all other times washed packed red blood cells should be used.

IgM Deficiency. Selective IgM deficiency is a rare primary disorder, and little information is available on its appropriate treatment. Certainly these patients have a markedly increased risk for infections with polysaccharide-encapsulated organisms and thus may benefit from prophylactic antibiotic administration. Since the other immunoglobulin isotypes are present in these patients, they should benefit from the polysaccharide vaccines (pneumococcal, meningococcal, and *Hemophilus influenzae* type B).

ISOLATED AND COMBINED T CELL DEFICIENCIES

In T cell disorders advances in treatment have been as impressive as those in B cell disorders, but treatment continues to be extremely complex and difficult and limited to a handful of research centers. This dichotomy is due largely to the nature of treatment protocols, with B cell disorders being adequately treated with products that deliver passive immunity, but T cell disorders by and large requiring immunologic reconstitutive efforts. We

will briefly outline some of the disorders principally affecting T cell and/or B and T cell systems as illustrations of treatment strategies.

DiGeorge's Syndrome. DiGeorge's syndrome (third and fourth pharyngeal arch syndrome) is characterized by progressive failure of the T cell system. Numerous treatments have been attempted, with the most successful being with fetal thymic transplants. Implantation of cultured thymic epithelial (CTE) fragments is the most recently evolved thymic transplant technique, but its success in DiGeorge's syndrome has yet to be assessed. Infection is rare during the first month of life with this syndrome unless there has been a number of invasive manipulations or procedures. Thus, the management of the patient's cardiac and endocrine disorders should receive the first priority. Assessment for the need of reconstitution efforts in these patients should be made over a period of time, since some of these patients have been reported to have spontaneous improvement in their immunologic function.

Several thymic hormones have been available for investigation, such as thymopoietin (TP-5), thymulin (FTS-Zn), and thymosin alpha-1. Treatment with these factors has been explored in a wide range of immunodeficiencies but is again passive replacement therapy rather than permanent reconstitution. Varying degrees of success have been reported, particularly with patients with DiGeorge's syndrome and with the combined immunodeficiency of ataxia-telangectasia.

Candidiasis. Chronic mucocutaneous candidiasis (CMC) is a heterogeneous disorder ranging from an isolated and partial T cell dysfunction in handling *Candida* to a disorder comprising candidiasis with polyendocrinopathy. Treatment of CMC is based upon aggressive use of antifungal agents and has been dramatically improved with the use of ketoconazole. Ketoconazole has few side effects, but signs of liver toxicity need to be monitored. Ketoconazole is best absorbed in an acid pH, so we generally recommend that it be taken with orange juice. We believe that the use of transfer factor (TF), a low molecular weight dialyzable leukocyte extract, has been shown to be useful in this disorder. Monthly injections of 1 IU (i.e., TF from 5×10^8 peripheral blood leukocytes) improved cell-mediated immunity responses to *Candida* in 70% of patients. Patients with Wiskott-Aldrich syndrome (WAS), characterized by eczema, thrombocytopenia, and a variable immunodeficiency marked by a progressive decrease in cell-mediated immunity, have been reported to improve clinically with TF but have no evidence of increased survival.

The treatment of choice for reconstituting the immune system of all patients falling into the category of severe combined immunodeficiency and other severe immunodeficiencies such as WAS is bone marrow transplantation. Successful use of this modality has been reported with a greater than 10-year survival. The major problems associated with this technique have been fatalities from infections and from the development of graft versus host disease. To minimize the latter danger, transplantation with histocompatible siblings who are HLA-D compatible by mixed lymphocyte reactions is clearly preferred; however, even this does not guarantee that there will be no development of graft versus host disease.

In patients who do not have compatible siblings, bone marrow transplantations have been attempted with parental donors, who must be haploidentical, in conjunction with pretreatment of the bone marrow to attempt to eliminate T cells. This major advancement in transplantation involves sedimentation of T cells by soybean agglutinin followed by either E rosetting and/or anti–T cell monoclonal antibody treatment with complement. Successful engraftment using these techniques has been reported but usually requires several transplant attempts and is often not as complete as histocompatible marrow transplants.

In patients with severe combined immunodeficiencies caused by adenosine deaminase deficiency, bone marrow transplantation remains the treatment of choice. However, some patients have responded to monthly partial exchange transfusions using irradiated red blood cells. Their immunologic function has improved, and a decrease in adenosine metabolites has been noted.

General Considerations

We believe that aggressive use of antibiotics in all patients with immunodeficiencies is indicated after appropriate cultures have been obtained. Indiscriminate use of antibiotics is not helpful and may only cloud issues at a later date. The corollary to aggressive antibiotic treatment is aggressive evaluation for opportunistic infections that might be amenable to treatment.

We seldom use antibiotics prophylactically except in the case of the patient with severe T cell abnormalities who should benefit from *Pneumocystis carinii* prophylaxis with trimethoprim-sulfamethoxazole. Similarly, as mentioned earlier, patients with IgM deficiencies or with asplenia syndromes are usually given prophylaxis with penicillin. For our patients with severe IgG deficiencies and chronic lung disease, we try to rotate our antibiotics and use periods of no antibiotics to decrease problems associated with the development of resistant organisms.

Routine pulmonary evaluation is essential in all immunodeficiencies but particularly in patients with the hypogammaglobulinemias, in which the development of chronic lung disease is a common occurrence. Annual pulmonary function tests and chest x-ray examinations are advisable in this setting. In the patient with chronic lung disease, education for the family and the patient on the techniques of postural drainage is mandatory.

Gastrointestinal discomfort and diarrhea are common complaints in the immunodeficient patient. Parasitic infections are often implicated, with the most common organism isolated being *Giardia lamblia*. However, other opportunistic infections may be seen in this population, such as Cryptosporidiosis, and therefore antibiotic treatment should be instituted only after microbiologic identification of a pathogen.

Immunization protocols in patients with immunodeficiencies are controversial. All would agree that patients with severe B or T cell abnormalities should not receive live virus vaccines. In addition, siblings or children of patients with immunodeficiencies should not receive live viral vaccines, particularly the oral polio vaccine, since the virus will be shed from the vaccinated subject and potentially infect the immunodeficient patient. We believe that patients with IgA deficiencies should not receive the oral polio vaccine until adequate secretory IgA can be demonstrated. Patients should be adequately protected by herd immunity, and if trips outside the protected population are anticipated, immunization with the killed polio vaccine can be planned. Of course, patients requiring IGIV are passively immunized to a wide range of bacterial and viral organisms.

All patients with severe immunodeficiencies should receive irradiated blood products (3000 R) until the nature of the immunodeficiency has been studied. At that time only patients with defects in T cell immunity need to have irradiated blood products, for the prevention of potentially lethal graft versus host disease. Our blood bank service irradiates whole blood, packed red blood cells, platelets, and neutrophils for patients identified as being at risk for the development of this disease. Some services also recommend irradiating plasma as well; however, the freezing step in fresh frozen plasma should be adequate to kill the remaining lymphocytes in that blood component.

All the immunodeficiency disorders that have been discussed carry an increased incidence of tumors, particularly of the lymphoreticular system. Health care providers for these patients need to be aware of this potential complication so that appropriate vigilance can be maintained both during routine examinations as well as during evaluations of patient complaints.

Although treatment of the primary immunodeficiencies is extremely important, attempts at their prevention must also be made. Genetic counseling and evaluation of the families of affected individuals should always be part of the diagnostic and management plans for those caring for immunodeficient patients. Recently, great advances have been made in the study of prenatal diagnosis of severe combined immunodeficiency disease, adenosine deaminase deficiency-severe combined immunodeficiency disease, x-linked agammaglobulinemia, and others. This allows identification of affected fetuses so that informed decisions may be made regarding the termination of the pregnancy or preparations for postnatal care to maximize the chances of survival.

ACQUIRED IMMUNE DEFICIENCY SYNDROME (AIDS)

Although not strictly a primary immunodeficiency, this devastating disease affects children; it occurs most commonly as a congenital infection. In addition, some neonates and children may become infected with the human T cell lymphocytotrophic virus (HTLV) III through blood products. AIDS in children, as in adults, can present as a range of illnesses from lymphadenopathy to a severe immunodeficiency marked by numerous opportunistic infections or tumors. The definition of pediatric AIDS by the Centers for Disease Control applies only to this later group, although it is clear that pediatric patients with AIDS have a much greater incidence of serious bacterial infections than their adult counterparts.

As in any severe disease the approaches to treatment need to be multidisciplinary. Accurate diagnosis is imperative for both social and scientific reasons. A child with risk factors and immunologic profiles suggestive of AIDS demands special vigilance and aggressive evaluation, when clinically indicated, for opportunistic infections that may be amenable to treatment. The myriad of opportunistic infections (fungal, protozoan, bacterial, and viral) seen in adults has similarly been reported in children. As in any immunocompromised host, early diagnostic procedures are important if these infections are to be recognized at a time when treatment may be of benefit.

Because of the profound immunodeficiency associated with AIDS, any successful treatment plan needs to include efforts to reconstitute or modulate the immune system. Attempts at this in adults have uniformly led to disappointing results. All of the modalities mentioned earlier have been tried, including bone marrow transplantation, cultured thymic epithelial fragment implants, thymic factors, and transfer factor, in addition to infusions with the lymphokines gamma interferon and interleukin 2. These discouraging findings probably result from reservoirs of HTLV-III still present in the patient that continue to infect and to kill T cells as they attempt to reconstitute the immune system. Active attempts at reconstitution seem futile at this point, but the development of reverse transcriptase inhibitors, such as suramin sodium, provides hope that combination protocols will be developed.

Some investigators routinely give passive protection with IGIV to their pediatric AIDS patients. We have used IGIV in selected patients without complications. The rationale is that although these patients most commonly have a polyclonal gammopathy, they have been demonstrated to be qualitatively deficient and respond very poorly to protein and polysaccharide vaccines. These patients need to be observed more closely than patients with hypogammaglobulinemia, since they are more likely to develop problems with immune complex formation.

The use of prednisone remains controversial, but we have found it to be beneficial in some circumstances. We use prednisone in the symptomatic treatment of the lymphoproliferative disease seen in pediatric AIDS, particularly in the marked lymphocytic pulmonary infiltrates. The use of steroids does not change the underlying illness in AIDS and should only be administered after tissue confirmation of lymphocytic pulmonary infiltrates with exclusion of other opportunistic infections. Marked improvements in pulmonary function tests can be monitored in those children old enough to cooperate; in younger children serial blood gas levels and chest x-rays may be needed to document the improvement in pulmonary function. We generally start steroids at a dose of 2 mg/kg/day for a couple of weeks, and then slowly taper that dose to the point at which the lymphoproliferative changes are just held in check. We do not recommend the use of steroids for subjective improvement of generalized adenopathy alone but do feel that in patients with progressive pulmonary infiltrates who have compromised pulmonary function a trial of steroids may be beneficial.

Equally as important as these issues is the need for early intervention by a social worker. Many of these patients come from disrupted families, to which the addition of this devastating illness would be overwhelming without further support systems. Of course, the parents and siblings of patients with pediatric AIDS not acquired by transfusions of contaminated blood products need to be evaluated for any AIDS-related illnesses as well.

Sudden Infant Death Syndrome (SIDS) and Near-Miss SIDS

WARREN G. GUNTHEROTH, M.D.

Sudden infant death syndrome (SIDS) is defined as sudden and unanticipated death in an infant, in whom, after postmortem examination, there is no recognized lethal disorder. By consensus, the neonatal period is excluded, and the first month of life is usually spared. The disease peaks between two and three months of age and is rare after six months of age.

The management of SIDS largely consists of family counseling. The unexpected nature of this disease, striking apparently healthy infants in their sleep, is capable of producing remarkable psychopathology, and the surviving family, including siblings, may require counseling. A good start is a thorough autopsy, which will establish whether there was an inherently lethal abnormality and allow an honest explanation to the family that the disorder was or was not SIDS. This should be followed by reassuring the parents that medical science has no way of preventing this tragedy in the vast majority of instances. (The few exceptions will be discussed under near-miss SIDS). Local parent organizations, which in the United States include the National Foundation for Sudden Infant Death Syndrome (8240 Professional Place, Landover, Maryland 20785; 800-221-SIDS, toll free), have branches in many communities throughout the country. The members include parents who have lost an infant through SIDS, and their support is remarkably helpful. In addition, the subsequent involvement of the bereaved parents in this positive organization is excellent therapy. Advice to the parents about the relatively low risk of recurrences in their family is important, and even the advice not to have a quick "replacement child" may be better understood if it comes from a sympathetic family who has undergone this experience.

Near-Miss SIDS

The observation of infants in the same age category as that affected by SIDS who have prolonged apnea with bradycardia suggests that there is a reversible stage before death in the SIDS infant. Although this concept has been heatedly debated, it seems unlikely that SIDS is 100% instantaneously fatal. If it were, it would be unique among all known diseases. In any case, the infant with prolonged apnea can be shown to be at increased risk of SIDS, and this group has the highest risk of SIDS of any living group of patients. The definition of near-miss SIDS applies simply to an infant discovered in a state that is perceived as moribund, and health professionals may find cyanosis, bradycardia, or marked pallor in addition to apnea.

Whether one describes these infants' condition as near-miss SIDS or prolonged apnea, there is consensus on certain aspects of their management. Of foremost importance is a medical work-up that excludes some of the treatable entities that can cause prolonged apnea. Infection, gastroesophageal reflux, seizure disorders, metabolic disorders

such as hypoglycemia, anemia (particularly in prematures), airway problems, and child abuse should be considered and ruled out. If any of these entities are discovered, they should be treated specifically. However, many of these infants appear to be healthy after they have recovered from the episode of prolonged apnea, and their further management is somewhat controversial. Many of us when confronted by anxious parents who have "dodged the bullet" will prefer to have that infant on a home monitor, if for no other reason than to permit the parents to sleep at night. It clearly makes no sense to do this, however, without training the parents and any other care givers in cardiopulmonary resuscitation. It has seemed reasonable to me in this circumstance to use the simplest form of monitor that is reliable, which is a heart rate monitor (particularly in areas remote from large support centers). These are relatively inexpensive and have few false alarms, and any episode of apnea that is long enough to produce hypoxia will slow the heart rate. On the other hand, monitors that record only respiration by chest movement are unreliable, since the relatively infrequent obstructive apnea would not be detected but would be detected by a drop in heart rate. The parents should be reassured at the outset that this is a problem of immaturity and that when the infant reaches 6 months of age the monitor will not be needed. This advice will prevent the parents and infant from becoming permanently "addicted" to the monitor.

Several centers have developed polygraphic techniques that are used in the decision regarding a home monitor. These diagnostic pneumocardiograms look for prolonged apnea, the frequency of shorter apnea, and periodic respiration. Although the protocols look very precise, these tests are not capable of sufficient predictability to rule out a fatal event, even the following day. Accordingly, if the history of prolonged apnea is unequivocal, particularly if it required resuscitation, monitoring would be prudent regardless of the pneumocardiogram. Following the experience with premature apnea, some centers use theophylline for infants sent home on monitors. The dose that has been advocated begins with 3–5 mg/kg as a loading dose and then 1–2 mg/kg every 8 hours. Blood levels should be in the range of 6–12 µg/ml. Theophylline can be demonstrated to improve the pneumocardiogram score, but blind studies have not shown it to be effective. There is some risk of forgetting to give the medication, which could result in deeper than normal sleep. In my opinion, theophylline should be used selectively and not routinely.

Other infants who are at increased risk of SIDS are also potential candidates for home monitors. This group includes the premature, twins, particularly if one has died of SIDS, and subsequent siblings of SIDS. The risk is not particularly high for any of these other groups, and the use of a home monitor is based less on the probability of a SIDS event than it is on the worry of parents who are in a situation in which the anxiety may be extreme. In those instances, a home monitor may be useful to reduce anxiety. The use of a diagnostic pneumocardiogram may be helpful in reassuring parents when the physician feels that the risk is trivial; but again, these diagnostic procedures are capable of false negatives as well as false positives.

The discontinuation of a home monitor depends upon whether apnea episodes have occurred at home. Obviously, if there have been fairly severe episodes requiring vigorous stimulation or even resuscitation, the monitor will be maintained in use for a longer period. In any case, everyone agrees that the infant should be free of apnea episodes for at least 2 weeks, and preferably 4 weeks, before a monitor is discontinued.

There are rare instances of more profound apneic disorders that are not transient, unlike the typical near-miss SIDS. Infants with infantile Ondine's curse, for example, will have respiratory difficulties for their entire life, and some infants with obstructive sleep apnea are apt to require special management that is not limited to the first 6 months of life. Regardless of the details of management of an infant with near-miss SIDS, the emotional impact on the mother, father, and older siblings may require considerable support and possibly counseling.

The Child and the Death of a Loved One

ROBERT ADLER, M.D.

For the child and the family, the experience of losing a loved one through either death or separation is traumatic. This is a time when the family often requests help and advice from a physician in dealing with the death or loss. In order to respond appropriately the physician must be aware of his own feelings about death and have a clear understanding of the child, the family, and the circumstances surrounding the loss. To respond to their grief, the focus must be on dealing with the bereaved family's feelings. The physician should avoid using these situations to deal with his own feelings about death.

The child's first experience with death may set the stage for further growth and development in dealing with other significant life events. This provides the physician with an opportunity to help the child learn about the inevitability of loss, separation, and death. The first experience of death and loss for a child may be the loss of parents, siblings, grandparents, other relatives and close friends, or even a beloved pet. In order to help the child, one needs to explore the child's own perception of the loss, previous experience with death, and ideas about death as well as level of cognitive development.

In our society, besides loss through death or illness, the child may experience loss of parents or siblings through separation or divorce. Although this will not be specifically addressed in this article, it should be understood that to a young child these separations may engender the same sense of loss that is felt upon the death of a loved one and can be dealt with in a similar framework. The child may need help in understanding that loss through death is permanent, whereas separation may only be temporary.

In discussions with the child, the physician should explore what experience the child has had with death and what he understands and knows about death. Discussing the events leading to and including the death of a loved one gives the physician an opportunity to clear up any misconceptions that the child may have about death and should create an atmosphere that allows the child to ask questions. The questions may reflect the child's stage of development. Regarding the death of a parent, the younger child may worry about who will care for him, while the older child may be more concerned about the pain of death and the circumstances surrounding the actual dying process. Young children may blame themselves for the death of a family member, attributing the death to their own negative feelings, thoughts, or behaviors. Physicians should explore these areas with an open, nonjudgmental approach, which will allow the child to express himself freely. In the continuing relationship with the family, physicians need to be alert to changes in the family dynamics, communication style, cultural background, and the family's approach to dealing with death in order to make sure that the counseling approach does not become irrelevant to the family's coping mechanisms.

Parents may raise specific questions about how to explain death to the child. Parents may wonder whether the child should view the body or attend the funeral. Death should be discussed truthfully and specifically, and it should not be treated ambiguously or easily confused with other life experiences. Explaining death by saying that someone "went to sleep" may raise fears in the child surrounding sleep. Saying "he went away for a long trip" may make the child fearful of trips. Explaining to the child that the person went to heaven when the family is not religious may be irrelevant and confusing.

If children desire to view the body or attend the

funeral, their wishes should be considered, but certain measures should be undertaken to protect them, especially younger children. A relative or close friend of the family should be asked to accompany the child throughout the process in order to comfort, explain, and if need be, remove the child from the ceremony if it becomes too uncomfortable. A child's imagination and perceptions of what happened may be worse than reality; viewing the body and attending the funeral can be reassuring.

After the acute events surrounding the death are settled, creating a supportive atmosphere in which the child feels comfortable expressing his emotions and asking questions is necessary for the grieving process. The physician can suggest that during the acute stages of grieving it may be helpful to ask a close friend or relative to be the supportive nurturing role model for the child until the parents or surviving family members have regained their ability to deal with their own emotions and feelings.

It is very useful for the physician to meet with the family 3 to 4 weeks after the death of the loved person. Physicians who find that they cannot comfortably do this may ask associated health professionals to initiate this conference, with the physician primarily reviewing the medical events leading up to the death. At the first meeting parents often express anger and hostility about the as yet unaccepted death in the family. This hostility is sometimes mistakenly perceived as directed toward the individual physician and should be handled with sensitivity. This session also gives the health care provider a chance to assess how the family is coping and to determine whether the grieving is proceeding normally or is maladaptive for the family or for individual members within the family. The practitioner can determine whether to recommend, to the entire family or to specific family members, further therapeutic intervention. This intervention can be in the form of additional psychological counseling or in the setting of an ongoing support group of other parents who have had similar losses.

This conference is also a good time to let the family know that the grieving process and the hurt associated with their loss will exist for a long period of time and will never fade completely. The severity of grieving may be surprising and disturbing to the family. It may raise doubts as to their emotional stability and should be addressed by the physician. Having dreams about the person, making plans for the person, or setting a place for him at the table is part of the normal grieving process and should be mentioned. Emotional responses associated with the death will often be manifested for at least a year thereafter and will become more acute on special days associated with the person

(e.g., anniversaries, birthdays, holidays). Some practitioners have taken to sending cards to the family on the anniversary of the death of the child, expressing understanding and offering help during this difficult time. It is important for the family to realize that this event will always have an impact on all of their lives, and the child will not forget the death of the loved one. The family can judge the psychological adjustment and resolution of the grieving process by the child's ability to remember the loved one with positive feelings without being overcome by grief. Losses and separations can be important maturational milestones for a child in which the physician plays a significant supportive and growth-promoting role.

Child Abuse

NAHMAN H. GREENBERG, M.D.

Abuse and injury to young children by their parents or caretakers, that is, nonaccidental violence and neglect, is a major health and social problem. Starvation, neglect, violence, and exploitation contribute to damaged minds and bodies of infants and children. The increased interest in child abuse today can be attributed to a greater awareness of the problem rather than to an actual increase in the incidence of abuse. Health professionals have become more attentive to these problems in compliance with state laws that mandate reporting of child abuse and neglect to designated public child protective agencies.

Estimates of the number of children abused yearly in the United States are as high as 5,000,000. As many as 5% of all children have histories of sexual abuse. From 75,000 to 100,000 children are battered or otherwise severely attacked each year in the U.S., and neglect is reported for many times that number. Combinations of these maltreatments can be assumed in 30 to 40% of cases. The most seriously maltreated and injured children are the very young, below the age of 2 years.

MALTREATED INFANTS AND CHILDREN
Some Methodological Problems

It is difficult to make general statements about short-term and long-term consequences of infant and child abuse since, for the most part, we lack careful and long-range follow-up data that include careful and systematic assessments of infant and child rearing and care practices and family conditions in which abuse occurs. There are no consistent criteria and conditions determining whether a child is removed from the family or when, if removed, reunion will take place. There is no apparent control over the number and durations of placements to which a child might be subjected.

There are added problems of sampling. While studies can be done of the maltreated children who are brought to our attention, we cannot study those who avoid attention and detection, or the many who are lost to follow-up. We are unable also to explain the effects of abuse on overall personality development, on the development of behavioral disturbances, or on correlations with personality, psychoneurotic and psychotic disorders, and psychophysiologic dysfunctions.

The clinical study of abused children is a scientific nightmare. The amount of data collected is limited by lack of time, money, and expertise. The more impersonal the study, the less reliable are the results. Data interpretation is difficult; even mortality rates and reinjury rates can be misinterpreted. Mortality rates include death from reinjury, the long-term consequences of abuse, and deaths from unrelated causes. The severity and incidence of reinjury need to be evaluated; reinjury rates are easily misconstrued, especially when related to intervention and its consequences. A large proportion of children are lost to follow-up for various reasons.

Difficulties in assessing psychologic consequences, including possible harm, are also related to inadequate conceptualization in selecting measurements that can test for specific effects. The effects of earlier abuses on the child's current and future functioning depend on the interactions of a number of factors. The understanding of consequences requires an examination of interactions of major determinants of the child's psychologic development, including predispositional variables and the stage and characteristics of the developmental processes during which specific painful events and experiences occurred. The seriousness of the outcome is also linked with other factors, including the age and developmental phase of the child, the duration of the adverse relationship, the quality of care and experiences with parents in other matters, and inherent vulnerabilities. These factors also influence the nature of the traumatic experience, its content and intensity.

Clinical Evaluations and Observations of Abused Children

The infant or young child victimized by parental brutality causing obvious bodily injuries may also have experienced combinations of less brutal abuse, neglect, and deprivation. The consequences of any one may appear different in form and degree than the interactional effects of any two or more occurring in the history of the infant or child.

Factors that correlate with psychiatric symptoms are not only the type or severity of the physical assault but also environmental factors: emotional disturbance in parents, family instability, number of home changes, punitiveness and rejection by caretakers, and the child's perception of lack of permanence in the home setting. The assumption that trauma is typical or inevitable with abusive experiences implies consequent pathology or dysfunction whether of short or lengthy duration. The persistence of dysfunction may well depend on later developmental experiences, on conditions that promote health, and on the assimilation of the traumatic experience. This perspective on consequences of childhood abuse holds the view that no truly abusive event, experience, or relationship is ever wholly assimilated or neutralized; some increased vulnerability persists even when there are no obvious indications of untoward consequences. There is no one classic or typical personality profile for abused children. It is difficult to predict the conditions or events that will sensitize a child's mind. Whether a child has mastered an early experience or been made more vulnerable by it generally is not obvious until a later time, when predispositions can be tested.

Abused and neglected children exhibit low self-esteem and often behave in ways that invite rejection. They are not happy and seem unable to enjoy themselves in play or in social interactions in a manner appropriate to their ages. Untreated abused children in later childhood seem bitter, hostile, and suspicious of adults; depression is common, although on the surface the children may seem apathetic and shallow. Behavioral disorders and psychiatric illnesses are observed as abused children enter their teens.

The mental harm from overwhelmingly painful, traumatic experiences predisposes to a sense of devastation and to disorganized mental function. The abused child feels "damaged" and vulnerable, and fears repetition of these painful states. Evidence of trauma is found in anxiety dreams or nightmares and in the propensity for helplessness, fright, disorganized thought, psychosomatic symptoms, and dread. In later years, there tend to be disturbances that include an overall impairment of ego functioning associated with intellectual and cognitive defects; traumatic reactions with acute anxiety states; pathologic object relationships characterized by failure to develop basic trust; excessive use of "pathologic" defenses such as denial, projection, introjection, and splitting; impaired control of aggressive impulses, damaged self-concept accompanied by self-destructive behavior; and low frustration tolerance. Many have been enuretic and hyperactive; bizarre behavior or atypical habits, school learning problems, withdrawal, and oppositional behavior are common.

Phobias, avoidance responses, inhibitions, maladjustment reactions, behavioral problems (including delinquent behavior and aggressivity), depression, and disturbed relationships are frequent. There is a chronic sense of low self-esteem, with feelings of inadequacy and inferiority; their sense of self is of being small and unprotected, with a hostile self-rejection when longings for care are felt. They are very sensitive to separation and quickly feel rejected.

Aside from the pediatric or medical findings, various clinical observations and studies have also shown language and general intellectual and development lag, atypical responses to maternal separation, and hypersensitivity of fear accompanied by avoidance responses. Data on speech and hearing development of abused children have shown them to have a much higher degree of language or speech delay. Children most affected are the younger ones who were seen during the critical periods of language development. Development in the older children seems to be less delayed. Many lack age-appropriate information such as knowing numbers and colors, and they also lack basic skills development. Children under 30 months may do well on motor skill items but perform less well in areas concerning object constancy, "means and end" relationships, and social relationships.

Where overt traumatic experiences are associated with an underlying fantasy, the imprint is probably more intense. For example, a neglected child left with intensified longings for nurturing care, touch, and affection will suffer physical punishment with even greater force and intensity and develop more enduring disturbing memories.

Attention must be given to the assessment of cognitive and attentional dev0pment to social responses, regulating functions, and stimulation tolerance. The breakdown of existing functions, the formation of unusual forms of behavior, the lag in development of or failure of emergence of functions are to be suspected as related to parental maltreatment. Neurologic studies are also indicated, particularly with evidence that children subjected to recurrent physical abuse during the first 2 years of life develop neurologic deficits in later years.

CHARACTERISTICS OF ABUSIVE PARENTS

It is important to separate abuse and neglect ascribed to cultural conditions from those due to the person responsible for child care or to interactions stimulated by the young child. If neglect is thought of in terms of deficiencies, restrictions, or the absence of specific environmental conditions, stimulations, and care needed for a child to thrive, then ignorance, famine, and poverty may result in child neglect. Faulty information combined with insufficient resources for educating an uninformed mother engaged in undesirable child care practices may also contribute to neglect. A withdrawn mother suffering from a serious mental disorder may neglect her child. Since experiences of the affected children in all three conditions may be similar, it is important to delineate cultural from subcultural or personal factors in planning treatment.

Parents who abuse their children have been characterized in many ways, even as "normal" if not healthy. Parents who beat their children often think of themselves as "disciplinarians"; some cite scripture to explain their use of physical pain. They think of corporal punishment as a desirable childrearing practice, as a positive force for a child's well-being and instrumental in socialization. Unfortunately, these views are common and contribute to the avoidance of discovering personal and more significant motives in using physical punishment on young children.

The use of corporal punishment to modify behavior is widely accepted as both appropriate and a parental prerogative. Many people fail to see the connection between the cultural sanctioning of mild physical pain to discipline children and the occurrence of child abuse resulting in physical trauma or death. Corporal punishment is particularly inappropriate not only because of the strong emotions accompanying its use but also because of its side effect of teaching children aggression. A common description of abusive parents is that of emotional immaturity, low frustration tolerance resulting in aggression, rigidity in thought patterns and behaviors, and low self-esteem. They are assumed to have been abused as children, and because they employ self-defeating defense mechanisms of regression, denial, and projection, they are prevented from realizing the consequences of their actions and from developing appropriate methods of expressing anger.

Our own studies indicate that most mothers of abused young children suffer from serious emotional disturbances. The majority qualified diagnostically as borderline, prepsychotic, severe character disordered, or psychotic. A predominance of their personalities were marked by a limited range of defenses: inflexibility, impaired judgment, and poor reality testing functions. Clinically, many seemed depressed, distant, apathetic, withdrawn, and emotionally impoverished. Little empathy and closeness were observed, and gratifying relations with other adults were uncommon. Their fantasy life appeared sparse and most often consisted of primitive notions and fears, with hostility and violence a principal theme. Their world was commonly portrayed as a cruel place where people get stung, neglected, gobbled up, hurt and taken advantage of even as they themselves sought for closeness and nurturance. Parents who abused young children were severely hostile, yet they seemed amazingly unaware of and unable to acknowledge hostile feelings or urges where very young children had been most violently abused.

These parents experienced strong negative attitudes toward the earlier pregnancy, a significant unawareness of the child's needs, a lack of clarity about their role as parents, and especially the importance of affection as a necessary ingredient in child care. The behavior of these mothers, observed in the presence of their children, revealed that they encouraged aggressive hostile acts between the children. They directed their child with strong, angry, verbal commands and abrupt harsh and painful hitting.

They never used gentle or simple physical restraint to alter the child's "objectionable" behavior. Impatience, unwarranted rejections, icy aloofness, and angry recriminations were often observed.

Parents who abuse their infants and children, including some who had committed infanticide, have been described as rigid, severely obsessive-compulsive, and "pseudoindependent," as well as demanding and aggressive toward the child, demanding strict compliance and obedience and physically punishing the child when frustrated by him. Low self-esteem and hypersensitivity to criticism, as well as a need for constant reassurance, have also been attributed to the personality of observed abusive parents. Crises involving severe attacks on the child have been correlated with the taxing of circumstances that evoked such conditions, such as an excessively crying infant. The backgrounds of these parents have been described as lacking in care and impoverished of love and self-esteem, with a childhood history of pain and punishment.

TREATMENT

Some General Conditions

The service needs of these parents and children are many and consist of different combinations according to living conditions, service resources, treatment indications, and treatability. The abusive parent often regards treatment as an intrusion. Therapists are perceived as unwelcome interlopers who exercise influence on the observed behavior of the family. A very punitive father who strongly considers beating children a necessary and legitimate right that serves the child well will strongly object to being informed that such practices not only are not acceptable but also are illegal.

It is not strange therefore that service plans include various emergency health and social services, individual and group therapies, parent groups, emergency and long-term foster homes, in-home services, and various health and child welfare agencies from the public and private sectors. It is important to not lose sight of the child

and to always include indicated diagnostic and treatment child services. No significant family member should be allowed to remain outside the therapeutic plans.

The awareness that children are helpless and suffering often intensifies the response of service providers, who may not readily accept not being able to bring prompt relief and remediation; it is difficult to not feel helpless and incompetent. The pressure to provide services is especially felt when the problems are more complicated and in greater numbers than previously assumed and of moral and social consequence. These problems do not yield to easy answers.

Crisis intervention and collaboration with social agencies are required when protection of the child is necessary, when trying to bring a family together, and when trying to prevent additional cases. Experienced therapists are reluctant to take on these difficult and complicated, stormy, crisis ridden problems, which disrupt the professional's orderly life, and for which services tend to be limited.

The decision of what treatment approach to use is frequently made on the often inadequate basis of availability. Treatment services are usually provided by those with less formal training and experience, and usually with fewer treatment skills and less sensitivity and psychological understanding, who are less prepared to do psychotherapy and who are inadequately trained in diagnostic and insight oriented skills. How many cases of abuse do we know of that receive an adequate diagnostic evaluation?

The specialized treatments and living conditions needed for adults and children involved in maltreatment are not so difficult to determine even with our limited knowledge. Since treatment services cannot be postponed until sufficient knowledge is developed to guide the design and application of specific treatment plans, we must keep an open mind on the selection of treatment approaches, recognize preferences and biases, and realize that "service plans" often reflect local resources, biases, economics, political considerations, or priorities. Intervention programs have often developed without prior testing or regulation but based on hunches and assumptions that intuitive responses are better than inaction. We reward innovativeness in procedures in the absence of controls, test data, and a sound rationale.

Most identified abusive parents are amenable to psychotherapy. Group and individual psychotherapy as well as psychotherapy augmented by child management information have shown clinical usefulness. The use of multiple family therapy as a treatment modality in child abuse cases requires that the family's interaction be observed and treated with all members present; emphasis is on the inter-relationship of family members; and therapeutic interventions are geared toward changes within the family rather than in individuals. Psychoeducational programs teaching more effective parental practices, crisis nurseries, and family developmental centers have come into being as approaches to modifying if not preventing faulty parental behavior.

Initiating Child Protective Services

Awareness of a wide occurrence of child maltreatment has stimulated the development of legal and social service mechanisms designed to intervene on behalf of a child whose health was endangered and who required protection from further maltreatment. The ability to intervene, although not necessarily to provide ongoing services, was enhanced through enactment of laws that gave child protective services legal authority to intervene in the lives of families to protect endangered children.

In the treatment of child abuse, there is a need to shift from the current reliance on placement to an emphasis on crisis intervention and comprehensive psychiatric and social services for the maltreated child and his or her family. The use of placement as a major intervention is recommended only as a last resort. Parents whose children have been placed or who were threatened with removal of their children respond with anger and frustration and question the genuineness of the offer of help. Sequelae of placement include depressive reactions in parents, the need to blame someone else, increased conflict with the spouse, and pregnancy within 1 year after placement.

Child protective services (CPS) responses to reported child abuse and neglect are a public promise of help through specialized social and mental health services. Intended to protect the "best interests of the child," they principally prevent further abuse by prompt intervention and introduction of services to assist the family in exercising responsibilities in the care and development of the children. Child protective services are in theory nonpunitive and noncondemning, and are an offer to help rehabilitate the family, to stabilize the home environment, and to treat the underlying factors causing child maltreatment. This depends on a study of presenting complaints, an adequate understanding of the persons and situational problems (i.e., a diagnostic work-up), a planning of the case's needs according to what requires changing and what services would bring that about, and finally, treatment proper, including arrangement and provision of services.

Services for abusive parents and abused children are founded on fundamental principles and practices of "helping relationships." The practices of professional social and mental health services are possible only insofar as certain conditions are met:

1. That clients or patients have the right to some degree of personal choice and decision on treatment.

2. That treatment be provided with respect; the patient is accepted as a worthy human being regardless of past actions, problems, and personal characteristics.

3. That the client has the right to have personal information treated with professional confidence.

4. That it is understood that the fundamental rights of patients cannot be violated by personal values or biases of the professional worker and there is an acceptance of the patient, so that evaluations are not influenced by personal opinions, differences, or personal values.

5. Time.

The severe increase in reports of abused and neglected children, causing caseloads that exceed the ability of professionals to provide adequate services, combined with the pressing into service of less well trained and experienced workers, decreases the amount and quality of services and promotes tougher management of administrative responses. Treatment skills and the influence of experience and professionalism are viewed as unaffordable luxuries, divorced from the realities of the situation. The situation encourages intercessions based on the power of coercion and threat, real and implied; changes are now to come about by demand and command. As the number of reported cases increases, as the child protective mandate is exercised in an increasingly narrow and legalistic way, the time for and expectation of understanding and use of skills essential to the development of working therapeutic relationships are reduced if not discarded. Initial interviews are no longer valued as crucial opportunities to assist families toward healthier futures; rather they become instruments to investigate without the commitment to bring about understanding and compassion.

With reduced options and increasing caseloads, immediate action is expected, and with less time for experience and education to develop and to improve skills. Protective custody and the placement of a young child in a foster home are the alternatives to professionalism and express the diversion into "removal of the problem" and the employment of an individualized form of "custodialism." This approach is relatively well oriented to management and narrow administrative ideas and to rigid and authoritarian individuals. Such legal devices reduce the demand and need for clinical skills and understanding to change behavior, to control and protect. They also reinforce the stereotype of the maltreating parent as someone who is inevitably dangerous and unpredictable, inferior and condemned; parents become vulnerable to attitudes and procedures of retribution and punishment. Psychotherapeutic and related clinical services become secondary if not tertiary in the hierarchy of methods to influence change.

The work of the therapist, the clinician, and the diagnostician involves an obligation to insure that no permanent physical or psychological harm will ensue from the procedures and that discomfort from such procedures or the loss of privacy will be remedied in an appropriate way during the course of treatment or at its completion.

The Initiation of Therapy and Collaboration in Child Abuse

The circumstances under which a person seeks treatment or is introduced to the need for treatment is very important to the initiation of psychotherapy and to the development of a treatment relationship. Likewise, the conditions under which a report is made of a child being abused and the characteristics of the response, usually by child protective service workers, can be powerful factors in the course of events and the quality of treatment services that follow. If we consider this phase of events a component of the initial phase of therapy, a phase concerned with the initiation of a treatment relationship leading to the establishment of a professional contractual involvement, then proper attention must be given to its difficulties, the technical skills required, the rationale underlying interventions, and a continuing attention to diagnosis. The initiation of child protective services and that of psychotherapeutic services differ even though the child protective services need to be employed to initiate treatment, fully recognizing that such interventions cannot always be performed with the neatness of a timed interpretation.

The nonvoluntary client or patient may or may not recognize the need for therapy or for change. The suggestion of a need for psychotherapeutic services based on a report of possible or actual child maltreatment is not a simple intervention to be carried out routinely without understanding the conditions and circumstances that will automatically influence the response to the suggestion and the possibility of bringing about a cooperative working relationship. The idea to seek treatment might originate in the patient or client, or it might be someone else's suggestion or wish; the idea to seek treatment might well have previously occurred in the nonvoluntary client.

Early contact with the social worker is essential for both diagnostic and treatment purposes, and in preparation for this, pediatricians and other specialists should maintain an honest relationship with the parents and keep them informed of the medical findings. An inquisitory or adversarial stature should be avoided. The earliest experiences in a psychotherapeutic relationship must be felt as helpful and as bringing about some lessening of distress, crises, and the sense of fear and anxiety. If an accusatory complaint, however valid, is made, the abuser can be expected to experience greater initial fear and threat as a period of uncertainty, isolation, and loneliness is entered. In the encouragement of open discussion and in the urging of a renunciation of concealment by abusive parents of the injurious behavior towards one or more of their children, there is an understanding in psychotherapy that the discussion will not bring about punishment or rejection. The assurance of nonrejection and of a nonpunitive response is most difficult when being given by an agent of a legal agency not provided with the privilege of professional confidence or by a law enforcement officer serving as a child protective service worker.

Individuals respond to external conditions perceived as dangerous or threatening and to internal conditions or inner drives, emotions, or fantasies perceived as unacceptable with fears of retaliation, rejection, and social isolation. The responses are typically those that will avoid the discomfort or pain of the anxiety reflecting or signaling danger and threat, whether from external or internal sources. In psychotherapy, the therapist also represents change and symbolizes an advocacy for change. In that context, the therapist is also seen as an authority and as an "authoritarian," dominating, fearsome, and hostile. These "transference" responses are expected and are treated for their underlying determinants and thereby reduce resistances against further exploration and learning. The revelation of ideas, relationships, feelings, and activities recognized as forbidden and punishable, or as shameful and humiliating, is difficult even when the patient or client is safe from punitive consequences or their threat. To assume that this is any less difficult under punitive conditions or their threat or where ordered by an authority under coercive circumstances approaches the incredible. A therapeutic relationship involves the search for understanding without rebuff.

There are unfortunate misunderstandings about "treatment motivation" or treatment participation and continuity. The abusive parent who is reluctant to talk openly or freely is unfairly compared with the adult who has requested psychotherapy. In fact, the patient who talks freely is a rarity, and many months of work might be necessary to secure a halfway sufficient degree of honesty. The abusive parent who is unwilling to talk freely and honestly, who might angrily protest complaints or accusations, and who might insult and depreciate child protective service worker efforts might in fact be more honestly expositive than one who readily confesses or admits to physical and/or sexual abuse of a child. The abusive parent, like most clients or patients, is seldom accessible to treatment in the beginning, is reluctant to "open up," and certainly does not have confidence in a total stranger, especially one initiating contact by means of a formal complaint even while offering services. A charge of maltreatment of a child cannot be expected to evoke initial responses of relief and calm in the parent so confronted.

The psychological treatment of members of a family with abusive relationships requires a dedication to interventions that initiate and aid in the development of a working relationship between the adult or child patient and the therapist. Genuine cooperation is vital during treatment sessions; the building of an effective treatment alliance is necessary if successful change is to be possible. A treatment alliance is not established immediately with first contacts and does not come about instantaneously. The alliance is, however, significantly facilitated or seriously obstructed by the quality of the earliest interactions during interviewing and other contacts. Abusive families are usually thought to be "hostile, concealing and rejecting the need of assistance." Participation in treatment also requires an understanding of the process and procedures of therapy, the expectations and purposes for some of the therapist's interventions. Confrontation, clarification, and the continuing encouragement of self-observation assisted by timed interpretations to facilitate the working alliance bring patients to a closer appreciation of why they resist assistance and change. Resistances cannot be ordered out of existence; they have developed for psychological reasons and they need to be treated.

The tendency in maltreatment is for chronic, however intermittent, patterns of abuse. Self-initiated treatment by abusive parents occurs and has been reported in the literature. The report of a family in which maltreatment of children is occurring probably involves persons who have not requested treatment, or at least not recently. Our experience with such families indicates a wide range of emotional disorders, including symptom neuroses and character neuroses, and such patients are well protected against insight, change, and intervention originating in the outer world.

Treatment of the Child

The dependency on parents is greater in abused children than in nontraumatized children, and the child's treatment itself is therefore dependent on the parent's attitudes toward treatment. A working alliance with parents is therefore essential not only to improve parent-child relationships but also to prevent the undermining of the child's therapy through failure of appointments or the child's perception of parental disinterest or disapproval and consequent fear of additional rejection and loss of care and hoped for affection.

The evaluation of children's emotional status or mental health is facilitated by assessments of mastery of age-appropriate tasks. Evaluations and treatment need to be carried out under appropriate conditions, including provisions for play, drawing, and testing. Very young children may have difficulty in separating from a parent, and flexibility is needed to allow a parent to be present until a relationship is established permitting separation for the period of the session. Play and drawings and their interpretations are significant avenues for the child to express feelings and conflicts about self and parents, about their life situation and the emotional climate at home.

Interviewing older children is very similar to interviewing adults. History, early memories, attitudes, anxieties, mood, and other aspects of mental status can be assessed. Complaints by the child freely offered become crucial in facilitating a working relationship through the reduction of tension and awareness of "help" as symptoms are revealed and underlying pathology considered. Many young children with histories of abuse and neglect become highly dependent on their therapist, and the treatment of longings for intimate and nurturing gratification in children who were in fact deprived and brutalized requires great inner strength and resiliency in therapists.

The Psychotherapeutic Situation in the Treatment of Childhood Abuse

Like every medical endeavor, psychotherapies are concerned with symptoms and with the ways and means of removing them. Like any healing art, the first and foremost interest is not in how good or how bad a person the patient happens to be, but primarily in how sick a person the patient is and in how the patient became ill, regardless of the origins of the illness. Psychotherapeutic methods are from the outset a method of empirical, cool, objective investigation; the therapist is braced against any feelings of horror, disgust, shame, or anxiety that might occur when dealing with human aberrations. As human beings, psychotherapists are not devoid of these feelings, but they learn to proceed without swerving and without diffidence, regardless of the aberrations they are faced with: murder, falsehood, theft, incest, intrigue, chicanery, or child abuse. All are grist to the mill of psychological study.

Child abuse work is conducted under conditions structured by legal, political, and social considerations. These are set against treatment that must remain strictly scientific, that is, objective, cool, rational, unmoralistic, nonpolitical, and equally indifferent toward and curious about social passions and political trends. Clinicians need to concentrate on the psychological dynamics that are set into play when humans kill each other, including young children. As a person, the clinician, including the pediatrician, is not at all immune to the torment of such inner queries but must maintain neutrality in his or her professional work and not get caught up in the decision-making and social action and experimentation that characterize the child protective system. Whether a person is allowed into treatment or whether the legal interventions are helpful are not the specific work of psychotherapy; however, the therapist cannot remain aloof from considerations about the conditions in which therapeutics are possible.

Fluid and Electrolyte Therapy

LEWIS A. BARNESS, M.D.

In health, fluid homeostasis is maintained by oral ingestion of fluids and foods that contain minerals, and fluid intake is regulated by thirst. Attention to fluid intake is necessary when the thirst mechanism is deranged, when fluid losses exceed intake, when the plasma volume is sub- or supranormal, or when the patient is unable to express his needs.

Water constitutes about 70% of lean body mass; 40 to 45% is intracellular, about 18% is interstitial, and 7% is intravascular. Intracellular cations are mainly potassium and magnesium; interstitial and intravascular mainly sodium (140–145 meq/l) and potassium (4–5 meq/l). Intracellular anions include phosphates, sulfates, bicarbonate, organic anions, and protein. Interstitial and intravascular cations are mainly chloride (95–105 meq/l) and bicarbonate (22–25 meq/l). Intravascular plasma also contains 6 to 7 gm of protein per dl (10 meq/l).

Maintenance water requirement, the volume required to replace insensible water loss (skin and respiratory tract) and water of urine and stool formation in an afebrile patient at bed rest, is approximately 100 ml/100 kcal expended. Calculations for fluid requirements may be based on metabolic rate, surface area, or weight (Table 1).

Hydrogen ion homeostasis is maintained by

Table 2. COMPOSITION OF ORAL SOLUTIONS (mM/l)

	Solution 1 (WHO)	Solution 2	Solution 3
Na^+	90	75	50
K^+	20	20	25
Cl^-	80	65	45
HCO_3^-	30	—	—
Citrate	—	30	30
Glucose	111	135	111
Osmolality	331	305	241

plasma buffers, by control of P_{CO_2} by the lung, and by renal excretion of acids or bases.

Maintenance Fluid Therapy. Maintenance fluids are used in conditions in which the child is in a normal state of hydration, such as in preoperative preparation. Such solutions should be made with sodium concentrations of 30 to 50 meq/l and potassium concentrations of 15 to 25 meq/l. Ordinarily, the anion can be entirely chloride, though basic anions (e.g., lactate, bicarbonate, acetate) may be used, up to one third of the total anions.

Dehydration. Assess the degree of dehydration. Volume depletion is estimated by weight loss as well as by blood pressure determination. Serum electrolytes and pH help determine status of individual ions. P_{CO_2} determination is useful in distinguishing pH abnormalities due to metabolic states in contrast to respiratory abnormalities. In respiratory acidosis the P_{CO_2} is high, and in respiratory alkalosis it is low. These are reversed in metabolic acidosis and alkalosis.

Oral Rehydration. If the patient is alert, awake, and not in shock, first attempt to correct dehydration by oral fluids. Compositions of three oral rehydration solutions are listed in Table 2.

The WHO solution (solution 1) has been successfully used worldwide for the treatment of diarrhea and dehydration but is little used here because of fear of causing hyperelectrolytemia. Solutions 1 and 2 should be supplemented with water or breast milk to compensate for insensible water losses. Solution 3 provides sufficient electrolytes and water for many deficiency states and is usually well taken by ill children.

For oral rehydration, give 50 ml/kg body weight within 4 hours for mild dehydration and 100 ml/kg over 6 hours for moderate dehydration. Amounts and rates should be increased if rehydration does not appear complete or if the patient continues to have excess losses, as with diarrhea. If the patient is nursing, these fluids should be supplemented with breast feeding. In other patients, plain water should be offered after treatment has been given for 4 to 6 hours, if solution 1 or 2 is used. Sufficient free water is available

Table 1. MAINTENANCE REQUIREMENTS

Weight (kg)	Surface Area (m^2)	Water (ml/kg)	Cal/kg	Na^+/kg (meq)	K^+/kg (meq)
3	0.20	100	40–50	3–4	3–4
5	0.27	90	50–70	3–4	2–3
10	0.45	75	40–60	2–3	2–3
15	0.64	65	40–50	2–3	2–3
30	1.10	55	35–45	2–3	1–2
50	1.50	45	25–40	1–2	1–2
70	1.75	40	15–20	1–2	1–2

Requirements/m^2: Water 1500 ml, Na^+ 60 meq, K^+ 45 meq.

Table 3. DEFICITS IN MODERATE DEHYDRATION

	H₂O (ml/kg)	Na⁺ (meq/kg)	K⁺ (meq/kg)	Cl⁻ (meq/kg)
Fasting	100–120	5–7	1–2	4–6
Diarrhea				
Isotonic	100–120	8–10	8–10	8–10
Hypotonic	100–120	10–12	8–10	10–12
Hypertonic	100–120	2–4	0–4	−2 to −6
Pyloric stenosis	100–120	8–10	10–12	10–12
Diabetic ketoacidosis	100–120	8–10	5–7	6–8

from solution 3. In many children with vomiting and diarrhea, vomiting will cease after 4 hours.

While diarrhea continues, an intake of 10 to 15 ml of electrolyte-containing solution per kg of body weight per hour is appropriate to compensate approximately for the stool losses. Maintenance therapy is added.

Parenteral Needs. Patients in shock, those with severe dehydration or with uncontrollable vomiting, those unable to drink for any reason including extreme fatigue or coma, and those with severe gastric distention require intravenous therapy.

Calculation of needs is similar to that above except that tolerance to intravenous fluids requires more frequent monitoring. Deficits of water and electrolytes can be estimated from Tables 3 and 4. Emergency management, especially if blood pressure is low, requires a central venous or pulmonary arterial catheter for more precise monitoring.

For severely dehydrated patients or those in shock, rapid intravenous administration of 20 to 40 ml/kg over 1 to 2 hours is given. Solution can be plasma, whole blood, human albumin, or other colloid. If these are not immediately available, start with a solution containing 75 meq/l of sodium and chloride in 5 to 10% glucose in water. A base such as lactate may be substituted for one third of the chloride. Next, the total volume of fluid to be administered over 24 hours is calculated. Half of this is given in the next 8 hours, and the remainder over the last 14 to 16 hours. This solution should contain 40–75 meq/l NaCl in 5 to 10% glucose.

Table 4. ELECTROLYTE CONTENT OF BODY FLUIDS (meq/l)

Source	Na⁺	K⁺	CL⁻
Gastric	20–80	5–20	100–150
Small intestine, pancreas, bile	100–140	5–15	90–130
Ileostomy	45–135	3–15	20–115
Diarrhea	10–90	10–80	10–110
Sweat			
Normal	10–30	3–10	10–35
Cystic fibrosis	50–130	5–25	50–110
Burns	140–145	4–5	110

Potassium, 20–30 meq/l, should be added as soon as the patient urinates.

For hypotonic or isotonic dehydration with adequate blood pressure, initial colloid can be eliminated, but calculations are similar. For hypertonic dehydration, similar solutions are used, but the rate of administration is decreased so that total fluids are given at a constant rate over 24 hours. Potassium concentration is 40 meq/l. Calcium gluconate, 10 ml of 10% solution, is added for each liter administered.

For acidosis with pH above 7.1, bicarbonate or other base is usually not necessary and, because H_2CO_3 traverses membranes including the CSF more rapidly than HCO_3^-, may be undesirable because the CSF pH will decrease while the blood pH is increasing. This is especially important when respiratory gas exchange is impaired. When the blood pH is 7.1 or less, bicarbonate, 15 to 25 meq/l, replaces an equal amount of chloride in the hydrating solution.

Diabetic Ketoacidosis. Elevations of blood sugar increase serum osmolality. Each 1000 mg/l has an osmolality of $1000 \div 180$ (the molecular weight) = 5.6 mosm. While each 100 mg glucose/dl would be expected to decrease serum sodium $5.6 \div 2 = 2.8$ meq, measurements have indicated that the true depression is about 1.6 meq/100 mg glucose. Serum sodium is decreased in hyperglycemic states. However, as the glucose is metabolized, water shifts out of the extracellular space, and the serum sodium rises. Therefore, even in the presence of a low serum sodium with hyperglycemia, calculations are similar as in isotonic dehydration unless the serum sodium is depressed more than 1.6 meq/100 mg/dl of elevated glucose.

Premature Infants—Maintenance. Maintenance requirements are 80 to 100 ml/kg/day. However, Na⁺ and K⁺ are not needed on the first day. Na⁺, 20 meq/l, is added on the second and third day and increased to 40 meq/l on the fourth day. K⁺, 2 meq/kg/day, is started on the second day. Fluids should be in 5 or 10% glucose, with careful monitoring of blood sugar and electrolytes and appropriate modifications made.

Infants under radiant warmers or under phototherapy require 25 to 50% increase in maintenance fluids.

Anuria. Fluids are restricted to insensible water loss, approximately one fourth maintenance requirements, plus any urine output as 5 to 10% D/W. Hyperkalemia or hyponatremia may occur and require correction.

Inappropriate Secretion of Antidiuretic Hormone. This may occur with CNS disease or trauma, or postoperatively. Serum osmolality is low, while urine osmolality is inappropriately elevated. Treat with fluid restriction to one fourth to one half maintenance. In those with CNS disease without apparent fluid abnormalities, treat expectantly at two thirds to three fourths maintenance.

Cardiac Disease with Failure. Restrict fluids and Na^+ to two thirds maintenance. Diuretics may be needed. Serum electrolytes must be monitored, especially for the development of low serum sodium.

Parenteral Nutrition. Any child requiring prolonged intravenous therapy requires calories other than those provided by glucose in the electrolyte/glucose mixtures. Principles of administration are similar to those described on pages 8–11. Caloric needs are those outlined in Table 1.

Malignant Hyperthermia

EUGENE K. BETTS, M.D.

Malignant hyperthermia (MH) is an abrupt and unexplained rise in body temperature above 40°C (104°F) from a fulminant hypermetabolic state triggered by anesthestic agents. MH predominantly occurs in children over 2 years of age and in young adults. The hypermetabolic state occurs in skeletal muscle and is induced by the combination of inhalation anesthetic agents and depo-

---

Table 1. MANAGEMENT OF MALIGNANT HYPERTHERMIA*

1. Prophylaxis
   a. Dantrolene,† 2.4 mg/kg intravenously, immediately before induction.
   b. "Clean" anesthesia machine and delivery circuit. Flow oxygen through machine 12 hours preoperatively. Remove halogenated agents from machine. Fresh CO_2 absorbent in cannister or a nonrebreathing system.
2. Monitoring
   a. Routine (MH suspected)
      (1) ECG, blood pressure, temperature, precordial stethoscope
   b. After presumed onset of MH
      (1) Arterial line: blood pressure and blood sampling for pHa, $Paco_2$, Pao_2, and electrolytes
   c. Foley catheter for urinary output
3. Supplies (have immediately available)
   a. Dantrolene‡ for IV administration
   b. Sodium bicarbonate (12 ampules)
   c. Iced saline (12 l)
   d. Furosemide
   e. Mannitol
   f. Procainamide
   g. Regular insulin and 50% glucose
   h. Ice chips
   i. Cooling blankets
   j. Extracorporeal perfusion apparatus in hospitals with experience in its use
4. Treatment
   a. STOP ANESTHESIA and SURGERY IMMEDIATELY. Change the breathing circuit and, if possible, the anesthesia machine.
   b. Hyperventilate with 100% O_2 at high flow rates.
   c. Administer the following:
      (1) Dantrolene‡: 1–3 mg/kg initial bolus with increments up to 10 mg/kg total
      (2) Sodium bicarbonate: 1–2 meq/kg increments guided by pHa and $Paco_2$. Bicarbonate will combat hyperkalemia by driving potassium into cells.
   d. ACTIVELY COOL PATIENT
      (1) IV iced saline (*not* lactated Ringer's) 15 ml/kg every 10 minutes for three times
      (2) Lavage stomach, bladder, rectum, and peritoneal and thoracic cavities with iced saline
      (3) Cool surface with ice and hypothermia blankets
      (4) Institute extracorporeal circulation and heat exchanger (femoral to femoral)
   e. Maintain urine output: Mannitol 0.25 gm/kg IV and furosemide 1 mg/kg IV (up to 4 doses each). Urine output >2 ml/kg/hr may help prevent subsequent renal failure.
   f. Procainamide for arrhythmias: Add 15 mg/kg to 100 ml normal saline and infuse over 10 minutes or until ventricular ectopy ceases. Do NOT use procaine HCl, as it may cause seizures in this dose.
   g. Insulin for hyperkalemia: Add 10 U of regular insulin to 50 ml of 50% glucose and titrate to control hyperkalemia.
   h. Postoperatively: Continue dantrolene‡ 1 mg/kg every 6 hours for 72 hours to prevent recurrence. Up to 10% of patients may have recurrence in first 8 hours postoperatively.

---

* Committee on Pediatric Anesthesia (Clinical Care): Technical bulletin for malignant hyperthermia. ASA Newsletter 46(11):5, 1982; 47(1):1, 1983.

† Flewellon E. H., Nelson T. E., Jones W. P., et al.: Dantrolene dose response in awake man: Implications for management of malignant hyperthermia. Anesthesiology 59:275–280, 1983.

‡ Manufacturer's warning: Safety of use of dantrolene in children under 5 years of age has not been established.

larizing muscle relaxants (e.g., succinylcholine) in a predisosed patient.

Table 1 outlines a plan of treatment for malignant hyperthermia. Dantrolene* is specific for the metabolic disorder occurring in the skeletal muscles. If regional or local anesthesia has been chosen for a patient predisposed to the syndrome, local anesthetics of the "ester" class (procaine, tetracaine, and chloroprocaine) probably should be selected because agents of the "amide" class (lidocaine, prilocaine, etidocaine, mepivacaine, bupivacaine) may have been implicated in triggering hyperthermia.

Colic

MARC WEISSBLUTH, M.D.

Determining whether crying is or is not colic helps determine how much therapeutic intervention is needed. Several published studies have diagnosed colic in otherwise healthy infants who had paroxysms of irritability, fussing, or crying lasting >3 hours a day, occurring >3 days in any one week, and continuing >3 weeks during the first three months. The criterion "more than three weeks" is important for two reasons. First, during the first few weeks, some infants have explosive outbursts of colicky-like behavior lasting less than three weeks. Apparent treatment successes, when this brief storm naturally passes, represent only placebo responses. The best treatment during these three weeks is watchful waiting. Most parents will accept this treatment if they know that the waiting period is definitely limited to three weeks. Second, infant crying always increases and peaks at about 6 weeks of age followed by a dramatic reduction. At this age, most babies do not cry >3 hours/day or >3 days/week but those that do, do so for less than 3 weeks. Placebo responses also occur after 6 weeks. Narrative diagnostic criteria tend to label too many babies. The importance of clear diagnostic criteria is that in most instances the crying is not diagnosed as colic and this fact sustains the parents in their wait for the crying to naturally disappear and in their resolve to avoid unproven remedies. Or, if the crying is determined to be colic, organized plans can be made to deal with a 3- to 5-month ordeal.

No treatment of a colicky infant leads to a symptom-free state as a light turned off leads to darkness. Some symptoms will always persist. Claims of treatment success are meaningless in the absence of clear entry criteria and explicit treatment outcome criteria. Exactly how much was the crying diminished and in what percentage of infants? Only when this information is available can a pediatrician or parent reasonably decide whether it is worthwhile to try a proposed treatment.

Many proposed so-called treatments are so simple that they probably will never be studied. These include hot water bottles, noises from vacuum cleaners or hair dryers, different nipple shapes, heart beat or intrauterine recordings, and lamb's wool pads. There is a subtle problem with encouraging parents to try these seemingly benign items. When parents repeatedly engage in minitreatment trials with initial high hopes for success, the inevitable failure to eliminate colicky crying reinforces the parental perception that something is fundamentally very unhealthy with the child, themselves, or both. This unwarranted perception of unhealthiness might persist long after the colic subsides and lead to beliefs and parenting practices that reinforce this false notion: My child is allergic; my child has a sensitive stomach; my child was ill his entire infancy and now needs special care; I could never calm my baby; I never had enough milk; he must have hated me then.

There are two older speculative ideas about causation and treatment of colic that have been supported and popularized by eminent physicians. These two nonempirical notions, "maternal anxiety" and "stimulus overload," are really only guesswork. Maternal anxiety as the cause of colic has been described in a famous pediatric psychiatry book (mother's "anxious overpermissiveness psychotoxically" disturbs the baby) and in a popular trade infant-care book (parents overreact and the tension around the infant builds up). Neither author really addressed the issue of directionality of effects but merely assumed that the dominant causative factor was parental or maternal emotionality.

Treating the mother or parents would be the logical conclusion, but it should be clearly understood: There is no study meeting contemporary standards of clinical behavioral research investigating the effects parents and children have on each other that supports this conclusion. In fact, contemporary research suggests that specific parenting patterns do not result from or cause colic. Also, when parents were observed to be trying many different ways to calm their colicky baby, it was assumed by older psychoanalytically inclined writers that parents were causing the colic in the first place by something called stimulus overload. This notion also has no basis in fact. Sensitivity to external stimulation may be a recognizable trait in some postcolicky infants, but the stimulus overload speculation does not fit well with the fact that paroxysmal colicky spells often occur in dark

---

* Manufacturer's warning: Safety for use in children under 5 years of age has not been established.

rooms only in the quiet evening hours. Treatment strategies built around the unsupported and, I think, erroneous notion that parents cause colic usually create unnecessary parental guilt, which lowers their self-esteem. If parents can accept the fact that they have a difficult temporary situation that is not their fault, they are better able to avoid feelings of helplessness or hopelessness. When they stop overintellectualizing, or practicing self-analysis, they can better carry out simple treatment strategies. Pediatricians should explicitly and repeatedly address this issue of parental nonculpability as part of the treatment process.

Treatment has progressed when parents know that their pediatrician is an ally, when they know what is meant by colic, when they know not to waste their energy and upset their emotional stability on useless gimmicks, and when they feel that they are unlucky but not guilty. What then can be done to reduce the crying? Three maneuvers tend to calm infants: (1) rhythmic motions, including rocking chairs, swings, cribs with springs attached to the casters, cradles, carriages and strollers, walking, bouncing, water beds, and automobile rides; (2) swaddling, including wrapping in blankets, snuggling, cuddling, and nestling; (3) sucking; including at breast, bottle, wrist, finger, or pacificer.

Parents should use other people to help care for the baby when the crying is most severe. Even if this break is only a few hours or a few days a week, it sustains morale because it is a rest period that the parents can anticipate. Tell parents that it is true no one can care for their baby as well as they can, but during their baby's inconsolable crying spell, their baby is probably unaware of who is doing the holding and rocking. Parents must understand that this break is for their pleasure and relaxation; it is not to do errands, chores, or housework. Parents need to be emphatically told that occasionally getting away from their crying baby is smart, not selfish. Taking care of themselves means that they will be better able to nurture their baby.

Parents inevitably want to know whether the constant attention will spoil the child, that is, create a crying habit. Data are available to support the contrary conclusion that consistent and prompt parental responsiveness in early infancy tends to reduce, not increase, crying at age 1 year. However, a potential complication of constant attention during the first few colicky months is that some parents do not change their strategies for the older postcolic child at bedtime and naptime, Thus, after the colic passes, the older child is never left alone at sleeptimes and is deprived of the opportunity to develop self-soothing skills. These children never learn to fall asleep unassisted. The resultant sleep fragmentation/sleep deprivation in the child, driven by intermittent positive parental reinforcement, leads to fatigue-driven fussiness long after the physiologic factors that had caused colic are resolved.

Therapeutic Educational Effort. Drug treatment is usually not needed when the parents are able to calmly learn about normal infant crying, and this learning process should occur before they leave the maternity hospital. Otherwise, after the delivery, the inevitable infant crying, commotion, excitement, inexperience, and fatigue combine to undermine parents' receptiveness to educational efforts. After the delivery, frequent visits, telephone calls, and lengthy conversations are usually required, and nothing will doom this educational effort faster than trying to limit it to a few glib responses hurriedly presented. There is no substitute for spending extra time with these families, and the pediatrician should be sensitive to his or her own feelings on this issue.

There may be situations when even a patient pediatrician might decide that an educational effort is not worth trying because the chances of success appear so dim. This might occur with some families when the infant crying ignites a fire storm of emotionality, fueled by unrelenting strident demands from parents and grandparents for diagnostic tests or drug treatments. "Colic is a medical problem; my child is sick with this problem. Therefore, doctor, give me the medicine to treat this problem." The pediatrician then has to decide whether to treat the child because of the severity of the parental response. Superficially, it seems unwarranted to consider drug treatment of the infant in order to primarily reduce parental anxiety and frustration over their inability to soothe their baby. But this does indirectly promote the health of the child by reducing the possibility of parental anger toward the child, child abuse, or infanticide. Not prescribing medicine in some instances will predictably lead to switching pediatricians, which, given the pediatrician's attitude toward the family, may or may not be in the child's best interest.

Drug Treatment. Dicyclomine hydrochloride* is the only drug of proven value in reducing colicky crying, but there are no widely accepted indications for initiating treatment. Presumably, a colicky infant should be considered a candidate for drug treatment if the spells of irritability, fussiness, or crying consist primarily of prolonged inconsolable crying or if the pediatrician senses that colic is creating a dangerous rift between child and parents. It should not be assumed that drug treatment

---

* Manufacturer's warning: Bentyl is contraindicated in infants less than 6 months of age.

Table 1. DOSAGE INSTRUCTIONS AND DOSES FOR DICYCLOMINE HYDROCHLORIDE*

Instructions
1. Start at lowest dose listed for age of your infant.
2. Give one dose in the morning, one at noon, and a third in the evening.
3. Increase the dose each day, if needed, to a maximum of $\frac{1}{2}$ tsp. four times daily, at morning, noon, afternoon, and evening.
4. Do not exceed the maximum dose of $\frac{1}{2}$ tsp. four times daily.
5. Reduce the dose to next lower dose if excessive drowsiness or infrequent urination (3 or fewer times per 24 hours) develops.
6. The medicine may be mixed with a small amount of juice or formula, which must then be finished by your baby.

Doses

Age less than 8 weeks
$\frac{1}{4}$ tsp. 3 times daily
$\frac{1}{4}$ tsp. 4 times daily
$\frac{1}{2}$ tsp. 3 times daily
$\frac{1}{2}$ tsp. 4 times daily

Age 8 weeks or older
$\frac{1}{2}$ tsp. 3 times daily
$\frac{1}{2}$ tsp. 4 times daily

* Manufacturer's warning: Bentyl is contraindicated in infants less than 6 months of age.

is needed to reduce pain in the infant. The presumption that colic is pain makes no more sense than assuming that a presocial smile represents pleasure. Nevertheless, parents find it easier to affectionately love their baby when crying is diminished, and this increased social contact is beneficial for both child and parents.

Dosage instructions are given in Table 1. Treatment with dicyclomine hydrochloride in one study eliminated colic in 63% of infants, and placebo was effective in 25% (corrected X^2 = 5.42, p = 0.02). Infants who responded to treatment had significantly fewer mean daily hours of crying than did nonresponders (mean ± 1 SD, 1.1 ± 0.8 versus 3.9 ± 1.4, p < 0.001). The mechanism of action is unknown but the assumption that it is effective by reducing gastrointestinal smooth muscle contractions is probably incorrect. Based on physiological studies of sleep-wake control and the drowsiness associated with excessive dicyclomine, it is likely that the reduction in crying and increased amount of calm/wakeful behaviors is due to central effects. Risks of drug treatment include accidental poisoning due to parental error and anticholinergic signs with overdosage. Also, there is a weak association with non–life-threatening apnea. Another risk is that parents might be encouraged to expect and demand prescription medicines for minor self-limiting illnesses when the child is older. In my practice, in which parents are from the middle social classes, I prescribe dicyclomine about once or twice a year. In similar practices, drug treatment may usually be avoided when educational efforts succeed.

Genetic Diseases

SUE Y. E. HAHM, M.D.
and HAROLD M. NITOWSKY, M.D.

Genetic disorders can be divided into 3 major groups: (1) chromosomal aberrations, (2) single gene disorders, and (3) polygenic or multifactorial disorders, which encompass many congenital malformation syndromes, such as cleft lip and palate, neural tube defects, pyloric stenosis, and certain common disorders such as diabetes mellitus. Although there are no precise data regarding the burden of genetic disorders in the population, it has been estimated that during their lifetime 10% or more persons will manifest some disorder reflecting an underlying genetic abnormality. Genetic diseases, although in most cases individually rare, are very common in aggregate. Large-scale studies of consecutive newborn infants have shown an incidence of chromosome aberrations of about 0.6%. Population surveys have shown that 2–3% of all neonates manifest some congenital malformation and birth defects. The infant mortality rate has been significantly reduced during the past decades, but deaths due to genetically related causes are relatively unchanged, accounting for $\frac{1}{3}$ of all infant mortality. Surveys of large teaching centers have shown that genetic disorders or diseases with some underlying genetic component account for about 30% of all pediatric admissions.

The approach to management of genetic disorders includes prevention, treatment or cure, and rehabilitation. A diagnosis of a genetic disorder can be made on clinical grounds or by specific laboratory tests such as enzyme analysis or cytogenetic studies. Early diagnosis is important because prompt intervention can prevent mental retardation and other serious sequelae in certain disorders (e.g., phenylketonuria, galactosemia, hypothyroidism) or neonatal death in other disorders (e.g., galactosemia, salt-losing form of congenital adrenal hyperplasia).

Prevention

Prevention of genetic diseases can be achieved through genetic counseling, carrier screening to detect at risk couples, and prenatal diagnosis. Genetic counseling has been defined as a process of communication to help the family to understand better the genetic and medical aspects of a genetic disorder in a family. This process involves an attempt by one or more appropriately trained persons to help the individual or family (1) to comprehend the medical aspects, including the diagnosis, the probable course of the disorder, and the available management; (2) to appreciate the way heredity contributes to the disorder and the risk of recurrence in specified relatives; (3) to understand the options for dealing with the risk of recurrence; (4) to choose the course of action that seems appropriate to them in view of their risk and the family goals and to act in accordance with that decision; and (5) to make the best possible adjustment to the disorder in an affected family member and to the risk of recurrence of that disorder.

Genetic counseling should be nondirective and focus upon the family's goals and values rather than reflect the counselor's subjective biases. Accurate diagnosis is necessary for correct counseling, since inaccurate diagnosis can lead to erroneous recurrent risks. A detailed family history and examination of other family members may be necessary to define the mode of inheritance and to offer appropriate counseling. With the advances in techniques for prenatal diagnosis and carrier detection, significant advances in counseling and prevention have become possible.

Carrier screening has been carried out successfully for Tay-Sachs disease in Ashkenazi Jews, sickle cell disease in blacks and other groups, beta thalassemia in persons of Greek and Italian decent, and alpha thalassemia for Southeast Asians. Reliable carrier testing may become available in the near future for cystic fibrosis, another common inherited disorder in Caucasians, with a carrier rate of 1/25.

Midtrimester amniocentesis is a safe and widely used procedure now routinely used in women who are 35 years and older to detect a fetus with Down syndrome or some other chromosomal abnormality. Amniocentesis is usually performed at 16–18 weeks of pregnancy; amniotic fluid obtained contains viable fetal cells, which then can be cultured in sufficient amount in approximately 3 weeks to allow cytogenetic or biochemical analysis. Most chromosomal and many metabolic defects are detectable in this way.

Alpha-fetoprotein is an albumin-like protein. It is produced early in gestation in the yolk sac and later by fetal liver and is first detectable in fetal serum 30 days after conception. Elevated alpha-fetoprotein in amniotic fluid is associated with open neural defect or ventral wall defects and fetal nephrosis. Amniotic fluid can be used for diagnosis of 21-hydroxylase deficiency of congenital adrenal hyperplasia using linkage analysis to the HLA locus or hormonal assay (170H progesterone) in amniotic fluid.

Prenatal diagnosis of hemoglobinopathies has been largely performed by globin chain analysis of fetal blood samples. With recent advances in recombinant DNA technology, including restriction endonuclease analysis, the molecular defect in many of the hemoglobinopathies has been clarified, and endonuclease analysis is now being used routinely in the prenatal diagnosis of hemoglobinopathies. Fetal DNA samples can be obtained from amniotic fluid cells by simple amniocentesis, and prenatal diagnosis can be done by direct DNA (globin gene) analysis or indirect DNA assays using linkage analysis between restriction fragment-length polymorphism and the globin gene locus. Restriction enzyme assay is also capable of recognizing many other disorders that may be difficult or impossible to diagnose during pregnancy (e.g., Lesch-Nyhan syndrome, alpha-1-antitrypsin deficiency, phenylketonuria, ornithine transcarbamylase deficiency, and Duchenne muscular dystrophy).

Recent application of chorionic villus sampling (CVS), which can be done at 9–11 weeks of pregnancy, permits an earlier approach to prenatal diagnosis. Developing chorionic villi can be obtained by passing a catheter through the cervix into the placenta, and chromosome analysis, biochemical diagnosis, and DNA analysis can be done. This procedure may be psychologically and socially more acceptable than mid-trimester amniocentesis because if a fetal abnormality is found, patients can opt for first-trimester termination, which is simpler, safer, and less psychologically stressful.

Another widely used method of prenatal diagnosis is fetal visualization by ultrasonography. As an adjunct to amniocentesis and CVS, sonography aids in dating gestation, in localizing the placenta, and in detecting multiple gestations. An ultrasound examination can assess amniotic fluid volume and fetal growth and detect specific abnormalities of the CNS, heart, gastrointestinal tract, genitourinary tract, and skeleton.

Direct visualization by fetoscopy and fetal blood or tissue sampling are other prenatal diagnostic methods that are used less often because of technical difficulties and enhanced fetal risk.

Prenatal diagnosis is usually offered only to families known to be at an increased risk for a fetal abnormality. Advanced maternal age with its increased risk for chromosomally abnormal progeny is the most common indication for prenatal studies. Couples known to be at risk for a detectable fetal condition by virtue of a previously affected child or positive family history are the next most common group. Other high risk couples may be discovered through carrier or prenatal screening programs. Maternal serum AFP determination has been used to identify fetuses with unsuspected fetal neural tube defects and may become a routine screening procedure during prenatal care. Recently, a very low level of maternal serum AFP has been found in association with fetal autosomal trisomy and fetal deaths. Thus, maternal serum AFP screening may be valuable in improving the prenatal detection of serious anomalies in the fetus. Prenatal diagnosis is one of the most important components in the control of genetic diseases.

It also provides an alternative for families who would otherwise choose not to have other children because of fear of recurrence of the problem in future progeny.

Treatment

Treatment of genetic disease includes restriction of a substance that the patient cannot metabolize, end-product replacement, vitamin supplement, induction and enhancement of enzyme activity, enzyme replacement, and surgical intervention (organ or marrow transplantation) (Table 1).

Genetic diseases in which symptoms are due to metabolic failures and subsequent accumulation of toxic substances are treated by dietary elimination (e.g., PKU, galactosemia). Genetic diseases that are characterized by inability to synthesize an essential substance due to an enzyme defect are treated with end-product replacement (e.g., thyroid hormone for patients with enzyme defects of thyroid hormone biosynthesis, corticosteroids or mineralocorticoids for congenital adrenal hyperplasia). The missing substance can be replaced to alleviate symptoms in genetic diseases in which symptoms are due to an inability to synthesize an essential gene product (e.g., hemophilia). A metabolic block can be overdriven by the supplementation of pharmacologic doses of the appropriate vitamin cofactor (e.g., B_{12}-responsive methylmalonic acidemia, thiamine or biotin for congenital lactic acidosis, B_6 for homocystinuria). Detoxifying therapies are used in Wilson disease (D-penicillamine to chelate copper accumulation).

Attempts to purify normal enzymes and then administer them to patients with lysosomal storage diseases (mucopolysaccharidoses, sphingolipidoses) that are due to missing lysosomal enzymes have been made. Recombinant DNA technology should make it possible to clone the gene for the normal enzymes and permit large scale production for replacement therapy. However, there is need for improvement in enzyme delivery to target tissues as well as the problem of the blood-brain barrier.

It is possible to replace organs that have been damaged as a result of a genetic defect (renal transplantations in patients with polycystic kidney disease, bone marrow transplantations in severe inherited immune deficiency disease). Bone marrow transplantation has also been used as a method of enzyme replacement in the lysosomal storage disorder. Recent experience shows that bone marrow transplantation may have a role in the management of genetic disorders of metabolism, particularly in patients with predominantly non-neurologic manifestations, although to date the clinical effects have been limited.

Since cure of genetic diseases is not possible, management has been primarily aimed at prevention and symptomatic treatment. However, with enormous recent advances in recombinant DNA technology, therapy at the gene level and cure of the diseases that are due to specific alterations in the patient's genome may become possible in the future. These approaches are called "gene therapy." In order to attempt gene therapy, (1) the genetic defect responsible for the disease has to be identified; (2) production of multiple copies of a specific, desired gene must be made; (3) insertion of the normal gene into the cell nuclei of the patient must be carried out; (4) incorporation of the inserted gene must be normally regulated and expressed; and (5) the inserted gene should not harm the cell.

The possibility of achieving a therapeutic benefit by using a drug to alter genetic expression temporarily to compensate for a genetic defect in humans has become feasible. With the hypothesis that DNA methylation is an important control mechanism in gene expression, 5-azacytidine, an inhibitor of DNA methylation, was tried on primates and found to cause an increased level of fetal hemoglobin. Subsequent studies of 5-azacytidine in patients with sickle cell disease and beta-thalassemia showed that tolerable acute and chronic doses led to increased fetal hemoglobin levels and evidence of hematologic and clinical improvement. Use of this and related agents may be limited to severely affected patients because of potential carcinogenicity. A less dangerous drug, hydroxyurea, which does not cause hypomethylation, has produced similar effects, suggesting that other mechanisms may be involved.

The timing of therapy is of critical importance for many inborn metabolic disorders. The pathologic consequences of prolonged metabolic disturbance may be irreversible. The necessity of prompt diagnosis has stimulated the widespread institution of neonatal screening programs. Such testing is practical in diseases that can be inexpensively and accurately detected presymptomatically and for which early therapy is available and effective. Neonatal screening began for phenylketonuria, and subsequently other disorders were included, such as galactosemia, homocystinuria, maple syrup urine disease, tyrosinemia, sickle cell disease, and other hemoglobinopathies. The recent advent of screening for congenital hypothyroidism has been of great importance, since this abnormality occurs at a frequency of 1:4000 newborns. Newborn screening is available or in the stage of development for 21-hydroxylase deficiency of CAH, alpha-1-antitrypsin deficiency, multiple carboxylase deficiency, and cystic fibrosis.

For some genetic diseases, even earlier recognition is required in order to minimize or avoid irreversible impairment. Prenatal surgical treatment has been carried out in fetal hydrocephalus

Table 1.   MODES OF GENETIC THERAPY

Dietary Elimination
1. PKU and other disorders of amino acid metabolism
2. Galactosemia
3. Lactose or fructose intolerance
4. Urea cycle defects
5. Organic acidemias

End-product Supplementation (distal to an enzymatic block)
1. Thyroid synthetic defects
2. Congenital adrenal hyperplasias
3. Glycogen storage disease (frequent or continuous carbohydrate feeding)

Replacement of Missing or Defective Gene Product
1. Hemophilia A and B
2. Growth hormone deficiency
3. Agammaglobulinemia

Metabolic Suppression via Feedback Mechanisms
1. Congenital adrenal hyperplasias
2. Acute intermittent porphyria (hematin therapy)

Avoidance of Drugs and/or Other Environmental Agents
1. G6PD deficiency
2. Porphyrias
3. Mastocytosis
4. Malignant hyperthermia
5. Pseudocholinesterase deficiency

Cofactor Supplementation
1. Methylmalonic acidemia (B_{12})
2. Propionic acidemia or multiple carboxylase deficiency (biotin)
3. Congenital lactic acidosis (thiamine, biotin)
4. Homocystinuria (B6)
5. "Infantile convulsions" (pyridoxine)
6. Vitamin D–dependent rickets

Enzyme Induction
1. Gilbert or Crigler-Najjar syndromes (induction of glucuronyl transferase with phenobarbital)
2. Methemoglobinemia (induction of NADPH dehydrogenase with methylene blue)

Metabolic Inhibition
1. Lesch-Nyhan syndrome (allopurinol)
2. Hyperlipoproteinemia, type III (clofibrate)
3. Nephrogenic diabetes insipidus (thiazide diuretics)

Detoxification by Depletion of Substrate
1. Wilson disease or cystinuria (D-penicillamine)
2. Familial hypercholesterolemia (cholestyramine)
3. Hemochromatosis (desferoxamine)
4. Gout (uricosuric agents)
5. Urea cycle defects (sodium benzoate)
6. Refsum disease (plasmapheresis)

Organ Transplantation
1. Immunodeficiency syndromes (marrow, fetal thymus, or fetal liver)
2. Osteopetrosis (bone marrow)
3. Polycystic kidneys (renal)
4. Mucopolysaccharidoses (fibroblasts questionably effective, bone marrow)

Surgery
1. Complete androgen insensitivity (malignant prophylaxis)
2. Retinoblastoma (extirpation)
3. Cleft lip (cosmetic)
4. Multiple epiphyseal dysplasia (hip replacement)
5. Hereditary spherocytosis (splenectomy)
6. Glycogen storage diseases (portacaval bypass)

Prenatal Therapy
1. Erythroblastosis fetalis (intrauterine transfusion)
2. Methylmalonic acidemia (maternal B_{12} administration)
3. Multiple carboxylase deficiency (maternal biotin administration)
4. Hydrocephalus (transcutaneous ventriculoamniotic shunt placement)
5. Urethral obstruction (transcutaneous vesicoamniotic shunt placement)
6. Fetal tachyarrhythmias (cardiac glycoside administration)
7. Congenital adrenal hyperplasia–21-hydroxylase deficiency (maternal dexamethasone suppression)

Gene Therapy
1. Beta-thalassemia and sickle cell disease (experimental administration of 5-azacytidine to derepress hemoglobin F synthesis)

Miscellaneous
1. Arthrogryposis (physical therapy)
2. Huntington disease (psychologic counseling)

and hydronephrosis by use of a drainage tube into the amniotic sac to decompress the obstruction. Prenatal treatment has also been tried by giving dexamethasone to the mother who is carrying a female fetus with classic 21-hydroxylase deficiency of CAH; this successfully suppresses the fetal adrenal gland and prevents virilization of external genitalia.

Thus, unlike the therapeutic mechanisms of the past, there are many approaches to the treatment as well as the prevention of genetic disorders. With the new developments in molecular genetics, it is likely that exciting new approaches for management of genetic disease will be available in the future.

Index

Page numbers followed by the letter t indicate tables.

773

BUSINESS REPLY MAIL

FIRST CLASS   PERMIT NO. 5152   NEW YORK, NEW YORK

POSTAGE WILL BE PAID BY ADDRESSEE

CBS Educational & Professional Publishing
W.B. Saunders Company
Order Fulfillment Department
383 Madison Avenue
New York, NY 10017

BUSINESS REPLY MAIL

FIRST CLASS   PERMIT NO. 5152   NEW YORK, NEW YORK

POSTAGE WILL BE PAID BY ADDRESSEE

CBS Educational & Professional Publishing
W.B. Saunders Company
Order Fulfillment Department
383 Madison Avenue
New York, NY 10017

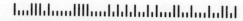